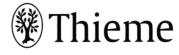

Vascular Medicine

Therapy and Practice

Thomas Zeller, MD
Professor
Head of the Department Angiology,
Clinic Cardiology and Angiology II
University Heart Center Freiburg-Bad Krozingen
Bad Krozingen, Germany

Thomas Cissarek, MD
Department of Angiology, Phlebology,
Vascular Surgery
Gefaesskrankheiten Rhein-Ruhr
Essen, Germany

Assistant Editor
Jerzy Wojciuk, MD, LRCP Edin,
LRCS Edin, LRCPS Glasg, MRCP (UK)
Lancashire Cardiac Centre
Blackpool
Lancashire, UK

William A. Gray, MD
Director, Endovascular Services
Associate Professor of Medicine
Center for Interventional Vascular Therapy at
Columbia University Medical Center
Presbyterian Hospital
New York, USA

Knut Kröger, MD
Professor
Head, Department of Angiology
HELIOS Hospital Krefeld
Krefeld, Germany

2nd edition

With contributions by
Jens Achenbach, Farzin Adili, Helene Arns, Ali Aydin, Jörn O. Balzer, Kai M. Balzer, Ulrich Beschorner,
Friedheim Beyersdorf, Hans-Georg Bone, Thomas Cissarek, Sebastian Debus, Curt Diehm, Uwe Dietrich,
Ali Dodge-Khatami, Arndt Dohmen, Christine Espinola-Klein, Jennifer Franke, Thomas Frieling,
Sophia Göricke, Ernst Gröchenig, Heinrich Hakuba, Jörg Heckenkamp, Bernhard Hellmich,
Joachim Hermanns, Philip Hilgard, Peter Horn, Verena Khan, Dietrich Koch, Manuela Koch,
Yskert von Kodolitsch, Tilo Kölbel, Marwan El-Koussy, Knut Kröger, Eric Lorenz, Felix Mahfoud, Erich Minar,
Shanti Naskar, Achim Neufang, Sigrid Nikol, Claus Nolte-Ernsting, Elias Noory, Georg Nowak,
Michael Offermann, Christoph Ozdoba, Wolfgang Peck, Michael Pillny, Roberta Pini, Siamak Pourhassan,
Maximilian J. A. Puchner, Reinhard Putz, Claudio Rabbia, Aljoscha Rastan, Marcus Rebel, Wilhelm Sandmann,
Frans Santosa, Dierk Scheinert, Tom Schilling, Marc Schlamann, Andrej Schmidt, Walther Schmiedt,
Thomas Schmitz-Rixen, Eva Schönefeld, Gerhard Schroth, Horst Sievert, Sebastian Sixt, Edda Spiekerkötter,
Matthias Thielmann, Giovanni Torsello, Dierk Vorwerk, Isabel Wanke, Werner Weber, Thomas Zeller

948 illustrations

Thieme
Stuttgart · New York · Delhi · Rio

Library of Congress Cataloging-in-Publication Data is available from the publisher.

This book is an authorized translation of the 2nd German edition published and copyrighted 2013 by ABW Wissenschaftsverlag, Berlin. Title of the German edition: Gefäßmedizin: Therapie und Praxis

Translator: Dr. Michael Robertson, Augsburg, Germany

Illustrator: brandnewdesign, Hamburg, Germany

Anatomical drawings: Karin Baum, Paphos, Cyprus

© 2010, 2014 ABW Wissenschaftsverlag GmbH
Altensteinstraße 42, 14195 Berlin, Germany
www.abw-verlag.de

Distributor:
Georg Thieme Verlag KG
Thieme Publishers Stuttgart
Rüdigerstrasse 14, 70469 Stuttgart, Germany,
+49 [0]711 8931 421
customerservice@thieme.de

Thieme Publishers New York
333 Seventh Avenue, New York, NY 10001, USA,
1-800-782-3488
customerservice@thieme.com

Thieme Publishers Delhi
A-12, second floor, Sector-2, NOIDA-201301, Uttar Pradesh, India,
+91 120 45 566 00
customerservice@thieme.in

Thieme Publishers Rio
Thieme Publicações Ltda.
Argentina Building, 16th floor, Ala A, 228 Praia do Botafogo, Rio de Janeiro
22250-040 Brazil, +55 21 3736-3631

Cover design: Thieme Publishing Group
Typesetting by medionet Publishing Services Ltd., Berlin
Printed in Germany by Media-Print Informationstechnologie, Paderborn

ISBN 978-3-13-176841-4

Also available as e-book:
eISBN 978-3-13-176851-3

Preface

The first edition of the interdisciplinary volume on *Vascular Medicine—Therapy and Practice* met with an extremely positive response from readers of both the German and the English editions. We have therefore decided to produce a new edition even though only four years have passed since the publication of the first. The advances that have been made in recent years have been tremendous, particularly in the area of endovascular therapy, and in this second edition we have two major aims.

Firstly, we updated and improved the content of the existing chapters. Improvements have mainly involved adding an introductory anatomy section to each of the major chapters. In addition, although the book's emphasis is still on treatment, a detailed duplex ultrasonography section has been added for each vascular region. This is because duplex ultrasound represents the fundamental method of imaging diagnosis in vascular medicine and is increasingly being carried out in every specialty field in vascular medicine. We hope in this way to contribute to a standardization of the method in everyday usage.

The second aim of the new edition is to achieve a substantial expansion of the content of the book by adding sections and main chapters that did not find their way into the first section for various reasons. This mainly involves the addition of the chapter on "Diseases of the lymphatic system," along with chapters on "Treatment of acute stroke" and "Renal sympathetic denervation"—two treatment fields that have acquired an increasing or new importance in recent years and in which tremendous progress in interventional therapy of the clinical fields involved can be expected in the future. We are particularly pleased that pioneers of each of these treatment methods have agreed to be co-authors for these sections. The section on the treatment of renal artery stenosis, "Surgical treatment of renal artery stenosis," is another important addition and comes from Prof. Sandmann's school in Düsseldorf, one of the most experienced international specialists in this field.

We would like to thank all of the authors for their valuable revisions and new contributions. We are also grateful to Dr. Bedürftig, Ms. Behle, and Ms. Sänger and to all the other staff, who along with the graphic designer Ms. Baum have once again given the book its excellent design.

Readers may notice that there has been a change in the order of the editors' names. We would like to continue this rotation in the coming years as well as to continue to keep readers informed about the very latest state of developments in the treatment of vascular diseases.

Thomas Zeller
Thomas Cissarek
William A. Gray
Knut Kröger

List of Contributors

Jens **Achenbach**, MD
Department of Angiology
Center for Vascular Diseases Rhein-Ruhr
Mülheim an der Ruhr / Essen, Germany

Farzin **Adili**, MD
Head, Department of Vascular and Endovascular Surgery
Darmstadt Hospital
Darmstadt, Germany

Helene **Arns**, MD
Department of Phlebology, Lymphology
Center for Vascular Diseases Rhein-Ruhr
Mülheim an der Ruhr / Essen, Germany

Ali **Aydin**, MD
Department of Cardiology, Electrophysiology
University Heart Center Hamburg
University Medical Center Hamburg-Eppendorf
Hamburg, Germany

Jörn O. **Balzer**, PD, MD
Head, Department of Radiology and Nuclear Medicine
Catholic Hospital Mainz
Mainz, Germany

Kai M. **Balzer**, MD
Associate Professor
Chief Resident
Department of Vascular Surgery and Kidney Transplantation
Universal Hospital Düsseldorf
Düsseldorf, Germany

Ulrich **Beschorner**, MD
Attending Physician
Department of Angiology and Cardiology
Heart Center Freiburg University
Bad Krozingen, Germany

Friedhelm **Beyersdorf,** MD, MD h.c.
Professor
Member of the Board of Medical Directors
Head, Department of Cardiovascular Surgery
University Heart Center Freiburg
Bad Krozingen, Germany

Hans-Georg **Bone**, MD
Professor
Head, Department of Anaesthesiology and
Intensive-Care Medicine
Clinicum Vest GmbH
Recklinghausen, Germany

Thomas **Cissarek**, MD
Department of Angiology, Phlebology, Vascular Surgery
Gefaesskrankheiten Rhein-Ruhr
Essen, Germany

Sebastian **Debus**, MD
Professor
Head, Department of Vascular
and Endovascular Surgery, Angiology
University Heart Center Hamburg
Hamburg, Germany

Curt **Diehm**, MD
Professor
Head, Department of Internal Medicine
Klinikum Karlsbad-Langensteinbach
Karlsbad, Germany

Uwe **Dietrich**, MD
Head, Department of Neuroradiology
Evangelic Hospital Bielefeld
Bielefeld, Germany

Ali **Dodge-Khatami**, MD
Professor of Surgery
Division of Pediatric and Congenital Heart Surgery
University of Mississippi Medical Center
Mississippi, USA

Arndt **Dohmen**, MD
Interdisciplinary Center for Vascular Medicine
University Heart Center Freiburg-Bad Krozingen
Bad Krozingen, Germany

Christine **Espinola-Klein**, MD
Professor
Head, Department of Angiology
University Medical Center of the
Johannes Gutenberg University Mainz
Mainz, Germany

Jennifer **Franke**, MD
Resident
Department of Internal Medicine
Heidelberg University Hospital
Heidelberg, Germany

Thomas **Frieling**, MD
Professor
Head, Department of Internal Medicine
HELIOS Klinikum Krefeld GmbH
Krefeld, Germany

Sophia **Göricke**, MD
Attending Physician
Department of Neuroradiology
Essen University Hospital
Essen, Germany

Ernst **Gröchenig**, MD
Head, Department of Internal Medicine
Kantonspital Aarau
Aarau, Switzerland

Heinrich **Hakuba**, MD
Head, Department of Lymphology
Hochrhein-Eggberg Hospital Bad Säckingen
Bad Säckingen, Germany

Jörg **Heckenkamp**, MD
Professor
Head,Department of Vascular and Endovascular Surgery
Niels-Stensen Hospital
Marienhospital Osnabrück
Osnabrück, Germany

Bernhard **Hellmich**, MD
Professor
Head, Department of Rheumatology and Clinical Immunology
Kirchheim Hospital
Kirchheim-Teck, Germany

Hans Joachim **Hermanns**, MD
Private Practice
Practice for Angiology
Krefeld, Germany

Philip **Hilgard**, PD, MD
Head, Department of Gastroenterology
Evangelic Hospital Mülheim
Mülheim an der Ruhr, Germany

Peter **Horn**, MD
Head, Department of Tranfusion Medicine
University Hospital Essen
Essen, Germany

Verena **Khan**, MD
Department of Radiology
Nuremberg Hospital
Nuremberg, Germany

Dietrich **Koch**, MD
Department of Vascular Surgery
Clinic for Vascular Diseases
Essen, Germany

Manuela **Koch**, MD
Department of Vascular Surgery
Clinic for Vascular Diseases
Essen, Germany

Yskert **von Kodolitsch**, MD
Professor
Chief Resident
Department of General and Interventional Cardiology
University Heart Center Hamburg
Hamburg, Germany

Tilo **Kölbel**, MD
Chief Resident
Department of Vascular Medicine
University Heart Center Hamburg
Hamburg, Germany

Marwan **El-Koussy**, MD
Chief Resident
Department of Diagnostic and Interventional Neuroradiology
Bern University Hospital
Bern, Switzerland

Knut **Kröger**, MD
Professor
Head, Department of Angiology
HELIOS Klinikum Krefeld GmbH
Krefeld, Germany

Eric **Lorenz**, MD
Department of Visceral and Vascular Surgery
St. Hedwig Hospital
Berlin, Germany

Felix **Mahfoud**, MD
Department of Cardiology, Angiology and Intensive Care
Saarland University Medical Center
Homburg/Saar, Germany

Erich **Minar**, MD
Professor
Angiologist
Private Practice
Vienna, Austria

Shanti **Naskar**, MD
Chief Resident
Department of Vascular Surgery
St. Marien Hospital Buer
Gelsenkirchen, Germany

Achim **Neufang**, MD
Head, Department of Vascular Surgery
Dr. Horst Schmidt Kliniken GmbH
Wiesbaden, Germany

Sigrid **Nikol**, MD
Professor
Head, Department of Angiology
Asklepios Hospital St. Georg
Hamburg, Germany

Claus **Nolte-Ernsting**, MD
Professor
Head, Department of diagnostic and interventional Radiology
Evangelic Hospital Mülheim
Mülheim an der Ruhr, Germany

Elias **Noory**, MD
Chief Resident
Department of Angiology
Heart Center Freiburg University
Bad Krozingen, Germany

Georg **Nowak**, MD
Director
Specialist in Surgery and Vascular Surgery
Marienhaus Klinikum
Krankenhaus Maria Hilf
Bad Neuenahr-Ahrweiler, Germany

Michael **Offermann**, MD
Phlebologist
Vascular Diseases Rhein-Ruhr
Private Practice
Essen/Mülheim, Germany

Christoph **Ozdoba**, MD
Chief Resident
Department of Diagnostic and Interventional Neuroradiology
University Hospital Bern
Bern, Switzerland

Wolfgang **Peck**, MD
Surgeon
Department of Vascular Surgery
University Heart Center Freiburg-Bad Krozingen
Bad Krozingen, Germany

Michael **Pillny**, MD
Head of Department
Department of Vascular Surgery
Elisabeth Krankenhaus
Recklinghausen, Germany

Roberta **Pini**, MD
Specialist for Interventional Radiology
Department of Vascular and Interventional Radiology
Molinette Hospital
Turin, Italy

Siamak **Pourhassan**, MD
General Surgeon
Private Practice for Vascular Diseases and Vascular Surgery
Oberhausen, Germany

Maximilian J. A. **Puchner**, MD
Head, Department of Neurosurgery
Klinikum Vest GmbH
Recklinghausen, Germany

Reinhard **Putz**, MD
Vice President
Ludwig-Maximilians-University Munich
Munich, Germany

Claudio **Rabbia**, MD
Department of Vascular and Interventional Radiology
Molinette Hospital
Turin, Italy

Aljoscha **Rastan**, MD
Department of Cardiology and Angiology II
University Heart Center Freiburg-Bad Krozingen
Bad Krozingen, Germany

Marcus **Rebel**
Green Lane Paediatric and Congenital Cardiac Service
Starship Children's Hospital
Auckland, New Zealand

Wilhelm **Sandmann,** MD
Professor
Head, Department of Vascular Surgery
Evangelical Hospital Duisburg North
Duisburg, Germany

Frans **Santosa**, MD
Head, Department of Angiology and Cardiology
Jakarta Vascular Center
Menteng, Indonesia

Dierk **Scheinert**, MD
Professor
Head, Department of Vascular Medicine
Park Hospital Leipzig
Leipzig, Germany

Tom **Schilling**, MD
Head, Department of Angiology
Wernigerode Hospital
Wernigerode, Germany

Marc **Schlamann**, MD
Head, Department of Neuroradiology
University Hospital Essen
Essen, Germany

Andrej **Schmidt**, MD
Department of Vascular Medicine
Park Hospital Leipzig
Leipzig, Germany

Walther **Schmiedt**, MD
Professor
Head, Department of Vascular Surgery
Catholic Hospital Mainz
Mainz, Germany

Thomas **Schmitz-Rixen**, MD
Professor
Head, Department of Vascular and Endovascular Surgery
Goethe-University Hospital Frankfurt
Frankfurt am Main, Germany

List of Contributors

Eva **Schönefeld**, MD
Department of Vascular Surgery
St. Franziskus-Hospital GmbH
Münster, Germany
and
Department of Vascular and Endovascular Surgery
Westfälische Wilhelms-Universität
University Hospital Münster
Münster, Germany

Gerhard **Schroth**, MD
Professor
Head, Department of Diagnostic
and Interventional Neuroradiology
University Hospital Bern
Bern, Switzerland

Horst **Sievert**, MD
Professor
Director, CardioVascular Center Frankfurt
Sankt-Katharinen
Frankfurt, Germany

Sebastian **Sixt**, MD
Private Practice
Angiologikum Hamburg
Hamburg, Germany

Edda **Spiekerkötter**, MD
Division of Pulmonary and Critical Care Medicine
Stanford University
Stanford, USA

Matthias **Thielmann**, MD
Department of Thoracic and Cardiovascular Surgery
Heart Center Germany West Essen
Essen, Germany

Giovanni **Torsello**, MD
Professor
Head, Department of Vascular Surgery
St. Franziskus-Hospital GmbH
Münster, Germany
and
Westfälische Wilhelms-Universität
University Hospital Münster
Center for Vascular and Endovascular Surgery
Münster, Germany

Dierk **Vorwerk**, MD
Professor
Head, Department of Diagnostic
and Interventional Radiology
Ingolstadt Hospital
Ingolstadt, Germany

Isabel **Wanke**, MD
Professor of Neuroradiology
Klinik Hirslanden
Zürich, Switzerland
and
University Hospital Essen
Department of Diagnostic
and Interventional Radiology and Neuroradiology
Essen, Germany

Werner **Weber**, MD
Head, Department of Radiology,
Neuroradiology and Nuclear Medicine
Hospital Vest GmbH
Recklinghausen, Germany
and
Treatment Center
Paracelsus-Hospital Marl
Marl, Germany

Thomas **Zeller**, MD
Professor
Head, Department of Angiology
Heart Center Freiburg University
Bad Krozingen, Germany

Contents

Contents

Contents

Contents

A

Diseases of the arteries

1 Supra-aortic vessels

1.1 Extracranial stenoses and occlusive processes

Anatomy of the extracranial arteries:
Reinhard Putz
Introduction: Jennifer Franke and Horst Sievert
Doppler/duplex ultrasonography: Tom Schilling
Conservative treatment: Horst Sievert and
Jennifer Franke
Endovascular treatment: Horst Sievert and
Jennifer Franke
Surgical treatment: Farzin Adili and
Thomas Schmitz-Rixen

1.1.1 Anatomy of the extracranial arteries

The external arterial supply to the head is provided by branches of the external carotid artery, which arises bilaterally from the common carotid artery at approximately the level of the fourth cervical vertebra or upper margin of the thyroid cartilage (Fig. 1.1-1). Its course is highly variable; it usually runs ventral and superficial to the internal carotid artery until it is behind the mandible. Its anterior branches pass to the thyroid gland, tongue and facial skin. A deep branch passes to the pharynx. Posteriorly, arteries branch off to the occiput and auricle. Behind the temporomandibular joint, the external carotid artery divides into its two terminal branches, the superficial temporal artery and the maxillary artery (Fig. 1.1-2). These two branches, like the occipital artery, may serve as collaterals to supply the brain in cases of occlusion of the internal carotid artery or vertebral artery. The lingual artery arises just above the hyoid bone and enters the tongue in an anterior direction behind the hyoglossus. One of its branches passes under the sublingual gland to the gingiva and mandibular muscles. The facial artery sometimes arises from a common trunk with the lingual artery and turns around the submandibular gland anteriorly to the edge of the mandible, through which it passes in a small ostium in front of the insertion of the masseter muscle. After giving off the inferior and superior labial arteries, it winds through the facial muscles lateral to the nose as far as the medial angle of the eye, where it connects with the superficial terminal branches of the ophthalmic artery—although this is rarely relevant in practice.

The posteriorly-directed occipital artery is important in that after crossing under the sternocleidomastoid and splenius muscles it supplies a dense vascular network rising at the occiput at the posterior margin of the trapezius muscle; this network has connections with the neighboring arteries. The superficial temporal artery is often visible on the surface at the temple; it divides at the level of the upper margin of the auricle into an often noticeably tortuous frontal branch and a parietal branch (Fig. 1.1-2).

The maxillary artery is the most important branch for the supply of the external parts of the head (Figs. 1.1-2, 1.1-3). After its origin (the mandibular part), it passes anterior or posterior to the lateral pterygoid muscle (pterygoid part) into the depth of the infratemporal fossa (pterygopalatine part), where the pterygoid venous plexus is also located. From it, branches pass to the teeth in both jaws, to the masticatory muscles, to the gingival and nasal mucosa, and—via the medial meningeal artery, which passes through the foramen spinosum—to the dura mater in the middle cranial fossa and part of the anterior cranial fossa.

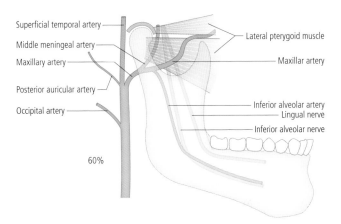

Fig. 1.1-1 Variants in the branching of the common carotid artery (60%, according to Lippert and Pabst 1985).

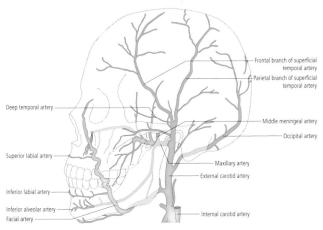

Fig. 1.1-2 Overview of the branches of the external carotid artery.

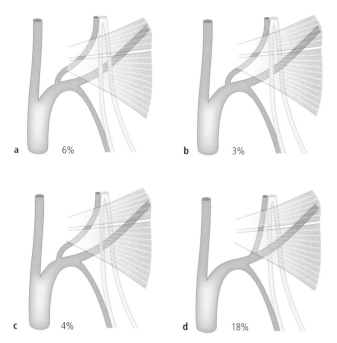

a   6%   b   3%

c   4%   d   18%

Fig. 1.1-3 Course of the maxillary artery (after Lippert and Pabst 1985).

1.1.2   Clinical picture (carotid artery, vertebral artery)

Cerebral ischemic events are the most frequent cause of stroke (80–85% of cases) and currently represent the third most frequent cause of death in the industrialized countries. Approximately 50% of the patients have significant mental or physical disturbances after a stroke. Stenoses of the internal carotid artery are the cause of nearly one-third of all cases of ischemic stroke. In stenoses of the internal carotid artery, nearly 80% of the clinical symptoms arise due to cerebral emboli from arteriosclerotic plaques. The remaining 20% of strokes arise due to hemodynamic compromise of cerebral circulation.

In approximately one-quarter of all cases of ischemic stroke, there is involvement of the posterior or vertebrobasilar circulation. Stenoses of the vertebral artery are the cause of up to 20% of all cases of ischemic stroke in the posterior flow region. Proximal stenoses of the vertebral artery are the second most frequent cause of ischemic stroke after stenoses of the internal carotid artery. As in the pathogenesis of internal carotid artery stenoses, stroke in the posterior flow region most often results from emboli from arteriosclerotic plaques. Hemodynamic compromise must be regarded as comparatively rare in the posterior flow region, as the basilar artery is supplied by two vertebral arteries. In contrast to the internal carotid artery, the vertebral artery also has many collateral vessels that are able to compensate cerebral perfusion when there is proximal constriction of a vertebral artery.

Good familiarity with the extracranial and intracranial anatomy is decisive for treatment of the relevant vascular occlusion processes. The left common carotid artery arises from the aortic arch, and the right one from the bifurcation of the brachiocephalic trunk. The common carotid artery does not have any side branches. At the level of the upper edge of the thyroid cartilage, it divides into the internal and external carotid arteries. The external carotid artery supplies the temporomandibular joint, the face, the neck, and the menin-

ges. It has two terminal branches—the superficial temporal artery and the maxillary artery. These two branches may also serve, along with the occipital artery, as collaterals if there is occlusion of the internal carotid artery or vertebral artery. The internal carotid artery ascends laterally behind the hypopharynx, where it can be palpated. It branches into the anterior and medial cerebral arteries. It has no visible side branches in its extracranial course up to the branching point. The first major intracranial branch is the ophthalmic artery. The vertebral artery arises from the subclavian artery and travels to the sixth cervical vertebra, where it passes through the transverse foramen in the transverse process of the sixth vertebra and courses in a sharply cranial direction in the same way through the corresponding foramina of cervical vertebrae C5 to C1. In this segment, the vertebral artery courses more or less parallel to the carotid artery. At C1, the vertebral artery turns posteriorly and arches around the posterior part of the vertebral arch. It then passes through the foramen magnum into the cranial cavity. At the lower margin of the pons, the left and right vertebral arteries unite to form the basilar artery, which in turn flows into the circle of Willis. Although generally the vertebral arteries make only a minor contribution to the overall cerebral circulation, they can be of significant importance when occlusion or stenosis of the internal carotid artery develops.

The circle of Willis is the most important intracranial collateral pathway. Via the anterior and posterior communicating arteries, the anterior, middle, and posterior cerebral arteries are connected in a circuit. In situations in which a proximal atherosclerotic process progresses slowly, the circle of Willis is able to compensate for vascular occlusions. However, the circle is not fully developed in all individuals. In patients with an incomplete circle of Willis, even brief occlusion of a vessel can lead to a stroke.

1.1.3   Clinical findings

The clinical symptoms of stenosis of the internal carotid artery or vertebral artery are characterized by ischemia in the corresponding region of cerebral flow. Symptomatic stenosis of the internal carotid artery is defined by syndromes in the ipsilateral hemisphere during the previous 6 months:

- Transitory ischemic attack (TIA) = focal neurological deficit for less than 24 h
- Amaurosis fugax = monocular amaurosis for less than 24 h
- Stroke = focal neurological deficit for more than 24 h

Symptomatic stenosis of the vertebral artery can become manifest in the form of:
- Syncope
- Vertigo
- Ataxia
- Ipsilateral TIA or stroke in the posterior region of flow

1.1.4   Differential diagnosis

Etiological differential diagnosis of ischemic stroke:
- Macroangiopathy of the supra-aortic vessels:
    - Atherosclerotic
    - Non-atherosclerotic (dissection, fibromuscular dysplasia, giant cell arteritis, Takayasu syndrome, bacterial or viral vasculitides)

- Cerebral microangiopathy:
  - Atherosclerotic
  - Non-atherosclerotic (vasculitides)
- Sources of cardiac emboli:
  - Atrial fibrillation, atrial myxoma, atrioseptal aneurysm, acute myocardial infarction, endocarditis, status post-cardiac valve replacement, dilated cardiomyopathy
- Paradoxical embolism:
  - Atrial septal defect, persistent oval foramen, in deep vein thrombosis in the lower extremity or pelvis, thrombophilia
- Atherosclerosis of the aortic arch
- Coagulation disturbances:
  - Genetic—e.g., in antithrombin III deficiency, protein S/protein C deficiency, activated protein C (APC) resistance, factor V Leiden mutation
  - Acquired in disseminated intravascular coagulation—e.g., in multiple trauma, sepsis
- Hematological diseases:
  - e.g., polycythemia, hemoglobinopathies, iron-deficiency anemia, leukemia, thrombocythemia

Differential diagnosis of acute focal neurological deficit:
- Intracerebral hemorrhage
- Subarachnoid hemorrhage
- Sinus thrombosis/cerebral venous thrombosis
- Migraine with aura
- Postictal hemiparesis (Todd paralysis)

In cases of suspected stenosis of the vertebral artery with no evidence of cerebral ischemia in the posterior region of flow, all of the differential diagnoses of syncope, vertigo, or ataxia also need to be considered.

1.1.5 Diagnosis

Carotid stenosis is diagnosed using color duplex ultrasonography, which is widely available and is low-cost. In addition to assessment of the grade of stenosis, the method also makes it possible to identify the plaque morphology (e.g., with an ulcerated surface).

Patients who should undergo duplex evaluation include those who have suffered a focal neurological deficit or amaurosis fugax. Cerebral computed tomography (CT) or magnetic resonance imaging (MRI) can also help exclude other causes of neurological symptoms, such as hemorrhage or tumor. In asymptomatic patients, there are no standard diagnostic recommendations, except when a bypass operation is planned. In this special situation, a duplex ultrasound examination is recommended in patients ≥ 65 years, patients with stenosis of the left main coronary artery, peripheral arterial occlusive disease, nicotine abuse, or a history including cerebral ischemia. Duplex ultrasound screening should also be carried out in asymptomatic patients who have a bruit over the internal carotid artery if the patient's general condition allows surgical or interventional treatment. When duplex ultrasound results are unclear, the diagnostic accuracy can be increased using supplementary computed-tomographic angiography or magnetic resonance angiography.

In the diagnosis of extracranial vertebral artery stenosis, a noninvasive duplex ultrasound examination is also the procedure of choice. More than 80% of vertebral arteries can be detected using duplex ultrasonography. Digital subtraction angiography is still the "gold standard" for assessing stenosis of the vertebral artery. However, it is associated with a certain rate of morbidity and mortality, albeit low.

1.1.5.1 Doppler/duplex ultrasonography

Examination technique

The examination is best carried out with the examiner positioned behind the patient's head, as this allows both hands to be used and functional tests can be carried out more easily. The examination is carried out at two levels using a high-frequency (≥ 7.5 MHz) linear probe, including the proximal vascular segments near the aortic arch (to detect any stenoses at the orifices for the common carotid artery, brachiocephalic trunk, subclavian artery, and vertebral artery). Supraclavicular and jugular insonation should be carried out, preferably using a microconvex probe (≥ 7.5 MHz). If this is not available, adapted programming of a low-frequency convex probe can be used, as well as insonation of carotid segments near the base of the skull. Although the bifurcation region is the most frequent site for pathological carotid processes, it is not the only one.

Examination of the carotid system

In addition to demonstration of any extracranial pathology, attention should be given to the Doppler velocities, as an indirect sign of proximal or distal pathologies. Side-to-side V_{mean} differences in the internal carotid artery showing ≥ 10% pulsatility differences or bilateral pulsatility changes should be assessed as follows:
- Increased pulsatility:
  - Distal circulatory pathway obstruction (stenosis, occlusion)—possibly unilateral in such cases
  - Cerebral microangiopathy (Binswanger disease)
  - Raised intracranial pressure (edema, bleeding)
  - Bradycardia
  - Aortic insufficiency
- Reduced pulsatility:
  - Proximal circulatory pathway obstruction (prolonged acceleration time)
  - Distal arteriovenous malformation or angioma (normal acceleration time)
  - Aortic stenosis, reduced ejection fraction

Transcranial Doppler/duplex ultrasonography should be carried out in cases of cerebral pathology with evidence of hemodynamically relevant extracranial processes. If it is not available, insonation of the supratrochlear artery with compression of the facial artery at the mandibular angle and of the superficial temporal artery in front of the tragus should be carried out (preferably at the same time). The findings at the supratrochlear artery reflect the cerebral hemodynamics along with the quality of intracerebral collateralization and can be predictive for watershed infarction.

Flow differences in the supratrochlear artery greater than 1:2 ratio may suggest:

- Proximal internal carotid artery stenosis on the side with lower flow
- External carotid artery stenosis on the side with higher flow
- Distal intracranial internal carotid artery stenosis after the origin of the ophthalmic artery or higher-grade T-fork/middle cerebral artery main trunk stenosis on the side with higher flow

False-negative compression tests may occur due to:

- Common carotid artery processes with similar compromise of flow in the internal and external carotid arteries
- Simultaneous internal carotid and external carotid processes
- Hypoplasia or aplasia of the supratrochlear artery

False-positive compression tests may occur due to:

- Wobbling: the most frequent error
- Anatomic variants (rare)

Examination of the subclavian/vertebral artery system

Demonstration of the orifice of the vertebral artery is obligatory, as this is the most frequent site for arteriosclerotic stenoses. Identification of vessels at the orifice using undulation at the mastoid is also necessary. Demonstration of the distal course (V2) allows better visualization of hypoplasia and aplasia, occlusions and dissections. The vertebral arteries are of equal size in only one-quarter of cases; when there are differences in diameter between the two sides, differences in pulsatility and amplitude between the two vertebral arteries are often seen and the Doppler velocities often differ due to an absent or hypoplastic connection between the vertebral and basilar arteries. It is incorrect to conclude from a bilaterally identical Dopplers of the distal vertebral artery that conditions are normal, although this frequently happens.

In cases of proximal occlusion, there is often distal collateral filling in the region of the atlas via occipital branches or other collaterals to the external carotid artery—and insonation should be carried out there as well, at least in these cases.

Differential diagnosis

Arteriosclerosis:

- Typical plaque morphology
- Classically localized at the carotid bifurcation and at the orifices of the vertebral artery, subclavian artery, and brachiocephalic trunk

Embolism:

- Hypoechoic to isoechoic occlusion material
- Otherwise unremarkable vascular system with no major atheroma

Arterial thrombosis:

- In addition to the hypoechoic occlusion, evidence of prior arteriosclerosis with sonographically complex plaques and structures creating acoustic shadows, possibly "older" echogenic occlusion components
- Involvement particularly of proximal vascular segments and vascular segments near the aortic arch and of branches of the external carotid artery (superficial temporal artery)

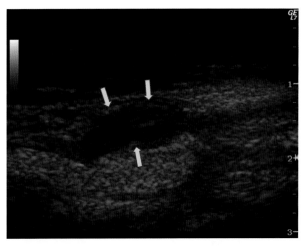

Fig. 1.1-4 Carotidynia: hypoechoic focal wall thickening, representing mural hematoma.

Table 1.1-1 The reaction pattern in the supratrochlear artery during compression of the external branches.

Increased flow	Evidence of normal orthograde flow
Reverse flow	Evidence of pathological retrograde flow
Reduced flow	Evidence of pathological retrograde flow; intracranial perfusion pressure probably poorer than with reverse flow
No reaction	If there are no notable external–internal carotid artery anastomoses or maxillary/ethmoidal artery collaterals → contralateral compression, and then alternatively a compression test in the supraorbital region → an increase in outflow resistance leads to reduced flow velocities, particularly diastolic → pulsatility increases
Zero flow, with evidence of flow only during compression	Pathological → equalized extracranial/intracranial pressure

Dissection:

- There may initially be a floating dissection membrane.
- The true lumen may be alternately compromised as far as the occlusion—possibly with a sharply tapering occlusion pattern (the string sign).
- The false lumen may thrombose.
- When there is a floating membrane, there may be a pathognomonic triphasic "splash signal."
- Circumscribed mural hematomas may occur ("carotidynia").
- Variants:
  - The vertebral artery in particular often shows hypoplasia and also aplasia.
  - Definition of vertebral artery hypoplasia: vascular diameter < 2.5 mm or diameter ratio > 1:1.7.
- Large-vessel vasculitis:
  - Typical homogeneous, hypoechoic and widened intima–media complex (macaroni sign)
- *Caution:* there are often respiratory-modulated buckling stenoses in the subclavian artery, particularly on the left side, which regress on inspiration.

Specific findings

Common carotid artery

The width of the boundary zone reflection (synonymous with the intima–media thickness, IMT) in the common carotid artery (CCA, and other vessels) has been found to be a parameter for assessing the atherosclerotic risk, and it correlates with the incidence of vascular events.

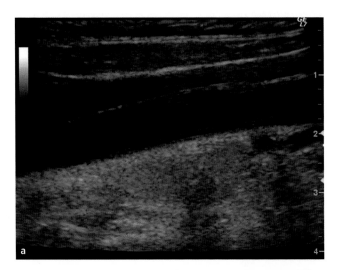

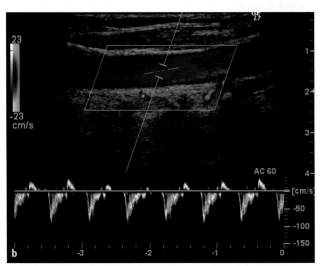

Fig. 1.1-5a, b Dissection of the internal carotid artery. (**a**) A visible dissection membrane in the area of the common carotid artery. (**b**) The typically altered polyphasic pulsed-wave Doppler signal.

There is no established classification based on maximum velocities for grades of stenosis in common carotid artery stenoses. In addition to the general characteristics of a stenosis (see under internal carotid artery stenoses), the peak velocity ratio (PVR) can be used.

Internal carotid artery

Various angiographic grading methods are available, with differing percentage figures. The residual diameter may refer either to the distal diameter of the internal carotid artery, with the local stenosis grade based on the North American Symptomatic Carotid Endarterectomy Trial (NASCET) criteria; or to the original proximal diameter, with the local stenosis grade based on the European Carotid Surgery Trial (ECST) criteria. An approximate formal conversion can be carried out:

> Local stenosis grade (based on ECST): ECST % = 0.6 × NASCET % + 40%
> Distal stenosis grade (based on NASCET): NASCET % = (ECST − 40%)/0.6

The traditional duplex ultrasound criteria used by the German Society for Ultrasound in Medicine (*Deutsche Gesellschaft für Ultraschall in der Medizin,* DEGUM) correlated with the ECST local stenosis grade (although the NASCET method was mainly used in radiography). The DEGUM criteria were revised in 2010 to establish comparability and transferred to NASCET (Table 1.1-3). The method used for duplex ultrasound classification must be clearly stated.

N.B.: Confusion may arise when the old and new stenosis grades for the internal carotid artery are compared or used in parallel.

Stenoses in other locations (external carotid artery, vertebral artery, common carotid artery, etc.) are generally continuing to be classified according to the local stenosis grade on the basis of previously customary hemodynamic criteria. Supra-aortic stenoses with the same local stenosis grade in other vascular territories may therefore

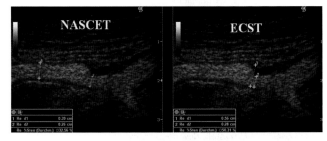

Fig. 1.1-6 NASCET–ECST: the principles of stenosis grading based on NASCET and ECST (B flow imaging).

Table 1.1-2 Age-dependent and gender-dependent normal values for intima–media thickness (IMT) in the common carotid artery (CCA), showing means, standard deviations, and 95% confidence intervals (Temelkova-Kurktschiev et al. 2001).

All data in mm	Men Age 40–54	Men Age 55–70	Women Age 40–54	Women Age 55–70
IMT$_{mean}$ – distal CCA	0.79 ± 0.13 (0.73–0.84)	0.87 ± 0.14 (0.81–0.93)	0.70 ± 0.11 (0.67–0.75)	0.82 ± 0.19 (0.75–0.90)
IMT$_{mean}$ – middle CCA	0.62 ± 0.10 (0.57–0.67)	0.69 ± 0.14 (0.62–0.76)	0.54 ± 0.07 (0.51–0.57)	0.64 ± 0.13 (0.57–0.71)
IMT$_{maximum}$ – CCA	0.90 ± 0.16 (0.83–0.93)	0.95 ± 0.16 (0.87–1.01)	0.78 ± 0.12 (0.74–0.84)	0.93 ± 0.20 (0.85–1.00)

be given as "higher" percentages than internal carotid artery stenoses, which are classified according to the distal stenosis grade.

In addition to hemodynamic criteria, new B-image optimization techniques and digital subtraction ultrasonography (B flow) provide effective assistance in demonstrating the morphology. Bifurcation stenoses in particular are often missed or incorrectly classified in angiographic procedures.

Cross-sectional planimetry correlates more with the local stenosis grade and is associated with error due to vascular remodeling of the internal carotid artery. A compensatory increase in the terminal diameter of the vessel occurs with increasing grades of stenosis, so that the percentage grade of stenosis is incorrectly raised. These values therefore need to be treated with caution.

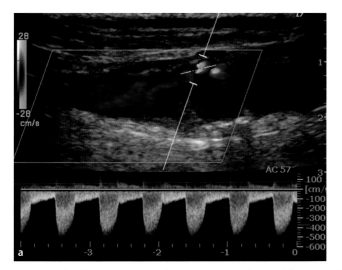 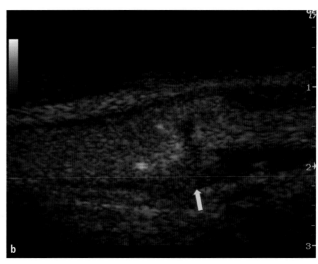

Fig. 1.1-7a, b Bifurcation stenosis of the internal carotid artery. (**a**) Imaging of a high-grade, eccentric internal carotid artery stenosis with apparently hypoechoic plaque material. (**b**) The bifurcation stenotic process is detected on the B-image/B-flow.

Table 1.1-3 Stenosis grading in the internal carotid artery based on NASCET (adapted from Arning et al. 2010).

Stenosis grade (NASCET definition) (%)		10	20–40	50	60	70	80	90	Occlusion
Stenosis grade, older (ESCT definition) (%)		45	50–60	70	75	80	90	95	Occlusion
Main criteria	1. B-image	+++	+						
	2. Color Doppler image	+	+++	+	+	+	+	+	+++
	3. Peak systolic velocity at maximum stenosis (cm/s), approx.			200	250	300	350–400	100–500	
	4. Peak systolic velocity, post-stenotic (cm/s)					> 50	< 50	< 30	
	5. Collaterals and preliminary stages (periorbital arteries/ACA)					(+)	++	+++	+++
Additional criteria	6. Diastolic flow deceleration, prestenotic (CCA)					(+)	++	+++	+++
	7. Post-stenotic flow disturbances			+	+	++	+++	(+)	
	8. End-diastolic flow velocity at maximum stenosis (cm/s), approx.			Up to 100	Up to 100	Over 100	Over 100		
	9. Confetti sign				(+)	++	++		
	10. Stenotic index ICA/CCA			[3] 2	[3] 2	[3] 4	[3] 4		

Notes on criteria 1–10 (see text for further explanations): stenosis grade based on NASCET (%): the figures given refer in each case to a 10% range (± 5%). Criterion 2: Evidence of low-grade stenosis (local aliasing effect) distinct from nonstenotic plaque, demonstration of flow direction in moderate to high-grade stenoses and evidence of vascular occlusion. Criterion 3: The criteria apply to stenoses with a length of 1–2 cm and only to a limited extent to processes affecting multiple vessels. Criterion 4: Measurement well distally, outside of the zone with jet stream and flow disturbances. Criterion 5: Possibly only one of the collateral connections may be affected: if only an extracranial examination is carried out, the value of the findings is lower. Criterion 9: Confetti sign can only be recognized when the pulse repetition frequency (PRF) is set low.
ACA, anterior cerebral artery; ICA, internal carotid artery; CCA, common carotid artery.

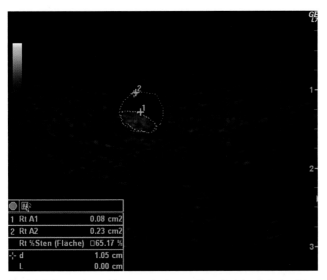

1	Rt A1	0.08 cm2
2	Rt A2	0.23 cm2
	Rt %Sten (Flache)	□65.17 %
-¦-	d	1.05 cm
	L	0.00 cm

Fig. 1.1-8 Internal carotid artery planimetry. The principle of planimetric stenosis grading. The limitations due to a compensatory increase in the external diameter should be noted.

Additional information on plaque status and on the prognostic assessment is particularly desirable for treatment decision-making in patients with asymptomatic stenoses. The aim is to detect stenoses that are associated with an increased risk of embolism, since at this stage it is usually an embolic source rather than a hemodynamically compromising structure that is removed (otherwise there is a very high number needed to treat in therapy for asymptomatic stenoses). Prognostic significance has not been conclusively evaluated for all of the parameters.

- Plaque echogenicity: hypoechoic plaques are prognostic for a 4–5-fold increase in the risk of stroke (Mathiesen et al. 2001).
- Plaque perfusion: the presence and extent of neovascularization of a plaque—demonstrated using ultrasound contrast enhancement with a low mechanical index (MI) technique—correlates positively with the risk of stroke and the general rate of cardiovascular events.
- Rate of spontaneous cerebral embolism (high-intensity transitory signals, HITS; see section A 1.2): for example, when there is evidence of HITS in asymptomatic 60% internal carotid artery stenosis, there is an approximately 15-fold increase in the risk of stroke in comparison with negative HITS (Spence et al. 2005).

Intracerebral collateralization/autoregulation reserve/CO_2 reactivity (see section A 1.2)—limited autoregulation reserve/CO_2 reactivity in intracerebral vessels correlates with hemodynamically caused watershed infarction.

There is a risk of overestimating stenoses in the internal carotid artery:

- When there is contralateral internal carotid artery occlusion or very high-grade stenosis with collateral function in the ipsilateral ICA (only with collateralization via the anterior communicating branch (transcranial Doppler examination required)
- When there are collaterals in the ICA via the posterior communicating branch in the flow area of the posterior cerebral circulation
- In cases of distal arteriovenous malformation
- Possibly in cases of elongation and kinking at the site of the stenosis

- Measurement of the relevant parameters during cardiac irregularities—e.g., after extrasystoles with a compensatory pause, or in absolute arrhythmia after a longer RR interval, or with an increased ejection volume in cases of aortic insufficiency or marked bradycardia

There is a risk of underestimating stenoses in the internal carotid artery:

- In cases of tandem stenoses of the internal carotid artery or high-grade flow obstructions in the area of the carotid "T" or main trunk of the middle cerebral artery
- With hyperventilation (intracerebral vasoconstriction)
- In cases of marked cerebral microangiopathy or raised intracranial pressure with disturbed distal outflow
- When measurements are carried out during hemodynamically compromising tachycardic heart action
- In cases of upstream high-grade flow obstructions

Occlusion can be differentiated from "pseudo-occlusion" or filiform stenosis by:

- Low flow–optimized setting of the device (PRF low, line thickness increased, etc.)
- Increasing the color enhancement appropriately (*caution:* artifacts)
- Using alternative color scales (mixed mode), color procedures (power mode), and imaging modes (B flow, color B flow)
- Optimizing the transducer head position and beam position
- Using ultrasound contrast enhancement
- Including the intracranial findings

Check-up examinations postoperatively or after stent angioplasty in the internal carotid artery:

- In both procedures: residual stenosis, recurrent stenosis, intimal hyperplasia in the internal carotid artery, intraluminal thrombi, flow conditions at the external carotid artery orifice?
- After surgery: intimal flap, proximal/distal step formation, aneurysmal dilation in the patch area (TEA)
- After internal carotid artery stenting: is the stent well opposed or is there flow behind it; is the stenotic area completely covered?

In-stent restenosis:

- Slightly altered velocity criteria have been described (by Armstrong et al. 2007, among others), partly due to reduced wall compliance in the stent area and loss of the luminal dilation ("bulb") often (but not always) located in the internal carotid artery orifice area.

External carotid artery

There is no established classification of stenosis grades for external carotid artery stenoses based on maximum velocities. In addition to general stenotic characteristics (see under internal carotid artery stenoses), the peak velocity ratio can be used.

The differential diagnosis should include distal arteriovenous malformations in the afferent areas for branches of the external carotid artery, as well as dural fistulas; flow acceleration/aliasing is then seen over long stretches and not only focally in the "stenotic area."

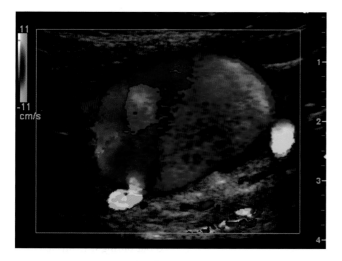

Fig. 1.1-9 An aneurysm in the internal carotid artery. A typical "coffee-bean" fragmented color pattern in an internal carotid artery aneurysm, with relative stenosis in the outflow area.

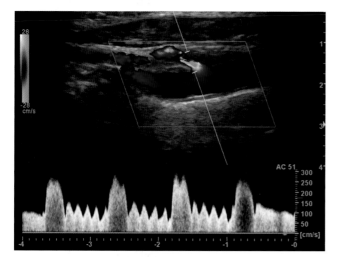

Fig. 1.1-10 Stenosis of the external carotid artery. A typical undulation phenomenon is seen in the external carotid artery, with evidence of moderate stenosis.

Table 1.1-4 Stenosis grades after stent angioplasty in the internal carotid artery.

	> 70%	> 50%
PSV (cm/s)	> 350	> 225
ICA–CCA ratio	> 4.75	> 2.5

CCA, common carotid artery; ICA, internal carotid artery; PSV, systolic velocity.

In cases of occlusion of the external carotid artery, side branches are often collateralized via the corresponding external carotid artery branches on the contralateral side or branches of the thyrocervical trunk or costocervical trunk.

Subclavian artery

See section A 4.1.

Vertebral artery

For findings involving the subclavian steal effect/syndrome, see section A 4.1.

There is no established classification of stenosis grades based on maximum velocities for vertebral artery stenoses. The criteria mentioned in connection with the internal carotid artery can be used, but it should be noted that minor flow disturbances in the obtusely angled orifice area of the vertebral arteries must be regarded as physiological. The velocities given should be lower, as the physiological maximum systolic flow velocity is approximately 60–100 cm/s. Values above 100 cm/s must be regarded as suspicious. The critical velocity after which the presence of a > 50% stenosis must be assumed is 120 cm/s (Baumgartner et al. 1999). The peak velocity ratio may also be used.

Differential diagnoses in cases of flow acceleration in the vertebral artery, with a risk of overestimating stenoses:

- Inadequate perfusion of the contralateral vertebral artery (e.g., due to aplasia, hypoplasia, stenosis, occlusion, dissection) with hyperperfusion of the artery being examined
- Hyperperfusion of the vertebral arteries when collaterals via the posterior communicating branch are compensating for obstructive carotid processes
- Arteriovenous malformations in the vertebrobasilar flow area
- Measurement of the relevant parameters, e.g., after extrasystoles, with a compensatory pause, or in cases of absolute arrhythmia after a longer RR interval, or with an increased ejection volume in patients with aortic insufficiency or marked bradycardia

Differential diagnoses in cases of flow deceleration in the vertebral artery, with a risk of underestimating stenoses:

- Distal vertebrobasilar flow obstruction (high pulsatility, and reduced diastolic flow in particular)
- Hypoplasia or dilatory arteriopathy in the vertebral artery
- Marked cerebral microangiopathy or raised intracranial pressure with disturbed distal outflow (with identical bilateral findings)
- When measurements are carried out during hemodynamically compromising tachycardic heart action
- In cases of proximal high-grade flow obstructions

Findings in occlusions of the extracranial vertebral artery:

- Vessel not identifiable (in continuous-wave mode, occlusion may only be suspected, however)
- Possible hyperperfusion of the contralateral vessel
- Arterial lumen definitely demonstrated on duplex ultrasound, without PW Doppler or color signals
- Demonstration of distal inflow collaterals possible

Findings in occlusions of the intracranial vertebral artery:

- Markedly increased extracranial pulsatility, with reduced diastolic flow in one vertebral artery that may amount to pendular flow (*caution:* outflow into a dilated PICA may lead to a normal Doppler signal when there is a distal vertebral artery occlusion)
- Possible hyperperfusion of the contralateral artery
- Course of the vertebral artery not capable of being imaged transnuchally

Vertebral artery compression syndrome (often suspected, but actually a rare finding) characterized by:

- Rotatory vertigo and nystagmus
- Capable of being reproducibly triggered by head rotation
- Can be stopped by a return movement
- Clear hypoplasia in one vertebral artery (duplex ultrasound evidence)
- Movement-dependent, hemodynamically compromising compression of a normal-lumen vertebral artery (Doppler and duplex ultrasound evidence possible), so that with relevant hypoplasia of a vertebral artery and suspicious clinical findings, an attempt should be made to provoke symptoms during Doppler/duplex ultrasound examination of various segments of the normal-lumen vertebral artery

1.1.6   Treatment

1.1.6.1   Conservative treatment

Medical treatment is indicated in both internal carotid artery stenosis and vertebral artery stenosis, in order to limit atherosclerotic progression and reduce the risk of a neurological event. This treatment recommendation is independent of the decision on whether to offer interventional or surgical revascularization therapy. Treatments currently available include inhibition of platelets using acetylsalicylic acid (ASA), dipyridamole plus acetylsalicylic acid, or clopidogrel. In addition, treatment with statins is advised due to their anti-inflammatory and thus plaque-stabilizing effect in other vascular territories. Medical treatment alone is recommended in patients with stenosis of the internal carotid artery who either have a low risk of stroke (symptomatic stenoses < 50%, asymptomatic stenoses < 60%) or who are at high perioperative or peri-interventional risk due to comorbid conditions, or who have a limited life expectancy.

Drug treatment was the only form of therapy available for cerebral ischemia in the posterior flow region prior to the advent of endovascular approaches. Unfortunately, there is still a lack of data from randomized studies comparing drug treatment with surgical or interventional therapy for extracranial stenoses of the vertebral artery. The results of the Vertebral Artery Stenting Trial (VAST), which is currently still recruiting, will probably be able to provide important information. At present, 180 patients with symptomatic vertebral artery stenosis > 50% have been randomly assigned either to endovascular treatment (stent implantation) or to the conservatively treated group in the study.

1.1.6.2   Endovascular treatment

Patient preparation

- General patient history
- Medication and allergy history
- Complete neurological evaluation, plus National Institutes of Health Stroke Scale (NIHSS)
- Cranial CT or MRI examination
- Duplex ultrasonography to exclude fresh thrombus formation
- ASA 100–300 mg/day and clopidogrel 75 mg/day, starting at least 5 days before a planned intervention, or bolus administration (ASA 500 mg, clopidogrel 600 mg) on the day before the procedure

Peri-interventional therapy

- Heparin (70–100 IU/kg) with an activated clotting time (ACT) of 250–300 seconds
- Electrocardiographic (ECG) monitoring due to potential bradycardia
- Blood pressure monitoring for possible hypotension related to carotid sinus stimulation by balloon inflation
- Intravenous administration of 1 mg atropine 2–3 min before implantation of the carotid stent, to prevent possible bradycardia or asystole (to be used with caution in patients with narrow-angle glaucoma)
- Infusions for marked or prolonged bradycardia/hypotension

Technique of carotid artery stenting (CAS)

Access route

It is important to establish a safe vascular access route in order to minimize complications during carotid stent implantation, and access via the femoral artery is the approach most often employed. The common femoral artery is punctured using a Seldinger needle, and a 12-cm long 5–6F sheath is placed. This initial sheath is then exchanged during the procedure for a 90-cm long sheath (e.g., Cook Shuttle sheath.). If a guiding catheter is to be used, a 12-cm long 8–9F sheath is needed. In patients in whom the pelvic arteries are occluded or who have high-grade stenosis, or in situations in which the access route via the femoral artery is unavailable for other reasons, access via the brachial or radial artery is obtained (Fig. 1.1-11). The right brachial artery is preferable for interventions on both the right internal carotid artery and the left internal carotid artery. If neither access route is possible, direct cervical common carotid access (percutaneous or open surgical) can be considered.

Engaging the common carotid artery

Angiography of the aortic arch is generally performed prior to any selective carotid angiography in order to identify possible difficult anatomic conditions that might make it necessary to exchange the typically employed diagnostic catheters (e.g., Berenstein, Judkins Right, Head Hunter, IMA, JB-1) for an alternative one (e.g., Simmons or Vitek catheter) (Fig. 1.1-12). To engage the common carotid artery, the 5F diagnostic catheter (e.g., Berenstein, Right Judkins, Head Hunter, IMA) is positioned over a 0.035-inch hydrophilic guidewire in the ascending aorta with the catheter tip pointing downward. This technique reduces the likelihood of embolization from aortic plaque or traumatic injury to the intima of the aortic arch and prevents the catheter from becoming caught in a vascular ostium. As soon as the catheter reaches the ascending aorta, it is rotated 180°. This places the tip of the catheter in a vertical, upright position on fluoroscopy. The catheter is then carefully withdrawn until it slides into the brachiocephalic trunk, and the hydrophilic wire is then advanced into the right common carotid artery and the catheter is advanced over this wire into the common carotid artery. To intubate the left common carotid artery, the catheter is slowly withdrawn from the ostium of the brachiocephalic trunk. It should be rotated 20° counterclockwise, so that the catheter tip points slightly anteriorly. When the aortic arch becomes unwound with advancing age, the origin of the left common carotid artery is lo-

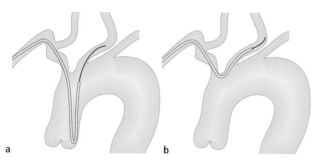

Fig. 1.1-11a, b Access via the brachial artery.

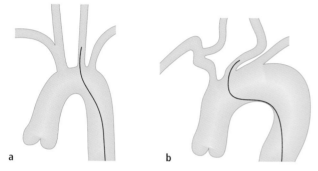

Fig. 1.1-12a, b (**a**) Simple anatomic conditions. (**b**) More difficult anatomic conditions. The catheter is capable of prolapsing into the ascending aorta.

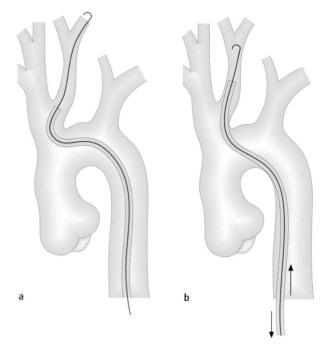

Fig. 1.1-13a, b The push-and-pull technique.

cated slightly further posterior. In these cases, it may be necessary to rotate the catheter posteriorly instead.

Once the left common carotid artery has been entered, the catheter should be rotated back 20° clockwise, so that the tip is once again pointing vertically or slightly posteriorly. The catheter position is checked by administering a small amount of contrast. This can exclude subintimal contrast flow or reduced blood flow. The hydrophilic wire is advanced to the distal common carotid artery, followed by the catheter.

Exploring the common carotid artery in difficult anatomy

If engagement of the common carotid artery is unsuccessful with the standard catheter, then a switch to a Simmons catheter is usually made. This type of catheter has a large reverse curve which must be re-shaped in the aorta after wire removal, usually in the ascending aorta. Moving the catheter backward slightly guides the tip into the brachiocephalic trunk, then into the left common carotid artery, and finally into the left subclavian artery. In contrast, Vitek or Mani catheters have smaller pre-formed curves and do not require shaping so these catheters are advanced from, rather than withdrawn toward, the distal aortic arch selecting the left subclavian artery first, and so on. Once the desired vessel is selected, the wire is advanced followed by the catheter. Advancement of the catheter is carried out slowly and with assistance from the pulsating blood flow. At the same time, the wire is withdrawn slightly, so that its position is maintained proximal to the carotid bifurcation. Advancement of the catheter and withdrawal of the guidewire are carried out alternately several times until the catheter is safely positioned in the vessel (push-and-pull technique) (Fig. 1.1-13).

Visualizing the vessels

Injections of contrast medium should be carried out manually or with a small amount of automated contrast administration (a maximum of 6 mL per injection). Larger amounts would lead to mixing of the arterial, intermediate, and venous phases, potentially leading to masking of early venous filling or other types of pathology. Some operators carry out four-vessel angiography to show the status of the collateral arteries. However, as this represents an additional procedural risk, the need for it is questionable, particularly in patients in whom magnetic resonance angiography has previously been carried out. During balloon dilation, the absence of collaterals may cause short periods of cerebral ischemia due to brief occlusion of the internal carotid artery. However, this reaction is reversible after deflation of the balloon and has no influence on the completion of the procedure. Once the anatomy of the target vessel has been defined, a hydrophilic guidewire is advanced into the external carotid artery so that the diagnostic catheter can be exchanged for a sheath or guide sheath. Bony landmarks can be used for guidance instead of road mapping to mark the origin of the external carotid artery during wire placement.

Vascular kinking

If the vessel is very tortuous, it can be straightened using a wire. It is also helpful to ask the patient to inhale deeply and hold the breath. An acute vessel angle can be negotiated by careful rotation and advancement of the catheter until it has reached the desired position (Fig. 1.1-14). If it is still not possible to advance the catheter, a Simmons III catheter should be used to introduce the guidewire into the external carotid artery. The Simmons III catheter can then be exchanged for a 4F multipurpose catheter. After this, the hydrophilic wire is exchanged for a 0.035-inch Amplatz wire or a softer wire. Finally, the 4F catheter is exchanged for a 5F catheter.

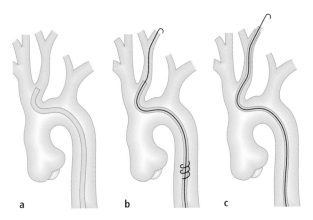

Fig. 1.1-14a–c (**a**) The technique of probing the left common carotid artery (CCA) and placing the guidewire in the external carotid artery (ECA) in the presence of a common trunk. (**b**) Placement of an IMA diagnostic catheter at the origin of the CCA. (**c**) Probing the ECA with a 0.035″ wire with antifriction coating (Terumo) and advancing the diagnostic catheter with slight right–left rotation as far as the ECA. Replacement with a more rigid uncoated wire (e.g., Supracor).

Placement of the guiding catheter

An 8F guiding catheter (e.g., a right coronary guiding catheter) is introduced into the ascending aorta via a hydrophilic 0.035-inch wire. In cases of difficult or abnormal anatomy, aortography of the aortic arch can be used to assist in selective exploration. Following angiography of the aortic arch and assessment of the anatomy, the guiding catheter is introduced into the common carotid artery. This should be followed by careful aspiration and flushing with saline to clear any possible atherosclerotic particles out of the catheter.

Placement of the long sheath

Engagement of the common carotid artery is carried out with a 5F diagnostic catheter and access to the external carotid artery obtained with an angled hydrophilic guidewire, and the diagnostic catheter introduced into the external carotid artery as described above. The wire is exchanged for a 0.035-inch wire, typically a stiff Amplatz wire. The diagnostic catheter is removed and a 6F 90-cm sheath placed using an over-the-wire technique into the common carotid artery below the bifurcation. The sheath should be handled very carefully, as trauma to the common carotid artery ostium or release of atherosclerotic deposits may occur leading to neurologic sequelae. The sheath should be meticulously aspirated and flushed to eliminate possible air or atherosclerotic debris.

Carotid access in occluded external carotid artery or common carotid artery stenosis

When the external carotid artery is occluded, or there is significant stenosis below the bifurcation, or a stenosis at the ostium of the common carotid artery, placing the 6F 90-cm sheath in the common carotid artery may represent a considerable challenge. If possible, crossing the stenosis with a stiff wire should be avoided, as this may dislodge necrotic plaque material and cause distal embolization. If necessary, the 5F diagnostic catheter is advanced over a 0.035- or 0.038-inch guidewire for placement further distally, slightly proximal to the stenosis. It can then be exchanged over a 0.035-inch Am-

platz wire (extra stiff). If there is an ostial/proximal stenosis of the common carotid artery, it may be necessary to treat this stenosis first in order to obtain access to the distal stenosis. However, if this stenosis is not severe, the bifurcation stenosis should be treated first and then the proximal stenosis on the "way back."

Predilation

Some operators predilate the stenosis using a small angioplasty balloon and a short inflation time of 5–10 seconds. This provides for better passage and positioning of the stent. The present authors would only recommend predilation if primary stent implantation has failed. In our view, primary stent implantation has a protective effect against distal embolization by fixing deposits on the vascular wall.

Protection against emboli

The possibility of procedural cerebral embolization is an important concern in carotid angioplasty. Balloon dilation, stent implantation, and manipulation of the vessels by the catheter and wire can easily release emboli, which if large enough can in turn cause severe cerebral damage. For this reason, emboli protection systems are routinely used in most centers. There are currently three different underlying principles on which protection against cerebral embolism is based: filter systems, distal occlusion balloons, and proximal occlusion balloons.

Distal occlusion balloons

Distal occlusion balloons (Fig. 1.1-15a) were the first embolism protection systems to become available, and were widely used in the initial carotid stent experience. It consists of a 0.014-inch guidewire with an occlusion balloon in the distal section, which is inflated and deflated through a very small channel in the guiding catheter (Guardwire® Temporary Occlusion and Aspiration System, Medtronic Vascular; TriActiv® ProGuard™ Embolic Protection System, Kensey Nash). After the guiding catheter is placed, the occlusion balloon is positioned distal to the stenosis and the balloon inflated until blood flow into the internal carotid artery stops. Stent implantation then follows. After the intervention, an aspiration catheter is introduced up to the occlusion balloon, and the blood in the occluded artery is aspirated. Any particles released during the intervention are thus removed. The advantages of the distal occlusion system are its low profile (2.2F), flexibility and good steerability. Disadvantages include the fact that balloon occlusion is not tolerated in 6–10% of patients, and that the vascular segment distal to the occlusion balloon cannot be imaged using contrast during the balloon occlusion procedure.

Filter systems

Most filter systems (Fig. 1.1-15b) consist of a metal framework that is covered with a polyethylene membrane or a nitinol mesh. The pore size can vary between 80 and 200 µm in diameter depending on the specific device. Filters are usually attached to the distal section of a 0.014-inch guidewire. In its closed state, the filter is sheathed by an introducer catheter, and it is introduced into the vascular seg-

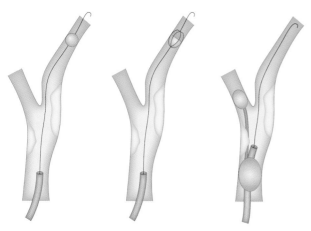

Fig. 1.1-15a–c Embolism protection system.

ment distal to the stenosis. Once the stenosis has been crossed, the filter is opened by withdrawing the outer catheter. Following stent implantation, the filter is closed by withdrawing it into a recovery catheter, and then removed from the vessel.

A wide range of second-generation and third-generation filter systems are currently available. The technical characteristics of a good filter consist of a low profile (< 3F), adequate steerability for maneuvering through highly tortuous vessels, and—when the filter is opened—good apposition to the vessel wall to allow the best possible protection against emboli.

Proximal occlusion systems

All distal protection systems, occlusion balloons and filters have the potential disadvantage that the stenosis has to be crossed before the system can be deployed and protection established. This unavoidable step carries a risk of distal embolization during the initial unprotected phase of the procedure. Proximal protection systems (Fig. 1.1-15c), such as the Gore Neuro Protection System (Gore) and the MO.MA System (Invatec), provide protection against cerebral embolism even before crossing the stenosis. This is particularly important in the case of stenosis with fresh thrombi where embolization with a distally placed system may be problematic. The use of a proximal protection system allows the operator to use any wire to negotiate difficult stenoses. These two systems consist of a long main sheath with a balloon on its distal end that is inflated in the common carotid artery to occlude forward carotid flow. A second balloon, which is inflated in the external carotid artery, prevents retrograde external flow, thus establishing complete arrest of antegrade flow into the internal carotid artery. The principle of proximal embolic protection systems takes advantage of the cerebral collateral system of the circle of Willis (Fig. 1.1-16). Following balloon occlusion of the external and common carotid artery, collateral flow via the circle of Willis produces what is known as reserve pressure. This prevents antegrade flow into the internal carotid artery. After stent implantation and before deflation of the occlusion balloon, blood in the internal carotid artery, which might contain released particles, is aspirated and removed. One disadvantage of the proximal protection system is that a small percentage of patients are unable to tolerate balloon occlusion due to incomplete intracranial collateralization.

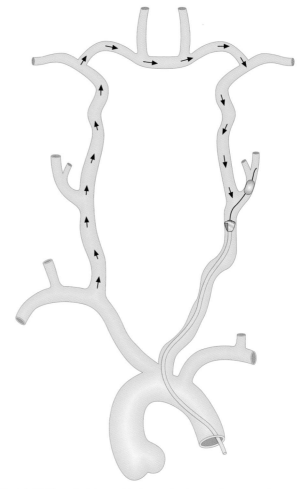

Fig. 1.1-16 The principle used in the proximal protection system (e.g., Gore Neuro Protection System), with reversal of flow in the internal carotid artery and continuous diversion of arterial blood via the protection system (with femoral venous return). This requires an intact anterior circle of Willis or other collateral support.

Stent implantation

Self-expanding stents are usually implanted in carotid stenting. Balloon-expandable stents are recommended in ostial stenoses of the common carotid artery, stenoses located in the distal internal carotid artery, and sometimes in severely calcified stenoses. The disadvantages of balloon-expandable stents are the repeated balloon dilations that are needed to implant the stent adequately, and stent compression that can occur during the long-term follow-up in areas vulnerable to external manipulation.

In vessels with the potential to bend or be manipulated, self-expanding nitinol stents are the best choice. They are designed to adapt to the shape of the vessel and therefore have little tendency to straighten it (Fig. 1.1-17). Stent-induced straightening of the vessel can give rise to a new stenosis distal to the stent due to kinking or folding of the vessel. Stents with a strong radial force are recommended for treatment of severely calcified stenoses. "Closed-cell" carotid stents usually have stronger radial force. Their cell structure may also provide better plaque coverage, which may be theoretically advantageous in stenoses with a high embolic risk. The clinical value of "open-cell" vs. "closed-cell" designs and the importance of the stent cell size is currently still unclear.

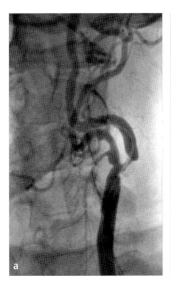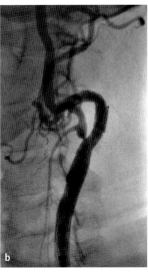

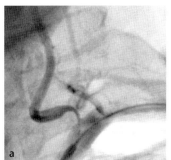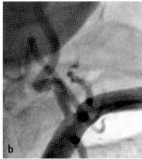

Fig. 1.1-18a, b (a) Outlet stenosis of the left vertebral artery before stent implantation. (b) After implantation of an expandable balloon stent.

Fig. 1.1-17a, b (a) Elongation of the internal carotid artery, with vascular kinking distal to the stenosis before stent implantation. (b) After implantation of a nitinol stent.

The authors recommend a stent diameter 1–2 mm larger than the largest vascular diameter to be stented. Carotid stents with a diameter of 6–8 mm are usually used if the stent is being implanted exclusively in the internal carotid artery, or with a diameter of 8–10 mm if the stent is to cross the bifurcation. Stenting across the external carotid artery is not a problem and priority should be given to the stent covering the entire stenosis, which in most cases will mean crossing the bifurcation to cover the distal common carotid artery plaque. While there are no data suggesting stent length is a determinant of restenosis in the carotid, a stent 20–30 mm longer is usually selected for discrete lesions, while for tandem stenoses, 40-mm stents are recommended.

Postdilation

Postdilation is usually carried out using a balloon with a diameter of ~5 mm, matched but not larger than the diameter of the internal carotid artery, but not referenced to the common carotid artery. A balloon with an unnecessarily large diameter might force particles through the stent cells and cause distal embolization. To prevent dissections, postdilation should be carried out at nominal pressure, and within the stent borders. A residual stenosis ≤ 30% is acceptable, since an adequate blood flow is established and the potentially emboligenic atherosclerotic deposits are compressed sufficiently to induce neointimal formation and eliminate the embolic potential of the lesion. The stent expands further during the following few hours. If contrast-enhancing ulcerations occur outside the stent edge, they do not need to be obliterated and can be left without any untoward effects. Postdilation of the stent segment in the common carotid artery is not necessary. If significant stenosis or occlusion of the external carotid artery develops following postdilation, it does not require treatment.

Following postdilation of the stent, angiography of the carotid arteries and intracranial vessels is carried out. Imaging of the intracerebral vessels should always include the venous phase, to allow objective comparison of conditions before and after stent implantation. For assessment of the intracerebral vessels and in preparation

for possible intracranial emergency intervention in case of cerebral embolism, angiography should be carried out with a lateral and anteroposterior 30° cranial (Towne) projection.

Technique of vertebral artery stent implantation

The vascular access route for vertebral artery interventions is the same as for carotid artery stent implantation, via the femoral or brachial artery. A contralateral oblique projection is best for demonstrating the ostium of the vertebral artery. The intracranial vertebrobasilar vascular system is best demonstrated in lateral and steep anteroposterior projections. A multipurpose 6F guiding catheter is suitable for the vertebral artery procedure. Balloon-expandable coronary stents should be used for ostial stenoses of the vertebral artery, and self-expanding stents can be used in extracranial vertebral artery stenoses that are located distal to the ostium in the body of the vessel. A 4-mm coronary balloon is usually used for dilation (Fig. 1.1-18). The embolic protection systems currently available cannot usually be recommended for vertebral artery procedures, as they still have relatively large diameters for this application.

Postinterventional follow-up and medication

Following the intervention, blood pressure has to be closely checked for at least 6 h. A neurological evaluation including the National Institutes of Health Stroke Scale (NIHSS) must be carried out before the patient is discharged. Lifelong ASA treatment (100 mg) and clopidogrel during the first month are recommended.

Clinical results

Clinical series/carotid stent implantation registry

A summary of the results in 12,392 carotid stent implantations in a total of 11,243 patients from 53 centers worldwide was published by Wholey et al. in 2003. Complications during the first 30 days included: TIA (3.1%), minor stroke (2.1%), major stroke (1.2%), and death (0.6%) (Wholey et al. 2003). In 2001, Roubin et al. published a series of 528 patients who had undergone carotid stent implantation. The major stroke rate was 1% (n = 6) and the minor stroke rate was 4.8% (n = 29). Overall, the rate of stroke/death after 30 days was 7.4% (Roubin et al. 2001).

In 2003, Cremonesi et al. published a series of 442 consecutive patients treated with carotid stent implantation with embolic protection. Stroke or death within the first month after the procedure occurred in 1.1% of these patients (Cremonesi et al. 2003).

Biasi et al. reported on the use of the echogenicity index, known as the gray scale median, as an indicator of the risk of stroke during carotid stent implantation. The authors concluded that low echogenicity in the carotid plaque, measured as a gray scale median ≤ 25, increased the risk of peri-interventional stroke (Biasi et al. 2004).

The German Association for Angiology and Radiology has developed a prospective registry for carotid stent implantations. The results for the first 48 months, from a total of 38 participating centers, were published in 2004. Carotid stent implantation was carried out in 3267 patients. The procedure was successful in 98% of the interventions. The peri-interventional mortality was 0.6%, the major stroke rate was 1.2%, and the minor stroke rate was 1.3% (Theiss et al. 2004).

In 2005, Bosiers et al. published the ELOCAS Registry, compiled retrospectively and prospectively from the results of four "high-volume centers." A total of 2172 consecutive patients were treated, and 99.7% of the procedures were technically successful. The stroke/death rate was 4.1% after 1 year, 10.1% after 3 years, and 15.5% after 5 years (Bosiers et al. 2005).

The CaRESS study was a nonrandomized multicenter study including 143 patients treated with carotid stent implantation and 254 patients who underwent carotid endarterectomy. No significant differences were observed with regard to the stroke/death rates either after 30 days (2.1% stent, 3.6% surgery) or after 1 year (10.0% stent, 13.6% surgery) (CaRESS 2005).

The ARCHeR study was published by Gray et al. in 2006 and consisted of three sequential multicenter studies. In ARCHeR 1, only the use of the Acculink (Guidant) carotid stent was evaluated; in the two subsequent studies (ARCHeR 2 and 3), adjuvant use of the Accunet embolic protection system (Guidant) was also tested. A total of 581 patients with high surgical risk from 48 centers were included between 2000 and 2003. The combined stroke/death/myocardial infarction rate was 8.3% after 30 days. The ipsilateral stroke rate after the first month and up to 1 year was 1.8%. The repeat stenosis rate was 2.2% within the first year (Gray et al. 2006).

The CAPTURE Registry (Carotid Acculink/Accunet Post-Approval Trial to Uncover Unanticipated or Rare Events) was published in 2007. A total of 3500 patients with high surgical risk and a stenosis grade > 50% (symptomatic) or > 80% (asymptomatic) were included. The stroke/death/myocardial infarction rate was 6.3% after 30 days. The major stroke/death rate after 30 days was 2.9%.

Embolism protection systems have been evaluated in several large, unrandomized multicenter studies. These include the European DESERVE study (Diffusion-Weighted MRI-Based Evaluation of the Effectiveness of the Mo.Ma System), which demonstrated that the Mo.Ma system, using diffusion-weighted magnetic resonance imaging (DW-MRI) during carotid stent implantation, is effective for protection against embolism. The cranial MRI examination was carried out before the procedure and 3–12 hours after carotid stent implantation in order to identify new ischemic lesions. In a total of 127 patients treated, new cerebral lesions were identified on DW-MRI in 38 (29.9%). However, clinically relevant stroke was only present in three patients (2.4%) (Rubino et al., paper presented at EuroPCR 2011).

In the EMPIRE Study, the Gore Flow Reversal System was evaluated in 29 centers with a total of 245 patients. The primary end point was the rate of myocardial infarction/stroke/death after 30 days. Thirty-two percent of the patients were treated for symptomatic carotid stenosis. Intolerance for balloon occlusion was noted in a total of six patients in the study (2.4%). The primary end point occurred in 3.7% of the patients (Clair et al 2011).

In the EMBOLDEN Study, the Gore Embolic Filter was evaluated in a total of 250 patients in 35 centers in 2009–2010. Fifteen percent of the patients included in the study were suffering from symptomatic carotid stenosis. After 30 days, 10 patients (4.0%) reached the primary end point, defined as myocardial infarction, stroke, and/or death (Gray et al., paper presented at the 23rd Annual International Symposium on Endovascular Therapy, 2011).

Randomized studies on carotid stent implantation

The Carotid and Vertebral Transluminal Angioplasty Study (CAVATAS I) was the first large-scale study in which carotid angioplasty (largely without stenting and embolic protection) was compared with carotid endarterectomy. The early stroke/death rate was 10% in both the carotid angioplasty and carotid endarterectomy groups. In the SAPPHIRE Study, carotid stent implantation using embolic protection was compared with carotid endarterectomy both in a randomized study and in a registry. The 30-day stroke/death rate was 4.5% in the group with randomized carotid stent implantations and 6.6% in the group of randomized patients who underwent surgical treatment. The registry also included patients who did not meet the inclusion criteria for the randomized study. The 30-day stroke/death rate in the registry among patients who underwent interventional treatment was 6.9%.

The EVA-3S study compared carotid stent implantation with carotid endarterectomy in patients with symptomatic stenoses ≥ 60%. The participation criteria for interventionalists were set very low; a participating interventionalist only had to have implanted 12 carotid stents beforehand. The stroke/death rate after 30 days was lower in the group of patients treated with embolic protection than in the group without embolic protection (18 of 227, 7.9% versus 5 of 20, 25%; P = 0.03). Randomization to the group with stent implantation without embolic protection was therefore prematurely stopped. The stroke/death rate after 30 days in the group with stent implantations with embolic protection was significantly higher (9.6%) in comparison with endarterectomy (3.9%). The relative risk was 2.5.

The SPACE (Stent-Protected Percutaneous Angioplasty of the Carotid versus Endarterectomy) study included patients with symptomatic stenoses ≥ 70% on duplex ultrasonography or ≥ 50% according to the NASCET criteria. The use of embolic protection systems was optional in this study. Many interventional centers had difficulties in meeting the participation criteria—at least 25 carotid stent implantations had to have been carried out previously. The 30-day ipsilateral stroke rate was 6.84% in the group of patients treated with carotid stent implantation, and in the surgical group, the rate was 6.34%. Although using embolic protection systems had already become a standard part of the procedure in most centers, 73% of the interventions in this study were carried out without embolic protection. Complications such as myocardial infarction, contralateral stroke, and cranial nerve lesions, which are almost exclusively complications of endarterectomy, were not evaluated. The study was designed as a non-inferiority study with a non-inferiority margin of < 2.5% which was based on a calculated complication rate of 5%. The one-sided P value for non-inferiority was 0.09. The study was terminated prematurely after inclusion of 1200 patients due to low patient recruitment and lack of finance when an analysis determined that including more than 2500 patients would have been necessary to reach a statistical power of at least 80%. According to the investigating physicians in the study, the study results were not capable of definitively demonstrating the non-inferiority of carotid stent implantation in comparison with carotid endarterectomy since the trial was not completed.

Overall, the results of the large randomized studies indicate that the differences between surgery and intervention were usually very small.

The Carotid Revascularization Endarterectomy vs. Stenting Trial (CREST) study started recruiting patients in 2000. Preliminary data from the introductory phase of the interventional arm of the study were published in 2004. The data so far indicate that the periprocedural risk increases significantly with increasing age. The stroke/death rate was 1.7% in the patient cohort under the age of 60; 1.3% in patients aged 60–69; 5.3% in those aged 70–79; and 12.1% in those aged 80 or over. The significant difference was independent of the patients' neurological status, grade of stenosis, or use of embolic protection systems.

Studies for which recruitment has already started include the International Carotid Stenting Study (ICSS) and the Asymptomatic Carotid Stenosis, Stenting versus Endarterectomy Trial (ACT-1). Studies already in the planning stage that are expected to provide new findings on the success of treatments for asymptomatic stenoses—e.g., with regard to neurocognitive function—include the Transatlantic Asymptomatic Carotid Intervention Trial (TACIT) and the Asymptomatic Carotid Surgery Trial 2 (ACST-2).

The Carotid Revascularization Endarterectomy vs. Stenting Trial (CREST), including a total of 2502 recruited patients, is the largest randomized study so far carried out to compare carotid stent implantation with carotid surgery. Data from the lead-in phase of the interventional arm of the study were published in 2004 (Hobson et al. 2004). In that report, the rates of stroke/death in the patient cohort were 1.7% in those under the age of 60, 1.3% in those aged 60–69, 5.3% in those aged 70–79, and 12.1% in patients aged 80 or over. The significant difference was independent of the patients' neurological status, the grade of stenosis, or the use of embolism protection systems. The full study results were published in 2010. No significant difference was seen between the two treatment methods with regard to the combined primary end point of periprocedural stroke, myocardial infarction or death, or ipsilateral stroke during the follow-up period. The event rates were 7.2% in the group of patients who were treated with stent implantation and 6.8% in the patients who underwent surgery (Brott et al. 2010). Studies still currently recruiting include the International Carotid Stenting Study (ICSS), the Asymptomatic Carotid Stenosis Stenting Versus Endarterectomy Trial (ACT-1), and the Asymptomatic Carotid Surgery Trial 2 (ACT-2).

An interim analysis of the ICSS study has been published for the first 120 days of follow-up. Patients with > 50% symptomatic carotid stenosis were randomly assigned either to endovascular or surgical treatment methods. It was not yet possible to analyze the study's primary end point (the 3-year stroke rate). Instead, the results of the analysis focused on the 120-day rate of stroke, death, or procedure-related myocardial infarction. In a total of 1713 randomized patients, a significantly higher rate was seen after carotid stent implantation at 8.5%, in comparison with 5.2% after carotid surgery (Ederle et al. 2010).

Clinical results—vertebral artery stent implantation

Sundt et al. first reported successful treatment of the vertebrobasilar system using angioplasty in 1980 (Sundt et al. 1980). Since then, many clinical series have been published on vertebral artery angioplasty/stent implantation, with high rates of technical success (98–100%) (Malek et al. 1999; Piotin et al. 2000; Mukherjee et al. 2001). However, there is still a lack of data from large clinical series and from controlled randomized studies to allow more precise assessments of the complication and restenosis rates during long-term follow-up. A subanalysis of the CAVATAS study compared a small group of 16 patients with symptomatic vertebral artery stenosis who received either endovascular treatment (PTA or stent implantation) or conservative drug therapy. Two of the eight patients who received endovascular treatment suffered a periprocedural TIA. No cases of stroke in the vertebrobasilar flow area occurred in either treatment arm during the long-term follow-up (mean 4.7 years). Three patients each in the drug-treated arm of the study and also in the group with endovascular treatment died due to myocardial infarction or stroke in the carotid flow area (Coward et al. 2007). In the VAST study, currently still in progress, 180 patients with symptomatic vertebral artery stenosis > 50% have been randomly assigned to groups receiving either endovascular treatment (stent implantation) or conservative therapy. The planned follow-up period is one year (Compter et al. 2008).

Prospects

The rapid developments in interventional treatment for carotid and vertebral artery stenoses, such as new stents with greater flexibility and smaller diameters, improved embolic protection systems with secure apposition on the vascular wall, and other technical innovations, are anticipated to improve the results of carotid and vertebral artery stent implantation in the near future.

1.1.6.3 Surgical treatment

Surgical removal of atherosclerotic obstruction in the carotid artery is the most frequently conducted vascular operation worldwide. In terms of the criteria of evidence-based medicine, it is also the best-studied surgical intervention that exists, with tens of thousands of patients documented in international prospective, randomized studies. Carotid endarterectomy (CEA) was first reported by Eastcott and colleagues in the treatment of a patient who had had 33 transitory ischemic attacks (TIAs) (Eastcott et al. 1954). The operation is now carried out in Germany, for example, over 25,000 times per year (BQS-Bundesauswertung 2007).

Indications for surgery

CEA is able to reduce the risk of stroke sevenfold in patients with TIAs, and in patients with 60–90% asymptomatic stenoses of the internal carotid it can achieve an absolute risk reduction of 5% over 5 years (Biller et al. 1998). The highest incidence of perioperative stroke is associated with the presence of high-grade bilateral internal carotid artery stenosis.

On the basis of large prospective, randomized multicenter studies (Anon. 1995; Anon. 1998; Ferguson et al. 1999), the American Heart Association formulated the following generally accepted guidelines for establishing the indication for carotid endarterectomy in an interdisciplinary consensus taking into account the natural history without surgery and thus the maximum acceptable perioperative rates of stroke and mortality (Biller et al. 1998):

- Asymptomatic stenoses of the internal carotid artery with a stenosis grade > 60%, with a combined perioperative stroke and mortality rate (major adverse cardiovascular event rate, MACE) of < 3% (evidence level 1b; recommendation grade A)
- Asymptomatic internal carotid artery stenosis > 60% and contralateral stenosis > 75% or occlusion, with a MACE of < 5% (evidence level 4; recommendation grade C)
- Symptomatic internal carotid artery stenoses > 50%, with a complication rate of < 6% (evidence level 1a; recommendation grade A)

The following groups of patients are particularly able to benefit from the operation:

- Those with hemispheric TIAs
- Those with crescendo TIAs—i.e., with the number and/or length of transitory ischemic attacks continually increasing
- Those with progressive stroke—i.e., patients with low-grade symptoms initially who show marked clinical deterioration within 6 h
- Those with stroke during the previous few weeks, as the risk of recurrent cerebral ischemia is particularly high in these cases
- Those with a subtotally occluded internal carotid artery but persistent residual flow (pseudo-occlusion)

CEA should be carried out without delay in these cases (Eckstein et al. 2004).

Despite the lack of level 1a evidence, differential treatment consideration for carotid artery stenting (CAS) appears to be justified, above all in the presence of a "high carotid bifurcation" (bifurcation of the carotid artery higher than C2); for repeat operations in the neck; when there is paralysis of the contralateral recurrent laryngeal nerve; and after cervical radiotherapy, as it avoids local complications (e.g., nerve injuries).

Contraindications

- Patients in poor general condition (American Society of Anesthesiologists IV, V) or with limited life expectancy (< 6 months)
- Fresh large cerebral infarction (major stroke), with no tendency to show clinical improvement (< 4 weeks)
- Following earlier disabling stroke (Rankin scale 5)

Patient preparation

- Specialist neurological examination to determine prior neurological symptoms or establish the patient's neurologic status
- B-imaging and duplex ultrasonography to determine the level of the carotid bifurcation, show whether the internal carotid artery is patent, and assess the grade of stenosis
- Cranial CT or MRI to identify older or more recent cerebral hemorrhage, infarct areas, and tumors
- Angio-CT, angio-MRI, or intra-arterial digital subtraction angiography only if there is a suspicion of supra-aortic multiple-vessel disease, poor definition of the stenosis on duplex ultrasound, contradictory duplex-ultrasound findings regarding the grade

of stenosis, suspected intracranial tandem stenoses, or extreme kinking or coiling of the vessel with ambiguous duplex findings
- Prophylaxis against thrombosis with low-molecular-weight heparin s.c. on the evening before the operation
- Fasting for at least 6 h before the operation; long-term medication may be taken with a little water on the morning of the operation. *Caution:* antidiabetic agents, clopidogrel, Coumadin

Preparations for the operation

The operation can be carried out either with regional anesthesia or general anesthesia, although a recent prospective randomized multicenter study (the GALA study) showed some advantages for regional anesthesia (Lewis et al. 2009).

- Positioning: modified beach-chair position—trunk raised, legs slightly lowered, head reclining/hyperextended and turned to the contralateral side, head positioned on a rubber ring, both arms juxtaposed (in regional anesthesia, the contralateral arm is laid free and a squeezing toy is placed in the patient's hand, which has to be rhythmically squeezed by the patient when requested and produces a loud sound)
- Sterile cleaning of the side of the neck that is being operated on to beyond the midline, laterally including the shoulder (acromion), caudally as far as the nipples, and cranially to include the mandible, chin, earlobe, and mastoid

Surgical access

The incision is made at the anterior margin of the sternocleidomastoid; preoperative assessment of the level of the carotid bifurcation can provide good guidance. The level of the palpable cricoid can also be used for guidance. The skin incision is usually approximately 7 cm long, and it is carried cranially toward the inferior margin of the earlobe. As far as possible, the incision should be made as little cranially or ventrally from the earlobe as possible, as injury to the oral branch of the facial nerve could occur, either directly or due to a subsequent retractor movement, leading to pareses in the ipsilateral corner of the mouth postoperatively.

After division of the skin, subcutaneous tissue, and platysma, the common carotid artery, which is usually easily palpated, is dissected and looped with a vascular sling. Following exposure of the common carotid artery, the internal carotid artery is exposed above the carotid bifurcation. Unnecessary manipulations of the vessel are avoided to avoid triggering embolizations ("no-touch" technique). During further dissection of the bulb in the direction of the internal carotid, the ansa cervicalis of the hypoglossal nerve is spared as much as possible. However, it may also be transected if necessary, usually without sequelae. Following it cranially leads to the hypoglossal nerve as it crosses the internal carotid artery. Particularly when there is a high carotid bifurcation, the hypoglossal nerve has to be mobilized, and the sternocleidomastoid branches of the occipital artery and vein attached to it have to be ligated. Circular exposure of the carotid bifurcation is only carried out after clamping of the internal carotid artery, in order to prevent embolization (Fig. 1.1-19a, b).

Surgical procedure

There are basically two procedures that can be used for plaque removal and reconstruction of the internal carotid artery or carotid bifurcation:

- Thromboendarterectomy (TEA) with a patch graft
- Eversion endarterectomy (EEA)

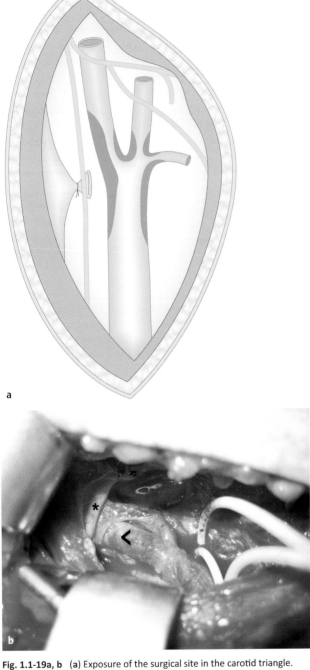

Fig. 1.1-19a, b   (a) Exposure of the surgical site in the carotid triangle. The common carotid artery, internal carotid artery, external carotid artery from its first branch, and superior thyroid artery have been exposed. The facial vein has been transected. Lateral to the stenotic carotid artery lies the ansa cervicalis, which courses cranial to the horizontally crossing hypoglossal nerve. (**b**) Photograph of the original surgical site. The common carotid artery has been looped with a yellow vascular sling. A hypoplastic external carotid artery is branching off in the medial direction (top). The internal carotid artery is marked with a black arrow (<). The hypoglossal nerve (*) crosses the internal carotid artery.

Thromboendarterectomy (TEA)

In classic TEA of the internal carotid artery, following clamping and dissection of the carotid bifurcation (Fig. 1.1-20a), a longitudinal arteriotomy is carried out on the anterolateral wall of the carotid bifurcation and is extended into the common and internal carotid artery. Using a dissector, the endarterectomy is then carried out, and any distal intima layers that may be present are fixed with a single or continuous attachment suture (polydioxanone 7–0). If there is significant stenosis of the external carotid artery, an EEA can also be carried out. The disengaged plaque is further smoothly transected proximally, in the common artery, preferably with scissors. After copious rinsing of the endarterectomized vascular segment and checking for possible residual tissue and thrombus, an alloplastic patch (polyester, Dacron, or expanded polytetrafluoroethylene) is trimmed to size and sutured in with a continuous nonresorbable monofilament suture (polypropylene, Prolene 5–0) (Fig. 1.1-20b, c). In delicate vessels, a patch obtained from autologous great saphenous vein can also be used. Comparative studies have not shown that autologous venous patches confer any significant advantages in comparison with alloplastic materials in routine use (Bond et al. 2004; Naylor et al. 2004) (Fig. 1.1-20c).

When there is symptomatic coiling or kinking, shortening can be carried out either with segmental resection of the internal carotid

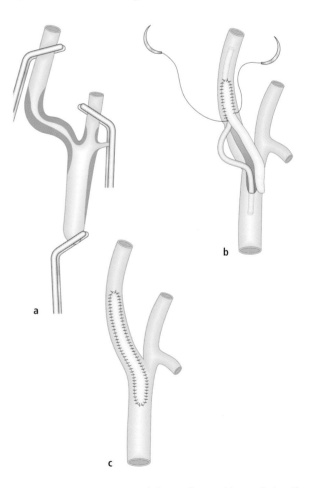

Fig. 1.1-20a–c   (a) Positioning of clips on the carotid artery before the arteriotomy. (**b**) Longitudinally arteriotomized common and internal carotid artery. An intraluminal shunt has been introduced. A Dacron patch is being sewn in with a continuous suture. (**c**) The Dacron patch has been sewn in with a continuous suture.

artery or proximalization (transposition) of the origin of the internal carotid. The advantage of TEA is that it provides a good overview of the operative vascular segment and of the distal layer of the intima. This allows safe treatment, particularly for long stenoses. In addition, it is technically easier to introduce a temporary shunt. However, the procedure is more time-consuming and usually leaves foreign material (the patch) in the artery.

Eversion endarterectomy (EEA)

In EEA, after clamping of the carotid bifurcation, transection of the internal carotid is carried out directly at its origin in the bifurcation. The correct dissection level is identified at the level of the external elastic lamina between the media and the intima before the internal carotid is rolled from inside out and the stenotic plaque is removed (Fig. 1.1-21a). At the distal end of the plaque, which usually terminates smoothly, the plaque cylinder normally breaks off without leaving a flap (Fig. 1.1-22). The internal carotid artery is rolled back into its original position and is then reattached with a resorbable monofilament continuous suture (polydioxanone 5–0) (Fig. 1.1-21b). To prepare a longer anastomosis, the arteriotomy can be extended cranially to a length of 15–30 mm in the internal carotid or proximally at the common carotid. Plaque removal of the bulb or of the common and external carotid artery can be carried out in the form of an open TEA or as an EEA at the external carotid artery. If a relevant distal intimal flap appears in the internal carotid, it can be secured with single fixation sutures stitched from the outside (tack sutures).

The technical advantage of EEA lies in the much shorter operating time required and the fact that there is no foreign material in the artery, provided resorbable suture material is used for reinsertion (Fig. 1.1-21c). As carotid stenoses often only appear in the bulb and in the area of the origin of the internal carotid, the limited extent of the vascular segment opened during eversion is usually adequate.

EEA also makes it possible to correct symptomatic coiling or kinking of the internal carotid artery much more easily using a shortening operation than with TEA; either a segment of the internal carotid is resected, or a longer, proximalized anastomosis can be created if there is only slight coiling. The EEA procedure only becomes more difficult in longer lesions or in extracranial tandem stenoses. Introducing a temporary shunt is also slightly more complicated. In this case, it is best to start with the suture in the internal carotid artery and to introduce the shunt only after the side further away from the surgeon has been completed.

The current data show that there are no relevant differences between the TEA and EEA procedures with regard to postoperative mortality, morbidity, or recurrent stenoses (Cao et al. 2004; Crawford et al. 2007).

Intraoperative neuromonitoring and temporary intraluminal shunt

To prevent procedure-related cerebral ischemia during CEA, systolic blood pressure should be raised to > 150 mmHg if possible and systemic heparinization with 50–100 IU heparin/kg body weight is obligatory.

The most reliable method of intraoperative neuromonitoring involves assessment of changes in the state of consciousness and in motor activity in cooperative, conscious patients under regional

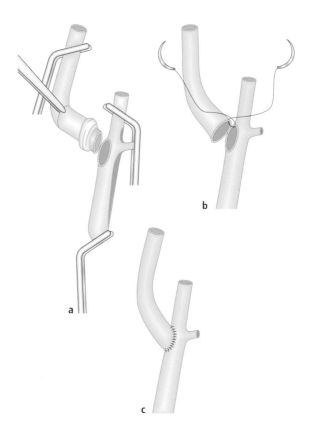

Fig. 1.1-21a–c (a) The surgical site in eversion endarterectomy of the internal carotid artery. The internal carotid artery has been transected obliquely at the common carotid artery. A dissection cylinder has been spatulated at the dissection level in the area of the external elastic membrane. The adventitia is now rolled up cranially until the cranial end of the dissected part tears spontaneously. (b) Reinsertion of the internal carotid artery into the common carotid artery using a continuous suture. (c) The surgical site after completion of the eversion endarterectomy.

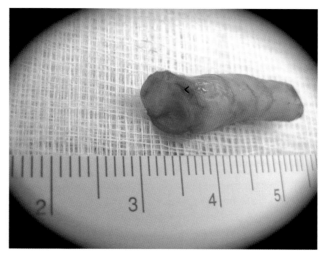

Fig. 1.1-22 The dissection specimen after eversion endarterectomy of the internal carotid artery. The arrow tip (<) marks the residual lumen of the artery before disobliteration.

anesthesia. These two checks can be carried out before and after clamping of the carotid artery by speaking to the patient and using rhythmic activation of a toy in the contralateral hand. If clouding of consciousness or loss of motor control *immediately* after clamping of the carotid artery occurs at high normal blood-pressure values, a temporary intraluminal or extraluminal shunt (e.g., a Javid or Pruitt shunt) should be placed. However, if the symptoms only occur after a *latency period* of several minutes, it is advisable—depending on the progress of the operation—either to complete the surgery quickly or to introduce a shunt. Optional shunt placement is needed in 5–10% of cases (BQS-Bundesauswertung 2007).

For placement of a temporary shunt in patients undergoing surgery with general anesthesia, there are basically two different approaches that have developed:

- Obligatory shunt placement
- Optional shunt placement after neuromonitoring

The advantages of general shunt placement have been reported to include in particular the safe maintenance of perfusion to the internal carotid artery, enlargement of the artery by the shunt, and educational and training considerations. Arguments in favor of optional shunt placement, by contrast, include the relatively infrequent need for shunting, the greater effort involved, and the risk of injury to or dissection of the distal internal carotid artery. However, the results with the two procedures in relation to perioperative mortality and morbidity are probably similar (Girn et al. 2008; Woodworth et al. 2007).

Methods of evaluating cerebral perfusion intraoperatively include measuring pressure in the stump of the internal carotid artery, assessment of somatosensory evoked potentials (SSEPs) or electroencephalography (EEG), and transcranial Doppler ultrasonography. However, there is controversy regarding the validity and practicality of these methods in the operating room. The use of such methods therefore depends on the preferences and experience of each surgical team.

Intraoperative quality control

Intraoperative quality control allows timely identification and correction of lesions capable of causing a cerebral insult. Such lesions include free-floating flaps > 2 mm and dissections with residual stenoses of more than 25%. Quality control can be carried out using the following methods:

- Duplex ultrasonography
- Continuous-wave (CW) Doppler
- Angioscopy
- Electromagnetic flowmetry
- Angiography at two levels

Postoperative follow-up

- Frequent checking of blood pressure and heart rate is needed. Normotensive blood-pressure values should be achieved before the patient is discharged from the hospital.
- Attention should be given to ipsilateral headaches/hyperperfusion (hemicephalalgia).
- A neurological status check by personnel managing postoperative care should be carried out to survey for defects.
- The patient should be allowed to drink clear fluids immediately. A normal diet can be resumed postoperatively after 6 h (or 3 h with regional anesthesia).
- The patient should be mobilized after 6 h—e.g., sitting in a chair or walking in the corridor (if this is possible in view of prior neurological deficits).

- A postoperative neurological examination should be carried out.
- Long-term inhibition of platelet function should be managed with aspirin (100 mg/d), plus clopidogrel (75 mg/d) for a period of 6 weeks.
- Plaque stabilization should be achieved with statins.
- Risk factors should be checked (hypertension, diabetes, etc.).
- For the period of the hospital stay, low-molecular-weight heparin should also be administered for prophylaxis against thrombosis (medium risk or higher due to other diseases).
- Duplex ultrasonography check-up examinations of the carotid vessels are performed before discharge, after 4 weeks, after 6 months, and then annually.

Clinical results

High-grade hemodynamically relevant recurrent stenoses > 70% occur much less frequently in the carotid artery (2%) than in other arteries such as the superficial femoral artery (BQS-Bundesauswertung 2007). If they develop within 1 year, they are most often caused by intimal hyperplasia, while luminal strictures occurring later are usually due to progression of the atherosclerosis. Since recurrent stenoses and those secondary to radiation injury are rarely embolic, invasive therapy is only required if they have hemodynamic effects. However, surgical correction and prior cervical surgery are associated with a much higher risk of neural injury (5%) due to adhesions in the wound area (Mozes 2005). Paralysis of the contralateral vocal cord significantly increases the perioperative morbidity. Carotid artery stenting (CAS) therefore offers theoretical advantages given the lack of cranial nerve injury with the percutaneous procedure.

False aneurysms are extremely rare surgical sequelae. They may be caused by incorrect surgical technique, such as an incorrect dissection level during endarterectomy, or by tearing or breakage of the patch suture. Very rarely, deep wound infection needs to be taken into consideration in aneurysms following alloplastic patch placement (with an incidence < 0.5%) (BQS-Bundesauswertung 2007). Treatment consists of complete removal of the patch and replacement with an autologous patch or bridging graft (from the great saphenous vein).

General complications

- Death (< 1%)
- Cardiovascular complications (decompensated cardiac insufficiency, severe cardiac dysrhythmia, cardiac infarction) (1.9%)
- Perioperative stroke (2.2%); 5–10% of cases are caused by intracerebral hemorrhage and the remainder are ischemic (BQS-Bundesauswertung 2007)

Local complications

- Postoperative hemorrhage requiring surgery (2.5%)
- Peripheral nerve lesions, mainly temporary (hypoglossal nerve, facial nerve, recurrent laryngeal nerve) (1.5%)
- Carotid occlusion (0.3%)
- Postoperative wound infection (0.2%)
- Hyperperfusion syndrome (hemicephalalgia) < 1% (BQS-Bundesauswertung 2007)

Internal carotid artery strictures can also be caused by *fibromuscular dysplasia,* in which constriction of the artery results from fibrous transformation of the media. Depending on the length of the vessel segment affected, the artery can be either patched or replaced. Segmental replacement of the carotid artery may be necessary in some cases for aneurysms, injuries, lesions resulting from prior radiation therapy, and after TEA with limited residual vascular wall. Autologous greater saphenous vein should be used for this purpose if possible. Replacement with a thin-walled polytetrafluoroethylene (PTFE) prosthesis is also possible in exceptional cases.

Prospects

CEA is currently the gold standard in the treatment of high-grade symptomatic and asymptomatic carotid stenoses. CAS has now entered clinical practice as a competitive procedure that is attractive for patients since it is less invasive, and may have some advantages over the established method of CEA in individual cases. While the trial data comparing the procedural safety of CAS to CEA are mixed due largely to probable methodological issues in individual trial conduct, there nevertheless is ample and growing data that long-term stroke prevention is equal between the two procedures out to at least 4 years and likely beyond. Several current studies nearing completion (the CREST, SPACE-2, and CAVATAS-2 trials) should provide a clearer picture as to the place CAS has in the management of carotid bifurcation disease. However, an indication for CAS may be considered after interdisciplinary consultation in individual cases in patients who are at high risk (e.g., with recurrent stenoses, radiogenic stenoses, contralateral recurrent nerve paralysis, etc.), or in the context of controlled studies.

References

ACCF/SCAI/SVMB/SIR/ASITN 2007 clinical expert consensus document on carotid stenting: a report of the American College of Cardiology Foundation Task Force on Clinical Expert Consensus Documents (ACCF/SCAI/SVMB/SIR/ASITN Clinical Expert Consensus Document Committee on Carotid Stenting). J Am Coll Cardiol 2007 Jan 2; 49 (1): 126–70. Erratum in: J Am Coll Cardiol 2007 Feb 27; 49 (8): 924.

Adams HP Jr, Bendixen BH, Kappelle LJ, et al. Classification of subtype of acute ischemic stroke. Definitions for use in a multicenter clinical trial. TOAST. Trial of Org 10172 in Acute Stroke Treatment. Stroke 1993 Jan; 24 (1): 35–41.

Al-Mubarak N, Roubin GS, Vitek JJ, et al. Effect of the distal-balloon protection system on microembolization during carotid stenting. Circulation 2001; 104: 1999–2002.

American Heart Association. Heart Disease and Stroke Statistics—2004 Update. www.americanheart.org.

Anonymous. Carotid endarterectomy for patients with asymptomatic internal carotid artery. JAMA 1995; 273: 1421–8.

Anonymous. Randomised trial of endarterectomy for recently symptomatic carotid stenosis: final results of the MRC European Carotid Surgery Trial (ECST). Lancet 1998: 1379–87.

Armstrong PA, Bandyk DF, Johnson BL, Shames ML, Zwiebel BR, Back MR. Duplex scan surveillance after carotid angioplasty and stenting: a rational definition of stent stenosis. J Vasc Surg 2007 Sep; 46 (3): 460–5; discussion 465–6.

Arning C, Widder B, von Reutern GM, Stiegler H, Görtler M. [Revision of DEGUM ultrasound criteria for grading internal carotid artery stenoses and transfer to NASCET measurement]. Ultraschall Med 2010 Jun; 31 (3): 251–7. Epub 2010 Apr 22. Review. German.

Bamford J, Sandercock P, Dennis M, Burn J, Warlow C. Classification and natural history of clinically identifiable subtypes of cerebral infarction. Lancet 1991; 337: 1521–6.

Bartels E, Flugel KA. Advantages of color Doppler imaging for the evaluation of vertebral arteries. J Neuroimaging 1993; 3: 229–33.

Baumgartner RW, Mattle HP, Schroth G. Assessment of >/=50% and <50% intracranial stenoses by transcranial color-coded duplex sonography. Stroke 1999 Jan; 30 (1): 87–92.

Berteloot D, Leclerc X, Leys D, Krivosic R, Pruvo JP. Cerebral angiography: a study of complications in 450 consecutive procedures. J Radiol 1999; 80: 843–8.

Biasi G, Froio A, Diethrich E, et al. Carotid Plaque Echolucency Increases the Risk of Stroke in Carotid Stenting: The Imaging in Carotid Angioplasty and Risk of Stroke (ICAROS) Study. Circulation 2004; 110: 756–62.

Biller J, Feinberg WM, Castaldo JE, et al. Guidelines for carotid endarterectomy: a statement for healthcare professionals from a Special Writing Group of the Stroke Council, American Heart Association. Circulation 1998; 97 (5): 501–9.

Bogousslavsky J, van Melle G, Regli F. The Lausanne Stroke Registry: analysis of 1,000 consecutive patients with first stroke. Stroke 1988; 19: 1083–92.

Bond R, Rerkasem K, Naylor R, et al. Patches of different types for carotid patch angioplasty. Cochrane Database Systematic Reviews 2004 (2).

Bosiers M, Peeters P, Deloose K, et al. Does carotid artery stenting work on the long run: 5-year results in high-volume centers (ELOCAS Registry). J Cardiovasc Surg (Torino) 2005 Jun; 46 (3): 241–7.

BQS-Bundesauswertung 2006 Karotis-Rekonstruktion. BQS-Qualitätsreport 2006. Düsseldorf: 2007: 1–75.

Cao P, De Rango P, Cieri E, et al. Eversion versus conventional endarterectomy. Semin Vasc Surg 2004; 17(3): 236–42.

Caplan LR, Amarenco P, Rosengart A, Lafranchise EF, Teal PA, Belkin M, DeWitt LD, Pessin MS. Embolism from vertebral artery origin occlusive disease. Neurology 1992; 42: 1505–12.

Caplan LR. Brain embolism, revisited. Neurology 1993; 43: 1281–7.

Caplan LR. Posterior Circulation Disease: Clinical Findings, Diagnosis, and Management. Cambridge MA, Blackwell Scientific Publishers: 1996.

CaRESS Steering Committee Carotid Revascularization Using Endarterectomy or Stenting Systems (CaRESS) phase I clinical trial: 1-year results J Vasc Surg 2005; 42: 213–9.

Clair DG, Hopkins LN, Mehta M, Kasirajan K, Schermerhorn M, Schönholz C, Kwolek CJ, Eskandari MK, Powell RJ, Ansel GM; EMPiRE Clinical Study Investigators. Neuroprotection during carotid artery stenting using the GORE flow reversal system: 30-day outcomes in the EMPiRE Clinical Study. Catheter Cardiovasc Interv 2011 Feb 15; 77 (3):420–9. doi: 10.1002/ccd.22789. Epub 2010 Nov 3.

Crawford RS, Chung TK, Hodgman T, et al. Restenosis after eversion vs patch closure carotid endarterectomy. J Vasc Surg 2007; 46 (1): 41–8.

Cremonesi A, Manetti R, Setacci F, et al. Protected carotid stenting: clinical advantages and complications of embolic protection devices in 442 consecutive patients. Stroke 2003 Aug; 34 (8): 1936–41.

Eastcott HH, Pickering GW, Rob CG. Reconstruction of internal carotid artery in a patient with intermittent attacks of hemiplegia. Lancet 1954; 267 (6846): 994–6.

Eckstein H-H, Heider P, Wolf O. Chirurgische Therapie extrakranieller Karotisstenosen. Schlaganfallprophylaxe auf höchstem Evidenzniveau. Deutsches Ärzteblatt 2004; 101 (41): A2753–62.

Endovascular versus surgical treatment in patients with carotid stenosis in the carotid and vertebral artery transluminal angioplasty study (CAVATAS): a randomized trial. Lancet 2001; 357: 1729–37.

Ferguson GG, Eliasziw M, Barr HW, et al. The North American Symptomatic Carotid Endarterectomy Trial: surgical results in 1415 patients. Stroke 1999; 30: 1751–8.

Girn HR, Dellagrammaticas D, Laughlan K, et al. Carotid endarterectomy: technical practices of surgeons participating in the GALA trial. Eur J Vasc Endovasc Surg 2008; 36 (4): 385–9.

Gray WA, Hopkins LN, Yadav S, et al. Protected carotid stenting in high-surgical-risk patients: the ARCHeR results. J Vasc Surg 2006 Aug; 44 (2): 258–68.

Gray WA, Yadav JS, Verta P, et al. The CAPTURE registry: predictors of outcomes in carotid artery stenting with embolic protection for high surgical risk patients in the early post-approval setting. Catheter Cardiovasc Interv 2007 Dec 1; 70 (7): 1025–33.

Hass WK, Fields WS, North RR, Kircheff II, Chase NE, Bauer RB. Joint study of extracranial arterial occlusion. II. Arteriography, techniques, sites, and complications. JAMA 1968; 203: 961–8.

Hobson RW 2nd, Howard VJ, Roubin GS, et al. Carotid artery stenting is associated with increased complications in octogenarians: 30-day stroke and death rates in the CREST lead-in phase. J Vasc Surg 2004 Dec; 40 (6): 1106–11.

Lewis SC, Warlow CP, Bodenham AR, et al. General anaesthesia versus local anaesthesia for carotid surgery (GALA): a multicentre, randomised controlled trial. Lancet 2009; 372 (9656): 2132–42.

Malek AM, Higashida RT, Phatouros CC, Lempert TE, Meyers PM, Gress DR, Dowd CF, Halbach VV. Treatment of posterior circulation ischemia with extracranial percutaneous balloon angioplasty and stent placement. Stroke 1999; 30: 2073–85.

Mas JL, Chatellier G, Beyssen B et al. Endarterectomy versus stenting in patients with symptomatic severe carotid stenosis. N Engl J Med 2006 Oct 19; 355 (16): 1660–71.

Mathiesen EB, Bønaa KH, Joakimsen O. Echolucent plaques are associated with high risk of ischemic cerebrovascular events in carotid stenosis: the tromsø study. Circulation 2001 May 1; 103 (17): 2171–5.

Mathiesen EB, Johnsen SH, Wilsgaard T, Bønaa KH, Løchen ML, Njølstad I. Carotid plaque area and intima-media thickness in prediction of first-ever ischemic stroke: a 10-year follow-up of 6584 men and women: the Tromsø Study. Stroke 2011 Apr; 42 (4): 972–8.

Mozes G. High-risk carotid endarterectomy. Semin Vasc Surg 2005; 18 (2): 61–8.

Mukherjee D, Roffi M, Kapadia SR, Bhatt DL, Bajzer C, Ziada KM, Kalahasti V, Hughes K, Yadav JS. Percutaneous intervention for symptomatic vertebral artery stenosis using coronary stents. J Invasive Cardiol 2001; 13: 363–6.

Naylor R, Hayes PD, Payne DA, et al. Randomized trial of vein versus dacron patching during carotid endarterectomy: long-term results. J Vasc Surg 2004; 39 (5): 985–93.

Piotin M, Spelle L, Martin JB, Weill A, Rancurel G, Ross IB, Rufenacht DA, Chiras J. Percutaneous transluminal angioplasty and stenting of the proximal vertebral artery for symptomatic stenosis. AJNR Am J Neuroradiol 2000; 21: 727–31.

Rabe K, Sugita J, Sievert H et al. Flow-Reversal Device for Cerebral Protection During Carotid Artery Stenting—Acute and Long-Term Results. J Interv Cardiol 2006 Feb; 19 (1): 55–62.

Roubin GS, New G, Iyer SS, et al. Immediate and late clinical outcomes of carotid artery stenting in patients with symptomatic and asymptomatic carotid artery stenosis: a 5 year prospective analysis. Circulation 2001; 103: 532–7.

SPACE Collaborative Group. 30 day results from the SPACE trial of stent-protected angioplasty versus carotid endarterectomy in symptomatic patients: a randomised non-inferiority trial. Lancet 2006 Oct 7; 368 (9543): 1239–47.

Spence JD, Tamayo A, Lownie SP, Ng WP, Ferguson GG. Absence of microemboli on transcranial Doppler identifies low-risk patients with asymptomatic carotid stenosis. Stroke 2005 Nov; 36 (11): 2373–8.

Spence JD, Pelz D, Veith FJ. Asymptomatic Carotid Stenosis: Identifying Patients at High Enough Risk to Warrant Endarterectomy or Stenting. Stroke 2011 Jul 28. [Epub ahead of print] No abstract available.

Sundt TM Jr, Smith HC, Campbell JK, et al. Transluminal angioplasty for basilar artery stenosis. Mayo Clin Proc 1980; 55: 673–80.

Temelkova-Kurktschiev T, Fischer S, Koehler C, Mennicken G, Henkel E, Hanefeld M. Intima-Media. Dicke bei Gesunden ohne Risikofaktoren. DMW 2001; 126: 1–5.

Theiss W, Hermanek P, Mathias K, et al. Pro-CAS: a prospective registry of carotid angioplasty and stenting. Stroke 2004 Sep; 35 (9): 2134–9.

Wholey MH, Al-Mubarek N. Updated review of the Global Carotid Artery Stent Registry. Catheter Cardiovasc Interv 2003 Oct; 60 (2): 259–66.

Wolf PA, Kannel WB, McGee PC. Epidemiology of strokes in North America. In: Barnet HJM, Stein BM, Mohr JP, Yatsu FM. Stroke: Pathophysiology, Diagnosis and Management Vol 1, New York: Churchill Livingstone, 1929 (1986).

Woodworth GF, McGirt MJ, Than KD, et al. Selective versus routine shunting during carotid endarterectomy: a multivariate outcome analysis. Neurosurgery 2007; 61 (6): 1170–6.

Yadav JS, Wholey MH, Kuntz RE, et al. Protected carotid-artery stenting versus endarterectomy in high-risk patients (the SAPPHIRE study). N Engl J Med 2004; 351: 1493–501.

1.2 Intracranial stenoses and occlusive processes

Basic anatomy of the intracranial arterial system: Reinhard Putz
Conservative treatment: Sophia Göricke, Marc Schlamann, Isabel Wanke
Doppler/duplex ultrasonography: Tom Schilling
Endovascular treatment: Sophia Göricke, Marc Schlamann, Isabel Wanke
Surgical treatment: Peter Horn

1.2.1 Basic anatomy of the intracranial arterial system

The interior of the cranium is supplied by two large paired arteries, in addition to several smaller afferents from the external carotid artery. The internal carotid artery, which flows without branches as far as the base of the skull, passes into the cranium through the carotid canal. Dorsally, the vertebral artery, after following a tortuous course in the vertebral artery groove, enters the vertebral canal through the atlanto-occipital membrane just under the foramen magnum.

Four segments of the internal carotid artery are distinguished along its course: a cervical part (this is described in more detail in section A 1.1), a petrous part, a cavernous part, and a cerebral part (Fig. 1.2-1).

The petrous part has a diameter of around 5 mm, is approximately 3–4 cm long; accompanied by a venous plexus and an autonomic nerve plexus, it courses in the double-curved carotid canal without giving off any branches.

The cavernous part starts as the artery enters the cavernous sinus; this part of the artery also has a double S-curve, although it is highly variable. A few very small arterial branches are given off by the internal carotid artery in the sinus and pass to the trigeminal nerve

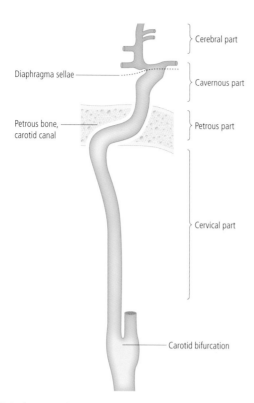

Cerebral part

Diaphragma sellae

Cavernous part

Petrous bone, carotid canal

Petrous part

Cervical part

Carotid bifurcation

Fig. 1.2-1 The parts of the internal carotid artery.

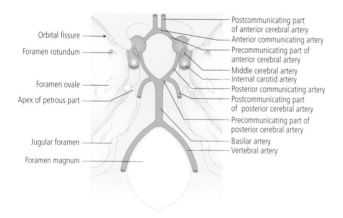

Orbital fissure

Foramen rotundum

Foramen ovale

Apex of petrous part

Jugular foramen

Foramen magnum

Postcommunicating part of anterior cerebral artery

Anterior communicating artery

Precommunicating part of anterior cerebral artery

Middle cerebral artery

Internal carotid artery

Posterior communicating artery

Postcommunicating part of posterior cerebral artery

Precommunicating part of posterior cerebral artery

Basilar artery

Vertebral artery

Fig. 1.2-2 The intracranial arterial supply.

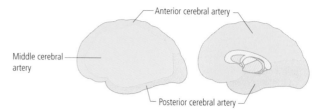

Anterior cerebral artery

Middle cerebral artery

Posterior cerebral artery

Fig. 1.2-3 Arterial supply to the telencephalon. Left: lateral view of the left hemisphere; right: medial view of the left hemisphere.

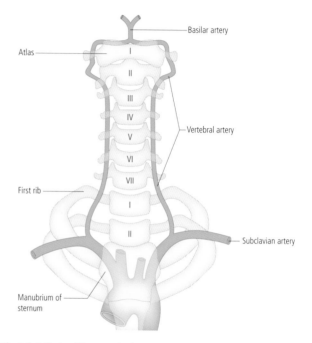

Basilar artery

Atlas

Vertebral artery

First rib

Subclavian artery

Manubrium of sternum

Fig. 1.2-4 Parts of the vertebral artery.

ganglion, the pituitary gland, and the dura mater. Embedded in the spongy sinus, the artery is partly also enclosed by endothelium externally. Laterally, it is obliquely crossed by the abducent nerve.

The cerebral part starts as it passes through the diaphragma sellae (Fig. 1.2-2). From this point on, the wall structure of the internal carotid artery and of all its intracranial parts changes. The elastic fibroreticulate structures in particular are less developed. The first branch after the artery emerges from the cavernous sinus is the ophthalmic artery, which—covered by the optic nerve—passes obliquely forward to the base of the optic canal. It then gives off a few very small branches to the upper part of the pituitary gland and the anterior choroid artery, as well as giving off the anterior cerebral artery, and after a very short course the artery then passes into the middle cerebral artery.

The middle cerebral artery bends in its sphenoid part (the M1 segment) almost at a right angle into the lateral cistern. Lenticulostriate branches from the M1 segment pass through the anterior perforated substance to enter the base of the telencephalon and supply large parts of the telencephalic nuclei. The insular part (the M2 segment), located in the lateral fossa, gives off multiple branches over a tortuous course and supplies the adjoining parts of the frontal and temporal lobes (Fig. 1.2-3a).

The right and left anterior cerebral artery are connected through the usually very short, thin anterior communicating artery, which rests directly in front of the pituitary stalk on the skull base. From the precommunicating part (the A1 segment), fine branches pass to the adjoining parts of the frontal lobe and to the hypothalamus and thalamus. The postcommunicating part (the A2 segment) follows the contour of the corpus callosum as far as its splenium, and branches arising from it supply the medial surface of the cerebral hemispheres to above their superior margin—with the exception of the corpus callosum itself.

Four parts of the vertebral artery are also distinguished (Fig. 1.2-4). The first segment, the prevertebral part, is generally given off dorsally as the last branch from the subclavian artery. Infrequently it arises directly from the aortic arch. In its transverse part, it enters the transverse foramen of the C6 vertebra from the caudal direction in 90% of cases and runs upward in the series of foramina as far as the transverse foramen of the atlas. Between C1 and C2, it always forms a loop, which often extends far laterally—a sign of the mobility of the atlantoaxial joint. The short atlantic part bends sharply at the posterior arch of the atlas and embeds itself there into the vertebral artery groove, surrounded by a dense venous plexus and lying

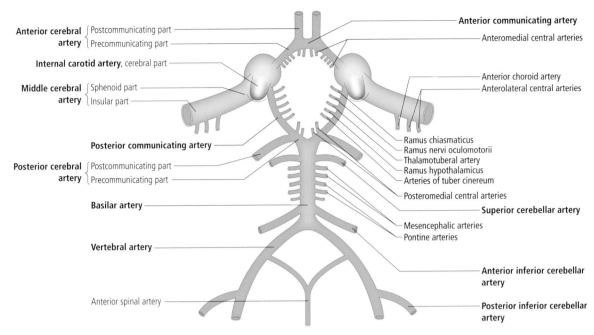

Fig. 1.2-5 The arterial circle.

tightly on the suboccipital nerve. At the medial end of the groove, which is sometimes closed to form a canal, it bends ventrally and—after penetrating the atlanto-occipital membrane and spinal dura mater—it reaches the subarachnoid space as the intracranial part. From the vertebral artery, which has a diameter of approximately 2.5 mm intracranially, the basilar artery forms in the pontocerebellar cistern, resting on the clivus, after the posterior inferior cerebellar artery has been given off (Figs. 1.2-2, 1.2-5). It is originally paired during embryonic development, and this explains some rare variations. From it emerge—in addition to the anterior inferior cerebellar artery and the superior cerebellar artery—numerous branches to the brain stem and inner ear, as well as to the meninges. Just before reaching the dorsum sellae, the basilar artery finally divides into the two posterior cerebral arteries, which in turn are connected to the two middle meningeal arteries via the posterior communicating arteries.

From the precommunicating part (the P1 segment), small branches enter the posterior part of the mesencephalon, parts of the hypothalamus and internal capsule, as well as the posterior part of the thalamus. Branches from the postcommunicating part (the P2 segment) pass to the anterior part of the mesencephalon and to the thalamus. Finally, the terminal branch of the artery (the P3 and P4 segments) supplies the medial surface of the parietal lobe and the inferior surface of the temporal lobe, as well as the posterior pole of the telencephalon (Fig. 1.2-3b).

The arterial circle lies centrally at the base of the skull or brain (Figs. 1.2-2, 1.2-5). It is formed bilaterally from the anterior cerebral artery, the trunk of the internal carotid artery, the middle cerebral artery, the posterior communicating artery, and the posterior cerebral artery. The ring is closed anteriorly by the anterior communicating artery. The sizes of the individual arteries involved differ widely even in normal conditions. The communicating arteries are usually very thin, and bilateral circulatory compensation is thus hardly possible. Almost every conceivable variant is also found, from a different origin of the cerebral arteries to a complete absence of individual arteries.

1.2.2   Clinical picture

In Europe, stroke is the third most frequent cause of early invalidity, after cardiovascular and malignant diseases. Ischemic stroke is the most frequent etiological and pathologic cause, representing 85% of cases. Arteriosclerosis in the intracranial vessels is the cause of approximately 8–10% of all cases of ischemic stroke. The annual risk of stroke in patients with intracranial stenosis of more than 50% who have already suffered stroke or a transient ischemic attack (TIA) lies in the range of 12–14% even with drug treatment. In high-risk patients (those with higher-grade stenoses > 70%, those with current symptoms, and women), the annual risk may be as high as up to 23%. Clinically asymptomatic stenoses are associated with a low annual risk of stroke (< 3.5%). Due to the narrow caliber of the intracranial vessels, the exact percentage of stenoses is difficult to assess. Strictures of approximately 50% of the vascular lumen may already lead to clinical symptoms. The findings of the Warfarin-Aspirin Symptomatic Intracranial Disease (WASID) study showed that stenosis greater than 70% markedly increased the relative risk of suffering a subsequent ischemic stroke. Three percent of patients with low-grade stenoses (50–69%) suffered a TIA within 1 year, in comparison with 14% of those with higher-grade stenoses (> 70%). Cases of manifest stroke within 1 year occurred in 8% of patients with low-grade stenoses and in more than 23% of those with high-grade stenoses. The most frequent locations for intracranial stenoses are the internal carotid artery at the level of the siphon, the main trunk of the middle cerebral artery, the distal vertebral artery and the middle segment of the basilar artery. The significance of tandem stenoses and multiple intracranial stenoses is as yet unclear, but there is considerable evidence to suggest that each individual stenosis carries the corresponding risk of infarction and that the risk is then increased.

Intracranial vascular occlusions often arise due to emboli that originate in the heart or aortic arch or from stenotic cervical arteries. Rarer causes include thrombotic occlusions of existing stenoses. The site of an intracranial occlusion is often influenced by wall changes and stenoses that are already present.

1.2.2.1 Clinical symptoms

Vascular occlusion can lead to loss of neurological function (hemiplegia, speech disturbance, visual disturbance, ataxia, and unconsciousness), but it can also produce nonspecific symptoms such as headache and vertigo. The clinical symptoms depend on the capacity of the intracranial collateral circulation and the extent and location of the occluded vascular segment.

Ischemic stroke is classified according to its temporal course. If the symptoms completely resolve within 24 hours, it is called a transient ischemic attack (TIA). Otherwise it represents ischemic stroke syndrome. However, magnetic resonance imaging shows diffusion disturbances as the correlate of cerebral ischemia in up to 50% of cases that are clinically classified as TIAs. Additional classifications into prolonged reversible ischemic neurological deficit (PRIND) and reversible ischemic neurological deficit (RIND) have been abandoned.

1.2.3 Differential diagnosis

Intracranial stenoses and occlusions need not always be caused by arteriosclerosis. Other causes may include dissection, vasculitis, vasculopathy (e.g., fibromuscular dysplasia, moyamoya), vasospasm and vascular compression by extravascular space-occupying lesions.

Dissection is the most frequent cause of ischemic stroke in young adults. However, it is not always possible to confirm intracranial dissection beyond doubt using imaging diagnosis, as intramural hematoma is difficult to confirm in these small vessels. This remains a diagnosis of exclusion, when there is no arteriosclerosis or no other risk factor for cerebral ischemia are present. Sites of predilection are the distal vertebral artery and main trunk of the middle cerebral artery.

In cases of vasculitis, magnetic resonance imaging usually shows multiple smaller subcortical ischemic areas in the white matter in both cerebral hemispheres. In some cases, typical irregularities in the vessel wall may already be seen on imaging (MRA, CTA, DSA), with stenotic and dilated segments. The final diagnosis is established by evidence of antibodies in serum and cerebrospinal fluid; a cerebral vessel biopsy is sometimes necessary. Treatment is determined by the underlying disease and may involve anti-inflammatory therapy or even immunosuppressive therapy.

One example of vasculopathy is moyamoya disease (*moyamoya* is Japanese for "foggy" or "smoky"), in which extremely fine, complex collateral networks form in the area of the perforating arteries when major cerebral arteries are occluded (see the section on surgical therapy below). Inflammatory diseases (e.g., meningitis) or neoplasia (e.g., meningioma at the base of the skull) may also lead to narrowing and occlusion of intracranial vessels. However, the main diagnosis in these cases is usually so obvious that differential-diagnostic considerations are secondary.

1.2.4 Imaging diagnosis

Ischemic cerebrovascular events present as transient, fluctuating, or permanent neurological deficits. Transient ischemic attack (TIA) has so far been defined clinically as a neurological deficit that lasts for up to a maximum of 24 hours. TIA leads to frank stroke within 90 days in over 10% of cases. In contrast to earlier approaches, rapid clarification and treatment within 24 hours are now recommended, and this reduces the risk of stroke to 2%. Imaging diagnosis must include either computed tomography (CT) or magnetic resonance imaging (MRI), or a combination of the two modalities. In patients with acute non-fluctuating deficit and significant loss of function, imaging should be carried out as quickly as possible in order to limit the damage caused by the ischemia.

To establish an indication for intravenous or intra-arterial thrombolysis or thrombectomy, noncontrast CT followed by CT angiography is usually sufficient. This makes it possible to distinguish hemorrhagic from ischemic stroke. In addition, treatment-relevant vascular occlusions can be quickly demonstrated (with an examination time of < 2 min). MRI is preferable to CT diagnosis in individual cases (e.g., unclear time window, young patient) in an acute setting, but it involves a longer examination time (approximately 15–20 min).

In addition to imaging of the area with diffusion disturbance or infarction and the underlying vascular pathology on MRI and CT, a perfusion study (CT and MRI) after bolus contrast administration may reveal underperfusion of the vascular territory involved.

Intracranial stenoses may lead to fluctuating neurological deficits as a result of recurrent emboli or underperfusion. When there is a drop in systemic blood pressure, stenoses often have hemodynamic effects as a sign of an inadequate collateral supply. Clarification of the hemodynamic components before a treatment decision is taken (for endovascular or surgical treatment) thus requires perfusion measurements in order to assess the quality of the cerebral collateral supply (described in the section on surgical therapy below) and the perfusion reserve.

1.2.4.1 Doppler/color duplex ultrasonography

Examination technique

Transtemporal insonation of the distal internal carotid artery, carotid T, middle cerebral artery (M1/2), anterior cerebral artery (A1), and posterior cerebral artery (P1/2) is obligatory. The latter may be confused with the superior cerebellar artery when pulsed-wave Doppler is used, therefore visual stimulation should be carried out as a check (the posterior cerebral artery shows increased flow in response to inert optic stimuli after prior closing of the eye, due to supply of the visual cortex; the superior cerebellar artery shows no reaction).

Optionally, transtemporal imaging of the internal carotid artery may be carried out at cerebral levels and toward the base of the skull, as well as in the basilar artery and clivus if needed. Transnuchal insonation of the vertebral artery bilaterally, as well as of the basilar artery, is also obligatory, with imaging of the posterior inferior cerebellar artery (PICA) if needed. Transtemporal insonation is difficult in approximately 30% of cases and impossible due to a widened calvaria in 20% of cases; an ultrasound contrast medium may then be used → initial saturation artifact ("blooming") can be corrected by reducing the transmission power (but not the gain; with a lower mechanical index, the contrast medium has a longer intravascular persistence). One milliliter of ultrasound contrast medium is often sufficient.

Differential diagnosis

- Arteriosclerosis: classic focal flow acceleration.
- Occlusion: no flow can be demonstrated even with ultrasound contrast medium, despite good imaging of other vessels at the skull base.
- Typical indirect preocclusive/postocclusive criteria.
- Vasculitis: there may be multifocal and serial focal or long flow acceleration.
- Vasospasm: there may be multifocal and serial focal or long flow acceleration.
- Findings may change over time.
- Dissection
- In cases of floating membrane, there may by a pathognomonic triphasic "splash signal"—otherwise, see stenosis/occlusion.
- Fibromuscular dysplasia.
- Beaded appearance.
- AVM feeder.
- Typical excess flow signal, particularly in diastole.
- Long increase in flow velocity.
- Possibly corresponding changes in the afferent extracranial vessels.
- Possibly pulsatile venous flow.
- Congenital variants.
- The vertebral artery often shows hypoplasia and also aplasia.
- The anterior/posterior communicating branch is often hypoplastic or aplastic.
- The P1 segment of the posterior cerebral artery is often hypoplastic (in up to 20% of cases)—then there is supply from P2 via the posterior communicating branch—i.e., from the internal carotid artery (*caution*: stenosis of the internal carotid artery may then be the cause of posterior infarction).

Specific findings

Middle cerebral artery

Unremarkable findings: maximum systolic velocity < 120 (−140) cm/s, with no flow disturbances detectable acoustically or in the spectral analysis.

Borderline findings: circumscribed maximum velocities around 140 cm/s (> 120 cm/s), but still with no flow disturbances.

Hyperperfusion: during recanalization after a stroke, there may be a phase of hyperperfusion. Signs arguing in favor of hyperperfusion and against a stenotic process in the middle cerebral artery are:

- Long increased flow velocities without circumscribed turbulence phenomena.
- Increased flow velocities, possibly also in medial branches.
- Flow velocities not exceeding 2 m/s.
- Quotients for maximum velocities in the middle cerebral artery/internal carotid artery < 2; values > 3 tend to suggest stenoses.
- The intra-individual course shows a tendency toward normalization.

Similar findings are seen after carotid surgery, with hyperperfusion (an increased flow velocity of > 50% in the middle cerebral artery on side-to-side comparison) also being observed in some patients—particularly those with poor preoperative collateralization and long clamping times (Widder 1999)—as a sign that autoregulation is still disturbed.

Low-grade stenosis (50 to < 70%): circumscribed increase in the maximum systolic flow velocity to values of 140–200 cm/s, as well as in middle and possibly diastolic flow velocities. The critical velocity after which the presence of a stenosis of more than 50% can be definitely assumed is 220 cm/s (Baumgartner et al. 1999).

Incipient flow disturbances, spectral widening, signs on the color Doppler signal of localized increases in flow velocity and turbulences, possibly a mixed signal with a normal main trunk signal and a stenotic signal in M2/middle artery stenoses.

Moderate stenosis (approximately 70% to < 80%): a focal increase in the maximum systolic flow velocity to values of 200–280 cm/s and also diastolic flow velocities. Clear flow disturbances, spectrum widening, blurred systolic window, retrograde flow components, marked signs on the color Doppler signal of a localized increase in flow velocity, reduced lumen size possibly visible in velocity mode and/or power mode.

High-grade stenosis (> 80%): a circumscribed increase in maximum systolic flow velocity to values of > 280 cm/s and of the diastolic flow velocities, marked flow disturbances, spectrum widening, blurred systolic window, marked retrograde flow components, clearly reduced post-stenotic flow velocity, marked signs on the color Doppler signal of a localized increase in flow velocity, also an increase in diastolic flow velocity visible particularly with variance coding (candle-flame phenomenon), lumen reduction visible in velocity mode and/or power mode, possible occurrence of musical murmurs.

Middle cerebral artery main trunk occlusion (M1): no demonstrable M1 signal despite good ultrasound imaging conditions, reduced flow velocities in the proximal vessels, possibly hyperperfusion of collaterals—e.g., the anterior and posterior cerebral arteries as afferent vessels for leptomeningeal anastomoses; in cases of occlusion distal to the origins of the lenticulostriate arteries, there may be a typical prestenotic highly pulsatile signal with low flow velocity in the proximal main trunk—confirmation using ultrasound contrast enhancement.

Middle cerebral artery branch occlusion (M2): lower flow velocity in the M1 segment in side-to-side comparison, possibly higher pulsatility in M1, absent M2 imaging, possible hyperperfusion of collaterals—e.g., the anterior and posterior cerebral arteries as afferent vessels for leptomeningeal anastomoses; possible retrograde perfusion of collaterals, occlusions of small vessels not detectable; flow differences in the proximal middle cerebral artery can be identified by detecting absolute systolic/diastolic velocities and by detecting pulsatility differences.

Carotid-T processes: these are often combined with distal internal carotid artery and outflow regions of the middle and anterior cerebral arteries; carotid-T occlusion processes are the hemodynamically most severe findings, since all collateralization pathways from the middle cerebral artery are blocked with the exception of leptomeningeal anastomoses. The anterior cerebral artery may be collateralized from the contralateral side via the anterior communicating branch.

Assessment of hemodynamic consequences:

- Demonstration of post-stenotic and postocclusive flow, assessment of the spectrum (steepness of increase, acceleration time, V_{max} systolic/diastolic)
- Demonstration of collateralization pathways (ideally using duplex ultrasonography)

- Possible compression test if the information provided is expected to have implications—e.g., for:
  - Clarifying the indication for surgery in multiple-vessel disease (e.g., internal carotid artery stenosis with contralateral occlusion)
  - Assessment of the afferent components of the various collateral pathways
  - Assessment of the hemodynamic consequences of a potential vascular occlusion (e.g., progressive asymptomatic internal carotid artery stenosis)
  - Testing the quality of the collateralization
  - Detecting any collateral pathways that cannot be spontaneously imaged (e.g., posterior communicating branch) by inducing hyperperfusion
  - Assessment of the risk of intraoperative clamping (see below) before or during carotid thromboendarterectomy or proximal embolic protection. Evidence for sufficient residual perfusion includes:
    - In cases of ≤ 80% stenosis of the internal carotid artery: mean residual flow velocity in the middle cerebral artery > 30–40% of the resting value
    - In cases of ≥ 80% stenosis of the internal carotid artery: mean residual flow velocity ≥ 30 cm/s
- Testing of CO_2 reactivity/autoregulation reserve:
  - Correlates with the risk of hemodynamic watershed infarction—corresponds to the remaining CO_2-induced dilation capacity in the intracerebral vessels
  - Methods:
    - Breath-holding index
    - Doppler CO_2 testing
    - Apnea–hyperventilation testing
    - Acetazolamide (Diamox) testing

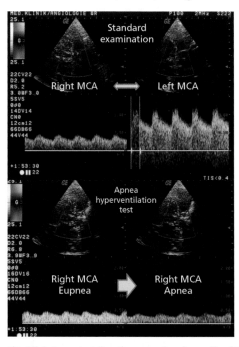

Fig. 1.2-6 Apnea test. Top: the power Doppler profile of the middle cerebral artery bilaterally, with massively reduced amplitude on the right, reduced pulsatility and prolonged acceleration time as signs of poor intracerebral collateralization in subtotal internal carotid artery stenosis. Bottom: inverse steal phenomenon in the apnea test as a sign of an absent autoregulation reserve and steal in a vascular area that is still capable of reacting.

The apnea–hyperventilation test is the fastest exploratory test in routine work: resting V_{max} is measured, followed by respiration for at least 30 seconds once a second or once per pulse and measurement of V_{max}, and finally an apnea phase induced at mid-respiration for a maximum duration, during which V_{max} is measured again. Standard: increase (apnea) and decrease (hyperventilation) by at least 15% in comparison with the resting values (Widder 1999).

Anterior cerebral artery

There are as yet no validated Doppler or duplex ultrasound criteria for grading stenoses of the anterior cerebral artery. The critical velocity from which a > 50% stenosis must be assumed to be present is 155 cm/s (Baumgartner et al. 1999). The criteria mentioned in connection with the middle cerebral artery can be used as an approximation. It is sometimes difficult to differentiate organically fixed stenoses from functional stenoses in collateral function: circumscribed flow accelerations argue more for localized stenoses, while longer flow accelerations—particularly in combination with other signs of collateralization (such as retrograde perfusion in the contralateral anterior cerebral artery, compression tests) suggest relative stenoses with collateral function.

Posterior cerebral artery

There are as yet no validated Doppler or duplex ultrasound criteria for grading stenoses of the posterior cerebral artery. The critical velocity from which a > 50% stenosis must be assumed to be present is 145 cm/s (Baumgartner et al. 1999). The criteria mentioned in connection with the middle cerebral artery can be used as an approximation. Particular sites of predilection for arteriosclerotic stenoses are the start of the P2 segment, the posterior arch, and more rarely the P1 outflow region. In the P1 segment, relative stenoses due to hyperperfusion in collateral function of the posterior cerebral artery via the posterior communicating branch or stenotic signals from the hyperperfused posterior communicating branch must be taken into consideration (*caution:* risk of possible confusion); color-coded imaging can be helpful for differentiation here.

Vertebral artery

See under extracranial occlusion processes.

Basilar artery

The head of the basilar artery is a site of predilection for arteriosclerotic lesions. There are as yet no validated Doppler or duplex ultrasound criteria for grading stenoses of the basilar artery. The critical velocity from which a > 50% stenosis must be assumed to be present is 140 cm/s (Baumgartner et al. 1999), but suspicion should already be raised at flow velocities of 100–120 cm/s. The criteria mentioned in connection with the middle cerebral artery can also be used as an approximation.

Basilar artery hypoplasia must be assumed when there is extracranial evidence of bilateral vertebral artery hypoplasia, particularly if the total diameter of the two vertebral arteries is less than 5 mm.

Occlusion of the basilar artery (basilar thrombosis) must be assumed with:

- High pulsatility (low or absent diastolic flow) in the extracranial segments of both vertebral arteries
- High pulsatility in the transnuchally visible vertebrobasilar pathway
- Inability to image the basilar artery on color-coded duplex ultrasound (signal enhancement may be needed)
- Noticeable postocclusive Doppler signal in the posterior cerebral arteries
- Possible collateral flow via the posterior communicating branch

Basilar occlusion cannot be definitively excluded only by evaluating the findings from the extracranial vertebral artery (particularly with older, collateralized occlusions that have developed gradually).

Other applications for transcranial Doppler and duplex ultrasonography

Evidence of spontaneous cerebral emboli/HITS analysis

High-intensity transient signals (HITS) with a relevant signal intensity and temporal latency in their occurrence in two sample volumes (multigating procedure) in the main trunk of the middle cerebral artery represent high-intensity signal peaks within the Doppler spectrum of blood components—i.e., spontaneous cerebral emboli. There is a 15-fold increase in the risk of stroke when there is evidence of HITS—e.g., in patients with 60% asymptomatic internal carotid artery stenosis—in comparison with negative HITS findings (Spence et al. 2005).

Testing for persistent patent foramen ovale (PFO)

An ultrasound contrast medium that will not enter the capillaries is injected into a large antecubital vein or the common femoral artery; after approximately 8 seconds, a Valsalva maneuver is carried out for approximately 4 seconds, possibly supported by compression in the abdominal area, with further ultrasound imaging for 5–10 seconds. When there is an intermittent cardiac right–left shunt due to PFO, there is a mean contrast appearance time of 9 ± 6 s (< 15 s) in comparison with 24 ± 9 s (> 15 s) with transpulmonary passage. A relevant shunt is present if more than 10 emboli appear at rest and/or more than 25 emboli appear after the Valsalva maneuver within the time stated. Larger persistent foramina lead to showers of emboli that can no longer be detected individually. Lower emboli rates are probably not relevant. The advantage of TCD in comparison with transesophageal echocardiography is that the procedure is not invasive, the patient can still cooperate (with the Valsalva), evidence of noncardiac shunts is also possible (explaining occasional differences), and the sensitivity is comparable for relevant shunts.

Intracranial pressure monitoring

Diastolic flow/pulsatility correlates with intracerebral pressure/outflow resistance; the parameters along the course are highly sensitive and measurement of absolute values is of course not possible (with the exception of diastolic zero flow, in which case intracranial pressure corresponds to the diastolic pressure, with phasic flow when there is a further rise in intracranial pressure).

Diagnosis of cerebral death

Transcranial Doppler ultrasound is an approved procedure used to shorten the waiting time before cerebral death is diagnosed. Prerequisites include not only availability of an examiner with the relevant expertise, but also confirmation that ultrasonography can be carried out in the patient and appropriate adjustment of the device settings (high gain, maximum transmission power, high reception speed, low wall filter, large measurement volume ≥ 15 mm). **Typical Doppler findings** in cerebral perfusion standstill:

- Phasic flow (biphasic flow with backflow components representing > 30% of the antegrade flow)
- No systolic peaks (maximum amplitudes 50 cm/s, duration < 200 ms)
- Passive breath-regulated signal amplitudes
- Absence of a diastolic signal
- No evaluable signal → *caution!* Check insonability, examination technique → possible use of ultrasound contrast enhancement

Prerequisites:
- Systemic blood pressure > 80 mmHg systolic
- Heart rate < 120/min
- No relevant calvarial defects

Criteria for brain death: evidence of phasic flow and/or small systolic peaks **twice** at an interval of at least 30 minutes, on each occasion **bilaterally** at the middle cerebral artery or intracranial internal carotid artery, or with duplex ultrasound in the internal carotid artery extracranially **and** in the basilar or vertebral artery intracranially, or with duplex ultrasound in the vertebral artery extracranially.

Doppler ultrasound can be used independently of the type of cerebral damage—i.e., even in cases of toxic injury. When an appropriate acoustic window is used, a false-positive finding cannot occur when an experienced examiner uses the above criteria. False-negative findings are possible:

- With cerebral arteriovenous malformations with shunt flow
- In the absence of raised intracranial pressure
- When perfusion re-starts (with intracranial pressure declining again)
- In infants with open fontanelles and sutures
- In the case of the proximal vertebral artery, due to branches not supplying the brain
- In a purely extracranial examination, due to residual perfusion of the internal carotid artery via the ophthalmic artery

Vasospasm monitoring in subarachnoid bleeding

The vasospasm that mainly occurs from days 4 to 10 can be recorded and monitored using transcranial Doppler (TCD) follow-up observations and by measuring velocities particularly in the middle cerebral artery main trunk:

- Borderline: $V_{mean} \geq 120$ cm/s
- Pathological: $V_{mean} \geq 160$ cm/s
- Critically raised: $V_{mean} \geq 200$ cm/s, $V_{max} \geq 300$ cm/s
- Suspicious: increases in flow velocities $\geq 50\%$ or ≥ 40 cm/s/d during the first 6–7 days (Grosset 1993)
- Pulsatility index (PI) > 1, resistance index (RI) > 0.6 (Klingelhöfer et al. 1991)

- Ratio of the maximum velocities in the middle cerebral artery and internal carotid artery (the middle cerebral artery/internal carotid artery index) ≥ 3

Caution:
- False-negative findings may occur when nonspastic vascular segments are examined.
- False-negative findings may occur with simultaneous raised intracranial pressure and consequently reduced flow velocities (pulsatility parameters should therefore also be used).
- Prior arteriosclerotic stenoses.
- Hyperperfusion (middle cerebral artery/internal carotid artery index < 2).

1.2.5   Treatment

1.2.5.1   Conservative treatment

The treatment strategy depends in principle on multiple factors and should be decided on an individual basis. Risk factors such as nicotine consumption, lipid disorders, hypertension, and diabetes should be eliminated or treated.

In patients with asymptomatic stenoses that are not hemodynamically relevant, invasive treatment is not currently recommended, but drug therapy with platelet inhibitors is recommended, possibly in combination with lipid-lowering agents.

Patients with symptomatic stenoses that are hemodynamically relevant initially receive drug treatment, and invasive therapy is only considered if symptoms recur. The WASID study found no benefit with warfarin administration in comparison with aspirin in patients with symptomatic intracranial stenoses. In comparison, the risk of stroke during the first year was 12% in the aspirin group and almost as high in the warfarin group at 11%; in the second year, the figures were 15% and 13%, respectively. However, as major hemorrhage only occurred in 3% of the patients in the aspirin group in comparison with 8% in the warfarin group, treatment with vitamin K antagonists is now obsolete. Treatment with dual platelet inhibition (e.g., aspirin and clopidogrel) should therefore be considered, particularly when an ischemic event has occurred during single antiplatelet treatment. Individual testing of drug efficacy is advisable in any case, as there is a high percentage (up to 30%) of low responders and nonresponders, although no data in this population that correlates responder rates and clinical events.

When ischemic symptoms recur during medication, the indication for PTA and, if appropriate, stent placement should be considered. A recently published study (the SAMMPRIS study) did not observe any clear benefits with an invasive approach using stenting—a finding that requires further research after optimization of patient selection and concomitant drug therapy.

As mentioned above, it is therefore absolutely imperative to differentiate between embolic and hemodynamically relevant stenoses. In stenoses that have hemodynamic effects, with clinical symptoms, conservative therapy is only appropriate in combination with endovascular therapy (PTA, possibly with stent assistance) in order to improve perfusion. If this is not technically possible, attention should be given to ensure that blood pressure is not reduced too much, to avoid negative effects on the collateral supply.

The treatment of intracranial vascular occlusions also depends on clinical symptoms. Conservative treatment for acute stroke includes normalization of general parameters (cardiovascular and pulmonary function, as well as fluid balance and metabolic parameters) and oxygenation. If a patient reaches hospital within the "thrombolysis window" (usually < 6 hours after the start of symptoms), systemic intravenous thrombolysis therapy (up to 4.5 hours after the initial symptoms) or local intra-arterial embolectomy or thrombolytic therapy can be carried out. The 4.5-hour time interval currently applies to systemic intravenous thrombolytic therapy (with recombinant tissue plasminogen activator, rt-PA). In all cases, the earlier the patient is treated, the better the clinical outcome is. In what is known as the "bridging approach," intravenous treatment (two-thirds of the total dosage, with 10% of that as a bolus) is combined with intra-arterial therapy. The initial intravenous thrombolysis allows rapid initiation of treatment and may optimize the efficacy of the endovascular intra-arterial therapy.

1.2.5.2   Endovascular intra-arterial therapy

Endovascular intra-arterial therapy is indicated and in most cases possible for hemodynamically relevant intracranial stenoses, or for stenoses that cause recurrent arterioarterial embolism in spite of adequate platelet function inhibition. The endovascular procedure consists of dilation (percutaneous transluminal angioplasty, PTA) (Fig. 1.2-7), which can be combined with stent implantation (Figs. 1.2-8, 1.2-9, 1.2-11). To prevent thromboembolic events during possible stent implantation, the patients should receive dual platelet inhibition (e.g., aspirin and clopidogrel), starting if possible several days before the procedure. It is advisable here to have the efficacy of platelet inhibition tested in the laboratory in order to identify nonresponders and poor responders, who may represent up to 30% of the patients. These patients then have to be treated with a correspondingly higher dosage. Following stent implantation, long-term monotherapy with aspirin or clopidogrel is required after temporary dual therapy.

Using expanding balloon stents to treat intracranial arteriosclerotic stenoses requires precise measurement of the vascular diameter in order to avoid possible overexpansion and rupture of intracranial arteries. However, precise measurement is not always technically reliable, and self-expanding stents were therefore developed that have markedly reduced the complication rate, as they are more flex-

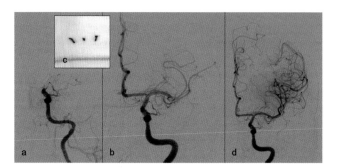

Fig. 1.2-7a–d A 71-year-old patient with unilateral symptoms on the right side in a case of left-sided carotid T-occlusion (**a**). During thrombus aspiration with a Penumbra® catheter, the left carotid flow area was recanalized (**b**). Multiple aspiration of small thrombus fragments (**c**). The vessels were successfully reopened (**d**).

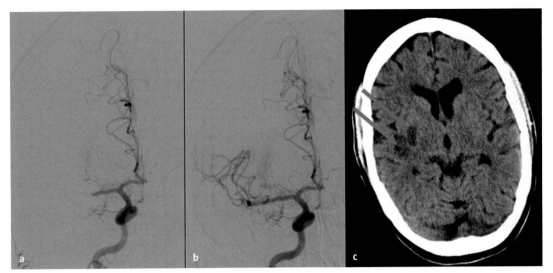

Fig. 1.2-8a–c A 57-year-old patient with unilateral brachiofacial symptoms on the left side in a case of right-sided occlusion of the main trunk of the middle cerebral artery (**a**). During intra-arterial abciximab (ReoPro®) administration, with stenting required for a subtotal internal carotid artery ostial stenosis on the left side and supplementary rt-PA administration, patency of the middle cerebral vessels was restored (**b**). Small areas of infarction are demarcated on the follow-up CT after 24 hours (**c**, arrows).

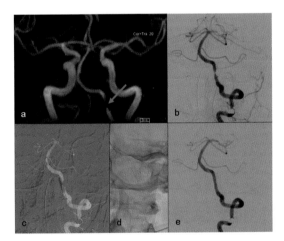

Fig. 1.2-9a–e A 56-year-old patient with high-grade stenosis of the vertebral artery on the left, on time-of-flight magnetic resonance angiography (MRA) (**a**, arrow), with recurrent TIAs and a hypoplastic vertebral artery on the right ending at the PICA. The corresponding digital subtraction angiography (DSA) image (**b**). A Pharos® stent at the level of the stenosis, with the balloon inflated (**c**). Imaging of the stent in the bone window (**d**). Normalization of the vascular caliber after complication-free stenting (**e**).

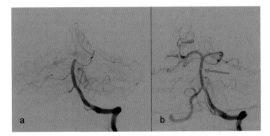

Fig. 1.2-10a, b A 72-year-old patient who suddenly became comatose, with distal occlusion of the basilar artery (**a**). Recanalization of the posterior flow area during thrombus aspiration using a Penumbra® catheter (arrow: catheter tip) (**b**).

ible and no balloon remodeling is needed. Self-expanding stents can adapt to varying vascular diameters and adjustment of critical stent radial forces allows secondary remodeling of the vessels after the vascular plaque has been broken through using PTA.

The intervention should be carried out with the patient under general anesthesia. Access is obtained via the route of least risk, usually the femoral artery. A microballoon catheter is introduced via a guide catheter positioned in the internal carotid artery or vertebral artery, the balloon positioned at the site of the stenosis, and percutaneous transluminal angioplasty (PTA) is carried out. In a second step, a self-expanding microstent catheter is advanced using a wire exchange maneuver. After optimal placement at the previously stenotic vascular segment, the stent is released by withdrawing the microcatheter. With balloon-mounted stents, prior PTA is not required, as this takes place during the stent deployment (Fig. 1.2-15).

A multicenter prospective study (the Wingspan study) reported good treatment results, with a fatal ipsilateral stroke rate of 7% within 6 months. During the same period, the repeat stenosis rate (with a stenosis grade of > 50%) was low at 7.5% and the patients affected remained without neurological symptoms. A multicenter study in the United States has also reported successful treatment, with technical success and a low periprocedural risk. The primary end point of stroke or death within 30 days after the intervention or ipsilateral stroke after 30 days was observed in 15.7% of the patients and in most cases was associated with withdrawal of platelet inhibition or recurrent stenosis.

In cases of acute vascular occlusion, local therapy nowadays consists of mechanical extraction of the embolus/thrombus.

The mechanical procedures mainly used today include aspiration via wide-lumen, highly flexible catheters that are advanced as far as the vascular occlusion (Fig. 1.2-10a) and a stent retriever system (Figs. 1.2-13, 1.2-14). The efficacy of these systems depends on the consistency of the thrombus/embolus and the arterial access. The systems are sometimes used in combination. Rapid mechanical recanalization of occluded intracranial arteries can be achieved in more than 90% of cases. All of the mechanical procedures can be combined with intra-arterial thrombolysis therapy or platelet inhibition with administration of glycoprotein receptor antagonists.

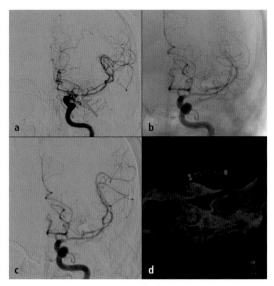

Fig. 1.2-11a–d A 77-year-old patient with high-grade stenosis of the middle cerebral artery trunk on the left side (**a**), with recurrent infarction in the middle cerebral artery flow area during dual medication. A Wingspan® stent at the level of the stenosis with an exchange wire in place in an M2 branch (**b**). Normalization of the vascular caliber after complication-free stenting (**c**). Three-dimensional imaging of the stent on Xper-CT (**d**).

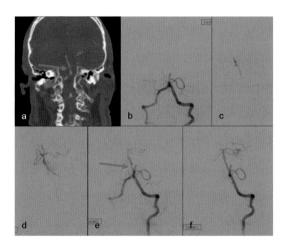

Fig. 1.2-12a–f An 82-year-old patient with multiple cervical and intracranial vascular stenoses, with recurrent TIAs in the posterior flow area and a principal finding of high-grade basilar artery stenosis (**a**, MPR on CTA, arrow). The patient had declined endovascular therapy. Three months later, there was acute hemiplegia on the right side, with dysarthria and bilaterally disturbed eye movements during dual medication. The cause was a proximal basilar artery occlusion (**b**) following earlier stenosis. It was only possible to pass the stenosis after balloon dilation, with contrast imaging of the distal occluded basilar artery (**c**). During local thrombolytic therapy with rt-PA, the posterior flow area reopened distally (**d**). Due to persistent relevant stenosis (**e**), stenting was carried out at the same time. The Wingspan® stent is seen at the level of the stenosis, with the exchange wire in place (**f**). In these conditions, there was normalization of the vessels in the posterior flow area and a tolerable occlusion of the right posterior cerebral artery with an anterior fetal supply.

If recanalization is successful and an underlying stenosis is identified (Fig. 1.2-12), it is beneficial due to the high rate of recurrent occlusion to treat the stenosis during the same session (with PTA alone or in combination with a stent). Unfortunately, the clinical outcome for the affected patients does not depend only on the re-

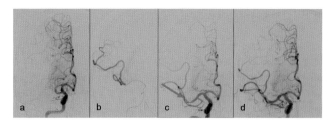

Fig. 1.2-13a–d A 72-year-old patient with right-sided occlusion of the main trunk of the middle cerebral artery (**a**) and acute left-sided hemiparesis. The thrombus was passed with a microcatheter (**b**) and introduction of a Solitaire® stent (**c**; arrow: distal stent marker), with revascularization with the opened stent lumen. Removal of the stent and successful thrombus extraction from the main trunk of the middle cerebral artery (**d**). It was not possible in this case to reopen an M2 branch, despite supplementary rt-PA administration and attempts at mechanical thrombolysis.

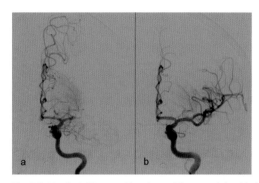

Fig. 1.2-14a, b A 51-year-old patient with acute right-sided hemiparesis and aphasia, with occlusion of the main trunk of the middle cerebral artery on the left (**a**). After the thrombus had been passed with a microcatheter and a Solitaire® stent had been introduced, the thrombus was successfully extracted from the main trunk and the flow area was revascularized (**b**).

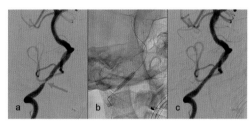

Fig. 1.2-15a–c A 52-year-old patient with high-grade stenosis of the vertebral artery on the right side (**a**, arrow), with recurrent TIAs and occlusion of the vertebral artery on the left. A Pharos® stent was placed at the level of the stenoses, with an inflated balloon (**b**). Normalization of the vascular caliber following complication-free stenting (**c**).

canalization of the vessels. The duration and location of the vascular occlusion, the collateral blood supply, the side of the affected brain area that has already suffered infarction, and concomitant diseases that the patient may have also play an important role.

In rare cases when there is persistent intermittent perfusion, recanalization treatment for non-acute, chronic vascular occlusion is indicated.

1.2.5.3   Surgical treatment

Surgical treatment for stenotic and occlusive processes in the region of the extracranial and intracranial circulation of the arteries supplying the brain represents a complementary strategy for preventing ischemia-related neurological deficits. In this approach, a further critical underperfusion event in circulation regions that are at risk for ischemia is avoided by carrying out surgical improvement in the exhausted cerebral collateral supply. This strategy is based on the results of studies in which symptomatic patients with signs of inadequate cerebral collateral supply—i.e., hemodynamic insufficiency or exhausted cerebral perfusion reserve—had a markedly higher annual risk of stroke, at 18–46%, in comparison with patients with an intact collateral supply. Patient selection—i.e., the choice of which patients should undergo targeted revascularization—therefore focuses on assessing what is known as the cerebral perfusion reserve. This can be measured using various functional examinations of regional cerebral blood flow (rCBF).

Determining cerebral perfusion reserve

This is based on carrying out paired examinations of the rCBF, with a baseline measurement being carried out in resting conditions. Following a vasodilatory stimulus—e.g., inhalation of carbon dioxide or administration of acetazolamide (15 mg/kg body weight i.v.)—the rCBF is measured again. After appropriate evaluation and application of various calculation algorithms, the perfusion reserve (cerebrovascular reserve capacity, CVRC, expressed as a percentage; also known as the vasomotor reserve) is calculated. For direct measurements of rCBF, methods that can be used include PET, stable Xe-CT, and quantitative SPECT; transcranial Doppler (TCD) ultrasonography only allows indirect estimates.

In physiological conditions, rCBF stimulation can be expected to produce at least a 30% increase in rCBF (CVRC > 30%—i.e., normal). Depending on the extent of hemodynamic restriction, there is then a reduction in reactive vasodilation, so that restricted CVRC is described as being present at a CVRC < 30%. At values < 10%, CVRC is regarded as having been eliminated. When there is a paradoxical reduction in rCBF (CVRC < –5%)—i.e., maximum vasodilation

before stimulation and consequent nonreaction of the resistance vessels—it is assumed that an intracranial steal phenomenon is present. This is the most severe grade of hemodynamic impairment and is associated with the highest risk of secondary ischemia (Fig. 1.2-16).

Indications for revascularization

The following criteria generally arise:
- Age < 70 years
- Clinical symptoms: recurrent TIA/PRIND
- Watershed infarction or normal findings in morphological diagnosis (MRI)
- Stenotic occlusive lesions (stenosis and/or occlusion) in the area of the anterior circulation that are not accessible to primary interventional treatment or vascular surgery/intervention
- Confirmed hemodynamic cerebrovascular insufficiency

With regard to the underlying pathology, there is considerable variability in the pathogenesis. In most cases, the patients have localized or systemic atherosclerosis. In a far smaller proportion of the patients, there is an indication for surgery due to inadequate collateral supply after carotid dissection or progressive tumor growth with resulting constriction or occlusion of the internal carotid artery, mostly in the area of the skull base. Patients with moyamoya disease or moyamoya syndrome represent a special case, which is discussed separately below.

Surgical technique

The aim of the surgical procedure is to normalize the CVRC and thus to "restore" physiological perfusion conditions. The technique used is a standard extracranial–intracranial (EC/IC) bypass. A donor vessel in an extracranial site, usually the superficial temporal artery (STA), is anastomosed with a cortically located branch of the middle cerebral artery (MCA) in the area of the lateral sulcus (sylvian fissure). The procedure is carried out with the patient under general anesthesia, with endotracheal intubation and neuroprotective measures to prevent ischemic complications. After preparation of the donor vessel (the STA), a craniotomy with a diameter of approximately 3 cm is carried out in the area of a defined target point over the lateral

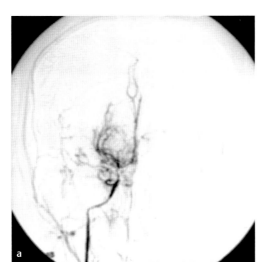

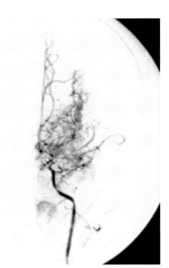

Fig. 1.2-16a, b A standard extracranial–intracranial (EC/IC) bypass in a patient with atherosclerotic occlusion of the right internal carotid artery. (**a**) Conventional angiography reveals insufficient collateral supply to the right hemisphere. Angiographic demonstration of the STA–MCA bypass using the right superficial temporal artery (STA), which was anastomosed with a distal branch of the middle cerebral artery (MCA). (**b**) Anteroposterior view.

sulcus. After opening of the dura mater and exposure of a suitable recipient vessel (the middle cerebral artery in the M2/M3 segment), the standard bypass is placed using an end-to-side technique with 10–12 interrupted sutures (Fig. 1.2-17). The patency of the bypass that has been created can usually be immediately documented intraoperatively using indocyanine green (ICG) video angiography. Thanks to improved perioperative treatment, more sophisticated surgical techniques, and the ability to check the success of the procedure immediately, it is now possible to carry out this procedure with only minor surgical morbidity (< 5%). The operation is only carried out after adequate inhibition of platelet aggregation (100 or 325 mg ASA/d p.o.). Among other things, this makes it possible to achieve a bypass patency of > 98%. Platelet aggregation inhibition starts before the operation and continues on a lifelong basis.

In addition, selective DSA and MRI are carried out postoperatively. Specific follow-up treatment for the patients is not necessary. When the indications described above are observed, the principles of microsurgery are rigorously applied, and the relevant expertise is pres-ent, it is possible to reduce the risk of secondary ischemia significantly in comparison with conservative treatment.

Special case: moyamoya disease and moyamoya syndrome

This is a rare, progressive steno-occlusive disease in which, due to unexplained causes, slowly progressive occlusion of the cerebral arteries in the region of the circle of Willis occurs. In parallel with this, spontaneous intracerebral and also extracranial–intracranial formation of collateral vessels is seen. These are regarded as outstanding examples of the way in which complex natural collaterals can develop on the basis of chronic ischemia. Both steno-occlusive changes with hemodynamically significant impairment of the cerebral blood supply along with spontaneous compensation mechanisms in the form of neoangiogenesis and arteriogenesis are therefore seen in patients with moyamoya disease. In addition to the impressive angiographic findings, the disease is distinct from other steno-occlusive diseases in relation to its epidemiology and clinical course (Fig. 1.2-18). The diagnostic characteristics of moyamoya disease (bilateral lesions,

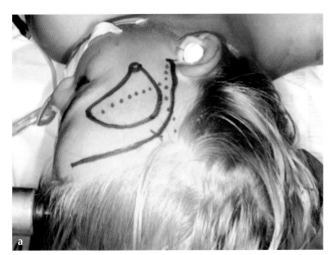
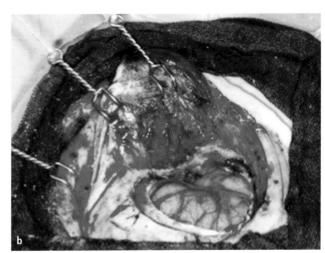

Fig. 1.2-17a, b Intraoperative view. (**a**) Positioning of the patient for planned placement of a superficial temporal artery (STA)–middle cerebral artery (MCA) anastomosis. The planning incision line (blue) is shown, along with the course of the superficial temporal artery (red) and the planned craniotomy. (**b**) Completed bypass in the area of the lateral sulcus (sylvian fissure).

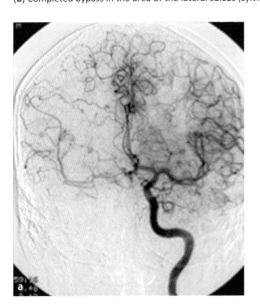
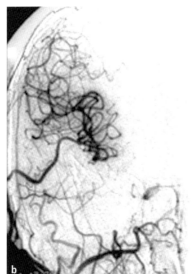
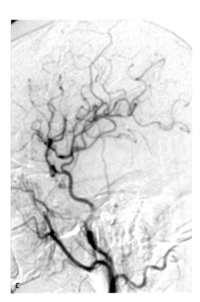

Fig. 1.2-18a–c Typical angiographic findings in adult moyamoya disease. There are bilateral steno-occlusive changes in the area of the intracranial carotid bifurcation, with simultaneous formation of extensive basal collaterals.

spontaneous collateral network) are more frequently associated with other diseases, sometimes systemic ones. In these cases, the condition is known as moyamoya syndrome. However, this does not generally lead to any changes in the treatment strategy. In central Europe, moyamoya disease and moyamoya syndrome occur sporadically and affect both children and adults. In contrast to the Asian form, which usually becomes manifest in adults in the form of intraparenchymal hemorrhage, cerebral ischemia is the major symptom in both age groups in Europe. Although it is mainly adult patients who suffer TIAs or stroke, the disease can also occur in children, often in the context of focal epilepsy or a cerebral organic psychological syndrome, resulting in inadequate formation of spontaneous collaterals and cerebral compensation mechanisms.

Indications for revascularization

In view of the poor results of conservative therapy and the underlying pathogenesis of the disease, revascularization surgery is an option for both children and adults. Surgical treatment is indicated in symptomatic adult patients when the diagnosis is confirmed, a reduced CVRC is demonstrated in the symptomatic hemisphere, and there is no severe focal neurological deficit. In children, surgical treatment in both hemispheres is recommended, due to the generally unfavorable natural course of the condition. This allows a marked improvement in the overall prognosis.

Surgical technique

The aim of surgical treatment is to improve the cerebral collateral supply. Various techniques are available for the purpose. In addition to the standard EC/IC bypass described above (STA–MCA anastomosis or STA–anterior cerebral artery anastomosis), which is preferred in adults, there are also a number of indirect procedures. These take advantage of the capacity for spontaneous collateralization. For example, extracranial "donor tissue" can be placed in contact with the arachnoid on the surface of the brain in order to induce spontaneous vascularization with new collateral vessels. This leads to effective revascularization approximately 3 months after the operation. Overall, more than 30 surgical modifications have been described, with indirect revascularization techniques being particularly effective in pediatric patients. Examples of potential "donor tissue" include the temporalis muscle, the epicranial aponeurosis, and the parietal side of the dura mater. In practice, a combination of direct and indirect techniques is used when possible, since in addition to immediate stabilization of perfusion conditions this can also allow delayed synergistic stabilization of regional perfusion. To improve bypass function and for secondary prophylaxis, lifelong medication with platelet aggregation inhibitors is also administered in moyamoya patients.

When combined revascularization is planned, the principles used in direct bypass surgery apply, and these can then be extended, depending on the planned procedure. Combining an STA–MCA anastomosis with encephalomyosynangiosis (EMS) requires an extended craniotomy (Fig. 1.2-19). In this procedure, the temporalis muscle is placed on the cerebral surface after a standard STA–MCA bypass has been created. Regular DSA and MRI examinations are then carried out during the postoperative follow-up. These are useful not only for checking the quality of the surgical procedure but also to assess the subsequent clinical course.

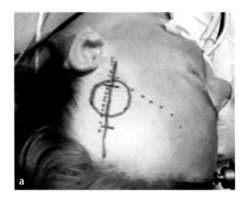

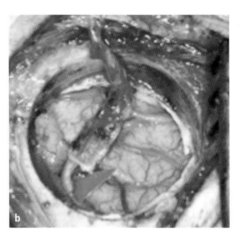

Fig. 1.2-19a, b (a) Positioning of the patient for planned combined revascularization. The planned incision line (blue), the course of the superficial temporal artery (red) and the planned craniotomy have been marked. (b) The intraoperative view after dissection of the temporal muscle, completion of the craniotomy, and resection of the dura mater before placement of the direct bypass.

References

Adams et al. Preview of a new trial of extracranial-to-intracranial arterial anastomosis: the carotid occlusion surgery study. Neurosurg Clin N Am 2001; 12 (3): 613–24, ix–x.

Baker WL, Colby JA, Tongbram V, Talati R, Silverman IE, White CM, Kluger J, Coleman CI. Neurothrombectomy devices for the treatment of acute ischemic stroke: state of the evidence. Ann Intern Med 2011; 154: 243–52.

Baumgartner RW, Mattle HP, Schroth G. Assessment of ≥ 50% and < 50% intracranial stenoses by transcranial color-coded duplex sonography. Stroke 1999; 30 (1): 87–92.

Bose A, Hartmann M, Henkes H, Liu HM, Teng MM, Szikora I, Berlis A, Reul J, Yu SC, Forsting M, Lui M, Lim W, Sit SP. A novel, self-expanding, nitinol stent in medically refractory intracranial atherosclerotic stenoses: the Wingspan study. Stroke 2007; 38: 1531–7.

Bose A, Henkes H, Alfke K, Reith W, Mayer TE, Berlis A, Branca V, Sit SP. For the Penumbra phase 1 stroke trial investigators. The penumbra system: a mechanical device for the treatment of acute stroke due to thromboembolism. AJNR 2008; 29: 1409–13.

Brekenfeld C, Schroth G, Mordasini P, Fischer U, Mono ML, Weck A, Arnold M, El-Koussy M, Gralla J. Impact of retrievable stents on acute ischemic stroke treatment. AJNR 2011; 32: 1269–73.

Chimowitz MI, Lynn MJ, Derdeyn CP, Turan TN, Fiorella D, Lane BF, Janis LS, Lutsep HL, Barnwell SL, Waters MF, Hoh BL, Hourihane JM, Levy EI, Alexandrov AV, Harrigan MR, Chiu D, Klucznik RP, Clark JM, McDougall CG, Johnson MD, Pride GL Jr, Torbey MT,

Zaidat OO, Rumboldt Z, Cloft HJ; SAMMPRIS Trial Investigators. Stenting versus aggressive medical therapy for intracranial arterial stenosis. N Engl J Med 2011 Sep 15; 365 (11): 993–1003. Epub 2011 Sep 7.

Derdeyn et al. Cerebral hemodynamic impairment: methods of measurement and association with stroke risk. Neurology 1999; 53 (2): 251–9.

Derdeyn et al. Re: Stages and thresholds of hemodynamic failure. Stroke 2003; 34 (3): 589.

Fiorella DJ, Turk AS, Levy EI, Pride GL Jr, Woo HH, Albuquerque FC, Welch BG, Niemann DB, Aagaard-Kienitz B, Rasmussen PA, Hopkins LN, Masaryk TJ, McDougall CG U.S. Wingspan Registry: 12-month follow-up results. Stroke 2011 Jul; 42 (7): 1976–81.

Gröschel K, Schnaudigel S, Pilgram SM, Wasser K, Kastrup A. A systematic review on outcome after stenting for intracranial atherosclerosis. Stroke 2009; 40: e340–7.

Gross et al. Use of transcranial Doppler sonography to predict development of delayed ischemic deficit after subarachnoidal hemorrhage. J Neurosurg 1993; 78: 183–7.

Grundmann K, Jaschonek K, Kleine B, Dichgans J, Topka H. Aspirin non-responder status in patients with recurrent cerebral ischemic attacks. J Neurol 2003; 250: 63–6.

Hacke W, Kaste M, Bluhmki E, Brozman M, Dávalos A, Guidetti D, Larrue V, Lees KR, Medeghri Z, Machnig T, Schneider D, von Kummer R, Wahlgren N, Toni D; ECASS Investigators. Thrombolysis with alteplase 3 to 4.5 hours after acute ischemic stroke. N Engl J Med 2008 Sep 25; 359 (13): 1317–29.

Horn et al. Moyamoya-like vasculopathy (moyamoya syndrome) in children. Child's nervous system: ChNS: official journal of the International Society for Pediatric Neurosurgery 2004; 20 (6): 382–91.

Horn et al. Risk of intraoperative ischemia due to temporary vessel occlusion during standard extracranial-intracranial arterial bypass surgery. J Neurosurg 2008; 108 (3): 464–9.

Kasner SE, Lynn MJ, Chimowitz MI, Frankel MR, Howlett-Smith H, Hertzberg VS, Chaturvedi S, Levine SR, Stern BJ, Benesch CG, Jovin TG, Sila CA, Romano JG; Warfarin Aspirin Symptomatic Intracranial Disease (WASID) Trial Investigators. Warfarin vs aspirin for symptomatic intracranial stenosis: subgroup analyses from WASID. Neurology 2006; 67: 1275–8.

Kasner SE. Natural history of symptomatic intracranial arterial stenosis. J Neuroimaging 2009; 19 (Suppl 1): 20S–1S.

Khan et al. Moyamoya angiopathy in Europe. Acta Neurochir Suppl 2005; 94: 149–52.

Klingelhöfer J, Sander D, Holzraefe M. Cerebral vasospasm evaluated by transcranial Doppler ultrasonography at different intracranial pressures. J Neurosurg 1991; 75: 752–8.

Kraemer et al. Moyamoya Disease in Europeans. Stroke 2008; 39: 3193.

Kuroda et al. Incidence and clinical features of disease progression in adult moyamoya disease. Stroke 2005; 36 (10): 2148–53.

Peña-Tapia et al. Identification of the optimal cortical target point for extracranial-intracranial bypass surgery in patients with hemodynamic cerebrovascular insufficiency. J Neurosurg 2008; 108 (4): 655–61.

Rothwell PM, Giles MF, Chandratheva A, Marquardt L, Geraghty O, Redgrave JN, Lovelock CE, Binney LE, Bull LM, Cuthbertson FC, Welch SJ, Bosch S, Alexander FC, Silver LE, Gutnikov SA, Mehta Z; Early use of Existing Preventive Strategies for Stroke (EXPRESS) study. Effect of urgent treatment of transient ischaemic attack and minor stroke on early recurrent stroke (EXPRESS study): a prospective population-based sequential comparison. Lancet 2007 Oct 20; 370 (9596): 1432–2.

Schmiedek et al. Improvement of cerebrovascular reserve capacity by EC-IC arterial bypass surgery in patients with ICA occlusion and hemodynamic cerebral ischemia. J Neurosurg 1994; 81 (2): 236–44.

So et al. Prediction of the clinical outcome of pediatric moyamoya disease with postoperative basal/acetazolamide stress brain perfusion SPECT after revascularization surgery. Stroke 2005; 36 (7): 1485–9.

Spence JD, Tamayo A, Lownie SP, Ng WP, Ferguson GG. Absence of microemboli on transcranial Doppler identifies low-risk patients with asymptomatic carotid stenosis. Stroke 2005; 36 (11): 2373–8. Epub 2005 Oct 13.

Weerakkody GJ, Brandt JT, Payne CD, Jakubowski JA, Naganuma H, Winters KJ. Clopidogrel poor responders: an objective definition based on Bayesian classification. Platelets 2007; 18: 428–35.

Widder B. Doppler- und Duplexsonographie der hirnversorgenden Arterien. Springer, 1999.

Woitzik et al. Intraoperative control of extracranial-intracranial bypass patency by near-infrared indocyanine green videoangiography. J Neurosurg 2005; 102 (4): 692–8.

1.3 Intracranial aneurysms, AV malformations, and other vascular malformations

Introduction and conservative treatment: Werner Weber, Uwe Dietrich
Interventional treatment: Werner Weber
Surgical treatment: Maximilian J.A. Puchner
Intensive care: Hans-Georg Bone

1.3.1 Aneurysms

1.3.1.1 Clinical picture

Intracranial aneurysms are bulges, usually saccular, in the arteries at the base of the brain that occur at vascular branching points, which represent a site of predilection for this disease. The vascular branching points must be regarded as a weak point at which the fibers of the tunica media—which is thinner in the intracerebral vessels than in the extracranial ones—diverge in order to divide into two vessels. This histological aspect means that the wall structure of aneurysms differs from that in normal cranial vessels. The tunica media is absent and the internal elastic lamina is very thin. The pathogenesis of the disease has not been fully explained. In addition to congenital factors such as hereditary connective-tissue diseases, factors such as degenerative vascular diseases, infection (in what are known as mycotic aneurysms, which are typically located mainly in the peripheral cerebral vessels) and hemodynamic factors (hypertension and downstream arteriovenous malformations) also need to be taken into account. In addition, there is an association of aneurysm with cystic renal degeneration.

The circle of Willis is the vascular circuit that connects the posterior and anterior circulation as well as linking the right and left halves of the brain circulation, and the circle has many variants. The connecting segments linking the two carotid flow areas are called the anterior communicating branch (usually unpaired, but with many variants, including even aplasia) and the posterior communicating branch, linking the carotid flow area with the posterior circulation (paired, with widely varying caliber and even paired or unpaired aplasia; hypoplasia of the segment of the posterior cerebral artery between the tip of the basilar artery and the orifice of the posterior communicating branch may also be seen here). It is not possible to describe all of the possible variants here, but to understand the frequency of aneurysms in these locations it is important to know that due to hypoplasia and aplasia, individual vascular segments in the circle of Willis may be subject to greater pressure at the remaining points; this is one reason for the frequency of aneurysms there. The most frequent location for aneurysms is in the anterior communicating branch, followed by the internal carotid artery/posterior communicating branch and the middle cerebral artery (together 60–70%). Aneurysms in the posterior circulation are much rarer; the most frequent there are aneurysms at the tip of the basilar artery, at about 10% (Fig. 1.3-1).

In addition to saccular aneurysms, there are also fusiform ones that affect the entire circumference of the vessel segment involved. These are caused by vascular wall dissection with bleeding into the wall and formation of what are known as "false aneurysms." Vascular dissections occur either spontaneously or due to trauma (Fig. 1.3-6).

On the basis of autopsy studies, the incidence of aneurysms is estimated at around 3–5% of the population. The incidence of intracranial aneurysmal bleeding varies regionally, and in Germany it is estimated at 10 cases per 100,000 population per year. The probability of bleeding increases with age; the patients' average age is approximately 50, and women are more often affected. The morbidity and mortality rates for these initial bleeds are very high. The outcome for the affected patients can be roughly estimated using the "rule of thirds": one-third of the patients die due to the acute effects of hemorrhage and complications during the course (spasm and hydrocephalus); one-third become handicapped as a result of the hemorrhage and are unable to return fully to normal everyday life; and one-third of the patients are able to return to their normal lives. The indications for the treatment of ruptured or space-occupying aneurysms (cranial nerve paralysis or other compression syndromes, e.g., in the brainstem with large fusiform basilar aneurysms) are based on the symptoms. Apart from emergency operations when there are acute symptoms of constriction, ruptured aneurysms should be treated promptly (within 24 h) in order to prevent an early second bleed. The indication for treatment of unruptured and asymptomatic aneurysms is much less clear. The bleeding risk in unruptured aneurysms is approximately 1–2% per year and is higher in patients with multiple aneurysms, large aneurysms, and those with aneurysms that have already ruptured. A growth tendency in the aneurysm, an irregular shape with daughter aneurysms, and a family history of subarachnoid bleeding can also be used as criteria for establishing the indication for treatment. The patients' psychological burden due to the diagnosis and their age and general condition, as well as comorbid conditions, should be taken into consideration when establishing the indication. Research on this topic is incomplete and unclear.

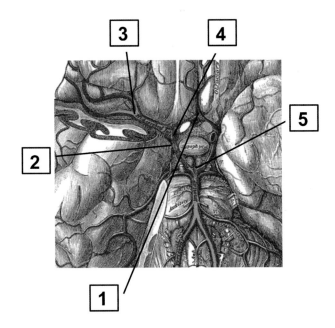

Fig. 1.3-1 Sites of predilection for saccular intracranial aneurysms. 1, anterior communicating artery (25%); 2, origin of the posterior communicating artery (20%); 3, division point of the middle cerebral artery (15%); 4, supraclinoid internal carotid artery (10%); 5, tip of the basilar artery (< 10%).

1.3.1.2   Clinical findings

Patients are at risk from intracranial aneurysms, as they may rupture, usually leading to what is known as subarachnoid bleeding. This may also be associated with intraparenchymal bleeding. The acute clinical symptoms of subarachnoid bleeding (SAB) are highly varied, depending on its extent. They range from mild headache to sudden coma. Typically, there is a sudden-onset headache (thunderclap headache), accompanied by nausea and stiff neck. Neurological deficits and various degrees of disturbance of consciousness may also occur. The Hunt and Hess scale (Table 1.3-1) describes the severity of SAB and the surgical mortality risk. Associated vascular spasm with consequent circulatory disturbances and imminent infarction, as well as disturbed cerebrospinal fluid resorption with resultant hydrocephalus, can aggravate the clinical findings as well as the outcome. In the worst case, the bleeding may be so extensive that immediate relief of cerebral pressure becomes absolutely necessary.

Unruptured aneurysms are asymptomatic, or may become apparent as a result of their space-occupying character (known as paralytic aneurysms). These are usually very large or medium-sized aneurysms in the corresponding locations; typical examples include aneurysms in the posterior communicating artery with compression of the oculomotor nerve and consequent paresis of the ocularmuscles, and large aneurysms in the anterior circulation in contact with cranial nerves. Figure 1.3-10 shows an aneurysm in the anterior communicating branch with space-occupying effects on the optic nerve. Figure 1.3-5 illustrates the state after surgical treatment.

In extremely rare cases, stroke may occur in association with very large, partly thrombosed aneurysms, due to thrombi embolizing of the aneurysm after forming at its neck when stenosis develop there, or simply due to the aneurysms' space-occupying effect.

Table 1.3-1 The Hunt and Hess (HH) scale for assessing the severity and surgical risk of subarachnoid bleeding, correlated with the Glasgow Coma Scale (GCS) and World Federation of Neurologic Surgeons scale (WFNS).

HH grade 1	Asymptomatic or slight head-ache, slight nuchal rigidity *(perioperative mortality 0–5%)*	GCS15	WFNS I
HH grade 2	Moderate to severe headache, nuchal rigidity, cranial nerve palsy *(perioperative mortality 1–10%)*	GCS 13–14	WFNS II
HH grade 3	Mild neurologic deficits, drowsi-ness, confusion *(perioperative mortality 10–15%)*	GCS 13–14	WFNS II
HH grade 4	Stupor, hemiparesis *(perioperative mortality 60–70%)*	GCS 7–12	WFNS IV
HH grade 5	Coma, decerebrate posturing *(perioperative mortality 70–100%)*	GCS 3–6	WFNS V

Table 1.3-2 The Fisher CT classification of subarachnoid bleeding (SAB).

Fisher 1	No bleeding
Fisher 2	SAB < 1 mm thick
Fisher 3	SAB > 1 mm thick
Fisher 4	*SAB of any thickness with intraventricular spread or intracranial bleeding*

1.3.1.3 Diagnosis

SAB is usually demonstrated using a noncontrast CT (Fig. 1.3-2). Typically, reversal of contrast is seen between the brain parenchyma and the subarachnoid space. The Fisher classification of SAB describes its extent in the brain and postulates a connection with the occurrence of vasospasm (large amounts of blood = extensive spasm). In questionable cases, and particularly when the bleeding was a considerable time before, lumbar puncture may be necessary in order to demonstrate blood or siderophages in the cerebrospinal fluid.

In the acute setting, the vessels are usually imaged using CT angiography (CTA) or digital subtraction angiography (DSA). Many incidental aneurysms are identified using magnetic resonance angiography (MRA).

However, the gold standard is still DSA, in which the aneurysm is displayed directly with a catheter, usually introduced via the femoral access route. Very small aneurysms in particular can be identified in this way with greater certainty. Modern DSA workstations are equipped with solid-state detectors that allow direct digital imaging for three-dimensional rotation angiography or for measuring the aneurysm. Biplanar examination systems that allow simultaneous radiography at two levels are usually used (Fig. 1.3-3). DSA also has the advantage that endovascular treatment can be added or vasospasm can be treated in the same session.

In some cases (approximately 10%), an aneurysm is not identified as the bleeding source in patients with clearly confirmed SAB. Two patterns need to be distinguished: in a typical case of perimesencephalic SAB (also known as a prepontine SAB), a little blood is seen on the CT immediately in front of the brainstem/mesencephalon.

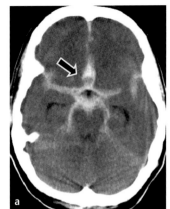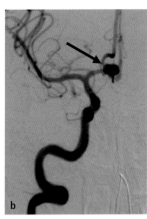

Fig. 1.3-2a, b Subarachnoid bleeding in a patient with an aneurysm in the anterior communicating artery. (**a**) The CT shows subarachnoid bleeding as a hyperdensity in the basal cisterns, with a spherical gap in the position of the anterior communicating branch (arrow). There is a typical reversal of contrast between the cerebrospinal fluid and brain parenchyma. (**b**) The gap corresponds to the angiographically demonstrated aneurysm in the anterior communicating artery (anteroposterior projection) (arrow).

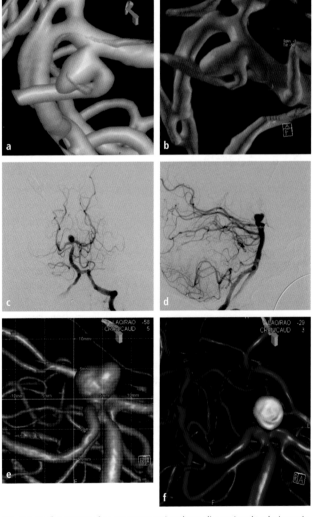

Fig. 1.3-3a–f Imaging of an aneurysm using three-dimensional techniques in digital subtraction angiography (DSA) and computed-tomographic angiography (CTA). (**a**) DSA imaging of a middle cerebral artery aneurysm on the right side. (**b**) CTA of the same aneurysm. (**c, d**) AP and lateral radiographic images of an aneurysm at the tip of the basilar artery. (**e, f**) 3D reconstruction of the aneurysm at the tip of the basilar artery before coiling (**e**) and after (**f**).

With this type of finding, no aneurysm is identified later either and the follow-up examination can be scheduled at a longer interval after the hemorrhage. When there is extensive SAB and an aneurysm is not identified, a repeat examination should be carried out at an early stage and further examinations should follow at appropriate intervals in order to exclude aneurysm with certainty.

1.3.1.4   Differential diagnosis

An SAB is considered to be excluded if the CT is negative and there is no evidence of erythrocytes on lumbar puncture. Differential-diagnostic considerations should then turn toward other causes of SAB, if there is no evidence of an SAB in connection with craniocerebral trauma.

Other vascular causes of spontaneous SABs include other types of cerebral or spinal vascular malformation (arteriovenous malformations, dural fistulas), vasculitides or dissections of intracranial vessels, rare brain tumors, coagulation disturbances, and thromboses in the venous sinuses.

When SAB occurs in connection with craniocerebral trauma, the following question always needs to be raised: did the accident occur because the patient had an SAB, or was the SAB exclusively a consequence of the trauma? In unclear cases, CTA, MRA, and/or DSA should be carried out.

Larger aneurysms may resemble a contrast-absorbing tumor of the skull base on imaging morphology and may be confused with meningioma or pituitary adenoma. This can usually be unambiguously clarified with modern diagnostic methods.

1.3.1.5   General treatment considerations

Ruptured aneurysms are usually treated in the first 24 hours after the hemorrhage, except when there is an accompanying space-occupying bleeding in which immediate decompression is required. Both treatment options—clipping and coiling—are usually now available in neurovascular centers. While it is beyond the scope of this chapter, decision-making on how to treat the aneurysm is best done in an interdisciplinary discussion that should include several variables: clinical findings, comorbidities, medication, spasm, location, anatomy of the aneurysm neck, and calcification in the aneurysm wall.

In patients with asymptomatic aneurysms, the indication for treatment is not clear and cases need to be considered on an individual basis. There have been no validated studies on this topic. To provide counseling for patients, data are available from large case series and in particular from a quite controversial study, the International Study of Unruptured Intracranial Aneurysms (ISUIA). When the indication is being established, the following criteria need to be taken into account: patient's age, comorbidities, medication, size and shape of the aneurysm, family history, and history of smoking. Space-occupying aneurysms and what are known as complicated aneurysms require particular individualized consideration. In addition to establishing the indication, the treatment technique—endovascular, surgical, or combined (e.g., with bypass)—also needs to be intensively discussed as well in these cases. New approaches to endovascular treatment have been developed recently (e.g., with flow diverters) and have allowed treatment of complicated aneurysms,

which had previously been associated with unsatisfactory results. While treatment considerations include vascular reconstruction or occlusion of the aneurysmal vessel, the aim should be to consider how the space-occupying effect of these usually large and/or fusiform and sometimes thrombosed aneurysms can be relieved.

Conservative treatment

As the clinical findings are usually clear, patients with an SAB are admitted to hospital as emergency cases. These patients should be in an intensive-care ward or, if the clinical findings are less severe, a monitoring ward. In the initial phase of the disease, the patients are at risk of secondary bleeding and possible hydrocephalus. Independently of the treatment for the aneurysm with a clip or coil, conservative treatments should also be started: pain treatment, possible sedation, and prophylaxis against vasospasm are the cornerstones when ventilation is not required. Additional information on this topic follows in the section on intensive-care medicine below.

Endovascular treatment

Endovascular treatment for cranial artery aneurysms has become established since the introduction of Guglielmi detachable coils (GDCs) in the early 1990s as an alternative to neurosurgical clipping operations. The preferred indications for interventional or endovascular procedures are aneurysms in the posterior cranial fossa. All accompanying conditions (advanced age, comorbidities) that may make an open surgical procedure problematic, including a prolonged recovery, tend to favor an endovascular intervention. There are also sequelae of SAB, such as extensive vascular spasm and cerebral edema, which argue against brain surgery. Endovascular approaches are usually more appropriate for aneurysms with its neck located in the bony base of the skull, and aneurysms of the anterior communicating branch that are large (approximately 1 cm in diameter) and with the dome directed dorsally. By contrast, surgery is better for very large, broad-based aneurysms, sometimes including branch orifices in the aneurysmal neck. Many aneurysms can be treated equally well using either technique, particularly as they have both undergone considerable further development in recent years. The following advances and innovations should be mentioned here in connection with the endovascular technique:

- Improvement and development of new coils
- Considerable improvements in catheters and wire systems
- Refinement of the balloon-assisted coil technique
- Introduction of highly flexible stents
- A general increase in interventionalists' degree of experience

Without an in-depth analysis of the International Subarachnoid Aneurysm Trial (ISAT), the following conclusions can be made: endovascular treatment has become established as an alternative and complementary form of treatment to surgery for cerebral artery aneurysms. A modern center for neurovascular treatment should have both capacities available. The prospective and randomized ISAT study showed a poor outcome (modified Rankin scale > 2) in approximately 24% of patients who received endovascular treatment, in comparison with 31% of those who underwent surgery for ruptured intracranial aneurysms. Generally speaking, the advantages of endovascular therapy lie in the fact that the intervention is less invasive, and this usually allows more rapid mobilization of the pa-

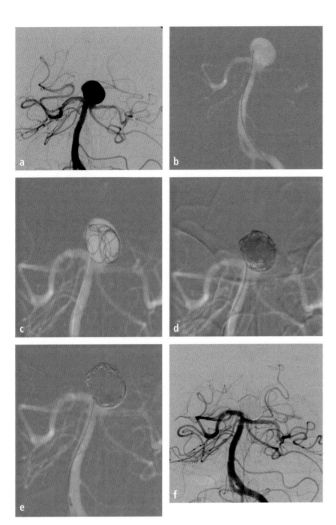

Fig. 1.3-4a–f Endovascular treatment of an aneurysm at the tip of the basilar artery. (**a–f**) DSA and road map images of the several steps involved in endovascular treatment of an aneurysm of the basilar artery tip. (**a**) AP projection before treatment. (**b**) Introduction of a catheter into the aneurysm. (**c**) During application of the first coil. (**d, e**) Imaging of the next treatment steps. (**f**) Final image after occlusion of the aneurysm with coils.

- In most centers, the interventions are carried out with the patient under general anesthesia and with heparin prophylaxis. Premedication with platelet inhibitors is increasingly being recommended for incidental aneurysms.
- Stents and balloons can support the treatment as permanent or temporary implants to protect the aneurysm-bearing vessel.

The typical complications of endovascular treatment consist of thrombus formation in the aneurysmal neck, with subsequent infarction, and perforation of the aneurysm. In experienced hands, both of these complications now occur only extremely rarely and they have also been minimized with premedication for the patients and as a result of improved devices. The combined mortality and morbidity rate in experienced centers is now at a low single-figure percentage.

In most centers, follow-up examinations with catheter angiography are carried out after 3 months or 6 months, and then with MRA at 1-year or 2-year intervals. Secondary bleeding is unusual with coiled aneurysms, but approximately 10% of these aneurysms receive secondary treatment when there is asymptomatic recanalization, in order to ensure long-term protection against bleeding.

Surgical treatment

Definitive occlusion of the aneurysm using a vascular clip is carried out with neurosurgery in order to prevent repeat bleeding. The timing of the operation depends on the patient's condition, on the interval between the SAB and diagnosis, and on the extent of vasospasm. To forestall repeat bleeding and provide thorough treatment for vasospasm, an attempt is usually made to obliterate the aneurysm as early as possible.

Space-occupying intracranial bleeding is an absolute indication for surgical treatment of an aneurysm. Relative indications include broad-based aneurysms (usually of the middle cerebral artery) and those that can only be treated interventionally with difficulty or at high risk. In patients with broad-based aneurysms or giant aneurysms, the vessel can be reconstructed by placing multiple aneurysm clips. Concomitant medical conditions may argue in favor of surgical treatment in cases of renal insufficiency and hyperthyroidism, and poor general condition due to various comorbidities is an argument against surgical therapy.

For achieving a definitive occlusion, the surgical approach is the most effective treatment method; a surgical vascular clip is placed directly on the neck of the aneurysm above the vessel in order to permanently occlude the aneurysm without impairing blood flow in the affected vessel (Fig. 1.3-5). Particular attention should be given here to ensure that blood flow definitely remains unaffected by the clip, both in the vessel bearing the aneurysm and also in vascular branches that originate from it. Intraoperative fluorescence angiography with indocyanine green (ICG), a fluorescent dye, allows reliable checking of blood flow after clip application. Any intracranial hematoma that is present is removed in the same session. An external ventricular drain is often placed before the actual occlusion of the aneurysm in order to treat coexistent hydrocephalus and relieve intracranial pressure. In highly selected cases, surgical placement of an extracranial–intracranial bypass may be indicated in advance of the neurosurgical aneurysmal occlusion.

tient. The general disadvantage, particularly with large, broad-based aneurysms, is that recanalization is possible as a result of aggregation of the platinum coils and that it may not be possible to achieve complete occlusion of the aneurysm in this anatomic situation. It is not clear whether such recanalization is associated with a relevant risk of bleeding. In general, the rate of secondary bleeding from aneurysms after SAB is extremely low both after surgery and after coiling, as demonstrated in the ISAT study.

Endovascular treatment for an aneurysm (known as "coiling," Fig. 1.3-4) can be described in outline as follows:

- Femoral arterial access with a 6F catheter system.
- Imaging of the aneurysm using 3D rotation angiography.
- Establishment of a suitable treatment position.
- Probing with a microwire and microcatheter.
- Selection of a coil with the appropriate size and length relative to the morphology of the aneurysm.
- After introduction of the first basket coil, the basket is filled with spirals of a suitable size and shape and the appropriate stiffness until no further flow into the aneurysm can be seen.

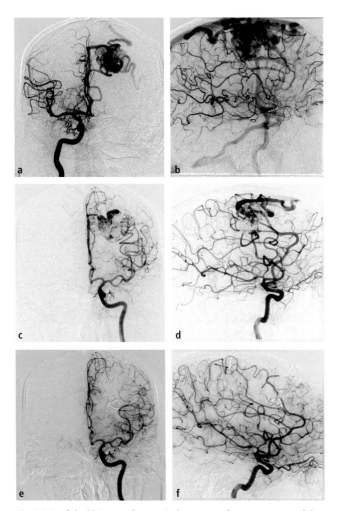

Fig. 1.3-5a–f **(a, b)** Status after surgical treatment for an aneurysm of the anterior communicating artery (see Fig. 1.3-10 for the preoperative image) and arteriovenous malformation (AVM) in the left frontal area. **(c, d)** Appearance after endovascular treatment of the AVM. **(e, f)** Appearance after surgical removal of the AVM.

The surgical mortality rate for unruptured aneurysms is approximately 2%, with a morbidity rate of around 7%. These complication rates increase dramatically with giant aneurysms. Following SAB, the outcome depends to a great extent on the patient's initial clinical state. The poorest postoperative results can be expected in patients who start with a Hunt and Hess grade of 4 or 5. The poor clinical outcome here is due to the preoperative condition and is not necessarily specific to the surgical procedure.

The course and prognosis after any form of treatment for aneurysms are affected by the following variables: secondary bleeding before occlusion of the aneurysm (5–10%), treatment-related complications (4–8%), occurrence of vasospasm-related infarction (27–31%), malabsorptive hydrocephalus (10–45%), and medical complications (10–15%). The long-term course is determined by the extent of neurological losses, as well as neuropsychological deficits and psychosocial environment.

Intensive-care medicine

Patients with acute intracerebral or subarachnoid bleeding due to intracranial aneurysms, arteriovenous malformations, and other vascular malformations should receive intensive-care treatment or monitoring until their vital parameters have stabilized until there is no further acute risk of secondary bleeding or vasospasm. In addition to the specific therapy for these patients in collaboration among neurologists, neurosurgeons, neuroradiologists, and intensive-care specialists, excellent basic intensive care is decisive for the prognosis. The intensive care includes optimization of respiration and oxygenation, hemodynamics, and of the blood glucose level, fluid and electrolyte balance.

Respiratory therapy. The aim should be to achieve adequate oxygenation of arterial blood ($Sao_2 > 92\%$), which can be critically important for metabolism in the critically perfused brain tissue. If adequate oxygenation cannot be achieved by supplying oxygen via a nasal probe or face mask, or if the patient has limited protective reflexes due to the bleeding, or a pathological respiratory pattern, he or she should be intubated and given controlled ventilation.

Cardiac treatment. Particularly after subarachnoid bleeding, cardiac arrhythmia and changes on ECG that meet the criteria for acute myocardial infarction are not rare, even in patients who do not have coronary heart disease. Cardiac enzymes may also be raised in these patients. Close monitoring during the first days after the bleeding is therefore obligatory in these patients.

Blood-pressure adjustment. Optimizing cardiac output, with systemic blood-pressure values in the high normal range, is also important. The patient should receive adequate volume substitution, and additional administration of catecholamines may also be required. Blood-pressure spikes must be fastidiously avoided in patients who have suffered subarachnoid bleeding with an aneurysm that has not yet been treated. However, drastic drops in blood pressure must also be avoided in these patients.

Glucose metabolism. In patients with acute cerebral pathology, hyperglycemia is an independent risk factor for a poor outcome. The raised glucose values that are often found in these patients should not be regarded merely as a stress response by the body but should be actively treated.

Control of fluid and electrolyte metabolism. Both disturbances of fluid metabolism and severe disturbances of electrolyte homeostasis are frequently observed after intracerebral and subarachnoid hemorrhage. In patients with acute cerebral pathology, hypernatremia may occur in cases of diabetes insipidus, as well as hyponatremia in patients with syndrome of inappropriate secretion of antidiuretic hormone (SIADH) or cerebral salt-losing nephritis.

Prophylaxis and treatment for vasospasm after SAB. The calcium antagonist nimodipine (Nimotop®) significantly reduces the risk of secondary neurological injury triggered by vasospasms after SAB and it should therefore be administered prophylactically. Adequate data are only available for oral administration of nimodipine (60 mg p.o. every 4 h, daily dosage 360 mg in all patients after day of admission for approximately 20 days). In patients who are unconscious and those with unclear enteral absorption, nimodipine can be started i.v. at a dosage of 1 mg/h (5 mL/h) in the first 6 h and after blood-pressure controls can be initially raised to 1.5 mg/h and after a further 6 h to the maintenance dosage of 2 mg/h (10 mL/h). Ensuring adequate (130–150 mmHg systolic) and stable blood pressure takes priority over nimodipine administration. Other pharmacological approaches for prophylaxis against cerebral vasospasm after SAB, such as administration of magnesium sulfate, statins, and endothelin receptor antagonists are still controversial. Hypertensive hypervolemic hemodilution (triple-H therapy) can be carried out when vasospasms are present after SAB, although the value of this form of treatment has so far not been demonstrated in larger randomized studies. For triple-H therapy, blood pressure and blood volume are raised by administering crystalloid or colloid infusion solutions and catecholamines. Triple-H therapy is not recommended for prophylactic treatment against cerebral vasospasms.

1.3.1.6   Special types of aneurysm

As mentioned initially, there are also special types of aneurysm—i.e., vascular abnormalities with a specific pathogenesis that does not fit the contexts described above. These special aneurysms may be caused by:

- Connective-tissue diseases, arteriosclerosis, and hypertension (dilatory arteriopathy)
- Inflammatory emboli
- Dissections
- Trauma and iatrogenic injury

Connective-tissue diseases, arteriosclerosis and hypertension, alone or in combination, lead to various degrees of dilatory arteriopathy that may lead to massive vascular changes.

The most frequent of these are large **fusiform aneurysms**—i.e., long, spindle-shaped dilation of the basal cranial arteries. The basilar artery is often affected (megadolichobasilar artery), or more rarely the internal carotid artery or middle cerebral artery (Fig. 1.3-6). These changes usually become apparent clinically as a result of thromboembolic ischemia or neurological deficits due to local pressure damage, or rarely through rupture and intracranial bleeding. Treatment therefore usually consists of drug-based secondary prophylaxis. Surgical and endovascular treatment approaches are associated with a high level of procedural risk. They are usually attempted if local pressure damage has led to disability. Recently, flow diverters—extremely closely-woven stents—have been used in these conditions in order to modulate flow in the diseased vessel and eventually seal off the aneurysm.

The old term **"mycotic aneurysms"** (Fig. 1.3-7) covers aneurysms with an infectious and embolic pathogenesis. These are usually located on peripheral branches of the intracranial arteries and may be either saccular or fusiform. Treatment is indicated in order to prevent intracranial bleeding. If selective occlusion of the aneurysm is not possible, the affected vessel has to be occluded endovascularly or surgically together with the aneurysm.

Dissecting aneurysms occur intracranially only rarely. Due to the narrow vascular caliber, dissection as the cause of this type of aneurysm can usually not be confirmed on MRI and it can only be postulated. Here again, the location and shape of the aneurysm suggest the diagnosis. Morphologically, these aneurysms tend to be fusiform rather than saccular. The last segment of the vertebral artery (V4) is frequently affected. In this location, endovascular occlusion is the treatment of choice if the contralateral vertebral artery is adequate. In other cases (Fig. 1.3-8), treatment with a flow diverter or stent may be considered.

Traumatic intracranial aneurysms are also rare. The "trauma" usually involves iatrogenic injury to the internal carotid artery near the base of the skull, or more rarely a skull base fracture (Fig. 1.3-9). As these aneurysms may cause life-threatening bleeding intra-

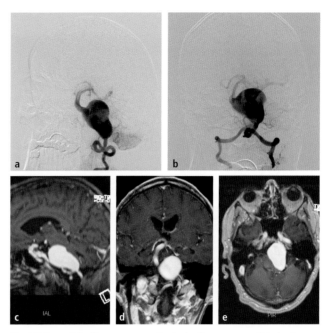

Fig. 1.3-6a–e A fusiform aneurysm in the basilar artery on digital subtraction angiography (**a, b**) and on a magnetization-prepared rapid gradient-echo (MP-RAGE) sequence after intravenous contrast administration, in three spatial directions (**c–e**).

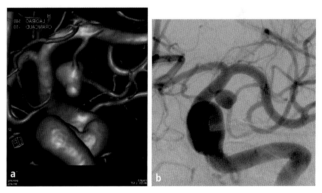

Fig. 1.3-7a, b "Mycotic aneurysm." Peripheral fusiform aneurysm in the left middle cerebral artery; a "mycotic aneurysm" may have this appearance.

cranially or into the nasopharynx, they should be identified and treated at an early stage. Due to their position inside the skull base, surgical treatment is not usually possible and an endovascular approach is preferable. Here again, vascular occlusion is the treatment of choice when there is an adequate collateral supply, especially if endovascular reconstruction of the vascular lumen is not possible. As mentioned above, high-density and conventional neurostents are available for the purpose. This group of aneurysms also includes aneurysms of the internal carotid artery that rupture into the cavernous sinus, as well as iatrogenic vascular injuries—e.g., during pituitary surgery.

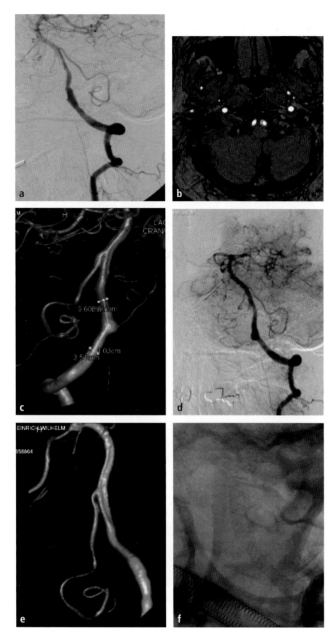

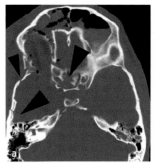
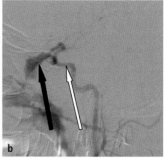

Fig. 1.3-9a, b Traumatic (false) aneurysm. (**a**) Fractures in the middle and anterior cranial fossa (arrowheads) were diagnosed on the right side on a CT 6 months previously. (**b**) Due to recurrent epistaxis, a "false" aneurysm on the right internal carotid artery was in the meantime occluded with coils. One month later, massive bleeding from the nasopharynx occurred. The DSA shows the aneurysm, with extravasation into the sphenoid sinus (black arrow). The coils can be seen at the lower edge (white arrow). The internal carotid artery was occluded with additional coils.

Table 1.3-3 Spetzler–Martin grading of surgical risk in arteriovenous malformations (1 point = no risk, 5 points = high risk).

Size	Small (< 3 cm)	1 point
	Medium (3–6 cm)	2 points
	Large (> 6 cm)	3 points
Site	Not "eloquent"	0 points
	"Eloquent"	1 point
Venous drainage	Superficial veins	0 points
	Deep cerebral veins	1 point

Fig. 1.3-8a–f Dissection-related aneurysm. (**a**) Digital subtraction angiography (DSA) of the left vertebral artery after subarachnoid bleeding, with evidence of slight wall irregularities. (**b**) At the follow-up examination, magnetic resonance angiography reveals dissection of the left vertebral artery. (**c, d**) A fusiform aneurysm at the level of the dissection, on DSA with 3D reconstruction and subtraction. (**e, f**) Findings after implantation of a flow diverter (**f**); 3D reconstruction of the check-up DSA (**e**).

1.3.2   Arteriovenous malformations and dural fistulas

1.3.2.1   Clinical picture in AVM

Vascular malformations in the brain and meninges are pathological shunts between the afferent arteries to the brain or dura and the efferent veins or venous sinuses.

AVMs are located in the cerebral parenchyma and are primarily supplied by afferent cerebral vessels; dural vessels may be recruited secondarily via transdural anastomoses. Drainage into the large venous sinuses takes place via parenchymal veins. The shunt (nidus) is located in the brain parenchyma and may have a plexiform, fistulous, or mixed structure. In the fistulous type, a very strong afferent artery opens directly into a vein without an intermediate vascular plexus.

AVMs occur much more rarely than aneurysms. They are congenital vascular malformations with a tendency to grow larger during the course of life. They can occur in any location in the brain. They are usually classified using the criteria included in the Spetzler and Martin score, which was developed in order to assess operability, with the risk being classified relative to the size, location and type of venous drainage (Table 1.3-3).

1.3.2.2   Clinical findings in AVM

AVMs usually become clinically manifest in middle age. The bleeding risk is estimated at approximately 2–4% per year. The leading diagnostic syndrome is intracranial bleeding (ICB; 50%), followed by headache and seizures at almost equal frequency. Neurological deficits without ICB as the first symptom are rare with these malformations. In children, ICB is the initial symptom more often. In contrast to aneurysmal bleeding, the course of bleeding from an AVM is clinically less severe and the risk of early secondary bleeding is much lower. Seizures occur particularly with large AVMs in supratentorial and cortical locations. Headache often occurs when the external vessels are involved. The clinical findings in patients with AVM are much more heterogeneous than in those with aneurysms and they depend much more on the size and position of the AVMs.

1.3.2.3 Diagnosis of AVMs

Starting from a size of at least 1 cm in diameter, there is no difficulty in diagnosing an AVM. Modern tomographic imaging procedures are all able to detect the lesions. A node of convoluted vessels with blood flowing through them is usually found, along with one or several large veins and hypertrophic afferent vessels. On CT, AVMs may show dilated vessels, calcification and hemorrhage. After contrast administration, there is strong enhancement of the vascular structures. MRI shows pathological vascular structures even before contrast administration (Fig. 1.3-10), particularly the angioma nidus and dilated efferent veins. For treatment planning, however, DSA with complete intracranial angiography is necessary, even after previous CTA or MRA. DSA not only identifies the afferent and efferent vessels in the vascular malformation, but also delineates the normal vascular supply to the brain, allowing assessment of the extent of the arteriovenous shunt and detection of aneurysms and stenoses in the vessels involved. In addition, DSA makes it possible to classify the malformation, and important treatment decisions usually depend on this. When there is spontaneous intracerebral bleeding, the following criteria should suggest a vascular malformation as the bleeding source: an "atypical" bleeding location (i.e., not in the white matter, basal ganglions, or cerebellum), age under 50, and no risk factors present (such as hypertension, coagulation disturbances, or amyloid angiopathy). Smaller AVMs showing bleeding or thrombosis can sometimes not be demonstrated during the initial diagnosis when there is intracerebral bleeding. In such cases, repeating CTA, MRA, or DSA after blood resorption can be recommended.

1.3.2.4 Indication for invasive therapy for AVMs

There is no conservative treatment approach for AVMs. Only supportive treatment, with anticonvulsant medication and symptomatic treatment for possible headache, is possible. A direct indication for invasive treatment is present when bleeding has taken place. The indication for invasive treatment in unruptured AVMs is a matter of debate.

1.3.2.5 General treatment considerations

There are three invasive treatment approaches for intracranial AVMs, which in principle can be used either alone or in combination in the framework of a multimodal concept. The decision for or against the various approaches is heavily dependent on local availability and expertise. In principle, endovascular occlusion, surgical removal, and stereotactic radiotherapy are available. The aim in all these procedures is to definitively eliminate the arteriovenous shunt in the AVM. With all of them, the difficulty of achieving this goal increases relative to the size and location of the AVM. It is certainly true to say "anyone can do the small ones." The neuroradiologist can occlude the vessels using embolization; the surgeon can expose the AVM, identify all of the arterial afferents and can remove the AVM completely; and the radiotherapist can induce sclerosis of the AVM vessels. Most medical centers will use a multimodal approach in which the first step consists of endovascular reduction in the size of the AVM, followed by removal of operable AVMs and radiotherapy for AVMs in inoperable locations. Endovascular treatment can only lead to obliteration of an

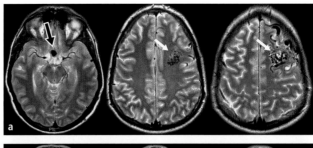

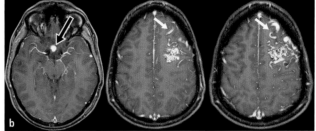

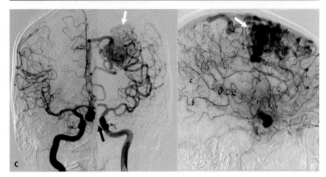

Fig. 1.3-10a–c MRI and DSA in the patient shown in Fig. 1.3-5 before treatment of either the aneurysm or the AVM. (**a**) T2-weighted and (**b**) T1-weighted images after intravenous contrast administration, showing the AVM (white arrow) and the aneurysm (black arrow). (**c**) DSA showing the aneurysm (white arrow) and the AVM in AP and lateral projections.

AVM to a limited extent. Depending on the location, radiotherapy or surgery are thus usually required. The advantage of radiotherapy is the lack of direct invasiveness, but the disadvantage is that the full effect of the treatment only follows after a latency period of 2–3 years and success rates of only 80–90% are possible, whereas incomplete surgical removal of AVMs tends to be the exception.

1.3.2.6 Endovascular treatment

In principle, endovascular treatment for AVMs is carried out in the same way as for aneurysms. However, the catheter materials are slimmer and different embolic agents are used. Corpuscular and liquid embolic agents are used.
Particulate embolic agents:

- Polyvinyl alcohol particles, etc.
- Very slim coils for injection

Liquid embolic agents:

- Ethylene vinyl alcohol copolymer (Onyx™)
- Acrylates (Histoacryl™, Glubran™)

The materials differ with regard to the level of occlusion (capillary or precapillary), the duration of the occlusion, and in their physical properties. For example, acrylates as a liquid embolic agent create a

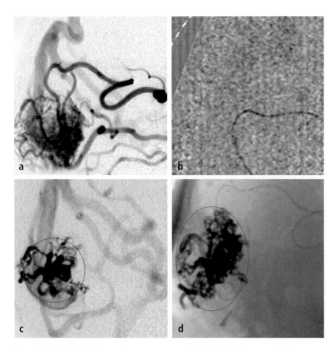

Fig. 1.3-11a–d Endovascular treatment of an AVM. (**a**) Superselective imaging of the AVM via the posterior cerebral artery. (**b**) Positioning of the microcatheter in the posterior cerebral artery. (**c, d**) Step-by-step embolization of the AVM.

capillary occlusion that is permanent and seals the vessels using a polymerization process. Particulate embolic agents create a precapillary occlusion that is not permanent. Onyx™ behaves like acrylate at the occlusion level, but it is not a glue and has other different properties. With all of the embolic agents, the initial aim is to advance the catheter as close as possible to the AVM. When embolizing with Onyx™, it is best to position the catheter tip intranidally so that the nidus can be filled from the center. The aim of embolization is to achieve compact occlusion of all the angioma structures (Fig. 1.3-11).

1.3.2.7   Surgical treatment

The indications for surgical removal of an AVM are prior bleeding, difficult-to-treat seizures, and prophylaxis against cerebral hemorrhage (Fig.1.3-5). In small and easily accessible AVMs (Spetzler grades 1–3), this is the method of choice for complete obliteration, and it can often be done without prior interventional treatment. However, surgery or radiotherapy can also be carried out at lower risk after previous—and if necessary multiple—sessions of interventional treatment. In large AVMs (Spetzler grades 4–5), the risk of postoperative neurological deficits needs to be weighed against the natural course (influenced by variables such as the bleeding risk and the patient's age and condition). Treatment is therefore contraindicated in older patients with multimorbid conditions with no history of bleeding but with extensive AVMs occupying large parts of the cerebral hemisphere. The view has become generally accepted in recent years that Spetzler–Martin grade 5 AVMs should only be treated in exceptional cases.

The aim of the operation is to excise the AVM completely. Partial removal is not useful and even increases the risk of bleeding. During the operation, all of the vessels leading to the AVM are initially coagulated and transected until finally the AVM is dissected free in a circular fashion. The mobilized AVM is then removed at the efferent vessel. Coexisting hemorrhage is controlled during the operation. Neuronavigation and intraoperative fluorescence angiography can be used as technical aids. The risks and complications depend on the Spetzler grade, with a global mortality rate of 1–5% and morbidity rate of 2–20%. If the postoperative control angiography shows a residual AVM, it must be removed promptly in a subsequent operation.

1.3.2.8   Radiotherapy

As mentioned above, radiotherapy is usually carried out when AVMs are in an inoperable location. Following the appropriate planning, the treatment is carried out using a linear accelerator or gamma knife with a stereotactic technique. One disadvantage of radiotherapy is the long latency period until the onset of effect—1–3 years are usually required before complete thrombosis takes place. In long-term follow-up, the rate of complete occlusions is much lower compared with surgery. The size of the AVM or residual AVM is a limitation for radiotherapy: good results are achieved with AVMs < 3 cm in size. Undirected and noncompact embolization before radiotherapy can actually have a negative effect on the treatment results. Embolization before radiotherapy is only useful if it compactly obliterates a defined part of the nidus.

1.3.2.9   Clinical picture in DAVFs

Dural arteriovenous fistulas (DAVFs) are acquired arteriovenous shunts on the wall of the dural sinus. In contrast to intracerebral pial AVMs, dural fistulas are mainly supplied by dural branches of the afferent cerebral vessels ("dural AVMs"). Pathophysiologically, it is assumed that there is a prior thrombosis in the affected sinus that has recanalized "incorrectly"—i.e., when the body attempts to recanalize the occluded vessel, arteries sprout into the sinus wall and the fistula arises when the sinus reopens.

The age at manifestation is 40–60 years. The symptoms depend on the location and type of venous outflow. A basic distinction should be made between three groups: fistulas at the large sinuses (transverse sinus and superior sagittal sinus); tentorial fistulas and ethmoidal fistulas; and thirdly, cavernous sinus fistulas.

The Cognard classification (Table 1.3-4) grades dural fistulas in relation to the type of venous outflow, from which the risk of bleeding is inferred depending on whether or not there is reflux of arterial blood into the cerebral veins. Such reflux is usually associated with obstruction of regular venous outflow, with stenosis or occlusion of the sinuses.

Tentorial and ethmoidal fistulas represent a rare and special form where the arterial supply and forms of venous drainage need to be managed on a case by case basis, since this type of DAVF is associated with a higher risk of bleeding.

The Barrow classification (Table 1.3-5) grades cavernous sinus fistulas in relation to their arterial afferents. Type A is a special form in which the pathogenesis mentioned above in connection with sinus thrombosis does not apply. Barrow type A fistulas arise as a result of rupture of an aneurysm in the cavernous course of the internal carotid artery or injury to the vessel in that area. They are also referred to as direct fistulas, in contrast to indirect fistulas, which are caused by the thrombosis described above.

Table 1.3-4 Cognard classification of dural arteriovenous fistulas relative to venous drainage (orthograde: no symptoms or only slight symptoms; reflux: raised intracranial pressure, bleeding risk 10% in type IIb, 40% in type III, 65% in type IV).

Type I	Orthograde drainage into the sinus
Type II	Retrograde drainage (reflux)
Type IIa	Reflux into the sinus
Type IIb	Reflux into cortical veins
Type IIc	Reflux into the sinus and cortical veins
Type III	Direct drainage into cortical veins
Type IV	Drainage into cortical veins with venous ectasia
Type V	Reflux into spinal veins

Table 1.3-5 Barrow classification of cavernous sinus fistulas.

Type A	Injury to the internal carotid artery or rupture of an aneurysm along the course of the cavernous sinus	Direct fistula	Traumatic
Type B	Supply to the fistula via dural branches of the internal carotid artery	Indirect fistula	Spontaneous
Type C	Supply to the fistula via dural branches of the external carotid artery	Indirect fistula	Spontaneous
Type D	Supply to the fistula via branches of the internal and external carotid arteries	Indirect fistula	Spontaneous

1.3.2.10 Clinical findings in DAVFs

In dural fistulas, the symptoms depend on the fistula's position and the extent to which venous drainage is compromised. Tinnitus and a pulse-synchronous bruit occur with lateral dural fistulas, and visual disturbances or double vision with cavernous sinus fistulas. Headache, hydrocephalus, neurological deficits, and even dementia have been attributed to chronic venous hypertension due to disturbance of intracranial venous drainage. However, the most severe clinical manifestation is spontaneous intracranial bleeding. As mentioned above, in dural fistulas the risk of spontaneous intracranial bleeding depends on the extent and type of venous reflux intracranially, as well as on the location of the fistula.

1.3.2.11 Diagnosis of DAVFs

Dural fistulas are rarely asymptomatic, incidental findings; as with cavernous sinus fistulas, it is more often the case the clinical findings tend to be incorrectly assessed. The typical situation is a patient with a pulse-synchronous bruit behind the ear that stops when the occipital artery is compressed, or which is position-dependent. The clinical examination already points the way here. DSA is the method of choice for diagnosis and classification. With cavernous sinus fistulas, the emphasis is on ocular symptoms, the leading ones

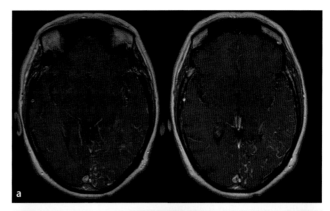
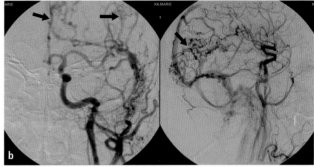
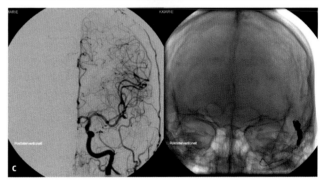

Fig. 1.3-12a–c Dural fistula in the transverse sinus (MRA and DSA). (**a**) The T1-weighted MRI after intravenous contrast administration shows extensive vascularization in the left occipital lobe, with an urgent suspicion of cortical drainage in the presence of a dural arteriovenous fistula. (**b**) The DSA shows a view over the left common carotid artery, with confirmation of the suspected fistula on the left transverse sinus and extensive cortical drainage (arrows). (**c**) Appearance after occlusion of the fistula site in the transverse sinus using platinum coils.

being exophthalmos, chemosis, ciliary injection and pareses of the extraocular muscles.

If vision is impaired as a result of venous drainage disturbances, there is an urgent indication for treatment. CT or MRI of the orbit can often reveal dilation of the superior ophthalmic vein. Here as well, however, DSA is the method of choice for diagnosis and classification. If the patients develop conspicuous symptoms as a result of intracranial bleeding or symptoms resembling infarction, a differential diagnosis of dural fistula needs to be considered on the basis of CT and/or MRI. Indicative signs here may include visible pathological vessels, signs of congestion in unusual locations such as the edge of the tentorium, or multiple collaterals, which can be well imaged using time-of-flight magnetic resonance angiography (TOF-MRA) (Fig. 1.3-12).

1.3.2.12 Indication for invasive treatment of DAVFs

Invasive therapy is indicated:

- When there are spontaneous fistulas at the transverse sinus and superior sagittal sinus in the venous drainage pattern, treatment is indicated when there is drainage into cortical veins. If there is no cortical drainage, the extent to which the patient is affected by the bruit in the ear may be an indication for therapy.
- Tentorial and ethmoidal fistulas represent an increased bleeding risk.
- In cavernous sinus fistulas with ocular symptoms, cosmetic effects and pareses of the eye muscles. Deteriorating vision represents an emergency indication.

1.3.2.13 General treatment considerations in DAVFs

In the most frequent dural arteriovenous fistulas—in the transverse sinus and cavernous sinus—treatment considerations are concerned with locating the fistulous segment on the wall of the sinus. Transvenous treatment of the fistula-bearing segment is the most widely used form of endovascular therapy. It is based on the assumption that this sinus segment is no longer required for normal drainage of the brain or eye. This is usually not critical in treatment of the cavernous sinus, but when fistulas of the transverse sinus are being treated, the anatomy of cerebral venous drainage needs to be analyzed carefully. All of the cerebral vessels have to be imaged with a long venous phase in order to delineate the anatomy of the intratentorial and supratentorial veins. Once the decision has been taken that the fistula-bearing segment can be occluded, then the location up to which this is to be carried out also has to be carefully assessed. Sinus segments that take up blood from the brain and are required for drainage must not be closed. Usually, coils are used to occlude the sinus. Recent developments have been based on a different approach: the aim is to preserve the sinus by inflating a balloon at a suitable point and then, via an arterial access route, injecting a liquid embolic agent that is modeled to the shape of the sinus wall by the balloon.

Surgical therapy and treatment of dural fistulas using stereotactic radiotherapy are unusual and are not discussed here in greater detail. Spontaneous healing has only rarely been reported with AVMs, but it does occasionally occur with dural fistulas. For example, manual compression of the occipital artery in patients with lateral dural fistulas and mild symptoms can be carried out in an attempt to reduce the shunt or even occlude the fistula by thrombosis. This procedure can also be used to achieve complete occlusion of fistulas that have already been treated but show a slight degree of residual flow.

1.3.2.14 Endovascular therapy for DAVFs

Tentorial and ethmoidal DAVFs

Tentorial and ethmoidal DAVFs are usually treated with arterial injection of liquid embolic agents in one or several sessions. This diverges from the considerations discussed above, because these fistulas are typically located in a circumscribed site and transvenous access is usually not possible due to the anatomic conditions. A surgical approach should also always be considered for these fistulas, and ethmoidal fistulas in particular are well accessible for surgical treatment.

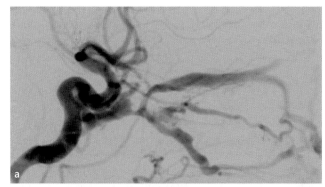
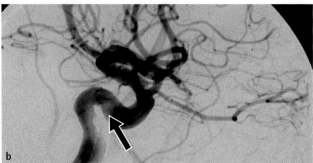
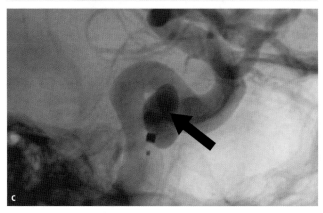

Fig. 1.3-13a–c Endovascular treatment of a traumatic fistula in the cavernous sinus. (**a**) DSA of the internal carotid artery, showing a fistula between the internal carotid artery and the cavernous sinus. (**b**) DSA after occlusion of the fistula with a detachable balloon (arrow). (**c**) Enlarged image of the balloon after opening at the fistula site in the cavernous sinus outside of the internal carotid artery (arrow).

Cavernous sinus fistulas (spontaneous, indirect, Barrow C–D)

These lie in the domain of endovascular therapy. In most cases, the fistula-bearing segment of the cavernous sinus is probed via the inferior petrosal sinus. If this is not possible, access via the facial vein is possible, with or without surgical exposure. The sinus is occluded with coils after arterial demonstration of the fistula; to secure the eye against any recurrence, the initial segment of the orbital veins should also be occluded.

Cavernous sinus fistulas (trauma or aneurysmal rupture, direct, Barrow A)

The fistulous connection consists of a hole in the internal carotid artery resulting from rupture of an aneurysm at that location, or due to direct injury. Endovascular therapy involves occluding the hole by coiling the aneurysm or using a detachable balloon that is

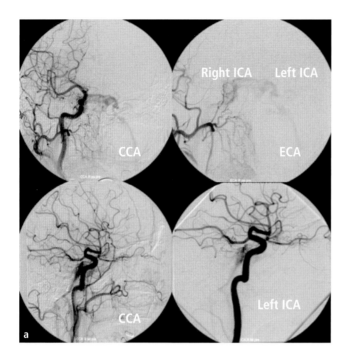

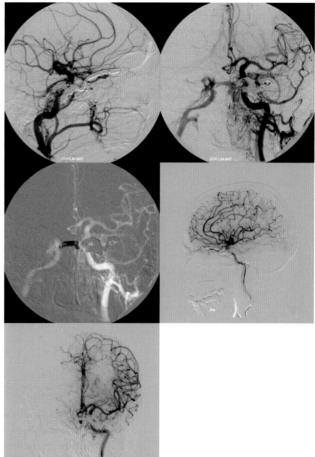

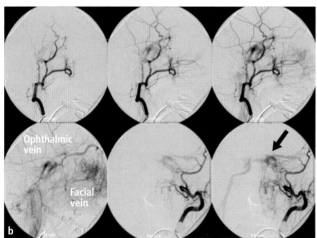

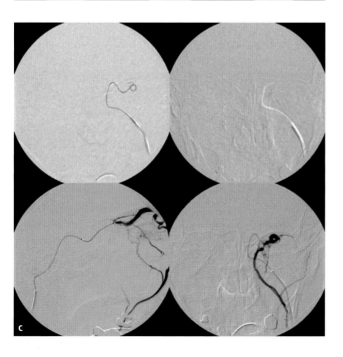

Fig. 1.3-14a–d Endovascular treatment of a spontaneous fistula in the left cavernous sinus. Angiographic analysis of the fistula using an injection into potentially afferent vessels. The fistula in the left cavernous sinus and intercavernous sinus is primarily supplied by the left external carotid artery. From the right, vessels from the external and internal carotid arteries are also involved (Barrow type D fistula). The vertical images (**a**) demonstrate the supply of the fistula from the carotid flow area from the right (right column). The image at the top left shows the afferent supply to the fistula from the right external carotid artery. Gaps in the cavernous sinus, which mark the course of the internal carotid artery, are clearly recognizable. The next six images (**b**) demonstrate the supply to the fistula from the external carotid artery, with the first four in a lateral projection with contrasting of the right superior ophthalmic artery in the first image in the lower row. The two last images in the lower row again show the cavernous sinus with gaps in the internal carotid artery (arrow). The following images (**c**) show access of the ophthalmic artery with a microcatheter, from top left to bottom right. The last five images (**d**) illustrate treatment using platinum coils; top row: filling of the ophthalmic vein and of the cavernous sinus; middle left: filling of the intercavernous sinus. The last two images show complete occlusion of the fistula.

opened at the rupture site outside of the carotid lumen, i.e. in the cavernous sinus, and released. Techniques involving stents and liquid embolic agents have also been described for the treatment of cavernous sinus fistulas, but are not discussed further here.

Transverse sinus and superior sagittal sinus fistulas

As mentioned above, these are usually treated endovascularly, but there are various techniques (see above) for closing the shunts in the sinus wall (see section 1.3.2.6). In addition to the methods mentioned, there is also a technique in which the fistulas in the sinus wall are probed directly from a transvenous or transarterial access route. Techniques involving releasing stents into the sinus have also been described.

1.3.3   Occult ("low-flow") cerebral vascular malformations

These are vascular malformations involving slow flow. There is no arteriovenous shunt. It is often not possible to demonstrate these malformations on angiography.

1.3.3.1   Cavernous hemangioma (cavernoma)

Cavernomas are congenital or acquired intracerebral vascular malformations with a cavernous venous structure that lie encapsulated in the cerebral parenchyma. Cavernomas are found as cerebral manifestations in approximately 10% of cases in patients with hereditary hemorrhagic telangiectasia (Rendu–Osler–Weber syndrome). In the familial form, there are usually multiple lesions. Seizures are the most frequent clinical manifestation, followed by neurological deficits due to spontaneous bleeding or space-occupying lesions. The risk of bleeding is approximately 2–3% per year, but it is assessed variously depending on whether or not clinically unremarkable blood deposits in the cavernoma are regarded as bleeding. Cavernomas may occur in combination with other vascular malformations, and are most often associated with venous malformation.

MRI is the examination method of choice, and it shows circumscribed areas with signal changes, which may resemble acute bleeding, fresh thrombosis, older bleeding, or only small punctate hemosiderin deposits, depending on the stage. A typical finding is a "popcorn-like" center with areas of bright and dark signal intensity, surrounded by a dark hemosiderin border (Fig. 1.3-15). CT only reveals larger cavernomas. Angiography is usually negative (cryptic or occult malformation).

There are no options for conservative treatment. Clinically silent cavernomas usually only receive observation. There is no endovascular treatment procedure. There is an indication for neurosurgical removal if the cavernoma increases in size or when there are focal neurological deficits, symptomatic bleeding, or seizures. Depending on the location, surgical removal may be considered in younger patients for prophylaxis to prevent bleeding. The lesion is removed *in toto*, and this can be safely accomplished even in critical locations such as the brainstem.

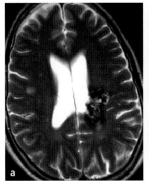
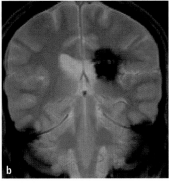

Fig. 1.3-15a, b Cavernoma. (**a**) The axial T2-weighted MRI sequences show a focal lesion in a deep parietal location on the left alongside the lateral ventricle, with a center formed by bright and dark points ("popcorn"), surrounded by a dark ring (hemosiderin deposits). (**b**) The hemosiderin-sensitive T2* gradient echo sequences, now with a coronal section, confirm the presence of blood breakdown products as dark signal losses.

1.3.3.2   Capillary telangiectasia

Capillary telangiectasia is another intracerebral vascular malformation with a cavernous venous structure. In contrast to cavernomas, however, the vessels are diffusely embedded in the cerebral parenchyma. These malformations are usually observed incidentally in the brainstem, thalamus, or basal ganglia during MRI examinations. There are no clinical symptoms associated with them. In individual patients with intracerebral bleeding, it has been debated whether this finding is coincidental or whether it occurs in combination with another vascular malformation that is not visible on imaging, such as a cavernoma or AVM.

On MRI, T1-weighted and T2-weighted images are usually normal, or only show discrete signal changes. Hemosiderin-sensitive sequences show slight signal fading, but not as marked as in cavernoma. After contrast administration, there is signal enhancement of small, striate vessels or of an extensive area, with no perifocal edema and no space-occupying characteristics (Fig. 1.3-16). The enhancement already declines again in late images—in contrast to most focal inflammatory or tumor findings. There is no indication for treatment.

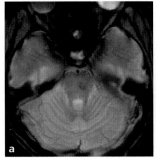
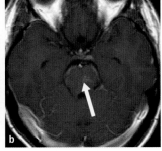

Fig. 1.3-16a, b Telangiectasia. (**a**) In a young woman with formication in the left arm, the hemosiderin-sensitive T2* gradient echo sequence on MRI shows flat signal fading in the left paramedian area in the pons, much weaker than in a cavernoma (see Fig. 1.3-12c). The T1-weighted and T2-weighted images were normal. (**b**) On the T1-weighted sequences after contrast administration, there is circumscribed enhancement of small vascular structures in this area, compatible with capillary telangiectasia as an incidental finding in the examination.

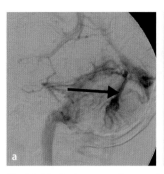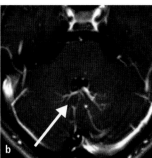

Fig. 1.3-17a, b Venous angioma or developmental venous anomaly (DVA). **(a)** Digital subtraction angiography identifies a venous malformation in the cerebellum solely in the venous phase, with small afferent veins ("caput medusae") and an efferent collecting vein (arrow). **(b)** Magnetic resonance imaging (T1-weighted sequence) after contrast administration shows a similar finding, with the small afferent veins contrasted (arrow). The collecting vein was imaged on adjacent sections (not shown).

1.3.3.3 Venous malformations (venous angioma)

Venous malformations are very often seen on MRI images. These represent a circumscribed persistent embryonic venous system consisting of small, spider-burst veins that flow into a dilated collecting vein ("caput medusae"). The term "developmental venous anomaly" (DVA) has therefore also been introduced to describe this type of vascular malformation. They often occur in combination with cavernomas, a radiographic search for which should therefore be carried out. Venous malformations usually have no clinical significance. An association with seizures or intracranial bleeding is more likely to be explained by small, radiographically undiagnosed cavernomas.

Venous malformations can be demonstrated angiographically. However, the venous structures are only first filled with contrast in the venous phase, as compared to arteriovenous malformations with early arteriovenous shunts. The MRI appearance is also typical, with small, confluent spider-burst veins and larger, efferent collecting veins becoming visible after contrast administration (Fig. 1.3-17). Treatment is not necessary and might be dangerous, as DVAs drain normal brain tissue.

References

Barrow DL, Spector RH, Braun IF et al. Classification and treatment of spontaneous carotid-cavernous fistulas. J Neurosurg 1985; 62: 248–56.

Barth M, Capelle HH, Weidauer S, et al. Effect of nicardipine prolonged-release implants on cerebral vasospasm and clinical outcome after severe aneurysmal subarachnoid hemorrhage: a prospective, randomized, double-blind phase IIa study. Stroke 2007; 38: 330–6.

Cognard C, Gobin Y, Pierot L et al. Cerebral dural arteriovenous fistulas: clinical and angiographic correlation with a revised classification of venous drainage. Radiology 1995; 194: 671–80.

Fisher C, Kistler J, Davis J. Relation of cerebral vasospasm to subarachnoid hemorrhage visualized by computerized tomographic scanning. Neurosurgery 1980; 6 (1): 1–9.

Forsting M, Wanke I. Intracranial vascular malformations and aneurysms. 2nd revised edition. Springer, Heidelberg, 2008.

Guglielmi G, Vinuela F, Dion J et al. Electrothrombosis of saccular aneurysms via endovascular approach. Part 2: preliminary clinical experience. J Neurosurg 1991; 75: 8–14.

Hunt WE, Hess RM. Surgical risk as related to time of intervention in the repair of intracranial aneurysms. J Neurosurg 1968; 28: 14–20.

Kassel NF, Torner JC, Haley C et al. The International Cooperative Study on the timing of aneurysmal surgery. Part 2: surgical results. J Neurosurg 1990; 73: 37–47.

Kis B, Weber W. Treatment of unruptured cerebral aneurysms. Clinical Neuroradiology 2007; 17 (3): 159–66.

Lasjaunas P, Burrows P, Planet C. Developmental venous anomalies (DVA): the so-called venous angioma. Neurosurg Rev 1986; 9: 233–44.

Lobato RD, Perez C, Rivas JJ et al. Clinical, radiological, and pathological spectrum of angiographically occult intracranial vascular malformations. J Neurosurg 1988; 68: 518–31.

Molyneux A, Kerr R, Stratton I et al. International Subarachnoid Aneurysm Trial (ISAT) of neurosurgical clipping versus endovascular coiling in 2134 patients with ruptured intracranial aneurysms: a randomised trial. Lancet 2002; 360: 1267–74.

Pelz DM, Fox AJ, Vinuela et al. Preoperative embolization of brain AVMs with isobutyl-2 cyanoacrylate. AJNR Am J Neuroradiol 1988; 9: 757–64.

Porter PJ, Willinsky RA, Harper W, Wallace MC. Cerebral cavernous malformations: natural history and prognosis after clinical deterioration with or without hemorrhage. J Neurosurg 1997; 87: 190–7.

Puchner MJA, Freckmann N, Herrmann HD. Familial subarachnoid hemorrhage in east Finland, 1977–1990 (letter). Neurosurgery 1994; 35: 173–4.

Raabe A, Beck J, Gerlach R, Zimmermann M, Seifert V. Near-infrared indocyanine green video angiography: a new method for intraoperative assessment of vascular flow. Neurosurgery 2003; 52: 132–9.

Spetzler RF, Martin NA. A proposed grading system for arteriovenous malformations. J Neurosurg 1986; 65: 476–83.

Stefani MA, Porter PJ, ter Brugge KG et al. Large and deep brain arteriovenous malformations are associated with risk of future hemorrhage. Stroke 2002; 33: 1220–4.

Tseng MY, Czosnyka M, Richards H, et al. Effects of acute treatment with pravastatin on cerebral vasospasm, autoregulation, and delayed ischemic deficits after aneurysmal subarachnoid hemorrhage: a phase II randomized placebo-controlled trial. Stroke 2005; 36: 1627–32.

Vajkoczy P, Meyer B, Weidauer S, et al. Clazosentan (AXV-034343), a selective endothelin A receptor antagonist, in the prevention of cerebral vasospasm following severe aneurysmal subarachnoid hemorrhage: results of a randomized, double-blind, placebo-controlled, multicenter phase IIa study. J Neurosurg 2005; 103: 9–17.

Vajkoczy P. Revival of extra-intracranial bypass surgery. Curr Opin Neurol 2009; 22: 90–5.

Wanke I, Doerfler A, Dietrich U et al. Endovascular treatment of unruptured intracranial aneurysms. AJNR Am J Neuroradiol 2002; 23: 756–61.

Westphal M, Cristante L, Grzyska U et al. Treatment of cerebral arteriovenous malformations by neuroradiological intervention and surgical resection. Acta Neurochir (Wien) 1994; 130: 20–7.

Wiebers D, Whisnant JP, Huston J et al. Unruptured intracranial aneurysms: natural history, clinical outcome, and risks of surgical and endovascular treatment. Lancet 2003; 362: 103–10.

Zimmerman RS, Spetzler RF, Lee KS et al. Cavernous malformations of the brain stem. J Neurosurg 1991; 75: 32–9.

1.4 Treatment for acute stroke

Gerhard Schroth, Christoph Ozdoba,
Marwan El-Koussy

1.4.1 Clinical picture

According to the definition established by the World Health Organization, stroke is characterized by the acute onset of focal or global disturbances of brain function due to vascular causes.

Synonyms for acute stroke include apoplexy, cerebrovascular accident, cerebral infarction, and ictus.

In Europe, cerebral infarction is the most frequent cause of disability among adults. After cardiac diseases and cancer, stroke is the third most frequent cause of death and it is one of the main causes of epilepsy and dementia in the elderly.

The incidence of stroke increases with age. Approximately two cases of stroke per year can be expected per 1000 population. In the over-50s age group, the incidence increases approximately two- to threefold in each decade of life.

Approximately 15–20% of stroke cases are caused by intracerebral or subarachnoid bleeding. The remaining 80% have ischemic causes, with occlusion of the cerebral arterial vessels. These two entities cannot be distinguished clinically; therefore every patient with stroke needs to undergo computed tomography (CT) or magnetic resonance imaging (MRI) as quickly as possible. If bleeding is excluded by the imaging examinations, then intravenous thrombolysis can be started on the CT/MRI table even while the location and effects of the vascular occlusion are demonstrated using CT angiography (CTA) or MR angiography (MRA).

The causes of acute vascular occlusion differ fundamentally between myocardial infarction and cerebral infarction, and require different treatment approaches. Heart attacks are due to local, and usually longstanding, arteriosclerotic changes in the vascular walls in over 90% of cases. This leads directly to acute occlusion of the coronary artery due to rupture of the plaque and secondary in situ thrombosis. In addition to rapid recanalization with thrombectomy and/or angioplasty, coronary stents are also used to stabilize the local vascular process.

By contrast, occlusions in the cerebral vessels are caused by arterio-arterial embolism in approximately 75% of cases. The aim of treatment for cerebral stroke is to remove the thrombus from an otherwise healthy cerebral vessel. Thrombi that are transported to the cerebral circulation often originate in the heart, but may also have formed on plaques in the aortic arch or cervical vessels. Thrombi that form in the pelvic and crural veins can be transported to the cerebral circulation via a right-to-left circulation defect such as a patent oval foramen. This phenomenon is termed "paradoxical" embolism.

The brain weighs approximately 1200 g, equivalent to around 2% of body weight, but it requires roughly 20% of cardiac output and oxygen consumption. The brain initially responds to a reduction in regional cerebral blood flow (CBF) with reversible cerebral dysfunction, which may progress to an irreversible defect—infarction—depending on the duration and extent of the drop in CBF (Fig. 1.4-1).

1.4.2 Clinical findings

A global interruption of blood supply to the brain (global ischemia)—e.g., due to cardiovascular arrest—leads to unconsciousness after approximately 10 seconds, and the cerebral tissue is already irreversibly damaged after only a few minutes. These intervals can be prolonged by hypothermia which acts as in a neuroprotective fashion.

In focal cerebral ischemia, cerebral blood flow is only reduced in the area supplied by the occluded cerebral vessel. The associated neuro-

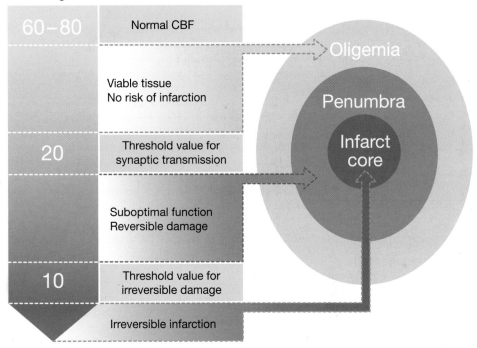

Fig. 1.4-1 Diagram showing threshold values for cerebral blood flow (CBF).

logical deficits depend on the size, location, and collateral supply in the underperfused areas of the brain.

Occlusion of the main trunk of the **middle cerebral artery** (M1 occlusion) or its proximal (M2) or peripheral (M3) branches is by far the most frequent form of cerebral infarction. The main symptoms are contralateral predominantly arm and facial hemiparesis along with speech disorders if the dominant hemisphere is affected (Fig. 1.4-2).

Circulatory disturbances in the **basilar artery** lead to infarction of the brainstem, cerebellum, and thalamus. The main symptoms are vertigo, ataxia, and gaze paralyses, which can quickly progress to coma, quadriplegia, or "locked-in syndrome," in which there is complete paralysis of the body and cranial nerves, but with preservation of cerebral cognitive function, and communication is only possibly using eye movements (Fig. 1.4-3).

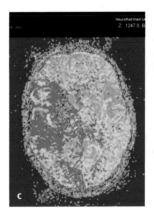
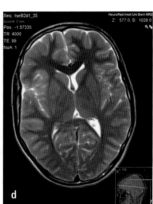

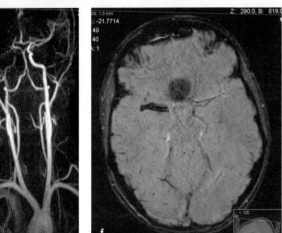

Fig. 1.4-2a–f Acute stroke with left-sided hemiparesis in a 13-year-old boy. The diffusion-weighted image (DWI) (**a**) and apparent diffusion coefficient (ADC) map (**b**) show cytotoxic edema in the anterior territory of the middle cerebral artery (MCA). (**c**) On the mean transit time (MTT) map, the entire MCA area and parts of the posterior territory show a perfusion deficit. (**d**) The T2-weighted spin-echo image only shows discrete signal enhancement in the right insula. (**e**) First-pass contrast magnetic resonance angiography reveals the cause as an occlusion of the MCA.
(**f**) On susceptibility-weighted imaging (SWI), the thrombus in the MCA leads to a flow void that demarcates the occlusion in an enlarged form (a round frontal artefact caused by the adjoining sphenoid sinus).

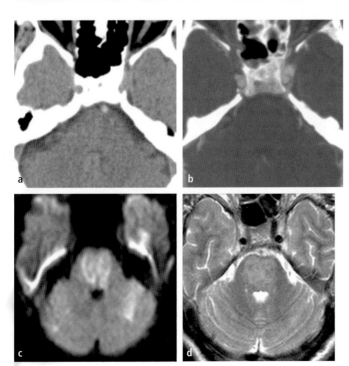

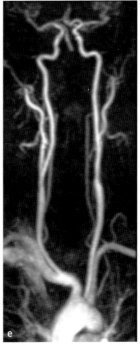

Fig. 1.4-3a–e A 64-year-old man with somnolence. The CT 85 minutes after the onset of symptoms shows an occlusion in the basilar artery. Intravenous thrombolysis was started 105 minutes after the onset of symptoms. The noncontrast CT (**a**) shows a hyperdense basilar artery that does not enhance after contrast administration (**b**). Magnetic resonance imaging 4 h 15 min after the onset of symptoms shows areas of acute ischemia in the brainstem and cerebellum on the diffusion-weighted image (**c**), which are already demarcated on the T2w image. Contrast-enhanced first-pass MRA of the cerebral arteries (**e**) shows the occlusion in the basilar artery.

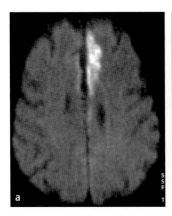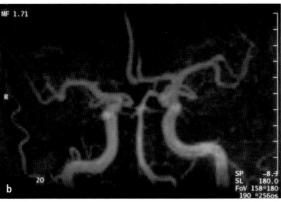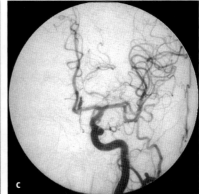

Fig. 1.4-4a–c Sudden paralysis of the right leg by a thromboembolic occlusion in the left anterior cerebral artery. (**a**) The diffusion-weighted MRI shows cytotoxic edema in the anterior cerebral artery territory. Occlusion of the left anterior artery was confirmed on MRA (**b**) and digital subtraction angiography (**c**) before endovascular mechanical removal of the thrombus.

In occlusions of the **anterior cerebral artery** (Fig. 1.4-4), the main symptom is central paralysis of the legs, while with **posterior infarction** (Fig. 1.4-5) the main symptom is narrowing of the visual field (homonymous hemianopia).

The symptoms of acute occlusion of the **internal carotid artery**, which is the cause of stroke in approximately 10% of cases, depend on the location of the occlusion and on the collateral vessels that are available to supply the downstream hemisphere. If the collateral supply is good, the carotid occlusion may be asymptomatic, whereas simultaneous occlusion of the middle and anterior cerebral artery (T occlusion) leads to death or extremely severe deficits in around 70% of cases.

Circulatory disturbances in the **ophthalmic artery** lead to monocular hemianopia due to retinal infarction that can be directly visualized on ophthalmoscopy. Acute occlusion of the central retinal artery may occur in isolation or as a partial symptom of carotid occlusion (Fig. 1.4-6).

The same applies to infarction of the **anterior choroidal artery**, which—after the ophthalmic artery and posterior communicating branch—originates as the third branch from the internal carotid artery, before the latter divides into the anterior and middle cerebral arteries. The main symptoms are sensory or, more rarely, motor hemisyndromes and homonymous hemianopia if the optic tract is affected after the optic chiasm.

The severity of stroke in the acute stage is classified using the **National Institutes of Health Stroke Scale** (NIHSS), in which points are assigned to neurological deficits and added, leading to maximum score of 42. These are summed up briefly in Table 1.4-1.

As a rule of thumb, thrombolysis is indicated starting from NIHSS 4. Up to NIHSS 9, the condition is described as minor stroke. From NIHSS 10, an occluded cerebral vessel is identified angiographically in over 95% of cases. From NIHSS 12, a large cerebral vessel is affected in over 90% of cases—such as the internal carotid artery (diameter 4–6 mm), the M1 segment of the middle cerebral artery (approx. 3 mm), or the basilar artery (3–4 mm). The recanalization rate with intravenous thrombolysis after occlusions of large cerebral vessels is relatively low.

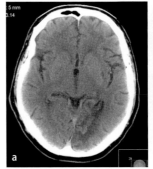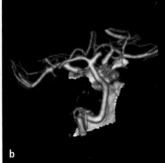

Fig. 1.4-5a, b The CT (**a**) shows a subacute, already partly demarcated left-sided posterior infarction due to occlusion of the posterior cerebral artery (**b**), displayed as a secondary 3D reconstruction from the CT angiogram.

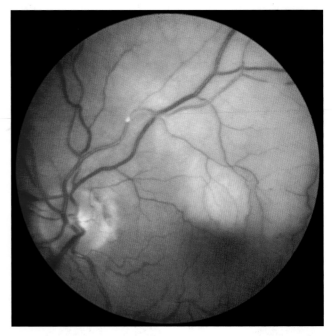

Fig. 1.4-6 Occlusion of the central retinal artery by a cholesterol crystal that is clearly visible on ophthalmoscopy, as is the occluded vessel and retinal edema due to an "ocular stroke." (Image kindly provided by Dr. Wolf, Dept. of Ophthalmology, University of Berne, Switzerland.)

Table 1.4-1 National Institutes of Health Stroke Scale (NIHSS).

1a Spontaneous level of consciousness	Alert	0	Coma	3
1b Level of consciousness—questions	Responses correct	0	No responses	2
1c Level of consciousness—commands	Tasks performed correctly	0	Not performed	2
2 Eye movements	Normal	0	Bilateral gaze paresis	2
3 Visual fields	Normal	0	Blindness	3
4 Motor function in face (facial nerve)	Symmetrical, normal	0	Complete paralysis	3
5a Motor function in right arm	Normal	0	No movement	4
5b Motor function in left arm	Normal	0	Paralysis	4
6a Motor function in right leg	Normal	0	Paralysis	4
6b Motor function in left leg	Normal	0	Paralysis	4
7 Ataxia	None	0	Marked	2
8 Sensory function	Normal	0	No sensation	2
9 Speech	Normal	0	Global aphasia	3
10 Dysarthria	Normal speech	0	Unintelligible	2
11 Neglect	No neglect	0	Hemineglect	2
NIH Stroke Scale (NIHSS) score				**XX/42**

1.4.3   Differential diagnosis

Approximately 20% of stroke cases are caused by bleeding, while the remainder (80–85%) are due to an acute onset of circumscribed hypoperfusion or ischemia. Approximately 60% of the cases of bleeding involve spontaneous **intracerebral hematoma** as a result of arterial or venous hemorrhage into the cerebral tissue. The remainder consist of subarachnoid bleeding, usually resulting from aneurysmal rupture (Figs. 1.4-7 and 1.4-8).

Approximately 3–5% of stroke cases are caused by bland or septic thrombosis of the cerebral veins or dural sinuses (sinus thrombosis). The symptoms have a wide range of severity and acuteness. The symptoms occur acutely in around 30% of cases, not rarely in the form of epileptic seizures—e.g., when the inferior anastomotic vein (Labbé vein) is affected, which opens into the transverse sinus and drains the ipsilateral temporal lobe. Treatment consists of heparin administration, even if signs of typical venous congestion and hemorrhagic infarction are already visible. Extensive sinus thromboses

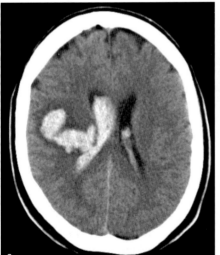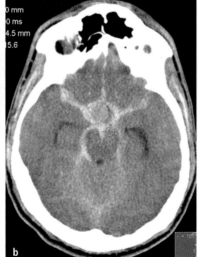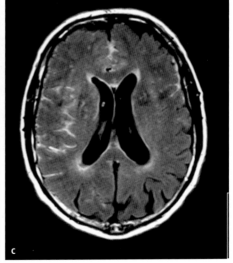

Fig. 1.4-7a–c (a) Intracerebral bleeding with ventricular penetration on CT. Subarachnoid bleeding is seen on CT (**b**) and MRI (**c**). In the fluid-attenuated inversion recovery (FLAIR) sequence, the MRI shows subarachnoid bleeding with a high level of sensitivity as a signal enhancement in the subarachnoid space in the right insular cistern.

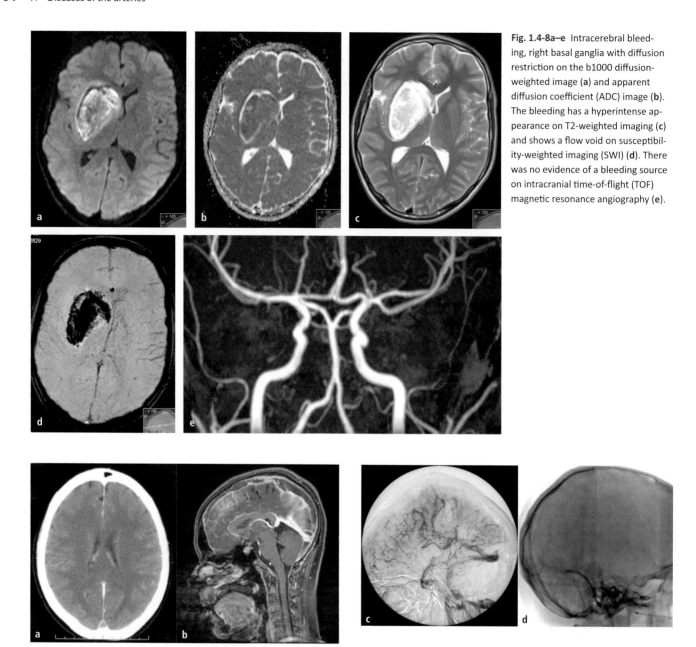

Fig. 1.4-8a–e Intracerebral bleeding, right basal ganglia with diffusion restriction on the b1000 diffusion-weighted image (**a**) and apparent diffusion coefficient (ADC) image (**b**). The bleeding has a hyperintense appearance on T2-weighted imaging (**c**) and shows a flow void on susceptibility-weighted imaging (SWI) (**d**). There was no evidence of a bleeding source on intracranial time-of-flight (TOF) magnetic resonance angiography (**e**).

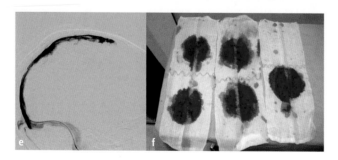

Fig. 1.4-9a–f Thrombosis in the superior sagittal sinus. (**a**) The CT shows a "negative triangle sign" (absence of contrast in the lumen, while the sinus wall takes up contrast). (**b**) The sagittal T1-weighted MRI shows the thrombus in the sinus. (**c**) The late venous catheter angiogram shows the congested cerebral veins and an absence of contrast in the superior sagittal sinus. (**d**) A 5F aspiration catheter (VASCO-ASP) in the transverse sinus. (**e**) Venogram showing the tip of the aspiration catheter in the anterior third of the partly recanalized superior sagittal sinus. (**f**) Thrombus material aspirated from the sinus.

that progress during systemic anticoagulation treatment represent an indication for local endovascular treatment. Large-lumen catheters can be used that allow aspiration (Fig. 1.4-9).

Dissections of the carotid artery (approximately 75% of all dissections) and vertebral artery (approximately 20%), which may also occur multiply and in intracranial locations (approximately 5%), are rare causes of infarction in children and adolescents. The resulting stenoses can lead to infarction directly by reducing blood flow, or indirectly due to arterioarterial transport of thrombi out the false lumen into the cerebral circulation. If the dissection expands intradurally, it can also lead to severe intracranial bleeding. When there are progressive symptoms in spite of anticoagulation and/or the dissection is expanding intracranially, stenting with several overlapping stents and/or a flow diverter may be able to stabilize the situation (Figs. 1.4-10 and 1.4-11).

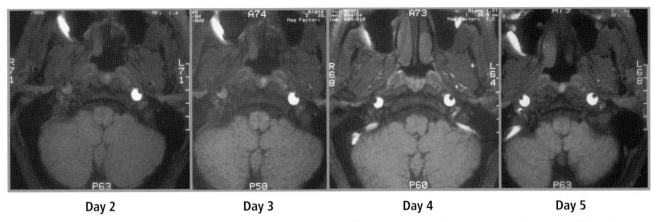

Day 2   **Day 3**   **Day 4**   **Day 5**

Fig. 1.4-10 Follow-up after a bilateral carotid dissection. Starting on day 4, the wall hematoma with the bright signal on the fat-saturated T1-weighted axial MRI can be easily distinguished from the dark residual lumen (flow void).

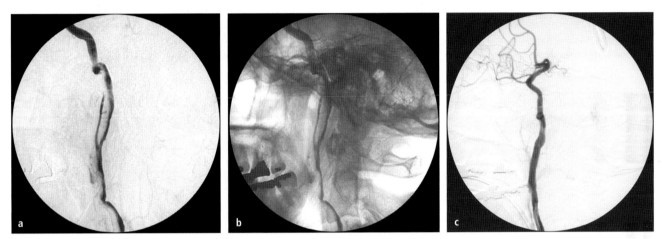

Fig. 1.4-11a–c Symptomatic dissection in the distal cervical segment of the internal carotid artery. (a) Digital subtraction angiography (DSA), (b) angiography without subtraction, (c) DSA after implantation of two carotid Wallstents.

Extremely rare causes of ischemic infarction include cerebral autosomal-dominant arteriopathy with subcortical infarcts and leukoencephalopathy (CADASIL), vasculitides such as temporal arteritis, Takayasu arteritis, and in particular central nervous system angiitis, which is difficult to diagnose.

1.4.4   Diagnosis

It is not possible to determine clinically whether a sudden neurological deficit is due to bleeding in the cerebral parenchyma or to a circulatory disturbance. Rapid imaging diagnosis is therefore key to decision-making.

If bleeding has been excluded using CT or MRI, it can be assumed that the cause of the acute neurological deficit is an ischemic cerebral infarction. In the second step, the imaging task is then to locate the vascular occlusion. Either CT angiography (CTA) or magnetic resonance angiography (MRA) methods can be used. Imaging of the cerebral vessels from the aortic arch to the peripheral branches of the cerebral arteries is obligatory, and with modern CT and MRI systems it takes less than a minute after contrast administration. Measurement of cerebral blood flow using perfusion CT or perfusion MR then follows, which also takes less than a minute.

When clinical and imaging diagnostic procedures have been completed, taking a maximum of 15–20 minutes, the following information must be available:

- That no cerebral bleeding is present
- Which cerebral vessel is occluded and where
- Whether the occlusion explains the clinical symptoms
- To what extent the cerebral tissue primarily supplied by the occluded vessel is already necrotic
- How extensive the ischemic penumbra is—i.e., the area in which cerebral blood flow is reduced but the brain tissue is not yet necrotic (Figs. 1.4-12 and 1.4-13).

For the purposes of targeted treatment planning, an attempt is also made to use multimodal datasets from the initial imaging procedures to obtain information about the chemical composition and biomechanics of the thrombus, as well as its length.

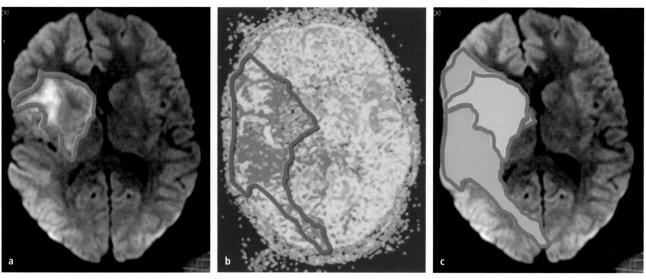

Fig. 1.4-12a–c Multimodal MRI with penumbra. (**a**) The cytotoxic edema in the diffusion-weighted MRI in the anterior middle cerebral artery (MCA) territory is outlined in blue. (**b**) In the perfusion image, almost the entire MCA territory shows delayed perfusion (outlined in red). (**c**) The hypoperfused but still uninfarcted area corresponds to the penumbra ("tissue at risk") and remains when area A is subtracted from area B.

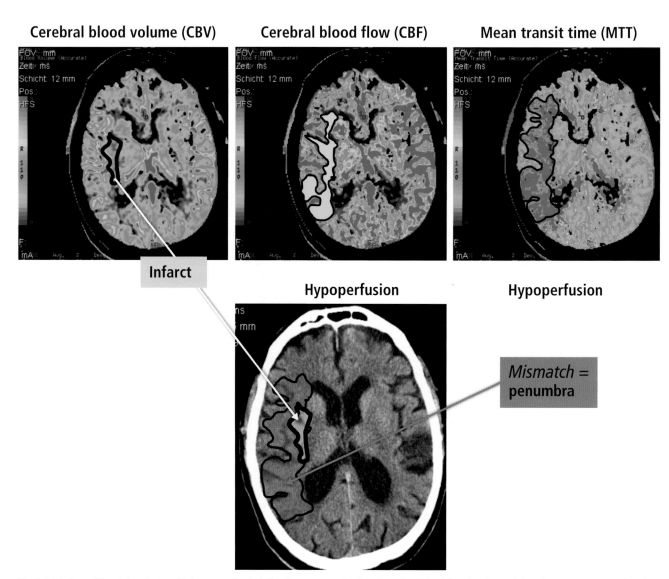

Fig. 1.4-13 On multimodal perfusion CT, the penumbra is defined as an area of reduced cerebral blood flow (CBF) or a delayed mean transit time (MTT), but still with a normal cerebral blood volume (CBV). The CBV is also reduced in the cerebral tissue that has already undergone irreversible infarction.

1.4.4.1 Computed tomography

Although the cerebral cortex (gray matter) has a higher water content at around 82% than the medullary layer (white matter, water content approximately 70%), it has greater X-ray absorption and is therefore displayed with greater hyperdensity. The reason for this is that there is a lower lipid concentration in the cerebral cortex (33% in comparison with 55% of the dry weight) and higher concentrations of protein (55% vs. 39%) and oxygen. The difference is approximately 8 Hounsfield units (HU). Good, neuro-optimized CT devices, technically accurate examinations and well-windowed images make visual differentiation of as little as 4 HU possible. The infarct leads to a continuous increase in water content, which can be recognized on CT as a decline in density. The infarct's hypodensity distinguishes it from the normal brain, but usually only after 2–4 hours.

At the same time, the density difference between the medulla and cortex declines. In the infarcted area, the basal ganglia are no longer distinguishable from the surrounding tracts (obscuration of the lentiform nucleus) (Fig. 1.4-14) and the contrast between the insula and the neighboring extreme capsule and external capsule disappears (insular ribbon sign; Fig. 1.4-15).

Slightly later, increasing water retention leads to local cerebral swelling, which becomes visible through compression of the adjacent sulci, with flattening of the relief of the cerebral gyri.

Large, compact thrombi are more dense and can be directly demonstrated on CT using the "hyperdense artery sign" in the absence of iodinated contrast (Fig. 1.4-16).

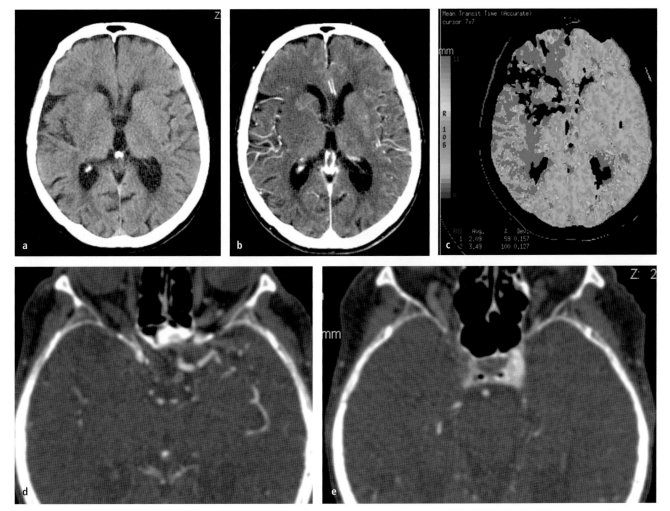

Fig. 1.4-14a–e (**a**) On the noncontrast CT, there is obscuration of the lentiform nucleus on the right side. (**b**) The hypodensity (ischemia) is better visualized with contrast enhancement. (**c**) Clear hypoperfusion, with the territory of the middle cerebral artery on the right. (**d, e**) Occlusion of the right internal carotid artery and middle and anterior cerebral artery (T occlusion) on the angio-CT.

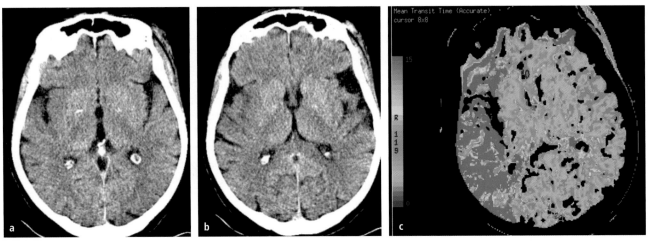

Fig. 1.4-15a–c Early signs of middle cerebral artery (MCA) infarction on a noncontrast CT 2 hours after thromboembolic occlusion of the MCA.
(**a, b**) There is hypodensity in the insula on the right, which is no longer distinguishable from the neighboring tracts of the external capsule and extreme capsule (insular ribbon sign). (**c**) The corresponding perfusion CT shows delayed perfusion in the entire circulation area of the middle cerebral artery on the right.

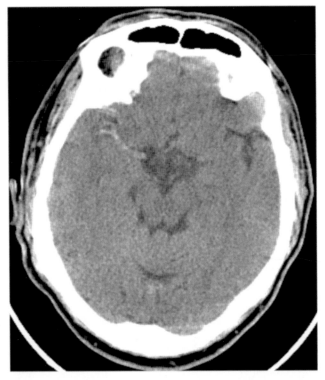

Fig. 1.4-16 Direct imaging of a large, hyperdense thrombus as the cause of acute middle cerebral artery infarction (dense artery sign).

1.4.4.2   Magnetic resonance imaging (MRI)

A diagnosis of cerebral infarction can be made within the first few minutes using multimodal MR techniques:

- On conventional spin echo imaging, there are no flow-related signal losses (flow voids).
- Time-of-flight (TOF) angiography displays the vascular occlusion directly, with no need for contrast administration.
- Diffusion-weighted imaging (DWI) even only a few minutes after the vascular occlusion can detect not only increased water retention in the hypoperfused cerebral tissue (vasogenic edema), but also redistribution of the water from the extracellular space to the intracellular space. This rapidly occurring cytotoxic edema results from failure of the cellular sodium-potassium pump due to oxygen and glucose deficiency in the territory. This leads to inflow of sodium and water into the neuroglia and neurons and thus to a redistribution of the water component from the extracellular to the intracellular space. The extracellular space, through which water can flow relatively unobstructed and which represents approximately 15% of the brain's volume, decreases in size. The intracellular space, in which water diffusion through the cell organelles and membranes is inhibited, expands. Calculating the apparent diffusion coefficient (ADC) value allows semiquantitative assessment of the extent of the cytotoxic edema and makes it easier to distinguish it from artifacts (known as "shining through").
- Susceptibility-weighted imaging (SWI) has a high level of sensitivity for detecting the thrombus in the vessel and hemostasis in the downstream arteries, as well as deoxygenated slowly flowing blood or thrombosed blood in the veins.

Comparison of conventional MR images with diffusion-weighted images makes it possible to narrow the time point of the infarction a bit better, which may be important if the stroke symptoms appear on waking ("wake-up stroke") or the patient is found unconscious or with global aphasia. If the DWI-marked infarct is not yet visible on T2 and/or FLAIR images, it is relatively fresh and there is more of an indication for acute thrombolytic or mechanical thrombectomy treatment.

1.4.4.3 CT angiography (CTA) and MR angiography (MRA)

Imaging of the cerebral arteries from the aortic arch up to the peripheral branches of the middle cerebral, anterior and vertebrobasilar territories is obligatory in cases of ischemic infarction, and with modern equipment it takes only a few minutes.

Intravenous contrast medium is injected to demonstrate the vessels, and imaging is started on the first passage of contrast through the aortic arch and cervical vessels. Standardized postprocessing programs allow selective three-dimensional display of the vessels (lumenography).

1.4.4.4 Perfusion CT imaging (PCT) and perfusion magnetic resonance imaging (PMRT)

Magnetic resonance and computed-tomographic perfusion imaging are procedures used for diagnostic demonstration and quantification of organ perfusion. They allow at least semiquantitative measurement of cerebral perfusion, can be carried out within a few minutes, and display hypoperfused areas of the brain immediately after vascular occlusion has occurred. Positron-emission tomography (PET) and single-photon emission computed tomography (SPECT), like ultrasound and Doppler ultrasonography, have no role in the modern diagnostic work-up for acute stroke.

Contrast-enhanced perfusion imaging is based on the indicator dilution theory: the passage of an intravenously administered contrast bolus, as compact as possible, through the cerebral circulation is displayed at a frame rate of no less than 1 image per second, if possible.

On the CT, the radiographic density of the normally perfused brain increases transiently during passage of the contrast (Fig. 1.4-17). On perfusion MRI, either T1-weighted imaging is used to determine the signal increase, or T2-weighted gradient imaging (T2*) is used to measure the signal decrease that occurs when the MR contrast flows through the capillaries, leading to local magnetic field changes (susceptibility disturbances) (Fig. 1.4-18).

Arterial spin labeling (ASL) is another elegant MR perfusion technique, and it does not require any contrast administration. Blood flowing into the brain is marked, and the blood itself serves as an endogenous marker during its passage through the brain. Due to the longer measurement time of approximately 5 minutes, in comparison with 1 minute for contrast-enhanced measurements, this technique is only used in special cases (contrast intolerance, renal problems) in patients with acute stroke (Fig. 1.4-19).

Functional parameters for cerebral perfusion are calculated from the signal curves using various mathematical models and algorithms and are presented in the form of parameter images. Changes in the mean transit time (MTT) and time to peak (TTP) parameters are the easiest to interpret and detect, and they allow perfusion to be described with a high level of sensitivity.

Cerebral blood flow (CBF) describes how much blood per unit of time is flowing through the cerebral tissue. Normal findings are 50–70 mL per 100 g tissue per minute. Neurological deficits occur starting from 20 mL/100 g/min. Irreversible cell damage occurs below a threshold of approximately 15 mL/100 g/min. This applies especially to the core of the infarct, although it is usually surrounded by tissue that is still temporarily receiving sufficient blood from collaterals. In a model that is not uncontroversial and which is of little assistance in treatment planning, this tissue is described as the penumbra, or "tissue at risk."

Cerebral blood volume (CBV) is the percentage proportion of the blood (arterial, capillary, and venous) within a defined quantity of brain (usually also 100 g).

In cases of acute stroke, autoregulation can initially keep the cerebral perfusion constant. A decline in perfusion leads to dilation of the cerebral vessels. This has the effect that during a stroke, the CBV increases as long as the affected cerebral tissue is still receiving blood via collaterals. Hemodynamically, the penumbra is characterized by a reduction in CBF but with normal or increased CBV, whereas in cerebral tissue that has already suffered infarction or in the core of the infarct, the CBV and CBF are both reduced—the latter to values below 15 mL/100 g cerebral tissue/min.

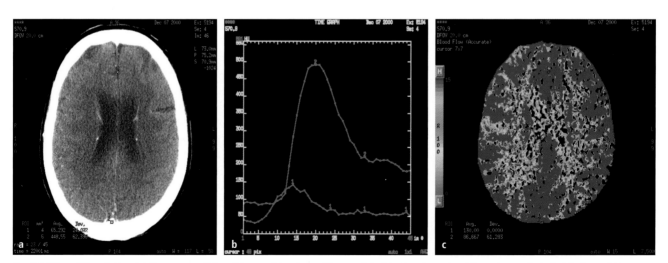

Fig. 1.4-17a–c CT perfusion. (**a**) Noncontrast CT in a 54-year-old patient with acute left-sided hemiparesis, with no clear pathological findings. (**b**) Interactive measurement of the arterial contrast increase in the anterior cerebral artery and of venous outflow in the superior sagittal sinus. (**c**) The CT perfusion image calculated from the data shows that hypoperfusion in the right central region is the cause of the left-sided hemiparesis.

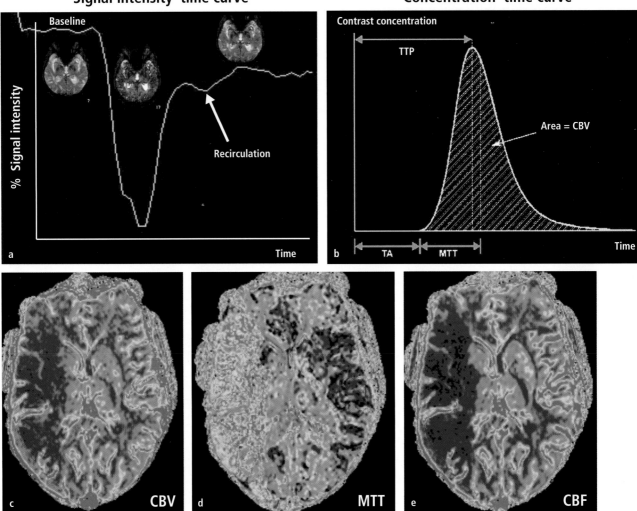

Signal intensity–time curve

Concentration–time curve

Fig. 1.4-18a–e Perfusion MRI. A signal intensity–time curve (**a**) is measured for each pixel, and on the basis of the indicator dilution theory a concentration–time curve (**b**) is adapted to it. The perfusion parameters are calculated using the concentration–time curve: the relative cerebral blood volume (RCBV) corresponds to the area under the concentration–time curve (**c**); the mean transit time (MTT) corresponds to the first moment of the concentration–time curve (**d**). The regional cerebral blood flow is calculated from the CBV and MTT (RCBF = RCBV / MTT) (**e**). The corresponding parameter maps are calculated for each of these parameters. The perfusion parameters (**c–e**) show hypoperfusion in the circulation area of the middle cerebral artery.

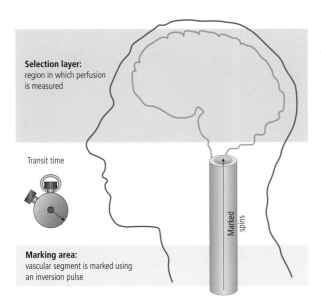

Fig. 1.4-19 The principle of arterial spin labeling (ASL).

1.4.4.5   Catheter digital subtraction angiography (DSA)

Catheter angiography is only used as a primary diagnostic tool in exceptional cases—e.g., to discover whether an occlusion or pseudo-occlusion is present, or to examine vessels using high spatial and temporal resolution—e.g., when vasculitis is the suspected cause of cerebral perfusion disturbances. On the other hand, imaging of the entire cerebral circulation is obligatory in the context of endovascular therapy in order to detect the morphology of the vascular occlusion and the extent of the collateral supply, particularly now that 3D images are available using rotation angiography and dyna-CT can be used on the angiography table as well to depict the brain parenchyma and measure CBV.

1.4.5   Treatment

Acute ischemic stroke is treatable. Rapid reopening of the occluded cerebral vessel leads to a reduction in the mortality rate and can help avoid disability in one in three patients. Spontaneous recanalization occurs in approximately 25% of cases, but mainly in occlusions of small cerebral vessels and usually too late to salvage the downstream cerebral tissue.

Many treatment approaches for revascularizing cerebral vessels have been borrowed from the field of cardiology. The main difference between infarction in the brain and in the heart is that cerebral infarction is usually caused by an embolism that occludes an otherwise healthy cerebral vessel. In contrast, occlusion in the coronary vessels usually takes place against the background of a local atherosclerotic vascular process. This difference has meant that interventional neuroradiology has had to find new and innovative ways of treating cerebral infarction different from that used to treat myocardial infarction.

Targeted, expert neurological care for stroke patients in specialized stroke units and protocol-driven basic measures beforehand have led to a significant reduction in the late sequelae of stroke. Optimizing respiration and blood-pressure management are decisive elements in this chain of treatment. After cerebral hemorrhage has been excluded as the cause of the symptoms, and when there is definitive evidence of vascular occlusion, blood pressure values above the normal level of a maximum of 200–220 mmHg systolic are targeted. The patient's temperature and blood glucose level have to be monitored and kept normal. Any form of excitement or agitation for the patient must be avoided, as the brain's oxygen consumption increases by up to 50% due to stress-related neuronal activation.

The primary goal of treatment for acute stroke is recanalization of the occluded cerebral vessel. Methods available included intravenous thrombolysis and endovascular, imaging-guided recanalization by interventional neuroradiologic methods. Treatment success is assessed at a clinical examination 3 months after the event, and the modified Rankin scale has become the internationally accepted standard for this (Table 1.4-2).

Table 1.4-2 Modified Rankin scale (mRS).

0	No symptoms, no disability in daily living
1	No significant disability, despite some symptoms: able to carry out all usual tasks and activities. Slight neurological impairment possible
2	Slight disability: unable to carry out all previous activities, but able to look after own affairs without assistance. Clear neurological deficit
3	Moderate disability: requires some help, but able to walk unassisted. Clear neurological deficit
4	Moderately severe disability: unable to walk unassisted, unable to attend to own bodily needs without assistance. Limited mobility, limited communication
5	Severe disability: bedridden, incontinent, requires constant nursing care and attention. Barely any communication

In some studies, death is scored as mRS 6.

1.4.5.1   Intravenous thrombolysis (IVT)

Thrombolytic agents were introduced for the treatment of stroke as early as the 1960s and 1970s. Patients were selected without any imaging procedures; the treatment was usually started too late, leading to very high rates of bleeding and mortality.

In the meantime, large studies totaling nearly 5000 patients have been carried out that have confirmed the efficacy of IVT within a time window of up to 4.5 hours after the onset of stroke. The National Institute of Neurological Disorders and Stroke (NINDS) study, published in 1995, included 624 patients with severe acute stroke (NIHSS 14). Within a 3-hour time window, half of the patients received a placebo and the other half were treated with intravenous administration of 0.9 mg rt-PA/kg body weight. A prior noncontrast CT examination excluded bleeding, but imaging evidence of a vascular occlusion was not required. No significant difference between the treatment group and the placebo group was observed within 24 hours. After 3 months, however, the patients treated with rt-PA showed a significantly better result than the placebo group (OR 1.7; 95% CI, 1.2 to 2.6; $P = 0.008$; number needed to treat: 7). Symptomatic intracerebral bleeding was observed in 6.4% of the treated patients, in comparison with 0.6% of the placebo patients. The publication of this study in 1995 led to approval in the United States for intravenous rt-PA administration at the above dosage within the 3-hour time window in the treatment of ischemic stroke.

Additional prospective, multicenter, and placebo-controlled studies in which the time window was extended to 6 hours achieved a significant improvement in the clinical outcome—the European Cooperative Acute Stroke Study (ECASS I and II) and the Alteplase Thrombolysis for Acute Noninterventional Therapy in Ischemic Stroke (ATLANTIS) trial. Patients treated with IVT within up to 4.5 hours (ECASS III) were found after 3 months to have significantly better clinical findings—defined as mRS scores of 0 and 1—in comparison with the placebo group (52.4% vs. 45.2%, $P = 0.04$; n = 821). However, if mRS 2 is also included as a "good outcome," the result is no longer significant, and the ECASS III study treated relatively mild cases of stroke (average NIHSS 9). The mortality rate also did not differ between the two groups, while symptomatic intracranial bleeding at 2.4% in the rt-PA group was very low, but significantly higher than in the control group (0.2%).

The disadvantage in the above studies is that no imaging documentation was available regarding the site of occlusion and the recanalization results. It is therefore clear that the studies must also have included patients in whom a vascular occlusion was not present or had already recanalized. The patients were therefore exposed to an unnecessary and indefensible risk of cerebral bleeding. Administering thrombolytic agents without positive CT, MRI, or angiographic evidence of vascular occlusion explaining the clinical symptoms is no longer acceptable given the currently available information.

When the initial findings and effect of intravenous treatment are documented with imaging or ultrasound methods, it is found that the efficacy of IVT declines with increasing vascular calibers. Adequate recanalization with IVT has been demonstrated using transcranial Doppler ultrasound 1 hour later in cases of occlusion of the internal carotid artery, middle cerebral artery, and anterior cerebral artery (carotid T occlusion) in 6% of cases, while recanalization of the main trunk of the middle cerebral artery (M1 occlusion) occurs in approximately 30% of cases and recanalization of branch occlusions (M2 occlusion) occurs in approximately 44% (Clotbust study). IVT-treated M1 occlusions that were reexamined using MRI after approximately 24 hours showed a persistent M1 occlusion in 30% of cases; minimal capillary recanalization was seen in 30% (TIMI 1); partial recanalization was found in 21% and complete recanalization (TIMI 3) in only 17%.

The advantage that IVT is rapidly and widely available stands in distinct contrast to the disadvantages of the low recanalization rate in large vessels, the associated bleeding complications, and the narrow time window of a maximum of 4.5 hours.

1.4.5.2   Endovascular stroke treatment

Local intra-arterial thrombolysis

Following pioneering studies by Zeumer, Mori, and Theron, it was the Prolyse in Acute Cerebral Thromboembolism (PROACT) I and II studies that subsequently confirmed the efficacy of intra-arterially administered prourokinase in the treatment of severe stroke (NIHSS 17). In both studies, angiographically documented occlusions of the middle cerebral artery were treated if it was possible to initiate the treatment within 6 hours of the start of symptoms. After documentation of the vascular occlusion, the treatment consisted of navigating a microcatheter into the M1 segment up to just in front of the occlusion. In 26 patients, 6 mg of prourokinase was injected locally for a period of up to 90 minutes, and in 14 patients only saline was injected (PROACT I). In the PROACT II trial, a maximum of 9 mg of prourokinase was injected for a maximum of 2 hours in front of the thrombus in 121 patients and the results were compared with 59 patients in whom only saline was injected as a placebo. Recanalization of the middle cerebral artery was observed in 66% of the patients who received intra-arterial thrombolysis, in comparison with 18% in the placebo group. After 3 months, only 25% of the patients in the placebo group had good clinical results (defined and measured as mRS 0–2), in comparison with 40% of those who were treated with prourokinase. The rate of symptomatic intracerebral bleeding among the patients who underwent thrombolysis was higher, at 10%, compared with the control group (2%).

Two other prospective studies have also confirmed the efficacy of local thrombolysis, although they were both ended prematurely. In the Middle Cerebral Artery Embolism Local Fibrinolytic Intervention Trial (MELT), urokinase was injected into the thrombus rather than in front of it, and mechanical fragmentation of the thrombus was also allowed. A recanalization rate of 74% was achieved in this way. A clear positive trend for thrombolysis therapy was also noted clinically: 49.1% of the patients treated with urokinase had a good clinical outcome (mRS 0–2), in comparison with 38.6% of those in the placebo group. The study, conducted in Japan, was prematurely stopped after the introduction of IVT in the country, and significance could therefore not be achieved due to the small numbers of patients included.

A third prospective and randomized study, the Australian Urokinase Trial (AUST), compared local thrombolysis with a placebo in patients with basilar artery occlusion, in the same way as in the PROACT study. The trial was stopped prematurely because the placebo group had an outcome (mRS 0–2) that was 38% poorer.

Table 1.4-3 Scales used to grade recanalization of an occluded cerebral vessel.

Thrombolysis in Myocardial Infarction (TIMI): assesses the local vascular findings	
TIMI 0	No recanalization
TIMI 1	Minimal, capillary recanalization
TIMI 2	Partial recanalization
TIMI 3	Vessel is completely patent
The Mori scale assesses cerebral perfusion after recanalization of the cerebral vessel	
Mori 0	No perfusion
Mori 1	Minimal reperfusion
Mori 2	Reperfusion area less than 50%
Mori 3	More than 50% reperfusion
Mori 4	Restoration of normal perfusion
The Thrombolysis in Cerebral Infarction (TICI) classification represents a combination of TIMI and Mori	
TICI 0	No perfusion, no anterograde flow distal to the occlusion
TICI 1	Capillary flow through the occlusion site, with minimal perfusion and with no contrast in the distal vascular tree
TICI 2	Partial perfusion; the arterial vascular tree distal to the occlusion shows contrast on angiography. However, inflow and/or wash-out are clearly delayed
TICI 2a	Only a maximum of two-thirds of the vascular territory after the occlusion is contrasted
TICI 2b	The entire vascular territory is contrasted, but with a marked delay as described under 2
TICI 3	Complete restoration of perfusion with no time delay in the arterial, capillary/parenchymal, and venous phases

In summary, these three studies show that patients with severe cerebral infarction benefit from local thrombolysis within a time window of 6 hours. In any comparison between the published results on intravenous thrombolysis and those for intra-arterial local thrombolysis, it needs to be taken into account that more severe cases of stroke (NIHSS around 17) were treated with the latter method, while in the intravenous studies strokes with severity grades of 14 (NINDS), 11 (ECASS II) and nine (ECASS III) were treated. The intra-arterial recanalization rates of 66–75% are notable, particularly as they were documented angiographically, with the advantage that the administration of the thrombolytic agent can be stopped once the vessel has become patent, and can checked approximately every 15 minutes by injecting contrast through the guide catheter. Local thrombolysis with a microcatheter, in front of or into the occlusion in the cerebral vessel, thus still represents a simple, relatively low-complication alternative to mechanical recanalization techniques when endovascular access to the occlusion site is difficult due to ectasia, kinking, or stenoses in the cervical vessels, expert interventional experience is lacking, or the diameter of the carotid artery or vertebral artery is too small for devices. The disadvantage is the relatively long time required for recanalization, and for this reason the available dosage (1 million units of urokinase, 0.6 mg rt-PA/kg body weight) is administered using a perfusion system for a period of 90–120 minutes. As the collateral supply to the brain tissue is not impaired by the microcatheter, however, this need not lead to enlargement of the infarction and a decrease in the penumbra provided that blood pressure is kept slightly elevated and stable.

A retrospective meta-analysis including 53 thrombolysis studies reporting recanalization rates within the first 24 hours after the start of symptoms also confirmed the good efficacy of endovascular thrombolysis. According to the data, spontaneous recanalization of an occluded middle cerebral artery occurs in approximately 22% of cases. After intravenous thrombolysis, this percentage can be raised to approximately 50%, while local intra-arterial thrombolysis led to recanalization in 67% of cases (PROACT) and 74% of cases (MELT). If additional mechanical recanalization techniques are used, the occluded cerebral vessel can be reopened in 80–90% of cases.

A retrospective comparison of two groups with clinically severe M1 occlusions (NIHSS 17), one of which received intravenous treatment while the other was treated intra-arterially, also showed significantly better clinical results in the group with endovascular treatment. Only 23% of the patients in the IVT arm had good results, in comparison with 53% of those who received endovascular treatment, with "good results" being defined as mRS 0–2 after 3 months. This finding is all the more remarkable in that the IVT was only allowed within a 3-hour time window, so that many stroke patients were excluded from the treatment who could still be treated with intra-arterial thrombolysis within the 6-hour time window.

Sonothrombolysis

The application of ultrasound during thrombolysis is intended to increase its effectiveness, although the precise mechanism involved is not known. In the Clotbust study, 126 patients with MCA occlusions received IVT within the 3-hour time window. The 63 patients in the treatment arm also received continuous transcranial ultrasound at 2 MHz during the infusion of the thrombolytic agent. Complete recanalization (TIMI 3) was significantly more frequent in the treatment arm (46% vs. 18%; $P < 0.001$). By contrast, the rate of symptomatic intracranial hemorrhage, the mortality rate, and the final clinical results did not differ significantly.

Another study, in which transcranial ultrasound (300 kHz) was used to supplement IVT within a time window of up to 6 hours, had to be stopped prematurely because symptomatic intracranial bleeding occurred in five of the 14 patients (36%) in the treatment arm.

In the Interventional Management of Stroke (IMS II) study, a combination of IVT/IAT and endovascular ultrasound applied using a 3.3F catheter led to complete recanalization in 69% of cases after a treatment period of 2 hours. However, six of the 33 patients (18%) suffered symptomatic intracranial hemorrhage. The catheter is only suitable for the treatment of large arteries (up to the M2 segment) and could not be advanced intracranially through an extremely tortuous internal carotid artery (ICA) in 9% of the patients.

Aspiration (Figs. 1.4-20, 1.4-21)

Recanalization by aspirating the thromboembolic foreign material for endovascular treatment of acute stroke is a particularly attractive method for several reasons:

- It is not necessary to pass the occlusion site and navigate the microwire and microcatheter in the occluded downstream vascular segment, which is not angiographically visible. This reduces the risk of vascular perforation, spasm, and dissection.
- In cerebral infarction, the vascular wall at the occlusion site has not undergone any arteriosclerotic changes, in contrast to myocardial infarction. The occlusion is caused by embolic transport of thrombi into the cerebral circulation, and the material is therefore less adherent to the vascular wall than in an arteriosclerotic occlusion of a peripheral or coronary vessel.
- Sophisticated neuroangiographic techniques allow a precise, imaging-guided procedure: the occlusion site is identified using 3D rotation angiography, or at least biplanar angiography with a resolution of less than 200 µm. The access route and occlusion site are "frozen" on the imaging display and the aspiration catheter is navigated to a point in front of the occlusion with imaging guidance (biplanar road map).
- Stabilization of the cerebral vessels at the skull base and meninges allows a precise approach with endovascular navigation, as the images are only slightly disturbed by pulse and respiratory artifacts.
- In contrast to the peripheral vessels, in which the effect of aspiratory negative pressure is limited due to collapse of the vessel, the cerebral vessels are fixed to the bone and hard meninges after they enter the skull base.

Aspiration techniques are mainly used to recanalize occlusions in the large vessels supplying the brain. Aspiration catheters with gauges of 5F and 6F are now available with a highly flexible distal third and with a curve at the tip that is pre-formed or can be shaped using steam or hot air. As they have a hydrophilic coating and reinforced proximal catheter shaft, they can be advanced using a telescoping technique through a 7F or preferably 8F catheter, sometimes without wire guidance, to occlusion sites in the M1 segment of the middle cerebral artery, or into the basilar artery. The siphon in the internal carotid artery usually offers the greatest resistance, as it is attached to bone and hard meninges and cannot be stretched. The tip of the aspiration catheter is advanced to the proximal end of the thrombus under imaging guidance (road map). As soon as the occlusion has been reached and blood stops flowing back through the aspiration catheter, a lockable 50-mL aspiration syringe is used to attach the thrombus to the tip of the aspiration catheter. The negative pressure that can be created with this technique at the tip of a 5F aspiration catheter is approximately 10 times greater than the suction pressure created by the Penumbra pump (see below), and it usually leads to deformation and fixation of the thrombus at the tip of the aspiration catheter. After approximately 1–2 minutes, with negative pressure being maintained and proximal flow arrest, the aspiration catheter is withdrawn. If spontaneous return flow from the guide catheter is not observed during this withdrawal maneuver, then it also has to be carefully aspirated; irrigation of the guide catheter must cease during this maneuver.

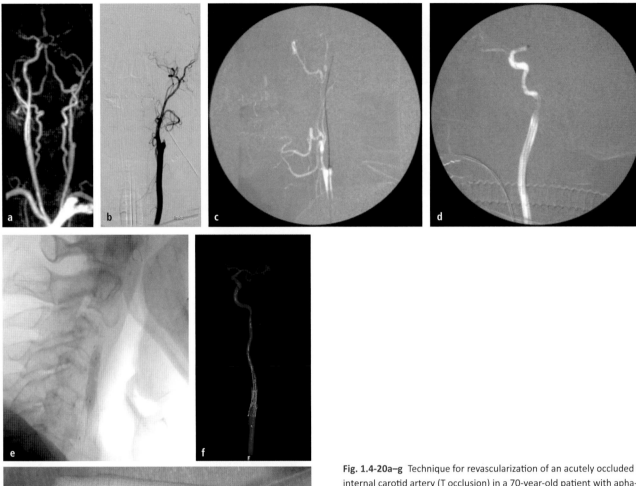

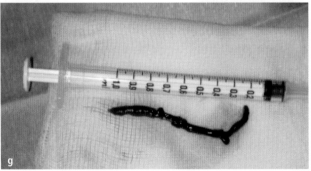

Fig. 1.4-20a–g Technique for revascularization of an acutely occluded internal carotid artery (T occlusion) in a 70-year-old patient with aphasia and right-sided hemiplegia (NIHSS 19). (**a**) The first-pass contrast magnetic resonance angiogram shows the occluded internal carotid artery on the left. (**b**) Common carotid angiogram on the left, with the stump of the left internal carotid artery. (**c**) The occlusion is passed with a long (3 m) 0.038″ wire using a biplanar road map. (**d**) Passage with a 5F aspiration catheter and the 8F guide catheter during continuous aspiration. (**e**) Stenting, with distal protection provided by a filter-wire protection system. (**f**) Checking with 3D rotation angiography after aspiration and stent placement. (**g**) The thrombus aspirated using the 8F catheter.

The disadvantage of this technique is that the withdrawal of the aspiration catheter causes loss of access, and the segment from the tip of the guide catheter up to the occlusion has to be traversed again if the thrombus cannot be removed on the first attempt.

The **Penumbra system** (Fig. 1.4-22) consists of an aspiration catheter that is navigated to the front of the vascular occlusion, with an aspiration pump that ensures continuous aspiration of the thrombus, which is simultaneously fragmented inside and outside the catheter tip by a wire with an olive-shaped tip. This means that the thrombus can be suctioned out piece by piece, with the aspiration catheter being kept clear. Despite higher recanalization rates of over 80%—which have usually been achieved in combination with administration of thrombolytic agents in bridging therapy—the clinical results are not satisfactory in all cases. This is because on the one hand, the negative pressure created by the pump is relatively low, while on the other the fragmentation movement of the separator

takes place outside of the aspiration catheter and thus in an area that is not visualized angiographically and/or by the road map. Although the separator wire is relatively soft, vascular injury, dissection, or spasm can occur quite rapidly if the tip of the aspiration catheter is directed at the vascular wall while passing a curve, so that the separator has no space available, or if the occlusion (as is often the case) is located in a vascular bifurcation towards which the tip of the aspiration catheter is directed. In addition, if there are small perforating branches that originate immediately in front of or inside the occlusion, thrombus fragments may be pressed by the separator itself into still-patent branches beyond the bifurcation, or may be washed back into reopened side branches during the recanalization procedure. The aspiration catheters supplied by Penumbra also had relatively small lumens, although there is now a 5F system recently added.

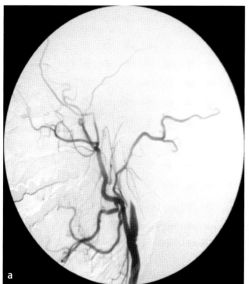
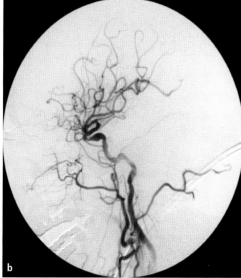
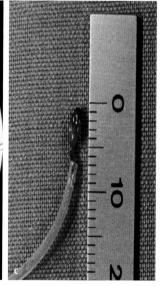

Fig.1.4-21a–c Acute occlusion of the internal carotid artery after heart surgery. (**a**) Lateral digital subtraction angiography image of the internal carotid artery. (**b**) The recanalized internal carotid artery after aspiration. (**c**) Deformation of the thrombus due to forced aspiration through the 5F aspiration catheter.

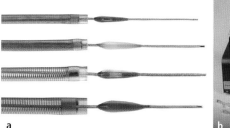
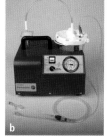

Fig. 1.4-22a, b The Penumbra aspiration system, with microcatheters in various sizes, corresponding separators, and the aspiration system. The thrombus is broken up by advancing and withdrawing the separator, and the fragments are continuously aspirated.

Mechanical retriever systems

Since 2000, there have been increasing numbers of publications describing small series and case reports of successful recanalization of cerebral vessels using microinstruments that were initially developed to manage complications during endovascular procedures. In individual cases, the grasping instruments developed for the purpose (such as microsnares and micro-alligator clips) can be used to grasp compact thrombi and remove them from the vessel. Numerous mechanical thrombectomy systems have been developed on the basis of this experience.

The retriever systems act at the distal end of the occlusion. It is therefore necessary to pass the occlusion site with a microwire and microcatheter, so that on the one hand there is a risk of vascular perforation and on the other a possibility of further distal migration of the thrombus. As a result these systems are increasingly being used in combination with proximal protection devices, and the following procedure is recommended for M1 occlusions:

- Imaging of the occlusion and collateral supply with a diagnostic 5F catheter.
- Placement of an 8F or 9F balloon catheter in the internal carotid artery, if necessary exchanging the catheter over a long wire.

- Preparation of a biplane road map, with the lateral projection also displaying the guide catheter balloon while the anteroposterior projection shows an enlarged image of the occlusion site.
- Navigation of a microcatheter and microwire through the occlusion, which should be achievable without difficulty in over 90% of cases.
- Careful injection of contrast through the microcatheter in order to ensure that the tip is positioned distal to the occlusion and that during the blind transit a vessel has been entered that is large enough for the retriever system to be opened inside it; positioning of the retriever through the microcatheter distal to the occlusion.
- Irrigation of the guide catheter must cease at this point, if not before.
- Arrest of flow by inflating the guide catheter balloon.
- Careful removal of the retriever system, with simultaneous aspiration of the guide catheter once the system is inside it.
- Removal of the retriever through the widely opened Tuohy valve and repeat aspiration if spontaneous backflow of blood from the guide catheter is not observed.
- Restoration of cerebral flow as quickly as possible by deflating the balloon.
- Careful inspection of both the retriever system and of spontaneous back-bleeding, or as a result of aspiration, from the guide catheter, in which fragments of thrombus can often be found.
- Follow-up angiography and if necessary a repeat procedure, or a move to a different technique.

The Catch system (Balt, Montmorency, France; Fig. 1.4-23) was one of the first to receive certification in Europe in animal trials and to be introduced into everyday clinical practice. The self-expanding basket, which is opened distal to the thrombus, is available in various diameters.

The Phenox Clot Retriever (Phenox Ltd., Bochum, Germany) consists of a soft wire with outward-pointing microfilaments woven into it, which are intended to grasp the whole length of the thrombus like

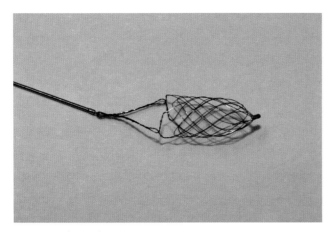

Fig. 1.4-23 The Catch retriever system.

a brush or pipe cleaner and mobilize it. Two systems can be used simultaneously for thrombi in the area of the middle cerebral artery bifurcation. The withdrawal maneuver has to be carried out with flow arrest and aspiration through the balloon-equipped guide catheter. The Merci retriever (Concentric Medical Inc., Fremont, California, USA; Fig. 1.4-24) is a nitinol wire, which after being extended from the microcatheter is designed to open like a corkscrew in order to catch and grasp the thrombus. It is delivered with an 8F or 9F balloon guide catheter, which blocks blood flow while the retriever is being withdrawn. The retriever is available in various diameters and with or without microfilaments (type L), which are intended to additionally attach the thrombus to the system. In a prospective registry study, recanalization rates of 43% were achieved with the initial system, which were increased to 64% when it was combined with local thrombolysis using rt-PA. In the Multi Merci Trial, including 131 patients with severe stroke (NIHSS 19), a recanalization rate (TIMI 2 and 3) of just under 70% was achieved with simultaneous intra-arterial rt-PA administration. Recanalization was achieved using the new Merci retriever alone in 57% of the cases.

In general, we regard these mechanical systems as providing an opportunity to force recanalization in rare, exceptional situations when the clinical and imaging findings show it to be necessary. Use of the systems requires experience not only with the instruments themselves, but also with the cerebral circulatory system, cerebral function, and neurophysiology. A careful review of the literature confirms the impression that the clinical improvement achieved cannot fully match the reported recanalization results, for several reasons:

- The results of recanalization are practically all classified using the Thrombolysis in Myocardial Infarction (TIMI) classification. It remains an open question whether the local reopening of the vessel also led to restoration of perfusion in the downstream cerebral tissue (TICI/Mori classification).
- Even brief flow arrest can completely destabilize the precarious hemodynamic situation in the penumbra, particularly when flow remains reduced by dissection or spasm after deflation of the balloon.
- We have observed in animal experiments that the thrombus is compressed by the mobilization procedure and parts of it can be pressed into side branches. When the thrombus is removed, these parts are sheared off and the side branches are occluded. This mechanism appears to play a role particularly during mechanical recanalization of the basilar artery, with its multiple small branches to the brain stem, and in the lenticulostriate branches to the middle cerebral artery.

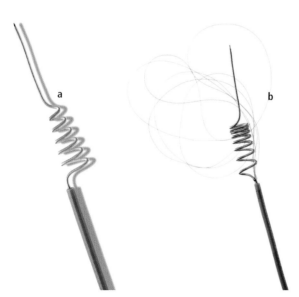
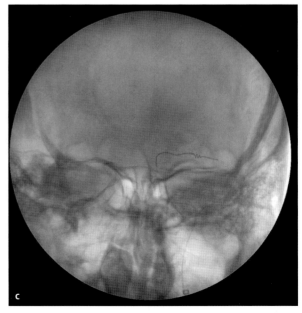

Fig.1.4-24a–c The Merci retriever. (**a**) Type A. (**b**) Type L with filaments. (**c**) Recanalization of an M1 occlusion using a Merci retriever, with the type X Merci in the M1 segment of the middle cerebral artery.

1.4.5.3 Percutaneous transluminal angioplasty (PTA) and stenting (Figs. 1.4-25, 1.4-26)

The principle of PTA and stent treatment involves pressing the thrombus into the wall and fixing it there with the stent if appropriate. It is known from animal experiments that the microcatheter does not penetrate the thrombus, but passes the occlusion site between the vascular wall and the thrombus. The thrombus is thus not attached to the vascular wall circumferentially, but attached to the part of the vessel opposite the point at which it has been passed with the wire or catheter. Attention therefore needs to be given to ensure that the microwire over which the stent will later be introduced passes the occluded basilar artery in the dorsal part of the vascular lumen, and this is only technically possible with the microcatheter when an enlarged lateral road map projection is used. Then, when the stent opens, the thrombus will be shifted ventrally and thus away from the branches to the pons that arise from the dorsal circumference of the basilar artery. Passage of an occluded M1 segment between the thrombus and the upper circumference of the middle cerebral artery is achieved analogously, so that the upward-directed origins of the lenticulostriate branches are kept open.

Animal studies and our own experience have confirmed that PTA can lead to rapid recanalization, but that the lumen closes again relatively rapidly if the thrombus is not fixed and compressed against the wall by a stent. The risk of fragmentation and embolization of the thrombus into distal branches is also greater with PTA alone. Rapid recanalization rates of up to 90% have been achieved with both balloon-mounted and self-expanding stents (Wingspan, Enterprise).

The disadvantage of stent recanalization is the relatively high rate of stent thrombosis, which requires a relatively aggressive form of management with double aggregation (i.v. aspirin and rapid titration of clopidogrel). The cause of these early stent occlusions is that the thrombus attached to the wall slowly expands back into the lumen through the mesh of the stent, and the lumen is then occluded again by thrombus. This observation has led to the development of a "removable stent", also known as "stentrievers".

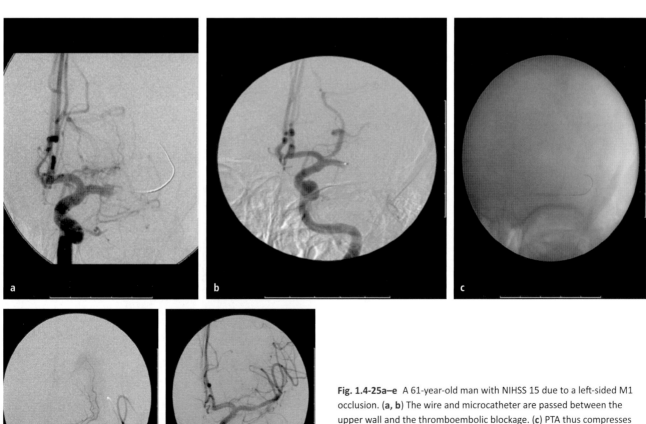

Fig. 1.4-25a–e A 61-year-old man with NIHSS 15 due to a left-sided M1 occlusion. (**a, b**) The wire and microcatheter are passed between the upper wall and the thromboembolic blockage. (**c**) PTA thus compresses the thrombus caudally. (**d**) The lenticulostriate end arteries arising from the upper wall, which supply the basal ganglia, are thus kept free or reopened. (**e**) Remodeling of the M1 lumen by secondary placement of a self-expanding stent.

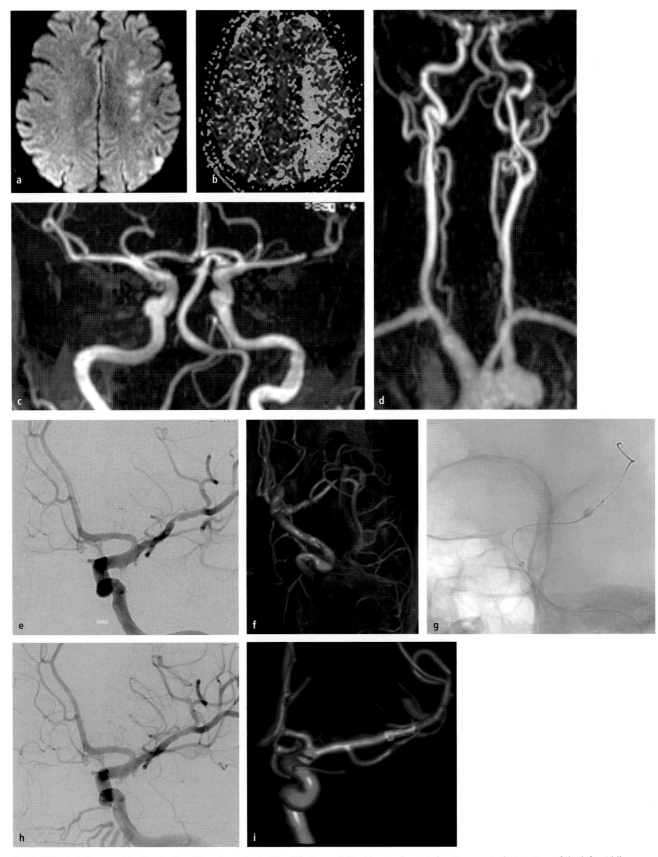

Fig. 1.4-26a–i A 62-year-old patient with mild motor aphasia. The diffusion-weighted image shows ischemic areas in the territory of the left middle cerebral artery (**a**), with delayed perfusion in the mean transit time perfusion image (**b**) and evidence of stenosis in the distal M1 segment of the left middle cerebral artery on time-of-flight magnetic resonance angiography (MRA) (**c**). (**d**) The first-pass contrast-enhanced MRA of the cervical vessels does not show any hemodynamically relevant stenoses in the cervical arteries. The acute, symptomatic stenosis was treated by placing a balloon-mounted neurostent. (**e, f**) Digital subtraction angiography (DSA) and 3D rotation angiogram of the stenosis. (**g**) Inflation of the balloon-mounted stent using a triple-catheter technique. (**h, i**) DSA and 3D rotation angiogram after stent placement.

1.4.5.4 Stent retriever device (Figs. 1.4-27, 1.4-28)

Initial attempts to achieve rapid, albeit transient, recanalization without definitive placement of a stent was accomplished by not fully releasing the self-expanding stent, so it could be withdrawn again into its sheath and retrieved when desired. The Solitaire stent (Covidien, ev3 Endovascular Inc., Plymouth, Minnesota, USA), which was originally developed for stent protection in endovascular treatment of broad-based aneurysms, proved to be particularly suitable. This is a laser-cut self-expanding stent that is attached to a guide wire with which it can be introduced and removed again through a 0.0021-inch microcatheter (Rebar, Prowler). As with coils for aneurysm treatment, the stent can be released from the wire electrolytically and can remain in place. The stents are available with various lengths and diameters, from 4 × 15 mm to 6 × 30 mm. When the stent is withdrawn in its opened state after approximately 5 minutes, animal experiments and small case series have shown that the thrombus is also removed in the stent mesh and that this leads to rapid recanalization of the vessel in around 90% of cases. Although the stent is withdrawn in its expanded state, spasm occurs rarely and dissections very rarely.

If possible, withdrawal of the stent retriever should be carried out in flow arrest through a large-lumen (8 or 9F) balloon guide catheter that is "parked" in the distal internal carotid artery and briefly opened during withdrawal of the stent.

Prospective single-center and multicenter registry studies have confirmed that using the stent retriever significantly reduces the time required for the intervention and achieves recanalization rates of 80–90%. This is paralleled by a marked improvement in the clinical results: 121 patients with acute stroke (NIHSS 18) were treated within the first 6 hours using the Solitaire retriever system in five centers in Europe. The recanalization rate was 90%, and 55% of the patients had good clinical results after 3 months, defined as mRS 0–2. This is much better than the results in the intravenous thrombolysis studies, although the latter only treated patients within a time window of 3–4.5 hours and only included patients with significantly milder cases of stroke with NIHSS scores of between 9 and 16.

Stent retriever systems are now being supplied by various companies, each with a slightly different design.

1.4.5.5 Combined intravenous thrombolysis and endovascular treatment (bridging approach)

This combined treatment approach is increasingly being used in stroke networks. In smaller hospitals, cerebral bleeding can be excluded as the cause of stroke using computed tomography, which is widely available, and intravenous thrombolysis can be started without delay. While this treatment is already taking effect, the patient can be moved to a center in which the technical facilities are then available for carrying out endovascular treatment if there is no improvement with the intravenous thrombolysis. If the patient's condition has changed on admission to the center, and/or more than 1–2 hours has passed, the center should carry out further imaging diagnosis in order to exclude bleeding into the infarct, or in any event to document successful recanalization using the intravenous bridging thrombolysis.

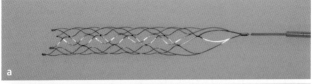

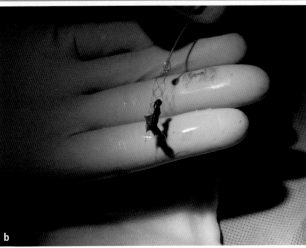

Fig. 1.4-27a, b (**a**) A retrievable stent. (**b**) Documentation of the thrombus in the stent after recanalization of a thromboembolic occlusion of the middle cerebral artery.

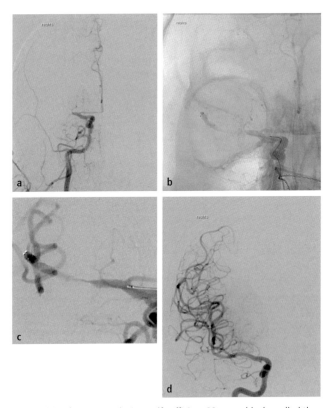

Fig. 1.4-28a–d Acute stroke in a self-sufficient 89-year-old who called the emergency physician herself (NIHSS 19). (**a**) Occlusion of the right middle cerebral artery. (**b**) Immediate capillary recanalization after initial deployment of the retrievable stent. (**c**) Detailed angiography (spatial resolution 0.1 mm) of the reopened capillary lumen after compression of the thrombus onto the wall by the stent, which is still in place. (**d**) Complete recanalization after removal of the stent. The patient wanted to go home again the next day to look after her husband and cat.

Studies on combined intravenous/intra-arterial thrombolysis have used lower intravenous dosages (0.6 mg rt-PA/kg body weight) in order to complete the intra-arterial thrombolysis with the remaining dose of rt-PA or urokinase. It also appears acceptable to administer the full dosage of rt-PA, 0.9 mg/kg body weight, followed by endovascular treatment if recanalization does not take place, as endovascular treatment is increasingly limited to the use of mechanical recanalization techniques.

1.4.5.6   Multimodal endovascular therapy

Modern approaches to the treatment of acute stroke take into account both the location of the occlusion and also the time between the start of symptoms and the therapeutic intervention. The treatment of vertebrobasilar infarctions begins with IVT within a 4.5-hour time window. The patients should be transferred without delay to a center in which mechanical recanalization can follow if needed. If the patient has in the meantime become comatose and is showing more extensive clinical symptoms of a brainstem lesion, multimodal magnetic resonance diagnosis should be carried out first in order to allow interdisciplinary assessment of the prognosis—e.g., imminent "locked-in" syndrome—and discussion of it with relatives.

Patients with an infarct in the carotid territory should receive IVT if they are within the 4.5-hour time window and there is no occlusion of the ICA or M1/M2 segment. For patients in whom the 4.5-hour window has already been exceeded, or who present with a larger vascular occlusion (ICA, M1, and M2), endovascular therapy is prepared, with or without bridging therapy, the time window for which is 6 hours for the middle cerebral artery. The endovascular procedure is carried out with anesthesia facilities on hand, through a wide-lumen port (8F), which keeps all options open for the subsequent procedure. After diagnostic imaging of both carotid territories and the posterior circulation, a 7F or 8F guide catheter is positioned in the relevant cervical artery. If there is a combined ICA/MCA occlusion, the ICA is initially recanalized using aspiration via the 8F catheter, with stent placement if needed. This improves perfusion of the collaterals and prevents re-occlusion. If the MCA is not already recanalized by the aspiration at this point, we follow this with IAT (< 6 h) or thromboembolectomy (< 8 h).

Depending on how much time has passed and upstream ICA conditions, occlusions of the MCA can initially be treated with IAT or aspiration (with a 4–5F catheter). IAT is carried out via a 2.4F microcatheter, the tip of which is placed in the thrombus. We infuse no more than 1 million IU urokinase via an infusion pump that distributes the dosage over a period of 90–120 minutes, with angiography being carried out via the guide catheter after 30 minutes and then every 15 minutes. The intra-arterial thrombolysis is then stopped once recanalization occurs. This makes it possible to reduce the rate of symptomatic intracerebral bleeding to less than 5%. Thrombolysis can be speeded up with careful passage and manipulation of the thrombus with the microwire and microcatheter. However, the risk of vascular perforation needs to be considered in all forms of manipulation. With persistent occlusions, or when IAT is contraindicated, mechanical procedures can be used for thrombectomy, PTA, and/or implantation of a stent as the last resort. The introduction of retrievable stents has changed the situation such that this technique can now be used as a primary form of endovascular therapy, with or without intravenous bridging treatment, since recanalization can be achieved rapidly and safely in a very high percentage of cases.

References

Alexandrov AV, Molina CA, Grotta JC, et al. Ultrasound-enhanced systemic thrombolysis for acute ischemic stroke. N Engl J Med 2004; 351: 2170–8.

Arnold M, Schroth G, Nedeltchev K, et al. Intra-arterial thrombolysis in 100 patients with acute stroke due to middle cerebral artery occlusion. Stroke 2002; 33: 1828–33.

Brekenfeld C, Remonda L, Nedeltchev K, et al. Symptomatic intracranial haemorrhage after intra-arterial thrombolysis in acute ischaemic stroke: assessment of 294 patients treated with urokinase. J Neurol Neurosurg Psychiatry 2007; 78: 280–5.

Brekenfeld C, Schroth G, Mattle HP, et al. Stent placement in acute cerebral artery occlusion: use of a self-expandable intracranial stent for acute stroke treatment. Stroke 2009; 40: 847–52.

del Zoppo GJ, Poeck K, Pessin MS, et al. Recombinant tissue plasminogen activator in acute thrombotic and embolic stroke. Ann Neurol 1992; 32: 78–86.

Furlan A, Higashida R, Wechsler L, et al. Intra-arterial proUK for acute ischemic stroke. The PROACT II study: a randomized controlled trial. Prolyse in Acute Cerebral Thromboembolism. JAMA 1999; 282: 2003–11.

Gralla J, Brekenfeld C, Mordasini P, Schroth G. Mechanical thrombolysis and stenting in acute ischemic stroke. Stroke 2012; 43: 280–5.

Hacke W, Kaste M, Bluhmki E, et al. Thrombolysis with alteplase 3 to 4.5 hours after acute ischemic stroke. N Engl J Med 2008; 359: 1317–29.

IMS Study Investigators. Combined intravenous and intra-arterial recanalization for acute ischemic stroke: the Interventional Management of Stroke Study. Stroke 2004; 35: 904–11.

Lewandowski CA, Frankel M, Tomsick TA, et al. Combined intravenous and intra-arterial r-TPA versus intra-arterial therapy of acute ischemic stroke: Emergency Management of Stroke (EMS) Bridging Trial. Stroke 1999; 30: 2598–605.

Mattle HP, Arnold M, Georgiadis D, et al. Comparison of intraarterial and intravenous thrombolysis for ischemic stroke with hyperdense middle cerebral artery sign. Stroke 2008; 39: 379–83.

Mattle HP, Arnold M, Lindsberg PJ, Schonewille WJ, Schroth G. Basilar artery occlusion (Review). Lancet Neurol 2011; 11: 1002–14.

Nedeltchev K, Arnold M, Brekenfeld C, et al. Pre- and in-hospital delays from stroke onset to intra-arterial thrombolysis. Stroke 2003; 34: 1230–4.

Nedeltchev K, Brekenfeld C, Remonda L, et al. Internal carotid artery stent implantation in 25 patients with acute stroke: preliminary results. Radiology 2005; 237: 1029–37.

Neumann-Haefelin T, du Mesnil de Rochemont R, Fiebach JB, et al. Effect of incomplete (spontaneous and postthrombolytic) recanalization after middle cerebral artery occlusion: a magnetic resonance imaging study. Stroke 2004; 35: 109–14.

Ogawa A, Mori E, Minematsu K, et al. Randomized trial of intraarterial infusion of urokinase within 6 hours of middle cerebral artery stroke: the middle cerebral artery embolism local fibrinolytic intervention trial (MELT) Japan. Stroke 2007; 38: 2633–9.

Rha JH, Saver JL. The impact of recanalization on ischemic stroke outcome: a meta-analysis. Stroke 2007; 38: 967–73.

Shaltoni HM, Albright KC, Gonzales NR, et al. Is intra-arterial thrombolysis safe after full-dose intravenous recombinant tissue plasminogen activator for acute ischemic stroke? Stroke 2007; 38: 80–4.

The National Institute of Neurological Disorders and Stroke rt-PA Stroke Study Group. Tissue plasminogen activator for acute ischemic stroke. N Engl J Med 1995; 333: 1581–7.

Theron J, Courtheoux P, Casasco A, et al. Local intraarterial fibrinolysis in the carotid territory. AJNR Am J Neuroradiol 1989; 10: 753–65.

Tomsick T, Broderick J, Carrozella J, et al. Revascularization results in the Interventional Management of Stroke II trial. AJNR Am J Neuroradiol 2008; 29: 582–7.

Zeumer H, Hacke W, Ringelstein EB. Local intraarterial thrombolysis in vertebrobasilar thromboembolic disease. AJNR Am J Neuroradiol 1983; 4: 401–4.

Zeumer H, Hündgen R, Ferbert A, et al. Local intraarterial fibrinolytic therapy in inaccessible internal carotid occlusion. Neuroradiology 1984; 26: 315–7.

2 Thoracic arteries

2.1 Arteriosclerotic and acquired inflammatory and congenital diseases of the thoracic aorta

Anatomy of the whole aorta: Reinhard Putz
Clinical findings: Friedhelm Beyersdorf and Thomas Zeller
Conservative treatment: Friedhelm Beyersdorf and Thomas Zeller
Endovascular treatment: Friedhelm Beyersdorf
Surgical treatment: Friedhelm Beyersdorf

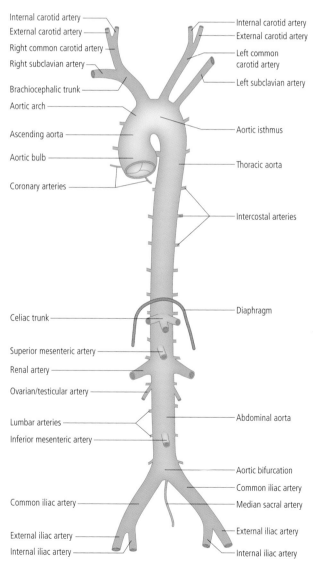

Fig. 2.1-1 Overview of the whole aorta.

2.1.1 Anatomy of the whole aorta

The body's main artery, the aorta, is divided into three parts (Fig. 2.1-1): the ascending aorta, the arch of the aorta and the descending aorta. The ascending aorta starts with the slightly dilated aortic bulb at the aortic valve, which with its three semilunar cusps (valvules) prevents backflow of blood during diastole (Fig. 2.1-2). The cusps consist of very firm, taut connective tissue and are covered with endothelium on both surfaces. They are attached to the inner wall of the junction between the left ventricle of the heart and the aorta and have small nodules (lunules) on their free edges. When blood is flowing back toward the heart, the cusps fill up (aortic sinus), pressing the lunules against each other and usually completely blocking backflow. These delicate edges interlock so finely that even slight changes due to various causes can unfortunately lead to insufficiency.

In the area of the aortic bulb, two arteries supplying the heart are typically already given off from the ascending aorta. The right coronary artery arises from the wall of the right sinus of the aortic valve, and the left coronary artery from the left sinus (Fig. 2.1-2).

The ascending aorta does not give off any branches along its subsequent course. It passes into the arch of the aorta without a clear boundary. The upper margin of the aortic arch projects onto the manubrium of the sternum. It has an oblique angle and passes dorsally into the descending aorta, lying in the inferior posterior mediastinum. Normally (in 70% of cases), three large vessels arise from the arch of the aorta in a cranial direction, with considerable variation (Fig. 2.1-3). With

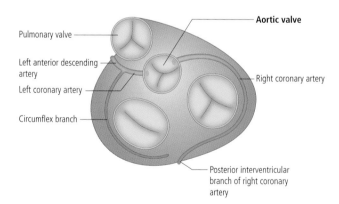

Fig. 2.1-2 The aortic valve from above, with the origins of the coronary arteries.

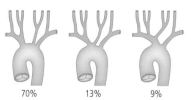

Fig. 2.1-3 Origins of the large arteries from the aortic arch (from Lippert and Pabst 1985).

the exception of branches to the chest, the entire right half of the head and right arm are supplied by the brachiocephalic trunk, which divides after a few centimeters into the right subclavian artery and right common carotid artery.

The left common carotid artery and left subclavian artery are given off separately on the left.

The most frequent variation is a separate origin, as early as at the aortic arch, of the two large arteries on the right side. Not infrequently, the right subclavian artery arises as the last branch from the aortic arch and then courses as the arteria lusoria behind the esophagus to the right side, where it branches further in the normal fashion. (This variant may seem surprising, but it is clearly explained by the development of the branchial arches.)

The subclavian artery leaves the deep cervical region on each side, lying on the first rib behind the scalenus anterior. The common carotid artery courses upward in a common connective-tissue sheath with the internal jugular vein in the carotid triangle.

The thoracic aorta, which is the initial part of the descending aorta, arises from the aortic arch without any clear boundary. It courses initially in a caudal direction in the posterior mediastinum, lying close to the vertebrae on the left, and gradually turns in the lower chest area toward the anterior side of the vertebral column. Apart from a few small branches to the mediastinum, it gives off nine intercostal arteries on each side, as well as a number of unpaired small arteries to the trachea, the bronchi, the esophagus, and the diaphragm. Small branches go off dorsally to the vertebral column and to the back muscles (Fig. 2.1-4).

The abdominal aorta, descending slightly obliquely from the left, lies anterior to the vertebral column together with the inferior vena cava and divides into the common iliac arteries directly in front of the lumbosacral joint. Like the thoracic aorta, just below the diaphragm it gives off the inferior phrenic artery on the right and left and four lumbar arteries to the dorsal body wall. Paired arteries pass to the adrenal glands, kidneys and ovaries or testicles. The latter ar-

teries descend steeply in the direction of the lesser pelvis. The right renal artery usually reaches the kidney along a course posterior to the inferior vena cava (Fig. 2.1-5).

Three arteries emerge ventrally from the aorta to the unpaired intestines. The celiac trunk already arises in the aortic hiatus and divides into the left gastric artery, the common hepatic artery, and the inferior gastric artery (Fig. 2.1-6). Approximately 1 cm caudal from it, the superior mesenteric artery arises. A further 1 cm caudally, approximately at the level of the lower margin of the second vertebra, the two renal arteries arise—the right renal artery in a ventrolateral direction and the left renal artery dorsolaterally. The inferior mesenteric artery arises at the left ventrolateral side of the aorta approximately at the level of the fourth lumbar vertebra.

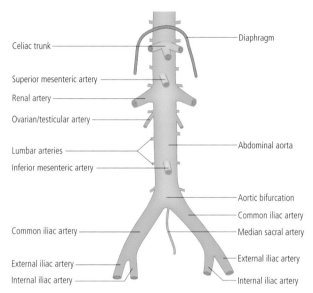

Fig. 2.1-5 Branches of the abdominal aorta.

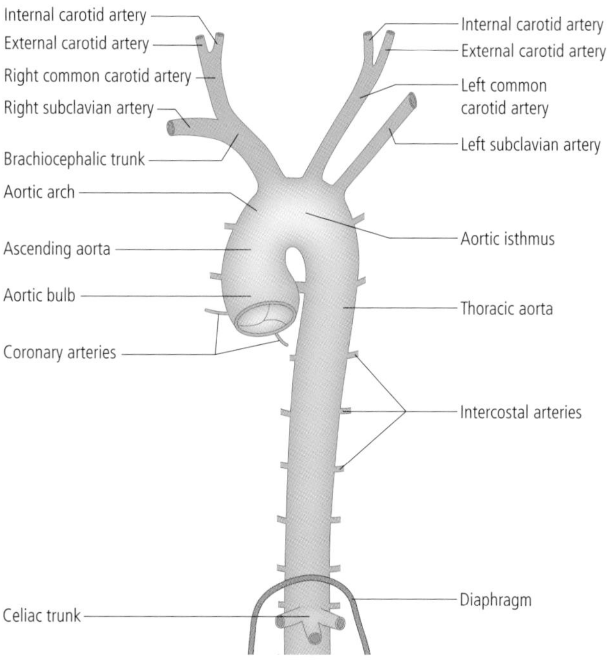

Fig. 2.1-4 Branches of the thoracic aorta.

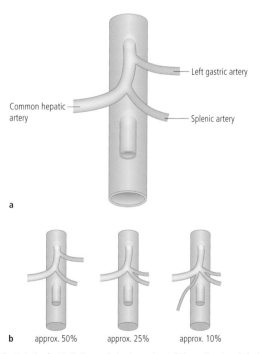

Fig. 2.1-6a, b Variations of the branches of the celiac trunk (adapted from Lippert and Pabst 1985).

The aortic bifurcation normally lies at the level of the fifth lumbar vertebra, but may also be slightly lower. The common iliac artery arises from it on the right and left sides, dividing further on each side after about 4–5 cm into the external and internal iliac arteries. In the area of the bifurcation, the unpaired median sacral artery arises from the posterior surface of the aorta and courses caudally along the anterior surface of the sacrum.

2.1.2   Clinical pictures and epidemiology of arteriosclerotic and acquired diseases of the thoracic aorta

2.1.2.1   Aortic aneurysms

The most frequent diseases of the aorta are aortic aneurysms. These may be limited to an isolated segment of the aorta (ascending aorta, aortic arch, descending aorta) or may affect several segments (ascending aorta and aortic arch; aortic arch and descending aorta; or thoracoabdominal aortic aneurysms). The Crawford classification is now usually used specifically for thoracoabdominal aortic aneurysms (Fig. 2.1-7).

The incidence of thoracic aortic aneurysms is estimated at 5.9 per 100,000 population per year. Among these, the ascending aorta segment is the one most frequently affected (approximately 50%), followed by the descending aorta (approximately 40%). The aortic arch is affected least often, at around 10% (Bickerstaff et al. 1982).

Multisegmental *degenerative aortic aneurysms* occur in approximately 12.6% of cases (Crawford and Cohen 1982). Some 1% of cases of sudden death are caused by aortic rupture (dissection 62%, aneurysm 37%, pseudoaneurysm 1%). Atherosclerosis is the principal cause of aortic aneurysms (90%).

The normal diameter of the ascending aorta in adults is < 3.5 cm; in the descending aorta, the normal diameter is < 3.0 cm. In asymptomatic patients, surgery (in the ascending aorta) or endoprosthesis implantation (in the thoracic aorta) is indicated at diameters of 5.0 cm or more.

2.1.2.2   Aortic dissection

Aortic dissection is a frequent disease of the thoracic aorta. It is nowadays usually divided into types A and B using the Stanford classification (Fig. 2.1-8). The frequency of aortic dissection is estimated at 10 per 100,000 population per year (Svensson and Crawford 1992). Aortic dissection involves a longitudinal split in the arterial wall, with separation of the intima–media complex from the adventitia. This gives rise to an original "true" lumen, lined with endothelium, and a "false" lumen surrounded by adventitia. It was earlier thought that aortic dissection was based on an aneurysm with additional Erdheim–Gsell cystic medial degeneration. However, an important role is now ascribed to arterial hypertension; 75% of the patients are hypertensive. Additional risk factors include nicotine abuse and hypercholesterolemia. Hereditary diseases such as Marfan syndrome, Ehlers–Danlos syndrome (with an incidence of one in 5000) and annuloaortic ectasia (5–10% of valve replacement operations in patients with aortic valvular regurgitation) are associated with an increased risk of dissection (Erbel et al. 2001). The prevalence is 0.5–3.0 per 100,000 population per year.

Intramural hematoma is an early stage of dissection. This involves hemorrhage into the media on the aortic wall, starting in the vasa vasorum. Dissection develops from this in 15–41% of patients, and rupture in 5–26% (Erbel et al. 2001). There is a high rate of mortality, at 20–80%. *Penetrating ulcer*, mainly in the descending aorta, can lead to the development of intramural hematoma and dissection, false aneurysm, and perforation.

In the acute stage, there is fluid blood in the dissection fissure, and this coagulates during the subsequent course within hours, or sometimes only after several weeks. The resulting thrombosis in the dissection fissure is the starting point for "spontaneous healing" of the dissection. When there is strong flow through the dissection channel, thrombosis may not take place, and the false lumen becomes endothelialized. The false lumen then often undergoes aneurysmal dilation and may compress the true lumen.

The aortic wall destroyed by the dissection may rupture either immediately or during the later course. Rupture occurs most often in the area of the ascending aorta, into the pericardium, leading to cardiac tamponade. However, rupture may also take place into the mediastinum or mediastinal organs (esophagus, trachea), into the pleura, retroperitoneum, or peritoneum. The branches of the

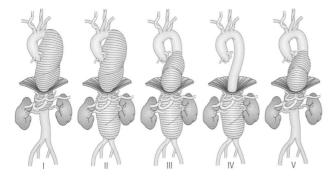

Fig. 2.1-7 The Crawford classification of thoracoabdominal aortic aneurysms. Type I starts distal to the subclavian artery and ends above the renal arteries; type II also starts distal to the subclavian artery and ends below the renal arteries; type III starts in the region of the distal descending aorta (below T6) and extends to underneath the renal arteries; type IV covers most of the abdominal aorta; type V stretches from the distal thoracic aorta to above the renal arteries.

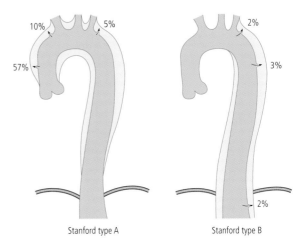

Stanford type A   Stanford type B

Fig. 2.1-8 The Stanford classification of acute aortic dissection.

aorta may be compromised or occluded, leading to a wide variety of ischemic organ symptoms. In dissection of the ascending aorta, the coronary arteries, carotids and brachial arteries are at risk, while in dissection of the descending aorta the renal arteries, celiac trunk, and pelvic arteries are affected. In dissection of the ascending aorta, the cusps of the aortic valve are often undermined, leading to acute aortic valve regurgitation of varying degrees of severity. The resulting acute volume loading of the left ventricle can cause left ventricular failure and lead to pulmonary edema. Left-sided heart failure is promoted by the perfusion disturbance in the coronary arteries that is often present at the same time if the right coronary or left coronary sinus of the aortic root is involved in the dissection.

The *prognosis* in this condition partly depends on the extent of the dissection. Signs of impending rupture such as pericardial effusion or pleural effusion and widening of the mediastinum, are associated with a mortality rate of more than 50% (Erbel et al. 2001).

2.1.2.3　Aortitis

Other diseases of the aorta include the appearance of inflammatory cells in the media or adventitia. This condition is known as *aortitis,* and again it can be divided into two major categories:

- Infectious aortitis
- Aortitis without known infectious pathogens

Infectious diseases of the aorta with confirmed pathogens can be divided into the following types:

- Chronic bacterial infections (not necessarily originating in the aorta per se, but often associated with chronic inflammatory changes in the aorta)
- Acute primary infections of the aorta (mycotic aneurysms)
- Infections of the aorta after prior surgery (usually involving prosthesis materials made of plastic)

In *aortitis without known infectious pathogens,* there is again a distinction into cases involving mainly:

- The aorta (Takayasu disease) or
- Other organ systems, with only secondary involvement of the aorta and other arteries (giant cell arteritis, rheumatoid arteritis, Behçet disease) (see also Part C, on vasculitides)

2.1.2.4　Traumatic aortic rupture

Traumatic changes in the aorta include primarily *traumatic aortic rupture* in typical locations—i.e., distal to the origin of the left subclavian artery.

2.1.2.5　Surgical anatomy

The aorta is divided into various segments. The segment above the aortic valve up to the sinotubular transition is known as the *aortic root.* The *sinotubular transition* marks the boundary between the aortic root and the ascending aorta. The *ascending aorta* extends from the sinotubular transition to the start of the brachiocephalic trunk. The *aortic arch* extends from a line lying at right angles proximal to the brachiocephalic trunk to a line lying at right angles distal

Table 2.1-1 Normal diameter of the aorta in adults (from Svensson and Crawford 1997).

Segment	Transverse diameter (mm)
Aortic root	31
Ascending aorta	32
Proximal aortic arch	32
Proximal descending aorta	28
Middle descending aorta	27
Distal descending aorta (at the level of the superior mesenteric artery)	26
Proximal infrarenal aorta	19
Distal infrarenal aorta	17
Common iliac artery	9
Common femoral artery	7

to the origin of the subclavian artery. The *descending aorta* is the segment from the left subclavian artery to the aortic hiatus in the diaphragm. The *abdominal segment of the aorta* is the final section, from the aortic hiatus to the aortic bifurcation.

Familiarity with the diameter of the healthy aorta plays an important role in correct decision-making regarding which type of operation is best suited to each patient. The diameters are listed in Table 2.1-1.

2.1.3　Clinical findings

The presentation is usually sudden in onset, sometimes in connection with severe physical or psychological stress (with an increase in blood pressure), and less often starting from a state of complete rest. The rupture event is usually associated with dramatic symptoms. The symptoms depend on the location and extent of the dissection, involvement of branching vessels and of the aortic valve, as well as the onset and location of the rupture. The latter can lead to sudden death that is only explained at autopsy. The major symptom is usually extremely severe chest pain radiating to between the shoulder blades.

2.1.4　Differential diagnoses

Common differential diagnoses include costovertebral syndrome (in which pain is position-dependent and can usually be induced by manual provocation), myocardial infarction (in which the pain center is retrosternal), pulmonary embolism (in which pain is respiration-dependent or there is dyspnea or hyperventilation), acute pleuritis (auscultation), and acute pericarditis (auscultation). More rarely, aortic dissection leads to stroke (with cerebral symptoms such as visual disturbances, syncope, coma, pareses, etc.), perfusion disturbances in the extremities, acute abdomen, or renal infarction (differential diagnosis: embolic occlusion).

2.1.5   Diagnosis

A careful clinical examination of the arterial vascular system usually leads to the first signs suggesting suspected aortic dissection. New systolic and diastolic noise phenomena over the aorta and differences in extremity blood pressure and peripheral pulse require further clarification.

Laboratory tests. Routine laboratory test parameters show only nonspecific findings (elevated erythrocyte sedimentation rate and C-reactive protein, leukocytosis, etc.). However, they are important for follow-up purposes, for recognizing hemorrhage and organ dysfunction. A specific marker that has recently come into use is an increase in smooth muscle myosin heavy chain (SMMHC) values.

ECG. The ECG can reveal nonspecific findings such as left ventricular hypertrophy, ischemic ST changes, and infarct patterns with coronary involvement (20%) or low voltage in pericardial effusions.

X-ray. Chest radiography plays a subordinate role nowadays, but can reveal elongation and/or widening of the ascending aorta and aortic arch, and in some cases also mediastinal widening. A tumor process, atelectasis, or pneumothorax can be excluded in the differential diagnosis.

Transthoracic and transesophageal echocardiography, duplex ultrasonography. Ultrasound diagnosis is the diagnostic method of choice, as it can be carried out at the bedside. Transthoracic and transesophageal echocardiography are complementary procedures. Two-dimensional imaging can detect the detached inner layer, and color Doppler can differentiate entries and reentries and thrombosed and perfused dissection lumina, and allows assessment of concomitant aortic regurgitation. The sensitivity and specificity of transthoracic ultrasound for recognizing a type A dissection are 77–80% and 93–96%, respectively. Biplanar transesophageal echocardiography (TEE) has a sensitivity and specificity of 99% and 89%, respectively. The distal extent of the dissection and compromise of the aortic side branches when there is infradiaphragmatic extension can be assessed using color duplex ultrasound.

Spiral computed tomography (CT). In addition to displaying the dissection as a double lumen, spiral CT also allows three-dimensional reconstruction, with precise depiction of the longitudinal extent—a prerequisite for planning endoprosthesis treatment. The sensitivity and specificity are both over 95%.

Magnetic resonance imaging (MRI) and magnetic resonance angiography. Like spiral CT, MRI allows three-dimensional reconstruction and identification of intramural hematoma, but it has several limitations in intensive care conditions (including the long examination time). The sensitivity and specificity of the method are both nearly 100%.

Conventional or digital subtraction angiography and coronary angiography. These procedures are now only carried out in exceptional cases and are indicated for assessing coronary heart disease before planned vascular surgery in type B dissections, for example.

2.1.6   Treatment

2.1.6.1   Conservative treatment

Aortic aneurysm

When the diameter of the aneurysm is not large enough for an intervention to be indicated, treatment essentially consists of secondary prophylactic medication, with a low-normal blood pressure level (< 120/85 mmHg) using β-blockers. Administering a statin to reduce inflammation of the vessel wall is generally recommended. Lifting of heavy weights (> 20 kg) is contraindicated.

Aortic dissection

In addition to symptomatic measures such as relieving pain (with morphine) and treating shock (with volume substitution), heart failure, and kidney failure, the classic treatment initially consists of reducing blood pressure, using negatively inotropic agents to reduce wall tension to prevent the dissection from progressing and leading to impending rupture. Sodium nitroprusside is the agent most frequently used for intravenous continuous infusion to achieve a controlled reduction in blood pressure; β-adrenoceptor blockers are used to reduce the speed of pressure increases (intravenous propranolol or esmolol). Blood pressure values should be reduced as much as possible both in the acute situation and during the subsequent course, ideally to 100–120 mmHg, and this usually requires multiple treatments. Even during initial treatment of the patient in the intensive care unit, noninvasive examinations have to be carried out and a cardiovascular surgery team (from the same institution or elsewhere) needs to be alerted. It is essential to ensure an adequate supply of blood, cross-matched if possible.

In type B dissections, the results of surgical treatment in the *acute stage* are not superior to those with conservative treatment. Most authors therefore recommend that immediate surgery, or alternatively percutaneous endoprosthesis implantation, should only be carried out when there are life-threatening complications such as rupture or ischemic kidney failure (Erbel et al. 2001). As the natural history is much better for type B dissections that are only diagnosed at the *chronic stage,* these should be treated electively with surgery or endoprosthesis placement, particularly when there are complications. If there are thromboses in the false lumen without substantial constriction of the aortic cross-section or branches, this can be regarded as a favorable course of spontaneous healing.

2.1.6.2   Endovascular and surgical treatment

The treatment options vary depending on which segment of the aorta is affected:

For diseases of the *aortic root and ascending aorta,* no endoluminal techniques are currently available. Open surgical procedures therefore predominate in this segment of the aorta.

In the area of the *aortic arch,* it is also mainly open surgical procedures that are used. However, specialized treatment for specific groups of patients is occasionally possible here using endoluminal stenting techniques, in combination with revascularization of the supra-aortic vessels (hybrid procedures).

In the area of the *descending aorta,* endoluminal treatment for aortic diseases has proved to be superior to open procedures and is now starting to predominate in the treatment of this segment of the aorta.

The *thoracoabdominal segment* can also be treated with endoluminal stents after debranching of the intestinal arteries in individual cases (hybrid procedure). Despite this, the majority of thoracoabdominal aortic aneurysms are still treated using conventional surgery.

Surgical treatment of the aortic root and ascending aorta in degenerative aneurysms

Supracoronary replacement of the ascending aorta

Supracoronary replacement of the ascending aorta is indicated in patients in whom the aortic root is not affected by disease and the aneurysm is restricted to the ascending aorta. In supracoronary replacement of the ascending aorta, the aorta is completely transected above the coronary arteries and proximal to the aortic clamp in the first step. Attention should be paid here to ensure, firstly, that there is a sufficient margin in the area of the supracoronary segment to allow the anastomosis to be created; and secondly, to ensure also that not too much of the diseased aortic wall remains. After resection of the aorta, both aortic stumps are initially strengthened with a 0.5-cm wide felt strip, which is sutured onto the aortic stump from outside with 4–0 Prolene using mattress sutures. The suture is not initially tied, to ensure that the diameter is not reduced.

The size of the presealed Dacron tube prosthesis is then selected using a folding measuring instrument. The proximal and distal anastomoses are created with 3–0 Prolene using a continuous technique. The proximal anastomosis is done first, and then the distal anastomosis. Air is removed from the prosthesis before blood flow is restored.

Aortic valve replacement and supracoronary replacement of the ascending aorta

Isolated aortic valve replacement in combination with supracoronary replacement of the ascending aorta is always applicable in the presence of significant aortic valve disease with an aneurysm of the ascending aorta, without marked dilation of the root. In this technique, attention should be given to ensuring that a sufficiently long border is left in the supracoronary aortic resection, since otherwise (e.g., when a biological valve is used) problems may arise when creating the proximal anastomosis. Otherwise, both the valve replacement and supracoronary aortic replacement are carried out using the same technique described above.

Replacement of the ascending aorta and aortic root with reconstruction of the aortic valve

In aortic root aneurysms with an intact, delicate aortic valve without structural defects, two surgical techniques are now available making it possible to do without valve replacement (replacement of the aortic root and ascending aorta, combined with reconstruction of the aortic valve). The surgical techniques that can be used in these cases are the David operation and the Yacoub operation.

David operation

There are numerous modifications and variations (David I–V) on the surgical technique first described by Tirone David. The technique preferred by this author is described here.

After administration of cardioplegia, the aortic root is initially dissected. The ascending aorta is then resected and the aortic root is further dissected, with the coronary ostia visible. As a rule of thumb, a 28-mm presealed Dacron tube prosthesis is used in men and a 26-mm presealed Dacron tube prosthesis in women. The size can be checked again using a folding measuring instrument, and it is best to do this at the still-preserved sinotubular junction. The two coronary ostia are then dissected out and the aortic root is dissected until the subannular sutures can be easily stitched. This is followed by stitching of around 12 subannular felt-supported retention sutures using a large needle (3–0 Ethibond, SH needle). Particularly in the area of the conduction system (the commissure between the right coronary sinus and the noncoronary aortic sinus), attention should be given to ensuring that the sutures are placed immediately underneath the aortic valve annulus (*caution:* atrioventricular block). Using Prolene suture material, the three commissures are then held up and the presealed Dacron tube prosthesis is placed over the aortic root. The subannular sutures are then distributed uniformly along the distal end of the prosthesis, followed by tying of the retention sutures. It is important that these sutures should not be hemostatic, so that here again the sutures should not be tied too tightly.

The next step in the operation involves attaching the three commissures to the prosthesis. This surgical step is extremely important, and the commissures should therefore be anchored anatomically correctly to the prosthesis. Once the commissures have been attached to the prosthesis with the previously stitched Prolene retention sutures, hemostatic suturing onto the prosthesis of the rest of the aortic border of the aortic root is carried out using 4–0 Prolene. This is best done with a 4–0 Prolene suture with a small needle (V7). The seal on the valve is then checked using saline.

In the next surgical step, first the left coronary ostium and then the right coronary ostium are reimplanted onto the prosthesis using the usual technique. In the final step of the operation, attachment of the distal row of sutures on the prosthesis to the distal ascending aorta is completed. After opening the aortic clamp, intraoperative TEE checking must be carried out in all cases to test the results of the aortic valve reconstruction.

Yacoub operation

The principle of reconstruction of the aortic valve and aortic root, as well as replacement of the ascending aorta, in the Yacoub operation also involves resection of the entire aortic root. The Dacron prosthesis is then trimmed in such a way that three new aortic sinuses are cut out of the prosthesis. After dissection of the aortic root, these neosinuses are then sutured directly onto the aortic valve annulus or residual aortic sinus using a continuous suture.

The *modified Yacoub operation* is a special form of the technique in which only the noncoronary aortic sinus is replaced with a tongue of the Dacron prosthesis. This is often possible when only the noncoronary aortic sinus shows aneurysmal dilation, while the right and left coronary sinuses have a normal caliber. It is then possible to carry out a supracoronary replacement of the ascending aorta in combination with complete replacement of the noncoronary aortic sinus.

Replacement of the ascending aorta, aortic root, and aortic valve

Mechanical valve conduit

In patients with significant structural aortic valve disease and/or dilation of the aortic annulus, or with aneurysm of the aortic root and ascending aorta, implantation of a valve-bearing conduit may be considered. The fundamental technique nowadays consists of excising the coronary ostia and using an end-to-end technique to reimplant them into the prosthesis (the button technique). After resection of the ascending aorta, dissection of the right and left coronary ostia, and excision of the aortic valve, implantation of the aortic conduit starts with the stitching of the valve sutures using an eversion technique with felt blocks. The sutures must be stitched very close together and distributed evenly along the ring. A sufficiently large valve can be implanted in almost all cases, and one should therefore make sure that not too large a conduit is used, as otherwise too much tension on the annulus is produced, and the sutures are then tied. After this, the coronary ostia are reimplanted—first the left ostium and then the right one. Depending on the quality of the wall, small felt rings can be used to support the 5–0 Prolene suture. One of the most important steps in this operation is correct localization of the site for the ostium anastomosis. It is sometimes advantageous to hold back the heart slightly to prevent later buckling of the coronary arteries. The final step in the operation is the distal aortic anastomosis, which is again created over a previously anastomosed felt strip with 3–0 Prolene.

Overall, this surgical technique can be carried out with excellent results. The Cabrol method (Cabrol et al. 1980) is hardly used any more, as direct reimplantation of the coronary ostia is in principle always possible and is associated with much better results than the Cabrol method. The same also applies to the original Bentall method.

Biological valve conduit (xenograft)

Biological valve conduits are now available (e.g., the Medtronic Freestyle®). In this method, swine aortic valve, aortic root, and proximal ascending aorta are used. In principle, the surgical method is comparable with the mechanical valve conduit, but the following points need to be taken into account:

- The suture ring in the biological valve conduit is much more fragile and is thinner than the strong ring used in the mechanical conduit.
- The resected and ligated coronary ostia in the swine valve conduit do not correspond to the anatomical position of the human coronary arteries. In most cases, only one coronary ostium can therefore be used for the human left coronary ostium. During implantation, rotation needs to be selected in such a way that the coronary ostia can be appropriately reimplanted.
- As the ligature provided by the manufacturer on the biological conduit does not hold 100% securely, it needs to be oversewn again with Prolene. In addition, the ascending aorta on the biological conduit is usually too short and has to be extended with a Dacron prosthesis.
- In addition, tube prostheses are available from various companies with integrated biological heart valve prostheses (Shelhigh, Carpentier–Edwards conduit with biological heart valve, etc.).

Allograft implantation

Implantation (actually transplantation) of fresh or cryoconserved heart valves and aortas (allografts) can also be used (like biological conduits) for aortic root replacement. One of the major limitations in using allografts is that they are difficult to obtain, however. In addition, the quality of biological valve conduits has improved markedly in recent years, so that allografts are now hardly ever used for aortic root replacement. There may be possible indications for allograft implantation in patients with endocarditis or in young patients. Data for the long-term results vary widely from center to center and depending on the surgical method used (the free-standing root or inclusion techniques). In contrast to aortic allografts, pulmonary allografts in the aortic position are unfavorable and should not be implanted.

Pulmonary autograft (Ross operation)

The principle of the Ross operation involves transferring an endogenous (autologous) pulmonary valve to the aortic position and using an allograft to replace the pulmonary valve. This surgical technique is based on the desire to replace the aortic valve with an endogenous valve (pulmonary valve). The hope is that this "biological" valve will be much more durable than all the other types of biological heart valve, particularly in younger patients. The disadvantage of the method is that it corrects a univalvular condition using a bivalvular heart-valve replacement. Despite this, the long-term results (see below) are excellent, and the rate of repeat surgery on the new aortic valve is extremely low. If repeat surgery is necessary, it is almost always the pulmonary graft that is needed (for details, see the Results section below). With the introduction of valvular prostheses that can be implanted transfemorally or transapically, this type of second valvular replacement will be associated with even lower risk in the future.

Special techniques for ascending aorta replacement in acute Stanford type A dissection

In acute type A dissections, numerous modifications are available in comparison with operations for degenerative aneurysms. These are based on the fact that the dissected aortic wall is extremely fragile in acute type A dissection, and in addition the aim must be to resect the primary tear. Provided that the primary tear is located in the ascending aorta (as is usually the case), replacing the ascending aorta is sufficient (Fig. 2.1-9). In the rare cases in which the tear is located in the aortic arch, the latter also needs to be replaced.

Both the proximal and distal aortic stumps have to be stabilized with a felt strip and biological glue in all cases. In addition, the distal anastomosis has to be created openly in all cases. Today, the subclavian artery is cannulated in most cases so that cerebral perfusion can be carried out during the procedure on the aortic arch, or while creating the open anastomosis in the area of the distal ascending aorta. If aortic arch replacement is necessary, the supra-aortic branches can be excised as a common island in most cases and reimplanted into the prosthesis later. If the dissection is to include the supra-aortic branches as well, aortic arch prostheses are available nowadays with prefabricated separate Dacron prostheses emerging from the prosthesis for the brachiocephalic trunk, the left common carotid artery, and the subclavian artery.

Another special form of aortic arch replacement is the "elephant trunk" technique. This is discussed with aortic arch surgery below.

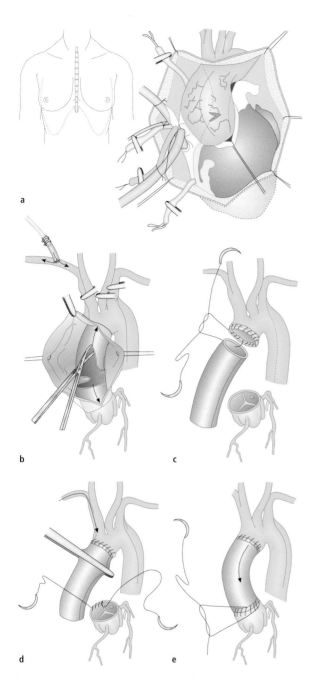

Fig. 2.1-9a–e Surgical steps in acute aortic dissection.

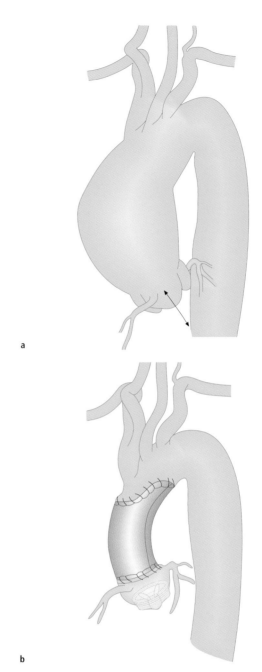

Fig. 2.1-10a, b Hemi-arch replacement with isolated valve replacement.

In acute dissections, particular attention should be given to the aortic root. Using biological glues and felt strips, it is often possible to carry out supracoronary ascending aorta replacement. However, if the dissection already includes the coronary ostia or has completely destroyed the aortic root, a David operation should be considered as well, possibly in combination with bypass treatment for dissected coronary arteries.

Conventional aortic arch replacement

Hemi-arch replacement

Hemi-arch replacement means replacement of the concave part of the aortic arch using an open anastomosis technique. This often-used procedure not only allows complete replacement of the ascending aorta, but also specialized arch replacement without the need to reimplant the supra-aortic branches. This surgical procedure can be used for both degenerative aneurysms and dissections (Fig. 2.1-10).

Replacement of the complete aortic arch

Replacement of the complete aortic arch is now carried out in combination with antegrade cerebral perfusion (usually via the right subclavian artery) (Fig. 2.1-11).

Replacement of the entire aortic arch can be carried out:

- By reimplanting the supra-aortic branches as an island into the Dacron prosthesis (Fig. 2.1-11)
- With prosthetic replacement of the three supra-aortic branches (Fig. 2.1-12)

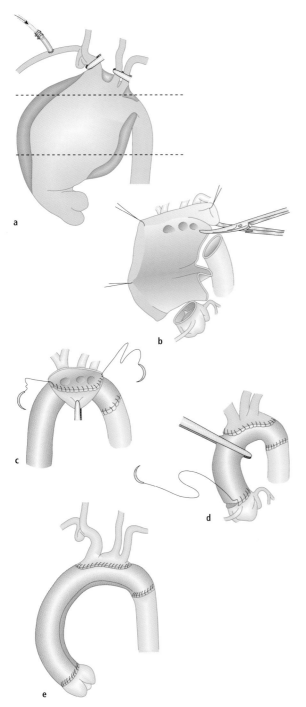

Fig. 2.1-11a–e Replacement of the aortic arch with a distal end-to-end anastomosis and reimplantation of the supra-aortic branches in an island.

Operations in the area of the aortic arch with antegrade cerebral perfusion are carried out with the patient in hypothermia (bladder temperature 22–25°C). During antegrade cerebral perfusion via the right subclavian artery, the brachiocephalic trunk, left carotid artery, and left subclavian artery are either clamped, closed with rubber bands, or blocked with catheters to prevent reverse bleeding from these vessels, resulting in a potential cerebral steal phenomenon, and to improve visibility in the surgical field. In most cases, a presealed Dacron tube prosthesis 24–30 mm in size is used as a substitute aortic arch, and the anastomoses are created with felt reinforcement. In the first step of the operation, the anastomosis to the descending aorta is carried out, and the island of the supra-aortic branches is then reimplanted into the prosthesis. Initially, a felt cuff is anastomosed onto the aortic stump using 4–0 Prolene with a mattress technique, to provide better quality in the aorta for later anastomoses. After exhaustive elimination of air, perfusion of the whole brain and lower half of the body is restored via the brachiocephalic trunk.

The proximal aortic anastomosis is carried out as the last step in the operation, either in a supracoronary position or as an anastomosis between two prostheses.

Protecting the myocardium is particularly important in these very large and often prolonged operations. The authors exclusively use cold antegrade/retrograde blood cardioplegia with terminal warm reperfusion. In addition, the surgical field is flooded with CO_2. The patient is warmed to a bladder temperature of 35°C. Subsequent stepwise warming up to 36–37°C is then carried out later in the intensive care unit with the appropriate warming mats.

Elephant trunk technique

Patients with aortic aneurysms extending from the aortic root over the ascending aorta and the entire aortic arch to the descending aorta represent a special problem. To minimize the problems in these large operations, Borst and colleagues (Borst et al. 1983, 1988) developed a two-step surgical technique in which the ascending aorta and aortic arch are initially replaced, with a segment of a distal Dacron graft being introduced into the descending aorta. The method

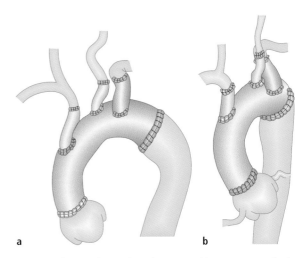

Fig. 2.1-12a, b Complete arch replacement with separate prosthetic use of the brachiocephalic trunk, left common carotid artery and left subclavian artery.

is known as the "elephant trunk" technique. Numerous modifications of the original technique now exist, such as that described by Svensson and Crawford (1997) (Fig. 2.1-13a–r).

Frozen elephant trunk technique

Another method of replacing the aortic arch and descending aorta via a median sternotomy involves a combined endovascular stent graft implantation with conventional aortic arch replacement (a hybrid technique). This technique was first described by Suto and colleagues (1996) and Usui and colleagues (1999). It was later named the "frozen elephant trunk" technique (Karck et al. 2003, 2005, 2008). In this technique, the entire aortic arch is first dissected free and opened. A special stented Dacron prosthesis with a Dacron prosthesis at its cranial end is then introduced via the aortic arch into the descending aorta. After previous measurement of the diameter of both the distal and proximal landing zones in the area of the descending aorta and of the desired length of the stent, the prosthesis can be implanted via the aortic arch under direct vision. The Dacron prosthesis attached to this Dacron-coated stent is then retracted and used to replace the aortic arch.

Replacement of the distal aortic arch

Operations to replace the distal aortic arch are usually carried out from a left lateral thoracotomy in the fourth intercostal space. These procedures are usually conducted using a heart–lung machine or a left heart bypass. Clamping of the aortic arch is usually done between the left common carotid artery and the left subclavian artery. Extreme care is needed here to protect the recurrent nerve and vagus nerve. In many cases, there is marked arteriosclerosis in these aneurysms, so that there is a relatively high risk of cerebral embolization. The surgical sequence does not differ from that in other aneurysm operations, with appropriate dissection of the proximal and distal aortic stump, suturing of the intercostal arteries, and replacement with a presealed Dacron tube prosthesis.

Endoluminal stent implantation into the aortic arch with prior revascularization of the supra-aortic vessels (hybrid operation)

Another form of treatment for aortic arch aneurysms involves a combination of endovascular stent graft implantation and open surgical revascularization of the supra-aortic branches. This hybrid operation is carried out via a median sternotomy. In the first step, an inverted Y Dacron prosthesis is used to revascularize the brachiocephalic trunk and left common carotid artery. The left subclavian artery is then revascularized with another separate prosthesis limb. Once revascularization of the supra-aortic branches has been ensured, a stent graft is advanced under radiographic guidance from the groin up to the distal ascending aorta. This not only eliminates the aortic arch aneurysm but also occludes the supra-aortic branches (the debranching operation).

Initial experience with this hybrid procedure has been positive, but the surgical effort and costs involved should not be underestimated.

Surgical techniques for replacing the descending aorta

Surgical replacement of the descending aorta

In recent years, surgical replacement of the descending aorta has clearly been overshadowed by endoluminal stent implantation. As discussed in the Results section below, the published results with endoluminal stent implantation are clearly superior to those with the surgical method (in terms of neurological complications, bleeding complications, and the overall postoperative course). The topic is therefore only mentioned here for the sake of completeness.

A clear indication for surgical replacement of the descending aorta is present in chronic type B dissections with aneurysm formation, in which the intestinal arteries originate in the false lumen. The dissection flap has to be generously resected here to ensure blood flow both into the true lumen and into the false lumen. In these cases, stent implantation is almost impossible and conventional surgery is the treatment of choice.

The patient is intubated with a dual-lumen tube and positioned for a left thoracotomy—i.e., at an angle of 80–90° on the table. Draping must be carried out in such a way that the left inguinal region remains free in order to connect the heart–lung machine or for an atriofemoral bypass (left heart bypass). The thoracotomy is carried out posterolaterally in the fourth intercostal space. The intercostal space selected depends on whether the operation is on the proximal or distal descending aorta. For the proximal descending aorta, the thoracotomy should be as high as possible, while the sixth intercostal space is usually used for the distal descending aorta. Following appropriate dissection of the descending aorta, the aorta is clamped with pressure control either distal to the subclavian artery or between the carotid and subclavian arteries. To prevent reverse bleeding from the intercostal arteries as much as possible, the descending aorta is clamped in the proximal third or in the middle, and the diseased aortic segment is dissected. All bleeding intercostal arteries are immediately sutured with 4–0 Prolene. The actual anastomosis is then carried out with 3–0 Prolene over felt strips (Fig. 2.1-14). Once the anastomosis has been created, the prosthesis is clamped and the sealing of the anastomosis is tested. The descending aorta is now clamped in a relatively healthy section and the rest of the descending aorta is opened. Arteries of Adamkiewicz or other large intercostal arteries are initially blocked with a red Fogarty catheter and then reimplanted into the prosthesis. All other intercostal arteries are also quickly sutured with 4–0 Prolene. The distal anastomosis is then carried out with 3–0 Prolene over felt strips.

With this anastomosis, special caution needs to be exercised relative to the esophagus, bronchus, and recurrent nerve, which must not be injured during this phase.

Endoluminal stent implantation into the descending aorta

Endovascular treatment is nowadays the treatment of choice for aneurysms in the descending aorta (including acute type B dissection). It requires precise measurement of the size of the aneurysm and of the proximal and distal landing zones for the endovascular stent. There are common sizes of up to 46 mm, but in individual cases larger stents can also be produced individually.

Preoperative clarification includes the issue of whether the stent can be securely anchored distal to the origin of the subclavian artery or whether the proximal landing zone will lie between the left com-

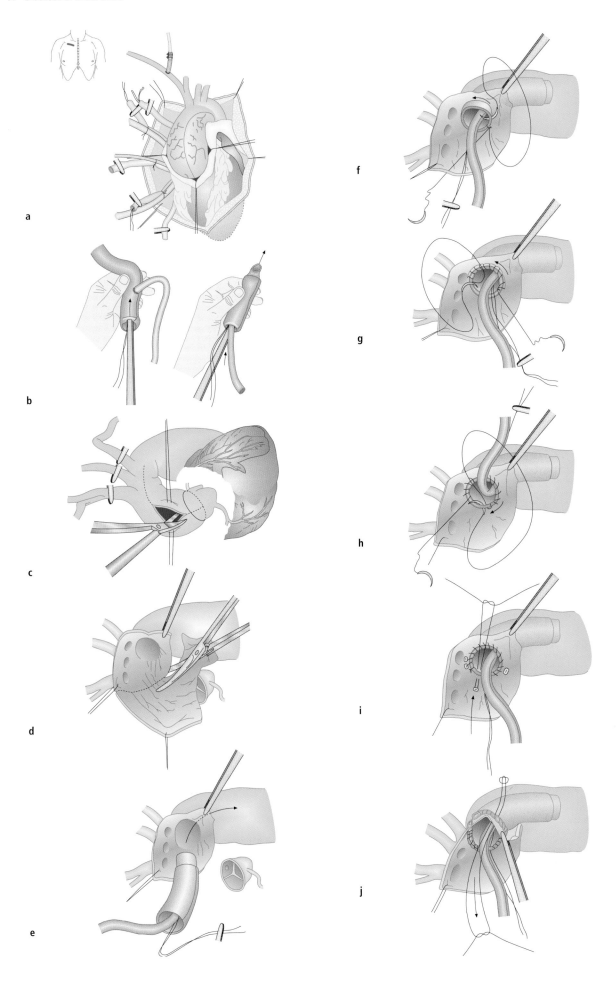

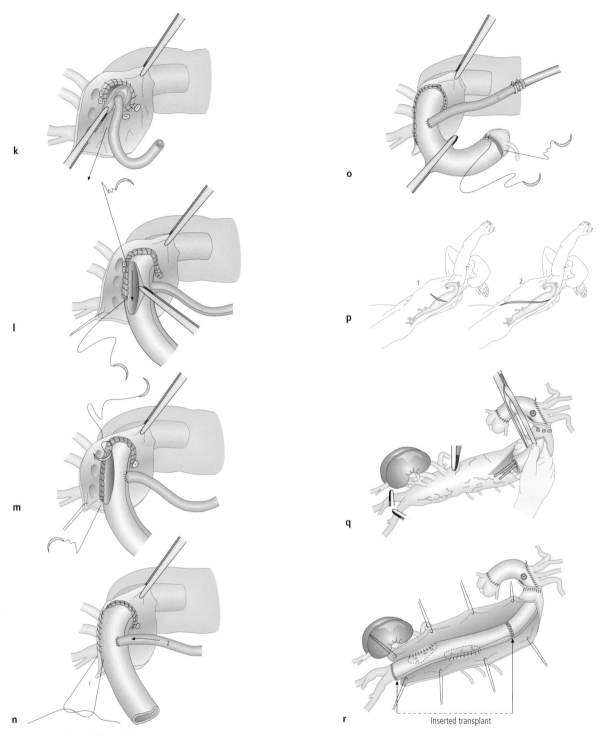

Fig. 2.1-13a–r The modified elephant trunk technique (Svensson and Crawford 1997). (**a**) Median sternotomy, connection to heart–lung machine via separate cannulation of the superior and inferior venae cavae, and cannulation of the right subclavian artery. Hypothermia and isolated antegrade cerebral perfusion. (**b**) Before the start of isolated cerebral perfusion, a 10-mm graft corresponding to the size of the distal aortic arch is anastomosed end-to-side to the larger Dacron prosthesis. In the next step, the proximal prosthesis is inverted into the distal prosthesis using the anastomosed side arm. (**c**) After exposure of the aorta, the proximal aorta is completely transected. (**d**) The distal aorta is also transected. (**e**) The inverted prosthesis is then placed in the descending aorta. (**f**) The prosthesis is anastomosed using a continuous Prolene suture in the region of the proximal descending aorta. (**g**) This anastomosis is usually sutured in an anticlockwise direction. (**h**) The two sutures are finally tied. (**i, j**) If there are any bleeding points, they are managed using felt-supported retention sutures. (**k**) The inverted prosthesis is now pulled out of the descending aorta prosthesis. (**l**) An opening for the arch vessels is cut into the prosthesis, and the posterior row of sutures is initially created. (**m**) The anterior row of sutures is then created. (**n**) 1. The sutures are tied. 2. Antegrade whole-body perfusion is then carried out via the side arm of the prosthesis. Alternatively, perfusion via the subclavian artery can be continued. (**o**) Completion of the proximal anastomosis after clamping of the distal ascending aorta prosthesis. (**p**) Several weeks or months after the operation, the patient is readmitted for replacement of the descending aorta (1) or thoracoabdominal aorta (2). (**q**) After exposure of the descending aorta, the elephant trunk prosthesis is grasped and clamped. (**r**) The descending aorta or thoracoabdominal aorta is replaced with the usual technique.

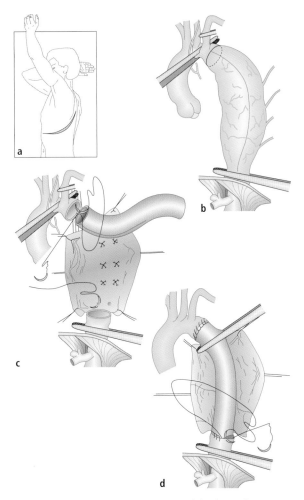

Fig. 2.1-14a–d Conventional replacement of the descending aorta.

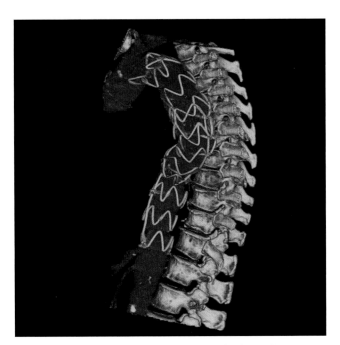

Fig. 2.1-15 Endovascular stent implantation into the descending aorta.

Specialized techniques in acute Stanford type B dissections

Endovascular stent implantation is currently the initial treatment of choice for acute type B dissections as well. It is possible in most cases to close the false lumen entrance and allow perfusion into the true lumen. Open surgery is now only rarely indicated for acute type B dissections.

Several prospective and randomized studies on the topic are currently in progress to assess the precise value of endovascular treatment for acute type B dissections.

Treatment for thoracoabdominal aortic aneurysms

Conventional surgical treatment

Conventional surgery for thoracoabdominal aortic aneurysms is one of the most elaborate interventions in cardiovascular surgery. The techniques that are in use today were developed by Crawford (Svensson and Crawford 1997), Svensson and colleagues (1993), De-Bakey and colleagues (1956), and Svensson and colleagues (1994).

The operation (Fig. 2.1-16) is carried out with neuroprotection (Weigang et al. 2007b) (cerebrospinal fluid drainage, derived motor-evoked potentials and sensory-evoked potentials) and using a heart–lung machine or atriofemoral bypass. The patient is intubated with a dual-lumen tube and positioned on the right side, so that the shoulders are at an angle of 60° and the pelvis is raised by 30°. The access route for the thoracoabdominal aorta has been described in detail elsewhere (Svensson et al. 1997).

In the first step, the aorta is clamped between the left carotid artery and the subclavian artery (Fig. 2.1-16). Following clamping of the aorta, special attention needs to be given to the proximal blood pressure. If it is too high, it can be reduced using the heart–lung machine and withdrawal of blood. To allow clamping of an as-small-as-possible section of the aorta, the descending aorta is optimally clamped proximally. However, clamping options need to be guided

mon carotid artery and subclavian artery. If it is necessary to cover the subclavian artery, it needs to be clarified preoperatively whether subclavian transposition should be carried out before the procedure in order to prevent later neurological complications (e.g., posterior cerebral infarction and left upper extremity ischemia). For this purpose, an exhaustive neurological examination needs to be carried out preoperatively to determine:

- Whether the two vertebral arteries are equally large
- Whether the common carotid arteries are open bilaterally
- Whether there are any stenoses in the circle of Willis

These data allow one to decide either for or against subclavian transposition (Weigang et al. 2007a).

The actual surgical procedure is preferably conducted in a hybrid operating room. Aortography is first carried out over the inguinal region. The stent, the diameter and length of which have previously been determined, can then be deployed. In most cases, the stent can be released relatively safely either between the carotid artery and subclavian artery or distal to the subclavian artery. Depending on the extent of the aneurysm, one or two additional stents then have to be introduced for lengthening purposes. After all of the stents needed have been implanted, a final aortography is carried out to assess whether there are any endoleaks. If a proximal or distal endoleak is identified, redilation can be carried out or lengthening of the stent may be needed in individual cases (Fig. 2.1-15).

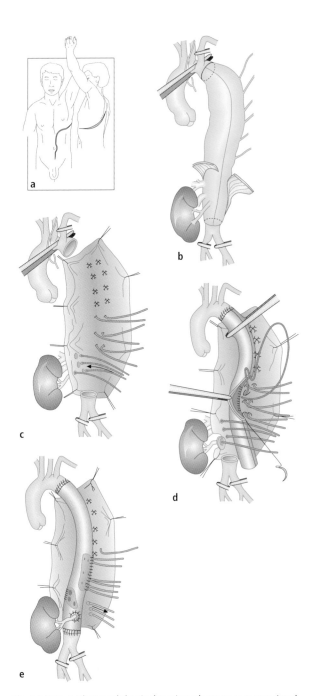

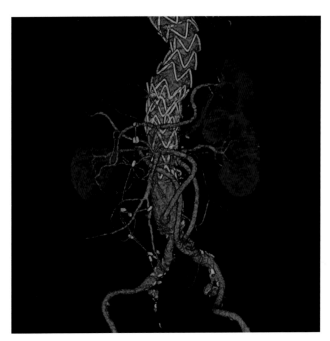

Fig. 2.1-17 Thoracoabdominal aortic replacement: hybrid technique with revascularization of the intestinal arteries and endovascular stent implantation.

Fig. 2.1-16a–e Thoracoabdominal aortic replacement: conventional surgical technique. For clarity, the illustration does not show the staged clamping of the aorta, but this needs to be taken into account during the surgical procedure. Particular attention needs to be given to avoid "reverse bleeding" from the intercostal arteries (caution: steal phenomenon from spinal perfusion).

by local conditions. After opening the aorta, the intercostal arteries are initially sutured and the proximal anastomosis is first created over felt strips with Prolene. In chronic dissections, the aorta has to be completely transected to ensure that a false lumen is not overlooked. Injuries to the esophagus in this area must be carefully avoided. After completion of the anastomosis, blood flow into the prosthesis is released to ensure reperfusion of the spinal cord via branches of the subclavian artery as quickly as possible. The distal clamp is then moved further distally (to the level of the aortic hiatus), and additional intercostal arteries are ligated or (after blocking

with a red Fogarty catheter) larger ones are sutured into the prosthesis. The prosthesis is then clamped again distally as well, so that antegrade perfusion is possible via the reimplanted intercostal arteries. In the next step, reimplantation of the intestinal arteries such as the celiac trunk, superior mesenteric artery, and renal arteries follows. The precise reimplantation technique depends on local conditions and the extent of the aneurysm or dissection. In individual cases, additional grafts (8-mm Dacron prostheses) also have to be placed to revascularize the intestinal arteries. The more distally the clamp is placed, the less the flow via the heart–lung machine will be. After completion of the entire aortic replacement, the clamps are removed and the patient is weaned from the heart–lung machine.

A very long phase of hemostasis then follows, which has to be conducted with extreme care to prevent postoperative bleeding. Administration of packed platelets, fresh frozen plasma, and application of fibrin glues, if necessary, are recommended.

Endoluminal stent implantation (hybrid procedures)

Another option for treating thoracoabdominal aortic aneurysms involves hybrid procedures—i.e., a combination of revascularization (by debranching) of the intestinal arteries and implantation of endovascular stents, with covering of the origins of the intestinal arteries (debranching) (Fig. 2.1-17).

2.1.7 Clinical results

In general, the results of surgical treatment in the thoracic aorta have markedly improved during the last 10 years—both in terms of the results of conventional surgical treatment and also endovascular stent implantation.

Supracoronary ascending aorta replacement can nowadays be carried out with minimal perioperative risk for degenerative aortic aneurysms. The risk is of course greater in patients with a type A dissection.

Table 2.1-2 Revascularization of the supra-aortic vessels with endovascular stenting of the entire aortic arch (hybrid procedure).

Authors	Year	Mortality
Weigang et al.	2008	4/26 (15.4%)
Szeto et al.	2007	1/8 (12.5%)
Ancona et al.	2007	0/4 (0%)
Melissano et al.	2007	2/14 (14.3%)
Shah et al.	2006	0/5 (0%)
Bergeron et al.	2006	2/15 (13.3%)

Table 2.1-3 The frozen elephant trunk operation (from Karck and Kamiya 2008).

Authors	Year	Mortality	Paraplegia
Baraki et al.	2007	5/39 (12.8%)	0/39 (0%)
Liu et al.	2006	2/60 (3.3%)	1/60 (1.6%)
Uchida et al.	2006	2/35 (5.7%)	0/35 (0%)
Flores et al.	2006	3/25 (12%)	4/25 (16%)

Due to the option of antegrade cerebral perfusion via the right subclavian artery, procedures requiring hemi-arch replacement or open distal anastomosis can also be carried out with very good short-term and long-term results. This is because:

- Extremely deep hypothermia is no longer needed for these procedures (24–26°C bladder or rectal temperature nowadays instead of 18°C).
- Antegrade perfusion also allows longer operating times on the aortic arch (i.e., over 30 min) without postoperative neurological complications.

However, operations on the aortic arch are still associated with considerable surgical risk. For this reason, not only conventional complete aortic arch replacement (with implantation of the supra-aortic branches as an island or separate prosthesis replacement for the supra-aortic branches), but also aortic arch replacement using a hybrid procedure can be carried out. The results of the hybrid aortic arch procedure are shown in Table 2.1-2.

Reliable data for the frozen elephant trunk operation are also available in the Ross Registry (Sievers et al. 2005). The study shows that the operation offers an excellent survival rate. The overall rate of repeat valvular surgery is very low with autografts, but the frequency of repeat surgery with allografts (in the pulmonary artery position) has been markedly increasing during the medium term among pediatric patients (Bechtel and Sievers 2005).

2.1.8 Prospects

Diseases of the thoracic aorta are likely to increase during the coming years. This is due to the general increase in life expectancy, as well as the fact that patients with arterial hypertension still do not yet have universal access to good treatment. Although tremendous advances have been made during the last 10 years in this field in particular, the short-term and long-term results are likely to improve even further as a result of innovations in surgical treatment in the thoracic aorta, with endovascular stent implantation and also improvements in the conventional surgical technique. Fenestrated and branched endovascular stents are particularly promising for further improvements in the aortic arch and at the thoracoabdominal junction. A new treatment approach, the implantation of, what is known as a Multilayer Aneurysm Repair System (MARS) stent, may in the coming years make it unnecessary to use branched endoprostheses or hybrid procedures with a debranching operation before endoprosthesis implantation. However, this approach involving modulation of the flow inside an aneurysmal sac, thereby inducing thrombosis of the aneurysm and local pressure reduction, will require further validation of its clinical value to be confirmed in the region of the abdominal aorta and thoracoabdominal aorta first, before it can be used to treat cerebral arteries. It is important that patients with these conditions should be referred to the relevant specialist centers in which the whole range of diagnosis and treatment is available, so that the best individual treatment strategy for each patient can be selected.

References

Antona C, Vanelli P, Petulla M, Gelpi G, Danna P, Lemma M, Inglese L. Hybrid technique for total arch repair: aortic neck reshaping for endovascular-graft fixation. Ann Thorac Surg 2007; 83: 1158–61.

Baraki H, Hagl C, Khaladj N, Kallenbach K, Weidemann J, Haverich A, Karck M. The frozen elephant trunk technique for treatment of thoracic aortic aneurysms. Ann Thorac Surg 2007; 83: S819–23.

Bechtel J FM, Sievers HH. Aortenklappenoperation bei jungen Erwachsenen. Dtsch Med Wochenschr 2005; 130: 669–74.

Bergeron P, Mangialardi N, Costa P, Coulon P, Douillez V, Serreo E, Tuccimei I, Cavazzini C, Mariotti F, Sun Y, Gay J. Great vessel management for endovascular exclusion of aortic arch aneurysms and dissections. Eur J Vasc Endovasc Surg 2006; 32: 38–45.

Bickerstaff LK, Pairolero PC, Hollier LH, et al. Thoracic aortic aneurysms: a population-based study. Surgery 1982; 92: 1103–9.

Borst HG, Frank G, Schaps D. Treatment of extensive aortic aneurysms by a new multiple-stage approach. J Thorac Cardiovasc Surg 1988; 95: 11–3.

Borst HG, Walterbusch G. Schaps D. Extensive aortic replacement using „elephant trunk" prosthesis. Thorac Cardiovasc Surg 1983; 31: 37–40.

Cabrol C, Pavie A, Grandjbakhch I, et al. Complete replacement of the ascending aorta with reimplantation of the coronary arteries. J Thorac Cardiovasc Surg 1980; 79: 388–401.

Crawford ES, Cohen ES. Aortic aneurysm: a multifocal disease. Arch Surg 1982; 117: 1393–400.

DeBakey ME, Creech O, Morris GC. Aneurysm of thoracoabdominal aorta involving the celiac, superior mesenteric, and renal arteries: report of four cases treated by resection and homograft replacement. Ann Surg 1956; 144: 549–73.

Erbel R, Alfonso F, Boileau C et al. Diagnosis and management of aortic dissection: recommendations of the Task Force on Aortic Dissection, European Society of Cardiology. European Heart Journal 2001; 22: 1642–81.

Flores J, Kunihara T, Shiliya N, Yoshimoto K, Matsuzaki K, Yasuda K. Extensive deployment of the stented elephant trunk is associated with an increased risk of spinal cord injury. J Thorac Cardiovasc Surg 2006; 131: 336–42.

Iida Y, Kawaguchi S, Koizumi N, Komai H, Obitsu Y, Shigematsu H. Thoracic endovascular aortic repair with aortic arch vessel revascularization. Ann Vasc Surg 2011 Aug; 25 (6): 748–51.

Karck M, Chavan A, Hagl C, Friedrich H, Galanski M, Haverich A. The frozen elephant trunk technique: a new treatment for thoracic aortic aneurysms. J Thorac Cardiovasc Surg 2003; 125: 1550–3.

Karck M, Chavan A, Nawid K, Friedrich H, Hagl C, Haverich A. The frozen elephant trunk technique for the treatment of extensive thoracic aortic aneurysms: operative results and follow up. Eur J Cardiothorac Surg 2005; 28: 286–98.

Karck M, Kamiya H. Progress of the treatment for extended aortic aneurysms; is the frozen elephant trunk the next standard in the treatment of complex aortic disease including the arch? Eur J Cardiothorac Surg 2008; 33: 1007–13.

Lippert H, Pabst R. Arterial variations in man. Bergmann, München, 1985.

Liu ZG, Sun LZ, Chang Q, Zhu JM, Dong C, Yu CT, Liu YM, Zhang HT. Should the „elephant trunk" be skeletonized? Total arch replacement combined with stented elephant trunk implantation for Stanford type A aortic dissection. J Thorac Cardiovasc Surg 2006; 131: 107–13.

Melissano G, Civilini E, Bertoglio L, Calliari F, Setacci F, Calori G, Chiesa R. Results of endografting of the aortic arch in different landing zones. Eur J Vasc Endovasc Surg 2007; 33: 561–6.

Shah, A, Coulon P, de Chaumaray T, Rosario R, Khanoyan P, Boukhris M, Tshiombo G, Gay J, Bergeron P. Novel technique: staged hybrid surgical and endovascular treatment of acute Type A aortic dissections with aortic arch involvement. J Cardiovasc Surg (Torino) 2006; 47: 497–502.

Shimamura K, Kuratani T, Matsumiya G, Shirakawa Y, Takeuchi M, Takano H, Sawa Y. Hybrid endovascular aortic arch repair using branched endoprosthesis: the second-generation "branched" open stent-grafting technique. J Thorac Cardiovasc Surg 2009 Jul; 138 (1): 46–52.

Sievers H-H, Stierle U, Hanke T, Bechtel M, Graf B, Rein J-G, Hemmer W, Botha C A, Böhm J O. Deutsches Ärzteblatt 2005; 102: A2090–7.

Suto Y, Yasuda K, Shiiya N, Murashita T, Kawasaki M, Imamura M, Takigami K, Sasaki S, Matsui Y, Sakuma M. Stented elephant trunk procedure for an extensive aneurysm involving distal aortic arch and descending aorta. J Thorac Cardiovasc Surg 1996; 112; 1389–90.

Svensson LG, Crawford ES. Cardiovascular and Vascular Disease of the Aorta. St. Louis, W. B. Saunders Company, 1997.

Svensson LG, Crawford ES. Aortic dissection and aortic aneurysm surgery: clinical observations, experimental investigations, and statistical analyses. Part II. Curr Probl Surg 1992; 29: 915–1057.

Svensson LG, Crawford ES, Hess KR, et al. Experience with 1509 patients undergoing thoracoabdominal aortic operations. J Vasc Surg 1993; 17: 357–70.

Svensson LG, Shahian DM, Davis FG, et al. Replacement of entire aorta from aortic valve to bifurcation during one operation. Ann Thorac Surg 1994; 58: 1164–6.

Szeto WY, Bavaria JE, Bowen FW, Woo EY, Fairman RM, Pochettino A. The hybrid total arch repair: brachiocephalic bypass and concomitant endovascular aortic arch stent graft placement. J Card Surg 2007; 22: 97–102.

Uchida N, Ishihara H, Shibamura H, Kyo Y, Ozawa M. Midterm results of extensive primary repair of the thoracic aorta by means of total arch replacement with open stent graft placement for an acute type A aortic dissection. J Thorac Cardiovasc Surg 2006; 131: 862–7.

Usui A, Tajima K, Nishikimi N, Ishiguchi T. Implantation of an endovascular covered stent-graft for distal aortic arch aneurysm via midsternotomy under pigtail catheter guidance. Eur J Cardiothorac Surg 1999; 16: 356–68.

Weigang E, Luehr M, Harloff A, Euringer W, Etz C, Szabo G, Beyersdorf F, Siegenthaler M. Incidence of neurological complications following overstenting of the left subclavian artery. Eur J Cardiothorac Surg 2007; 31: 628–36.

Weigang E, Sircar R, von Samson P, Hartert M, Siegenthaler M, Luehr M, Richter H, Szábo G, Czerny M, Zentner J, Beyersdorf F. Efficacy and frequency of cerebrospinal fluid drainage in operative management of thoracoabdominal aortic aneurysms. Thorac Cardiovasc Surg 2007; 55: 73–8.

Weigang E, Parker J. Czerny M, Peivandi A, Dorweiler B, Beyersdorf F, Siegenthaler M. Endovascular aortic arch repair after aortic arch debranching. Ann Thorac Surg 2009; 87: 603–7.

ter Wolbeek C, Hartert M, Conzelmann LO, Peivandi AA, Czerny M, Gottardi R, Beyersdorf F, Weigang E. Value and pitfalls of neurophysiological monitoring in thoracic and thoracoabdominal aortic replacement and endovascular repair. Thorac Cardiovasc Surg 2010 Aug; 58 (5): 260–4.

2.1.9 Marfan syndrome and aortic diseases determined genetically

Yskert von Kodolitsch, Tilo Kölbel, Sebastian Debus

2.1.9.1 Clinical pictures and epidemiology

Marfan syndrome is an autosomal-dominant hereditary disease of connective tissue that occurs in one per 10,000 of the population. The disease is caused by mutations in the fibrillin-1 gene (*FNB1*), which is located in chromosome region 15q21.1 and codes for an important microfibril in connective tissue. The changes in the connective tissue caused by this mutation lead to a risk of early death due to rupture or acute dissection of the aorta, particularly in the area of the aortic root. Marfan syndrome is by far the most frequent genetically determined disease of the aorta and is regarded as a model disease for a wide range of genetically determined aortic diseases that continue to be newly identified (von Kodolitsch and Robinson 2007). This section presents the clinical findings, differential diagnoses, diagnosis and treatment of Marfan syndrome and discusses common features and differences in comparison with other genetically determined aortic diseases.

2.1.9.2 Clinical findings

The prognosis and course of Marfan syndrome are mainly determined by the aortic condition. Untreated patients mainly die due to dissection or rupture of the aorta. With comprehensive care in Marfan centers, the mean life expectancy has increased from only 32 years to over 60 years. By avoiding cardiovascular, orthopedic, and ophthalmologic complications, the patients' life expectancy and probably also their quality of life can be improved as long as their ability to work and maintain independence are preserved (Silverman et al. 1995; von Kodolitsch et al. 2002; Manow et al. 2010).

Marfan syndrome represents a multiple-system disease. Typical symptoms of the syndrome are above all skeletal changes such as

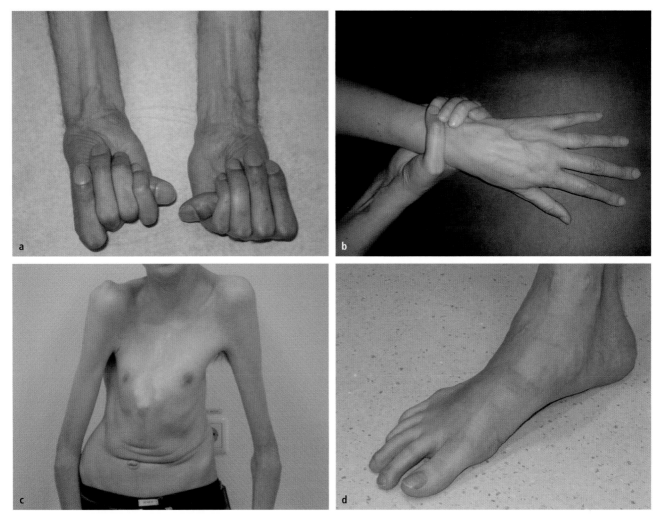

Fig. 2.1-18a–d Typical clinical signs of Marfan syndrome. (**a**) The Steinberg thumb sign is positive if the entire thumbnail extends beyond the ulnar edge of the hand when the thumb is bent over (De Paepe et al. 1996). (**b**) The hand joint sign or Murdoch sign is positive if the thumb overlaps the terminal phalange of the fifth finger when grasping the contralateral wrist (De Paepe et al. 1996). (**c**) A patient with severe skeletal involvement in Marfan syndrome, with marked scoliosis, asymmetric chest and sternal deformity, which had already led to impaired respiration. (**d**) The simple pes planus shown here can be scored according to the recent Ghent classification; talipes valgus, which is given two points on the scale, is not present here (Loeys et al. 2010).

gigantism, altered physical proportions with a comparatively short trunk and long lower and upper limbs, scoliosis and pectus carinatum or pectus excavatum (Figs. 2.1-18 and 2.1-19). Ophthalmological manifestations include lens luxation, myopia, amblyopia, strabismus, secondary glaucoma development and retinal detachment, which can lead to severe visual impairment or complete blindness. Involvement of pulmonary structures can lead to the development of emphysema with acute pneumothorax. Another typical manifestation is dural ectasia, which often causes chronic back pain and can lead to complications in peridural anesthesia or spinal surgery; it can also cause characteristic orthostatic headache as a result of rare dural fistula formation. Hernia formation is observed more often in Marfan patients than in the general population (Sheikhzadeh et al. 2011a). Skin changes are usually only seen in the form of clinically "harmless" striae cutis distensae, although these are quite typical in congenital connective-tissue diseases (Fig. 2.1-19 and 2.1-20).

With the improved prognosis for patients with Marfan syndrome, a number of additional health problems have emerged. These include ventricular cardiac arrhythmia with sudden cardiac death, mitral insufficiency, endocarditis, sleep apnea syndrome and terminal heart failure (von Kodolitsch et al. 2008).

a

Skeletal manifestations in 176 patients with Marfan syndrome (%)

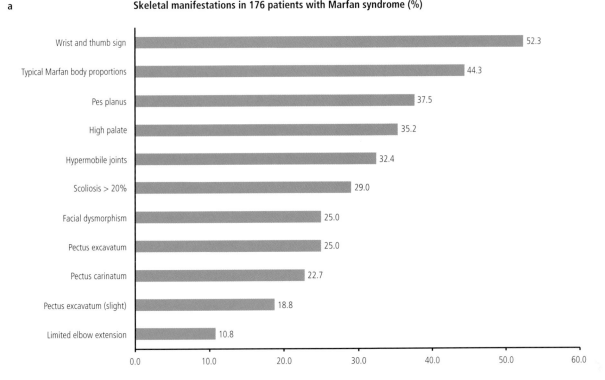

b

Extraskeletal manifestations in 176 patients with Marfan syndrome

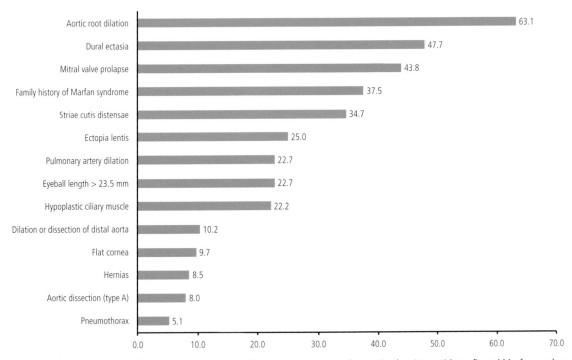

Fig. 2.1-19a, b The frequency of typical Marfan manifestations in 176 consecutively examined patients with confirmed Marfan syndrome, classified by skeletal manifestations (**a**) and extraskeletal manifestations (**b**) in the group studied by Sheikhzadeh et al. (2011a).

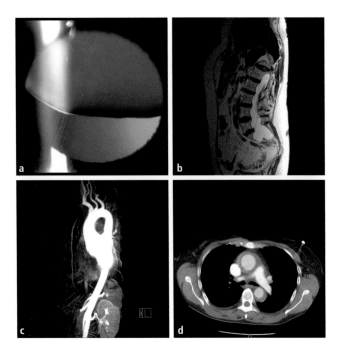

Fig. 2.1-20a–d Typical imaging findings in Marfan syndrome. (**a**) The slit-lamp examination shows the left eye in a Marfan patient in whom the lens has dislocated in an upper temporal direction. Dilated zonular fibers of the suspensory ligament of the lens are visible at the lower edge of the lens. (**b**) The magnetic resonance image (MRI) of the lumbosacral joint in a patient with classic Marfan syndrome shows marked dural ectasia, which in an erect posture is usually particularly clear in the distal region of the dural sac, due to hydrostatic pressure in the cerebrospinal fluid (Sheikhzadeh et al. 2011b; Habermann et al. 2005). (**c**) The contrast MRI of the entire aorta shows typical Marfan aortic pathology with a clear, pear-shaped distension of the aortic root but a normal-caliber aorta in the arch and descending thoracic and abdominal parts of the vessel. (**d**) The contrast computed tomogram taken due to acute chest pain shows acute intramural hemorrhage marked by acute bleeding into the middle layer of the aortic wall, seen here in both the ascending and descending aorta and often leading to progression of the classic aortic dissection and development of a false lumen in the aortic wall. When there is intramural hemorrhage with involvement of the ascending aorta, emergency surgery is indicated in the same way as in a classic aortic dissection (Hiratzka et al. 2010; von Kodolitsch et al. 2003).

2.1.9.3   Differential diagnoses

Typical reasons for a suspicion of Marfan syndrome include an aortic aneurysm or aortic dissection in young adults, manifestations of Marfan in a patient's family, connective-tissue weakness or hypermobility in the extremities and Marfan-like skeletal manifestations (Fig. 2.1-21). Interestingly, Marfan syndrome is only actually confirmed in 28% of individuals with skeletal changes, while the confirmation rate in patients with suspicious eye manifestations is 70% and in those with a positive family history it is 44% (Fig. 2.1-21). Overall, the tentative diagnosis is only confirmed in approximately half of patients with suspected Marfan syndrome. Despite this, Marfan-like changes may also be seen in patients in whom the syndrome has been "excluded" (Fig. 2.1-22). It is extremely important to be unsatisfied with a diagnosis of "Marfan syndrome excluded" in these patients and to conduct a search for other differential diagnoses. Figure 2.1-22 shows the alternative syndromes which are diagnosed and their relative frequency. These syndromes are described below.

Other FBN1-associated diseases

The range of diseases that can be caused by mutations in the area of the *FBN1* gene is very wide, ranging from neonatal Marfan syndrome, with an average life expectancy of less than 1 year, to a Marfan-like appearance that is not associated with aortic disease or with any reduction in life expectancy. Only a few forms of isolated thoracic aneurysms and dissections (i.e., with no other extra-aortic manifestations) are associated with *FBN1*. The mitral valve, aorta, skin and skeletal features (MASS) phenotype is a mild form of manifestation of Marfan syndrome. Mitral valve prolapse syndrome is associated with Marfan-like skeletal manifestations, but mutations in the *FBN1* gene and aortic disease have not yet been reported with it. Particularly in pediatric groups of patients, Shprintzen–Goldberg syndrome and Weill–Marchesani syndrome are diagnosed in association with *FNB1* gene mutations. *Aortic phenotype:* the MASS phenotype should not show any progression in the dilation of the aortic bulb, while in neonatal Marfan syndrome aortic dissections are already noted at the intrauterine stage.

Loeys–Dietz syndrome (LDS)

Loeys and Dietz have described a Marfan-like syndrome caused by mutations in the *TGFBR1/2* genes, showing aortic disease with syndromal changes that differ clearly from Marfan syndrome in both the aortic and extra-aortic findings (Fig. 2.1-23). Type 1 Loeys–Dietz syndrome is characterized by cardiovascular, craniofacial, neurocognitive and skeletal manifestations (Mizuguchi et al. 2004). The cardinal craniofacial symptoms consist of hypertelorism, cleft palate, cleft or wide uvula, blue sclera and craniosynostosis. Rare manifestations include atrial septal defect, patent ductus arteriosus, type 1 Arnold–Chiari malformation, hydrocephalus, developmental retardation and club foot (Loeys et al. 2005). Type 2 Loeys–Dietz syndrome was first described in 2006 in patients with mutations in the *TGFBR1* and *TGFBR2* genes who met the clinical criteria for vascular Ehlers–Danlos syndrome, but without having the changes in type III collagen typical of that syndrome. Type 2 Loeys–Dietz syndrome is characterized by the development of arterial aneurysms, hypermobility and at least two additional symptoms that are typical for vascular Ehlers–Danlos syndrome such as intestinal rupture in the viscera, uterine rupture particularly during pregnancy, translucent, silky, brittle, or hyperelastic skin, and atrophic cicatricial tissue. *Aortic phenotype:* although more than 80% of the affected patients develop aneurysms in the proximal aorta in type 1 and 2 Loeys–Dietz syndrome, there are also often aneurysms in the distal aorta, in side branches of the aorta, in the cervical arteries or head—in contrast to Marfan syndromes. An additional feature of Loeys–Dietz syndrome is pathological elongation and tortuosity in the arteries. Furthermore, the age of manifestation of Loeys–Dietz syndromes is lower, acute vascular complications are located in multiple vascular regions and the risk of rupture and dissection does not depend on the diameter of the aorta.

Aneurysm–osteoarthritis syndrome (AOS)

The clinical presentation of this aortic syndrome is similar to that of Loeys–Dietz syndrome, and it is caused by mutations in the *SMAD3* gene. There are mild signs of craniofacial dysmorphia bifid uvula,

Reasons for suspected Marfan syndrome in 300 patients

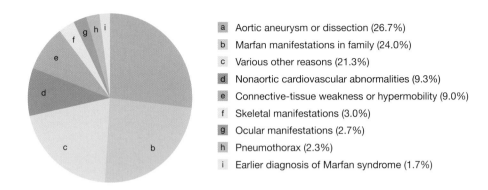

a | Aortic aneurysm or dissection (26.7%)
b | Marfan manifestations in family (24.0%)
c | Various other reasons (21.3%)
d | Nonaortic cardiovascular abnormalities (9.3%)
e | Connective-tissue weakness or hypermobility (9.0%)
f | Skeletal manifestations (3.0%)
g | Ocular manifestations (2.7%)
h | Pneumothorax (2.3%)
i | Earlier diagnosis of Marfan syndrome (1.7%)

a

Percentage confirmation of Marfan syndrome per reason for suspicion

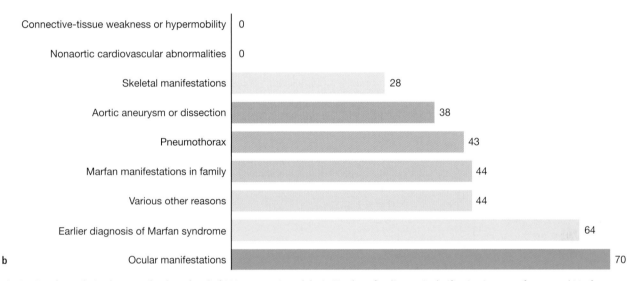

b

Fig. 2.1-21a, b Analysis of reasons for the referral of 300 consecutive adults in Hamburg for diagnostic clarification in cases of suspected Marfan syndrome. The methods with which these data were obtained are described in Sheikhzadeh et al. (2011a). (**a**) The reasons why the referring physicians raised a suspicion of Marfan syndrome. (**b**) The relative frequency with which the diagnosis was actually confirmed in patients with a specific reason for suspected Marfan syndrome. It is notable that "signs of connective-tissue weakness or joint hypermobility" and patients with "typical Marfan skeletal manifestations" were rarely in fact found to have Marfan syndrome.

skeletal changes resembling those in Marfan syndrome, dural ectasia, involvement of the inner organs and skin changes (van de Laar et al. 2011). Osteoarthritides are typical in this syndrome and are not observed in the other aortic syndromes. In addition to vascular complications, mitral valve diseases, pulmonary valve stenoses, septal defects, and patent ductus arteriosus may occur. *Aortic phenotype:* aneurysms and dissection mainly occur in the aortic root, but can also develop in all of the other vascular segments of the aorta and extra-aortic arteries. The arteries also often have a severely tortuous course.

Vascular Ehlers–Danlos syndrome (VEDS)

The Ehlers–Danlos syndromes are diseases of connective tissue that are characterized by increased elasticity in the skin, hypermobility in the joints and involvement of internal organs (Beighton et al. 1998). The vascular form of Ehlers–Danlos syndrome is caused by mutations in the type 3 collagen gene *(COL3A1)*. *Aortic phenotype:*

aortic complications occur starting from the mid-20s onward and often affect the aortic arch, descending aorta and abdominal aorta. Dissections and ruptures of the medium-sized arteries often occur. Aortic ruptures during pregnancy and intraoperative complications during vascular procedures are also frequent.

Bicuspid aortic valve disease (BAVD)

Isolated bicuspid aortic valve disease is a relatively frequent cause of aortic dissection (Homme et al. 2006). Aortic dissection associated with the bicuspid aortic valve usually affects relatively young patients with no other cardiovascular risk factors. Bicuspid aortic valve disease is one of the most frequent forms of cardiovascular malformation, with a prevalence of around 1–2%. There is an increased risk of aortic stenosis and aortic insufficiency, infectious endocarditis and aortic dissection. *NOTCH1* mutations are only identified as the cause of the disease in a small proportion of the families affected. Aortic phenotype: in contrast to Marfan syn-

No. of Marfan-typical manifestations (Ghent 1) in 300 patients with suspected Marfan syndrome

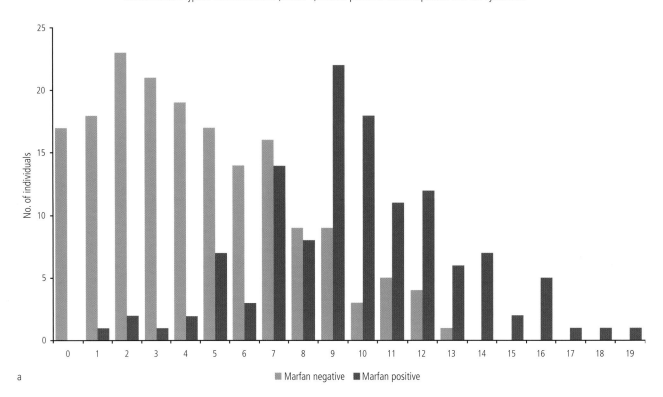

a   ■ Marfan negative ■ Marfan positive

Final diagnosis in 300 patients with suspected Marfan syndrome (%)

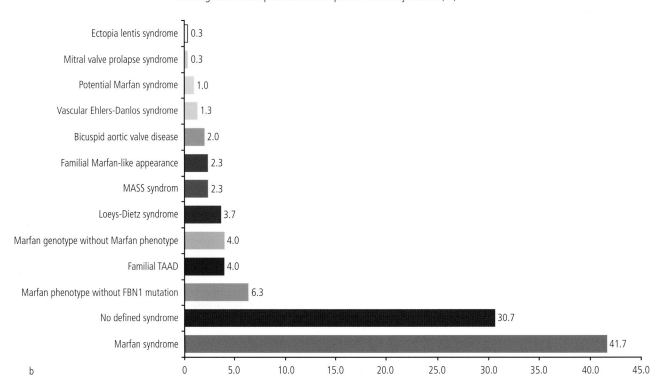

Fig. 2.1-22a, b Typical manifestations of Marfan syndrome per person according to the Ghent-1 classification (De Paepe et al. 1996). As discussed in detail by Sheikzadeh et al. (2011a), 300 adults with suspected Marfan syndrome were examined. (**a**) It was found that a considerable proportion of the patients in whom Marfan syndrome was excluded had a large number of typical Marfan manifestations. (**b**) The range of final diagnoses in these 300 adults.

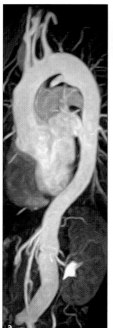
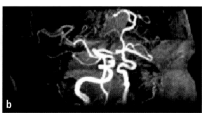
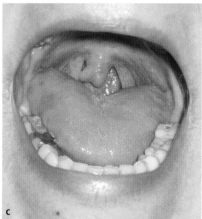

Fig. 2.1-23a–c Typical findings in Loeys–Dietz syndrome that should raise doubts regarding a diagnosis of "Marfan syndrome." (**a**) Contrast magnetic resonance angiography shows a typical Loeys–Dietz aorta. Although the pear-shaped distension of the aortic root is indistinguishable from aortic pathology in Marfan patients, a patent ductus arteriosus is also visible here, which is atypical in Marfan syndrome. In addition, the abdominal aorta has been replaced with a tubular prosthesis from the renal arteries downward. The development of aneurysms in the abdominal aorta is atypical in Marfan patients. (**b**) The CT angiography in a patient with confirmed Loeys–Dietz syndrome shows noticeable elongation and contortion in the cerebral vessels. (**c**) The discretely bifid uvula shown here was noticed during the clinical examination and raised a suspicion of Loeys–Dietz syndrome, which was confirmed by evidence of a mutation in the *TGFBR2* gene.

drome, a bicuspid aortic valve with stenosis leads to dilation of the ascending aorta above the sinotubular junction. In cases of insufficiency, Marfan-like dilation of the aortic root may occur, and in rare cases aneurysm formation is possible even without stenosis or insufficiency in the aortic valve (Aydin et al. 2011a). Aortic changes distal to the proximal aorta are typical, particularly when there is a simultaneous aortic isthmus stenosis. Aneurysms can also form after successful replacement of the aortic valve or aortic coarctation repair (Aydin et al. 2011b, 2002; Cotrufo and Della Corte 2009).

Extremely rare hereditary thoracic aortic aneurysms and dissections (TAADs)

There is no established definition of what TAADs should include. We would use it to cover all of the very rare (prevalence in the general population ≤ 1 per 100,000) monogenic aortic diseases that occur with or without syndromally defined extra-aortic manifestations (von Kodolitsch et al. 2010; Milewicz et al. 2008). The syndromal aortic diseases include dermatochalasis (cutis laxa), caused by mutations in the *FBLN4* gene; arterial tortuosity syndrome, caused by mutations in the *GLUT10* gene and TAAD with patent ductus arteriosus, caused by mutations in the *MYH11* gene. TAAD due to mutations in the *ACTA2* gene is associated with marked livedo reticularis and early occurrence of coronary heart disease. Aortic phe-

notype: depending on the gene involved, this may vary widely. In TAAD associated with *ACTA2* gene mutations, dissections occur in both the proximal and distal aorta, but the overall aortic prognosis is similar to that in Marfan syndrome.

2.1.9.4   Diagnosis

Diagnosis of Marfan syndrome

A revised version of the classification, intended to allow easier diagnosis, has been available since 2010 (Table 2.1-4) (Sheikhzadeh et al. 2011a; Loeys et al. 2010). In patients who do not have a confirmed family history of Marfan syndrome, the syndrome is diagnosed if there is evidence of aortic dilation with ectopia lentis or with a causative *FBN1* mutation, or with a systemic score ≥ 7 points (Loeys et al. 2010). Evidence of ectopia lentis with an *FBN1* mutation known to be the cause of aortic disease is not sufficient to confirm a diagnosis of Marfan syndrome. If there is a family history including confirmed Marfan syndrome, the diagnosis of Marfan is confirmed if there is evidence of aortic dilation or a systemic score ≥ 7 points or ectopia lentis. The systemic score and criteria for a causative *FBN1* mutation are specified in the revised Ghent classification (Loeys et al. 2010). Marfan syndrome should not be diagnosed without excluding the clinical signs of alternative diagnoses. The revised Ghent classification provides a list of the criteria (Table 1.2-5).

Diagnosis of alternative aortic syndromes

From our point of view, three diagnostic rules need to be observed. Since Marfan syndrome is by far the most frequent cause of genetically determined aortic syndromes and many of its extra-aortic manifestations also occur in other aortic syndromes, the first rule is, when there is a suspicion of a genetically caused aortic disease, that one must always evaluate whether the clinical criteria for Marfan syndrome are present. If extra-aortic signs of Marfan syndrome are present in addition to thoracic aortic disease, sequencing of the *FBN1* gene should be carried out primarily. If the evaluation shows typical manifestations of alternative aortic syndromes, then—particularly if they are typical of Loeys–Dietz syndrome—sequencing of the *TGFBR1/2* genes or *SMAD3* gene should be carried out first, or other alternatives should be considered if there are relevant clinical signs (see Table 2.1-5 and Fig. 2.1-24). The introduction of next-generation sequencing technology is likely to lead to the establishment of a sequencing strategy that allows diagnosis of all the typical genes responsible for aortic diseases (Baetens et al. 2011).

Another diagnostic rule is that a specific aortic syndrome should not be diagnosed, even if there is evidence of a gene sequence change in one of the potentially causative genes, unless the relevant phenotypic criteria are met. This has been firmly established for Marfan syndrome for a long time and is regulated by internationally recognized classifications (Loeys et al. 2010; De Paepe et al. 1996). The current Ghent classification also defines diagnostic criteria for MASS syndrome, ectopia lentis syndrome and mitral valve prolapse syndrome (Loeys et al. 2010). By contrast, vascular Ehlers–Danlos syndrome is diagnosed using the criteria set out in the revised Villefranche classification (Beighton et al. 1998). The diagnostic signs of Loeys–Dietz syndrome are listed in the new Ghent classification (Table 2.1-5) (Loeys et al. 2010), while the presence of aneurysm–osteoarthritis

Table 2.1-4 Diagnosis of Marfan syndrome according to the criteria of the revised Ghent classification (Loeys et al. 2010).

A diagnosis of Marfan syndrome is made with the following findings:	
A No confirmed family history of Marfan syndrome:	
1. Aortic root dilation (Z ≥ 2) or aortic dissection and lens luxation[1]	
2. Aortic root dilation (Z ≥ 2) or aortic dissection and *FBN1* mutation	
3. Aortic root dilation (Z ≥ 2) or aortic dissection and systemic involvement (≥ 7 points)[1]	
4. Lens luxation and *FBN1* mutation previously noted in an individual with aortic dilation	
B At least one relative meeting one of the four criteria above independently of the individual being examined (positive family history):	
5. Positive family history and lens luxation	
6. Positive family history and systemic involvement (≥ 7 points)[1]	
7. Positive family history and aortic root dilation (Z ≥ 2 > 20 years, Z ≥ 3 ≤ 20 years)[1]	
C Systemic score[2]:	
Systemic characteristic:	*Score points:*
Positive wrist and thumb sign	3
Positive wrist or thumb sign	1
Pectus carinatum	2
Pectus excavatum or chest asymmetry	1
Talipes valgus	2
Pes planus	1
Pneumothorax	2
Dural ectasia	2
Otto disease (protrusio acetabuli)	2
Reduced leg–body ratio and arm length–height ratio > 1.05 (with exclusion of high-grade scoliosis)[3]	1
Scoliosis or thoracolumbar kyphosis[4]	1
Reduced elbow extension (170° or less)	1
Facial characteristics (at least three of the five signs)[5]	1
Striae cutis distensae	1
Myopia > 3 diopter	1
Mitral valve prolapse	1

1 Requires exclusion of relevant differential-diagnostic clinical signs of Shprintzen–Goldberg syndrome, Loeys–Dietz syndrome, or vascular Ehlers–Danlos syndrome and after *TGFBR1/2* mutation analysis, collagen biochemistry examination and *COL3A1* analysis if indicated (see Table 2.1-5).
2 Systemic involvement is present at ≥ 7 points (maximum 20).
3 The leg–body ratio, measured from the upper edge of the pubis, is considered abnormal from < 1 at an age of 0–5 years, < 0.95 at age 6–7, < 0.9 at age 8–9, and < 0.85 at age ≥ 10 in whites and < 0.78 in blacks.
4 Scoliosis is present with a Cobb angle ≥ 20° or a height difference between the right and left dorsal halves of the chest ≥ 1.5 cm when the patient is leaning forward.
5 Signs of facial dysmorphia are dolichocephalism, enophthalmos, laterally sloping eyelid axes, malar hypoplasia and retrognathism.
Z = Aortic root Z score.

syndrome has to be tested using the phenotypical abnormalities described in the original publication (van de Laar et al. 2011).
In our experience, there are many patients in whom it is not possible to diagnose a syndrome despite clear evidence of a genetically determined aortic disease. There are also patients who have nucleotide sequence changes in the "aortic genes" who do not have any manifestation of aortic disease. Substantial diagnostic difficulties may arise in chil-

dren in particular, as many extra-aortic and cardiovascular changes have age-dependent manifestations. In addition, there are no established criteria for recording many signs of dysmorphia and assessing aortic changes, therefore clinical experience is vital. Due to multiple-organ involvement in many syndromes, collaboration between several medical disciplines is always essential. A third diagnostic rule should be that diagnostic assessment of patients with genetically determined

Table 2.1-5 Clinical signs relevant to the differential diagnosis in the revised Ghent classification (Loeys et al. 2010).

Differential diagnosis	Gene	Clinical signs
Loeys–Dietz syndrome (LDS)	TGFBR1/2	Cleft palate/bifid uvula, arterial tortuosity, hypertelorism, diffuse aortic and arterial aneurysms, craniosynostosis, talipes equinovarus, unstable cervical vertebrae, silky and brittle skin, bleeding tendency
Shprintzen–Goldberg syndrome (SGS)	FBN1 and others	Craniosynostosis, mental retardation
Congenital contractural arachnodactyly (CCA)	FBN2	Wrinkled ears, contractures
Weill–Marchesani syndrome (WMS)	FBN1, ADAMTS10	Microspherophakia, brachydactyly, stiff joints
Ectopia lentis syndrome (ELS)	FBN1, LTBP2, ADAMTSL4	Exclusion of aortic dilation
Homocystinuria	CBS	Thromboses, mental retardation
Familial thoracic aortic aneurysm (FTAA) syndrome	TGFBR1/2, ACTA2	Exclusion of marfanoid skeletal manifestations, livedo reticularis, iris flocculi
FTAA with bicuspid aortic valve (BAV)		
FTAA with patent ductus arteriosus (PDA)	MYH11	
Arterial tortuosity syndrome (ATS)	SLC2A10	Generalized arterial tortuosity, arterial stenoses, facial dysmorphia
Ehlers–Danlos syndromes (vascular, valvular, kyphoscoliotic types)	COL3A1, COL1A2, PLOD1	Aneurysms in the medium-sized arteries, severe cardiac valvular regurgitation, translucent skin, atrophic scars, facial characteristics

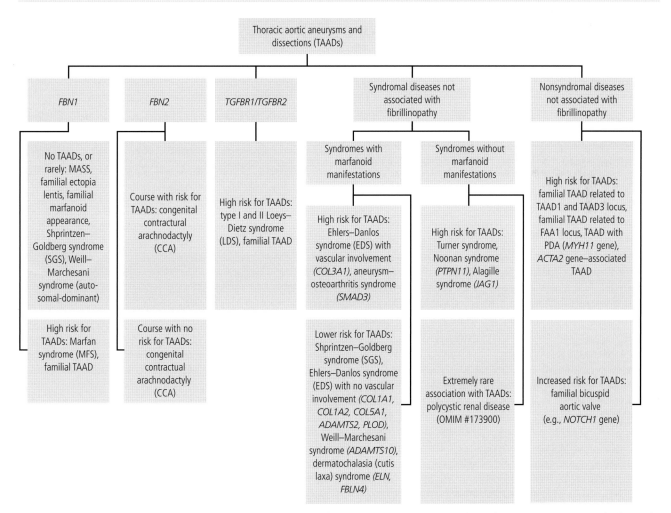

Fig. 2.1-24 Diagram of the differential diagnosis in patients with thoracic aortic aneurysms and dissections (TAADs) with a suspected genetic background. The involvement of a specific gene regarded as being causative of TAADs in principle makes it possible to develop specific phenotypes, which are shown in the diagram under each gene. The arrangement of the various syndromes runs from left to right according to declining phenotypic similarity with Marfan syndrome, and on the right shows the TAADs that typically occur without any extravascular manifestations (von Kodolitsch and Robinson 2007). Abbreviations are explained in the text.

aortic diseases should take place in specialized centers (von Kodolitsch et al. 2002). These centers are approved in Germany as part of "out-patient hospital treatment" (Book V, Para. 116b of the German Social Code) (Bekanntmachungen 2007). This regulation permits specialized hospitals to carry out comprehensive diagnosis, including gene sequencing, while approximately covering costs (Manow et al. 2010).

2.1.9.5   Treatment

Conservative treatment

The principles used in the medical management of Marfan syndrome have hardly changed during the last 25 years (Pyeritz and McKusick 1979). From the internal-medicine and cardiology point of view, there are five important measures (von Kodolitsch et al. 2008): 1, detailed consultation with the patient regarding lifestyle adjustments and planning for ways of living with moderate impairment of physical activities; 2, administering prophylactic antibiotic treatment against endocarditis; 3, serial cardiological examinations including tomographic assessment of the aorta and if appropriate serial ophthalmological and orthopedic check-ups; 4, prescribing a β-blocker for protection of the aorta; and 5, prophylactic replacement of the aortic root in accordance with the current criteria (Table 2.1-6).

Adults with Marfan syndrome should avoid emotional stress and dynamic exercise such as that involved in running, tennis or volleyball with preference for static exercise such as weightlifting, water-skiing or gymnastics, as dynamic exercise can lead to moderate blood-pressure increases. Contact sport and activities that lead to too-rapid acceleration or abrupt deceleration of movement sequences such as soccer, martial arts, or basketball should be avoided, as should scuba diving with oxygen apparatus or amateur flying in planes that lack pressurized cabins. However, diving with a snorkel and flying in pressurized commercial aircraft are possible without any problems. With regard to competitive sports, participation in billiards, cricket, curling, golf, bowling and sports shooting is possible. With children, the focus is on setting life goals for adulthood that take into account the impaired health resulting from Marfan syndrome, while strict bans on sports are not generally required (von Kodolitsch et al. 2008; von Kodolitsch and Rybczynski 2006). Detailed and individualized counseling for patients with Marfan syndrome is particularly important. In our view, this should include not only detailed discussions but also mention of published self-help guides for patients (Marfan Hilfe [Deutschland] e.V. 2007); information about the support provided by Marfan Hilfe Deutschland e.V. (see http://www.marfan.de/) has also proved helpful.

According to the current guidelines, endocarditis prophylaxis should only be considered if patients have already developed endocarditis or have received an artificial cardiac valve or have valvulopathy after heart transplantation (Wilson et al. 2007). Among 1000 patients with Marfan syndrome, 15 will develop mitral valve endocarditis up to the age of 35 and 84 will develop it by the age of 60 (Rybczynski 2010). The risk of endocarditis in Marfan patients is thus much higher than in patients with idiopathic mitral valve prolapse, for example (Avierinos et al. 2002). In the opinion of experts, endocarditis prophylaxis is therefore also indicated, in addition to the information given in the official guidelines, if the native cardiac valve shows signs of any dysfunction, frequently in the form of aortic or mitral valve insufficiency (von Kodolitsch et al. 2008).

Table 2.1-6 Classic principles of medical management in patients with Marfan syndrome (von Kodolitsch and Robinson 2007).

General measures in adults with Marfan syndrome
Moderate restriction of physical activity
Endocarditis prophylaxis*
Echocardiography and MR angiography of the aorta at annual intervals
β-blockers to protect the aorta
Measures during family planning and pregnancy
Providing information about the 50% risk of inheritance of Marfan syndrome by children
High-risk pregnancy in patients with aortic root diameter > 40 mm or status post heart surgery and cases of severe heart disease
When pregnancy is planned in women with an aortic root diameter ≥ 40 mm, prophylactic replacement of the aortic root should be carried out
Serial (e.g., 3-monthly) echocardiographic check-ups for up to 3 months after delivery
Indication for prophylactic replacement of the aortic root in adults (≥ one criterion)
Aortic root diameter ≥ 45 mm
Aortic ratio ≥ 1.5 (normal size, i.e., 20–37 mm divided by actual measurement, corrected by age, gender and body surface area)
Ratio for diameter of aortic root and descending aorta ≥ 2
Increase in diameter of aortic root ≥ 5 mm/year
Indication for prophylactic replacement of the aortic root in children
The operation should be delayed if possible until completion of growth
Assessment of the aortic root diameter is based on the criteria for adults
Aortic root diameters above the upper confidence intervals move further upward during the course of echocardiographic check-ups
Indication for mitral valve surgery
The indication is established in accordance with the current AHA recommendations

* In addition to the indications given in the current AHA guideline recommendations, the view of experts is that endocarditis prophylaxis should be carried out in all Marfan patients in whom any relevant dysfunction of the natural cardiac valve has been diagnosed (von Kodolitsch et al. 2008).

Drug treatment for protection of the aorta previously consisted exclusively of β-blocker administration. The effectiveness of this has been confirmed in a prospective and randomized study which demonstrated a slowing in the rate of aortic root dilation in pediatric patients (Shores et al. 1994). However, animal experiments have shown that angiotensin II receptor blockers such as losartan and matrix metalloproteinase inhibitors also have stabilizing effects on the metabolism of the aortic wall (Habashi et al. 2006). A large study in the United States is therefore currently testing whether the protective effect of losartan on the aorta is superior to the effects of β-blockers in patients with Marfan syndrome.

Pregnancy

There is thought to be a high risk of aortic complications during pregnancy in Marfan patients. According to the current guidelines, the risk of aortic rupture or aortic dissection during pregnancy must be regarded as high if the diameter of the aortic root is ≥ 40 mm or an aortic dissection has already occurred beforehand (Hiratzka et al. 2010). Several authors have reported an increased risk only from 45 mm upwards (Meijbook et al. 2005). Women at increased risk who wish to have children should be advised against pregnancy, or prophylactic aortic root replacement should be discussed with them.

Surgical treatment

The improved life expectancy in patients with Marfan syndrome is mainly achieved by prophylactic replacement of the aortic root, which prevents spontaneous rupture or dissection of the aortic root. The standard operation on a typical aorta with Marfan changes until recently consisted of complete replacement of the aortic root with a valve-bearing conduit (Gott et al. 1999a). The Bentall technique or several of its variants were used in this procedure (von Kodolitsch et al. 1998).

There are two important trends in aortic root surgery for Marfan patients. Firstly, the criteria for prophylactic replacement of the aortic root have become increasingly generous during the last 25 years and the current criterion is a diameter ≥ 45 mm. Continuing improvements in the results, with very low mortality rates in elective operations, have played a role in this, along with a recognition that even slightly dilated aortae with a diameter of 40–45 mm involve a risk of acute complications, while the postoperative course in patients who have survived an aortic dissection is in principle associated with higher complication rates and a poorer quality of life (von Kodolitsch et al. 2008; Gott et al. 1999b).

Secondly, the view is currently becoming accepted that the conduit operation with complete replacement of the aortic root must not be regarded as the standard operation; instead, the primary aim should be to achieve a valve-preserving reconstruction of the aortic root. This changed approach has also been reflected in the current guidelines (Hiratzka et al. 2010). Valve-preserving surgical techniques are derived from Yacoub, along with a modified technique by David. They both developed techniques for reconstructing the aortic root by preserving the physiological valvular apparatus while still keeping a radical resection of the entire proximal aorta. Yacoub's remodeling techniques have not become established, due to unfavorable long-term results with higher rates of aortic valve insufficiency and therefore reimplantation techniques must currently be regarded as the standard (Fig. 2.1-25). Reconstruction of the aortic root can be carried out with good early and medium-term results, avoiding the disadvantages of valvular replacement with the associated increased risk of thromboembolism and endocarditis (Bernhardt et al. 2011a). The aim in mitral valve surgery is currently to use a valve-preserving approach, and although present experience with mitral valve reconstruction in Marfan patients is not based on a large number of cases, it is highly promising (Gillinov et al. 1994; Bernhardt et al. 2011b).

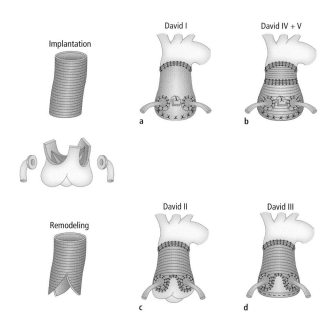

Fig. 2.1-25 In the current variants of the David operation, the aortic tissue is completely excised along the crown-shaped upper annulus of the aortic sinus. The tissue from the aortic sinus, with the valve-bearing tissue, is preserved. However, this approach removes the aortic tissue from the coronary orifices, and reimplantation of the coronaries into the tubular prosthesis that replaces the aorta is therefore an integral component of all David operations. The illustration shows different variants of the David operation, dividing into David I–V types, proposed by Miller (2003). The upper row in the illustration shows the variants of the operation that are described as David reimplantation techniques. The basic principle in these techniques involves suturing the natural valve-bearing sinus into the aortic prosthesis and attaching the aortic prosthesis both to the base of the sinus and along the upper crown-shaped annulus. The David I operation consists of this basic technique. In the David IV and V operations, the ascending aorta is replaced with an additional, narrower tubular prosthesis and the aortic sinus is formed by a wider tubular prosthesis into what is known as a neo-sinus. The lower row in the illustration shows the variants of the operation that are known as David remodeling techniques. The basic variant in this technique is the David II operation, in which as in the Yacoub procedure the upper, crown-shaped annulus of the aortic sinus is directly sutured to a correspondingly trimmed tubular prosthesis. David uses this surgical method only in patients with no dilation of the lower annulus. In the David III variant, the lower annulus is also stabilized externally with a felt strip that is sutured in.

Treatment for other genetically determined aortic diseases

The principles of medical management of genetically determined aortic diseases, excluding Marfan syndrome, are based on the management of Marfan syndrome. However, there are signs that the practical approach used may be starting to diverge from that used in management of Marfan syndrome, depending on the underlying syndrome and the gene mutation causing the condition. These differences mainly affect the indication for surgical intervention, which sometimes used to be very substantial. It will also be conceivable in the future for specific aortic diseases to be treated with drugs in different ways, depending on the pathological mechanism involved (von Kodolitsch et al. 2010; Milewicz et al. 2008). Table 2.1-7 sums up the surgical treatment recommendations that are taylored to a relevant gene defect or the presence of a specific aortic syndrome (Table 2.1-6).

Table 2.1-7 Treatment recommendations for genetically caused aortic diseases (von Kodolitsch et al. 2010).

Disease	Causative gene*	Published recommendations for the treatment of the aortic disease
Syndromal aortic diseases		
Marfan syndrome (MFS)	*FBN1*	See Table 2.1-6
Type 1 Loeys–Dietz syndrome (LDS 1)	LDS 1a: *TGFBR1* LDS 1b: *TGFBR2*	Prophylactic aortic surgery in: Children in whom the diameter of the ascending aorta is > 99th percentile or annulus > 18 mm Adolescents and adults in whom the diameter of the ascending aorta is ≥ 40 mm
Type 2 Loeys–Dietz syndrome (LDS 2)	LDS 2a: *TGFBR1* LDS 2b: *TGFBR2*	Same recommendations as for LDS 1
Vascular Ehlers–Danlos syndrome (VEDS)	*COL3A1, COL1A2, PLOD1*	Due to higher rates of intraoperative and postoperative complications, the indication for surgery should be considered cautiously in patients with unruptured aortic dissections
Ehlers–Danlos syndrome, with periventricular heterotopia	*FLNA* (X-chromosome-linked)	Treatment recommendations have so far only been issued for the treatment of convulsive seizures (Sheen et al. 2005)
Aneurysm–osteoarthritis syndrome (AOS)	*SMAD3*	*SMAD3*-associated aneurysms are aggressive and require early diagnosis, monitoring of the entire arterial system and prophylactic vascular surgery intervention
Arterial tortuosity syndrome (ATS)	*SLC2A10/GLUT10* (autosomal-recessive)	No specific treatment recommendations are so far available
Dermatochalasis (cutis laxa syndrome, CLS)	*FBLN4* (autosomal-recessive)	Patients with CLS require lifelong monitoring for cardiovascular complications (Szabo et al. 2006)
	ELN	Patients with CLS require lifelong monitoring for cardiovascular complications (Szabo et al. 2006)
Turner syndrome (TS)	45,X karyotype (women with complete or partial monosomy in the X chromosome)	Treatment recommendations in the literature: Patients with an aortic anomaly or dilation must be examined regularly by a cardiologist and require blood-pressure adjustment Patients with significant aortic valve dysfunction and dilation of the ascending aorta should undergo surgery Patients with an aortic size index > 2.0 cm/m^2 require tight cardiological monitoring Patients with an aortic size index ≥ 2.5 cm/m^2 have a much higher risk for aortic dissections
Noonan syndrome (NS)	Type 1 NS: *PTPN11*	No specific treatment recommendations are so far available
	KRAS *SOS1*	
Autosomal-dominant polycystic kidney disease (ADPKD)	*PKD1, PKD2*	No specific treatment recommendations are so far available
Osteogenesis imperfecta (OI)	*COL1A1* *COL1A2*	Due to the fragility of the vessels and bleeding tendency, special surgical measures are required, such as reinforcement of every vascular suture
Alagille syndrome (AGS)	*JAG1*	No specific treatment recommendations are so far available
Genetically caused thoracic aortic aneurysms or dissections (TAADs)		
TAAD2 locus	*TGFBR2*	Patients with *TGFBR2* mutation R460 should undergo surgery with aortic diameters of 40–42 mm
TAAD3 locus		No specific treatment recommendations are so far available
TAAD with persistent ductus arteriosus 16p locus	*MYH11*	No specific treatment recommendations are so far available
TAAD4 locus	*ACTA2*	No specific treatment recommendations are so far available

continued on p. 99

Table 2.1-7 Continuation.

Disease	Causative gene*	Published recommendations for the treatment of the aortic disease
Bicuspid aortic valve disease		
	Causative gene unknown	The current European Society of Cardiology (ESC) guidelines make the following recommendations: Elective aortic surgery if the diameter of the ascending aorta is > 50 mm First-degree relatives, even without a bicuspid aortic valve, should undergo echocardiography at regular intervals
	NOTCH1	No specific treatment recommendations are so far available

* Unless otherwise specified, heredity is autosomal-dominant.

Endovascular therapy in genetically determined aortic diseases

Endovascular treatment has become established for nongenetic diseases of the descending aorta and infrarenal aorta, due to the lower rates of perioperative morbidity and mortality in comparison with open surgery (Svensson et al. 2008). However, this basically requires the presence of an undilated, healthy vascular segment in which the radial force of the stent graft can achieve a seal. This prerequisite for safe anchoring of the stent graft is certainly present in Marfan syndrome and other hereditary diseases of the aorta if the end of the stent graft is positioned in a vascular segment that has already been replaced during open surgery. Which segments of the aorta are affected varies so widely with the numerous genetic diseases described above that it is hardly possible to make any general statements regarding the possibility of endovascular treatment. However, implantation of rigid stent grafts, particularly proximal bare stents into the aortic arch should be viewed critically in all patients with genetically determined diseases, since excessive pressures at the stent tips can occur in a highly pulsatile vascular segment and can lead to vascular erosion, dilation and rupture.

The use of stent grafts for endovascular treatment of aneurysmal or dissected aortic segments has not yet been sufficiently investigated in these patients. Only case reports and case series with small numbers of patients have been published, which in summary describe the technical feasibility of the procedure with a low rate of periprocedural mortality, but without any long-term results (Baril et al. 2006; Botta et al. 2009; Geisbusch et al. 2008; Nordon et al. 2009). The published results are also inconsistent with regard to the success of the treatment (Botta et al. 2009). A common feature in the published case series is the high proportion of patients who have undergone previous surgery with replacement of the ascending aorta or aortic arch, presence of distal dissection with dilation of the false lumen and a high rate of secondary interventions (Fig. 2.1-26). With the increasing life expectancy and frequent previous operations in patients with Marfan syndrome, for example, the endovascular treatment options in principle represent an attractive and less invasive alternative.

2.1.9.6 Prospects

The increasingly wide range of different drug-based, surgical and interventional treatment options available is likely to lead to growing differentiation in the criteria for using them. Highly individualized decision-making criteria will apply. Molecular genetics will play a

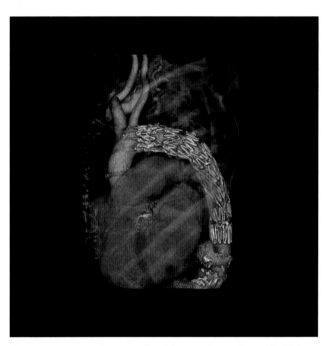

Fig. 2.1-26 Computed tomography of the aorta in a patient with classic Marfan syndrome, showing the prosthesis in the ascending aorta after treatment with a bio-conduit for an aortic root aneurysm with high-grade aortic valve insufficiency when the patient was aged 71. Due to a progressive false-lumen aneurysm with a chronic Stanford type B aortic dissection, with an overall diameter of the aorta of 71 mm, repeat treatment was carried out when the patient was aged 74, with placement of an aortic stent graft following initial stent graft implantation in the aortic arch and descending aorta when the patient was 69. The current CT shows good results with the stent treatment, with successful exclusion of the aneurysm. However, renewed aneurysm formation can be seen at the distal end of the stent graft.

progressively important role here (von Kodolitsch et al. 2010). In addition, with the normalization of life expectancy for the affected patients, the issue of quality of life for young patients will also become paramount. The affected patients want to be able to live with as much freedom from prohibited behaviors as possible and to take part in all aspects of occupational and social life, sports and leisure activities. This area will require further research on care provision and the development of programs for rehabilitating patients with Marfan syndrome and other hereditary aortic diseases.

References

Avierinos JF, Gersh BJ, Melton LJ, 3rd, Bailey KR, Shub C, Nishimura RA, et al. Natural history of asymptomatic mitral valve prolapse in the community. Circulation 2002; 106 (11): 1355–61.

Aydin A, Desai N, Bernhardt AM, Treede H, Detter C, Sheikhzadeh S, et al. Ascending aortic aneurysm and aortic valve dysfunction in bicuspid aortic valve disease. Int J Cardiol 2011a.

Aydin A, Mortensen K, Rybczynski M, Sheikhzadeh S, Willmann S, Bernhardt AM, et al. Central pulse pressure and augmentation index in asymptomatic bicuspid aortic valve disease. Int J Cardiol 2011b; 147(3): 466–8.

Aydin MA, Koschyk DH, Karck M, Cremer J, Haverich A, Berger J, et al. Prädiktoren der Aneurysmaentwicklung nach chirurgischer Korrektur einer Aortenisthmusstenose. Z Kardiol 2002; 91 (Suppl 1): I/338 (A).

Baetens M, Van Laer L, De Leeneer K, Hellemans J, De Schrijver J, Van De Voorde H, et al. Applying massive parallel sequencing to molecular diagnosis of Marfan and Loeys-Dietz syndromes. Medline vom 02.07.2012: Hum Mutat 2011 May 3. doi: 10.1002/humu.21525 [Epub ahead of print].

Baril DT, Carroccio A, Palchik E, Ellozy SH, Jacobs TS, Teodorescu V, et al. Endovascular treatment of complicated aortic aneurysms in patients with underlying arteriopathies. Ann Vasc Surg 2006; 20 (4): 464–71.

Bekanntmachungen. Beschluss des Gemeinsamen Bundesausschusses gem. § 91 Abs. 4 SGB V vom 15. August 2006. Deutsches Ärzteblatt 2007 Januar; 34.

Bernhardt A, Treede H, Rybczynski M, Sheikzadeh S, Detter C, von Kodolitsch Y, et al. Mitral valve surgery in patients with Marfan syndrome. J Thorac Cardiovasc Surg 2011b; under review.

Bernhardt AM, Treede H, Rybczynski M, Sheikhzadeh S, Kersten JF, Meinertz T, et al. Comparison of aortic root replacement in patients with Marfan syndrome. Eur J Cardiothorac Surg 2011a Nov; 40 (5): 1052–7.

Botta L, Russo V, La Palombara C, Rosati M, Di Bartolomeo R, Fattori R. Stent graft repair of descending aortic dissection in patients with Marfan syndrome: an effective alternative to open reoperation? J Thorac Cardiovasc Surg 2009; 138 (5): 1108–14.

Geisbusch P, Kotelis D, von Tengg-Kobligk H, Hyhlik-Durr A, Allenberg JR, Bockler D. Thoracic aortic endografting in patients with connective tissue diseases. J Endovasc Ther 2008; 15 (2): 144–9.

Cotrufo M, Della Corte A. The association of bicuspid aortic valve disease with asymmetric dilatation of the tubular ascending aorta: identification of a definite syndrome. J Cardiovasc Med (Hagerstown) 2009; 10 (4): 291–7.

De Paepe A, Devereux RB, Dietz HC, Hennekam RC, Pyeritz RE. Revised diagnostic criteria for the Marfan syndrome. Am J Med Genet 1996; 62 (4): 417–26.

Gillinov AM, Hulyalkar A, Cameron DE, Cho PW, Greene PS, Reitz BA, et al. Mitral valve operation in patients with the Marfan syndrome. J Thorac Cardiovasc Surg 1994; 107 (3): 724–31.

Gott VL GP, Alejo DE, et al. Replacement of the aortic root in patients with Marfan syndrome. N Engl J Med 1999b; 340: 1307–13.

Gott VL, Greene PS, Alejo DE, Cameron DE, Naftel DC, Miller DC, et al. Replacement of the aortic root in patients with Marfan's syndrome. N Engl J Med 1999a; 340 (17): 1307–13.

Habashi JP, Judge DP, Holm TM, Cohn RD, Loeys BL, Cooper TK, et al. Losartan, an AT1 antagonist, prevents aortic aneurysm in a mouse model of Marfan syndrome. Science 2006; 312: 117–21.

Habermann CR, Weiss F, Schoder V, Cramer MC, Kemper J, Wittkugel O, et al. MR evaluation of dural ectasia in Marfan syndrome: reassessment of the established criteria in children, adolescents, and young adults. Radiology 2005; 234 (2): 535–41.

Hiratzka LF, Bakris GL, Beckman JA, Bersin RM, Carr VF, Casey DE, Jr., et al. 2010 ACCF/AHA/AATS/ACR/ASA/SCA/SCAI/SIR/STS/SVM guidelines for the diagnosis and management of patients with Thoracic Aortic Disease: a report of the American College of Cardiology Foundation/American Heart Association Task Force on Practice Guidelines, American Association for Thoracic Surgery, American College of Radiology, American Stroke Association, Society of Cardiovascular Anesthesiologists, Society for Cardiovascular Angiography and Interventions, Society of Interventional Radiology, Society of Thoracic Surgeons, and Society for Vascular Medicine. Circulation 2010; 121 (13): e266–369.

Homme JL, Aubry MC, Edwards WD, Bagniewski SM, Shane Pankratz V, Kral CA, et al. Surgical pathology of the ascending aorta: a clinicopathologic study of 513 cases. Am J Surg Pathol 2006; 30 (9): 1159–68.

Loeys BL, Chen J, Neptune ER, Judge DP, Podowski M, Holm T, et al. A syndrome of altered cardiovascular, craniofacial, neurocognitive and skeletal development caused by mutations in TGFBR1 or TGFBR2. Nat Genet 2005; 37: 275–81.

Loeys BL, Dietz HC, Braverman AC, Callewaert BL, De Backer J, Devereux RB, et al. The revised Ghent nosology for the Marfan syndrome. J Med Genet 2010; 47 (7): 476–85.

Manow ML, Paulsen N, Rybczynski M, Mir T, Bernhardt AM, Treede H, et al. [Analysis of Costs and Profits of Ambulatory Care of Marfan Patients after Initiation of a Novel German Legal Directive (section sign 116 b SGB V).]. Med Klin (Munich) 2010; 105 (8): 529–37.

Marfan Hilfe (Deutschland) e.V. (Hrsg.). Marfan-Syndrom: Ein Ratgeber für Patienten, Angehörige und Betreuende. Steinkopff Verlag, Darmstadt, 2007.

Meijboom LJ, Vos FE, Timmermans J, Boers GH, Zwinderman AH, Mulder BJ. Pregnancy and aortic root growth in the Marfan syndrome: a prospective study. Eur Heart J 2005; 26(9): 914–20.

Milewicz DM, Guo DC, Tran-Fadulu V, Lafont AL, Papke CL, Inamoto S, et al. Genetic basis of thoracic aortic aneurysms and dissections: focus on smooth muscle cell contractile dysfunction. Annu Rev Genomics Hum Genet 2008; 9: 283–302.

Miller DC. Valve-sparing aortic root replacement in patients with the Marfan syndrome. J Thorac Cardiovasc Surg 2003; 125 (4): 773–8.

Mizuguchi T, Collod-Beroud G, Akiyama T, Abifadel M, Harada N, Morisaki T, et al. Heterozygous TGFBR2 mutations in Marfan syndrome. Nat Genet 2004; 36: 855–60.

Nordon IM, Hinchliffe RJ, Holt PJ, Morgan R, Jahangiri M, Loftus IM, et al. Endovascular management of chronic aortic dissection in patients with Marfan syndrome. J Vasc Surg 2009; 50 (5): 987–91.

Pyeritz RE, McKusick VA. The Marfan syndrome: diagnosis and management. N Engl J Med 1979; 300: 772–7.

Rybczynski M, Mir TS, Sheikhzadeh S, Bernhardt AM, Schad C, Treede H, et al. Frequency and Age-Related Course of Mitral Valve Dysfunction in the Marfan Syndrome. Am J Cardiol 2010; 106 (7): 1048–53.

Sheen VL, Jansen A, Chen MH, Parrini E, Morgan T, Ravenscroft R, et al. Filamin A mutations cause periventricular heterotopia with Ehlers-Danlos syndrome. Neurology 2005; 64 (2): 254–62.

Sheikhzadeh S, Kade C, Keyser B, Stuhrmann M, Arslan-Kirchner M, Rybczynski M, et al. Analysis of phenotype and genotype information for the diagnosis of Marfan syndrome. Clin Genet 2011a; in press.

Sheikhzadeh S, Rybczynski M, Habermann CR, Bernhardt AM, Arslan-Kirchner M, Keyser B, et al. Dural ectasia in individuals with Marfan-like features but exclusion of mutations in the genes FBN1, TGFBR1 and TGFBR2. Clin Genet 2011b; 79 (6): 568–74.

Shores J, Berger KR, Murphy EA, Pyeritz RE. Progression of aortic dilatation and benefit of long-term β-adrenergic blockade in Marfan's syndrome. N Engl J Med 1994; 330: 1335–41.

Silverman DI, Burton KJ, Gray J, Bosner MS, Kouchoukos NT, Roman MJ, et al. Life expectancy in the Marfan syndrome. Am J Cardiol 1995; 75: 157–60.

Svensson LG, Kouchoukos NT, Miller DC, Bavaria JE, Coselli JS, Curi MA, et al. Expert consensus document on the treatment of descending thoracic aortic disease using endovascular stent-grafts. Ann Thorac Surg 2008; 85 (1 Suppl): S1–41.

Szabo Z, Crepeau MW, Mitchell AL, Stephan MJ, Puntel RA, Yin Loke K, et al. Aortic aneurysmal disease and cutis laxa caused by defects in the elastin gene. J Med Genet 2006; 43 (3): 255–8.

van de Laar IM, Oldenburg RA, Pals G, Roos-Hesselink JW, de Graaf BM, Verhagen JM, et al. Mutations in SMAD3 cause a syndromic form of aortic aneurysms and dissections with early-onset osteoarthritis. Nat Genet 2011 Feb; 43 (2): 121–6 [Epub 2011 Jan 9].

Beighton P, De Paepe A, Steinmann B, Tsipouras P, Wenstrup RJ. Ehlers-Danlos syndromes: revised nosology, Villefranche, 1997. Ehlers-Danlos National Foundation (USA) and Ehlers-Danlos Support Group (UK). Am J Med Genet 1998; 77 (1): 31–7.

von Kodolitsch Y, Arslan-Kirchner M, Vogler M, Rybczynski M. Das Marfan-Syndrom – eine Übersicht. Internistische Praxis 2008; 48: 233–47.

von Kodolitsch Y, Csösz K, Koschyk DH, et al. Intramural hematoma of the aorta: predictors of progression to dissection and rupture. Circulation 2003; 107: 1158–63.

von Kodolitsch Y, Raghunath M, Karck M, Haverich A, Nienaber CA. The Marfan syndrome: therapeutic approach to cardiovascular manifestations. Z Kardiol 1998; 87: 173–84.

von Kodolitsch Y, Robinson PN. Marfan syndrome: an update of genetics, medical and surgical management. Heart 2007; 93 (6): 755–60.

von Kodolitsch Y, Rybczynski M, Bernhardt A, Mir TS, Treede H, Dodge-Khatami A, et al. Marfan syndrome and the evolving spectrum of heritable thoracic aortic disease: Do we need genetics for clinical decisions? VASA 2010; 39 (1): 17–32.

von Kodolitsch Y, Rybczynski M, Detter C, Robinson PN. Diagnosis and management of Marfan syndrome. Future Cardiol 2008; 4 (1): 85–96.

von Kodolitsch Y, Rybczynski M, Trivic V, Hofmann T, Meinertz T. In Kompetenzzentren behandeln: Lebensqualität und Lebenserwartung beim Marfan-Syndrom verbessern. Klinikarzt 2002; 31: 201–6.

von Kodolitsch Y, Rybczynski M. Marfan-Syndrom: Sport und Fitness. In: Marfan-Syndrom. Ein Ratgeber für Patienten, Angehörige und Betreuende. Herausgeber: Marfan Hilfe (Deutschland) e.V. Steinkopff Verlag, Darmstadt, 2006.

Wilson W, Taubert KA, Gewitz M, Lockhart PB, Baddour LM, Levison M, et al. Prevention of infective endocarditis: guidelines from the American Heart Association: a guideline from the American Heart Association Rheumatic Fever, Endocarditis, and Kawasaki Disease Committee, Council on Cardiovascular Disease in the Young, and the Council on Clinical Cardiology, Council on Cardiovascular Surgery and Anesthesia, and the Quality of Care and Outcomes Research Interdisciplinary Working Group. Circulation 2007; 116 (15): 1736–54.

2.1.10 Adults with congenital aortic isthmus stenosis

Marcus Rebel, Ali Dodge-Khatami, Ali Aydin, Yskert von Kodolitsch

2.1.10.1 Clinical pictures and epidemiology

Congenital aortic isthmus stenosis is also known as aortic coarctation and is a classic clinical picture in pediatric medicine. In most cases, adults with congenital aortic isthmus stenosis have undergone surgical correction while they were children. However, adults with corrected aortic isthmus stenosis have a number of medical problems and a first diagnosis of aortic isthmus stenosis is often only made in adults. This section aims to describe the specific vascular-medicine problems that arise in adults with corrected aortic isthmus stenosis or with a late first diagnosis of the condition. This approach is in accordance with current efforts to treat the situation faced by adults with congenital cardiac defects as a separate medical challenge (Schmaltz et al. 2008).

Aortic isthmus stenosis is defined as a congenital narrowing of the aorta in the area of the distal aortic arch, up to the start of the thoracic aorta at the level of the origin of the left subclavian artery and orifice of the ductus arteriosus; the isthmus is a physiological narrowing of the aorta in this area. The ductus arteriosus is the fetal "diversion" of the pulmonary circulation and links the pulmonary trunk with the aorta; within a few days to weeks of birth, it closes physiologically and regresses to a connective-tissue structure, the ligamentum arteriosum.

With an incidence of 0.2–0.6 per 1000 live births, aortic isthmus stenosis represents 5–8% of all congenital cardiac defects (Brickner et al. 2000; Krieger and Stout 2010). Boys are affected approximately twice as often as girls. The location of the aortic isthmus stenosis is postductal in 75% of cases, while 25% are in preductal locations. The classification of aortic isthmus stenosis into pediatric and adult anatomic forms is now no longer used, as the two types of anatomy occur without any strict age-dependence. Aortic isthmus stenosis is often associated with other congenital malformations; bicuspid aortic valve, patent ductus arteriosus, and cardiac septal defects are the most frequent (Table 2.1-8).

No familial predisposition is present in many patients with aortic isthmus stenosis. In familial cases, there is usually multifactorial inheritance, and autosomal-dominant inheritance is reported more rarely. A family has been described in which aortic isthmus stenoses were inherited over four generations, probably with an autosomal-dominant mode of inheritance, and a high degree of gene penetrance with variable phenotype expression was observed (Beekman and Robinow 1985). Aortic isthmus stenoses often occur in the context of complex syndromes, with Turner syndrome being the one most frequently associated with aortic isthmus stenosis (Table 2.1-9).

There are two hypotheses regarding the cause of aortic isthmus stenosis. In the hemodynamic hypothesis, it is assumed that aortic isthmus stenosis develops on a localized shelf on the posterior wall of the aorta opposite the orifice of the ductus arteriosus. When the ductus arteriosus closes, an obstruction gradually develops in the area of the duct's orifice ("juxtaductal"), leading to increased resistance (Rudolph et al. 1972). This theory above all explains isthmus stenoses in defects involving left ventricular obstruction such as bicuspid aortic valve, mitral stenosis and subaortic stenosis. However, it does not explain all forms of aortic isthmus stenosis, and in particular does not account for isolated aortic isthmus stenosis with no intracardiac malformations. By contrast, Skoda considered as long ago as 1855 that scattered ductal tissue was responsible for the development of aortic isthmus stenosis. This hypothesis has in the meantime been confirmed by histological analyses (Fig. 2.1-27) (Ho and Anderson 1979). More recent discussion has focused on defective development of cells of the neural crest as the cause of isthmus stenosis (Kappetein et al. 1991).

Table 2.1-8 Malformation associated with congenital aortic isthmus stenosis.

Malformation	Frequency in aortic isthmus stenosis (%) (Kappetein et al. 1991; Becker et al. 1970; Beekman et al. 1981; Campbell et al. 1980; Clarkson et al. 1983; Hesslein et al. 1981; Lerberg et al. 1982; Liberthson et al. 1979; Pennington et al. 1979; Pinzon et al. 1991)
Bicuspid aortic valve	15–65
Aortic valve stenosis or regurgitation	2–9
Patent ductus arteriosus (PDA)	10–45
Ventricular septal defect (VSD)	7–47
Hypoplastic aortic arch*	22–63
Atrial septal defect (ASD)	1–18
Mitral valve anomaly (parachute)	4
Intracranial aneurysms	~10

* The aortic arch is defined as hypoplastic relative to the diameter of the ascending aorta:
- Proximal arch of the brachiocephalic trunk to the left carotid artery: < 60%
- Distal arch of the left carotid artery to the left subclavian artery: < 50%
- Aortic isthmus from the left subclavian artery to the insertion of the duct: < 40% of the diameter of the ascending aorta (Moulaert et al. 1976)

Table 2.1-9 Syndromes associated with a risk of congenital aortic isthmus stenosis.

Turner syndrome
Noonan syndrome
DiGeorge syndrome
Loeys–Dietz syndrome
Williams–Beuren syndrome
Down syndrome
Rubella syndrome
Trisomy 18
McCune–Albright syndrome
Klippel–Feil syndrome
Camptomelic syndrome
Shone syndrome
Goldenhar syndrome
Scimitar syndrome
Pierre Robin syndrome
Roberts syndrome
Type 1 neurofibromatosis
Kabuki syndrome
Alagille syndrome

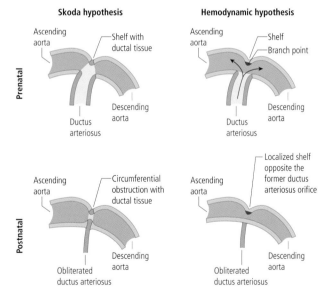

Fig. 2.1-27 In the hemodynamic hypothesis, it is assumed that aortic isthmus stenosis develops on a localized shelf on the posterior wall of the aorta opposite the orifice of the ductus arteriosus. By contrast, Skoda believed that scattered ductal tissue was responsible for the development of aortic isthmus stenosis.

2.1.10.2 Differential diagnosis of aortic isthmus syndrome

Pseudocoarctation refers to elongation and folding of the aorta in the thoracic segment, particularly of the aortic arch and proximal descending thoracic aorta, with no significant pressure gradients. However, there may be an indication for surgery if adjacent organs such as the esophagus are displaced or compressed, or if aneurysmal dilation of the aorta occurs.

Abdominal coarctation, also known as "mid-aortic syndrome" (MAS), is locally circumscribed in two-thirds of the cases. In one-third, however, it may also involve extensive changes. These are usually caused by inflammatory changes such as those seen in Takayasu arteritis or granulomatous vasculitis. The condition is also observed in patients with fibromuscular dysplasia, neurofibromatosis, retroperitoneal fibrosis, extensive atherosclerosis and congenital malformation (Connolly et al. 2002). Typical findings are renal artery stenosis with severe arterial hypertension, while stenoses of the celiac trunk or mesenteric arteries occur less frequently.

2.1.10.3 Clinical findings and course

Children: Two clinical groups are distinguished. Firstly, those with preductal aortic isthmus stenosis, which manifests in the first week of life. In this form of isthmus stenosis, the perfusion of the lower half of the body is dependent on the ductus arteriosus. When the duct closes, acute hypoperfusion of the lower half of the body results. Due to a lack of collateral circulation, afterload increases with acute cardiac and renal failure that require urgent correction of the aortic isthmus stenosis in severely affected neonates. An infusion of prostaglandin E_1 can reopen the ductus arteriosus to stabilize the neonate clinically until emergency surgery can be carried out.

The second group of children with aortic isthmus stenosis remain asymptomatic for a longer period. These children become conspicuous due to hypertension in the upper half of the body and hypotension in the lower half. Typical times for first diagnosis in these children are pediatric check-ups and pre-school medical examinations. At the physical examination, the inguinal pulse may be only weakly palpable, if at all, in comparison with the pulse in the radial artery, depending on the severity of the stenosis. Symptoms include headache, epistaxis and intermittent claudication.

Untreated adults: Untreated adults usually become symptomatic due to their untreated hypertension. Typical symptoms with late diagnosis are headache, epistaxis, intermittent claudication, heart failure and acute aortic dissection. The annual mortality rate in untreated patients with aortic isthmus stenosis is age-dependent and shows a peak frequency in the first year of life. According to data from the first half of the twentieth century, the mean life expectancy for individuals with untreated aortic isthmus stenosis is 34 (Abbott 1928; Campbell and Baylis 1956). Reasons for the high mortality rate include frequent accompanying anomalies with severe cardiac insufficiency (Table 2.1-10). Another extremely important factor is the risk of rupture or dissection of the aorta, which must be regarded as high in the presence of a simultaneous bicuspid aortic valve and due to systemic weakness in the wall of the aorta, particularly in patients with untreated or inadequately controlled hypertension.

Table 2.1-10 Causes of death in patients with untreated aortic isthmus stenosis (Campbell 1979).

Cause of death	%	Average age (years)	Decade of life
Decompensated cardiac failure	26	39	3rd–5th
Rupture or dissection of the aorta	21	25	2nd–3rd
Bacterial endocarditis	18	29	1st–5th
Intracranial bleeding	12	29	2nd–3rd
Aortic isthmus stenosis not the cause of death	24	47	4th–6th

2.1.10.4 Diagnosis

Clinical examination

Blood pressure and pulse: A classic sign of aortic isthmus stenosis both in adults and children is a difference in systolic pressure between the upper and lower extremities. In contrast to the systolic pressure, diastolic blood pressure often shows no differences between the upper and lower extremities (Brickner et al. 2000). Blood pressure is usually the same in the right and left arm, corresponding to a location of the aortic isthmus stenosis distal to the original of the left subclavian artery. When the subclavian artery arises distal to the isthmus stenosis, blood pressure in the left arm may be lower than in the right. Very rarely, when both subclavian arteries arise distal to the isthmus stenosis, it is possible for similarly reduced blood pressures to be present in all four extremities. The current guidelines for diagnostic clarification of hypertension therefore recommend that pulse and blood pressure should be examined and compared in the upper and lower extremities (Warnes et al. 2008).

Auscultation: In addition to cardiac murmurs in associated malformations, a typical finding in aortic isthmus stenosis is a short midsystolic murmur that can also be heard for longer than the second heart sound and is best heard in a left paravertebral position. In addition, continuous flow murmurs may be heard over collateral vessels.

Electrocardiography: In children with aortic isthmus stenosis, there are often signs of right ventricular hypertrophy, while signs of left ventricular hypertrophy are typical in adults.

Exercise tests: Ergometric exercise with electrocardiographic or echocardiographic monitoring may be useful, particularly for recognizing exercise hypertension or diagnosing a raised transisthmic gradient (Warnes et al. 2008). However, these examinations are not recommended as a general routine for follow-up in patients with aortic isthmus stenosis.

Imaging

The entire diagnostic work-up for an aortic isthmus stenosis can be carried out noninvasively. For diagnosis and follow-up in patients with aortic isthmus stenosis, the classic chest x-ray has been abandoned for echocardiography and other tomographic methods. Even

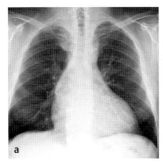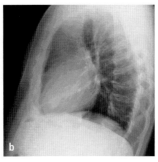

Fig. 2.1-28a, b Posteroanterior (**a**) and lateral (**b**) radiographs in a 37-year-old patient with aortic isthmus stenosis. Rib defects can be seen as typical radiographic signs of aortic isthmus stenosis, as well as a notch in the descending aorta. Left ventricular hypertrophy is present as a secondary sign. A localized luminal constriction in the aorta can be seen in the area of the aortic isthmus on the lateral image.

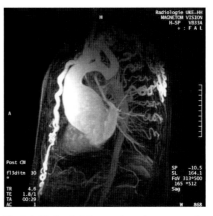

Fig. 2.1-29 Aortic isthmus stenosis on magnetic resonance imaging, with marked collateral formation and development of an aneurysm in the ascending aorta. Sagittal image with gadolinium contrast.

though a chest x-ray is still a frequently used screening procedure, particularly for acute diagnosis, it cannot provide important information about the presence of aortic pathology (von Kodolitsch et al. 2004; Hiratzka et al. 2010). Although changes in the ascending aorta often cannot be recognized in the mediastinal shadow, larger aneurysms in the descending thoracic aorta are often surprisingly well demonstrated (Hiratzka et al. 2010). On a sagittal noncontrast image, an isthmus stenosis may be demarcated as a notch-like dent in the aorta at the junction of the aortic arch and descending aorta, known as the "3 sign" of aortic isthmus stenosis. When one is assessing aortic isthmus stenosis radiographically, it should be borne in mind that the characteristic defects from the third to eighth ribs (notching on the underside of the ribs) usually appear only after the age of 8. These defects arise as a result of dilated intercostal arteries (known as Dock's sign; Fig. 2.1-28). In general, a chest x-ray only has very limited diagnostic reliability, with a sensitivity of < 20% for detecting re-stenoses after correction of an aortic isthmus stenosis (Therrien et al. 2000).

Echocardiography: The aortic valve, ascending aorta and aortic arch with the origins of the supra-aortic branches can usually be well assessed with transthoracic echocardiography. It is important to carry out the examination from a suprasternal direction, which allows Doppler echocardiographic assessment of the gradient across the aortic isthmus stenosis (Warnes et al. 2008). Both Doppler echocardiography and invasive measurement of pressure gradients may underestimate the severity of an isthmus stenosis when there is good collateral flow (Warnes et al. 2008). Echocardiography has a sensitivity of 87% and a specificity of 78% for diagnosing recurrent stenoses of the aortic isthmus, while its sensitivity and specificity for diagnosing aneurysms in adults after correction of an aortic isthmus stenosis are only 29% and 98%, respectively (Therrien et al. 2000). It is important to carry out a search for malformations typically associated with aortic isthmus stenosis during the echocardiographic examination (Table 2.1-8) (Warnes et al. 2008). Transesophageal echocardiography is rarely used to identify an aortic isthmus stenosis.

Magnetic resonance imaging (MRI) or computed tomography (CT) with three-dimensional reconstruction: According to the current guidelines, all adults with aortic isthmus stenosis should undergo an initial examination with demonstration of the entire aorta and intracranial vessels (Warnes et al. 2008). MRI produces high-quality,

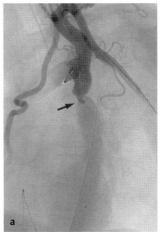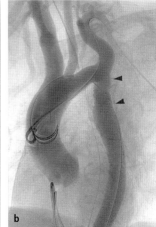

Fig. 2.1-30a, b Angiographic imaging of an aortic isthmus stenosis before (**a**) and after balloon angioplasty with successful stent placement (**b**, arrows).

high-resolution images that show the anatomy very well and it can also be used to quantify the flow in collateral vessels (Fig. 2.1-29) (Warnes et al. 2008). It provides all the information required for surgical correction, and it is also used for follow-up imaging examinations in patients who have undergone surgery for aortic isthmus stenosis. Several studies have confirmed that MRI can also be used in infants and neonates.

Intracardiac catheter examination: Invasive diagnosis is by today's standards only indicated in the context of interventional therapy for the aortic isthmus stenosis or to clarify complex cardiac defects, or in adults for preoperative exclusion of coronary heart disease (Fig. 2.1-30) (Warnes et al. 2008; Marek et al. 1995).

2.1.10.5 Treatment

Conservative treatment and general principles

Official recommendations are only available for control of arterial hypertension with medications. β-Blockers, angiotensin-converting enzyme (ACE) inhibitors and sartanes are the agents of choice (Warnes et al. 2008). In patients with aneurysm formation, β-blockers and vasodilators are particularly recommended (Warnes et al. 2008). The effect of statins is currently being tested for reducing atherosclerotic complications in adult patients with congenital heart defects (Krieger and Stout 2010). In accordance with the recommendations of the 36th Bethesda Conference, patients with significant re-stenosis or untreated isthmus stenosis, associated bicuspid aortic valve with aortic stenosis and those with dilation of the aortic root are advised not to take part in contact sports, isometric exercise, weightlifting, or sports involving abrupt starting and stopping (Graham et al. 2005). There has often been critical discussion of pregnancy in women with aortic isthmus stenosis. However, the published data suggest that relatively few complications occur and in particular that the risk of aortic dissection only appears to be slightly increased (Warnes et al. 2008; Pourmoghadam et al. 2002). According to the current guidelines, endocarditis prophylaxis is only indicated if surgical correction or stent placement has taken place during the previous 6 months, while uncomplicated and untreated aortic isthmus stenoses and uncomplicated re-stenoses do not require endocarditis prophylaxis (Warnes et al. 2008).

Correction of aortic isthmus stenosis

An indication for correction is basically established at the first diagnosis of aortic isthmus stenosis. In adults with previously undiagnosed aortic isthmus stenosis, an intervention is indicated according to the current guidelines if the peak-to-peak gradient over the isthmus stenosis on invasive measurement is $\geq 20\,mmHg$, or with smaller gradients if there is evidence on noninvasive imaging of severe isthmus stenosis with clear collateral formation (Warnes et al. 2008). If the noninvasively measured gradient already shows clear evidence of high-grade aortic isthmus stenosis, invasive measurement is not absolutely necessary.

Choice of technique

Surgical and percutaneous interventional procedures are available as alternatives for treating aortic isthmus stenosis. There are two indications for which one of these two options is clearly preferable. Firstly, surgical treatment for primary correction of aortic isthmus stenosis is currently recommended in neonates, since balloon angioplasty leads to re-stenosis or aneurysm formation in 10–70% of cases in this age group (Pourmoghadam et al. 2002). On the other hand, primary balloon angioplasty is also a good treatment option in this age group as well if the patient is at high surgical risk due to severe systemic diseases. Secondly, balloon angioplasty is regarded as the procedure of choice for the treatment of re-stenoses after corrected aortic isthmus stenosis in older children and young adults. In all other patients, there are currently no recommendations regarding the preference for a surgical or interventional correction procedure. However, in many centers surgical correction for aortic isthmus stenosis in adults is now only carried out when percutaneous interventional procedures do not appear appropriate (Warnes et al. 2008). It is recommended

Table 2.1-11 Typical criteria for choice of the correction technique in patients with aortic isthmus stenosis.

Technique	Typical indication
End-to-end anastomosis/extended end-to-end anastomosis; Waldhausen subclavian flap plasty*	Age 0–2 years
Patch enlargement plasty*	Age 2–16 years
Tube prosthesis interposition	Age > 16 years Long or atypically located stenoses Re-stenosis Local aneurysm formation
Balloon angioplasty/ stent placement	Method of choice in adults with re-stenosis of the aortic isthmus (Warnes et al. 2008)

* Methods now only rarely used.

that the decision regarding which procedure to use should be made in a center for adults with congenital heart defects in collaboration between cardiologists, interventionalists and surgeons (Warnes et al. 2008). The choice of surgical technique is mainly based on the patient's age (Table 2.1-11). In women who wish to have children, the advice tends to be to carry out primary treatment for aortic isthmus stenosis using a direct surgical approach with complete resection of the paraisthmic tissue (Warnes et al. 2008).

Surgical treatment for aortic isthmus stenosis

The following principles should be followed with surgical procedures. Firstly, to prevent re-stenoses from occurring, the resection or bridging of the aortic isthmus stenosis is always carried out at a wide distance from the immediate constriction. The aim here is particularly to achieve complete resection of scattered ductal tissue. Secondly, simultaneous continuous invasive arterial blood pressure measurement should be carried out at the radial artery and femoral artery intraoperatively. Thirdly, the mean arterial blood pressure in the upper half of the body should always be kept in the high normal range in order to avoid spinal cord ischemia and paraplegia. Fourthly, young adults and older patients are ventilated with a double-lumen tube so that the left lung can be immobilized for the duration of the surgical procedure.

End-to-end anastomosis

The technique for resection of aortic isthmus stenosis and end-to-end anastomosis described by Craoford and Nylin (1945) is mainly used in small children and is currently regarded by many surgeons as the preferable correction method (Schmid and Asfour 2009; Karck et al. 2003). The technique can also be used with an "enlarged" end-to-end anastomosis to correct aortic arch hypoplasia. After mobilization of the aorta and ligation and transection of the ductus arteriosus, the aorta is adequately clamped well proximally and distally to the aortic isthmus stenosis. The stenotic area is resected and the distal and proximal aortic stumps are anastomosed. To keep the anastomosis as tension-free as possible, the aorta has to be adequately mobilized during this process. In the enlarged end-to-end anastomosis described by Amato et al. (1977), the small cur-

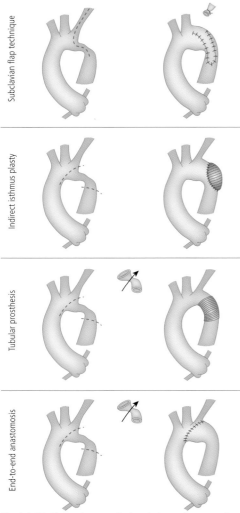

Fig. 2.1-31 The various surgical techniques for correcting an aortic isthmus stenosis.

vature of the aortic arch is further incised in order to enlarge a hypoplastic segment of the aortic arch. The distal segment of the aorta is connected to the lower side of the aortic arch, as in a side-to-end anastomosis (Fig. 2.1-31) (Amato et al. 1977).

Indirect isthmus plasty (patch enlargement plasty)

The technique of isthmus plasty, in which the area of the aortic isthmus is enlarged using a patch, was introduced by Vossschulte in 1957 (Vossschulte 1956/1957). After proximal and distal clamping of the aorta, the vessel is split lengthwise over the area of the stenosis, followed by cross-suturing. In this process, a diamond-shaped or rhomboid patch of polytetrafluoroethylene (PTFE), also known as Gore-Tex or Teflon, is introduced using a continuous suture. This procedure is only suitable for very short stenoses in aortae with few degenerative changes. The advantages of the indirect isthmus plasty procedure are that there is no need to mobilize the aorta, the intercostal arteries are preserved and the technique is suitable for correcting re-stenoses. Disadvantages include residual ductal tissue, use of a synthetic material, and local aneurysm development, which occurs frequently even without the use of Dacron, which is associated with a particularly high risk for localized aneurysm formation (Schmid and Asfour 2009; Karck et al. 2003; von Kodolitsch et al. 2002).

Waldhausen subclavian flap plasty

In the subclavian flap plasty technique, developed by Waldhausen and Nahrwold in 1966, the left subclavian artery is used as a patch to bridge the aortic isthmus stenosis (Waldhausen and Nahrwold 1966). The left subclavian artery is removed distally, so that the blood supply to the left arm is ensured only if there is adequate collateral circulation. The advantages of this procedure are that it can be used with a long stenosis and that foreign material is avoided (Schmid and Asfour 2009). However, malperfusion with trophic disturbances or growth retardation in the left arm occurs in some patients. A subclavian steal phenomenon is also observed if the vertebral artery is not ligated. The technique is nowadays hardly used any more due to these complications.

Interposition of a tubular prosthesis

After resection of the stenotic aortic segment, a vascular prosthesis can be inserted. This consists of synthetic material such as Dacron, Teflon, or Gore-Tex; an aortic homograft is rarely used. The technique is used when an end-to-end anastomosis is not possible—e.g., with long stenoses or stenoses in atypical locations, when there is a prestenotic or post-stenotic aortic aneurysm, when the vascular wall has been lacerated during attempted end-to-end anastomosis, for primary correction of an aortic isthmus stenosis in adults, when the aorta has massive atherosclerotic changes, or in surgery for recurrences of the stenosis. As the tubular prosthesis used has a rigid diameter, this procedure should be used only in older adolescents, in order to avoid disparities between the prosthesis diameter and the aortic diameter.

Interventional therapy for aortic isthmus stenosis

Balloon angioplasty is an alternative to surgical treatment for isolated aortic isthmus stenosis. The procedure for dilating an aortic isthmus stenosis was first used in a postmortem case by Sos et al. (1979); in 1982, Singer et al. carried out balloon angioplasty successfully for the first time to treat re-stenoses in patients with aortic isthmus stenoses that had previously been operated on. Sperling et al. (1983) used balloon angioplasty in previously untreated aortic isthmus stenoses. Since then various research groups have reported on primary dilation of a previously untreated aortic isthmus stenosis, with varying success rates. The American Heart Association recommends this procedure only as the primary treatment option for adults with aortic isthmus stenosis in cases of re-stenosis, while a surgical approach is still recommended for longer re-stenoses and in patients with a simultaneous hypoplastic aortic arch (Warnes et al. 2008). To reduce the risk of re-stenosis, balloon angioplasty with stent placement can be carried out in patients whose body weight is over 25 kg (Warnes et al. 2008). In smaller patients, there are no advantages with primary stent placement. Of note, stents can be dilated further later on, therefore can be used in children in whom growth has not yet been completed. The indication for using stents to treat long stenoses is a matter of controversy and this is not currently recommended (Warnes et al. 2008).

Results in adults after corrected aortic isthmus stenosis

Successful correction of an aortic isthmus stenosis is currently regarded more as a palliative procedure, rather than as a cure for the condition (Krieger and Stout 2010). In a series of 248 patients who underwent successful surgery for an aortic isthmus stenosis, for example, a 25-year follow-up period showed a 12% mortality rate, with a mean age at death of 34 years (Maron et al. 1973). The main causes of death were coronary heart disease, sudden cardiac death, cardiac insufficiency, and stroke (Krieger and Stout 2010).

Typical long-term complications after correction of an aortic isthmus stenosis are listed in Table 2.1-12. Arterial hypertension and atherosclerotic complications are the main factors involved in an unfavorable long-term prognosis. When aortic isthmus stenosis is corrected later than the neonatal period, there is an increased risk for the development of chronic hypertension. This "paradoxical" or "rebound" hypertension may first occur immediately postoperatively, typically after an interval of 24–36 hours, with an increase in mean arterial pressure. This early hypertension is caused by activation of sympathicotonia and is best treated with β-blockers (Warnes et al. 2008). Secondly, the hypertension may occur at a late postoperative stage, with an increase in diastolic blood pressure in particular, even years after successful correction of the aortic isthmus stenosis. This type of hypertension is caused by activation of the renin–angiotensin–aldosterone system and occurs independently of re-stenosis of the aortic isthmus (Hager et al. 2007). Disturbed tissue elasticity in the aortic wall is also an important factor in the pathogenesis here.

Table 2.1-12 Typical long-term complications after correction of an aortic isthmus stenosis.

Complications	Frequency (after Krieger and Stout 2010) (%)
Persistent arterial hypertension or arterial hypertension developing during subsequent course	Correction during childhood: < 5% Correction in adults: > 25%
Re-stenosis of the aortic isthmus	Correction in neonates: 2.4–5.5% Correction at a later age: < 1%
Aortic aneurysm/aortic dissection	5–16%

Re-stenosis is defined as the recurrence of a peak-to-peak gradient ≥ 20 mmHg, and is often associated with symptoms of uncontrolled arterial hypertension. Re-stenosis may remain asymptomatic for a long period and then can only be diagnosed using a targeted examination. The main risk factor for re-stenosis developing is correction of the aortic isthmus stenosis in neonates and children aged under 1 year. Re-stenosis is an important risk factor for recurrent arterial hypertension. A second procedure is indicated when the peak-to-peak gradient is ≥ 20 mmHg, or with smaller gradients if hypertension cannot be controlled with drugs or collateral circulation circuits have developed (Krieger and Stout 2010; Warnes et al. 2008). The treatment primarily involves the use of interventional procedures (Warnes et al. 2008). Successful elimination of the re-stenosis usually also leads to a reduction in blood pressure (Krieger and Stout 2010).

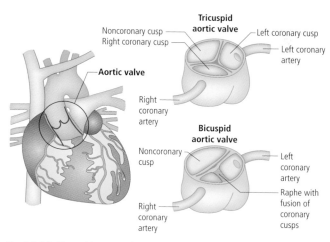

Fig. 2.1-32 Bicuspid aortic valve is an independent risk factor for the development of aneurysms, particularly in the area of the ascending aorta (Aydin et al. 2011). Patients who have undergone successful correction of an aortic isthmus stenosis, particularly with a bicuspid aortic valve, always require lifelong follow-up with imaging including the ascending aorta (von Kodolitsch et al. 2002; 2010).

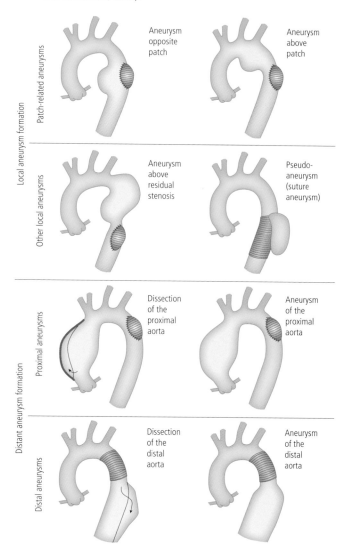

Fig. 2.1-33 Anatomic types of aneurysm development in the aorta after primary correction of an aortic isthmus stenosis.

Table 2.1-13 Aneurysm development after surgical correction of aortic isthmus stenosis (von Kodolitsch et al. 2002).

	Cases of aneurysm development after surgical correction of aortic isthmus stenosis/ cases of correction of aortic isthmus stenosis					Deaths with postoperative aneurysm	
	Correction technique					With aneurysm surgery	
Reference	All procedures	Subclavian flap plasty	Patch aortoplasty	Tube interposition	End-to-end anastomosis	Not carried out	Attempted/ completed
Pennington et al. 1979	4/164	–	–	2/59	2/92	1/4	–
Sorland et al. 1980	1/138	–	–	–	1/138	1/1	–
Clarkson et al. 1985	8/73	–	5/52	3/21	–	1/5	–
Hehrlein et al. 1986	18/303	–	18/285	0/8	0/10	2/3	2/15
Del Nido et al. 1986	3/63	–	3/63	–	–	–	0/3
Rheuban et al. 1986	8/79	0/5	8/45	0/3	0/26	–	–
Koller et al. 1987	5/343	–	–	5/47	0/296	–	1/5
Ala-Kulju and Heikkinen 1989	22/67	–	22/67	–	–	–	0/22
Bromberg et al. 1989	7/29	–	7/29	–	–	–	–
Kron et al. 1990	10/197	0/58	9/56	1/7	0/76	–	0/5
Pinzon et al. 1991	64/215	29/92	9/26	–	26/97	–	–
Bogaert et al. 1995	33/73	–	33/73	–	–	1/33	–
Parks et al. 1995	20/39	–	20/39	–	–	6/20	–
Knyshov et al. 1996	48/891	0/10	43/494	1/32	4/333	18/18	4/30
Heger et al. 1997	0/37	–	0/9	0/7	0/21	–	–
Total (%)	251/2711 (9)	29/165 (17)	177/1238 (14)	12/184 (6)	33/1089 (3)	30/84 (36)	7/80 (9)

– = information not available.

Aneurysm formation is another complication and is associated with a high mortality rate (Table 2.1-13) (von Kodolitsch et al. 2002, 2010; Oliver et al. 2004; Aydin et al. 2002). Aneurysms may develop independently of the technique used, the patient's age and the success of the aortic isthmus stenosis correction. Local aneurysms have even been observed in 8% of cases after balloon angioplasty (Fawzy et al. 2004). The development of local aneurysms is noted postoperatively particularly after patch enlargement plasty (Karck et al. 2003), while aneurysms in the ascending aorta appear particularly in patients with a bicuspid aortic valve (Aydin et al. 2002; von Kodolitsch et al. 2002). Depending on the pathological mechanism and location, true, false, and dissecting aneurysms may occur (Figs. 2.1-32 and 2.1-33). Treatment for local aneurysms is generally surgical, although it can also be carried out using stent grafts in individual cases (Warnes et al. 2008).

Follow-up

Due to the high complication rates and even higher mortality after correction of aortic isthmus stenosis, the affected patients need lifelong follow-up with cardiologists with expertise in caring for adult patients with congenital heart disease (Schmaltz et al. 2008; Krieger and Stout 2010; Warnes et al. 2008). Follow-up examinations should be carried out at least at annual intervals. At each follow-up examination, a physical examination should be carried out with measurement of blood pressure and an ECG recording (Krieger and Stouth 2010). Measurement of blood pressure in both arms with the patient supine, simultaneous palpation of the radial and femoral pulse, and auscultation at precordium and left paravertebral position to detect any re-stenosis are obligatory elements in the physical examination (Krieger and Stout 2010). Ophthalmoscopy of the fundus of the eyeball to note any chronic hypertension, are also recommended at each follow-up consultation.

Measurement of blood pressure over 24 hours and ergometry testing to identify exercise hypertension are recommended by many authors, but these are not obligatory. Imaging of the entire aorta every 2–5 years is recommended (Krieger and Stout 2010).

References

Abbott ME. Coarctation of the aorta of the adult type. Am Heart J 1928; 381: 574.

Ala-Kulju K, Heikkinen L. Aneurysms after patch graft aortoplasty for coarctation of the aorta: long-term results of surgical management. Ann Thorac Surg 1989; 47 (6): 853–6.

Amato JJ, Rheinlander HF, Cleveland RJ. A method of enlarging the distal transverse arch in infants with hypoplasia and coarctation of the aorta. Ann Thorac Surg 1977; 23 (3): 261–3.

Aydin A, Desai N, Bernhardt AM, Treede H, Detter C, Sheikhzadeh S, et al. Ascending aortic aneurysm and aortic valve dysfunction in bicuspid aortic valve disease. Medline vom 02.07.2012: Int J Cardiol 2011 Jul 29 [Epub ahead of print].

Aydin MA, Koschyk DH, Karck M, Cremer J, Haverich A, Berger J, et al. Prädiktoren der Aneurysmaentwicklung nach chirurgischer Korrektur einer Aortenisthmusstenose. Z Kardiol 2002; 91 (Suppl 1): I/338 (A).

Beauchesne LM, Connolly HM, Ammash NM, Warnes CA. Coarctation of the aorta: outcome of pregnancy. J Am Coll Cardiol 2001; 38 (6): 1728–33.

Becker A, Becker M J, Edwards JE. Anomalies associated with coarctation of the aorta: particular reference to infancy. Circulation 1970; 41: 1067–75.

Beekman RH, Robinow M. Coarctation of the aorta inherited as an autosomal dominant trait. Am J Cardiol 1985; 56 (12): 818–9.

Beekman RH, Rocchini AP, Behrendt DM, et al. Reoperation for coarctation of the aorta. Am J Cardiol 1981; 48: 1108–14.

Bogaert J, Gewillig M, Rademakers F, Bosmans H, Verschakelen J, Daenen W, et al. Transverse arch hypoplasia predisposes to aneurysm formation at the repair site after patch angioplasty for coarctation of the aorta. J Am Coll Cardiol 1995; 26 (2): 521–7.

Brickner ME, Hillis LD, Lange RA. Congenital heart disease in adults. First of two parts. N Engl J Med 2000; 342 (4): 256–63.

Bromberg BI, Beekman RH, Rocchini AP, Snider AR, Bank ER, Heidelberger K, et al. Aortic aneurysm after patch aortoplasty repair of coarctation: a prospective analysis of prevalence, screening tests and risks. J Am Coll Cardiol 1989; 14 (3): 734–41.

Campbell J, Delorenzi R, Brown J, Girod D, Hurwitz R, Caldwell R, King H. Improved results in newborns undergoing coarctation repair. Ann Thorac Surg 1980; 30: 273.

Campbell M, Baylis JH. The course and prognosis of coarctation of the aorta. Br Heart J 1956; 18: 475–95.

Campbell M. Natural history of coarctation of the aorta. Br Heart J 1970; 32 (5): 633–40.

Clarkson PM, Brandt PW, Barratt-Boyes BG, Rutherford JD, Kerr AR, Neutze JM. Prosthetic repair of coarctation of the aorta with particular reference to Dacron onlay patch grafts and late aneurysm formation. Am J Cardiol 1985; 56 (4): 342–6.

Clarkson PM, Nicholson MR, Barratt-Boyes BG, Neutze JM, Whitlock RM. Results after repair of coarctation of the aorta beyond infancy: a 10 to 28 year follow-up with particular reference to late systemic hypertension. Am J Cardiol 1983; 51 (9): 1481–8.

Hesslein PS, McNamara DG, Morriss MJ, Hallman GL, Cooley DA. Comparison of resection versus patch aortoplasty for repair of coarctation in infants and children. Circulation 1981; 64 (1): 164–8.

Connolly JE, Wilson SE, Lawrence PL, Fujitani RM. Middle aortic syndrome: distal thoracic and abdominal coarctation, a disorder with multiple etiologies. J Am Coll Surg 2002; 194 (6): 774–81.

Craafoord C, Nylin F. Congenital coarctation of aorta and its surgical treatment. J Thorac Surg 1945 (14): 347–61.

del Nido PJ, Williams WG, Wilson GJ, Coles JG, Moes CA, Hosokawa Y, et al. Synthetic patch angioplasty for repair of coarctation of the aorta: experience with aneurysm formation. Circulation 1986; 74 (3 Pt 2): I32–6.

Fawzy ME, Awad M, Hassan W, Al Kadhi Y, Shoukri M, Fadley F. Long-term outcome (up to 15 years) of balloon angioplasty of discrete native coarctation of the aorta in adolescents and adults. J Am Coll Cardiol 2004; 43 (6): 1062–7.

Graham TP, Jr., Driscoll DJ, Gersony WM, Newburger JW, Rocchini A, Towbin JA. Task Force 2: congenital heart disease. J Am Coll Cardiol 2005; 45 (8): 1326–33.

Hager A, Kanz S, Kaemmerer H, Schreiber C, Hess J. Coarctation Long-term Assessment (COALA): significance of arterial hypertension in a cohort of 404 patients up to 27 years after surgical repair of isolated coarctation of the aorta, even in the absence of restenosis and prosthetic material. J Thorac Cardiovasc Surg 2007; 134 (3): 738–45.

Heger M, Gabriel H, Koller-Strametz J, Atteneder M, Frank H, Baumgartner H, et al. [Aortic coarctation—long-term follow-up in adults]. Z Kardiol 1997; 86 (1): 50–5.

Hehrlein FW, Mulch J, Rautenburg HW, Schlepper M, Scheld HH. Incidence and pathogenesis of late aneurysms after patch graft aortoplasty for coarctation. J Thorac Cardiovasc Surg 1986; 92 (2): 226–30.

Hiratzka LF, Bakris GL, Beckman JA, Bersin RM, Carr VF, Casey DE, Jr., et al. 2010 ACCF/AHA/AATS/ACR/ASA/SCA/SCAI/SIR/STS/SVM guidelines for the diagnosis and management of patients with Thoracic Aortic Disease: a report of the American College of Cardiology Foundation/American Heart Association Task Force on Practice Guidelines, American Association for Thoracic Surgery, American College of Radiology, American Stroke Association, Society of Cardiovascular Anesthesiologists, Society for Cardiovascular Angiography and Interventions, Society of Interventional Radiology, Society of Thoracic Surgeons, and Society for Vascular Medicine. Circulation 2010; 121 (13): e266–369.

Ho SY, Anderson RH. Coarctation, tubular hypoplasia, and the ductus arteriosus. Histological study of 35 specimens. Br Heart J 1979; 41: 268–74.

Kappetein AP, Gittenberger de Groot AC, Zwinderman AH, Rohmer J, Poelmann RE, Huysmans HA. The neural crest as a possible pathogenetic factor in coarctation of the aorta and bicuspid aortic valve. J Thorac Cardiovasc Surg 1991; 102: 830–36.

Karck M, Leyh R, von Kodolitsch Y, Haverich A. Patcherweiterungsplastik bei Aortenisthmusstenose. Gefahr von lokalen Spätaneurysmen. Dtsch Ärztebl 2003; 100: A416–19.

Knyshov GV, Sitar LL, Glagola MD, Atamanyuk MY. Aortic aneurysms at the site of the repair of coarctation of the aorta: a review of 48 patients. Ann Thorac Surg 1996; 61 (3): 935–9.

Koller M, Rothlin M, Senning A. Coarctation of the aorta: review of 362 operated patients. Long-term follow-up and assessment of prognostic variables. Eur Heart J 1987; 8 (7): 670–9.

Krieger EV, Stout K. The adult with repaired coarctation of the aorta. Heart 2010; 96 (20): 1676–81.

Kron IL, Flanagan TL, Rheuban KS, Carpenter MA, Gutgesell HP, Jr., Blackbourne LH, et al. Incidence and risk of reintervention after coarctation repair. Ann Thorac Surg 1990; 49 (6): 920–5; discussion 25–6.

Lerberg DB, Hardesty RL, Siewers RD, Zuberbuhler JR, Bahnson HT. Coarctation of the aorta in infants and children: 25 years of experience. Ann Thorac Surg 1982; 33 (2): 159–70.

Liberthson RR, Pennington DG, Jacobs ML, Daggett WM. Coarctation of the aorta: review of 234 patients and clarification of management problems. Am J Cardiol 1979; 43 (4): 835–40.

Marek J, Skovranek J, Hucin B, Chaloupecky V, Tax P, Reich O, et al. Seven-year experience of noninvasive preoperative diagnostics in children with congenital heart defects: comprehensive analysis of 2,788 consecutive patients. Cardiology 1995; 86 (6): 488–95.

Maron BJ, Humphries JO, Rowe RD, Mellits ED. Prognosis of surgically corrected coarctation of the aorta. A 20-year postoperative appraisal. Circulation 1973; 47 (1): 119–26.

Moulaert AJ, Bruins CC, Oppenheimer-Dekker A. Anomalies of the aortic arch and ventricular septal defects. Circulation 1976; 53 (6): 1011–15.

Oliver JM, Gallego P, Gonzalez A, Aroca A, Bret M, Mesa JM. Risk factors for aortic complications in adults with coarctation of the aorta. J Am Coll Cardiol 2004; 44: 1641–47.

Parks WJ, Ngo TD, Plauth WH, Jr., Bank ER, Sheppard SK, Pettigrew RI, et al. Incidence of aneurysm formation after Dacron patch aortoplasty repair for coarctation of the aorta: long-term results and assessment utilizing magnetic resonance angiography with three-dimensional surface rendering. J Am Coll Cardiol 1995; 26 (1): 266–71.

Pennington DG, Liberthson RR, Jacobs M, Scully H, Goldblatt A, Daggett WM. Critical review of experience with surgical repair of coarctation of the aorta. J Thorax Cardiovascular Surg 1979; 77: 217–29.

Pinzon JL, Burrows PE, Benson LN, Moes CA, Lightfoot NE, Williams WG, et al. Repair of coarctation of the aorta in children: postoperative morphology. Radiology 1991; 180 (1): 199–203.

Pourmoghadam KK, Velamoor G, Kneebone JM, Patterson K, Jones TK, Lupinetti FM. Changes in protein distribution of the aortic wall following balloon aortoplasty for coarctation. Am J Cardiol 2002; 89 (1): 91–3.

Rheuban KS, Gutgesell HP, Carpenter MA, Jedeikin R, Damman JF, Kron IL, et al. Aortic aneurysm after patch angioplasty for aortic isthmic coarctation in childhood. Am J Cardiol 1986; 58 (1): 178–80.

Rudolph AM, Heymann MA, Spitznas U. Hemodynamic considerations in the development of narrowing of the aorta. Am J Cardiol 1972; 30 (5): 514–25.

Schmaltz AA, Bauer U, Baumgartner H, Cesnjevar R, de Haan F, Franke C, et al. [Medical guideline for the treatment of adults with congenital heart abnormalities of the German-Austrian-Swiss Cardiology Specialty Society]. Clin Res Cardiol 2008; 97 (3): 194–214.

Schmid C, Asfour B. Aortenisthmusstenose. Leitfaden Kinderherzchirurgie. Steinkopff Verlag, Stuttgart, 2009: 155–62.

Singer MI, Rowen M, Dorsey TJ. Transluminal aortic balloon angioplasty for coarctation of the aorta in the newborn. Am Heart J 1982; 103 (1): 131–2.

Sorland SJ, Rostad H, Forfang K, Abyholm G. Coarctation of the aorta. A follow-up study after surgical treatment in infancy and childhood. Acta Paediatr Scand 1980; 69 (1): 113–8.

Sos T, Sniderman KW, Rettek-Sos B, Strupp A, Alonso DR. Percutaneous transluminal dilatation of coarctation of thoracic aorta post mortem. Lancet 1979; 2 (8149): 970–1.

Sperling DR, Dorsey TJ, Rowen M, Gazzaniga AB. Percutaneous transluminal angioplasty of congenital coarctation of the aorta. Am J Cardiol 1983; 51 (3): 562–4.

Therrien J, Thorne SA, Wright A, Kilner PJ, Somerville J. Repaired coarctation: a "cost-effective" approach to identify complications in adults. J Am Coll Cardiol 2000; 35: 997–1002.

von Kodolitsch Y, Aydin AM, Bernhardt AM, Habermann C, Treede H, Reichenspurner H, et al. Aortic aneurysms after correction of aortic coarctation: A systematic review. VASA 2010; 39 (1): 3–16.

von Kodolitsch Y, Aydin AM, Koschyk DH, et al. Predictors of aneurysm formation after surgical correction of aortic coarctation. J Am Coll Cardiol 2002; 39: 617–24.

von Kodolitsch Y, Aydin AM, Koschyk DH, Loose R, Schalwat I, Karck M, et al. Predictors of aneurysm formation after surgical correction of aortic coarctation. J Am Coll Cardiol 2002; 39: 617–24.

von Kodolitsch Y, Nienaber CA, Dieckmann C, Schwartz AG, Hofmann T, Brekenfeld C, et al. Chest radiography for the diagnosis of acute aortic syndrome. Am J Med 2004; 116 (2): 73–7.

Vossschulte K. Isthmusplastik zur Behandlung der Aortenisthmusstenose. Thoraxchirurgie 1956/1957; 4: 443.

Waldhausen JA, Nahrwold DL. Repair of coarctation of the aorta with a subclavian flap. J Thorac Cardiovasc Surg 1966; 51: 532–33.

Warnes CA, Williams RG, Bashore TM, Child JS, Connolly HM, Dearani JA, et al. ACC/AHA 2008 Guidelines for the Management of Adults with Congenital Heart Disease: a report of the American College of Cardiology/American Heart Association Task Force on Practice Guidelines (writing committee to develop guidelines on the management of adults with congenital heart disease). Circulation 2008; 118 (23): e714–833.

2.2   Diseases of the pulmonary arteries

2.2.1   Pulmonary artery embolism

Clinical findings: Edda Spiekerkötter and Thomas Zeller
Anatomy of the pulmonary arteries: Reinhard Putz
Conservative treatment: Edda Spiekerkötter and Thomas Zeller
Endovascular treatment: Thomas Zeller
Surgical treatment: Matthias Thielmann

2.2.1.1   Anatomy of the pulmonary arteries

The right and left pulmonary arteries originate in a shallow bifurcation from the pulmonary trunk, which is approximately 5 cm long and 3 cm wide and lies in an oblique cranial position. The start of the trunk is marked by the pulmonary valve, which like the aortic valve is formed by three semilunar cusps. The three pockets formed in this way do not lead to any distension of the initial part of the trunk, however, since the systolic pressure in the pulmonary system is much lower than in the aorta. The walls of the large pulmonary arteries are accordingly slightly less robust comparatively and only contain a strong elastic fibrous lattice instead of an internal elastic membrane.

The trunk initially lies anterior to the ascending aorta and then ascends on the left side of it where it then divides under the aortic arch, which is then already located outside of the pericardium. The slightly longer and slightly wider right pulmonary artery passes behind the ascending aorta and superior vena cava, but in front of the right mainstem bronchus and esophagus, in an oblique dorsal course to the hilum of the right lung. The left pulmonary artery also crosses at a slightly oblique angle on the short path into the hilum of the left lung. Just after the division of the two pulmonary arteries, the ligamentum arteriosum connects the left pulmonary artery

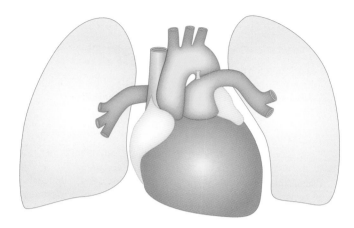

Fig. 2.2-1 Anterior view of the pulmonary arteries.

with the inner contour of the aortic arch. This "ligament," which has highly variable alignments, is the rudimentary residue of the fetal ductus arteriosus (Fig. 2.2-1).

Before the division into the lobar branches, the trunk of the right pulmonary artery reaches its furthest cranial point in the hilum; on the left side, this occurs at the left mainstem bronchus. The primary branches of the two pulmonary arteries cross the bronchial tree ventrally and then enter the pulmonary lobes centrally along with the bronchi. Along with the bronchi, they divide further into the segmental arteries, which also lie centrally.

2.2.1.2   Clinical picture

The pathoanatomic correlate for pulmonary artery embolism is occlusion of the pulmonary arteries by thrombi (or rarely by fat, air, foreign bodies, tumor, or amniotic fluid) from another vascular region. The extent of the vascular obstruction and underlying cardiopulmonary function determine the severity and thus the mortality of pulmonary artery embolism.

Acute pulmonary embolism is the third most frequent cardiovascular disease; in the U.S. alone, it has an annual incidence of approximately 500,000 and is responsible for 200,000 deaths per year. In Germany, pulmonary embolism has a reported incidence of approximately 100,000 per year (one to three per 1000 inhabitants), with 20,000–30,000 of these cases having a fatal course, and it affects 0.1–0.4% of hospitalized patients, 12–14% of postoperative deaths and 45–90% of all deaths within 2 h.

Massive and fulminant acute pulmonary embolism (Grosser stages III and IV) as a sequela of deep venous thrombosis is life-threatening and has an overall mortality rate of more than 30%, with 50% of deaths occurring within the first 30 min, 70% within the first hour, and more than 85% within the first 6 h after the onset of symptoms. Particularly in patients requiring resuscitation, the prognosis without immediate revascularization treatment is unfavorable. Rapid diagnosis and appropriate therapy are therefore decisive for saving the patient's life. Developments in fibrinolytic and percutaneous treatment have increasingly pushed surgical treatment for acute massive and fulminant pulmonary embolism into the background.

For chronic recurrent pulmonary embolism, see section A 2.2.2.

2.2.1.3   Diagnosis

Clinical findings

The clinical probability of pulmonary embolism and deep venous thrombosis is estimated as described above.

ECG

- Right axis deviation
- Sinus tachycardia: 50%
- ST segment changes (particularly V1–V4): 40%
- Right bundle-branch block: 15%
- S_IQ_{III} type: 15%
- P pulmonale: 5%

Laboratory findings

- Blood gas analysis (BGA): hypoxemia despite hyperventilation ($Po_2 \downarrow$, $Pco_2 \downarrow$)
- D-dimers (microplate ELISA, VIDAS ELISA, Simpli-RED®):
  - Negative findings (< 500 µg/L) practically exclude pulmonary embolism; i.e., in 30% of patients with emergency admission, but fewer than 10% of inpatients, pulmonary embolism can be excluded using D-dimer assessment.
  - *Caution:* D-dimers are also raised in infection, inflammation, carcinoma, status post surgery, cardiac insufficiency and renal insufficiency, acute coronary syndrome, pregnancy, and sickle-cell crisis.
  - Troponin: evidence of hemodynamically significant pulmonary embolism, right ventricular enlargement, right cardiac ischemia
- Coagulation tests:
  - Protein C
  - Protein S
  - Angiotensin III
  - APC resistance
  - Rheumatism serology, including anticardiolipin

Chest x-ray

Nonspecific changes include:
- Atelectasis/infiltrate: 80%
- Pleural effusion: 50%
- Elevation of the diaphragm (unilateral): 30%
- Vascular asthenia: 20%
- Prominent pulmonary artery segment: 15%
- Hilar vessel truncation (Westermark sign): 10%
- Wedge-shaped solidification near the pleura (pulmonary infarction): 10%

An unremarkable chest x-ray does not exclude pulmonary embolism.

Diagnosis of deep venous thrombosis

- B-image ultrasound with compression testing, color duplex ultrasonography (see section B 1.2, diagnosis of DVT)
- Phlebography

Table 2.2-1 Pathophysiology of pulmonary embolism.

Pulmonary artery obstruction → afterload increase for RV → wall tension ↑, RV ischemia, RV decompensation, acute cor pulmonale → RV output ↓, RV volume ↑, septal deviation → LV preload ↓, cardiac output ↓ → RV coronary perfusion ↓ → right heart failure
Inhomogeneous perfusion → wasted ventilation → hypoxemia
Released mediators (thromboxane A2, serotonin, fibrinopeptides, leukotriene) → vasoconstrictio

RV, right ventricle; LV, left ventricle.

Table 2.2-2 Clinical probability of pulmonary embolism (adapted from Perrier).

High (80–100%)	Risk factor present, otherwise unexplained dyspnea, pleuritic pain, gas exchange disturbance or abnormalities on chest x-ray
Intermediate (20–79%)	Neither high nor low probability of pulmonary embolism
Low (0–19%)	No risk factors present, clinical symptoms and findings explicable by other causes

Table 2.2-3 Severity of pulmonary embolism (adapted from Grosser).

	I	II	III	IV
Clinical findings	Mild dyspnea, chest pain	Acute dyspnea, tachypnea, tachycardia, chest pain	Acute severe dyspnea, cyanosis, restlessness, syncope, chest pain	Additional shock symptoms, possible cardiovascular arrest
Blood pressure	Normal	Reduced	Reduced	Shock
PAP$_{mean}$	Normal	16–25 mmHg	25–30 mmHg	> 30 mmHg
Po$_2$	Approx. 80 mmHg	70 mmHg	60 mmHg	< 60 mmHg
Vascular occlusion	Peripheral branches	Segmental arteries	One pulmonary arterial branch	Main pulmonary artery trunk or several lobar arteries

Massive	Submassive	Not massive
Shock, BP$_{syst}$ < 90 mmHg, BP drop of > 40 mmHg for > 15 min without other cause, catecholamine requirement	No shock, but echocardiographic signs of right ventricular dysfunction	All other types of pulmonary embolism

BP, blood pressure.

Echocardiography (transthoracic echocardiography, transesophageal echocardiography)

- Acute right ventricular load:
  - Dilated, hypokinetic RV
  - Raised RV/LV ratio
  - Deviation of the intraventricular septum in LV
  - Dilated proximal pulmonary arteries
  - Regurgitation via the tricuspid valve (jet: 2.5–2.8 m/s)
  - Dilated inferior vena cava without collapse on inspiration
- Evidence of an embolus in transit
- Exclusion of differential diagnoses:
  - Myocardial infarction
  - Valvular insufficiency
  - Hypovolemia
  - Endocarditis
  - Aortic dissection
  - Pericardial tamponade

Ventilation–perfusion scintigraphy

Only applicable with normal findings (15%) → exclusion of pulmonary embolism, high-probability finding (13%) → treatment. When ventilation–perfusion scintigraphy is not diagnostic—i.e., in approximately 70% of cases—further diagnostic procedures are necessary.

Spiral CT

- High sensitivity (94%) and specificity (94%) in embolism of the main trunk of the pulmonary artery and segmental arteries
- Evidence of right ventricular dilation

It is recommended that spiral CT should be used in combination with the clinical findings, laboratory test data, and compression ultrasonography. The advantage of spiral CT is that it is not invasive and allows differential diagnoses to be excluded.

Magnetic resonance imaging (MRI)

Imaging of the central vessels, with sensitivity and specificity comparable to those with spiral CT.

Advantages: noninvasive, exclusion of differential diagnoses, contrast administration not necessary.

Disadvantages: long examination time (with breathing pauses).

Pulmonary artery catheter

- Complete data on pressure conditions and hemodynamics
- Increased PAP$_{mean}$ > 25 mmHg: obstruction of pulmonary bloodstream in only 50%
- Increased PAP$_{mean}$ > 40 mmHg: only with a previously preloaded right ventricle

Caution: bleeding complications in planned lysis. Pulmonary angiography is the gold standard for massive and submassive pulmonary embolism and planned treatment (lysis). Definite signs include vascular abruption and filling defects. Catheter fragmentation of thrombi can be carried out in the same session if appropriate.

2.2.1.4 Treatment

Conservative treatment

General measures

- Bed rest
- Oxygen administration: nasal probe, oxygen glasses or mask up to 10 L O_2/min. When there is hypoxemia despite O_2 administration ($SaO_2 < 80\%$): intubation and ventilation
- Analgesia and sedation: morphine 5 mg i.v./s.c., diazepam (e.g., Valium®) 5–10 mg i.v.
- Heparin 5000–10,000 IU i.v. as a bolus, followed by therapeutic heparinization (20 IU/kg/h) aiming for 1.5–2.5 times partial thromboplastin time (PTT)

Initial care

- Volume administration:
  - Caution when there is severe right ventricular dysfunction; 500 mL "fluid challenge" (e.g., HAES-steril® 10%) with cardiac output ↓ and normal blood pressure (BP)
- Catecholamines:
  - Mild hypertension: dobutamine (Dobutrex®) 2.5–12.0 µg/kg/min. Effect: cardiac output ↑, oxygen transport ↑, peripheral vasodilation (β_2 receptors), peripheral vascular resistance ↓, possible deterioration of ventilation–perfusion mismatch with Po_2 ↓
  - Severe shock: norepinephrine (Arterenol®) 0.05–0.30 µg/kg/min. Effect: mean arterial pressure ↑ (α_1 receptors), right ventricular coronary perfusion ↑, right ventricular ischemia ↓, cardiac output ↑ (β_1 receptors)

Systemic fibrinolytic therapy

Indications. Massive pulmonary embolism (it is currently being debated whether this type of treatment can also be used in submassive pulmonary embolism—i.e., when there is right ventricular dysfunction without shock and with no contraindications for lysis). The pulmonary embolism should be confirmed by CT in submassive pulmonary embolism before lysis treatment is started, or there should be a high clinical likelihood of acute cor pulmonale (TTE, TEE) without prior cardiorespiratory disease.

Contraindications. The same contraindications as those for systemic lysis apply:

- Absolute:
  - Active internal bleeding
  - Spontaneous intracranial bleeding
- Relative:
  - Larger operation
  - Pregnancy, labor
  - Organ biopsy
  - Puncture of noncompressible vessels < 10 days
  - Cerebral ischemia < 2 months
  - Gastrointestinal bleeding < 10 days, severe trauma < 15 days
  - Neural or ophthalmic surgery < 1 month
  - Severe hypertension, BP_{syst} > 180 mmHg, BP_{diast} > 110 mmHg
  - Bacterial endocarditis
  - Diabetic hemorrhagic retinopathy, thrombocytes < 100,000/µL
  - Status post resuscitation

Procedure:

- rt-PA (Actilyse®): short-term lysis: 10 mg bolus i.v., 90 mg over 2 h, bolus lysis: 50 mg bolus i.v., second bolus after 30 min, always with simultaneous full heparinization
- Urokinase (Actosolv®, Corase®): short-term lysis: 1 million IU as bolus i.v., 2 million IU over 2 h, bolus lysis: 3 million IU as a bolus i.v., always with simultaneous full heparinization
- Streptokinase (Streptase®): short-term lysis: 1.5 million over 30 min, 1.5 million/h over 3–4 h, repetition after 24 h possible

Limitations of systemic fibrinolytic therapy. The Management Strategies and Prognosis in Patients with Pulmonary Embolism (MAPPET) registry has shown that 40% of patients with acute pulmonary embolism have at least one contraindication against fibrinolytic therapy. In the International Cooperative Pulmonary Embolism Registry (ICOPER), it was clearly shown that 17.4% of the patients included died within 90 days; 21.7% of patients who received fibrinolytic therapy had severe bleeding complications, and 3% developed intracerebral hemorrhage. It must therefore be assumed that fibrinolysis treatment actually has a higher complication rate than has been postulated in controlled and therefore fairly selective and artificial individual studies. Some 15–25% of patients who receive lysis have only partial dissolution of the emboli in the pulmonary vascular circulation. However, persistent pulmonary hypertension after pulmonary embolism is associated with increased mortality. Meneveau et al. (2003) showed that the "residual embolism burden" after incomplete fibrinolytic reopening of the pulmonary vascular bed is an independent prognostic factor for the long-term results in these patients. When there was a residual obstruction of more than 30% of the pulmonary vascular bed, the multivariate analysis showed a relative risk of 2.2, with a 95% confidence interval of 1.7 to 2.7, for long-term mortality. While it was previously assumed that chronic thromboembolic pulmonary hypertension only develops in very few patients after acute pulmonary embolism, Meneveau et al. suggest that the numbers of patients affected may have been underestimated and propose more careful follow-up for patients with residual obstruction so that they can then undergo pulmonary thromboendarterectomy if appropriate. A flow model (Fig. 2.2-2) may provide a flow-physiological explanation for the incomplete thrombolysis. Proximal to the occlusion,

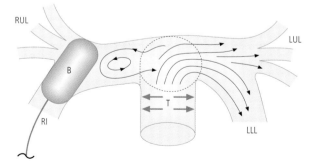

Fig. 2.2-2 Flow model for flow-physiological explanation of incomplete systolic thrombolysis. Turbulence proximal to the occlusion (B) and diversion of the blood flow into the unoccluded left pulmonary artery. The turbulence in front of the thrombus leads to poor contact between the thrombolytic agent and the thrombus (Uflacker 2004). RUL, right upper pulmonary arteries; RI, right inferior pulmonary arteries; B, thrombus; T, main pulmonary artery trunk; LUL, left upper pulmonary arteries; LLL, left lower pulmonary arteries.

there is turbulence with diversion of the blood flow into nonoccluded vascular segments, so that the contact between the thrombolytic agent and the thrombus is often only inadequate. Thabut et al. (2002) thus confirmed in a meta-analysis of nine randomized and controlled studies including 461 patients that fibrinolytic therapy provides no advantages in comparison with intravenous heparin administration in unselected patients, although it is associated with an increased risk of severe bleeding complications.

Endovascular therapy

Indications for endovascular therapy

The same indications apply as for systemic lysis treatment—massive pulmonary embolism in which more than 50% of the pulmonary circulation is obstructed, with the patient showing hemodynamic instability.

Contraindications against endovascular therapy

In contrast to systemic lysis, there are no real contraindications here. Any patient, including those in resuscitation conditions, can receive percutaneous endovascular treatment.
In principle, the general contraindications against the use of iodine-containing radiographic contrast media apply (e.g., hyperthyroidosis, previous severe reaction to contrast medium, advanced renal insufficiency), with no option available for using an alternative contrast agent (e.g., gadolinium in DSA-capable x-ray equipment).

Patient preparation

As this is usually an emergency procedure, patients must have the basic aspects of the planned procedure explained to them if they are conscious, and the legally prescribed waiting period of 1 day does not need to be observed.

Medication

With unstable hemodynamic indices, all patients have already received therapeutic heparinization. Administration of platelet aggregation inhibitors has not been confirmed in controlled studies, but is recommended (with an intravenous bolus dose of 50 mg acetylsalicylic acid). After placement of the femoral sheath, a heparin bolus of 2500–5000 IU is administered, depending on the patient's body weight and the expected length of the procedure.

Access route

The most frequently used access route is transvenous femoral access, or less frequently brachial access via the basilic vein or cephalic vein. Jugular access is reserved for special large-lumen catheter systems.

Femoral access

Femoral access is the standard route. The femoral artery pulse can serve for guidance; the femoral vein lies approximately 1.0–1.5 cm medial to the artery. Due to the potential need for local lysis, detailed attention should be given to ensure that the artery is not punctured. It may be helpful to carry out the puncture with fluoroscopy, as the artery can be identified radiographically if there is calcification of the arterial walls. The size and length of the sheath depend on the selected interventional technique and can vary from 5F to 11F and from 11–90 cm, respectively. Reaching the right ventricle or pulmonary arteries is easiest using a flow-directed balloon-tipped catheter that has a guidewire lumen. After the flow-directed balloon-tipped catheter has been positioned in the right ventricle, the guidewire (0.035-inch Glidewire®, Terumo) is introduced, and the flow-directed catheter is exchanged over the guidewire for a pigtail catheter (5F or 6F) for diagnostic angiography.

Brachial access

A 5F or 6F sheath is placed in the basilic vein or alternatively in the cephalic vein, and a pigtail catheter is advanced into the right ventricle or main pulmonary arterial trunk for diagnosis, as in femoral access.

Preinterventional angiography

Either conventional angiography or DSA (15 mL/s contrast injection at 600 psi, total amount 30 mL) is carried out via the pigtail catheter. It is possible to distinguish between submassive and massive pulmonary embolism using the Miller score. With a maximum score of 34 (central obstruction of the right pulmonary artery, 9 points; left pulmonary artery, 7 points; peripheral obstruction of the upper, middle, and lower lobe of the lung, each with no flow, 3 points; severely reduced flow, 2 points; moderately reduced perfusion, 1 point), a score > 10 signifies a massive pulmonary embolism.

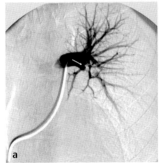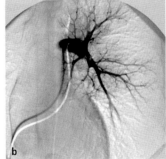

Fig. 2.2-3a, b Angiographic image of an embolism (arrow) in the pulmonary artery supplying the left lower lobe, **(a)** 15 min after 8-mm PTA and 15 mg rt-PA locally as a bolus **(b)**.

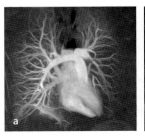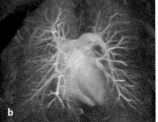

Fig. 2.2-4a, b **(a)** Embolism in the left main pulmonary artery trunk (MRI). **(b)** Image 6 months after local lysis treatment.

Interventional techniques

Various catheter-based interventional techniques are available, although none of these except local thrombolysis can be regarded as generally valid.

Local thrombolysis

Only some 60–70% of patients with massive pulmonary embolism are able to undergo lysis treatment; the remaining 30–40% have contra-indications such as a recent history of surgery, trauma, or carcinoma. In local catheter thrombolysis, a 5F Cragg–McNamara lysis catheter with side holes over a length of 5–10 cm (ev3 and Boston Scientific, etc.) is placed in the thrombus over a hydrophilic-coated 0.035-inch guidewire. As a lytic agent, either urokinase (4500 IU/kg body weight as a bolus, followed by 2000 IU/kg body weight/h) or rt-PA (25–50 mg as a bolus, followed by 25–50 mg/h) is used. When rt-PA is used, heparin with PTT guidance needs to be infused to reduce reocclusion rates. The patient either remains in the catheter laboratory so that the success of the lysis treatment can be documented with serial angiography or, if there is adequate circulatory stability, can be returned to the intensive care unit, where lysis can be continued until hemodynamic improvement is seen.

According to the International Cooperative Embolism Registry (ICOPER), relevant bleeding complications occur with lysis treatment in up to 21% of cases, and intracranial hemorrhage in up to 3% of cases.

Ultrasound-enhanced local thrombolysis. For this procedure, a catheter with several ultrasound-emitting probes attached to its sides (EkoSonic™; Ekos Corporation, Bothell, Washington, USA) is placed in the pulmonary artery and the thrombolytic agent is infused via the catheter during the application of ultrasound waves. The ultrasound waves are intended to separate the fibrin bridges and thus allow better penetration of the drug into the thrombus, shortening the time required for thrombolysis. Controlled studies on the technique are in progress.

Mechanical catheter thrombus fragmentation and local catheter lysis

In central obstruction of the major pulmonary artery trunk, simple mechanical thrombus fragmentation with the guidewire or by rotating the pigtail catheter used for diagnostic angiography in the thrombus can already lead to significant hemodynamic improvement. Mechanical thrombus fragmentation can also be achieved using balloon dilation. However, the contrary effect of further hemodynamic deterioration can occur due to shifting of the thrombi into the peripheral vascular region (Fig. 2.2-5). Mechanical thrombus fragmentation should therefore always be combined with subsequent local lysis over a 5–10-cm sidehole catheter.

Thrombus aspiration

Pulmonary thrombus aspiration was first reported by Greenfield et al. in 1971 using a 10F aspiration catheter. This system is currently the only aspiration catheter approved by the U.S. Food and Drug Administration (FDA). It is now possible to use large-lumen catheters (minimum 8F), which are available in various configurations. These allow clots to be aspirated even from the segmental pulmonary branches (with suction using a 50-mL syringe).

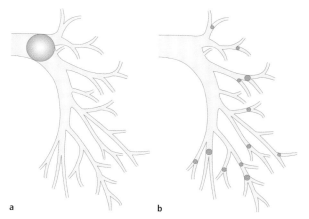

Fig. 2.2-5a, b Dispersion of small thrombi into the peripheral branches of the pulmonary artery after mechanical fragmentation.

Mechanical and rheolytic catheter thrombectomy

No mechanical thrombectomy systems are currently approved for use in patients with major pulmonary embolism. Ideally, the system should be very flexible, allowing easy passage into the right heart and pulmonary artery system with high suction, with no risk of damaging the pulmonary arteries.

Various systems that are used on an off-label basis at the moment, such as the AngioJet™ (Possis, Fig. 2.2-6), Amplatz Clot Buster™ (BARD), and Hydrolyser™ (J&J Cordis), were not designed for use in vessels with large lumina and therefore have to be used in combination with local fibrinolytic therapy.

Potential side effects of these catheter systems include mechanical hemolysis, macroembolization, and microembolization. According to the current literature, only 5% of patients with a major pulmonary embolism are treated with a mechanical catheter thrombectomy system. Thrombectomy catheters that have been used to date are:

- *Hydrolyser™*. This is a 6F or 7F triple-lumen catheter with a narrow injection lumen, a larger emission lumen, and a 0.020-inch guidewire lumen. The system is available in various lengths and is activated using a standard contrast injection pump filled with 0.9% saline. The catheter can be used safely without related vascular wall reactions in vessels with a diameter of 3–8 mm. It is a rheolytic catheter that takes advantage of the Venturi effect. A jet of saline is injected in a retrograde direction through the insertion lumen under high pressure, directed toward the catheter's central emission lumen. This fluid jet shatters and removes the thrombus.
- *Amplatz Clot Buster™* system. This is a 100-cm long 7F catheter, at the tip of which a propeller fragments the thrombus without removing it.

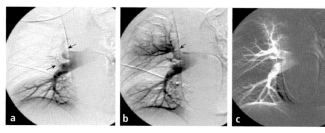

Fig. 2.2-6a–c (a) Embolic occlusion of the pulmonary artery supplying the right upper lobe and middle lobe. (b, c) After AngioJet™ thrombectomy and local urokinase thrombolysis.

■ *AngioJet™.* The catheter consists of a 3.2F to 6F double-lumen tube that has a narrow injection lumen and a larger emission lumen. Saline is injected at high pressure through multiple side holes at the distal tip into the emission lumen, fragmenting and removing the thrombus. The device requires a special pump that produces a pressure of 70,000–105,000 kPa.

■ *Trerotola thrombectomy system.* This is a 5F sheath-compatible rotation catheter primarily designed for the treatment of venous dialysis shunt occlusions. After passing the occlusion in a closed position, a self-expanding nitinol basket attached to the tip of the catheter is opened. The catheter is activated and withdrawn through the occlusion with the basket slowly rotating. This mechanically fragments the thrombus, without removing it.

Postprocedural follow-up and medication

Despite successful revascularization, pulmonary infarction and subsequent infarction pneumonia can be expected. Close clinical and radiographic follow-up, with antibiotic treatment if necessary, are indicated. Postprocedural anticoagulation treatment is essential, initially with fractionated or unfractionated heparin at therapeutic dosages, followed by overlapping oral anticoagulation treatment with coumarin at a target INR of 2.5–3.0 after hemodynamic stabilization. The duration of the anticoagulation therapy depends on the cause of the pulmonary embolism, but in accordance with the general guidelines should continue for at least 1 year.

Potential risks of endovascular treatment

In percutaneous mechanical thrombectomy and thrombolysis, smaller thrombi are scattered into the peripheral branches of the pulmonary artery, and this can lead to residual obstruction (Fig. 2.2-5). Other possible complications include vascular perforation or dissection, pericardial tamponade, pulmonary bleeding, and recurrent embolism.

Course and prognosis

The 30-day mortality with massive pulmonary embolism, defined as cardiogenic shock or systemic systolic blood pressure < 90 mmHg, is up to 30%. There is still a lack of systematic studies on the extent to which catheter interventions for revascularization are able to improve the prognosis for patients with this clinical picture.

Prospects

A rotational thrombectomy system specifically designed for percutaneous use in patients with pulmonary embolism, the Aspirex® catheter (Straub Medical; Fig. 2.2-7) has been clinically tested in an international multicenter study, but the study had to be prematurely stopped due to more frequent local bleeding. A modified system was to be clinically tested again in 2012. The system consists of a highly flexible 10F thrombectomy catheter that can be introduced via the port, with a diameter of 6–14 mm, developed for use in the pulmonary arteries. As in the Rotarex® catheter described elsewhere, a spiral rotating at high frequency (32,000 rpm) inside the catheter creates negative pressure at the L-shaped catheter tip. Thrombi are sucked inside the catheter tip, where they are fragmented and removed.

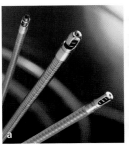 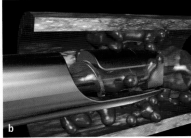

Fig. 2.2-7a, b (a) The Aspirex® catheter family, with an 11F system for pulmonary applications in the center. **(b)** Diagram showing the catheter tip.

The catheter is introduced via the femoral or jugular access route over a 0.035-inch Glidewire™ (Terumo). An 80-cm long sheath has proved useful. In animal studies, the pulmonary artery was largely free of thrombi after activation of the system for 1 min, with blood loss of approximately 200 mL.

Ultrasound-enhanced local thrombolysis using the EkoSonic system is already being clinically tested, but studies confirming a benefit (with a shorter thrombolysis time and lower dosage of the thrombolytic agent) with this more expensive form of combination treatment are still awaited.

Surgical treatment

Surgical treatment for acute pulmonary embolism

Open surgical pulmonary artery embolectomy was first carried out in 1908 by Trendelenburg, without a heart–lung machine, and by Cooley in 1961 for the first time with a heart–lung machine (Trendelenburg 1908; Cooley 1961). It has increasingly become a last-resort treatment for patients requiring resuscitation—with correspondingly poor results. However, against the background of the limitations of fibrinolytic and percutaneous therapy and a lack of data showing clear advantages for these treatments, there has been a renaissance in the use of open surgery for pulmonary artery embolectomy.

Indications for surgery

Surgical pulmonary artery embolectomy is indicated in patients with a central, massive, or fulminant pulmonary embolism (grade III and IV pulmonary embolism). Surgical pulmonary embolectomy should be considered in patients with a diagnosis of acute pulmonary embolism who meet certain criteria. These eight criteria are as follows:

■ Life-threatening shock
■ Arterial hypotension
■ Circulatory arrest requiring cardiopulmonary resuscitation
■ Echocardiographic evidence of right heart strain and/or pulmonary hypertension
■ Precapillary pulmonary hypertension
■ Increased arterial–alveolar oxygen gradient (> 50 mmHg)
■ Clinically severe pulmonary embolism in which thrombolysis has already failed
■ Patients in whom thrombolysis is contraindicated

As a suspected clinical diagnosis of acute pulmonary embolism is often uncertain or even incorrect, a definitive diagnosis should be established or excluded before the patient is brought into the operating room. This can be provided by echocardiography, or, if a hybrid operating room is available, the diagnosis can be confirmed or excluded using acute pulmonary angiography before emergency surgery. Echocardiography provides excellent assessment of volume status in the right heart cavity, of contractility in the right ventricle, and of the presence of tricuspid incompetence. In addition, a large thrombus caught in the right atrium or ventricle can often be identified using transesophageal echocardiography in hemodynamically unstable patients.

Preoperative risk stratification

Thanks to more reliable risk stratification, critical patients who are at high risk can today be identified more quickly. Patients with acute pulmonary embolism often maintain a normal systemic blood pressure even when there is marked dysfunction of the right heart. The central importance of right heart dysfunction has been demonstrated in many clinical studies. The ICOPER registry clearly showed that right echocardiographic evidence of right ventricular hypokinesis was associated with a doubling of the risk of death within 90 days—underlining the validity of echocardiography. In patients with acute pulmonary embolism confirmed on CT, Schoepf et al. showed that a right to left ventricular ratio of more than 0.9 increased the risk of dying within 30 days by a factor of 5.2 (Schoepf et al. 2004). Preoperative assessment of cardiac biomarkers (troponins, BNP) can also provide helpful evidence of existing myocardial stress and cardiac damage. A recently published meta-analysis of 20 studies including 1985 patients clearly confirmed the significance of cardiac troponins for the short-term and long-term prognosis in patients in this situation.

Surgical technique

Access is through a median sternotomy and longitudinal opening of the pericardium. Open surgery pulmonary artery embolectomy is carried out in principle in the warm, beating heart using a heart–lung machine. To achieve this, the ascending aorta and superior and inferior venae cavae are selectively cannulated following systemic heparinization (20,000 IU heparin i.v. or i.a., ACT > 400 s). Femoral cannulation of emergency patients under cardiopulmonary resuscitation does not reduce the time required to attach the heart–lung

machine. This method of cannulation should therefore only be used in patients who have previously undergone cardiac surgery. Cardioplegia-induced cardiac arrest is generally not required, as this would further damage the already strained right ventricle.

In Essen, Germany, a modified pulmonary artery embolectomy technique was developed, first described by Jakob et al. (1995). Separate incisions are made in the right and left pulmonary arteries (Fig. 2.2-9) using a specially miniaturized (2–6 mm) suction system, as used in the classic pulmonary embolectomy. This allows complete thrombectomy of the pulmonary arteries up to the subseg-

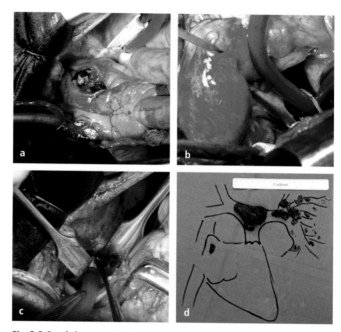

Fig. 2.2-9a–d Separate incisions in the left (**a**) and right (**b**) pulmonary artery. (**c**) Using specialized miniature (2–6 mm) aspiration systems allows complete disobliteration of the vascular bed of the pulmonary artery up to the subsegmental arterial level (**d**).

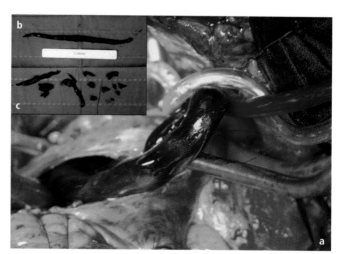

Fig. 2.2-10a–c (**a**) Opening of the right atrium, with an open inferior vena cava, and extirpation of a large outflow thrombus (**b**) from the pelvis–leg venous circulatory pathway after intraoperative unwrapping of the legs and repeated abdominal compression during extracorporeal circulation. (**c**) Emboli removed from the vascular bed of the pulmonary artery up to the subsegmental arterial level.

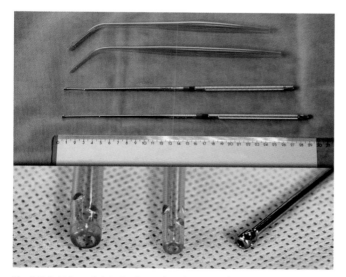

Fig. 2.2-8 Using miniaturized metal aspirators with 2–6-mm tips allows complete disobliteration up to the subsegmental level.

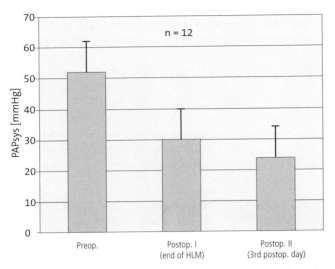

Fig. 2.2-11 Perioperative course of pulmonary artery pressure after selective surgical embolectomy.

mental arteries. In addition, both pleural cavities are opened so that additional small thrombi can be pressed out of the peripheral vasculature using cautious compression on both lungs, and suctioned out. It is extremely important to avoid blind instrumentation of the pulmonary artery bed, as damage to the pulmonary vessels can be fatal. After complete embolectomy, the pulmonary artery is closed with a continuous suture. Thrombectomy and inspection of the right ventricle, right atrium, vena cava and large peripheral veins then follow. For this purpose, with an open inferior vena cava and use of three suction systems, the legs are unwrapped in a central direction while the abdomen is repeatedly compressed, so that mobilized thrombus material in the pelvic and leg veins can be removed from the right atrium, reducing the risk of a recurrent pulmonary embolism (Fig. 2.2-10). Depending on right heart function, appropriate reperfusion should be carried out on the heart–lung machine until the patient can be weaned from the machine without problems.

The rationale of this operation involves effective reduction of right ventricular afterload and prevention of intraoperative or early postoperative recurrent thromboembolism. Among the patients treated by the authors, it was possible to measure systolic pulmonary artery blood pressure in the case of 12 hemodynamically stable patients immediately before the start of extracorporeal circulation and to repeat the measurements after selective pulmonary artery embolectomy. The pulmonary artery pressures were almost normal immediately after the operation, and a further reduction in pulmonary artery pressures was observed up to the third postoperative day, when the Swan–Ganz catheter was removed.

Postoperative follow-up

Immediately after the operation, while the patient is still in the operating room, the legs should be wrapped with elastic compression stockings. Postoperative intensive-care treatment in these patients is much the same as the management of postoperative cardiac surgery patients. Hemodynamic monitoring using a Swan–Ganz catheter and controlling cardiac and renal function using appropriately tailored drug treatment are therefore of the utmost importance. Postoperatively, renal failure and cerebral injury due to phases of inadequate cardiopulmonary resuscitation before the operation can

be expected. Broad-spectrum antibiotic treatment should be administered, particularly in patients who have undergone emergency sternotomy during cardiopulmonary resuscitation. Following the operation, CT angiography or duplex ultrasonography are carried out, and anticoagulation medication with vitamin K antagonists (INR 2.0–3.0) is administered for at least 6 months. In patients in whom oral anticoagulation therapy is contraindicated and those with recurrent pulmonary embolism despite adequate anticoagulation treatment, implantation of a vena cava filter system is indicated.

Results of surgical treatment

The wide variation in the results of surgical pulmonary artery embolectomy needs to be seen against the background of the extremely heterogeneous patient population, ranging from patients who are still hemodynamically stable patients despite massive pulmonary embolism to those with fulminant pulmonary embolism requiring preoperative cardiopulmonary resuscitation. The mortality rates reported in the medical literature range from 11% to 55%, depending on the preoperative risk profile and the patient's hemodynamic status. In emergency surgical embolectomy in resuscitation conditions, mortality rates of 45–75% are reported, or 8–36% in hemodynamically stable patients. The main cause of death is hypoxic brain damage, heart failure, severe bleeding, and postoperative sepsis, as well as recurrent pulmonary embolism. However, nearly 80% of patients who undergo successful surgical treatment can be expected to experience a long-term reduction in pulmonary hypertension and normalized physical exercise capacity. Aklog et al. reported a 30-day survival rate of 89% with surgical treatment for acute pulmonary embolism within the first 24 h after diagnosis, using an interdisciplinary approach with a surgical team constantly available (Aklog 2002). However, the inclusion of hemodynamically stable patients with massive pulmonary embolism and the use of liberal indications for surgery certainly contributed to these favorable results.

The modified technique for surgical pulmonary artery embolization described by Jakob et al. was used in 35 patients in Essen, Germany, up to 2008. The patients' average age was 49 ± 18 years (range 27–71 years). Eighteen patients had a deep vein thrombosis diagnosed preoperatively, and nine underwent preoperative thrombolysis treatment. Ten patients (29%) were delivered to the operating room during ongoing cardiopulmonary resuscitation. Seven of these 10 patients survived the postoperative phase. With the exception of one patient, the operation was carried out in normothermic beating-heart conditions. The bypass time was 137 ± 51 min. Intraoperative venous thrombectomy was successful in 17 of the 35 patients after unwrapping of the legs. Five patients died within the first 30 days, and a further three patients died during the long-term follow-up. There were no cases of recurrent pulmonary embolism.

Surgical treatment for chronic pulmonary embolism

Clinical picture

Patients with a mixture of fresh and chronic pulmonary embolism are particularly problematic. If an acute pulmonary embolism is given sufficient time to become organized and recurrent emboli are already occurring, the time window of approximately 10–14 days available to carry out a pulmonary embolectomy will be missed. Suction or removal of the thromboembolism from the vascular intima is no longer possible at this stage, and the classic thrombectomy procedure carries a risk of vascular wall perforation due to the instability of vascular media. In this case, one should wait at least 6 months for the thromboembolism to mature—i.e., with increasing connective-tissue organization and incorporation of the former thromboembolus into the vascular wall, creating a stable media, before the patient undergoes pulmonary artery thromboendarterectomy with deep hypothermia and circulatory arrest.

Without the appropriate surgical treatment, chronic recurrent pulmonary embolism leading to the development of pulmonary hypertension is associated with a very poor prognosis for the patient, depending on the severity of the pulmonary hypertension (5-year survival with a mean pulmonary pressure PAP > 33 mmHg: 30%; 5-year survival with a mean PAP > 50 mmHg: 10%). Surgical treatment with pulmonary thromboendarterectomy makes it possible to reduce the pulmonary hypertension over the longer term, improving the patient's capacity for physical exercise and the long-term prognosis. However, this specialized operation is nowadays only carried out in a few centers that have the relevant experience, and it is associated with a perioperative mortality rate of 10–20%. In view of the increased surgical mortality rate associated with pulmonary thromboendarterectomy, lung transplantation or heart–lung transplantation if appropriate should be considered in specialized centers for selected patients with a favorable risk profile.

References

Aklog L, Williams CS, Byrne JG, Goldhaber SZ. Acute pulmonary embolectomy: a contemporary approach. Circulation 2002; 105: 1416–9.

Becattini C, Vedovati MC, Agnelli G. Prognostic value of troponins in acute pulmonary embolism: a meta-analysis. Circulation 2007; 116: 427–33.

Chitwood WR Jr, Lyerly HK, Sabiston DC Jr. Surgical management of chronic pulmonary embolism. Ann Surg 1985; 201: 11–26.

Cooley DA and Beall AC Jr. A technic of pulmonary embolectomy using temporary cardio-pulmonary bypass. Cardiovascular Surg 19961; 2: 496.

Dauphine C, Omari B. Pulmonary embolectomy for acute massive pulmonary embolism. Ann Thorac Surg 2005; 79: 1240–4.

Dörge H, Schöndube FA, Voss M, Seipelt R, Messmer BJ. Surgical therapy of fulminant pulmonary embolism: early and late results. Thorac Cardiovasc Surg 1999; 47: 9–13.

Fedullo PF, Auger WR, Kerr KM, Rubin LJ. Chronic thromboembolic pulmonary hypertension. N Engl J Med 2001; 345: 1465–72.

Goldhaber SZ, Visani L, De Rosa M. Acute pulmonary embolism: clinical outcomes in the International Cooperative Pulmonary Embolism Registry (ICOPER). Lancet 1999; 353: 1386–9.

Goldhaber SZ. Pulmonary embolism. Lancet 2004; 363: 1295–1305.

Greenfield LJ, Proctor MC, Williams DM, et al. Long-term experience with transvenous catheter pulmonary embolectomy. J Vasc Surg 1993; 18: 450–7.

Guidelines on diagnosis and management of acute pulmonary embolism. Tasc Force on pulmonary embolism, European Society of Cardiology. Eur Heart J 2000; 21: 1301–6.

Gulba DC, Schmid C, Borst HG, Lichtlen P, Dietz R, Luft FC. Medical compared with surgical treatment for massive pulmonary embolism. Lancet 1994; 343: 576–7.

Jakob H, Vahl C, Lange R, Micek M, Tanzeem A, Hagl S. Modified surgical concept for fulminant pulmonary embolism. Eur J Cardiothorac Surg 1995; 9: 557–60.

Jamieson SW, Kapelanski DP, Sakakibara N, Manecke GR, Thistlethwaite PA, Kerr KM, Channick RN, Fedullo PF, Auger WR. Pulmonary endarterectomy: experience and lessons learned in 1,500 cases. Ann Thorac Surg 2003; 76: 1457–62.

Konstantinides S, Geibel A, Olschewski M, Heinrich F, Grosser K, Rauber K, Iversen S, Redecker M, Kienast J, Just H, Kasper W. Association between thrombolytic therapy and the prognosis of hemodynamically stable patients with major pulmonary embolism. Circulation 1997; 96: 882–8.

Kramm T, Mayer E, Dahm M, Guth S, Menzel T, Pitton M, Oelert H. Long-term results after thromboendarterectomy for chronic pulmonary embolism. Eur J Cardiothorac Surg 1999; 15: 579–84.

Kucher N, Goldhaber SZ. Cardiac biomarkers for risk stratification of patients with acute pulmonary embolism. Circulation 2003; 108: 2191–4.

Kucher N, Windecker S, Banz Y, Mettler D, Schmitz-Rode T, Meier B, Hess O. Percutaneous catheter thrombectomy device for acute pulmonary embolism. Radiology 2005; 236: 852–8.

Kucher N. Catheter embolectomy for acute pulmonary embolism. Chest 2007; 132: 657–63.

Leacche M, Unic D, Goldhaber SZ, Rawn JD, Aranki SF, Couper GS, Mihaljevic T, Rizzo RJ, Cohn LH, Aklog L, Byrne JG. Modern surgical treatment of massive pulmonary embolism: results in 47 consecutive patients after rapid diagnosis and aggressive surgical approach. J Thorac Cardiovasc Surg 2005; 129: 1018–23.

Meneveau N, Ming LP, Séronde MF, Mersin N, Schiele F, Caulfield F, Bernard Y, Bassand JP. In-hospital and long-term outcome after submassive and massive pulmonary embolism submitted to thrombolytic therapy. Eur Heart J 2003; 24: 1447–54.

Perrier A. et al. Non-invasive diagnosis of venous thrombembolism in outpatients. Lancet 1999; 353: 190–5.

Schmitz-Rode T, Janssens U, Schild HH, et al. Fragmentation of massive pulmonary embolism using a pigtail rotation catheter. Chest 1998; 114: 1427–36.

Schoepf UJ, Kucher N, Kipfmueller F, Quiroz R, Costello P, Goldhaber SZ. Right ventricular enlargement on chest computed tomography: a predictor of early death in acute pulmonary embolism. Circulation 2004; 110: 3276–80.

Tapson VF. Acute pulmonary embolism. N Engl J Med 2008; 358: 1037–52.

Thabut G, Thabut D, Myers RP, Bernard-Chabert B, Marrash-Chahla R, Mal H, Fournier M. Thrombolytic therapy of pulmonary embolism: a meta-analysis. J Am Coll Cardiol 2002; 40: 1660–7.

Trendelenburg, F. Über die operative Behandlung der Embolie der Lungenarterie. Langenbecks Arch klin Chir 1908; 86: 686.

Uflacker R. Treat the clot. Endovascular Today 2004; 3: 23–32.

Uflacker R. Interventional therapy of pulmonary embolism. J Vasc Interv Radiol 2001; 12: 147–64.

Voigtlander T, Rupprecht HJ, Nowak B, et al. Clinical application of a new rheolytic thrombectomy catheter system for massive pulmonary embolism. Cath cardiovasc Intervent 1999; 47: 91–6.

Wood KE et al. Major pulmonary embolism. Chest 2002; 121: 877–905.

Yalamanchili K, Fleisher AG, Lehrman SG, Axelrod HI, Lafaro RJ, Sarabu MR, Zias EA, Moggio RA. Open pulmonary embolectomy for treatment of major pulmonary embolism. Ann Thorac Surg 2004; 77: 819–23.

2.2.2   Pulmonary artery hypertension (PAH)

Edda Spiekerkötter and Thomas Zeller

2.2.2.1   Clinical picture

A diagnosis of PAH is made when there is evidence of increased pulmonary vascular resistance after exclusion of chronic thromboembolic pulmonary hypertension (CTPH), pulmonary venous hypertension in the context of heart disease, and secondary pulmonary hypertension in lung diseases. A distinction is made in PAH between:

- Idiopathic pulmonary artery hypertension (IPAH), familial pulmonary artery hypertension (FPAH), sporadic pulmonary artery hypertension; and
- Associated forms (APAH)

A mean pulmonary arterial pressure (PAP_m) > 25 mmHg at rest and > 28–30 mmHg during exertion is required for the diagnosis of pulmonary hypertension.

The classification of pulmonary hypertension agreed at the Venice Conference in 2003 is currently used:

1	Pulmonary arterial hypertension (PAH)
1.1	Idiopathic pulmonary arterial hypertension (IPAH)
1.2	Familial pulmonary arterial hypertension (FPAH)
1.3	Pulmonary arterial hypertension in association with other diseases (APAH), i.e.:
1.3.1	Collagen vascular disease
1.3.2	Congenital cardiac defects
1.3.3	Portal hypertension
1.3.4	HIV infection
1.3.5	Drugs and toxins
1.3.6	Other diseases or disorders
1.4	Pulmonary arterial hypertension with significant venous or capillary involvement
1.5	Persistent pulmonary arterial hypertension of the newborn (PPHN)
2	Pulmonary hypertension associated with left heart disease
3	Pulmonary hypertension associated with lung disease and/or hypoxemia
3.1	Chronic obstructive lung disease (COLD)
3.2	Interstitial lung disease (ILD)
3.3	Sleep apnea
3.4	Alveolar hypoventilation
3.5	Chronic altitude sickness
3.6	Developmental lung abnormalities
4	Pulmonary hypertension due to chronic thrombotic and/or embolic disease (CTEPH)
5	Miscellaneous forms of pulmonary hypertension

Epidemiology

Pulmonary hypertension is a rare disease, with an incidence of approximately one per 1 million population per year. Some 6–12% of primary pulmonary hypertension (PPH) cases are familial, and the condition is inherited in an autosomal-dominant fashion, with reduced penetrance. It usually occurs sporadically, with a male to female ratio of 3:1.

Pathogenesis

- Mutations of the bone morphogenetic protein receptor type II (BMPR II) in cases of familiar PPH and in up to 30% of sporadic PPH → abnormal proliferation of pulmonary vascular cells (endothelial proliferation, media hypertrophy, intima fibrosis)
- Endothelial dysfunction with increased vasoconstrictors (endothelin, thromboxane) predominating the vasodilators (prostaglandins, nitric oxide)
- Excessive "thrombosis in situ" in chronic recurrent pulmonary thrombosis
- Monoclonal endothelial cell proliferation ("plexiform lesions")
- Functional disturbance of potassium channels → vasoconstriction
- Increased elastase and matrix metalloproteinase levels in the adventitia, with resulting proliferation of smooth muscle cells
- Exogenous triggering factors: HIV, appetite suppressants, toxic oil syndrome

2.2.2.2   Clinical findings

Pulmonary hypertension often presents with nonspecific symptoms that are recognized too late by both the patient and the physician. The mean latency period between the start of symptoms and the establishment of a diagnosis is 2 years. Typical symptoms are:

- Exertional dyspnea
- Chronic fatigue
- General weakness
- Dizziness, especially when walking upstairs or when standing up
- Fainting
- Reduced left ventricular filling
- Low cardiac output
- Angina pectoris (right heart angina)
- Edema and ascites due to right heart failure
- Raynaud phenomenon in approximately 10–20% of cases

2.2.2.3   Differential diagnosis

Pulmonary venous hypertension:
- Diseases of the left atrium or left ventricle
- Left heart valve diseases
- Extrinsic compression of the pulmonary veins
- Pulmonary veno-occlusive disease

Pulmonary hypertension due to respiratory disease and/or hypoxemia:
- Chronic obstructive lung diseases
- Interstitial lung diseases
- Sleep-related respiratory disturbances
- Hypoventilation syndromes
- Long stays at high altitude
- Congenital lung diseases

Pulmonary hypertension as result of chronic thromboembolic and/or embolic processes:
- Chronic recurrent thromboembolism
- Obstruction of the distal pulmonary arteries:
  - Embolic (clots, tumor particles, parasites, foreign bodies)
  - In situ clots
  - Sickle cell disease

Pulmonary hypertension due to diseases of the pulmonary vasculature:
- Inflammatory:
  – Schistosomiasis
  – Sarcoidosis
  – Other forms
- Pulmonary capillary hemangiomatosis

2.2.2.4 Diagnosis

Clinical history: The following risk factors should be looked for when taking the clinical history (relative to the various forms of pulmonary hypertension):
- Appetite suppressants
- Drug consumption
- HIV infection
- Liver diseases
- Splenectomy
- Sleep-related respiratory diseases
- Chronic obstructive lung disease
- Thyroid or connective tissue diseases
- Thrombosis
- Pulmonary embolism
- Coagulation disorders

Some 6–10% of patients with primary pulmonary hypertension have a positive family history.

Physical examination:
- Central cyanosis in hypoxia, due to a right–left heart shunt (patent foramen ovale)
- Visible jugular venous pulse
- Elevated jugular venous pressure
- Leg edema
- Ascites
- Auscultation:
  – Emphatic pulmonary component of the second heart sound (P2)
  – Early systolic click
  – Holosystolic murmur in tricuspid insufficiency

Laboratory tests: Laboratory diagnosis includes assessment of TSH, ANA, anti-DNS, anti-scl-70, anticardiolipin antibody, rheumatoid factor, urea, hepatitis serology, and HIV testing.

ECG: There are signs of right ventricular hypertrophy:
- Vertical type to right axial deviation
- P pulmonale
- Leftward R/S shift
- Right ventricular Sokolow–Lyon index > 1.05 mV
- Incomplete or complete right bundle-branch block
- ST-segment depression in V2–V6

Chest x-ray (anteroposterior and lateral): common but nonspecific findings are the following:
- Enlargement of the central pulmonary vessels
- Normally wide or constricted peripheral vessels
- Caliber changes from central to peripheral
- Enlarged heart silhouette, with a prominent enlarged pulmonary segment

- Prominent atrial configuration on the right heart
- Widening of the retrosternal space on lateral x-ray
- Exclusion of secondary causes of pulmonary hypertension such as pulmonary emphysema and pulmonary fibrosis

Blood gas analysis: rarely hypoxemia, only in the case of shunting or patent foramen ovale.

Echocardiography: Echocardiography plays a very important role in the diagnosis of pulmonary hypertension. Right atrium and right ventricle size and function can be assessed or examined, as well as the possibility of valvular disease.

Doppler sonography can be used to assess right ventricular systolic pressure in patients with tricuspid incompetence and to identify intracardiac or intrapulmonary shunts using the bubble contrast technique.

Ventilation–perfusion scintigraphy: Scintigraphy is used to measure the extent of thromboembolic pulmonary hypertension, but it has been replaced in most cases by spiral CT. Most cases of pulmonary hypertension demonstrate either normal pulmonary scintigrams, or inhomogeneous perfusion distributions with subsegmental perfusion defects.

Spiral computed tomography: Spiral CT has become the gold standard for excluding central, segmental, or subsegmental clots, as well as excluding interstitial lung disease.

Right heart catheterization: Right heart catheterization is indicated in all cases of pulmonary hypertension to establish the diagnosis and to help in the planning of medical treatment. Pulmonary vascular resistance (PVR), mean pulmonary artery pressure (PAP_m), and stroke volume can be measured, as well as vasoconstriction/dilation testing.
- Testing is carried out with:
  – Nitric oxide (NO, 10–80 ppm)
  – Prostacyclin analogue inhalation (Ilomedin®, 5–17 μg per inhalation, depending on the inhalation system)
  – Intravenous prostacyclin (Flolan®, starting at 2 ng/kg/min, increasing by 2 ng/kg/min depending on tolerance usually up to a maximum of 10 ng/kg/min)
  – Adenosine (beginning with 50 μg/kg/min, increasing every 2 min, depending on tolerance, by 50 μg/kg/min).

Responders to the treatment have a decrease in PVR and PAP by at least 20%. Calcium-channel blockers are only useful in patients who show a 50% reduction in PVR and near-normalization of the PAP_m immediately after the first administration.

Spirometry/6-min walking test: This is useful for evaluating the patient's exercise capacity and response to treatment.

2.2.2.5 Treatment

General approaches to medical treatment

- Anticoagulation treatment (INR 2.0–2.5) improves life expectancy and should be administered to all patients in whom it is not contraindicated
- Oxygen therapy only has prognostic value in patients with chronic obstructive lung diseases
- Calcium antagonists (high-dose: 4–6 × nifedipine ret. 20 mg, diltiazem 6 × 120 mg, amlodipine 2 × 10 mg) in approximately 10% of patients (very good responders in the acute setting)

- Healthy lifestyle
- Infection treatment/prophylaxis
- Diuretics if there is an increase in central venous pressure, signs of right heart insufficiency with edema and ascites
- Avoidance of hypoxia at high altitudes > 1500 m without supplemental oxygen, also during air travel
- Effective contraception in women

Treatment with prostanoids

Prostanoids have a vasodilatory, antiproliferative, anti-inflammatory, and antiplatelet aggregation effect. They are indicated in patients in New York Heart Association (NYHA) stages III and IV.
Continuous intravenous administration of prostacyclin (Flolan®) and iloprost (Ilomedin®):
- Flolan®: half-life: 1–2 min, dosage: initially 2–4 ng/kg/min, increasing by 1–2 ng/kg/min until clinical symptoms improve or signs of side effects appear
- Ilomedin®: half-life: 20–30 min, dosage: initially 0.5–1.0 ng/kg/min, maintenance dose 2–4 ng/kg/min (up to 8 ng/kg/min)

Potential side effects include flushing, headache, jaw pain, diarrhea, nausea and burning feet syndrome.
Iloprost aerosol (Ilomedin®): daily inhaled dosage 12–17.5 μg 6–9 times daily (depending on the nebulizer). The advantage of the inhaled route is selective vasodilatation. Disadvantages are side effects such as the intermittent administration with overnight breaks, flushing, headache, and the high cost of treatment.
Subcutaneous treprostinil (Remodulin®) is administered using a subcutaneous delivery pump system, with titration depending on the effect and side effects. A dosage of > 13.8 ng/kg/min shows the greatest clinical advantage. The advantage of subcutaneous administration is continuous delivery, while disadvantages are pain in the area of administration, generally the stomach, and the limited ability to increase the dosage.
Oral beraprost (Procyclin®): daily dosage of 4 × 120 μg.

Endothelin receptor antagonists

Indications for use are NYHA stages (I)–II–III. Bosentan (Tracleer®) is a dual endothelin A and B receptor antagonist. The dosage is 2 × 62.5/day to 2 × 125 mg/day. Selective endothelin A receptor antagonists are:
- Ambrisentan (Volibris®) (dosage: 5–10 mg/per day)
- Sitaxsentan (Thelin®) (dosage: 100 mg/per day)

These drugs have the advantage that they can be given orally and are generally well tolerated, except for the potential side effect of raised liver enzymes. A liver enzyme check is necessary every 4 weeks.

Other medical treatments

Phosphodiesterase inhibitors can also be used:
- PDE-5/6-inhibitor: sildenafil (Viagra®, Revatio®), dosage 3 × 20–40 mg
- PDE-3/4-inhibitor: tolafentrine

These agents lead to prolongation and intensification of the effect of prostanoid.

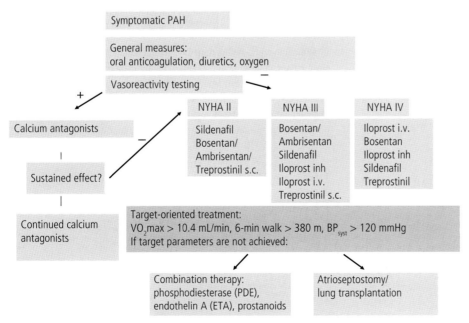

Fig. 2.2-12 Treatment algorithm in pulmonary artery hypertension (PAH).

Surgical treatment

Atrial septostomy. The aim of this operation is to create an artificial right-to-left heart shunt from the atrium to increase the systemic circulation and ease the burden on the right ventricle. This procedure is indicated in patients with severe right heart failure despite maximal medical treatment, and oxygen saturation > 90%. The operation is associated with a mortality rate of 10% and can only be carried out in specialized centers.

Pulmonary endarterectomy (PEA) for the treatment of chronic thromboembolic pulmonary hypertension. This form of treatment is useful in a small group of patients with secondary pulmonary hypertension, to reduce the pulmonary resistance or even restore normal hemodynamic function. It is important to carry out a careful angiographic evaluation of the degree of obstruction before establishing the indication for surgery. It is possible that medical therapy may be as effective in CTEPH as in PAH. Medical treatment may be useful for patients who are not suitable for surgery, or before and after PAH, and further studies are necessary to establish criteria for specific treatment of CTEPH.

Lung transplantation. This is can be regarded as a last resort when all other treatment options have failed.

2.2.2.6 Course and prognosis

Without treatment, the mean survival after the diagnosis of primary pulmonary hypertension is 2.8 years. Controlled studies on the long-term effects, side effects, quality of life, and costs of the various medical treatments have yet to be carried out. The choice of medical treatment depends on the clinical situation, the experience of the medical team, and the patient's preferences.

References

Archer S, Rich S. Primary pulmonary hypertension. A vascular biology and translational research "Work in Progress". Circulation 2000; 102: 2781–91.

Archibald C, Auger WR, Fedullo PF, Channick RN, Kerr KM, Jamieson SW, Kapelanski DP, Watt CN, Moser KM. Long-term outcome after pulmonary thromboendarterectomy. Am J Resp Crit Care Med 1999; 160: 523–8.

Barst RJ, Rubin LJ, Long WA, et al. A comparison of continuous intravenous epoprostenol (prostacyclin) with conventional therapy for primary pulmonary hypertension: the Primary Pulmonary Hypertension Study Group. N Engl J Med 1996; 334: 296–302.

Bonderman D, Wilkens H, Wakounig S, Schäfers HJ, Jansa P, Lindner P, Simkova I, Martischnig AM, Dudczak J, Sadushi R, Skoro-Sajer N, Klepetko W, Lang IM. Risk factors for chronic thromboembolic pulmonary hypertension. Circulation 2007; 115 (16): 2153-8.

Channick RN, Simonneau G, Sitbon O, Robbins IM, Prost A, Tapson VF, Badesch DA, Roux S, Reinisio M, Bodin F, Rubin LR. Effects of the dual endothelin-receptor antagonist bosentan in patients with pulmonary hypertension: a randomised placebo-controlled study. Lancet 2001; 358: 1119–23.

Grünig E, Janssen B, Mereles D, Barth U, Borst MM, Vogt IR, Fischer C, Olschewski H, Kuecherer HF, Kübler W. Abnormal pulmonary artery pressure response in asymptomatic carriers of primary pulmonary hypertension gene. Circulation 2000; 102: 1145–50.

Kemp K, Savale L, O'Callaghan DS, Jaïs X, Montani D, Humbert M, Simonneau G, Sitbon O. Usefulness of first-line combination therapy with epoprostenol and bosentan in pulmonary arterial hypertension: An observational study. J Heart Lung Transplant 2011 Dec 2; [Epub ahead of print].

Long J, Russo MJ, Muller C, Vigneswaran WT. Surgical treatment of pulmonary hypertension: Lung transplantation. Pulm Circ 2011 Jul; 1 (3): 327–33.

McGoon M, Gutterman D, Steen V, et al. Screening, early detection, and diagnosis of pulmonary arterial hypertension. Chest 2004; 126: 14S–34S.

Olschewski H, Ghofrani HA, Schmehl T, et al. Inhaled iloprost to treat severe pulmonary hypertension: an uncontrolled trial: German PPH Study Group. Ann Intern Med 2000; 132: 435–43.

Pauwaa S, Machado RF, Desai AA. Survival in pulmonary arterial hypertension: A brief review of registry data. Pulm Circ 2011 Jul; 1 (3): 430–1.

Rich S, Kaufmann E, Levy PS. The effect of high doses of calcium channel blockers on survival in primary pulmonary hypertension. N Engl J Med 1992; 327: 76–81.

Rubin LJ. Diagnosis and management of pulmonary arterial hypertension: ACCP evidence-based clinical practice guidelines. Introduction. Chest 2004; 126: 7S–10S.

Wensel R, Opitz CF, Ewert R, Bruch L, Kleber FX. Effects of iloprost inhalation on exercise capacity and ventilatory efficiency in patients with primary pulmonary hypertension. Circulation 2000; 101: 2388–92.

Wilkens H, Guth A, König J, Forestier N, Cremers B, Hennen B, Böhm M, Sybrecht GW. Effect of inhaled iloprost plus oral sildenafil in patients with primary pulmonary hypertension. Circulation 2001; 104: 1218.

Wilkens H. Therapie der chronischen Thromboembolie. Pneumologe 2007; 4: 30–8.

2.2.3 Pulmonary arteriovenous malformations (PAVMs)

Edda Spiekerkötter, Thomas Zeller

2.2.3.1 Clinical picture

Definition

PAVM is an abnormal connection between pulmonary veins and pulmonary arteries, usually congenital, leading to the formation of a right-to-left shunt.

Synonyms include:

- Pulmonary arteriovenous fistulas
- Pulmonary arteriovenous aneurysms
- Pulmonary hemangioma
- Cavernous angioma of the lungs
- Pulmonary telangiectasia

Epidemiology

PAVM is a very rare disease, and precise figures for its incidence are not available. Approximately 500 cases have been described in the literature. The incidence is approximately two to three per 100,000 population, the ratio of women to men is approximately 2:1, while in newborns there is a male predominance. Ten percent of PAVM cases are identified in childhood, with most cases being identified before the age of 30.

Up to 70% of cases are associated with hereditary hemorrhagic telangiectasia (HHT). Approximately 15–35% of patients with HHT go on to develop PAVM. Although it is already present at birth, PAVM in patients with HHT does not become apparent until adulthood (after the vessels have withstood a certain degree of perfusion pressure over a period of decades).

Etiology

The etiology of the disease is unknown, and up to 80% of cases are congenital. There is an association with HHT. Mutations in the endoglin gene (chromosome 9q3), activin receptor-like kinase 1 (chromosome 12q), and transforming growth factor-β (TGF-β) II receptor genes (chromosome 3q22) lead to changes in the ligands of transforming growth factor-β, leading to angiogenesis and vascular remodeling after vascular damage. In rare cases, the malformations are acquired—e.g., after chest trauma, after thoracic surgery, liver cirrhosis, mitral valve stenosis, infections (schistosomiasis, actinomycosis), Fanconi syndrome, metastases from thyroid carcinoma, and in the case of systemic amyloidosis.

An increase in PAVM has been described in pregnancy (increased blood volume and cardiac output, increased pulmonary blood flow, particularly in cases of PAVM with low pulmonary vascular resistance, resulting in dilation of the PAVM).

Pathology

Some 50–70% of PAVMs are located in the inferior pulmonary lobes. In 75% of patients, the disease presents unilaterally. Thirty percent of patients have multiple lesions, 50% of which are bilateral. The typical size is 1–5 cm.

PAVM is divided into two subgroups:

- Simple PAVM: a single feeding artery connects to a drainage vein
- Complicated type: there are two or more afferent vessels or efferent veins

Altogether, there are three characteristic types: a saccular plexiform arrangement due to dilated vessels, and either wide or narrow direct arteriovenous connections.

2.2.3.2   Clinical findings

The clinical symptoms depend on the size and number of the PAVMs, as well as the size of the right-to-left shunts. Isolated PAVMs < 2 cm are often asymptomatic. Neurological symptoms are common, due to paradoxical embolization.

Major symptoms include:

- Epistaxis (nosebleeds)
- Dyspnea
- Hemoptysis
- Chest pain
- Cough

PAVM-induced complications include:

- Hypoxia/orthopnea/paroxysmal nocturnal dyspnea: 80–100%
- Migraine, headaches: 43%
- Transient ischemic attacks (TIAs): 37%
- Polycythemia: 25%

- Stroke: 18%
- Anemia: 17%
- Brain abscess: 9%
- Epileptic seizure: 8%
- Hemothorax: 8%
- Hemoptysis: 8%
- Life-threatening hemoptysis: rare
- Heart failure: rare
- Pulmonary hypertension: rare

2.2.3.3   Differential diagnosis

- Right-to-left heart shunts (patent foramen ovale, septal defects)
- Hepatopulmonary syndrome and portal hypertension
- Vascular tumors
- Atelectasis causing a right-to-left shunt
- Microvascular telangiectasia

2.2.3.4   Diagnosis

Clinical examination

The typical clinical triad of dyspnea, cyanosis, and clubbed nails occurs only in 10% of patients. Telangiectasias (on the face, mouth, breast, and upper extremities), are common, as they are associated with HHT. On auscultation, the murmur is loudest in the sitting position and during inspiration.

Arterial blood gas analysis at rest

Hypoxia at rest is defined as a Pao_2 < 104 (0.24 times age). Orthostatic: Pao_2 or Sao_2 fall when the patient sits up after lying down (increased shunt flow during sitting down; PAVMs are more prevalent in the lower pulmonary regions).

Chest x-ray on two planes

Round or oval nodules are visible, 1–5 cm in size, demarcated with smooth walls. A single nodule is present in approximately 70% of cases; multiple PAVMs usually have two to eight nodules, or in rare cases 10–100. In the case of microvascular telangiectasia, a normal chest x-ray is possible.

Evaluating right-to-left shunts

1. Measurement of Pao_2 during inhalation with 100% oxygen for 15–20 min:

- Evaluating the shunt fraction using nomograms (requires measurement of arterial Po_2 and calculation of alveolar Po_2 using the alveolar gas equation)
- Physiological shunt ≤ 5% (admixture of proportions of bronchial arterial blood to pulmonary venous blood, inflow of thebesian veins into the left atrium)
- Pathological shunt > 5%: further clarification needed

2. Contrast echocardiography:

- No right-to-left shunt: bubbles appear in the right atrium and are quickly captured by the pulmonary circulation.

- Cardiac right-to-left shunt: bubbles appear in the left atrium within a cardiac cycle.
- Pulmonary right-to-left shunt: bubbles appear in the left atrium with a latency of three to eight cardiac cycles.

Chest CT (contrast CT, spiral CT)

- High sensitivity, noninvasive procedure
- False-positive findings in vascular tumors
- Good follow-up possible

Pulmonary artery angiography

- Gold standard for PAVMs
- Best assessment of the angioarchitecture of individual PAVMs (superior to CT)
- Necessary before surgical intervention or embolization

2.2.3.5 Treatment

Conservative approach: observation

There have been no controlled studies comparing conservative therapy with intervention. In general, slow growth can be expected in 25% of PAVMs. With observation alone, the mortality rate is 0–16%, with death mainly being due to cerebral abscess, stroke, hemoptysis, or hemothorax.

The morbidity is high, due to the major symptoms and complications (see above).

Accepted indications for treatment for PAVMs are:

- Increase in size
- Paradoxical embolisms
- Symptomatic hypoxemia
- Size of the afferent segmental arteries $\geq 3\,mm$ (neurological complications $\uparrow$), size of the PAVMS $\geq 2\,cm$

Rigorous prophylaxis against endocarditis is important before abdominal surgery and dental procedures to minimize the risk of bacterial colonization of the PAVM and cerebral abscesses.

Embolization treatment

The principle of treatment consists of closure of the arteries feeding the PAVM, using steel coils, removable balloons, or an occluder. Embolization is the preferred treatment for PAVMs, and particularly for multiple or bilateral PAVMs (sparing the lung parenchyma) and in patients at high surgical risk. At diameters $\geq 3\,mm$, endovascular treatment is indicated due to the possibility of paradoxical embolisms.

Technique

- Angiographic localization of the PAVM, usually via transfemoral venous access (or alternatively via the cubital vein or jugular vein), usually via DSA with a 5F pigtail catheter
- Selective catheterization of the feeding artery—e.g., with a 3F microcatheter (Tracker™, Boston Scientific)
- Superselective positioning of the catheter tip near the neck of the PAVM

- Advancing one or more coils—e.g., electrolytically detachable GDC™ platinum coils (Boston Scientific) or Tornado™ (Cook; or balloon or occlude)—through the catheter and placing it, repeating the procedure until blood flow in the PAVM ceases.

The clinical success rate is > 90% (oxygenation $\uparrow$, shunt fraction $\downarrow$, dyspnea $\downarrow$). It may be necessary to repeat the procedure at a second session.

Possible complications include pleural pain, pulmonary infarction (rare), and migration of the device.

Surgical treatment

The principle is to resect the PAVM. The scale of the surgical procedure depends on the extent of the PAVM and includes simple ligation, local excision, segmentectomy, lobectomy, or pneumectomy. As a last resort in individual cases, there may be an indication for lung transplantation. Minimal morbidity and mortality rates are reported, and postoperative recurrence of PAVMs is rare.

Despite the relatively low complication rate, the disadvantages of a surgical approach lie in the morbidity and surgical risk due to thoracotomy, and the long hospital stay of 4–7 days in comparison with embolization.

References

Bauer de Torres A, Leppien A, Eckert B. „High-flow" pulmonale arteriovenöse Malformation – endovaskuläre Therapie mit Vena-Cava-Filter. Fortschr Röntgenstr 2008; 180: 148–50.

Dutton JA, Jackson JE, Hughes JM, Whyte MK, Peters AM, Ussov W, et al. Pulmonary arteriovenous malformations: results of treatment with coil embolization in 53 patients. AJR Am J Roentgenol 1995; 165: 1119–25.

Ference BA, Shannon TM, White RI, Zawin M, Burdge CM. Life-threatening pulmonary hemorrhage with pulmonary arteriovenous malformations and hereditary hemorrhagic teleangiectasia. Chest 1994; 106: 1387–90.

Gossage JR, Kanj G. Pulmonary arteriovenous malformations. A state of the art review. Am J Respir Crit Care Med 1998; 158: 643–61.

Guttmacher AE, Marchuk DA, White RI. Hereditary hemorrhagic teleangiectasia. N Engl J Med 1995; 333: 918–24.

Haitjema T, Westermann CJ, Overtoom TT, Timmer R, Disch F, Hauser H, et al. Hereditary hemorrhagic teleangiectasia (Osler-Weber-Rendu disease): new insights in pathogenesis, complications, and treatment. Arch Intern Med 1996; 156: 714–19.

Kress O, Wollstein AC; Wagner H-J, Folz BJ; Werner JA; Klose KJ; Alfke H. Embolisation pulmonaler arteriovenöser Malformationen bei hereditärer hämorrhagischer Teleangiektasie mittels elektrolytisch ablösbarer Spiralen. Rofo. Fortschritte auf dem Gebiet der Röntgenstrahlen und der bildgebenden Verfahren 2004; 176: 1501–5.

Lee DW, White RI Jr, Egglin TK, Pollak JS, Fayad PB, Wirth JA, Rosenblatt MM, Dickey KW, Burdge CM. Embolotherapy of large pulmonary arteriovenous malformations: long term results. Ann Thorac Surg 1997; 64: 930–40.

Moussouttas M, Fayad P, Rosenblatt M, Hashimoto M, Pollak J, Henderson K, Ma TYZ, White RI. Pulmonary arteriovenous malformations—cerebral ischemia and neurologic manifestations. Neurology 2000; 55: 959–64.

Puskas JD, Allen MS, Moncure AC, Wain JC, Hoilgenberg AD, Wright C, Grillo HC, Mathisen DJ. Pulmonary arteriovenous malformations: therapeutic options. Ann Thorac Surg 1993; 56: 253–7.

Rastogi N, Kabutey NK, Kim D, Norbash A. Percutaneous management of segmental pulmonary artery aneurysm in a patient without pulmonary artery hypertension. Vasc Endovascular Surg 2011 Apr; 45 (3): 283–7.

Ritscher D, Igual M, Rüttimann S, Turina J, Russi EW. Pulmonale arteriovenöse Malformationen. Schweiz Med Wochenschr 1999; 129: 1970–7.

Swanson K, Prakash U, Stanson A. Pulmonary arteriovenous fistulas: Mayo Clinic experience 1982–1997. Mayo Clin Proc 1999; 74: 671–80.

Ueki J, Hughes JM, Peters AM, Bellingan GJ, Mohammed MA, Dutton J, et al. Oxygen and 99mTc-MAA shunt estimations in patients with pulmonary arteriovenous malformations: effects of changes in posture and lung volume. Thorax 1994; 49: 327–31.

3 Abdominal vessels

3.1 Diseases of the abdominal aorta

Eva Schönefeld and Giovanni Torsello
Doppler/duplex ultrasonography: Tom Schilling

3.1.1 Abdominal aortic aneurysm

3.1.1.1 Clinical picture

Dilation of the abdominal aorta to a size of more than 3 cm is defined as an aneurysm. Infrarenal aortic aneurysms are found with an incidence of 0.3–2.8% in men over the age of 65 (Ruppert et al. 2005; Torsello et al. 2005a). Men are affected more often than women, at a ratio of 6:1.

In 98% of cases, the *pathogenesis* involves atherosclerosis, and there is also a high frequency of concomitant conditions, including pulmonary and renal insufficiency. Additional *risk factors* are nicotine consumption and, less often, a positive family history, coronary heart disease, peripheral arterial occlusive disease (PAOD), hypercholesterolemia, hypertension, and cerebrovascular insufficiency. Rarer forms of aneurysm include the traumatic, mycotic, septic, and congenital types (Marfan syndrome, Ehlers–Danlos syndrome). The *locations* of abdominal aneurysms are:

- 95% infrarenal aorta
- 10–30% extension to the pelvic arteries
- 5% extension to the thoracoabdominal aorta
- 5% juxtarenal
- Up to 20% with additional aneurysm locations
- Rare: generalized aneurysmosis (cystic medial necrosis, segmental mediolytic arteriopathy)

Inflammatory aneurysm represents a special morphological type. It is not frequent, with an incidence of 5%, and it is limited to the infrarenal aorta and pelvic arteries. Two hypotheses have been proposed for its etiology: on the one hand, it may be a primary inflammatory disease of the retroperitoneum, while on the other retroperitoneal fibrosis (Ormond disease) has been considered as a possible explanation. Macroscopically, there is a fibrous aortic wall with a slightly reddish to gray-white surface. Neighboring structures (ureters, small bowel, sigmoid, transverse colon, left renal vein) are usually adherent to the aortic wall and are challenging during dissection.

3.1.1.2 Clinical findings

Three different forms of aortic aneurysm are distinguished clinically:

- *Asymptomatic* aortic aneurysm
- *Symptomatic* aortic aneurysm
- Aortic aneurysm at the *rupture* stage

In the majority of cases, abdominal aneurysm may be asymptomatic. The diagnosis is nowadays often made incidentally (60–80% of cases), due to the increasing use of abdominal ultrasound diagnosis. If there are symptoms without rupture, the clinical findings tend to be nonspecific, resulting from expansion and displacement of other organs:

- Back pain, in rare cases as a result of the erosion of the vertebrae
- Diffuse abdominal symptoms, which may or may not radiate into the pelvis
- Flank pain (to be distinguished from urological clinical pictures)
- Sciatic/paresthesia (with differential diagnosis from orthopedic conditions)
- Peripheral embolization of vessels in the lower extremities and renal and mesenteric vessels
- Septic phenomena in mycotic aneurysm

In acute rupture, the following classic triad appears (Morasch 2009; Torsello et al. 2005a):

- Acute back and/or abdominal pain
- Hypovolemic shock
- Pulsating tumor

When there is penetration into the gastrointestinal tract, the patient has the clinical signs of hyperacute gastrointestinal bleeding. Fistula formation into the vena cava leads to acute cardiac decompensation. Sequelae may include renal failure and intestinal ischemia, with the clinical picture of "acute abdomen."

3.1.1.3 Diagnosis

The diagnostic approach depends on the urgency of treatment for the aneurysm, and begins with taking a medical history if the patient is conscious and responsive, and/or with indirect history from observers/relatives.

- In very slim patients, the examination will show a visible abdominal aortic aneurysm.
- On palpation, there may be a pulsating mass in the navel region that is painful on pressure. If the mass can be distinguished from the costal border, an infrarenal location is very probable.
- An absent peripheral pulse may suggest complete thrombosis of the aneurysm, or rupture if there are symptoms of shock.

The principal diagnostic method is *color duplex ultrasonography,* which allows diagnosis both in the asymptomatic stage and also after rupture. Its sensitivity and specificity in experienced hands are more than 90% (Kranokpiraksa and Kaufman 2008; Ruppert et al. 2005; Sternbergh et al. 2008). Ultrasonography is a noninvasive technique that is suitable for use as a screening method and also makes it possible to monitor the course (Kranokpiraksa and Kaufman 2008; Torsello et al. 2005b). The ability to diagnose an abdominal aneurysm is limited both in obese patients and when there is massive superimposition of bowel gas.

Computed tomography is still the standard method for detailed assessment of the morphology of an aneurysm (Figs. 3.1-1 and 3.1-2). The sensitivity and specificity of the procedure are superior, particularly in comparison with color duplex ultrasound. Despite the radiation exposure involved for the patient, computed tomography (CT) is recommended, as multiplanar reconstructions allow precise treatment planning.

After clarification of renal function and allergies, computed tomography is indicated:

■ For basic diagnosis in asymptomatic and symptomatic patients with stable circulation
■ For treatment planning (with slices ≤ 3 mm) when an endovascular procedure is planned
■ For monitoring the course after endovascular treatment

Computed tomography and ultrasonography are the essential components of diagnosis in abdominal aortic aneurysm.
Imaging provides the following information:

■ Type and shape of the aneurysm (true, false, saccular, fusiform)
■ Location
■ Size (length, transverse diameter, ventrodorsal diameter vertical to the *vessel!* axis—otherwise overestimation is possible)
■ Vessel diameter proximal and distal to the aneurysm, for treatment planning

■ Relation to the origins of the renal arteries, distance of the ostia from the start of the aneurysm
■ Relationship to the iliac arteries and distance from the internal iliac artery
■ Grade of thrombosis, breadth of the residual lumen
■ Signs of instability in the wall
■ Coincidental aneurysms
■ Assessment of impairment of neighboring structures
■ Evidence of an inflammatory origin
■ Differential diagnosis versus aortic dissection
■ Free intra-abdominal fluid

Magnetic resonance imaging may offer an alternative diagnostic method if the patient is allergic to contrast medium. Disadvantages are that magnetic resonance angiography is not universally available, more expensive, and involves longer examination times. Precise measurement of an endovascular prosthesis is not possible (Ruppert et al. 2005). Contraindications include implanted cardiac pacemakers and claustrophobia on the part of the patient.

Magnetic resonance imaging is particularly suitable for special investigations on soft-tissue pathology, such as retrograde fibrosis or para-aortic lymph-node enlargement.

Intra-arterial digital subtraction angiography (DSA) depicts the perfused lumen of the vascular system and is therefore not indicated on its own for detecting an abdominal aneurysm (Leurs et al. 2005). The *indications for angiography* are:

■ Planning of complex vascular and endovascular procedures—often simultaneous with implantation of an endovascular prosthesis
■ Suspected juxtarenal or suprarenal abdominal aortic aneurysm

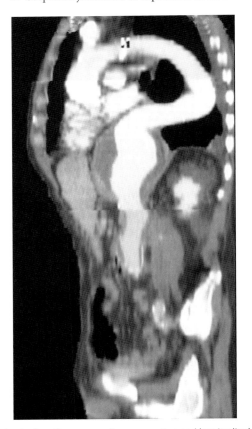

Figs. 3.1-1 and 3.1-2 Computed-tomographic appearance of an infrarenal abdominal aortic aneurysm in cross-section and longitudinal section; contrast imaging of the perfused residual lumen.

- Thoracoabdominal aneurysm
- Assessment of the aortic branches (kidneys, mesenteric arteries, pelvic and leg vessels), with a specificity of 100%

Doppler/duplex ultrasonography

Examination technique

A 3.5–5.0 MHz sector probe is typical. Color imaging is usually with a suboptimal Doppler angle, with the pulse repetition frequency (PRF) set low so that stenoses, ectasias, and aneurysms are not overlooked. The examination is carried out with the necessary pressure on the probe required to compress bowel contents etc. and improve the image quality. During diagnostic imaging of atherosclerosis and peripheral vascular disease, and particularly for confirmation of a popliteal artery aneurysm, the aorta should always be included as part of the examination.

Differential diagnosis

- Atherosclerosis:
  - Typical plaque morphology
  - Classically located in the infrarenal aorta
- Embolism:
  - Hypoechoic to isoechoic occlusive material at the aortic bifurcation, possibly with a demonstrable coupling phenomenon—i.e., a convex configuration of the occlusive material toward the free lumen; possible unremarkable vascular system otherwise, with no major atheroma
- Large-vessel vasculitis:
  - Characterized by a homogenous, hypoechoic widened intima–media complex (macaroni sign)
  - Frequently associated with Ormond disease
- Dissection:
  - Dissection flap may be visible

Specific findings

Infrarenal aortic aneurysm

Questions that need to be answered on Doppler/duplex ultrasonography:

- Location of the aneurysm
- Type and shape of the aneurysm (fusiform, saccular, combined)
- Size of the aneurysm: length, transverse diameter, ventrodorsal diameter (should always be measured perpendicular to the vascular axis, not to the body axis, as this might lead to divergence from tomographic standards)
- Vascular diameter proximal and distal to the aneurysm (for treatment planning)
- Relationship of aneurysm to branching vessels, particularly to the renal arteries; measurement of the distance between renal artery branching and the start of the aneurysm
- Relationship to the iliac vessels—involvement? → If so, then assessment of the iliac vessels according to the criteria listed here as well
- Thrombosis? (Extent, distribution, consistency, pulse-synchronous behavior)
- Signs of emboligenicity in endoluminal thrombi (floating structures, niches), signs of distal embolization
- Diameter of the residual lumen; occlusion by thrombosis?

- Signs of wall instability: thrombi with flow behind, hypoechoic vascular wall structures as signs of dissection, perivascular hypoechoic structures as signs of rupture, leakage (Fig. 3.1-3)
- Signs of impairment of neighboring structures (compression effects)
- Evidence of an inflammatory pathogenesis (hypoechoic, thickened wall structures, Fig. 3.1-4)
- Differentiation of aortic dissection from dissecting aneurysm
- Other aneurysms: e.g., simultaneous aortic, iliac, and popliteal

Duplex ultrasound risk markers for rupture:

- Diameter > 5 cm (UK Small Aneurysm Study: 76% of all ruptured aneurysms > 5 cm)
- Increase in diameter > 1 cm/year
- Eccentric or absent thrombus margin
- Inflammation/mycotic aneurysm
- Burst calcium deposits in the aneurysmal wall
- Saccular bulges

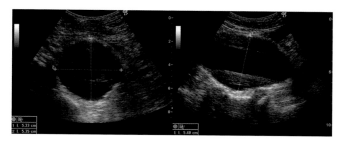

Fig. 3.1-3 An infrarenal aortic aneurysm with a circular, fragmented thrombus margin.

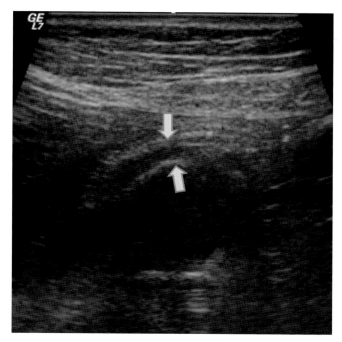

Fig. 3.1-4 An inflammatory abdominal aortic aneurysm, with typical hypoechoic and concentric widening of the wall.

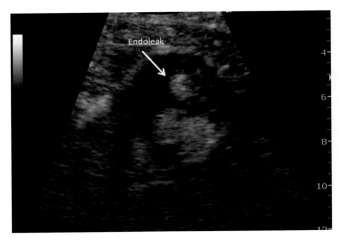

Fig. 3.1-5 Clear evidence of an endoleak with ultrasound contrast enhancement (SonoVue®). Recent studies have shown that duplex ultrasonography with contrast enhancement, rather than conventional color-coded duplex ultrasound, is at least as good as CT for checking the results after endovascular treatment for abdominal aortic aneurysm.

In patients who have previously undergone endovascular treatment for an aortic aneurysm:
- Change in the aneurysm's diameter over time.
- Evidence of endoleak? According to recent data, contrast ultrasonography with a low-MI technique is at least as good as CT; color-coded Doppler ultrasound is much less sensitive (Fig. 3.1-5).
- Aneurysm formation in other locations?

In patients who have previously undergone surgical treatment for an aortic aneurysm:
- Change in the aneurysm's diameter over time
- Aneurysm formation in other locations?
- Is there any evidence of stenosis/ectasia/pseudoaneurysm in the area of the anastomoses?

Aortic stenosis and occlusions

The site of predilection for arteriosclerotic aortic stenoses is the distal abdominal aorta, including the transition to the aortic bifurcation. Embolic occlusions mainly affect the bifurcation region, potentially with ascending thrombosis.
Stenoses are graded using the peak velocity ratio and generally applicable grading criteria (turbulence phenomena, acoustics, indirect prestenotic/post-stenotic criteria). When the iliac arteries or aortic bifurcation are/is occluded, an incorrectly high proximal starting-point for the occlusion may be artifactually created by reduced pre-occlusive flow; a low flow-optimized display should therefore be selected in order to avoid this reading (Fig. 3.1-6).
The following need to be distinguished in the differential diagnosis:
- Stenoses caused by thrombotic aneurysms (duplex ultrasound signs of aneurysm).
- Emboli straddling the bifurcation, embolic occlusions (hypoechoic occlusive material, possibly with no or only slight atherosclerotic changes, pulse-synchronous deformation of the occluding material when it still has a soft consistency).
- Vasculitic stenoses: hypoechoic wall thickening → macaroni sign.
- Aortic coarctation: in an abdominal location (suprarenal, intrarenal, infrarenal), the B-image may show evidence of a preexisting segmental hypoplastic/aplastic vessel.

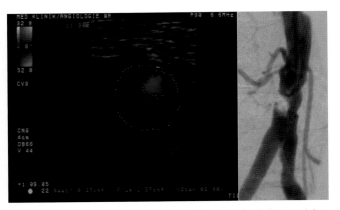

Fig. 3.1-6 Stenosis of the infrarenal abdominal aorta. It should be noted that on intra-arterial digital subtraction angiography (DSA), the stenosis grade can appear less severe despite high-grade stenosis on duplex ultrasonography with cross-sectional planimetry and on pulsed-wave Doppler ultrasound.

Additional diagnostic clarification on ultrasound:
- Involvement of aortic branches
- Collateralization pattern (e.g., retrograde perfusion of the inferior mesenteric artery as an afferent collateral due to hypoperfusion of the superior mesenteric artery when pathology is located between the branch origins; increased flow in the inferior mesenteric artery when there is a distal process as well)
- Signs of emboligenicity in the stenotic or occlusive material; signs of distal embolization
- Occlusion pressure in the lower leg arteries
- Simultaneous distal stenotic and occlusive processes

Aortic dissection and rupture

Optimal B-mode imaging and color adjustment must always be "enforced." When insonation is difficult, the color M-mode should be used; this shows different flow characteristics in the various lumens, as well as the dynamics of the dissection membrane, with high temporal resolution. Color B-flow imaging also shows areas of slow flow and perfusion even with poor insonation angles; alternatively, ultrasound contrast enhancement may also be used.
Questions that need to be answered by Doppler/duplex ultrasonography:
- Where are the sites of entry and reentry?
- If possible, clarification of whether a type A or type B dissection is present (insonation of the aortic arch) (Fig. 3.1-7).
- What are the longitudinal extent and maximum diameter?
- What shape does the dissection membrane have? *Caution:* reverberation echoes may mimic delicate dissection membranes in a hurried examination.

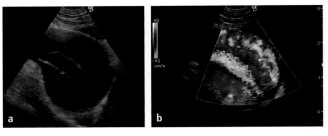

Fig. 3.1-7a, b After initial evidence of dissection of the abdominal aorta (a), immediate insonation of the aortic arch (with a 7.5-MHz microconvex probe) confirms dissection (b).

Table 3.1-1 Comparison of procedures.

	Screening	Diagnosis	Measurement	Checking size of findings	Checking of stent graft
CD ultrasound	+++	++	(+)	++	+
DSA	0	+	(+)	0	(+)
MRI	++	++	+	++	(+)
CT	++	+++	+++	++	+++

CD, color Doppler; CT, computed tomography; DSA, digital subtraction angiography; MRI, magnetic resonance imaging.

Table 3.1-2 Rupture rates in abdominal aortic aneurysms.

Diameter (cm)	Rupture risk/year
4.0–4.9	3%
5.0–5.9	10%
6.0–6.9	15%
> 7.0	> 60%

- Perfusion conditions in the lumens should be checked for evidence of partial thrombosis.
- Perfusion should be checked in branches that are given off (supra-aortic, mesenteric, renal) and the afferent lumen should be differentiated in each case.
- Is there any evidence of critical perfusion disturbances in each of the areas supplied?
- Differentiation between aortic dissection and dissecting aneurysm (evidence of preexisting aneurysm).
- Are there any signs of rupture?
- Is there any extension to the iliac vessels?

3.1.1.4 Differential diagnosis

See Table 3.1-3.

3.1.1.5 Indication

The aim of surgery is to eliminate the aortic aneurysm in order to prevent rupture. The risk of rupture is associated with:
- The size of the aneurysm, or its diameter and growth rate
- Patient-specific risk factors, such as:
  - Sex; women are at higher risk for aortic rupture
  - Hypertension
  - Chronic occlusive pulmonary disease (COPD)
  - Family history

The decision on whether to carry out an intervention depends on the expected risk of rupture relative to the patient's life expectancy and the procedure-related mortality rate.

In addition to the diameter of the aneurysm, its *annual growth rate* plays an important role in the risk of rupture. At a growth rate of less than 0.3 cm per year, the risk of rupture is slight; a mean of 0.5 cm or greater than 0.5 cm per year portends a higher risk of rupture. Independently of the above considerations, treatment of a *symptomatic aneurysm* is indicated without delay, and urgent intervention is required within 24 hours.

Covert and freely *ruptured abdominal aortic aneurysms* are emergencies that require immediate treatment.

Table 3.1-3 Differential diagnosis of unruptured symptomatic abdominal aortic aneurysms.

Symptoms	Cause	Differential findings
Back/gluteal pain	Lumbar and sciatic pain Intervertebral disk prolapse	Neurological findings (sensorimotor function)
Diffuse abdominal symptoms	Intraperitoneal inflammation, peritonitis	Pain on pressure, generalized signs of inflammation, overflow incontinence
Flank pain	Urolithiasis, pyelonephritis	Generalized signs of inflammation, pain on percussion in the renal bed
Paresthesias in the pelvic region and lower extremities	Orthopedic and neurological clinical presentations	Reduced reflexes, normal pulses
Peripheral embolization in the legs, kidneys, and mesenteric vessels	PAOD, formation of cardioembolic thrombus	Abnormal echocardiography, intermittent claudication, no acute events
Septic appearance in mycotic aneurysm	Intra-abdominal inflammatory processes, abscesses, urosepsis, meningoencephalitis	Etiologic evidence required

PAOD, peripheral arterial occlusive disease.

3.1.1.6 Treatment

Conservative treatment

Conservative treatment usually involves monitoring of the course of small, asymptomatic abdominal aortic aneurysms (Ruppert et al. 2005; Torsello et al. 2005a). This requires additional measures, including for example antihypertensive medication, administration of statins, and avoidance of heavy physical exercise or work.

Findings in which a conservative approach is preferable include asymptomatic, fusiform small aneurysms with a diameter of less than 5 cm and only a low growth tendency. Surgery in very severely ill patients with terminal tumor disease, treatment-resistant cardiorespiratory insufficiency, or severe dementia should be considered inappropriate except in rare circumstance.

The goals of conservative treatment are to:
- Minimize cardiovascular risk factors
- Avoid extreme physical activities
- Ensure regular check-ups using ultrasound, or CT if appropriate
- Inform the patient

Endovascular therapy

The mortality rate resulting from the rupture of an abdominal aneurysm can be reduced using two strategies:

- Ultrasound screening allows timely diagnosis and thus reduces rupture-related mortality.
- When indicated, endovascular therapy as a minimally invasive form of treatment with a low perioperative mortality rate can prevent aneurysmal rupture.

Technique

The endovascular procedure has been increasingly used since 1991 as a means of minimizing the invasiveness of aneurysm treatment, the length of the hospital stay involved, and the convalescent period (Torsello et al. 2005b, 2006). Implantation of a Dacron-coated or polytetrafluoroethylene(PTFE)-coated stent is carried out without laparotomy via the transfemoral access route, usually with a bi-iliac endoprosthesis. When a monoiliac system is used, implantation of a femorofemoral crossover bypass is required. A straight tube prosthesis can only be used for circumscribed aneurysms with an adequate proximal and distal neck. Suitable anatomy is an important prerequisite in such cases and is infrequent (Table 3.1-4) (Norwood et al. 2007). Patients with configurations that differ from the above should not be considered for endovascular therapy using standard prostheses. Hybrid operations and fenestrated (side branch) stent graft systems can be used as supplementary procedures. There is experience in some centers with both of these methods, suggesting that they are associated with minor perioperative mortality. Implantation of special stent graft systems should be reserved for experienced *endovascular specialists*.

Anesthesia

The procedure can be carried out with locoregional or endotracheal anesthesia.

Indication for endovascular aneurysm repair (EVAR)

In the early period of endovascular treatment, the indication for endovascular elimination of an infrarenal abdominal aortic aneurysm consisted of a contraindication to conventional reconstruction. This included patients at *increased surgical risk* who were unfit for surgery, as well as those with *abdominal adhesions*, an unfavorably positioned artificial anus, or a urinary fistula.

Treatment for infrarenal aneurysms with a stent graft depends on the *anatomical configuration* of the aorta and pelvic arteries (Table 3.1-4).

This leads to the following *contraindications:*

- Substantial kinking or high-grade stenosis of the pelvic arteries, preventing passage of the introduction system
- Proximal infrarenal aneurysm neck < 1 cm long
- High-grade PAOD with severe calcification in the pelvic circulatory pathway
- Aneurysm neck that is conical or acutely angled

Prosthesis selection initially involves a choice between a one-piece endograft (unibody) or one with several individual parts (modular).

Table 3.1-4 Optimal anatomy for endovascular aneurysm repair.

Anatomy	Size
Length of aneurysm neck	> 15 mm
Diameter of aneurysm neck	< 30 mm
Neck angle	< 50°
Wall thrombus in neck	< 2 mm
Diameter of external iliac artery	> 7 mm
Iliac angle	< 90°
Diameter of common iliac artery	< 18 mm

A stent graft system that has a long main body is preferable. Additional anchorage with hooks or barbs in the suprarenal region is now possible and useful (Torsello et al. 2006).

Technical procedure

Implantation of a stent graft system is carried out in the operating room with the assistance of a high-quality DSA-capable C-arm or stationary DSA equipment. The patient lies on a radiopaque operating table. Following sterile cleaning and draping of the abdomen and inguinal region, the common femoral artery is exposed surgically or directly punctured using a percutaneous technique (Fig. 3.1-8). In the latter technique, an endovascular suture (e.g., with Prostar XL 10F with a Perclose technique) is made in the vessel (12–14F) even before placement of a large-caliber sheath. The Terumo wire then passes through the vessel up to the thoracic aorta. The Terumo wire is exchanged for a stiff wire (e.g., Lunderquist) using a pigtail catheter. An angiography catheter is advanced to the level of the visceral arteries via a contralateral sheath. A rotation check is carried out under fluoroscopic guidance with the help of the markings.

After removal of the 14F sheath, the endograft is advanced over the Lunderquist wire, which is kept under tension. If this maneuver is

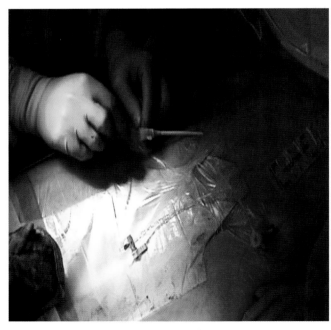

Fig. 3.1-8 Transfemoral access in endovascular aneurysm repair.

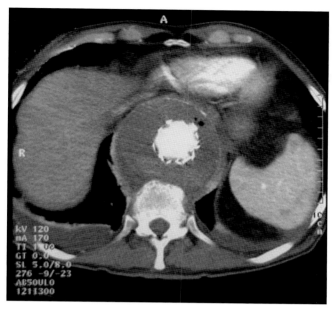

Fig. 3.1-9 Cross-section of an abdominal aortic aneurysm after endovascular treatment, with no signs of endoleaks.

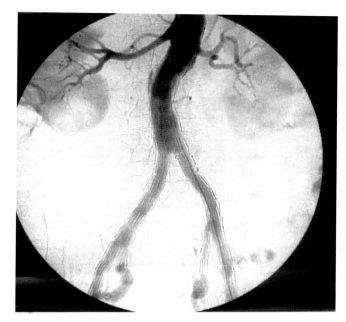

Fig. 3.1-10 Final angiography after introduction of a stent graft system.

not possible due to severely contorted and calcified pelvic vessels, the wire can be led out transbrachially (with the "through-and-through" technique), to allow the endoprosthesis to be advanced with the wire under tension.

When the upper end of the stent graft has reached the level of the visceral arteries, angiography is carried out with the maximum possible enlargement, centered on the renal arteries. After marking of the renal artery, with its inferior origin, the proximal part of the main body of the prosthesis is released. The introduction system is withdrawn until the markings on the first part of the coated stent series lie just underneath the ostia of the renal arteries. Withdrawing the sheath of the endoprosthesis then releases the remaining stent series in the main body and contralateral leg. An angiographic check is now carried out to ensure that the renal arteries are patent, and the prosthesis can still be pulled down if needed.

The pigtail catheter is straightened with a Terumo wire and pulled down alongside the partly expanded prosthesis. Complete release of the stent graft is only carried out after wire probing of the contralateral limb. Once the precise positioning of the wire in the prosthesis has been ensured, the Terumo wire is exchanged for a stiff wire. The contralateral limb is advanced over the stiff wire and precisely positioned using the marks provided. Retrograde angiography of the contralateral sheath should be carried out to avoid inadvertent stenting over the internal iliac artery. Depending on the system used, the ipsilateral iliac limb can be extended in the same way as the contralateral side, with care being taken to protect the internal iliac artery. After the whole prosthesis has been released and adapted to shape with inflations using the latex balloon provided, a final angiographic check is made (Fig. 3.1-10).

Complications

Wound infection, embolization, and (temporary) deterioration in renal function have been reported at similar frequencies for the endovascular operation in all controlled studies in which it has been compared with the open procedure (Ruppert et al. 2005). The in-

Table 3.1-5 Classification of endoleaks after endovascular aneurysm repair (White et al. 1997).

Endoleak type	Cause (of perigraft flow)
Type I	Landing zones for the prosthesis on the original vascular wall
IA	Proximal landing zone
IB	Distal
IC	Iliac limb
Type II	Persistent inflow and outflow in the aneurysmal sac from branch vessels
Type III	Modular leaks in the connections between endograft sections (including suture sites)
Type IV	Porosity in the graft wall/material failure

traoperative blood loss is significantly lower, as well as the need for blood transfusions. Cardiac events are much rarer than with open aortic reconstruction, with a maximum incidence of 3.3%. Pulmonary complications are also less frequent.

The following late complications are observed at rates of 8–35%:

- Failure of the graft material
- Stent migration
- Endoleaks
- Occlusion of a limb of the prosthesis

Failure of the graft material and migration occurred particularly with older-generation stent prostheses (up to 1999). The risk of endoleak is still high. However, the indications for secondary intervention have changed. On the basis of the observation that type II endoleaks are associated with a benign course, with a chance of spontaneous regression, an expectant approach with frequent checks is now often justified (Blankenstein et al. 2005; EVAR Trial Participants 2005; Go et al. 2008).

The *follow-up* after EVAR allows complications to be identified in a timely fashion and is currently undergoing changes (Figs. 3.1-11 and 3.1-12).

- The time schedule for follow-up examinations includes a check-up before discharge (Fig. 3.1-9), which should include peripheral Doppler measurement, duplex examination of the aorta, biplanar spot-film radiography, and CT angiography.
- This examination is repeated after 3, 6, and 12 months.
- It has been proposed that the follow-up examinations can be reduced when the course is uncomplicated—e.g., by eliminating the 6-month check-up (Go et al. 2008; Kranokpiraksa and Kaufman 2008; Sandford et al. 2008).
- More individualized scheduling of follow-up examinations could reduce the burden for the patient, work for staff, and also costs.

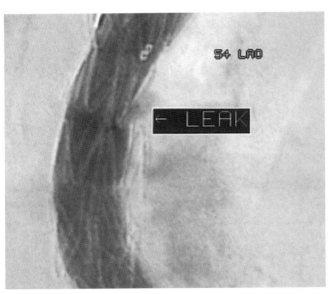

Fig. 3.1-11 Porosity of the graft is seen here, indicating a type IV endoleak.

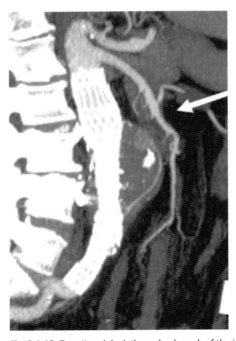

Fig. 3.1-12 Type II endoleak through a branch of the inferior mesenteric artery (arrow). There is contrast leaking into the eliminated aneurysmal sac.

Surgical treatment

Preparation for elective surgery

Diagnosis of risk factors/concomitant diseases and optimization of treatment

- Doppler examination of the peripheral arteries
- Duplex ultrasonography of the peripheral arteries to exclude peripheral aneurysms
- Cardiac risk assessment: electrocardiography (ECG), echocardiography, stress ECG, internal-medicine consultation, coronary angiography
- Duplex ultrasonography of the supra-aortic branches to exclude carotid stenosis requiring treatment, or a subclavian process
- Chest x-ray and chest CT if needed, pulmonary function; breathing exercises, reducing nicotine consumption, mucolytics, spasmolytics
- Renal scintigraphy if there is hypertension and raised creatinine, hydration, renal protection
- Neurological consultation if there are abnormalities
- For *endovascular therapy,* preoperative measurement angiography may be necessary in complex cases (Fig. 3.1-13).

Specialized preparation includes *laboratory tests* immediately before the operation to establish blood group, urinary findings, and Hemoccult. It should be discussed with the patient at an early stage whether *autologous blood* or *fresh frozen plasma* (FFP) donation is desired. Packed cells should be available in open aortic reconstruction. In consultation with the family practitioner, the patient should also stop taking *platelet inhibitors* and *anticoagulants. Bowel preparation* is with a 2-day liquid diet and a cleansing enema on the day before the procedure.

Due to the high mortality rate with aneurysmal rupture (50–80%), the indication for surgery should be established at the asymptomatic stage. If rupture should occur, the procedure is carried out immediately.

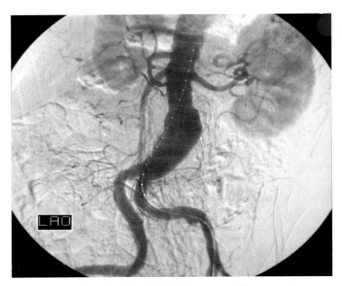

Fig. 3.1-13 Angiography of an abdominal aneurysm. The measuring points visible on fluoroscopy are used to select the size of the endograft.

Technique

Via a laparotomy, interposition of a tube or bifurcation prosthesis made of Dacron material or PTFE is carried out. A bifurcation prosthesis is implanted when there are aneurysmal or severe atherosclerotic changes in the iliac arteries (Fig. 3.1-14).

Positioning

- Dorsal position
- Slight reclination of the torso
- Left arm positioned free
- Cushioning of the heels

Anesthesia

The conventional aneurysm operation is usually carried out with endotracheal anesthesia. Placing an epidural catheter may also be helpful to reduce postoperative pain.

Incision

Median laparotomy provides fast and clear access to the abdominal cavity, and to the aortoiliac circulatory pathway, including the renal arteries, after dissection.

Transverse laparotomy and *extraperitoneal access* are intended to reduce the incidence of incisional hernia and respiratory insufficiency, but the intraoperative view is limited. With the extraperitoneal approach, it is also not possible to assess the intestinal circulation without opening the peritoneum.

Surgical procedure

Following the laparotomy, the retractor system is placed and the greater omentum is inspected, with mobilization and exploration of all the abdominal organs. After this, the small bowel is displaced to the right, and a longitudinal incision is made into the retroperitoneal fascia parallel to the inferior vena cava and abdominal aorta. Depending on the findings, the *left renal vein,* which usually has a transverse course at the level of the neck of the aneurysm, is dissected and preserved. In some cases, the vein has to be ligated due to the anatomic conditions. The *aneurysm neck* is dissected, and depending on the distance to the renal arteries it is exposed. The iliac arteries are sparingly exposed.

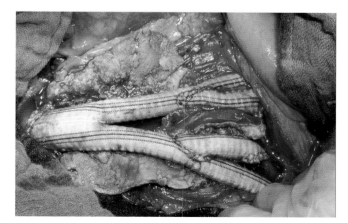

Fig. 3.1-14 Status post implantation of an aortic prosthesis in a patient with an aneurysm.

In inflammatory aneurysms, the aorta should be exposed subdiaphragmatically so that cranial clamping can be carried out if there are bleeding complications. The pelvic arteries can be blocked with balloon catheters. After pressure-sensitive clamping of the aorta, the aneurysm is opened in an H shape. If the inferior mesenteric artery shows reverse bleeding, it can be temporarily closed with a vessel clamp and then later treated with a ligature. Closure of the inferior mesenteric artery depends on adequate intestinal perfusion, which can be assessed macroscopically during the subsequent course of the operation. Bleeding lumbar arteries can be grasped with stitches. The sac of the aneurysm is thrombectomized and serves as a coating for the vascular prosthesis after it has been introduced.

An end-to-end anastomosis of the proximal aorta to the presealed Dacron or expanded polytetrafluoroethylene (ePTFE) prosthesis is then carried out. The anastomosis is sutured with a monofilament nonresorbable suture, size 3–0 for the aortic anastomosis and 4–0 for the iliac one. Heparin rinsing, de-airing and checking of afferent and efferent flow are necessary before the blood flow is restored. After restoration of blood flow, peripheral and intestinal perfusion is assessed. When antegrade flow to the internal iliac arteries is maintained, reinsertion of the *inferior mesenteric artery* is usually unnecessary and a purse-string ligation is performed.

Complications

The mortality rate with the open conventional operation for infrarenal aortic aneurysm is in the range of 3.5–8.4% (Blankensteijn et al. 2005; EVAR Trial Participants 2005; Torsello et al. 2005a).

The morbidity rate with the open operation is one of the reasons why it was possible for endovascular treatment to become established. Early complication rates of 46–96% for systemic complications and 37–58% for local complications have been reported (Ruppert et al. 2005; Torsello et al. 2005b):

- Intraoperative and postoperative bleeding 4.8%
- Bleeding requiring transfusion, with a 1.4% rate of revision surgery
- Prolonged ventilation
- Reduced renal function—a risk factor for increased mortality
- Increase in cardiac arrhythmia requiring treatment and infarction, 9.1%
- Peripheral ischemia 1–25%
- Intestinal ischemia 1.1–10%
- Sexual dysfunction 30–83%

Late complications include:
- Suture aneurysm
- Aortoenteric fistula
- Prosthesis occlusion
- Infection
- Incisional hernia

Suture aneurysms are associated with a risk of rupture and should be eliminated. Like aortoenteric fistulas, they present a considerable surgical challenge. Incisional hernias develop in one-third of the patients. *Follow-up examinations after open aortic reconstruction* need to be carried out on a long-term basis in the same way as for endovascular reconstructions (Torsello et al. 2005b). Annual ultrasound check-ups are indicated. If there are any suspicious findings, the follow-up schedule needs to be extended.

Ruptured aortic aneurysms

In the case of ruptured abdominal aortic aneurysms in an unstable condition, open reconstruction should be used as the standard procedure (Morasch 2009). Research conducted to date has not demonstrated any advantages here with the endovascular technique.

In patients who are still hemodynamically stable, the two treatment approaches (open and endovascular reconstruction) can be carried out with equivalent effectiveness. The anatomic criteria for endovascular reconstruction (see Table 3.1-4) need to be taken into account. Another limitation is the need for immediate availability of the endoprosthesis required and for an adequately trained team. If an endovascular procedure with local anesthesia is possible, it makes it possible to avoid the circulatory fluctuations caused by general anesthesia with the open procedure. In terms of time, the procedure is also shorter and associated with less blood loss in most cases. The overall hospital stay and the period of intensive-care unit treatment are also shorter, even with ruptured aneurysms (Blankensteijn et al. 2005; Leurs et al. 2005; Morasch 2009).

Prospects

Endovascular treatment to eliminate an infrarenal aortic aneurysm significantly reduces the postoperative mortality rate. The procedure is likely to become increasingly established, as better endografts have been developed since 2000.

Positive results with the endovascular procedure at the rupture stage have been reported (Morasch 2009). The development of fenestrated stent graft systems and the combination of open and endovascular procedures (hybrid operations) are allowing new approaches to be developed in the treatment of complex clinical pictures and complex anatomy.

3.1.2   Aortic stenosis

3.1.2.1   Clinical picture

Isolated occlusive disease in the region of the infrarenal aorta occurs less frequently in comparison with aneurysmal dilation.

Four different types of aortic stenosis are distinguished, depending on their morphology, and the treatment options relate to the different types (Table 3.1-6).

The suprarenal type A aortic stenosis is extremely rare and has an atherosclerotic pathogenesis (Fig. 3.1-15). With regard to type B, it should be mentioned that the etiology of these stenoses may vary; in most cases, there is coarctation of the abdominal aorta, or less frequently "coral reef" aorta (Fig. 3.1-16).

Table 3.1-6 Aortic stenosis.

Type A	Suprarenal location, with no involvement of the visceral or renal arteries
Type B	Aortic stenosis with involvement of the renal and visceral vessels, renovascular hypertension due to reduced renal perfusion
Type C	Infrarenal aortic stenosis with no involvement of the iliac arteries
Type D	Aortic stenosis with involvement of the iliac arteries (the most frequent form)

Coarctation of the abdominal aorta is a unique manifestation and is not located in the usual site, the aortic isthmus. It represents 0.5–3.0% of cases of aortic coarctation (Stelter et al. 1976). Renovascular hypertension is a sequela of underperfusion or inadequate perfusion of the kidneys. The patients are often young (under the age of 30) and already show hypertension during adolescence. This leads to a high rate of early mortality in these patients, before the age of 50, due to marked heart failure and stroke.

Interestingly, there appears to be an association between coarctation and Takayasu arteritis, neurofibromatosis, and viral diseases (such as rubella) during pregnancy (Stelter et al. 1976).

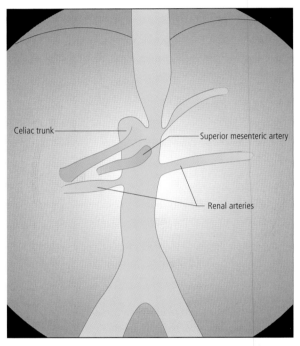

Fig. 3.1-15 Type A aortic stenosis (suprarenal involvement).

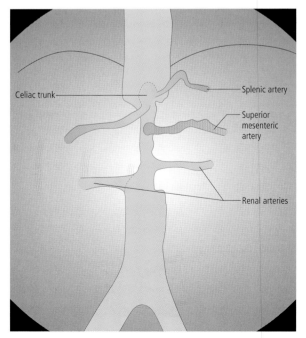

Fig. 3.1-16 Type B aortic stenosis (with complex findings).

Takayasu arteritis is a form of chronic inflammatory arteriopathy that can affect the aorta and its neighboring branches. The pulmonary arteries are also involved in the vasculitic process (see section C 3). The resulting stenoses are notably rigid and lead to secondary contraction of the vascular lumen (Klonaries et al. 2008; Uberoi and Tsetis 2007).

Type C aortic stenosis with isolated infrarenal luminal narrowing is seen more frequently in women (Fig. 3.1-17). These female patients are usually aged between 30 and 50, with extremely high nicotine consumption and raised blood lipid concentrations.

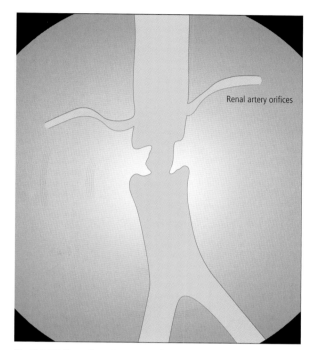

Fig. 3.1-17 Type C aortic stenosis (infrarenal location).

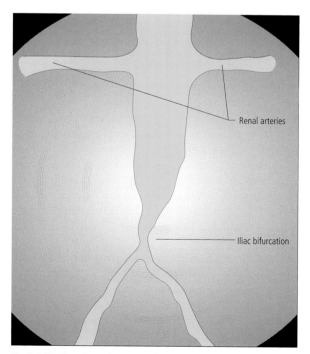

Fig. 3.1-18 Type D aortic stenosis (infrarenal with iliac circulatory pathway).

Type D aortic stenosis, resulting from atherosclerosis, is the most frequent form (Fig. 3.1-18). This type and types A and C are easily accessible for endovascular procedures and can be successfully treated.

Type B aortic stenoses undergo open reconstruction, depending on the extent of further vascular involvement.

The *causes* of aortic stenosis principally include atherosclerosis, which obstructs the vascular lumen. Other flow obstructions arise due to a reduced diameter in the aorta—e.g., with coarctation of the abdominal aorta (see above), which may also be associated with Takayasu disease.

3.1.2.2 Clinical findings

Patients with aortic stenosis present due to intermittent claudication of both legs, with walking distances that are usually less than 100 m. Intermittent claudication is often associated with gluteal pain and back or hip symptoms. Back pain is rarely reported; nonhealing ulcerations of the lower leg and foot, as well as "blue toe" syndrome, are among the possible symptoms.

Secondary hypertension may suggest the diagnosis. Particularly in younger patients, and often in women, nonspecific symptoms without any suggestive findings are observed. The patients often have a palpable foot pulse at rest and often describe pain only during exertion (Vallabhaneni et al. 2005).

The patients are often in considerable mental distress and feel unable to deal with stress in their social environment. A reduced ability to cope with physical exertion can be a disadvantage at work, and impotence can cause family difficulties.

3.1.2.3 Diagnosis and differential diagnosis

Following the patient history, staged noninvasive diagnostic investigations should be carried out:

- Local findings in the lower extremities
- Measurement of walking distance
- Pulse status
- Peripheral Doppler measurement to assess the ankle-brachial index
- Ankle-brachial index with exercise, because it is often unremarkable at rest
- Color duplex ultrasonography, particularly of the aortoiliac circulation
- Magnetic resonance imaging (MRI) or CT (noncontrast, to assess the extent of sclerosis) if duplex ultrasound is not diagnostically useful
- Intra-arterial pressure measurement

If duplex ultrasound does not provide sufficient diagnostic information—e.g., in extremely obese patients or when examination conditions are difficult (e.g., with artificial anus)—computed-tomographic angiography (CTA) or magnetic resonance angiography (MRA) should be considered. MRA is preferable if very severe calcification appears to be present, as this leads to artifacts on both ultrasound and CTA. In addition, MRA allows easier assessment and is easier to use in obese patients with limited renal function or those with contrast allergy.

Table 3.1-7 Differential diagnosis in aortic stenosis.

Symptoms	Cause	Differential findings
Hypertension	Primary form (secondary: renovascular)	Idiopathic, atherosclerosis, fibromuscular dysplasia, congenital dysplasias, strictures, aneurysm, dissections
Back/gluteal pain	Lumbar and sciatic pain, intervertebral disk prolapse	Neurological findings in sensorimotor function
Flank pain	Urolithiasis, pyelonephritis	Generalized signs of inflammation, pain on percussion in the renal bed
Hip symptoms	Coxarthrosis	Radiographic and clinical signs of coxarthrosis
Paresthesias in the pelvic region and in the lower extremities	Orthopedic and neurological clinical presentations	Reduced reflexes, pulses normal even during exercise
Peripheral embolization	PAOD, cardiac thrombus	Pathology on echocardiography, acute event

PAOD, peripheral arterial occlusive disease.

3.1.2.4   Treatment

Endovascular therapy

Angioplasty

The endovascular procedures are usually carried out with regional anesthesia. Facilities for endotracheal anesthesia should be available during treatment for lesions that are at high risk for rupture or dissection.

Access is percutaneous and may be unilateral or bifemoral, depending on the findings and the treatment planned. Surgical exposure of the common femoral artery is rarely necessary. Duplex ultrasonography or an ultrasound-guided aspiration needle can help locate the common femoral artery. Alternatively, brachial access is possible.

The lesion to be treated is initially passed with a hydrophilic guidewire, which is then replaced with more rigid wires. In a few cases, (supplementary) brachial access may be helpful for managing technically difficult stenoses. In stenoses that are located immediately at the aortic bifurcation and/or include the outlets of the common iliac artery, the "kissing balloon" technique is used (Figs. 3.1-19–3.1-21). Isolated aortic stenoses further proximally are dilated with a single percutaneous transluminal angioplasty (PTA) catheter.

The size of the balloon used depends on the preprocedural imaging findings or intraoperative measurement, but it should be narrower than the maximum diameter of the aorta. The sizes of the distal aorta and iliac arteries need to be taken into account in the "kissing balloon" technique. The patient should be asked about any pain symptoms during inflation of the balloon. For safety reasons, one can start with a smaller balloon and then gradually adjust the diameter used.

Stent release

Stenting can be used as a primary or secondary procedure. In most cases, stents are implanted following preliminary dilation. The indications include:

- (Almost) complete aortic occlusion
- Persistent transstenotic pressure gradient > 5 mmHg (or > 10 mmHg with pharmacologically induced vasodilation)
- ≥ 30% residual stenosis after angioplasty
- Occurrence of a dissection

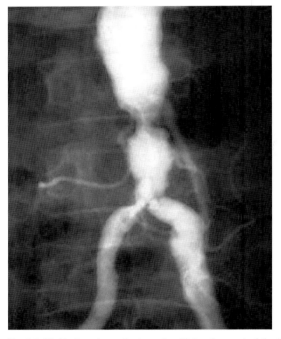

Fig. 3.1-19 Findings in aortic stenosis with involvement of the bifurcation.

Self-expanding nitinol stents with a strong radial force are used in the great majority of cases (Lastovickova and Peregin 2008; Morris-Stiff et al. 2008; Simons et al. 2006). Balloon-expanding stents are used less often, due to the greater risk of rupture. In addition, a larger-lumen sheath is needed for these. Balloon-mounted stents are less flexible, leading to reduced adaptation to the vessel wall and consequently an increased risk of dissections and ruptures. Covered stents or stent grafts should be available for this type of complication.

The stent implantation procedure corresponds to the course of an angioplasty; here again, the lesion is traversed using a sheath system with wires. The stents are positioned and opened under fluoroscopic guidance. Repeat dilation after stent release is often required, as self-expanding materials in particular need to be completely adapted to the vessel wall.

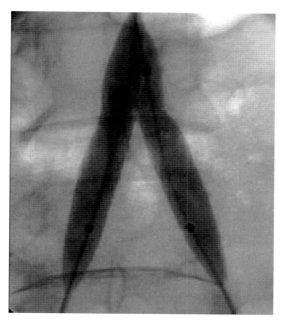

Fig. 3.1-20 The "kissing stents" technique.

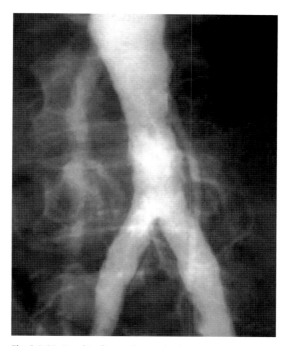

Fig. 3.1-21 Results after endovascular treatment.

The *"kissing stents" technique* involves simultaneous release of two stents at the level of the aortic bifurcation in order to reconstruct it. Both stents should ideally extend 5–15 mm into the distal aorta. The percutaneous access is closed by compression and/or with the help of an arterial sealing system (Angio-Seal, Perclose, etc.) (Torsello et al. 2002). Bed rest for 4–6 hours follows. Preinterventional antiplatelet treatment is continued, with lifelong treatment with acetylsalicylic acid (ASA) 100 and also clopidogrel for 2–3 months.

Clinical results

The primary technical success rate with PTA and stent placement in patients with stenotic aortic vascular disease is 96% (Uberoi and Tsetis 2007).

Endovascular treatment is capable of reducing the periprocedural morbidity and mortality significantly in comparison with conventional surgery. The 30-day mortality rate with the endovascular procedure is only 0.5%, with complication rates of 0.4–3.6%.

Reported *complications* include:

- Aortoiliac dissection
- Distal embolization
- Iliofemoral thrombosis
- False aneurysm
- Access-route hematoma
- Local infection

Surgical treatment

The open procedure is the treatment of choice for type B aortic aneurysms. The indication for surgery is hypertension, in view of the unfavorable prognosis and life expectancy of the untreated condition.

Thromboendarterectomy (TEA) is carried out in atherosclerotic stenoses. TEA is not possible due to the sclerotic, hypoplastic wall in coarctation and Takayasu arteritis. Patch plasty or a bypass procedure can be recommended for these lesions. An *extra-anatomic bypass* can be implanted as an axillobifemoral conduit in patients with multiple morbidities. The aim is to achieve antegrade reconstruction. Depending on the involvement of the visceral and renal vessels, elaborate reconstruction procedures may be required.

Clinical results

All of the conventional procedures show excellent patency rates: 90% of the reconstructions are patent after 5 years and 75% after 10 years (Uberoi and Tsetis 2007; Vallabhaneni et al. 2005). Disadvantages are high rates of early complications, ranging from 9% to 27%, and a 30-day mortality rate of 1–7% (Klonaris et al. 2008). This shows the effect of the invasiveness of the procedure on at least one central vessel.

Prospects

Endovascular therapy has clear advantages in comparison with the surgical procedure, and the minimally invasive approach will therefore become increasingly established in the coming years. The patient groups reported in publication to date are small and retrospective. Prospective multicenter studies would be needed, but due to the low incidence of the disease it is difficult to conduct them.

The open surgical procedure is still the standard for the complex clinical picture of type B aortic stenosis.

In summary, the endovascular procedure provides low mortality and morbidity rates, avoids the need for endotracheal anesthesia and laparotomy, and leads to shorter hospital stays. Sexual function is preserved, particularly in male patients.

References

Blankensteijn JD, de Jong SE, Prinssen M, van der Ham AC, Buth J, van Sterkenburg SM et al. Two-year outcomes after conventional or endovascular repair of abdominal aortic aneurysms. N Eng J Med 2005; 352: 2398–405.

EVAR Trial Participants. Endovascular aneurysm repair versus open repair in patients with abdominal aortic aneurysm (EVAR 1 Trial): randomised controlled trial. Lancet 2005; 365: 2179–86.

Go MR, Barbato, JE Rhee, RY Makaroun, MS. What is the clinical utility of a 6-month computed tomography in the follow-up of endovascular aneurysm repair patients. J Vasc Surg 2008; 47: 1181–7.

Klonaris C, Katsargyris A, Tsekouras N, Alexandrou A, Giannopoulos A, Bastounis E. Primary stenting for aortic lesions: From single stenoses to total aortoiliac occlusions. J Vasc Surg 2008; 47: 310–7.

Kranokpiraksa P, Kaufman JA. Follow-up of endovascular aneurysm repair: plain radiography, ultrasound, CT/CT angiography, MR imaging/MR angiography, or what? J Vasc Interven Radiol 2008; 19 (6) (Suppl 1): S27–S36.

Lastovickova J, Peregrin JH. Primary self-expandable Nitinol stent placement in focal lesions of infrarenal abdominal aorta: long term results. Cardiovasc Intervent Radiol 2008; 31: 43–8.

Leurs LJ, Laheij RJ, Buth J, EUROSTAR Collaborators. What determines and are the consequences of surveillance intensity after endovascular abdominal aortic aneurysm repair? Ann Vasc Surg 2005; 19: 868–75.

Morasch M. EVAR for the Treatment of Ruptured AAA. Perspect Vasc Surg Endovasc Ther 2009, January 27; published online first.

Morris-Stiff G, Ogunbiyi S, Winter RK, Brown R. Aortic replacement in aorto-occlusive disease: an observation study. BMC Surg 2008; 8: 19.

Norwood MGA, Lloyd GM, Bown MJ, Fishwick G, London NJ, Sayers RD. Endovascular abdominal aortic aneurysm repair. Postgrad Med J 2007; 83: 21–7.

Ruppert V, Umscheid T, Steckmeier B. Elektive Therapie des asymptomatischen infrarenalen Aortenaneurysmas. DMW 2005; 130: 1330–6.

Sandford RM, Bown MJ, Sayers RD, Fishwick G, London NJ, Nasim A. Endovascular abdominal aortic aneurysm repair: 5-year follow-up results. Ann Vasc Surg 2008; 22 (3): 372–8.

Simons PCG, Nawijn AA, Bruijninckx CMA, Knippenberg B, deVries EH, vanOverhagen H. Long-term results of primary stent placement to treat infrarenal aortic stenosis. Eur J Vasc Endovasc Surg 2006; 32: 627–33.

Stelter WJ, Becker HM, Zumtobel V, Schildberg FW, Heberer G. Die atypische Coarctatio aortae mit Hypertonie. VASA 1976; 5 (1): 5–8.

Sternbergh WC, Greenberg RK, Chuter TAM, Tonnessen BH, Zenith Investigators. Redefining postoperative surveillance after endovascular aneurysm repair: Recommendations based on 5-year follow-up in the US Zenith multicenter trial. J Vasc Surg 2008; 48: 278–85.

Torsello G, Can A, Schumacher S. Das Bauchaortenaneurysma. Gefäßchirurgie 2005a; 10: 139–53.

Torsello G, Schumacher S, Osada N, Teßarek J, Torsello GF. Lebensqualität nach Behandlung eines Bauchaortenaneurysmas – Ein Langzeitvergleich der endovaskulären und der konventionellen Therapie. Gefäßchirurgie 2005b; 10: 85–92.

Torsello G, Osada N, Florek HJ, Horsch S, Kortmann H, Luska G, Scharrer-Pamler R, Schmiedt W, Umscheid T, Wozniak G. Long-term outcome after talent endograft implantation for aneurysms of the abdominal aorta: A multicenter retrospective study. J Vasc Surg 2006; 43: 277–84.

Torsello G, Teßarek J, Kasprzak B, Klenk E. Aortenaneurysmabehandlung mit komplett perkutaner Technik. Eine Zwischenbilanz nach Behandlung von 80 Patienten. DMW 2002; 127: 1453–7.

Uberoi R, Tsetis D, Standards for the endovascular management of aortic occlusive disease. Cardiovasc Intervent Radiol 2007; 30: 814–9.

Vallabhaneni SR, Björses K, Malina M, Dias NV, Sonesson B, Ivancev K. Endovascular management of isolated infrarenal aortic occlusive disease is safe and effective in selected patients. Eur J Vasc Endovasc Surg 2005; 30: 307–10.

White GH, Yu W, May J et al. Endoleaks as a complication of endoluminal grafting of abdominal aortic aneurysms: classification, incidence, diagnosis, and management. J Endovasc Surg 1997; 4 (2): 152–68.

3.2 Diseases of the branches of the abdominal aorta

Anatomy of the mesenteric and renal arteries:
Reinhard Putz
Acute and chronic mesenteric occlusive disease:
Claudio Rabbia, Roberta Pini, Thomas Zeller
Duplex ultrasonography: Tom Schilling

3.2.1 Anatomy of the mesenteric and renal arteries

The celiac trunk arises ventrally from the abdominal aorta as it passes through the diaphragm in the aortic hiatus, at the level of T12. Less than 1 cm further on, the superior mesenteric artery is given off. The third unpaired artery, the inferior mesenteric artery, also arises ventrally, but a few centimeters further caudally.

The celiac trunk divides after barely 1 cm into its three branches, which supply the upper abdominal organs (see Fig. 2.1-6 in section A 2.1.1). The left gastric artery courses in the hepatogastric fold to the lesser curvature of the stomach. The common hepatic artery courses along the upper edge of the pancreas toward the liver, and before entering the porta hepatis it divides into the proper hepatic artery and the gastroduodenal artery, which descends caudally. The latter in turn supplies the head of the pancreas and the duodenum, anastomoses with a branch of the inferior mesenteric artery, and gives off the gastro-omental artery to the greater curvature of the stomach. Embedded in the upper edge of the pancreas, the splenic artery after a tortuous course reaches the splenic hilum. It supplies the body and tail of the pancreas and gives off the left gastro-omental artery to the greater curvature of the stomach.

The superior mesenteric artery, a similarly large vessel, arises immediately caudal to the celiac trunk (Fig. 3.2-1). After giving off the inferior pancreaticoduodenal artery, the superior mesenteric artery descends behind the head of the pancreas and then enters the mesentery, where it branches to the jejunum (jejunal arteries) and ileum (ileal arteries) and also supplies the colon (right and left middle colic arteries and ileocolic artery). Arising from the trunk of the superior mesenteric artery, the superior pancreaticoduodenal artery forms anastomosis with the inferior pancreaticoduodenal artery, which comes from the gastroduodenal artery, to supply the head of the pancreas and the duodenum.

The inferior mesenteric artery arises from the abdominal aorta near the bifurcation (Fig. 3.2-2), and immediately after its origin turns left to the final third of the transverse colon, the descending colon

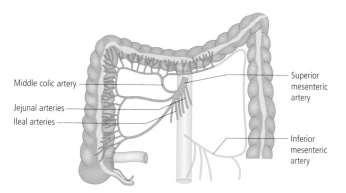

Fig. 3.2-1 Branches of the superior mesenteric artery.

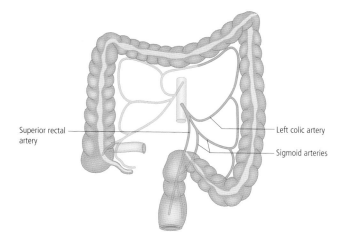

Fig. 3.2-2 Branches of the inferior mesenteric artery.

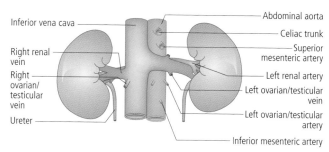

Fig. 3.2-3 Paired visceral branches of the abdominal aorta.

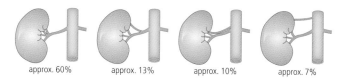

approx. 60%   approx. 13%   approx. 10%   approx. 7%

Fig. 3.2-4 Variants in the arterial supply to the kidneys (adapted from Lippert and Pabst 1985).

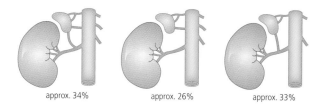

approx. 34%   approx. 26%   approx. 33%

Fig. 3.2-5 Variants in the arterial supply to the suprarenal gland.

(left colic artery) and sigmoid (sigmoid arteries). The furthest caudal branch that it gives off is the superior rectal artery, the branches of which form an arterial plexus in the wall of the rectum and finally also supply the corpus cavernosum.

The renal arteries arise from the abdominal artery at the level of L2 slightly below the origin of the superior mesenteric artery (Fig. 3.2-3). The left renal artery passes on a short course behind the left renal vein on an oblique dorsal course to the hilum of the kidney. In very rare cases (less than 1%), the left renal vein lies posterior to the abdominal aorta and thus also posterior to the left renal artery. The right renal artery arises slightly higher than the left one and turns, crossing the vertebral column, and descends slightly obliquely behind the inferior vena cava to the hilum of the right kidney. The two renal arteries are covered by the pancreas, with the head of the pancreas on the right and the body of the pancreas on the left.

In the hilum of the kidney, the renal arteries usually branch along with the renal veins into anterior and posterior main branches. An inferior main branch is sometimes also present.

Variants of the renal arteries are relatively common. Aberrant arteries to one of the poles of the kidney or duplications of the main trunk (accessory arteries) are found in more than 20% of cases. Polar renal arteries, passing to one of the poles of the kidney as separate additional arteries, are also not uncommon (Fig. 3.2-4).

The suprarenal glands (adrenal glands) are generally supplied from three sources. From the cranial direction, the superior suprarenal artery passes to the gland from the inferior phrenic artery. The middle suprarenal artery arises directly from the aorta. In most cases,

there is an inferior suprarenal artery that ascends from the renal artery to the suprarenal gland from below (Fig. 3.2-5).

The situation at the origins of the ovarian or testicular arteries is also important. Although they normally arise a few centimeters below the renal arteries from the anterolateral side of the aorta, their site of origin may be directly below each renal artery in up to 20% of cases. In these cases, they may pass caudally anterior to the associated renal vein. (The left ovarian or testicular vein always enters the renal vein directly from below, while the right ovarian or testicular vein flows into the inferior vena cava before the renal vein.)

3.2.2 Acute and chronic mesenteric occlusive disease

3.2.2.1 Acute mesenteric ischemia

Acute mesenteric ischemia is a life-threatening disease associated with a very high mortality rate. The most frequent cause of acute bowel ischemia is arterial occlusion due to an embolus of cardiac origin, from an upstream arterial segment, or (less frequently) acute local thrombosis due to a ruptured atherosclerotic plaque. Only early and rigorous treatment is able to reduce mortality.

Acute mesenteric ischemia is a rare disease, representing around 0.1% of hospital admissions. It may be caused by sudden occlusion of arteries or veins or by vasoconstriction and it leads to inadequate resting perfusion in the intestines. The most frequent cause is a car-

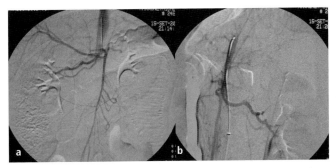

Fig. 3.2-6a, b Acute mesenteric ischemia in a young patient with Marfan syndrome and cocaine abuse, who had previously undergone surgery with replacement of the aortic arch and ascending thoracic aorta due to acute aortic dissection. The abdominal aorta has a thin true lumen, which is being compressed by the false lumen, with consequent visceral hypoperfusion. **(a)** Anteroposterior angiogram. **(b)** Lateral angiogram.

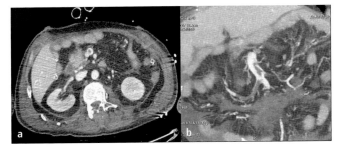

Fig. 3.2-7a, b Postoperative thrombosis of the superior mesenteric vein. Contrast computed tomography.

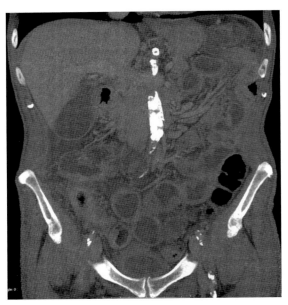

Fig. 3.2-8 Coronary computed tomography in a patient with intestinal ischemia: intestinal hyperdistention, wall thickening, intra-abdominal fluid.

diac embolus or embolus from a proximal artery. The vessel most frequently affected is the superior mesenteric artery (50%). Arterial embolism is suspected particularly when there is simultaneous atrial fibrillation or the patient has had a previous myocardial infarction or percutaneous vascular intervention in which plaque material may have been released from the suprarenal aortic wall. Other causes include arterial thromboses from arteries that have previously had atherosclerotic stenoses, thrombotic occlusion as a sequela of procoagulant diseases, and acute aortic dissection (Fig. 3.2-6).

The early symptoms of acute mesenteric occlusive disease are usually nonspecific. Initially, abdominal pain that is often severe and persistent occurs in the periumbilical region. An early abdominal examination is often unremarkable, and this is the main reason why the diagnosis is often only made at a very late stage. Additional symptoms include nausea, vomiting, transient diarrhea, and blood-coated feces. If the blood supply to the intestines is not restored, peritonitis with a generalized systemic inflammatory response and multiple-organ failure develop within hours or days. Laboratory tests show leukocytosis and lactic acidosis, and approximately half of the patients have raised amylase levels.

Arterial occlusions are the main cause of acute impairment of the mesenteric circulation, while venous thromboses are only responsible for 5–10% of cases. The main causes of venous occlusion are procoagulant diseases, intra-abdominal inflammations such as pancreatitis or diverticulitis, and postoperative conditions (Fig. 3.2-7). Nonocclusive mesenteric infarction (NOMI) is the cause in the remaining 25–30% of cases. The latter condition occurs in patent arteries and intact vessels and is caused by intestinal vasospasm due to low blood flow—e.g., in the context of cardiogenic shock, sepsis, hy-

povolemia, dehydration, and use of vasoactive agents or agents such as cocaine. The prognosis in patients with acute mesenteric occlusive disease is unfavorable, with overall mortality rates of 32–90%, depending on the cause. The highest mortality rates are associated with NOMI and cases of arterial thrombosis of a vessel supplying a larger proportion of the intestines. Rapid diagnosis is extremely important in order to avoid intestinal infarction and multiple-organ failure, which are the main reasons for the high mortality rate.

3.2.2.2   Chronic mesenteric occlusive disease

Chronic mesenteric arterial occlusive disease is rare, representing approximately 1–2% of all cases of bowel disease. Ischemic symptoms occur when the blood supply to the bowel is impaired due to lesions in one or more of the three mesenteric arteries: the celiac trunk, superior mesenteric artery, and inferior mesenteric artery. Atherosclerotic lesions are by far the most frequent cause (95%), and the lesion is typically found at the orifices of the mesenteric arteries. Other rare diseases include Buerger syndrome, Takayasu arteritis, fibromuscular dysplasia, intestinal dissections, aortic dissection, Dunbar syndrome (caused by eccentric compression of the celiac trunk by the median arcuate ligament, Fig. 3.2-9), and Leriche syndrome, in which a mesenteric steal phenomenon may occur. Most patients with chronic mesenteric occlusive disease have multiple cardiovascular risk factors. They are mainly female (70%) and are often heavy smokers. Atherosclerotic changes are also found in other vascular territories such as the coronaries, carotids, and leg arteries.

There are large gaps in our knowledge of mesenteric arterial occlusive disease. In particular, there is no information about the overall frequency of arterial mesenteric stenoses or occlusions, or what the patients' symptoms are. Although arteriosclerosis in the celiac trunk and superior and inferior mesenteric artery has often been reported—with significant arteriosclerotic lesions in 14–24% of patients undergoing angiography—revascularization procedures are only carried out in 2%. The celiac trunk and superior and inferior

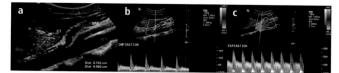

Fig. 3.2-9a–c Dunbar syndrome: longitudinal Doppler ultrasound. (a) The B-image shows proximal stenosis of the celiac trunk by a hypertrophic crus of the diaphragm, with post-stenotic ectasia. (b) The pulse wave Doppler shows a normal flow velocity during inspiration. (c) During expiration, there is significant stenosis, with an increase in the systolic and diastolic flow velocity.

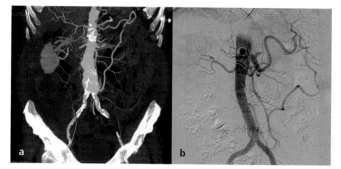

Fig. 3.2-10a, b Collateral network between the superior and inferior mesenteric arteries. (a) Coronal CT section, (b) angiography.

mesenteric artery are closely interconnected, and blood may flow in one direction or the other depending on where a relative stenosis is located. The celiac trunk and superior mesenteric artery are primarily connected via the pancreaticoduodenal arteries. The inferior and superior mesenteric arteries are connected with each other via the Riolan anastomosis and marginal artery of the colon (artery of Drummond) (Fig. 3.2-10). In addition, when there is occlusion of the inferior mesenteric artery, it can be filled from the hypogastric artery by reverse flow. A proximal arterial stenosis or occlusion in one of the three mesenteric arteries can thus often be well tolerated. It is therefore generally assumed that the clinical syndrome of chronic mesenteric ischemia must require occlusion or stenosis of at least two or three of the bowel arteries. Despite this, patients with one diseased vessel sometimes feel pain, while other patients with occlusions or stenoses in all three arteries may be asymptomatic—so that the mechanism of mesenteric ischemia does not strictly correlate with the number of vessels involved. Other factors may play a role, such as the location of the stenosis below the anastomoses, interruption of the normal collaterals as a result of previous abdominal surgery, or the speed at which the stenosis develops and the resulting degree of collateralization. In addition, complex hormonal and autonomic autoregulation systems such as cardiac output may play a role in the ischemia and may interact with the disease in the bowel arteries. Nonocclusive mesenteric ischemia (NOMI), with chronic or recurrent intestinal hypoperfusion, is a very rare form of chronic mesenteric disease in which a reduced effective blood volume and vasoconstriction in the bowel arteries with subsequent ischemia occur simultaneously. The patients affected typically have severe concomitant diseases such as chronic cardiac insufficiency or terminal renal insufficiency with low blood pressure at the end of the dialysis session.

Clinical presentation

The frequent and characteristic symptom of chronic mesenteric occlusive disease is postprandial abdominal pain, also known as abdominal or intestinal angina, with weight loss. The typical abdominal pain starts 15–30 minutes after eating and continues for around 1–3 hours. The symptoms arise because the intestines' metabolic demand on cardiac output rises from 10–20% in the resting period to 35% postprandially. Over time, the patients develop a fear of meals and start to eat less. Constant nausea, intermittent diarrhea, and otherwise unexplained gastric ulcers or even gastroparesis also occur. The diagnosis is typically not made immediately, since mesenteric arterial occlusive disease is rare and there are many causes of abdominal pain and weight loss. Before diagnosis, many patients have therefore been symptomatic for several months or even years and have often undergone an intensive search for cancer. When the disease progresses, the pain may even be triggered by a small drink or at rest. Vascular abdominal pain at rest or persistent abdominal pain unconnected with eating are important prognostic markers and often indicate imminent acute bowel ischemia. There are still no laboratory markers available to allow diagnosis at present. Possible laboratory findings include anemia, leukopenia or lymphopenia, as well as electrolyte disturbances and reduced serum albumin as a result of malnutrition.

3.2.2.3   Diagnosis

Duplex ultrasonography is used as a screening method. Although duplex ultrasound can often demonstrate visceral artery occlusion and stenosis in patients with acute ischemia, the examination is usually of little diagnostic value due to dilated bowel loops and associated tympanites. In cases of chronic mesenteric ischemia, it is able to diagnose visceral artery stenoses, which are typically located at the orifice, usually involving plaque from the aorta. The examination is easily carried out and provides both structural and functional information. The anatomy of the vessel is demonstrated on B-imaging, and blood flow and flow velocity can then be recorded (Fig. 3.2-11). Duplex ultrasonography of the visceral arteries is technically difficult, but an experienced examiner can carry it out successfully in approximately 85–90% of the patients. In specialized departments, the sensitivity of the examination method is 90% for stenoses > 70% and for vascular occlusion. Significant stenosis is characterized by increased flow velocity and turbulent flow, with an increase in the systolic and diastolic flow velocity and a change in color on color-coded duplex ultrasound (Fig. 3.2-12, Table 3.2-1).

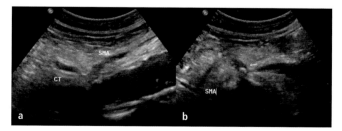

Fig. 3.2-11a, b B-imaging ultrasound: a hyperechogenic atheroma at the orifice of the superior mesenteric artery (arrow). (a) Longitudinal section, (b) axial section.

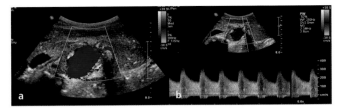

Fig. 3.2-12a, b Stenosis at the orifice of the superior mesenteric artery, with axial Doppler ultrasound. (**a**) Color-coded Duplex ultrasound shows a color switch at the orifice of the artery. (**b**) The pulse wave Doppler shows high systolic and diastolic flow velocities, with a maximum systolic flow velocity > 300 cm/s as evidence of significant stenosis.

Table 3.2-1 Duplex criteria for significant visceral artery stenosis (fasting).

Vessel	Duplex criterion for > 70% stenosis or occlusion
Celiac trunk (Moneta et al. 1993)	PSV ≥ 200 cm/s or no flow signal
Superior mesenteric artery (Moneta et al. 1993)	PSV ≥ 275 cm/s or no flow signal
Inferior mesenteric artery (Pellerito et al. 2009)	PSV > 200 cm/s, EDV > 25 cm/s, and MAR > 2.5

EDV, end-diastolic velocity; MAR, mesenteric to aortic ratio; PSV, peak systolic velocity.

3.2.2.4   Duplex ultrasound examination technique

This should be carried out with the patient fasting if possible, in order to optimize the ultrasound conditions and exclude prandial modulations when the visceral vessels are being examined. If appropriate, an examination in the postprandial state can follow to allow assessment of physiological flow changes. The examination should be carried out with appropriate application pressure from the scanner in order to compress bowel contents etc. and improve the imaging quality. Constant pressure is better than applying pressure briefly, with "relapsing" of the bowel contents.

Differential diagnosis

- Arteriosclerosis:
  - Typical plaque morphology
  - Classically located in the regions of origin
  - No respiratory modulation (celiac trunk)
- Celiac trunk compression syndrome: see special findings
- Embolism: there is hypoechoic to isoechoic occlusive material on B-imaging, absence of flow, markedly reduced imaging sensitivity in patients with acute abdomen due to guarding of muscles, pain, and meteorism
- Large-vessel vasculitis: may also be present when there is aortic involvement, with a typical finding being a homogenously hypoechoic, widened intima–media complex (macaroni sign)
- Hyperperfusion:
  - When there are arteriovenous malformations or inflammation in the vascular area
  - Increased flow with diastolic emphasis
- Dissection: may also be present when there is aortic dissection, possibly with demonstration of a dissection membrane and in that case a typical triphasic "splash phenomenon"

Specific findings

Celiac trunk

Normally V_{max} systolic 1.0–2.4 m/s, V_{max} diastolic 0.2–0.6 m/s. Postprandial increase in flow velocities up to 20%. As a normal variant occurring in up to 30% of cases, the celiac trunk may be constricted by the arcuate ligament in celiac trunk compression syndrome (also known as arcuate ligament syndrome or Dunbar syndrome), with an increase in flow velocities on exhalation that may even involve functional high-grade stenosis or occlusion. This is only pathologically relevant in exceptional cases, and the classification of stenosis is not based on set threshold velocities; the general direct criteria for stenoses apply.

Superior mesenteric artery

There is a common trunk with the celiac trunk in 5–7% of cases. When the patient is fasting, the flow profile may be triphasic, with V_{max} systolic up to 1.8 m/s. Postprandially, there is an increase in flow volume and then a monophasic flow signal with a high diastolic flow component. Up to around 45 min postprandially, V_{max} systolic may be up to a maximum of 2.4 m/s. The classification of stenosis is not based on set threshold velocities; the general direct criteria for stenoses apply.

Inferior mesenteric artery

Duplex ultrasound imaging is possible in approximately 80% of cases. Various functional states are seen as in the superior mesenteric artery, with a fasting V_{max} systolic rate of 1.5 m/s. The classification of stenosis is not based on set threshold velocities; the general direct criteria for stenoses apply.

Specialized examination methods

Magnetic resonance imaging (MRI) using gadolinium contrast is a good method of imaging atherosclerotic lesions at the orifices of the visceral arteries. MRI has high sensitivity and specificity in comparison with digital subtraction angiography as the "gold standard." However, although it is in widespread use, it cannot be regarded as the gold standard for examining the vascular anatomy.

Computed tomography (CT) is the examination method most often carried out in patients with acute abdominal pain. When intestinal ischemia is suspected, CT can make it possible either to diagnose or exclude arterial and venous occlusions. In addition, it can diagnose intestinal changes such as hyperdistention, wall thickening, intra-abdominal fluid, and perforation (Fig. 3.2-8). In addition, computed tomography can identify a combination of intestinal pneumatosis and air in the portal vein, which raises an urgent suspicion of severe bowel ischemia. In patients with chronic mesenteric ischemia, CT angiography is an appropriate method for imaging the visceral arteries, veins, and collaterals. With the introduction of thin-section computed tomography, with a section thickness of less than 2 mm, CT angiography can now provide detailed imaging of the vessels (Fig. 3.2-13). Angiographic multiple-slice CT can reveal proximal occlusive disease, the distal vascular bed, and also the type of plaque involved. Multiple-slice CT with multiplanar reconstruction and three-dimensional reconstruction is also important for planning of the interventional approach and particularly for selecting the best access route. In ad-

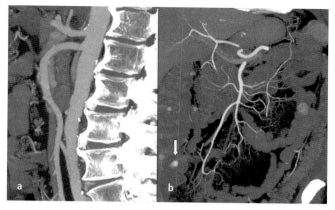

Fig. 3.2-13a, b Thin-slice computed tomography after contrast injection. (a) Sagittal reconstruction: good documentation of the proximal segment of the intestinal artery. (b) Maximum intensity projection (MIP) on coronal imaging: the coronal MIP format provides very good imaging of the distal vascular bed of the superior mesenteric artery. As an incidental finding, bleeding is seen in the right colon (arrow).

dition, it can diagnose or exclude other vascular diseases, bowel involvement, and other diseases in patients with abdominal pain.

The gold standard for the examination of the visceral arteries is still intra-arterial digital subtraction angiography. The method's accuracy in angiographic imaging of the anatomy, stenoses or occlusions, collaterals, and anatomic variants is unsurpassed. Although the procedure has been used less often more recently, it is still the first step for any endovascular procedure. The combination of high diagnostic accuracy with the option of carrying out an intervention makes angiography the method of choice in symptomatic patients.

Tonometry of the gastrointestinal tract is another method of detecting bowel ischemia. Mucosal perfusion is measured by quantifying the luminal P_{CO_2}. In selected patients, exercise tonometry in the stomach is a functional test that can be carried out in addition to imaging examinations. It appears to have a sensitivity of 78% and a sensitivity of 92% for identifying ischemia. In addition, the test is helpful for treatment decision-making in patients with vascular disease, as there is a strong correlation between normalization of a pathological P_{CO_2} and the disappearance of symptoms after successful revascularization.

3.2.2.5　Treatment for acute mesenteric ischemia

Conservative treatment

Aggressive drug treatment is essential, including antibiotics, systemic anticoagulation, vasodilators, and rehydration. In general, the treatment is aimed at restoring blood flow via surgical or endovascular access and resection of infarcted areas of bowel.

In patients with nonocclusive mesenteric ischemia, drug treatment for the underlying disease (cardiogenic shock, hypovolemia) should be administered first. If interventional treatment is still required in addition to the drug therapy, it usually consists of administering an intra-arterial infusion of papaverine and nitroglycerin via a guide catheter.

Surgical treatment

Surgical treatment consists of laparotomy with embolectomy or placement of an arterial mesenteric bypass, followed by examination of the intestines for infarction after revascularization has been carried out

and resection of necrotic bowel segments. As the vitality of the bowel may be difficult to assess at the start of the treatment, a "second-look" procedure 24–48 hours after the first is usually required, particularly if lactate levels in the blood rise and clinical deterioration occurs.

Endovascular therapy

The endovascular treatment options after angiography depend on the cause of the ischemia. They may include local intra-arterial catheter administration of vasodilators or thrombolytic agents, followed by angioplasty and stent implantation if appropriate. Mechanical thrombectomy is also an option. A subsequent laparotomy is important for assessing bowel integrity.

In patients with occlusive intestinal artery ischemia, thrombolysis treatment alone or in combination with mechanical thrombectomy is a good option, in view of the poor results with purely surgical treatment. Thrombolytic agents that can be used include urokinase, streptokinase, and tissue plasminogen activator (TPA), and these can be administered directly into the occluded vessel via a catheter with multiple side holes. Vasodilators and intra-arterial heparin should be administered at the same time.

Theoretically, endovascular treatment should be able to achieve reperfusion more rapidly than surgical treatment, so that the primary area of ischemia should be smaller. However, there are very few data available on this approach. The most convincing report was a study including 70 patients who were treated over a 9-year period, 56 of whom were treated with endovascular methods. TPA infusions in combination with mechanical thrombectomy were used in 12% of the patients, and 88% were treated exclusively with thrombolytic agents. Eighty-seven percent of the interventions were successful, with a significant reduction in the mortality rate (36%) and need for surgical procedures (50%). Laparotomy was necessary after endovascular therapy in 69% of the cases. The segments of bowel resected were smaller than in the patients who underwent surgical revascularization, and multiple-organ failure occurred more rarely. Another treatment option, described in a few recently published case reports, is a less invasive hybrid technique known as retrograde stent implantation in the superior mesenteric artery. This combines open surgical and endovascular methods, with laparotomy and demonstration of the superior mesenteric artery for retrograde cannulation and stent implantation. This approach makes it possible to inspect bowel integrity without the risks involved in surgical bypass such as clamping of the aorta or infection of a vascular prosthesis.

No guidelines are available on the treatment of ischemia caused by intestinal vein thrombosis. If the patient is clinically unstable, abdominal laparotomy and resection of the infarcted bowel segment are required. If the patient's course is clinically stable, systemic anticoagulation is indicated in order to limit further spread of the thrombus.

3.2.2.6　Treatment for chronic mesenteric ischemia

Only symptomatic patients with chronic mesenteric arterial occlusive disease require treatment. The only exception to this rule is in patients who are undergoing aortic or renovascular surgery for other indications. The aim of treatment is to eliminate symptoms, improve the nutritional situation, and prevent intestinal infarction. There is continuing debate as to whether surgical or endovascular treatment is better initially. As mesenteric occlusive disease is rare, very few vascular surgeons or interventionalists have broad experience with the treatment of these diseases, and the choice between surgical and endovascular therapy depends very much on the institution in which the patient is being treated. The decisive elements in the choice of treatment procedure should be the patient's clinical situation, the anatomy of the affected vessel, and whether endovascular therapy is appropriate in the patient. For example, a simple stenosis is better treated with the less invasive endovascular method. A large number of surgical techniques have been described for open surgery on the bowel arteries, including reimplantation, transarterial and transaortic endarterectomy, and antegrade and retrograde aortovisceral bypass placement with veins, arteries, or vascular prostheses. Surgical release of the triangle of the diaphragm and reconstruction of the celiac trunk are indicated in patients with symptomatic compression syndrome.

Angioplasty in the visceral arteries was first described in 1980, but larger series of patients have been reported during the last 10 years and endovascular therapy has become the preferred method in many centers. Endovascular angioplasty and stent implantation are safe and effective, and above all have advantages in patients with severe co-morbid conditions that would make open surgery difficult. Most endovascular procedures have been carried out in cases of intestinal arterial stenosis, fewer in cases of complete occlusion.

The number of vessels that should be treated is an open question. The chances of clinical improvement are already very good when an affected bowel artery is revascularized. Despite this, more than one vessel is reconstructed in patients who undergo surgical treatment, in order to reduce the likelihood of a symptomatic recurrence. The strategy with endovascular therapy is variable, but in most cases only one artery is treated, starting with the artery that is technically easiest to approach. For example, it is logical in the case of patients with two occluded arteries and one stenotic one to treat the stenosis first instead of the occlusions. The artery preferred for interventional treatment is the superior mesenteric artery, followed by the celiac trunk, but if both of these arteries are occluded, the best short-term and long-term results can be expected from treatment of a stenotic inferior mesenteric artery. If there are two stenotic arteries, treating both stenoses would improve the blood flow and prevent symptomatic recurrence. This therapy approach is significantly better than carrying out treatment for a single vessel (Fig. 3.2-14).

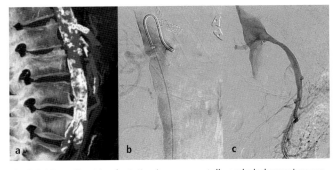

Fig. 3.2-14a–c Stent implantation in a segmentally occluded superior mesenteric artery in a patient with no significant clinical improvement after stent implantation in a celiac trunk with high-grade stenosis. (**a**) Diffuse calcification of the aortic wall and a large calcified plaque at the orifice of the superior mesenteric artery. (**b**) Selective catheterization of the superior mesenteric artery, which is completely occluded for a length of 1 cm starting from the orifice. (**c**) Concluding angiogram after stent implantation.

Endovascular approach

As soon as an indication for interventional therapy has been established, it should be ensured that the patient always receives antiplatelet treatment with acetylsalicylic acid or clopidogrel before the intervention.

Access route

A femoral access route is suitable in most cases, but when there are steep vessels off-takes it is repeatedly necessary to switch to transbrachial access. Access via the left arm (brachial or radial) may be necessary if the visceral artery being treated cannot be reached from the aorta via a femoral route. Despite the longer overall distance, this route is more direct in comparison with the femoral access route. Longer sheaths and guide catheters are used, and a curved catheter (e.g., Multipurpose or Headhunter) is used for selective catheterization of the superior mesenteric artery and celiac trunk.

Preinterventional angiography

Diagnostic angiography is first carried out using a pigtail catheter inserted into the abdominal aorta at the level of T12 or L1. Lateral aortography is the best projection for demonstrating the typical proximal stenosis in the bowel arteries, or a short stump in case of an occlusion. These lesions are often not visible on a frontal view. Anteroposterior aortograms can reveal the distal vascular bed and show indirect signs of a proximal visceral artery occlusion such as the presence of an enlarged Riolan anastomosis. Selective aortography of the visceral vessels is not always successful, as it is not always possible to place the catheter in a suitable position.

Intervention

During the procedure, systemic heparin administration should be administered with an activated clotting time (ACT) of 250–300 s as the target. A curved 6F (7F) guide catheter, typically 55 cm long, can be advanced over a 0.035" wire, or alternatively a long sheath can be advanced into the aorta up to the level of the target vessel. The orifice of the visceral artery is probed with catheters of various configurations (e.g., Simmonds, Hook, Sos-Ombi, or Cobra). A hydrophilic wire (e.g., Radiofocus®, Terumo) is then advanced into the lesion, particularly in cases of occlusion, or a J-wire in cases of stenosis. The guide catheter is then advanced in front of the orifice, with attention being given to ensure that the vessel is not closed. A 0.014" or 0.018" extra support wire is then advanced instead of the 0.035" wire. This procedure provides good stability in the interventional system and arteriographic checking at any time during the procedure. Predilation of the lesion is carried out with a low-profile balloon, typically 3 mm in diameter, in order to prevent dislocation of the stent during the subsequent intervention in case of high-grade stenosis or occlusion. Semiselective injections of contrast via the guide catheter can allow precise release of a balloon-expandable stent. The results should be documented on a concluding angiogram (Fig. 3.2-15).

The length of the stent used depends on the lesion that needs to be crossed, and attention should be given to ensure that the stent projects 1–2 mm into the aorta. Balloon-expandable stents are normally preferable due to their greater radial force in calcified lesions and because they are usually easier to release. In nonatheromatous

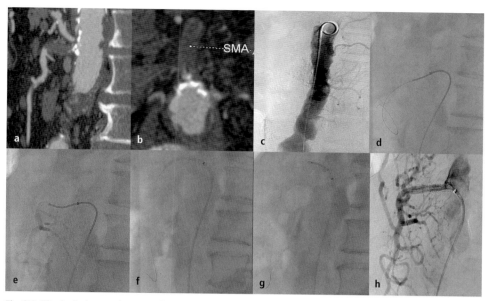

Fig. 3.2-15a–h Endovascular recanalization of the superior mesenteric artery (after a previous failed attempt to recanalize the celiac trunk). (**a**) High-grade stenosis of the celiac trunk and a long occlusion in the superior mesenteric artery (on a sagittal CT). (**b**) Close-up of an occlusion in the mesenteric artery (axial CT). (**c**) Lateral aortogram: the splanchnic arteries are not imaged. (**d**) Selective catheterization of the mesenteric artery using a 0.035″ straight hydrophilic wire (deep intubation). (**e**) Check-up angiography to determine the intraluminal position of the catheter. (**f**) Predilation of the lesion with a low-profile balloon via a 0.018″ extra support wire. (**g**) After release of a long self-expanding stent, a balloon-expandable stent is also implanted proximally. (**h**) The final angiogram shows a good result: the entire lesion is covered by the two stents to reduce the risk of distal embolization.

lesions, angioplasty (without stent implantation) shows the best results, but stent implantation is reserved for cases with relevant residual stenosis or complications such as dissection. If there is a longer occlusion of the superior mesenteric artery, a combination of balloon-expandable and self-expanding stent is preferable, so that the entire length of the occlusion can be treated and the stents can be adapted to the curvature that usually follows the post-orifice segment of the vessel. In addition, complete coverage of the occlusion by the stent also reduces the risk of distal embolization. The risk is extremely low in the treatment series that have so far been reported; nevertheless, several authors suggest that a distal embolic protection system should be used. Another method of reducing the risk of embolism is the "no-touch technique," particularly in patients with pronounced plaques in the abdominal aorta. The critical step in this technique requires a J-shaped bent wire above the tip of the guide catheter in order to prevent direct contact with the aortic wall while a second guide wire is advanced into the visceral artery.

Endovascular recanalizations can be carried out with a conventional 0.035″ wire, but the current trend is toward use of 0.014″ or 0.018″ wires with a low profile and quickly exchangeable materials in order reduce the invasiveness and complications. The examiner's level of experience is the main factor involved in reducing complications.

Postinterventional follow-up

Following recanalization, all patients should receive long-term anti-platelet therapy with acetylsalicylic acid and/or clopidogrel. The accompanying risk factors for arteriosclerosis should be treated. Most authors recommend dual antiplatelet therapy for 1 month after stent implantation.

During the first few days after revascularization, special attention should be given to the possibility of a reperfusion syndrome developing. After 2–3 days, patients may experience symptoms such as

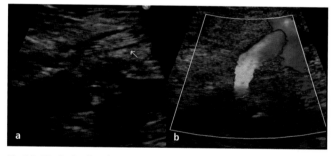

Fig. 3.2-16a, b Duplex ultrasound check-up in the case shown in Fig. 3.2-10. Three days after the procedure, the symptoms suddenly recurred due to reperfusion syndrome, rather than a recurrent vascular occlusion. (**a**) B-image: stent (arrow). (**b**) Color-coded duplex ultrasound: an intact vessel with no recurrent stenosis is seen (monochromatic signal without color switching).

nausea, diarrhea, and abdominal pain, similar to or worse than before the treatment. These patients must receive parenteral nutrition and should receive proton-pump inhibitors. They generally recover completely within a few weeks. When these symptoms start, it is important to use imaging (duplex ultrasound or computed tomography) to distinguish between a reperfusion syndrome and recurrent occlusion of the vessel that has been treated.

Complications

Most of the complications affect the access route. Local complications such as hematoma, pseudoaneurysm, or thrombotic occlusion are more frequent after a brachial artery access route. Pseudoaneurysms can be treated with ultrasound-guided compression or a thrombin injection. Arterial occlusions usually occur when there are additional local anatomic variants or atherosclerotic changes, and in some cases they require surgical thrombectomy. If there is

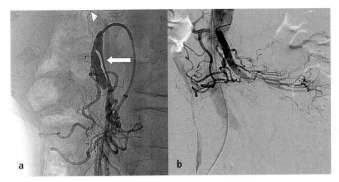

Fig. 3.2-17a, b Dissection of the superior mesenteric artery during attempted revascularization in a woman with a medical history including partial resection of the colon and recurrence of chronic mesenteric occlusive disease, despite previous stent implantation in the celiac trunk. (**a**) The lateral selective angiogram provides good visualization of the intima flap (arrow). (**b**) Anteroposterior angiogram: the hemodynamic importance of the intima flap—with no filling of the mesenteric arcades above the jejunal orifices on contrast imaging—should be noted.

bleeding in the vicinity of the brachial artery, with development of a hematoma that compresses the neurovascular plexus on the inner side of the upper arm, early surgical relief is necessary in order to prevent severe and lasting neurological damage.

Complications affecting the artery that has been treated are rare, but potentially very dangerous. Dissection or thrombotic occlusion can lead to acute ischemia (Fig. 3.2-17). If it is not possible to treat the occlusion endovascularly (with stent implantation, thrombolysis, or thrombus aspiration), an emergency surgical intervention may be necessary in order to restore flow. However, in this case the results are often unsatisfactory.

Hemorrhage occurs very rarely in connection with intestinal reperfusion and can usually be controlled with percutaneous embolization. Other complications include blue toe syndrome and acute renal failure due to embolizations of plaque material from the aorta into the leg arteries and renal arteries during manipulation of the catheter and wires in the atheromatous aorta.

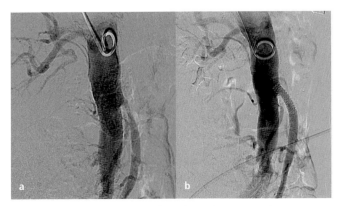

Fig. 3.2-18a, b Stenosis in a reimplanted superior mesenteric artery. (**a**) Diagnostic angiogram, showing a stenotic reimplanted artery on the infrarenal abdominal aorta. (**b**) Good result after stent implantation.

Results

The data in the literature show that endovascular therapy is associated with a significantly lower rate of hospital mortality and with a lower rate of perioperative morbidity (6% vs. 11% and 50% vs. 47%, respectively), and with a shorter hospital stay (5 vs. 16 days) in comparison with surgery. In addition, symptomatic improvement in patients with chronic mesenteric arterial occlusive disease with endovascular therapy is similarly good in comparison with surgical treatment. The technical success rate is high with both forms of treatment. Long-time studies have shown that the clinical benefit of surgical therapy lasts longer than with endovascular therapy, with lower rates of recurrence of symptoms (7% vs. 25%), re-stenosis (13% vs. 23%), and repeat interventions (9% vs. 18%). The primary patency rate after 1 year and 5 years is better with surgical therapy (89% vs. 74% and 69% vs. 32%, respectively), with comparable secondary patency rates with the two treatment methods. However, despite the lack of randomized studies, percutaneous revascularization has largely replaced surgery and is now accepted as the treatment of choice both for chronic mesenteric occlusive disease and for re-stenosis after surgical treatment (Fig. 3.2-18). In interventional therapy—as in open surgical revascularization—two-vessel treatment is preferable, as the probability of symptomatic recurrence afterwards is reduced. The open surgical procedure is still the best form of treatment for low-risk patients and for relatively young patients with a long life expectancy.

After treatment, a careful follow-up examination is necessary with both forms of therapy. Duplex ultrasound check-ups are recommended after 1, 3, 6, and 12 months and at 12-month intervals thereafter.

Summary

Since the first percutaneous treatment for chronic mesenteric arterial occlusive disease in 1980, endovascular techniques have increasingly been used as the treatment of choice. This is because of their lower invasiveness and lower rates of perioperative mortality and morbidity in comparison with surgery. However, surgical treatment still has an important role in younger, healthier patients with longer life expectancy, due to the better long-term results. Surgical revascularization is still the best treatment approach in cases of acute mesenteric ischemia, as it allows the integrity of the intestines to be evaluated at the same time. Hybrid procedures combining endovascular treatment methods with open surgery may be an alternative, but further data are needed on this topic.

References

AbuRahma AF, Stone PA, Bates MC, Welch CA. Angioplasty/stenting of the superior mesenteric artery and celiac trunk: early and late outcomes. J Endovasc Ther 2003 Dec; 10 (6): 1046–53.

Armstrong PA. Visceral duplex scanning: evaluation before and after artery intervention for chronic mesenteric ischemia. Perspect Vasc Surg Endovasc Ther 2007 Dec; 19 (4): 386–92; discussion 93–4.

Babu SC, Shah PM. Celiac territory ischemic syndrome in visceral artery occlusion. Am J Surg 1993 Aug; 166 (2): 227–30.

Biebl M, Oldenburg WA, Paz-Fumagalli R, McKinney JM, Hakaim AG. Surgical and interventional visceral revascularization for the treatment of chronic mesenteric ischemia—when to prefer which? World J Surg 2007 Mar; 31 (3): 562–8.

Cademartiri F, Palumbo A, Maffei E, Martini C, Malago R, Belgrano M, et al. Noninvasive evaluation of the celiac trunk and superior mesenteric artery with multislice CT in patients with chronic mesenteric ischaemia. Radiol Med 2008 Dec; 113 (8): 1135–42.

Cleveland TJ, Nawaz S, Gaines PA. Mesenteric arterial ischaemia: diagnosis and therapeutic options. Vasc Med 2002; 7 (4): 311–21.

Cognet F, Ben Salem D, Dranssart M, Cercueil JP, Weiller M, Tatou E, et al. Chronic mesenteric ischemia: imaging and percutaneous treatment. Radiographics. 2002 Jul–Aug; 22 (4): 863–79; discussion 79–80.

Davies RS, Wall ML, Silverman SH, Simms MH, Vohra RK, Bradbury AW, et al. Surgical versus endovascular reconstruction for chronic mesenteric ischemia: a contemporary UK series. Vasc Endovascular Surg 2009 Apr–May; 43 (2): 157–64.

Dietrich CF, Jedrzejczyk M, Ignee A. Sonographic assessment of splanchnic arteries and the bowel wall. Eur J Radiol 2007 Nov; 64 (2): 202–12.

Ghosh S, Roberts N, Firmin RK, Jameson J, Spyt TJ. Risk factors for intestinal ischaemia in cardiac surgical patients. Eur J Cardiothorac Surg 2002 Mar; 21 (3): 411–6.

Hellinger JC. Evaluating mesenteric ischemia with multidetector-row CT angiography. Tech Vasc Interv Radiol 2004 Sep; 7 (3): 160–6.

Horton KM, Fishman EK. Multidetector CT angiography in the diagnosis of mesenteric ischemia. Radiol Clin North Am 2007 Mar; 45 (2): 275–88.

Laissy JP, Trillaud H, Douek P. MR angiography: noninvasive vascular imaging of the abdomen. Abdom Imaging 2002 Sep–Oct; 27 (5): 488–506.

Laghi A, Iannaccone R, Catalano C, Passariello R. Multislice spiral computed tomography angiography of mesenteric arteries. Lancet 2001 Aug 25; 358 (9282): 638–9.

Lee RW, Bakken AM, Palchik E, Saad WE, Davies MG. Long-term outcomes of endoluminal therapy for chronic atherosclerotic occlusive mesenteric disease. Ann Vasc Surg 2008 Jul–Aug; 22 (4): 541–6.

Liberski SM, Koch KL, Atnip RG, Stern RM. Ischemic gastroparesis: resolution after revascularization. Gastroenterology 1990 Jul; 99 (1): 252–7.

Mell MW, Acher CW, Hoch JR, Tefera G, Turnipseed WD. Outcomes after endarterectomy for chronic mesenteric ischemia. J Vasc Surg 2008 Nov; 48 (5): 1132–8.

Mensink PB, van Petersen AS, Geelkerken RH, Otte JA, Huisman AB, Kolkman JJ. Clinical significance of splanchnic artery stenosis. Br J Surg 2006 Nov; 93 (11): 1377–82.

Moawad J, Gewertz BL. Chronic mesenteric ischemia. Clinical presentation and diagnosis. Surg Clin North Am 1997 Apr; 77 (2): 357–69.

Moneta GL, Lee RW, Yeager RA, Taylor LM, Jr., Porter JM. Mesenteric duplex scanning: a blinded prospective study. J Vasc Surg 1993 Jan; 17 (1): 79–84; discussion 5–6.

Otte JA, Huisman AB, Geelkerken RH, Kolkman JJ. Jejunal tonometry for the diagnosis of gastrointestinal ischemia. Feasibility, normal values and comparison of jejunal with gastric tonometry exercise testing. Eur J Gastroenterol Hepatol 2008 Jan; 20 (1): 62–7.

Pellerito JS, Revzin MV, Tsang JC, Greben CR, Naidich JB. Doppler sonographic criteria for the diagnosis of inferior mesenteric artery stenosis. J Ultrasound Med 2009 May; 28 (5): 641–50.

Schaefer PJ, Schaefer FK, Hinrichsen H, Jahnke T, Charalambous N, Heller M, Mueller-Huelsbeck S. Stent placement with the monorail technique for treatment of mesenteric artery stenosis. J Vasc Interv Radiol 2006 Apr; 17 (4): 637–43.

Schermerhorn ML, Giles KA, Hamdan AD, Wyers MC, Pomposelli FB. Mesenteric revascularization: management and outcomes in the United States, 1988–2006. J Vasc Surg 2009 Aug; 50 (2): 341–8 e1.

Silva JA, White CJ, Collins TJ, Jenkins JS, Andry ME, Reilly JP, Ramee SR. Endovascular therapy for chronic mesenteric ischemia. J Am Coll Cardiol 2006 Mar 7; 47 (5): 944–50.

Taylor LM, Jr., Moneta GL. Intestinal ischemia. Ann Vasc Surg 1991 Jul; 5 (4): 403–6.

Thomas JH, Blake K, Pierce GE, Hermreck AS, Seigel E. The clinical course of asymptomatic mesenteric arterial stenosis. J Vasc Surg 1998 May; 27 (5): 840–4.

van Bockel JH, Geelkerken RH, Wasser MN. Chronic splanchnic ischaemia. Best Pract Res Clin Gastroenterol 2001 Feb; 15 (1): 99–119.

Wilson DB, Mostafavi K, Craven TE, Ayerdi J, Edwards MS, Hansen KJ. Clinical course of mesenteric artery stenosis in elderly Americans. Arch Intern Med 2006 Oct 23; 166 (19): 2095–100.

Zeller T, Rastan A, Schwarzwälder U, Schwarz T, Frank U, Bürgelin K, Sixt S, Müller C, Rothenpieler U, Flügel PC, Pochert V, Neumann FJ. Endovascular therapy of chronic mesenteric ischemia. Eurointervention 2007; 2: 444–51.

Zerbib P, Lebuffe G, Sergent-Baudson G, Chamatan A, Massouille D, Lions C, et al. Endovascular versus open revascularization for chronic mesenteric ischemia: a comparative study. Langenbecks Arch Surg 2008 Nov; 393 (6): 865–70.

Zwolak RM. Can duplex ultrasound replace arteriography in screening for mesenteric ischemia? Semin Vasc Surg 1999 Dec; 12 (4): 252–60.

3.2.3 Renal artery stenosis

Thomas Zeller
Color-coded duplex ultrasonography: Tom Schilling
Surgical treatment: Kai Balzer, Wilhelm Sandmann

3.2.3.1 Clinical picture

Epidemiology, etiology, and course

Atherosclerotic renal artery stenosis, the most frequent form of renal artery stenosis, is a condition usually located at an ostium with a tendency to progress, while the rarer forms of renal artery stenosis seen in fibromuscular dysplasia, arteritis, and external compression are usually located in the distal main renal arteries or segmental arteries.

The exact prevalence of renal artery stenosis (RAS) is still unclear. Early autopsy studies reported a frequency of up to 25% for stenosis of over 50% of the diameter in patients of the age of 50. Current estimates show that the frequency is less than 5% in patients with high blood pressure. In an angiographically controlled duplex ultrasonography study, we found RAS ≥ 40% in 19.6% and ≥ 70% in 7.5% of 500 patients examined. An ultrasound study in patients with end-stage renal disease reported evidence of RAS > 60% at the start of dialysis in 22% of the patients.

Atherosclerotic RAS is typically a disease of older men, with only one-third of the patients being women. It is usually one of several manifestations of generalized atherosclerosis; up to 95% of patients have concomitant coronary heart disease, 56% have cerebral arterial occlusive disease, and 74% have peripheral arterial occlusive disease (PAOD) in the lower extremities. RAS ≥ 50% has been observed in 28% of patients with PAOD, 34% of older patients with coronary disease, and 15% of patients undergoing coronary angiography. The risk factors most frequently associated with RAS, in addition to arterial hypertension (99%), are dyslipidemia (89%), nicotine consumption (61%), and less frequently diabetes mellitus (41%).

Atherosclerotic RAS, particularly with stenoses greater than 60%, is a progressive disease that leads to occlusion in 18% of cases, with subsequent development of a contracted kidney. In a prospective study, 3% of patients affected by unilateral atherosclerotic RAS, 18% of those with bilateral RAS and 55% of those with contralateral renal artery occlusion had nonfunctional kidneys after 2 years.

Life expectancy is substantially reduced in patients with end-stage renal disease. The 5-year mortality rate for patients aged 65–74 years is 80%, while for those aged 75 or over it is 91%; patients with atherosclerotic RAS have the poorest prognosis. However, life expectancy is also reduced in patients with atherosclerotic RAS without terminal renal insufficiency. A follow-up study after stent angioplasty in patients with atherosclerotic RAS showed a 2-year mortality rate of 5% with a preinterventional serum creatinine concentration < 1.2 mg%, 11% with a creatinine level of 1.2–2.5 mg%, and as high as 70% with a creatinine level higher than 2.5 mg%.

The course of fibromuscular dysplasia (FMD), which leads to classic secondary renovascular hypertension and is therefore curable, is much more benign. This form of renal artery sclerosis is rarely progressive (with the exception of superimposed atherosclerosis) and leads only extremely rarely to renal artery occlusion or progressive renal insufficiency.

Clinical findings

Atherosclerotic RAS usually exacerbates preexisting arterial hypertension, and can lead to recurrent pulmonary edema, mainly in older patients with bilateral stenoses and diastolic left ventricular function disturbances. However, in contrast to fibromuscular dysplasia in younger patients, it rarely causes the classic secondary form of hypertension. Along with FMD, Takayasu aortoarteritis is the second most frequent cause of secondary renovascular hypertension. Arterial hypertension, and also activation of the renin–angiotensin–aldosterone system, can lead to multiple end-organ injuries such as left ventricular hypertrophy with subsequent diastolic and congestive heart failure. Bilateral RAS in particular often leads to acute myocardial pump failure with pulmonary edema and progressive renal failure.

In economic terms, the most significant condition is ischemic nephropathy, marked by intermittent focal intrarenal vascular obstructions and inflammation, with increasing numbers of cases of end-stage renal failure requiring dialysis treatment. There is a connection between the grade of stenosis in atherosclerotic RAS and evidence of renal atrophy, which in turn correlates with an increase in the serum creatinine concentration as a sign of ischemic nephropathy.

3.2.3.2 Anatomy and positional variants

See also section A 3.2.1 on the anatomy of the abdominal aorta and its side branches.

The kidney is a paired organ that is usually supplied by a single artery, although multiple arteries, usually symmetrical, may be present in up to 20% of cases (Fig. 3.2-19). Accessory renal arteries may originate in some cases from the distal infrarenal aorta or from the common iliac artery (Fig. 3.2-20). In a cross-section of the aorta at the level of the origins of the renal arteries, the right renal artery usually arises at the 10–11-o'clock position and the left renal artery at the 4–5-o'clock position (Fig. 3.2-21a).

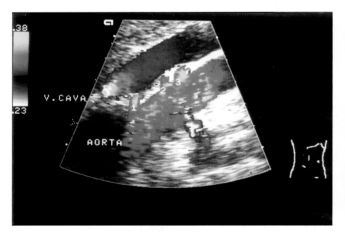

Fig. 3.2-19 Color duplex ultrasonography of the abdominal aorta in a lateral longitudinal section, showing three renal arteries on the right side (courtesy of Prof. B. Kumme).

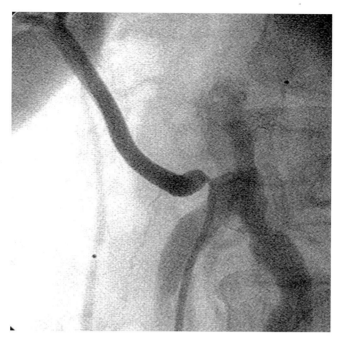

Fig. 3.2-20 An atypical right accessory renal artery, originating in the distal abdominal aorta.

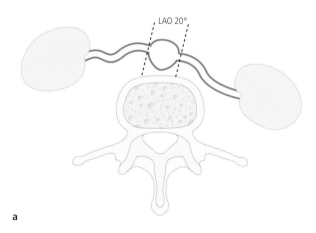

a

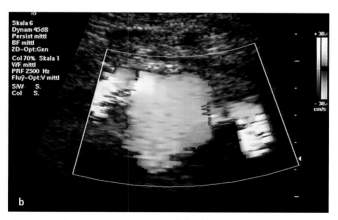

b

Fig. 3.2-21a, b The anatomic course of the renal arteries in cross-section. (**a**) Diagram. (**b**) Color duplex ultrasonography.

3.2.3.3　Diagnosis

Clinical examination

In slim patients, abdominal auscultation between the xiphoid and the navel may identify a bruit (in up to 40% of cases). However, this is a nonspecific finding that can also occur with plaques or stenoses of the aorta or mesenteric arteries.

Imaging diagnosis

Color-coded duplex ultrasonography

Color duplex is currently the best diagnostic method for distinguishing between stenoses that are hemodynamically relevant ($\geq$ 70%) and those that are not relevant. In unilateral renal artery stenosis, a side-to-side difference in the mean intrarenal resistance index (RI) > 0.05 is regarded as a reliable sign of stenosis of at least 70%. This parameter cannot be used when there is significant bilateral renal artery stenosis, however, and a prolonged acceleration time (> 0.07–0.10 s) in the intrarenally measured Doppler spectrum has to be used instead (Fig. 3.2-22). All other parameters—particularly what are known as direct duplex parameters, such as a systolic intrastenotic peak flow velocity > 200 cm/s and a renal–aortic velocity ratio > 3.5—are not suitable for use as isolated evaluation parameters for diagnosing hemodynamically relevant renal artery stenosis, as they were defined using an angiographic stenosis grade of 50% or 60%, which was regarded as hemodynamically relevant in the studies concerned. Provided that the duplex examination is carried out by an experienced examiner with adequate equipment, this should be the preferred diagnostic screening method for renal artery stenosis. The advantages of the method are its lack of invasiveness, the avoidance of radiation exposure and radiographic contrast administration, local flexibility (as a bedside method), the ability to repeat the examination at any time, and its low cost.

Examination technique

A 3.5–5-MHz sector scanner is usually used. The examination should be carried out with an appropriate application pressure from the scanner in order to compress bowel contents etc. and improve the imaging quality. Constant pressure is better than applying pressure briefly, with "relapsing" of the bowel contents. The typical monophasic flow signal in the renal artery is V_{max} systolic 1.8 m/s and V_{max} diastolic 0.2–1.0 m/s.

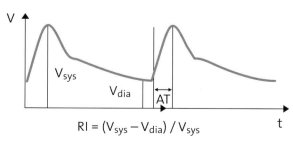

Fig. 3.2-22 Intrarenal Doppler flow profile, with definition of the intrarenal resistance index (RI) and acceleration time (AT).

Table 3.2-2 Age-related normal values for the resistance index (RI) in the intrarenal segmental arteries (adapted from Karasch et al. 1993).

Age (years)	21–30	31–40	41–50	51–60	61–70	71–80
Mean RI	0.63 ± 0.088	0.65 ± 0.05	0.67 ± 0.04	0.67 ± 0.06	0.72 ± 0.05	0.78 ± 0.07
RI benchmark values	0.54–0.73	0.58–0.70	0.59–0.73	0.56–0.81	0.61–0.85	0.70–0.87

In addition to the systolic/diastolic velocities, intrarenal flow conditions are also described using the resistance index (RI), for which age-related standard values are available (Table 3.2-2).

Differential diagnosis

Arteriosclerosis:
- Usually located in more proximal segments of the renal artery
- Ostial (0–5 mm from the origin): approx. 30%
- Proximal (5–10 mm from the origin): approx. 50%
- Truncal (> 10 mm from the origin): approx. 20%

Fibromuscular dysplasia:
- Localized disease is usually in the distal third.
- A bead-like stenotic picture may be visible.

Large-vessel vasculitis:
- May also be present when there is aortic involvement, with a typical finding being a homogenously hypoechoic, widened intima–media complex (macaroni sign)

Dissection:
- May be present when there is aortic dissection, possibly with demonstration of a dissection membrane and in that case a typical triphasic "splash phenomenon"

Occlusion:
- Hypoechoic to isoechoic occlusive material on B-imaging, absence of flow, marked intrarenal flow disturbances (slight residual perfusion via collaterals, mainly from the suprarenal arteries, is possible)

Specific findings

Criteria for renal artery stenosis

Direct criteria for stenosis:
- Hemodynamically relevant renal artery stenosis shows a V_{max} systolic of more than 2–2.5 m/s. However, there is no fixed threshold velocity; the lower the threshold velocity used, the better the sensitivity, at the cost of reduced specificity.
- Renal–aortic ratio (RAR; V_{max} kidney/V_{max} aorta): with a renal artery stenosis of more than 50–60%, the ratio is > 3.5.
- Peak velocity ratio (PVR; V_{max} intrastenotic/V_{max} prestenotic): can be used with distal renal artery stenoses.
- In cases of proximal renal artery stenosis, an adjusted PVR can be used (V_{max} intrastenotic/V_{max} post-stenotic). *Caution:* insonation should not be carried out in a segment showing post-stenotic dilation.
- Usual stenosis phenomena/spectral widening.

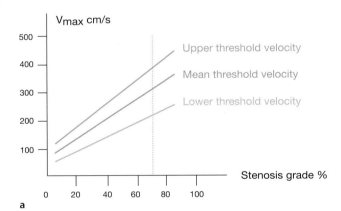

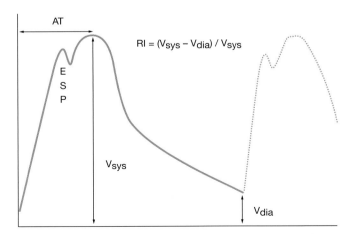

Fig. 3.2-23 Intrarenal duplex ultrasound measurement parameters: imaging of the relevant measurement parameters for assessment of renal artery perfusion. AT, acceleration time; ESP, early systolic peak; RI, resistance index; V_{dia}, end-diastolic flow velocity; V_{sys}, systolic peak velocity.

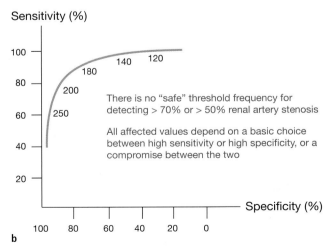

Fig. 3.2-24a, b Threshold velocity (**a**) and sensitivity–specificity relationship (**b**). For example, a 70% stenosis may involve various maximum velocities—there is always an inverse relationship between sensitivity and specificity when a defined threshold velocity is selected.

Indirect criteria for stenosis:

- With unilateral renal artery stenosis, the post-stenotic RI is reduced > 0.05 (V_{max} systolic – V_{max} diastolic/V_{max} systolic).
- With bilateral renal artery stenosis, the RI on both sides is below the standard value for the age.
- Intrarenal acceleration time > 0.07 s (> 0.10 s).
- Flattened systolic pack, absent early systolic peak.

Criteria for a transplant renal artery stenosis

- V_{max} systolic > 220 (250) cm/s
- Local flow increase > 50%
- Renal–iliac ratio > 2.6–3.0
- Widened frequency range
- Retrograde flow components/turbulences

Increased RI → differential diagnosis

- Interstitial renal changes (e.g., Kimmelstiel–Wilson disease)
- Preeclampsia (edema–proteinuria–hypertension gestosis)
- Hemolytic–uremic syndrome
- Obstructive pyelocaliceal dilation (RI > 0.7)
- Liver cirrhosis—imminent hepatorenal syndrome due to vasoconstriction
- Kidney transplant complication (with an intra-individual course)
- Bradycardia

Decreased RI → differential diagnosis

- Upstream renal artery stenosis (main trunk, pole of kidney stenosis or segmental artery stenosis—with only segmental RI changes in the latter case, so that measurements in the cranial, middle, and caudal segments of the kidney are needed)
- Intrarenal arteriovenous malformations (segmental RI usually ≤ 0.52)
- Drug effects
- Aortic valve insufficiency
- Tachycardia

Kidney transplant vascularization

Normal:

- Transplant artery with RI less than 0.71 (does not safely exclude rejection)
- RI in transplant 0.6–0.7 (–0.75)

Rejection reaction:

- Increasing reduction in diastolic flow ranging up to retrograde flow; intra-individual course (differential diagnosis: renal vein thrombosis)
- RI above 0.80 → poor prognosis
- RI above 0.90 in studies sometimes used as cut-off value for repeat surgery
- Acute and chronic conditions are not distinguishable
- Differential diagnosis: urinary obstruction, arteriosclerosis/arteriolosclerosis, acute tubular necroses

Arterial angiography

Selective arterial angiography is still regarded as the gold standard for diagnosis. The parameter most often used for quantifying a stenosis is the ratio of the minimum lumen diameter (MLD) in the stenosis and the reference vessel diameter (RVD): % stenosis = (MLD/

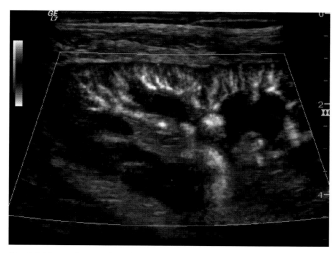

Fig. 3.2-25 Duplex renal perfusion. Low flow–sensitive color imaging (color B-flow here) makes it possible to visualize perfusion in the renal parenchyma—e.g., in order to detect a perfusion deficit in cases of embolism.

RVD) × 100. However, angiography has considerable technical limitations; the main disadvantage of the method is its invasiveness, with a potential risk of local vascular access route complications such as hematoma, including pseudoaneurysm formation and infection (in cases of obesity), as well as renal embolization and contrast nephropathy. In addition, the accuracy of measurements with the planar examination method is questionable, particularly since most stenoses are located near the orifice. There is therefore a lack of a proximal reference segment of the vessel to determine the grade of stenosis. Using the vascular segment located distal to the stenosis to obtain a reference diameter has limitations, particularly in high-grade stenoses, because the segment usually shows post-stenotic dilation, inevitably leading to overestimation of the grade of stenosis.

Magnetic resonance angiography (MRA)

This method has come into widespread use during the last 5 years due to its noninvasiveness and avoidance of radiation exposure and radiographic contrast medium. Gadolinium-enhanced three-dimensional volume acquisition techniques with 1.5-Tesla machines and measurement of pressure gradients using the Doppler technique have made the procedure much more reliable. The amount of contrast needed has proved to be tolerable for the kidney. The main limitations of the method are the fact that signal loss occurs after stainless-steel stents have been implanted, as well as its cost.

Computed-tomographic angiography (CTA)

As in MRA, the use of multi-slice technology makes it possible to produce excellent three-dimensional reconstructions of vessels, including depiction of calcified plaques, without the limitations resulting from stent artifacts. The disadvantages of the method, particularly for serial screening and follow-up of the course of disease, include its cost and the need to use x-rays and radiographic contrast medium. The latter also involves a potential risk of causing further deterioration when renal function is already impaired.

3.2.3.4   Treatment

Conservative treatment

There are certain limitations of drug treatment for arterial hypertension in patients with RAS. In the first place, the willingness of the patient to take regular medication may be limited, leading to often inadequate blood-pressure levels; secondly, angiotensin-converting enzyme (ACE) inhibitors and diuretics in particular, as well as other groups of antihypertensive agents, can lead to acute or chronic ischemic renal failure, particularly in older patients. Despite this, randomized studies have all so far shown that supervised antihypertensive drug treatment can lead to blood-pressure levels as good as those with endovascular therapy. In principle, all groups of antihypertensive medications are suitable in the treatment of renal hypertension, with the exception of high-grade bilateral RAS, in which there is a contraindication for ACE inhibitors. The goal of treatment is to achieve a normotensive blood-pressure level, which is ideally monitored using outpatient 24-h blood-pressure assessment.

Endothelial dysfunction is an important factor contributing to renal damage following revascularization of a stenotic renal artery. Nebivolol, a new-generation β-blocker, induces endothelium-dependent NO-controlled relaxation of the arterial wall and may improve endothelial dysfunction. In patients with > 70% renal artery stenosis, a small randomized pilot study investigated the effect of nebivolol on the estimated glomerular filtration rate (eGFR) after revascularization. The eGFR improved significantly in the nebivolol group and remained unaltered in the placebo group. Proteinuria also declined more strongly in the verum group (Duranay et al. 2009).

In atherosclerotic RAS, rigorous drug treatment is also necessary for secondary prophylaxis, with reduction of the low-density lipoprotein (LDL) level to below 100 (70) mg/dL, cessation of nicotine consumption, and hemoglobin A_{1c} adjustment to < 6.5 g%.

Endovascular treatment

Prior to the stenting era, catheter treatment for RAS was limited to fibromuscular dysplasia and atherosclerotic truncal RAS, and the primary success rates for percutaneous transluminal renal angioplasty (PTRA) for ostial atherosclerotic RAS (24–91%) were as disappointing as the rate of recurrent stenoses (25–45%). However, stent PTRA has become the treatment of choice since smaller randomized studies and single-center registry data demonstrated the superiority of stent angioplasty over conventional PTRA, with primary success rates of 88–100% and recurrent stenosis rates of 10–18%.

Indications for PTRA

- Hemodynamically relevant ($\geq$ 70%) unilateral and bilateral RAS with arterial hypertension and normal or preterminally restricted renal function, with a life expectancy of at least 2 years after the intervention
- Hemodynamically relevant unilateral and bilateral RAS or renal artery occlusions in acute or subacute terminal renal insufficiency

Contraindications against PTRA

- Hemodynamically relevant RAS < 70%
- Life expectancy markedly reduced due to concomitant diseases
- Chronic dialysis

Patient preparation

The following examinations should be carried out before the procedure, before the patient is discharged, and during the follow-up:

- Renal function parameters (serum creatinine concentration, serum urea, at least an estimated creatinine clearance rate (evaluated glomerular filtration rate, GFR), or preferably creatinine clearance measured using 24-h urine)
- 24-h blood-pressure monitoring
- Color duplex ultrasonography of the renal arteries with measurement of renal–aortic flow velocity quotients and Pourcelot intrarenal resistance index
- Analysis and documentation of antihypertensive medication
- The patient should provide informed consent at least 1 day before the procedure
- Fasting 6 hours before the procedure
- Prehydration with intravenous isosmotic saline or orally (mineral water, tea) in patients with advanced renal insufficiency (GFR < 60 mL/min)

Medication before the procedure

- Pretreatment with ASA 100 mg/d as long-term therapy, or 500 mg ASA as a bolus before the procedure, clopidogrel 600 mg as a loading dose on the day of the procedure or the day before
- After placement of the sheath, administration of a heparin bolus of 5000 IU
- There is controversy regarding the administration of acetylcysteine to capture free radicals, at a dosage of 2 × 600 mg (1200 mg) on the day before the procedure and on the day of the procedure

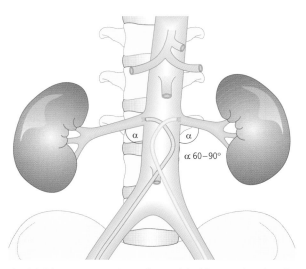

Fig. 3.2-26 Anatomic position of a renal double curve (RDC) guide catheter from the right femoral and left femoral approaches.

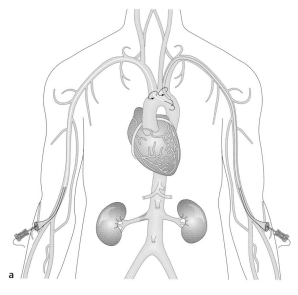

a

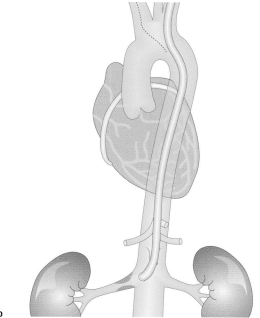

b

Fig. 3.2-27a, b Anatomic position of a multipurpose (MP) guide catheter introduced via the left transbrachial approach.

Access route

Femoral access

Femoral access is the standard access route if there are no untreated stenoses or occlusions in the infrarenal abdominal aorta or pelvic or femoral arteries (in the inguinal region) and there is no marked tortuosity of the pelvic arteries or a steeply angled caudal origin of the renal artery. The guiding catheter technique has replaced the original guidewire technique, as it is easier and safer to use. The sequence is as follows:

■ After local anesthesia, a 6F or 7F sheath (11 cm long) with a hemostatic valve is placed in the common femoral artery. If there is tortuosity in the iliac arteries, a 23-cm sheath may be helpful.

■ Introduction of a 0.035" or 0.038" standard J guidewire into the thoracic aorta.

■ Via the guidewire, the guide catheter (55 cm long) is positioned at the level of the L1/L2 intercostal space and, with the wire in place, the renal artery origins are non-selectively imaged for guidance.

■ After identification of the origin of the renal artery that is to be treated, the catheter tip is positioned, with the wire in place, slightly above the renal artery ostium. The guidewire is then gradually withdrawn. The guide catheter tip then usually "falls" into the ostium, with only slight correction movements being needed. After the catheter has been positioned, and before the first selective injection of contrast, the guide catheter should be cleared of any plaque and thrombus material that may have collected in its tip during the probing process. To do this, free aspiration via Tuohy can be carried out, or it can simply be allowed to bleed back with pulsation for a few cardiac cycles. Selective contrast injection should only be carried out after this step. Depending on the anatomy, a guide catheter with a renal double curve (RDC), hockey stick, IMA, or Judkins right (JR) configuration is used.

■ Alternatively, a Vista BriteTip IG™ "guide sheath" can be used, combining a 55-cm long guide catheter with a hemostatic valve. This saves 1F in the sheath size.

Brachial access

The brachial access route can be used on both sides, but the left side is preferable in order to avoid passage into the cerebral arteries. In most cases, a 6F sheath or alternatively a 7F guide sheath is placed in the brachial artery in retrograde fashion. After placement of a 0.035" guidewire with antifriction coating at the level of L1, nonselective imaging of the origins of the renal arteries is carried out, followed by placement of the guide catheter as described above.

Materials required are: a 7F guide sheath, 90 cm long, with a multipurpose configuration; guidewire: 6F, 90 cm long, with a multipurpose (MP) or right Amplatz configuration; and a Terumo 0.035" stiff J wire.

Preprocedural angiography

Before the procedure, the renal artery stenosis has to be selectively and non-selectively imaged using angiography. With normal aortic anatomy, the renal artery ostia are best assessed using a 20° left anterior oblique (LAO) projection. In approximately 15% of the normal population, the kidneys have multiple afferent arteries, and the accessory arteries sometimes have atypically positioned origins (e.g., the distal abdominal aorta, proximal common iliac artery). Attention should therefore be given to ensure that the angiographically demonstrated renal artery does supply the entire renal contour; otherwise, accessory arteries should be sought.

Procedure

■ After selective exploration of the renal artery, a guidable 0.014" extra support guidewire is introduced through the RAS as far as the segmental arteries (*caution:* the parenchyma should not be damaged).

■ Markedly calcified RAS and stenoses ≥ 90% are predilated with a 3-mm coronary balloon catheter. Alternatively, the premounted stent/balloon systems can also be used for primary stenting.

■ If there is an ostial stenosis (defined as ≤ 10 mm distal from the origin), the stent should completely cover the renal artery ostium and extend 1–2 mm into the aortic lumen.

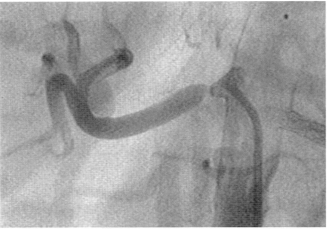
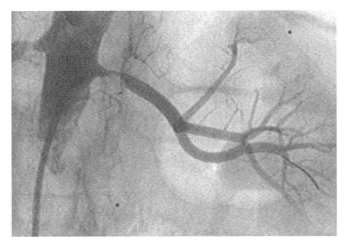
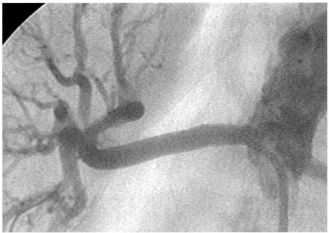
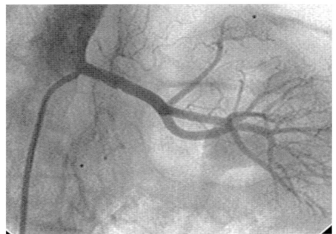

Fig. 3.2-28 The normal origin and proximal course of the renal arteries.

- The ratio of the stent/balloon to the diameter of the renal artery should be 1:1–1.0:1.2. *Caution:* oversizing can lead to aortic wall rupture or aortic dissection.
- There is controversy regarding the use of distal protection systems, and in the present author's view, this should not be done routinely until manufacturers are able to supply systems specially developed for PTRA.

Postprocedural follow-up and medication

Monitoring of cardiovascular parameters for 12 hours is recommended, as excessive drops in blood pressure may occur in individual cases. Particularly in patients with renal insufficiency before the procedure, regular postprocedural checking of renal function parameters is indicated, at least 48 hours after exposure to contrast media. Postprocedural medication consists of long-term treatment with ASA 100 mg/d, plus clopidogrel 75 mg/d for 4 weeks.

Potential risks of the procedure

- Renal (cholesterol) embolization with subsequent deterioration in renal function, potentially progressing to terminal renal insufficiency
- Contrast-induced nephropathy: the risk increases along with the initial degree of renal dysfunction

- Renal artery and aortic dissection or rupture
- Incorrect stent placement
- Local vascular complications at the puncture site, such as false aneurysm, arteriovenous fistula, hematoma requiring transfusion, etc.

Surgical treatment for renal artery stenoses and renal artery aneurysms

Introduction

The connection between arterial hypertension and renovascular occlusive disease was established by Goldblatt in 1934. He showed that renal artery constriction leads to atrophy of the affected kidney and hypertension, and noted that in patients with hypertension or high blood pressure, the vessels are damaged and that the renal arteries are affected particularly frequently. He concluded that the vascular condition occurs first and that hypertension appears as soon as the renal arteries are affected by it; he also suspected that the reduced renal perfusion results in high blood pressure. In addition, he showed that hypertension caused by renal artery stenosis can be successfully treated using nephrectomy (Goldblatt 1934). On the basis of these findings, Leadbetter and Burkland carried out a nephrectomy of an atrophic kidney in a 5-year-old child in 1938 and were thereby able to cure the hypertension (Leadbetter and Burkland 1938).

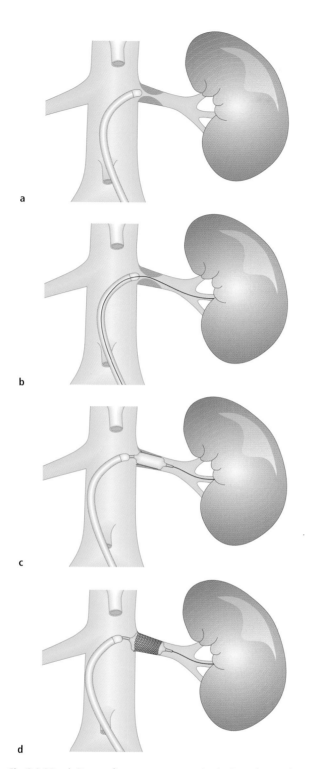

a

b

c

d

Fig. 3.2-29a–d Stages of percutaneous transluminal renal angioplasty (PTRA) stenting from the transfemoral approach.

In the years that followed, many patients were treated using nephrectomy in cases of hypertension and renal atrophy confirmed by intravenous pyelography. In 1956, Smith reviewed the treatment results in 575 patients who had been treated in this way. He found that only 26% of the patients were cured, and called for stricter indications to be established for nephrectomy (Smith 1956).

In 1954, Freeman reported that thromboendarterectomy in the renal arteries resolved the hypertension in a patient with hypertension and chronic infrarenal aortic occlusion.

Despite these initial successes, the rate of cure for hypertension did not rise above 50%. It was only a precise clarification of the pathophysiological basis and the implementation of the results in clinical practice that made it possible to assess precisely whether a renal artery stenosis is inducing renovascular hypertension. Accordingly, publications on surgery for renal artery revascularization now report rates of improvement in hypertension of 40–80%. In a prospective randomized study, our own group reported that hypertension was cured following surgery in 7% of the patients and that improvement was noted after surgery in 74% (Balzer et al. 2009).

In addition to the development of hypertension, stenosis of the renal artery also contributes to renal insufficiency, in a condition known as ischemic nephropathy. In 1962, Morris reported improvements in renal function after surgical revascularization of the renal artery in eight patients (Morris 1962). Various retrospective studies have demonstrated a positive effect of surgical revascularization in patients with impaired renal function; patients in whom renal function improves after surgical revascularization appear to benefit particularly in relation to freedom from dialysis and dialysis-free survival (Hansen et al. 2000). A review of a total of 21 publications (1979–2004; 2314 patients, four prospective non-randomized studies, and 17 retrospective evaluations) reported a benefit from surgical revascularization with regard to renal function and lower rates of deterioration in renal function in comparison with interventional studies (Abela et al. 2009). Despite this, it is still an open question whether surgical revascularization of the renal arteries contributes to an improvement in ischemic nephropathy, as there are currently no criteria for predicting recovery of renal function and there is a lack of prospective randomized studies on the topic.

Although randomized studies have not shown any advantage with interventional therapy for atherosclerotic renal artery stenosis in comparison with optimal drug treatment, it is possible to identify patients who are capable of benefiting from revascularization therapy. Close interdisciplinary collaboration is needed here in order to develop criteria for identifying these patients. Surgical treatment will continue to play a role, particularly in younger patients who can benefit from the much longer patency following surgical revascularization, and also in patients in whom interventional therapy has failed. In addition to purely atherosclerotic stenosis of the renal arteries, dysplastic and aneurysmal processes in the renal arteries also represent an indication for surgical treatment.

Indications for surgical treatment

Arterial hypertension is often the first diagnostic sign of the presence of renal artery stenosis. The patient's age and a history of high blood pressure already suggest the probable etiology of the stenosis. In formal terms, processes at the renal arteries can be classified according to their causes into degenerative stenoses with atherosclerotic causes, stenoses due to dysplasia or dissection, and aneurysmal processes. Renal artery stenoses in combination with renal artery aneurysms represent a special form. During the diagnostic work-up for renovascular hypertension, distinctions need to be made between screening procedures for clarifying arterial hypertension or renal insufficiency, examinations assessing the hemodynamic relevance of the stenosis and the prognosis for resolving hypertension, and procedures for morphological imaging of the stenosis in order to plan the treatment procedure.

Renal artery stenoses can be recognized using color-coded duplex ultrasonography. The procedure is also suitable for postoperative check-ups. Tomographic methods such as CTA and MRA are also suitable for detecting renal artery stenoses and aneurysms. Intra-arterial digital subtraction angiography is regarded as the gold standard for diagnosing renal artery stenoses and is usually required for treatment planning.

The aims in treatment for renal artery stenosis are to improve or cure the hypertension and improve or stabilize renal function. The indications for surgical treatment are basically the same as those for interventional therapy. Interventional or surgical revascularization should be considered particularly in patients who meet the following criteria:

- Low co-morbidity
- Age
- Kidney size > 8 cm
- Bilateral stenoses or unilateral stenosis when there is only one kidney (unilateral in cases of fibromuscular dysplasia as well)
- Blood pressure no longer controllable with more than three drugs
- Stenosis > 70%
- Presence of risk factors
- Mild proteinuria
- Rapid deterioration in renal function (particularly during ACE inhibitor treatment)
- Recurrent pulmonary edema
- RI < 0.8

Distinctions needed to be made among the indications and diagnostic algorithms, due to the various forms of renovascular hypertension—which can appear even in young individuals due to fibromuscular dysplasia with predominant hypertension, on the one hand, while on the other it may also occur in those of advanced age due to atherosclerosis with hypertension and ischemic nephropathy.

Arteriosclerotic renal artery stenoses

Atherosclerotic renal artery stenoses show a tendency to progress. Significant renal artery stenoses lead to hypoperfusion of the kidney, activation of the renin–angiotensin system with hypertension, and progressive renal insufficiency. In this process, renal ischemia and thus disturbed renal function are usually exacerbated by a reduction in hypertensive blood pressure, since for hemodynamic reasons this results in an additional reduction in perfusion in the affected kidney. Treatment with ACE inhibitors in this context can lead to deterioration in renal function. Morphologically, renal ischemia leads to cortical atrophy, with irreversible damage to glomeruli, tubules, vessels, and interstitium. Preventing the progression of ischemic nephropathy requires a kidney that is still sufficiently large, so that there is a borderline zone in which revascularization is still useful depending on the penumbra. A longitudinal diameter of 8 cm is often given as a borderline value for effective revascularization. Against the background of efforts to preserve the organ and improve hypertension, all cases of hemodynamically effective atherosclerotic renal artery stenosis should be evaluated on an interdisciplinary basis in relation to treatment options. Patients who

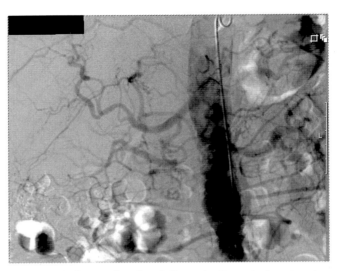

Fig. 3.2-30 Angiogram of a subtotal atherosclerotic renal artery stenosis on the right side, with a renal artery stenosis on the left, in a patient with a marked atherosclerotic process in the aorta and ischemic nephropathy and hypertension.

only have slight impairment of renal function and blood pressure, which is well controlled with drug treatment, hardly have any benefit from revascularization. Rapid progression of ischemic nephropathy, increasingly uncontrollable blood pressure, and recurrent left ventricular decompensation are indications for revascularization. Patients in whom an atherosclerotic cause of a renovascular occlusive condition is suspected should undergo function tests (captopril scintigraphy or captopril ultrasonography), depending on the examiners' expertise, if the withdrawal of the relevant antihypertensive drugs appears defensible. Noninvasive procedures such as duplex examinations are very valuable, but MRA or CTA can also be used to confirm a diagnosis. Invasive angiography should be used when it is intended to carry out an intervention or to investigate unclear findings in the distal renal arteries (Fig. 3.2-30).

Fibromuscular dysplasia (FMD)

Fibromuscular dysplasia in the renal arteries, the second most frequent cause of renal artery stenosis, is markedly different from arteriosclerotic lesions with regard to the age of predilection, angiographic findings, prognosis, and treatment indications. The condition has widely varying manifestations due to various types of distribution. Intra-arterial angiography is therefore required in order to confirm the diagnosis (Fig. 3.2-31).

Five main types of FMD can be distinguished (Pfeiffer et al. 2004; van Dongen 1988):

- Medial fibroplasia: the stenoses are usually not high-grade, show little progression, and can be well treated with drugs.
- Intimal fibroplasia: the stenosis is progressive, hypertension can rarely be well treated with drugs, and there is therefore an indication for revascularization of the renal artery.
- Perimedial fibroplasia: the stenoses are progressive, hypertension can rarely be well treated with drugs, and there is therefore an indication for revascularization of the renal artery.
- Medial hyperplasia, pseudoatherosclerotic form: the stenosis is rapidly progressive, drug control of hypertension is not possible, and revascularization of the renal artery is indicated (Fig. 3.2-32)

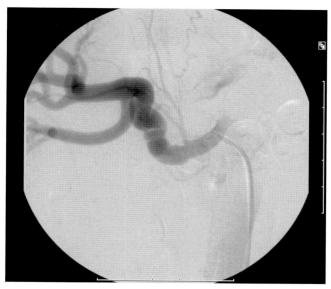

Fig. 3.2-31 Angiogram showing right-sided fibromuscular dysplasia with hypertension.

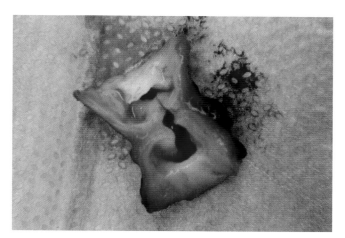

Fig. 3.2-32 Resection specimen, with medial hyperplasia in the renal artery (same patient as in Fig. 3.2-31).

- Pseudohypoplastic form: the whole kidney is affected; hypertension should be treated with drugs, and it may be necessary to consider nephrectomy.
- Medial dissection: a complication of FMD in which the segmental arteries are usually also affected and the results with revascularization are unsatisfactory.

In patients with a suspected fibromuscular cause of renovascular hypertension, after a noninvasive examination—preferably with duplex ultrasound of the renal arteries and kidneys if the relevant expertise is available—angiography should be considered, to allow clear imaging above all of any involvement of the segmental arteries.

Renal artery dissections

Spontaneous renal artery dissection is a rare disease of middle age. Intramural bleeding in the vasa vasorum, primary intimal lacerations, or fibromuscular dysplasia are thought to be the causes (Fig. 3.2-33); traumatic causes are rare (12% among our own patients).

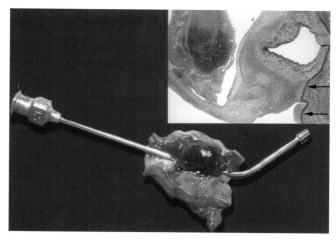

Fig. 3.2-33 Resected renal artery with a cannula in the stenotic true lumen and thrombus in the false lumen. The histological image shows a typical dissection, with laceration of the media (from Müller et al. 2003).

Among our own patients, revascularization surgery, which is a technically demanding procedure, was carried out using a venous graft in 83% of cases. In more than 50% of the cases, distal revascularization as far as the segmental arteries was required. With regard to hypertension, healing or improvement were observed in 38% of the patients and 32% of the patients suffered loss of function in the affected kidney during the subsequent course (Müller et al. 2003). Ex situ reconstruction with autotransplantation is an alternative to orthotopic surgery. Long-term preservation of the kidney and healing or improvement of hypertension appear possible with surgical reconstruction, but they require critical preoperative evaluation. When there are unilateral findings, a large preoperative renal infarction, shrunken kidney, and severely limited renal function on isotope nephrography, attempts of revascularization do not appear to be justified and primary nephrectomy should be considered in order to optimize hypertension control.

Renal artery aneurysm

Patients with a renal artery aneurysm are often asymptomatic, and the diagnosis is an incidental finding due to unclear abdominal symptoms or clarification of renovascular hypertension. The incidence of renal artery aneurysms when angiography of the renal arteries is carried out for various reasons may be up to 1% (Edsmann 1957). The reported proportion of patients with ruptures in larger cohorts with renal artery aneurysms is up to 5.3% (Pfeiffer et al. 2003). Hypertension is present in up to 90% of patients with renal artery aneurysms, and causative factors such as macroembolization, microembolization, and kinking have been considered in addition to simple co-occurrence (Youkey et al. 1985). There is an indication for treatment of the aneurysm starting from a size of 2 cm, but rupture has already been reported in individual cases at sizes of 1.5 cm. Pregnant patients in particular appear to be at higher risk for rupture of a renal artery aneurysm during the third trimester and during birth (Graff et al. 2003); however, the overall incidence of aneurysms in pregnant women is not increased. Women of child-bearing age should therefore have reconstructive treatment for a renal artery aneurysm carried out before a planned pregnancy. Treatment for renal artery aneurysm is carried out in order to prevent rupture, preserve the organ, and improve any hypertension that may be present. For diagnosis, noninvasive imaging methods such as CTA or MRA are often sufficient, and angiog-

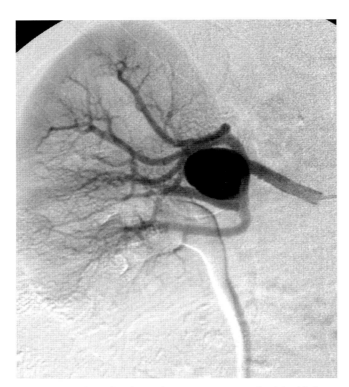

Fig. 3.2-34 Angiography of a renal artery aneurysm on the right side in a patient with arterial hypertension.

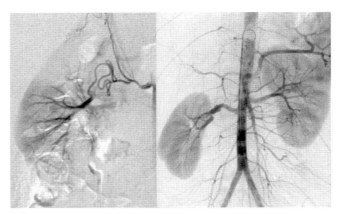

Fig. 3.2-35 Preoperative and postoperative findings in a girl aged 14 in 1999, with occlusion of the right renal artery due to fibromuscular dysplasia. Reconstruction with an aortorenal venous graft was carried out.

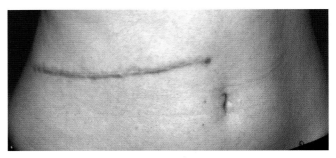

Fig. 3.2-36 Scar after a right-sided transverse upper abdominal laparotomy (same patient as in Fig. 3.2-35).

raphy is occasionally required with unclear findings or questionable involvement of the segmental branches (Fig. 3.2-34).

Interventional therapy is currently only possible in exceptional cases, and it is not a real alternative at the moment in view of the excellent results with surgical treatment. The results with reconstruction of renal artery aneurysms show very low mortality rates and excellent function rates of 75–95% (Pfeiffer et al. 2003). In addition to aortorenal bypass, surgical reconstruction methods also include local reconstruction techniques. Ex situ reconstruction with autotransplantation may be necessary, but in our own group of patients this is hardly necessary any more due to a technique developed by Sandmann.

Pediatric renal artery stenoses

Fibrodysplastic changes in the renal arteries and aortic coarctation are the main causes of renovascular hypertension in children. There is always an indication for treatment if blood pressure is inadequately controlled with drug therapy; if there is left cardiac damage and changes in the fundus of the eyeball due to hypertension; when renal function deteriorates; and when shrinking of growth disturbances are noted. Isolated stenoses can be reconstructed using bypass procedures in the majority of cases, and local reconstructive procedures are occasionally possible. Due to the potential development of aneurysmal dilations after autologous vascular replacement and of recurrent stenoses when alloplastic and autologous material is used, tightly scheduled follow-up examinations are necessary. Arterial reconstructions can lead to good long-term results in children with regard to graft patency, renal function, and blood pressure adjustment (Pourhassan et al. 2010). In view of the fact that life expectancy is severely limited due to organ complications in children with longstanding uncontrolled renovascular hypertension, elaborate revascularization procedures are justified at an early stage (Fig. 3.2-35).

Surgical procedures and results

In principle, local disobliteration procedures, bypass techniques, and local reconstructive procedures are available for surgical treatment of renal artery stenoses and renal artery aneurysms.

In addition to median or transverse laparotomy, which is preferable for bilateral renal artery processes and when there is involvement of the aorta (arterial occlusive disease, aneurysm), possible access routes include transverse upper abdominal or mid abdominal incisions, even with unilateral processes (Fig. 3.2-36).

Local disobliteration procedures

Transaortic renal artery disobliteration

This procedure is usually carried out via a median laparotomy. After exposure of the aorta and mobilization of the left renal vein, the origins of the two renal arteries are demonstrated, possibly with partial transection of the diaphragmatic crus. After suprarenal clamping of the aorta, a longitudinal incision is made in the vessel. Disobliteration of plaque is carried out circularly, starting in the aorta in the external lamina of the media, with cautious eversion disobliteration of plaques projecting into the renal arteries; the ends of the plaques often tear off smoothly. The incision is closed with a continuous suture using nonresorbable suture material (Fig. 3.2-37). Another advantage of this procedure is that the visceral arteries can also be reconstructed simultaneously while the aorta is clamped, leading—in contrast to PTA and stenting—to local removal of the atherosclerosis. Alternatively, a transverse arteriotomy of the aorta can be carried out as far as the origins of the renal arteries, which can improve the

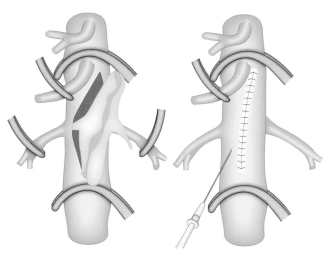

Fig. 3.2-37 Transaortic renal artery disobliteration (adapted from Wylie et al. 1969).

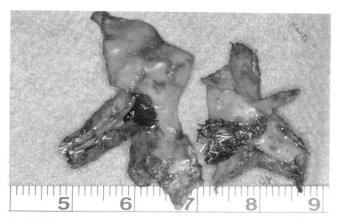

Fig. 3.2-38 Surgical specimen from a transaortic renal artery disobliteration in a 59-year-old patient with status post bilateral percutaneous transluminal angioplasty and stenting.

overview of the outlines of the plaque in the renal arteries. To avoid suture-related stenosis, this procedure should always be combined with a local patchplasty. The kidneys' tolerance for ischemia can be increased with local infusion of cold saline with the addition of heparin and alprostadil. It is important to check renal perfusion after blood flow to the renal arteries has been released again, and this can be done with Doppler ultrasound, duplex ultrasound, or intraoperative angiography. In addition, intensive-care supervision for the first 24 hours is necessary in order to monitor vital parameters and urination; regular postoperative duplex ultrasound check-ups should be carried out.

Among our own patients, this procedure has been used in approximately 90% of those with atherosclerotic renal artery stenosis. The secondary patency rate after 4 years is 90%; in a randomized study, this led to healing of the hypertension in 7% of the patients, improvement in 74%, and failure of surgical therapy relative to blood pressure in 19% in accordance with the criteria defined by Rundback (Rundback et al. 2002). Reliable stabilization of renal function was generally observed in the patients (Balzer et al. 2009). Other studies have reported a better outcome relative to the end points of hypertension and death, particularly in the subgroup of patients with creatinine levels of 2.0–4.0 mg/dL (Uzzo et al. 2002). The 30-day mortality rate after renal artery reconstruction with simultaneous aortic reconstruction was 3.1%, and after exclusion of simultaneous aortic surgery the mortality rate after purely renal revascularization was only 0.18% higher than that for interventional techniques (Abela et al. 2009).

Among our own patients, it was possible to use this procedure in over 80% of the renal arteries requiring reconstruction, even in patients with atherosclerotic renal artery stenoses who had previously undergone interventional treatment (Fig. 3.2-38). The procedure can stabilize renal function, can reduce hypertension significantly in comparison with the preoperative value, and can reduce drug requirements. Despite this, disappointing results are seen when the healing and improvement rates are assessed using the Rundback criteria, with only a 22% rate of improvement or healing of hypertension. In addition, there is a high rate of permanent renal failure (9.3%), reconstruction proved to be no longer possible in 6% of the renal arteries that were to be treated, and the re-stenosis rate after a

mean follow-up period of 4.16 years was 16.3% (Balzer et al. 2012). If the relevant expertise is available, reconstruction of renal arteries that have previously undergone interventional treatment is possible, but the results are poorer in comparison with primary surgical reconstruction—a fact that should be taken into account when the indication for interventional treatment is being assessed.

Bypass procedures

Aortorenal bypass

This reconstruction can be carried out via a median laparotomy or unilateral transverse upper abdominal or mid abdominal laparotomy. In atherosclerotic renal artery stenosis, the aortorenal bypass is used when transaortic reconstruction does not appear possible due to the morphology of the stenosis (e.g., changes extending far into the renal artery, recurrent stenoses), or is not possible due to incomplete tearing of plaque. This technique is the method regularly used in patients with fibromuscular dysplasia (Fig. 3.2-39). In patients who have previously undergone interventional treatment for an atherosclerotic renal artery stenosis, the procedure is used more often than in primary surgical treatment for an atherosclerotic renal artery stenosis.

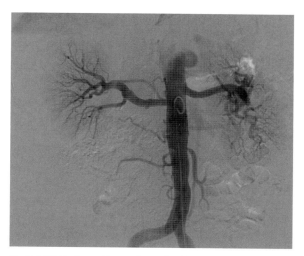

Fig. 3.2-39 Postoperative angiography after an aortorenal bypass to the right renal artery in a patient with fibromuscular dysplasia (same patient as in Fig. 3.2-31).

The technique is also used primarily in cases of inflammatory stenoses, dissections of the renal artery, and processes caused by elastosis. The preferred bypass material is great saphenous vein from the groin, which almost always has an adequate lumen for reconstruction. Alternatively, the internal iliac artery or prosthetic material (Dacron or PTFE) can be used unilaterally, and these are indicated particularly in inflammatory processes and elastoses. In a unilateral procedure with transverse access, dissection of the renal artery, kidney, and aorta is carried out retroperitoneally. The aorta is clamped infrarenally and the proximal part of the bypass is inserted and led without tension to the renal artery. This is usually possible via an anatomic route, but it can also be done on the right in front of the vena cava. The distal anastomosis with the renal artery is carried out at the level of the hilum of the kidney, usually with interrupted sutures and with patched extension of both incisions.

Excellent results with the aortorenal bypass were already reported 20 years ago, with a secondary patency rate of 97% after 2 years (Weibull et al. 1993). Among our own patients, preference is given to transaortic disobliteration of atherosclerotic renal artery stenosis, but the procedure is used on an individual basis in patients with fibromuscular dysplasia, for reconstructions after previous interventional treatment, and in patients with renal artery aneurysms. Other centers carry out aortorenal bypasses regularly in up to 60% of cases, also with excellent results (Hansen et al. 2000). Particularly in children and adolescents, use of the great saphenous vein can lead to aneurysmal dilation, and regular monitoring of these patients using ultrasound or tomographic procedures is therefore necessary.

Extra-anatomic bypass

If it is not possible to use the aorta as a donor vessel for various reasons, the iliac or visceral arteries are available as alternative donor vessels. In addition to an iliacorenal bypass (Fig. 3.2-40), a hepaticorenal bypass on the right (Fig. 3.2-41) and a splenorenal bypass on the left are possible. These procedures can be carried out both with great saphenous vein and also with prosthetic material. A precise familiarity with the anatomy and careful dissection and anastomotic techniques are obligatory to ensure that perfusion in the vascular territories of the donor vessels is not impaired.

Extra-anatomic revascularization techniques were mainly used in the only study so far published comparing surgical and drug treatment for renal artery stenoses. In the 25 randomized patients who received surgical treatment, eight hepatorenal bypasses, six iliacorenal bypasses, and three splenorenal bypasses were carried out. Advantages for the patients who underwent surgery were observed mainly in those who had preoperative creatinine levels of 2.0–4.0 mg/dL (Uzzo et al. 2002).

Local reconstructive procedures

New implantation/transposition

In this technique, the nonstenotic distal part of the renal artery is directly reimplanted into the aorta, usually slightly distally from the previous insertion site. Due to the only slight variability in the length of the renal artery, this procedure is therefore suitable only for very localized processes near the aorta and renal artery orifice, such as fibrotic or membranous stenoses. Atherosclerotic processes exclude this procedure due to their morphology and fact that the plaques frequently start in the aorta. Interrupted sutures

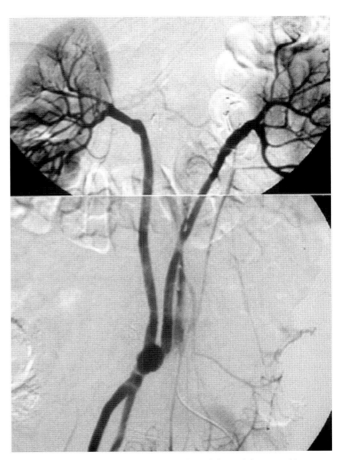

Fig. 3.2-40 Postoperative angiography after a bilateral iliacorenal bypass in a patient with an acute type B dissection (with reconstruction material from the great saphenous vein).

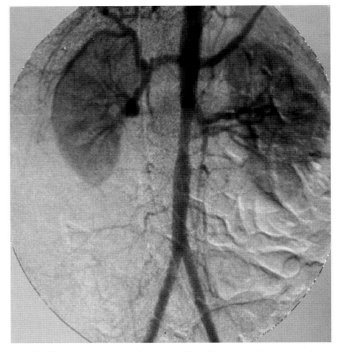

Fig. 3.2-41 Postoperative angiography after a hepatorenal bypass and coarctation of the abdominal aorta.

should be used for reimplantation of the renal artery, and resorbable suture material is particularly useful in young patients who are still growing.

Resection and end-to-end anastomosis

Local aneurysmal or dysplastic processes, particularly in the middle third of the renal artery, may allow local resection of the diseased segment of the renal artery, with direct end-to-end suturing. Failed disobliteration with a local intimal lip can also be treated using local end-to-end anastomosis, with fixation of the distal intimal lip. Interrupted sutures are also recommended here as the suturing technique.

Aneurysmorrhaphy / tailoring

The authors have focused on local treatment with autologous reconstruction in the treatment of renal artery aneurysms—a procedure developed by Sandmann in our own institution. These aneurysms often arise in a berry-like shape from the original lumen of the main renal artery or segmental artery. After local exposure—usually carried out in patients with unilateral findings via a flank incision, with extraperitoneal access to the kidney—the aneurysm is grasped with purse-string sutures, the main trunk of the renal artery is clamped, the aneurysm is incised between the sutures, and the kidney is flush-perfused via this access route using a perfusion catheter with Ringer solution at 4°C with alprostadil and heparin added. After this, the aneurysm is locally resected, with healthy renal artery wall and the neck of the aneurysm being left in place, and the continuity of the renal artery is restored either with continuous sutures or interrupted sutures at the aneurysm neck. If the lumen is insufficient, a patchplasty using great saphenous vein can also be used here.

We have used this technique in our own patients both for aneurysms in the main artery and also in the segmental arteries and pole arteries. Among 95 patients with 104 renal artery aneurysms, the technique was possible in 76.7% of the patients (74.7% with tailoring, 2.1% with tailoring and patch) and in 76.9% of the aneurysms (75% with tailoring, 1.9% with tailoring and patch). The primary technical success rate for patients with tailoring was 91.5%, and the secondary success rate after successful repeat surgery in two patients was 94.4%. The long-term patency rate with this reconstruction technique after more than 5 years was 95.7% in our patients, and ex situ reconstruction with autotransplantation was needed in less than 4% of cases. A combination of different procedures in patients with complex findings is sometimes necessary (Fig. 3.2-42).

Postoperative follow-up

In the early postoperative period after surgical reconstruction, it is easy to demonstrate the patency of the reconstruction. Regular duplex ultrasound check-ups should be carried out initially, and in our hospital these are carried out immediately postoperatively following intraoperative Doppler ultrasound of the renal artery, after 12 and 24 hours, and regularly during the subsequent course. In addition, urination and kidney-specific laboratory parameters such as lactate dehydrogenase (LDH), creatinine, and urea have to be checked at short intervals (every 6 hours during the first 24 hours). Blood-pressure monitoring is also needed, with appropriate countermeasures if it falls too abruptly. This often makes it necessary to place the patient in the intensive-care or intermediate-care unit for monitoring during the first 24 hours postoperatively. Any unclear changes

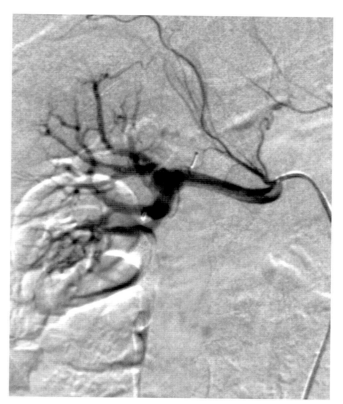

Fig. 3.2-42 Postoperative angiography after tailoring of a renal artery aneurysm on the right side (same patient as in Fig. 3.2-34).

in urination or an increase in retention parameters make a duplex ultrasound check-up necessary. If there is any suspicion of a distal intimal lip remaining after disobliteration, angiography with PTA and stent implantation may be an option for diagnosis and treatment. Due to the kidney's low tolerance for ischemia, the indication for surgical revision can be liberal if there are any relevant abnormal findings on duplex ultrasonography. Anticoagulation treatment is administered with low-dose heparin perioperatively, and a purely renal artery reconstruction does not in our view require any effective anticoagulation. Over the longer term, secondary prophylaxis with platelet inhibitors (e.g., acetylsalicylic acid 100 mg daily) should be administered if the patient has generalized arteriosclerosis.

Long-term checking of renal function, hypertension, and blood-pressure control are usually carried out by the patient's family physician, but regular check-ups in the center that carried out the surgery should also take place, with duplex ultrasound to detect any recurrent stenoses. If recurrent stenosis is suspected, an indication for repeat imaging diagnosis should be established on the basis of the patient's condition, renal function, and hypertension.

Prospects

Prospective randomized studies, including the Angioplasty and Stenting for Renal Artery Lesions (ASTRAL) trial, have called into question the principle of interventional therapy for renal artery stenosis in comparison with optimal drug therapy. Despite its good results in both the past and present, surgical treatment is also affected by this trend, with patient numbers already declining in competition with interventional therapy. It should be noted here that patients who would certainly benefit from the relevant interventional revascularization therapy were not included in the ASTRAL study. A point open to criticism here is that PTA with stent implantation was carried out in the framework of other interventional procedures without adequate prior interdisciplinary diagnostic clarification for the patient. In the future, relevant criteria (which may still need to be defined) will be used to identify patients who are able to benefit from revascularization of the renal arteries. In the present authors' view, there is therefore no reason for pessimism regarding revascularization therapy in the renal arteries; instead, there is a challenge to carry out more intensive interdisciplinary observation, evaluation, and treatment of patients with renal artery diseases. Younger patients in particular and possibly patients with renal artery stenosis in whom interventional treatment is unfavorable or not possible will continue to benefit from individualized surgical treatment. In view of the variability of the reconstruction options available, this must be carried out in centers that have the relevant expertise.

3.2.3.5　Current state of research (Zeller et al. 2011)

Effect of angioplasty on blood-pressure control

The clinical value of endovascular revascularization is still a matter of controversy. Up to 2007, 21 uncontrolled cohort studies including 3368 patients had been published. The rates of blood-pressure normalization, improvement, and deterioration were in the ranges of 4–18%, 35–79%, and 0–13%, respectively. Two studies reported significant improvement in the New York Heart Association (NYHA) score in patients with global renal ischemia (renal artery stenosis with functional individual kidney or bilateral renal artery stenosis). Three small randomized studies in the 1990s that compared balloon angioplasty with drug therapy found no significant differences with regard to blood pressure behavior, although in both cases there were significantly lower amounts of antihypertensive medication in the PTA group. However, a meta-analysis of these three studies also showed significantly improved systolic and diastolic blood-pressure values (Nordmann et al. 2003). This is a rather remarkable finding, since the studies—including the DRASTIC study (van Jaarsveld et al. 2001)—featured elementary methodological flaws to the disadvantage of the angioplasty groups. The study has a high rate of patients receiving drug therapy who underwent dilation during the follow-up period due to uncontrollable blood-pressure values (44%), but who continued to be evaluated as receiving drug treatment in the intention-to-treat analysis. At the conclusion of the study, due to the high cross-over rate to angioplasty in the conservatively treated group and the high rate of re-stenosis of 48% after 12 months in the angioplasty group, the groups being compared were practically identical with regard to vascular status. Another weakness of the study was the inclusion of a high proportion of patients with renal artery stenoses of between 50% and 70%, which cannot be regarded as hemodynamically relevant.

The two randomized studies comparing stent angioplasty and conservative therapy published in 2009 suffer from similar limitations. The ASTRAL trial (ASTRAL 2009) and the Stent Placement in Patients with Atherosclerotic Renal Artery Stenosis and Impaired Renal Function Trial (Bax et al. 2009) ended with practically identical systolic and diastolic blood-pressure values. However, the amount of antihypertensive medication in the stent cohort was significantly reduced in the ASTRAL study.

Influence of angioplasty on renal function

The effect of the intervention on renal function has not been conclusively clarified. The meta-analysis of three randomized balloon angioplasty studies showed no effect of the intervention on the course of serum creatinine, but these studies were also not powered relative to that end point. Interestingly, however, the DRASTIC study showed impressively that balloon angioplasty can improve renal function, although the result was not significant due to the small number of patients in the group. In the PTA group, a slight persistent increase in creatinine clearance occurred immediately after the intervention, whereas it initially declined in the conservatively treated group. After 3 months, however, creatinine clearance also improved in the latter group, since nearly half of the patients initially randomized to receive conservative treatment underwent revascularization after the 3-month check-up due to inadequate blood-pressure control or deterioration in renal function.

In contrast to earlier balloon angioplasty studies, the STAR and ASTRAL studies defined renal function as the primary end point. ASTRAL is by far the largest study, with 806 patients. The study only recruited patients in whom it was unclear whether revascularization of the renal artery stenosis was appropriate at all. Forty-one percent of the patients had renal artery stenoses < 70%, and 60% already had limited renal function. On average, two patients per center and year were included in the study, suggesting a relevant degree of selection bias. After a mean of 34 months, there were no significant differences either in renal function or in clinical events, even in subgroups of patients with high-grade stenoses. The primary end point of the study, a decline in renal function during the study period, only showed a slightly lower trend after stent angioplasty (-0.07×10^{-3} vs. -0.13×10^{-3} L/μmol/year; $P = 0.06$).

The STAR study included 140 patients, with the primary end point being a decline in creatinine clearance of at least 20%. The end point did not occur significantly less often in the stent group than in the conservative group (16% vs. 22%). More than 50% of the patients in the stent cohort had renal artery stenoses < 70%, and 28% of the patients in the stent cohort did not actually receive a stent, as the CTA or MRA diagnosis of renal artery stenosis was not confirmed on angiography. However, these patients were still included in the intention-to-treat analysis as having received stents! It may be suspected that in the conservative group, as in the stent group, nearly half of the patients did not have hemodynamically relevant renal artery stenoses. The reason for this is that the screening method was based on MRA or CTA, and both methods overestimate the grade of stenosis particularly in patients with renal artery stenosis. This has an effect on the outcome of the study: due to the absence of relevant renal artery stenosis in the conservative group, there is no noticeable decline in renal function during the course, and revascularization of irrelevant renal artery stenoses does not lead to any improvement in renal function, while exposing the patient to the risks associated with the intervention (contrast administration, embolization, etc.). This study, inadequately powered in relation to the primary end point, shows that renal insufficiency may progress despite successful revascularization, since the perfusion disturbance is not the sole cause of the clinical picture of ischemic neuropathy, which is still not fully understood. In addition, the study shows that stent angioplasty for renal artery stenosis, despite considerable technical advances, is associated with a relevant rate of complications and mortality (4.3%) when carried out by inexperienced practitioners.

In an analysis of two consecutive registries in England and Germany, including a total of 908 patients, it has been demonstrated that above all patients with already advanced renal insufficiency (clearance < 60 mL/min) benefit markedly from revascularization, with an improvement in renal function (Kalra et al. 2010).

Influence of angioplasty on mortality

To date, no controlled studies, including the STAR and ASTRAL trials, have confirmed any survival advantage for endovascular therapy. By contrast, the analysis of the two consecutive patient cohorts showed a 45% reduction in the 1-year mortality rate for the endovascular group; the only independent predictive factor for this was revascularization (Kalra et al. 2010). A reduction in left ventricular mass—a major predictive factor for mortality—after endovascular therapy for renal artery stenosis has been demonstrated in echocardiographic studies (Zeller et al. 2007). The CORAL study, which is currently in the follow-up phase, features a combined clinical event end point and may provide information about the influence of revascularization on the mortality rate over the long-term course.

In summary, there is a general consensus that in patients with hemodynamically relevant renal artery stenosis and recurrent myocardial decompensation, as well as those with progressively deteriorating renal function, there is a clear indication for revascularization, as is also the case with all renal artery stenoses with a nonarteriosclerotic pathogenesis. Clinical predictive factors for successful revascularization include a pulse pressure of 50 ± 10 mmHg (Dieter et al. 2009), raised diastolic blood pressure, a raised B-type natriuretic peptide (BNP) level (Staub et al. 2010), and renal insufficiency. Invasive predictive factors for successful invasive treatment include a ratio of pressure distal to the stenosis to the resting aortic pressure < 0.9 (Kapoor et al. 2010) and a hyperemic systolic pressure gradient > 20 mmHg (Mangiacapra et al. 2010).

Negative predictive factors include any marker for advanced renal parenchymal damage, such as proteinuria > 1 g/24 h, renal atrophy, and severe intrarenal arteriolar sclerosis.

3.2.3.6　Prospects

The negative results of the ASTRAL and STAR studies have currently led to a drastic reduction in the numbers of cases in which renal artery angioplasty is regarded as indicated—to the disadvantage of patients who still have a good indication for intervention. The European/South American RADAR study (with a primary end point of creatinine clearance) had to be stopped after inclusion of one-third of the patients, as the recruitment numbers were too low. The decisive element in establishing the indication for the intervention is evidence of the hemodynamic relevance of the renal artery stenosis. Unfortunately, the most recent study, the CORAL study in the United States (with a combined end point of "major adverse event," free survival) did not take this into account and it must therefore be expected that this study will also not demonstrate the true benefit of correctly indicated renal artery revascularization.

References

Abela R, Ivanova S, Lidder S, et al. An analysis comparing open surgical and endovascular treatment of atherosclerotic renal artery stenosis. Eur J Vasc Endovasc Surg 2009; 38: 666.

Balzer KM, Neuschäfer S, Sagban TA, Grotemeyer D, Pfeiffer T, Rump LC, Sandmann W. Renal artery revascularization after unsuccessful percutaneous therapy: a single center experience. Langenbecks Archi Surg 2012; 397: 111.

Balzer KM, Pfeiffer T, Rossbach S, et al. Prospective randomized trial of operative vs interventional treatment for renal artery ostial occlusive disease (RAOOD). J Vasc Surg 2009; 49: 667.

Balzer KM, Pfeiffer T, Rossbach S, Voiculescu A, Mödder U, Godehardt E, Sandmann W. Prospective randomized trial of operative vs interventional treatment for renal artery ostial occlusive disease (RAOOD). J Vasc Surg 2009 Mar; 49 (3): 667–74; discussion 674–5.

Bax L, Woittiez A-JJ, Kouwenberg HJ et al. Stent placement in patients with atherosclerotic renal artery stenosis and impaired renal function: a randomized trial. Ann Intern Med 2009; 150: 840–8.

Caps MT, Zierler RE, Polissar NL, Bergelin RO, Beach KW, Cantwell-Gab K, et al. Risk of atrophy in kidneys with atherosclerotic renal artery stenosis. Kidney Int 1998; 53: 735–42.

Chi YW, White CJ, Thornton S, Milani RV. Ultrasound velocity criteria for renal in-stent restenosis. J Vasc Surg 2009 Jul; 50 (1): 119–23.

Dieter RS, Darki A, Nanjundappa A, Chhokar VS, Khadim G, Morshedi-Meibodi A, Freihage JH, Steen L, Lewis B, Leya F. Usefulness of wide pulse pressure as a predictor of poor outcome after renal artery angioplasty and stenting. Am J Cardiol 2009 Sep 1; 104 (5): 732–4.

Dorros G, Jaff M, Mathiak L, Dorros II, Lowe A, Murphy K, et al. 4-year follow-up of Palmaz-Schatz stent revascularisation as treatment for atherosclerotic renal artery stenosis. Circulation 1998; 98: 642–7.

Duranay M, Kanbay M, Akay H, Unverdi S, Sürer H, Altay M, Kırbaş I, Covic A, Zoccali C. Nebivolol improves renal function in patients who underwent angioplasty due to renal artery stenosis: A pilot study. Nephron Clin Pract 2009 Nov 28; 114 (3): c213–7.

Edsmann G. Angionephrography and suprarenal angiography: a roentgenologic study of the normal kidney, expansive renal and suprarenal lesions and renal aneurysms. Acta Radiol 1957; 155 (Suppl): 1.

Freeman NE, Leeds FH, Elliott WG, et al. Thromboendarterectomy for hypertension due to renal artery occlusion. JAMA 1954; 157: 1077.

Goldblatt H. Studies on experimental hypertension. J Exp Med 1934; 59: 346.

Grabensee B, Voiculescu A. Nierenarterienstenose (NAST) und renovaskuläre Hypertonie (RVH). Klinikarzt 2003; 32: 334.

Graff J, Schälte G, Jovanovic V. Rupture of a renal artery aneurysm during delivery. Aktuelle Urol 2003; 34: 350.

Hansen KJ, Cherr GS, Craven TE, et al. Management of ischemic nephropathy: Dialysis-free survival after surgical repair. J Vasc Surg 20003; 1: 472.

Hansen KJ, Cherr GS, Craven TE, Motew SJ, Travis JA, Wong JM, et al. Management of ischemic nephropathy: dialysis-free survival after surgical repair. J Vasc Surg 2000; 32: 472.

Hricik DE, Browning PJ, Kopelman R, Goorno WE, Madias NE, Dzau VJ. Captopril-induced functional renal insufficiency in patients with bilateral renal-artery stenoses or stenosis in a solitary kidney. N Engl J Med 1983; 308: 373–6.

Kalra PA, Chrysochou C, Green D, Cheung CM, Khavandi K, Sixt S, Rastan A, Zeller T. The benefit of renal artery stenting in patients with atheromatous renovascular disease and advanced chronic kidney disease. Cath Cardiovasc Intervent 2010; 75: 1–10.

Kapoor N, Fahsah I, Karim R, Jevans AJ, Leesar MA. Physiological assessment of renal artery stenosis: Comparisons of resting with hyperemic renal pressure measurements. Catheter Cardiovasc Interv 2010; 76: 726–32.

Krijnen P, van Jaarsveld BC, Deinum J, Steyerberg EW, Habbema JD. Which patients with hypertension and atherosclerotic renal artery stenosis benefit from immediate intervention? J Hum Hypertens 2004; 18: 91–6.

Krumme B, Blum U, Schwertfeger E, Flügel P, Höllstin F, Schollmeyer P, Rump L. Diagnosis of renovascular disease by intrarenal and extrarenal Doppler scanning. Kidney Int 1996; 50: 1288–92.

Leadbetter WFG, Burkland CE. Hypertension in unilateral renal disease. J Urol 1938; 39: 611.

Lin J, Li D, Yan F. High-resolution 3D contrast-enhanced MRA with parallel imaging techniques before endovascular interventional treatment of arterial stenosis. Vasc Med 2009 Nov; 14 (4): 305–11.

MacDowell P, Kalra PA, O'Donoghue DJ, Waldek S, Mamtora H, Brown K. Risk of morbidity from renovascular disease in elderly patients with congestive heart failure. Lancet 1998; 352: 13–6.

Mahmud E, Smith TW, Palakodeti V, Zaidi O, Ang L, Mitchell CR, Zafar N, Bromberg-Marin G, Keramati S, Tsimikas S. Renal frame count and renal blush grade: quantitative measures that predict the success of renal stenting in hypertensive patients with renal artery stenosis. JACC Cardiovasc Interv 2008 Jun; 1 (3): 286–92.

Mangiacapra F, Trana C, Sarno G, Davidavicius G, Protasiewicz M, Muller O, Ntalianis A, Misonis N, Van Vlem B, Heyndrickx GR, De Bruyne B. Translesional pressure gradients to predict blood pressure response after renal artery stenting in patients with renovascular hypertension. Circ Cardiovasc Interv 2010 Dec; 3 (6): 537–42. Comment in: Circ Cardiovasc Interv 2010 Dec; 3 (6): 526–7.

Morris GC, DeBakey ME, Cooley DA. Surgical treatment of renal failure of renovascular origin. JAMA 1962; 182: 609.

Müller BT, Reiher L, Pfeiffer T, et al. Surgical treatment of renal artery dissection in 25 patients: Indications and results. J Vasc Surg 2003; 37: 761.

Nordmann AJ, Woo K, Parkes R, Logan AG. Balloon angioplasty or medical therapy for hypertensive patients with atherosclerotic renal artery stenosis? A meta-analysis of randomized controlled trials. Am J Med 2003; 114: 44–50.

Pfeiffer T, Müller BT, Huber R, Reiher L, Häfele S, Sandmann W. Therapie der Nierenarterienstenosen. Herz 2004; 29: 76.

Pfeiffer T, Reiher L, Grabitz K, Grünhage B, Häfele S, Voiculescu A, Fürst G, Sandmann W. Reconstruction for renal artery aneurysm: Operative technique and long-term results. J Vasc Surg 2003; 37: 292.

Pourhassan S, Sandmann W (Hrsg.). Gefäßerkrankungen im Kindes- und Jugendalter. Springer, 2010.

Radermacher J, Chavan A, Bleck J, Vitzthum A, Stoess B, Gebel MJ, et al. Use of Doppler ultrasonography to predict the outcome of therapy for renal-artery stenosis. N Engl J Med 2001; 334: 410–7.

Rundback JH, Sacks D, Kent KC, Cooper C, Jones D, Murphy T, et al. Guidelines for the reporting of renal artery revascularization in clinical trials. J Vasc Interv Radiol 2002; 13: 959.

Rundback JH, Sacks D, Kent KC, et al. Guidelines for the reporting of renal artery revascularization in clinical trials. Circulation 2002; 106: 1572–85.

Safian RD, Textor SC. Renal-artery stenosis. N Engl J Med 2001; 344: 431–2.

Silva JA, Chan AW, White CJ, Collins TJ, Jenkins JS, Reilly JP, Ramee SR. Elevated brain natriuretic peptide predicts blood pressure response after stent revascularization in patients with renal artery stenosis. Circulation 2005; 111: 328–33.

Smith HW. Unilateral nephrectomy in hypertensive disease. J Urol 1956; 76: 685.

Staub D, Zeller T, Trenk D, Maushart C, Uthoff H, Breidthardt T, Klima T, Aschwanden M, Socrates T, Arenja N, Twerenbold R, Rastan A, Sixt S, Jacob AL, Jaeger KA, Mueller C. Use of B-type natriuretic peptide to predict blood pressure improvement after percutaneous revascularisation for renal artery stenosis. Eur J Vasc Endovasc Surg 2010; 40: 599–607.

Tendera M, Aboyans V, Bartelink ML, Baumgartner I, Clement D, Collet JF, Cremonesi A, De Carlo M, Erbel R, Fowkes FGR, Heras M, Kownator S, Minar E, Ostergren J, Poldermans D, Riambau V, Roffi M, Röther J, Sievert H, van Sambeek M, Zeller T. ESC Guidelines on the diagnosis and treatment of peripheral artery diseases: Document covering atherosclerotic disease of extracranial carotid and vertebral, mesenteric, renal, upper and lower extremity arteries. European Heart Journal 2011; 32: 2851–906, doi:10.1093/eurheartj/ehr211.

The ASTRAL Investigators. Revascularization versus medical therapy for renal-artery stenosis. N Engl J Med 2009; 361: 1953–62.

Uzzo RG, Novick AC, Goormastic M, Mascha E, Pohl M. Medical versus surgical management of atherosclerotic renal artery stenosis. Transplantation Proceedings 2002; 34: 723.

Van Dongen RJ. Renal and intestinal artery occlusive disease. World J Surg 1988; 12: 777.

Van Jaarsveld BC, Krijnen P, Pieterman H, Derkx FHM, Deinum J, Postma CT, et al for the Dutch Renal Artery Stenosis Intervention Cooperative Study Group. The Effect of Balloon Angioplasty on Hypertension in Atherosclerotic Renal-Artery Stenosis. N Engl J Med 2000; 342: 1007–14.

Weibull H, Berqquist D, Bergentz SE, Jonsson K, Hulthén L, Manhem P. Percutaneous transluminal renal angioplasty versus surgical reconstruction of atherosclerotic renal artery stenosis: a prospective randomized study. J Vasc Surg 1993; 18: 841.

Wylie EJ, Perloff DL, Stoney RJ. Autogenous tissue revascularization technics in surgery for renovascular hypertension. Ann Surg 1969; 170: 416.

Youkey JR, Collins GJ Jr, Orecchia PM, Brigham RA, Salander JM, Rich NM. Saccular renal artery aneurysm as a cause of hypertension. Surgery 1985; 97: 498.

Zeller T, Frank U, Müller C, Bürgelin K, Sinn L, Bestehorn HP, Cook-Bruns N, Neumann FJ. Predictors of improved renal function after percutaneous stent-supported angioplasty of severe atherosclerotic ostial renal artery stenosis. Circulation 2003; 108: 2244–9.

Zeller T, Müller C, Frank U, Bürgelin K, Horn B, Cook-Bruns N, Schwarzwälder U, Neumann FJ. Stent-angioplasty of severe atherosclerotic ostial renal artery stenosis in patients with diabetes mellitus and nephrosclerosis. Cath Cardiovasc Interv 2003; 58: 510–5.

Zeller T, Müller C, Frank U, Bürgelin K, Schwarzwälder U, Horn B, Roskamm H. Survival after stent-angioplasty of severe atherosclerotic ostial renal artery stenoses. J Endovasc Ther 2003; 10: 539–45.

Zeller T, Noory E, Rastan A. Nierenarterienstenose. Kardiologie Up-2date 2011; 7: 125–39.

Zeller T, Rastan A, Schwarzwälder U, Müller C, Frank U, Bürgelin U, Sixt S, Schwarz S, Noory E, Neumann FJ. Regression of left ventricular hypertrophy following stenting of renal artery stenosis. J Endovasc Ther 2007; 14: 189–97.

3.2.4 Renal sympathetic denervation

Felix Mahfoud

3.2.4.1 Clinical picture (treatment-refractory arterial hypertension)

With its high prevalence, arterial hypertension is one of the most frequent chronic diseases in Western industrialized countries and is a major risk factor for cardiovascular morbidity and mortality. It is known from meta-analyses that every increase in blood pressure (systolic/diastolic) by 20/10 mmHg is associated with a doubling of cardiovascular risk. Approximately 5–15% of patients with high blood pressure have treatment-refractory arterial hypertension. A distinction needs to be made here between **true resistance to treatment** and **pseudoresistance**—e.g., resistance due to inadequate treatment compliance or situationally raised blood pressure values such as those seen in white coat hypertension. A secondary cause is often present in patients with treatment-refractory hypertension, with a potentially reversible pathogenesis for the high blood pressure, so that systematic exclusion of an organic cause is an obligatory component of any treatment. Resistant hypertension is defined as blood-pressure control inconsistent with guideline values (**> 140/90 mmHg generally, > 130–139/80–85 mmHg in patients with diabetes mellitus, > 130/80 mmHg in patients with chronic renal disease**) despite antihypertensive triple therapy at a maximum or maximum tolerated dosage, including a diuretic. Pseudoresistance is present when there is insufficient treatment compliance, inadequate antihypertensive medication, incorrect measuring methods, and in white coat hypertension. White coat hypertension is present when blood pressure measured in the office or in hospital is > 140/90 mmHg and values measured at home do not exceed 140/90 mmHg.

3.2.4.2 Clinical findings

The etiology of resistant arterial hypertension is multifactorial. However, a number of risk factors and co-morbid conditions are associated with treatment resistance:

- Advanced age, high systolic blood pressure, obesity, high levels of salt consumption, chronic renal disease (creatinine > 1.5 mg/dL), diabetes mellitus, left ventricular hypertrophy, and female sex

A suboptimal combination of hypertensive drugs is a frequent cause of inadequate blood pressure control. Existing co-medication can also increase blood pressure or reduce the effect of antihypertensive medication. Special attention needs to be given here to frequently used nonsteroidal anti-inflammatory drugs, as these agents can lead to hypervolemia with a subsequent increase in blood pressure due to increased sodium retention. Other important drugs that lead to an increase in blood pressure include:

- Nonsteroidal anti-inflammatory drugs, sympathomimetics (diet pills, amphetamines), glucocorticoids, estrogens in contraceptive drugs, antidepressive agents, immunosuppressive agents (ciclosporin, tacrolimus, etc.), and erythropoietin

3.2.4.3 Diagnosis

Diagnosis of resistant arterial hypertension

Reversible or organic causes must be systematically excluded before the presence of resistant hypertension can be established (Table 3.2-3).

Table 3.2-3 Secondary causes of hypertension that have to be excluded before renal sympathetic denervation.

Frequent	Rare
Obstructive sleep apnea syndrome	Pheochromocytoma
Chronic renal diseases	Cushing syndrome
Primary hyperaldosteronism	Hyperparathyroidism
Renal artery stenosis	Aortic coarctation

The most frequent forms of secondary hypertension are obstructive sleep apnea syndrome, chronic renal diseases, primary hyperaldosteronism, and renal artery stenosis. There is a high prevalence of obstructive sleep apnea syndrome in patients with resistant arterial hypertension. The guidelines therefore recommend sleep apnea screening if there is any suspicion. Chronic renal insufficiency is not only a cause of resistant hypertension, but also often a complication of it, with hypertensive end-organ injury. As a result of a bidirectional pathological mechanism between renal insufficiency and high blood pressure, fewer than 15% of patients with chronic renal disease reach the target values (< 130/80 mmHg) despite multiple drug combinations. Hyperaldosteronism is present in 10–20% of patients with resistant arterial hypertension. Hypokalemia is often suggestive here, although up to 50% of patients with confirmed primary hyperaldosteronism have normokalemia. A hemodynamically relevant renal artery stenosis (> 70%) is present in approximately 10% of patients with resistant arterial hypertension aged over 65. Renal angiography examinations during coronary angiography show a higher prevalence of renal artery stenosis of up to 20%. Particularly in women under the age of 50, fibromuscular dysplasia should be considered. Rare causes include pheochromocytoma, Cushing syndrome, hyperthyroidism, and aortic coarctation.

Diagnosis before renal sympathetic denervation

The following therapeutic and diagnostic measures should be carried out before renal sympathetic denervation:

- Lifestyle modification (weight reduction, physical exercise, alcohol abstinence, reduced salt intake)
- Optimization of antihypertensive therapy and withdrawal of drugs that raise blood pressure
- Detailed medical history (including drug history), physical examination
- Ambulatory blood-pressure measurement to confirm treatment resistance (daily average for systolic blood pressure > 135 mmHg)
- Laboratory analyses of serum electrolytes, glucose, and creatinine, and urinary diagnosis with protein measurement and urinary sodium excretion

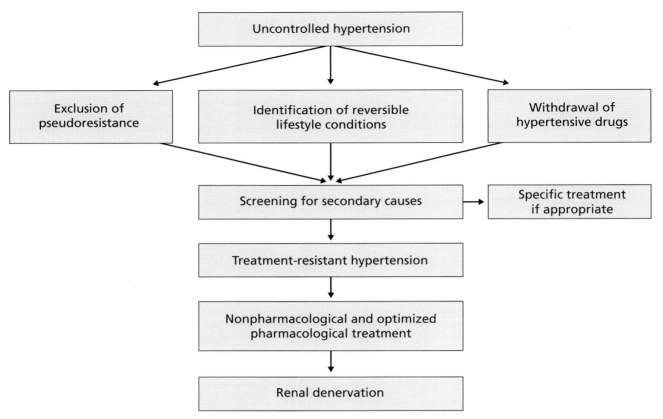

Fig. 3.2-43 Procedure in patients with uncontrolled hypertension (adapted from Mahfoud et al. 2011).

- Exclusion of secondary hypertension:
  - Screening for primary hyperaldosteronism by measuring with aldosterone–renin ratio. Attention must always be given to possible interactions with antihypertensive agents here. If primary hyperaldosteronism is suspected, further imaging examinations or separate suprarenal vein blood samples on each side are necessary.
  - If there are episodic, critical increases in blood pressure, pheochromocytoma should be excluded.
  - Ultrasound diagnosis of the renal arteries is recommended in younger patients with suspected fibromuscular dysplasia and patients who are at increased atherogenic risk, to exclude atherosclerotic renal artery stenosis.

3.2.4.4   Endovascular therapy

The sympathetic nervous system, and particularly hyperactivity in it, play a decisive role in the development of high blood pressure and the development of co-morbidities. The renal sympathetic nerve fibers arise from the sympathetic ganglion at the thoracolumbar transition (T10–L1). They surround the renal vessels like a net and penetrate into the adventitia. A distinction is made between **afferent** sympathetic fibers, on the one hand, which link the kidneys to the central nervous system and are activated when there are raised concentrations of adenosine and nitrogen monoxide, as well as in renal ischemia. It is known from animal experiments that central sympathetic activity is decisively influenced by these fibers. The **efferent** sympathetic fibers, on the other hand, which pass from the central nervous system to the end organs (Fig. 3.2-44), among other things stimulate:

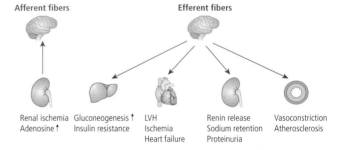

Fig. 3.2-44 Afferent and efferent sympathetic nerve fibers (adapted from Mahfoud and Böhm 2010).

- Renin release in the juxtaglomerular complex
- Tubular resorption of sodium
- Renal vasoconstriction, with a resulting decline in renal blood flow
- Gluconeogenesis in the liver
- Left ventricular hypertrophy and cardiac ischemia and arrhythmia

They also mediate vasoconstriction and atherosclerosis in the vessels.

State of research

The interventional renal denervation procedure was investigated in the multicenter Symplicity HTN-1 study and in the randomized and controlled Symplicity HTN-2 study in patients with treatment-resistant arterial hypertension.

Clinical data—Simplicity HTN-1 and HTN-2 (summary)

- The Symplicity HTN-1 study investigated the effect of renal denervation in 45 patients with treatment-resistant hypertension (systolic blood pressure > 160 mmHg).
- At the start of the study, the patients' mean blood pressure was 177/101 mmHg, despite treatment with a mean of 4.7 antihypertensive agents.
- Primary end points: antihypertensive effect and periprocedural and long-term safety of the procedure.
- Even after 1 month, there was a significant reduction in blood pressure by 14/10 mmHg (systolic/diastolic blood pressure) during office measurements. The values increased again during the 12-month follow-up period to 27/17 mmHg ($P = 0.026$). The reduction in sympathetic activity due to renal artery denervation was confirmed by a significant decline in the renal norepinephrine spillover rate by 47% (n = 10).
- The Symplicity HTN-2 study (randomized and controlled) investigated the effect of renal denervation on blood-pressure behavior in 106 patients with treatment-refractory hypertension (systolic blood pressure ≥ 160 mmHg; ≥ 150 mmHg in patients with type 2 diabetes). At the start of the study, the patients' mean blood pressure was 178/96 mmHg despite treatment with a mean of 5.2 antihypertensive agents.
- Six months after renal denervation, a reduction in office-measured blood pressure by 32/12 mmHg ($P < 0.0001$) was observed, while blood pressures in the control group did not change.
- Blood pressure measured at home also declined by 20/12 mmHg ($P < 0.001$, n = 32), while in the control group there was a slight increase in blood pressure values by 2/0 mmHg (n = 40).
- The reduction in blood pressure led to a reduction in drug intake or dosage in 20% of the patients.

Limitations of the studies

- Evaluable long-term blood-pressure measurements (> 70% successful measurements) were only available in the study for around half of the patients at the start of the investigation and 6 months after renal denervation.
- As expected, the reduction in blood pressure was less marked in the 24-hour measurements than in the office measurements, and at 6 months was –11/–7 mmHg (P for systolic blood pressure = 0.006; P for diastolic blood pressure = 0.014).

Long-term effects

- The reductions in office blood pressure measurements (systolic/diastolic blood pressure) after 12, 18, and 24 months were 23/11, 26/14, and 32/14 mmHg, respectively (Fig. 3.2-45). The sustained reduction in blood pressure makes functional reinnervation or regeneration of the kidneys with sympathetic nerve fibers unlikely, and it can therefore be assumed that there is a longer-term effect on blood pressure.
- It was possible to de-escalate antihypertensive medication in 27 patients who had a marked reduction in blood pressure, but in 18 patients antihypertensive therapy was intensified.
- No significant changes in creatinine clearance were observed 12 months after the intervention (–2.9 mL/min; 95% confidence intervals, –6.2 to + 0.3 mL; n = 63).

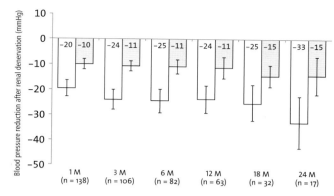

Fig. 3.2-45 Systolic (white) and diastolic (gray) blood pressure reduction over a period of 24 months after renal denervation (adapted from Symplicity HTN-1 Investigators 2011).

Response rate (systolic ≥ 10 mmHg) and criteria for response and nonresponse

- Response rates to the procedure were in the range of 84–92%.
- Independent predictive factors for a marked reduction in blood pressure were:
  - Higher systolic blood pressure at the examination time point ($P < 0.001$)
  - Intake of sympatholytic agents with central nervous system effects ($P = 0.018$)
  - Low heart rate ($P < 0.004$)
- Due to the small number of nonresponders, no predictive factors can currently be identified for a lack of response.

Safety of the procedure

The intervention did not cause any severe complications in the 206 patients included in the studies. Pain requiring conscious sedation occurred during the application of high-frequency energy. Complications reported during or after renal denervation were:

- Peri-interventional bradycardia (n = 7)
- Postinterventional pseudoaneurysms in the femoral artery (n = 4)
- Renal artery dissection during insertion of the guide catheter (n = 1)
- Progression of prior renal artery stenosis 6 months after renal denervation (n = 1)

It was shown that there were no signs of chronotropic incompetence after renal denervation. Spiroergometry examinations repeatedly carried out in 46 patients following renal denervation showed a significant reduction in resting blood pressure and exercise blood pressure and sustained adaptation of blood pressure.

Indication for renal denervation

The following criteria should be met before renal denervation:

- Office-measured systolic blood pressure ≥ 160 mmHg or ≥ 150 mmHg in patients with type 2 diabetes mellitus
- Intake of three or more antihypertensive agents (genuine treatment resistance with treatment compliance)
- Exclusion of secondary causes of hypertension
- Normal to slightly reduced renal function (glomerular filtration rate ≥ 45 mL/min/1.73 m^2)

■ Suitable renal artery anatomy: no prior interventions in the renal arteries, no significant stenosis or other abnormalities in the renal arteries.

Patient preparation

■ In elective procedures, the patient should receive information and provide written consent at least 24 hours before the intervention.
■ The patients should fast for at least 6 hours before the intervention.
■ Coagulation status, serum electrolytes, and renal function should be checked.

Medication

■ After the catheter has been placed, administration of 5000 IU heparin (target activated clotting time between 200 and 250 s).
■ Conscious sedation—e.g., with midazolam and morphine before radiofrequency ablation:
– Due to the common course of C pain fibers and sympathetic nerve fibers, diffuse visceral pain occurs during radiofrequency ablation. The pain stops immediately after the ablation.

Access route

■ Puncture of the femoral artery and introduction of a 6F catheter.

Intervention

■ Angiography of the renal arteries to inspect the vascular morphology and exclude any relevant renal artery stenosis or duplicate supply/pole artery via a femoral 6F catheter.
■ The renal artery should be > 20 mm long and have a diameter of > 4 mm. These sizes are important for ensuring that blood flow and thus cooling in the vessel are sufficient during the high-frequency ablation.
■ Probing of the renal arteries using a guide catheter—e.g., renal double curve (RDC), internal mammary artery (IMA), renal long (RE-L), and multipurpose (MP) (Fig. 3.2-46).
■ Insertion of the ablation catheter (Symplicity® Flex-Catheter, Medtronic/Ardian Inc., USA) (Fig. 3.2-47), with fluoroscopic guidance, distally to approximately 5 mm in front of the first bifurcation (Fig. 3.2-48).
■ Connection of the catheter to the generator, which measures temperature and impedance during the procedure.
■ Irrigation (500 mL NaCl 0.9% + 2500 IU heparin) is provided via a T-connector to prevent clotting.
■ High-frequency energy is administered via the tip of the catheter, leading to focal warming of the vascular wall to a maximum of 70°C.
■ Cooling of the vessel by the intraluminal blood flow.
■ The quantity of energy is determined and administered using the measured temperature and impedance with an algorithm stored in the generator. The maximum energy delivery is 8 W and it is limited to 120 s per ablation point.
■ As the probe is withdrawn from distal to proximal, at least four ablations (preferably more) are carried out at intervals of at least 5 mm (see shaft markings) in each renal vessel (Fig. 3.2-49).
■ The points are distributed through the vessel in anterior, superior, posterior, and inferior positions in the form of an interrupted

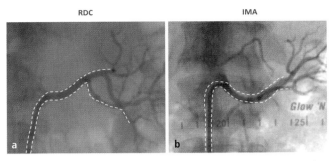

Fig. 3.2-46a, b Selection of the guide catheter depends on the origin of the renal arteries (**a**, RDC; **b**, IMA).

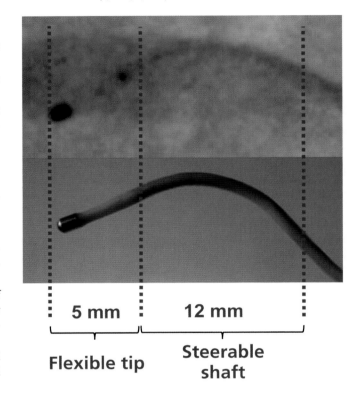

5 mm **12 mm**

Flexible tip **Steerable shaft**

Fig. 3.2-47 The Symplicity ablation catheter.

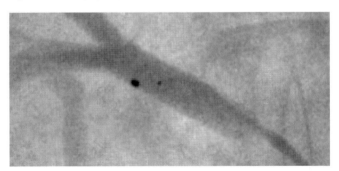

Fig. 3.2-48 Placement of the ablation catheter distally in the renal artery, approximately 5 mm in front of the first bifurcation.

spiral (Fig. 3.2-49). To denervate the entire circumference of the renal arteries, as many ablation points as possible should be applied in accordance with the above criteria. Due to the high density of the fibers, particularly afferent sympathetic nerve fibers, the last ablation point should be applied in a superior position at a distance of 3 mm from the orifice.

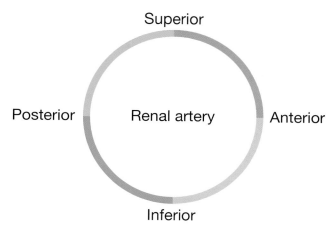

Superior

Posterior   Renal artery   Anterior

Inferior

Fig. 3.2-49 The ablation points are distributed along the vessel in a spiral pattern at intervals of at least 5 mm. An attempt should be made to achieve superior, anterior, inferior, and posterior positions.

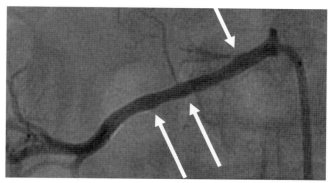

Fig. 3.2-50 After radiofrequency ablation, areas of edematous swelling that do not limit blood flow may occur, but these usually resolve spontaneously.

- Ablation should be avoided in areas of atherosclerotic plaque or calcification.
- After radiofrequency ablation small, edematous swellings that do not limit blood flow may appear at the points treated (Fig. 3.2-50). These usually resolve spontaneously. Alternatively, intra-arterial administration of nitroglycerin may be necessary.
- The intervention takes approximately 40–60 min for a bilateral procedure.
- The arterial sheath is usually removed using an occlusion system.

Potential risks of the intervention

- Inguinal complications
- Hypotension and airway complications due to conscious sedation
- Peri-interventional vascular spasms
- Renal artery dissection
- Mobilization of atherosclerotic plaque
- Contrast-induced nephropathy (the risk increases along with the degree of renal function impairment and amount of contrast administered)

Postinterventional follow-up and medication

- Postinterventional platelet inhibition with acetylsalicylic acid 100 mg/day for at least 4 weeks
- Continued administration of antihypertensive medication:
  - Antihypertensive medication should only be reduced if there is symptomatic hypotension or there are signs of reduced organ perfusion (creatinine increase, vertigo, orthostatic dysfunction).
  - Reducing antihypertensive medication is only possible in 20% of the patients.
- Regular follow-up examinations—e.g., after 3, 6, 12, 24, 48, and 60 months. Minimum requirements:
  - Medication check, physical examination
  - Office and long-term blood-pressure measurement
  - Laboratory tests (creatinine/cystatin C, electrolytes, spot urine test: albumin, creatinine, sodium)
  - Renal artery imaging (duplex ultrasound, MRA or CTA)

3.2.4.5   Prospects

Initial research results suggest that glucose metabolism can be favorably influenced by renal denervation. In a study including 50 patients, interruption of the bidirectional pathological mechanism between sympathetic hyperactivity and insulin resistance with subsequent hyperinsulinemia led to a significant reduction in glucose and insulin concentrations and a marked improvement in insulin sensitivity after renal denervation. In a pilot study including 10 patients with treatment-refractory hypertension and a diagnosis of obstructive sleep apnea syndrome, renal denervation led not only to a significant reduction in blood pressure but also to improvement in the severity of the obstructive sleep apnea syndrome, measured using the apnea–hypopnea index. There was a significant reduction in the hemoglobin A_{1c} concentration and 120-minute glucose value in the oral glucose tolerance test after renal denervation. In addition to the diseases mentioned above, chronic renal insufficiency and chronic cardiac insufficiency are also characterized by increased sympathetic activity. The influence of renal denervation on these two entities is currently being examined in clinical studies.

References

Calhoun DA, et al. Resistant hypertension: diagnosis, evaluation, and treatment: a scientific statement from the American Heart Association Professional Education Committee of the Council for High Blood Pressure Research. Circulation 2008; 117 (25): e510–26.

Calhoun DA, et al. Hyperaldosteronism among black and white subjects with resistant hypertension. Hypertension 2002; 40 (6): 892–6.

Esler MD, et al. Renal sympathetic denervation in patients with treatment-resistant hypertension (The Symplicity HTN-2 Trial): a randomised controlled trial. Lancet 2010; 376 (9756): 1903–9.

Goncalves SC, et al. Obstructive sleep apnea and resistant hypertension: a case-control study. Chest 2007; 132 (6): 1858–62.

Krum H, et al. Catheter-based renal sympathetic denervation for resistant hypertension: a multicentre safety and proof-of-principle cohort study. Lancet 2009; 373 (9671): 1275–81.

Krum H, et al. Device-based antihypertensive therapy: therapeutic modulation of the autonomic nervous system. Circulation 2011; 123 (2): 209–15.

Mahfoud F, et al. Expert consensus statement on interventional renal sympathetic denervation for hypertension treatment. Dtsch Med Wochenschr 2011; 136 (47): 2418.

Mahfoud F, et al. Treatment strategies for resistant arterial hypertension. Dtsch Arztebl Int 2011; 108 (43): 725–31.

Mahfoud F, et al. Effect of renal sympathetic denervation on glucose metabolism in patients with resistant hypertension: A pilot study. Circulation 2011; 123 (18): 1940–6.

Mahfoud F, Böhm M. [Interventional renal sympathetic denervation—a new approach for patients with resistant hypertension]. Dtsch Med Wochenschr 2010; 135 (48): 2422–5.

Sobotka PA, et al. Sympatho-renal axis in chronic disease. Clin Res Cardiol 2011; 100 (12): 1049–57.

The Symplicity HTN-1-Investigators. Catheter-based renal sympathetic denervation for resistant hypertension: durability of blood pressure reduction out to 24 months. Hypertension 2011; 57 (5): 911–7.

Ukena C, et al. Cardiorespiratory response to exercise after renal sympathetic denervation in patients with resistant hypertension. J Am Coll Cardiol 2011; 58 (11): 1176–82.

Witkowski A, et al. Effects of renal sympathetic denervation on blood pressure, sleep apnea course, and glycemic control in patients with resistant hypertension and sleep apnea. Hypertension 2011; 58 (4): 559–65.

Wolf-Maier K, et al. Hypertension prevalence and blood pressure levels in 6 European countries, Canada, and the United States. JAMA 2003; 289 (18): 2363–9.

3.2.5   Aneurysms of the branches of the abdominal aorta

Thomas Frieling
Endovascular treatment: Thomas Zeller

3.2.5.1   Clinical picture

Aneurysms of the splanchnic vessels are responsible for most abdominal arteriovenous fistulas. In autopsy studies, their frequency is estimated at around 0.07–10%. Splanchnic aneurysms often appear in multiple forms and are located preferentially at the bifurcations. The frequency of abdominal aneurysms peaks at the age of 56, and they affect men more frequently, while splenic artery aneurysms are more frequent in men than in women (with a ratio of 3:1) and mainly appear in the fifth to seventh decades of life. After splenic artery aneurysms (60%), the second most frequent manifestation of aneurysms of the splanchnic vessels is hepatic artery aneurysm (20%). Twenty percent of hepatic artery aneurysms are intrahepatic, and the aneurysms are multiple in 20% of cases; 10% of all cases of hemobilia are caused by rupture of a hepatic artery aneurysm.

The most frequent cause of hepatic artery aneurysms is traumatic intrahepatic aneurysms (37%), caused by liver biopsies, biliary drains, or infusion catheters in the hepatic artery. By contrast, aneurysms of the splenic artery most often have an atherosclerotic pathogenesis. Other etiologies include, in addition to atherosclerosis (30%), medial vascular wall degeneration (21%), liver transplantation with local infection (17%), mycotic aneurysms (4%), and vasculitides. In addition, splenic artery aneurysms may be caused by portal hypertension, pancreatitis and congenital vascular anomalies. Spontaneous hepatic artery aneurysms occur preferentially in the region of the common hepatic artery or right hepatic artery.

Arteriovenous splenic fistulas are rarities, with only 91 cases reported up to 1995. They are caused by atherosclerotic aneurysmal ruptures (44%), congenital malformations (20%), and prior splenectomy (13%).

3.2.5.2   Clinical findings

Aneurysms of the hepatic arteries are typically asymptomatic. The most frequent complications of hepatic artery aneurysms are rupture and bleeding into the biliary tract (hemobilia), peritoneal cavity (acute abdomen), or portal vein (portal hypertension). Large hepatic artery aneurysms can compress the biliary tract and lead to extrahepatic cholestasis. In symptomatic aneurysms, abdominal pain (55%) and gastrointestinal hemorrhage or hemobilia (46%) are the leading clinical signs. The classic triad (of Quincke) consists of epigastric pain, hemobilia, and obstructive jaundice (30%). The most frequent symptoms of arteriovenous splenic fistulas are gastrointestinal bleeding (48%) and portal hypertension (65%).

3.2.5.3   Diagnosis and differential diagnosis

The clinical examination is usually unremarkable. Large aneurysms may lead to pulsatile areas of resistance and bruits in the upper abdomen. Calcification is sometimes seen on scout films. On ultrasonography, hypoechoic lesions are found inside one lobe of the liver, between the porta hepatis and the pancreas, or along the splenic artery. These can sometimes also be seen on endosonography. Hyperechoic peripheral areas represent thrombi, and separate pulsations are regarded as a vascular criterion. A hypoechoic border or space-occupying mass, or free fluid in the abdomen, are found in cases of rupture (hematoma). In rare cases, evidence of a dissection membrane may be seen.

In hemobilia, there may be endoscopic evidence of bleeding from the papilla. Imaging of the bile duct on endoscopic retrograde cholangiography (ERC) or magnetic resonance cholangiography (MRC) shows contrast gaps in the bile duct or biliary dilation. Large aneurysms can cause impressions on and deformation of the duodenum during upper gastrointestinal x-ray series. Extensive aneurysm in the splenic artery may have the appearance of submucous gastric tumors. Arteriovenous splenic fistulas may cause portal hypertension. On color duplex ultrasonography, a typical arterial pulsation curve is seen. There are often areas of turbulent flow. Imaging is not possible with endoluminal thrombosis.

On conventional computed tomography and three-dimensional spiral CT, a hypodense or hyperdense space-occupying lesion is seen. In partly thrombosed aneurysms, this appearance may be overlooked if insufficient contrast is administered or if small aneurysms are overlooked when the CT slices are too thick.

In the differential diagnosis, it should be recalled that extravasation of contrast is seen in cases of rupture. The aneurysm may be underestimated or may not be seen if there is an extensive endoluminal thrombus. Circumscribed fluid collections, hepatic cysts, and pseudocysts (pancreas) may resemble an aneurysm. Angiography is the method of choice for treatment planning, showing a typically saccular dilation of the affected vascular segment.

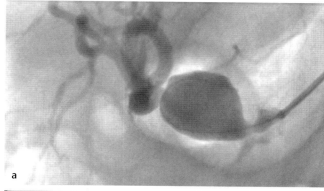

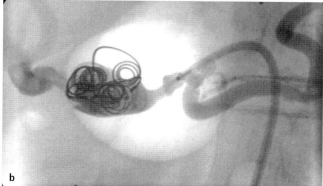

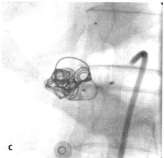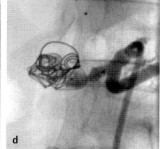

Fig. 3.2-51a–d Elimination of an aneurysm in the hepatic artery proper using two-stage coil embolization and implantation of an occluder. (**a**) Selective angiography before the procedure. (**b**) After placement of several coils via a 5F diagnostic catheter. (**c, d**) After additional proximal placement of an Amplatz occluder via a 45-cm long sheath (Destination, Terumo).

3.2.5.4 Treatment

Endovascular treatment

Nonsurgical procedures include catheter embolization of intrahepatic hepatic artery aneurysms (with Gelfoam, Ivalon, or coils) and endovascular stenting of extrahepatic aneurysms using covered stents. However, most of the extrahepatic hepatic artery aneurysms described in the literature have been treated surgically. Embolization of pregastroduodenal aneurysms is not recommended, because of the risk of hepatic necrosis.

Due to the often sinuous access route, endovascular treatment for splanchnic aneurysms is challenging, particularly if endoprostheses are to be implanted.

Embolization treatment

The access route is usually transfemoral, and less often transbrachial. A 5F sheath is usually adequate for embolization therapy, and access to the aneurysm is usually obtained with a diagnostic catheter with antifriction coating (Glidecath, Terumo) or special support catheters that are introduced using a coaxial technique via a guide catheter or a long sheath.

Particularly in splenic artery aneurysms, it must be ensured that the artery distal to the aneurysm is coiled to begin with, to prevent retrograde reperfusion of the aneurysm. However, placing embolized material distal to the splenic hilum should be avoided, as there is otherwise a risk of splenic infarction. Alternatively, if the vascular course is not too tortuous, the aneurysm can be occluded with two occluders (Amplatzer® Vascular Plug, AGA Medical).

Endoprosthesis implantation

Placement of covered stents is limited by the diameters of the hepatic artery and splenic artery, which are usually 6–7 mm. Covered stents of the appropriate size have little flexibility and require large sheaths or guide catheter diameters. In addition, it must be ensured that there are adequate landing zones for the stent anchor and seal proximal and distal to the aneurysm. The most flexible devices are self-expanding endoprostheses (e.g., Viabahn, Gore), but these require a sheath of at least 7F, as in balloon-expanding systems like the Jostent graft (Abbott Vascular). These systems can usually only be implanted in the proximal parts of the hepatic artery or splenic artery if it is possible to advance a long sheath into the celiac trunk and stabilize it there.

Prospects

Promising initial results have been reported with the implantation of what are known as multilayer stents (Henry et al. 2008; Ferrero et al. 2011; Ruffino et al. 2011). These are two-layered or three-layered nitinol stents that are used to cover the aneurysm and cause it to thrombose within a few hours or days. If there are side branches emerging from the aneurysm, they are preserved, but the aneurysm itself gradually thromboses due to a change in the flow dynamics (Fig. 3.2-52a–f).

Controlled studies on the prevention of aneurysmal rupture with this type of stent are still awaited. The main limitation of the existing systems (e.g., MARS®, Cardiatis) at present is their axial rigidity, which makes implantation in vessels with coiled and elongated courses difficult.

Surgical treatment

Diagnosed hepatic artery aneurysms require treatment because of the risk of rupture. The treatment is usually surgical. The extent to which the size of the aneurysm correlates with the risk of rupture is unclear. Dilation of the splenic artery larger than 2 cm should be treated with surgical excision of the aneurysm, with ligation of the proximal and distal ends of the splenic artery. Splenic perfusion is provided by the short gastric arteries and veins. Arteriovenous splenic fistulas can be treated with splenectomy, fistula excision, or percutaneous embolization.

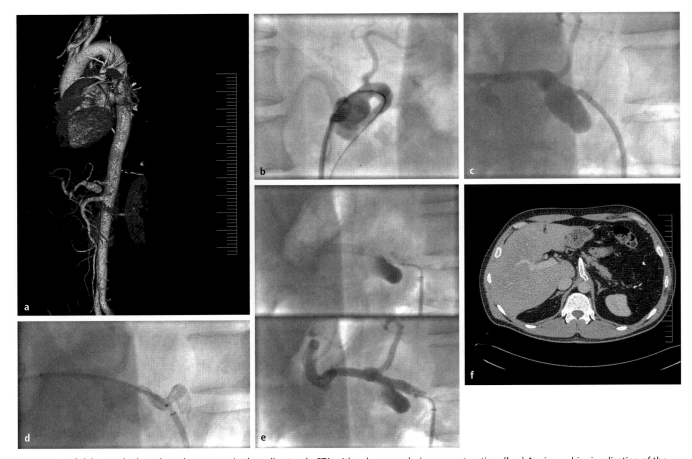

Fig. 3.2-52a–f (a) A partly thrombosed aneurysm in the celiac trunk. CTA with volume rendering reconstruction. (b, c) Angiographic visualization of the aneurysm, also showing an upstream stenosis. (d) Placement of the Cardiatis® multilayer stent. (e) Motionless contrast medium in the aneurysm after stent placement. (f) CTA 3 months after multilayer stent implantation. The stent is perfused and the aneurysm has thrombosed.

When rupture of a hepatic artery aneurysm occurs, exploratory laparotomy is carried out, with ligation of the hepatic artery or segmental lobectomy if there is massive bleeding into the free abdominal cavity. Depending on the findings and initial situation, aneurysm reduction, arterial reconstruction or liver transplantation may be necessary.

Liver-transplant patients who have extrahepatic hepatic artery aneurysms usually undergo surgery (with local infections as the cause and with a risk of donor artery occlusion resulting from catheter embolization).

References

Abbas MA, Fowl RJ, Sone WM, Panneton JM, Oldenburg WA, Bower TC, Cherry KJ, Gloviczki P. Hepatic artery aneurysm: factors that predict complications. J Vasc Surg 2003; 38: 41–5.

Chisci E, Setacci F, de Donato G, Cappelli A, Palasciano G, Setacci C. Renal aneurysms: surgical vs. endovascular treatment. J Cardiovasc Surg (Torino) 2011 Jun; 52 (3): 345–52. Review.

Croner RS, Anders K, Uder M, Lang W. Visceral arterial aneurysm. (article in German) Dt Ärztebl 2006; 1003: 1161–5.

Ferrero E, Ferri M, Viazzo A, Robaldo A, Carbonatto P, Pecchio A, Chiecchio A, Nessi F. Visceral artery aneurysms, an experience on 32 cases in a single center: treatment from surgery to multilayer stent. Ann Vasc Surg 2011 Oct; 25 (7): 923–35. Epub 2011 Aug 10.

Gehling G, Balzer K. Diagnostik des Aneurysmas der Arteria hepatica. DMW 1994; 119: 701–4.

Hiramoto JS, Messina LM. Visceral artery aneurysms. Curr Treat Options Cardiovasc Med 2005; 7: 109–17.

Henry M, Polydorou A, Frid N, Gruffaz P, Cavet A, Henry I, Hugel M, Rüfenacht DA, Augsburger L, De Beule M, Verdonck P, Bonneau M, Kang C, Ouared R, Chopard B. Treatment of renal artery aneurysm with the multilayer stent. J Endovasc Ther 2008 Apr; 15 (2): 231–6.

O'Driscoll D, Olliff SP, Olliff JFC. Pictorial Review. Hepatic artery aneurysm. Br J Radiology 1999; 72: 1018–25.

Ruiz-Tovar J, Martinez-Molina E, Morales V, Sanjuanbenito A, Lobo E. Evolution of therapeutic approach of visceral artery aneurysms. Scand J Surg 2007; 96: 308–13.

Ruffino M, Rabbia C; Italian Cardiatis Registry Investiagtors Group. Endovascular treatment of visceral artery aneurysms with Cardiatis multilayer flow modulator: preliminary results at six-month follow-up. J Cardiovasc Surg (Torino) 2011 Jun; 52 (3): 311-21.

Sessa C, Tinelli G, Porcu P, Aubert A, Thony F, Magne JL. Treatment of visceral artery aneurysms: description of a retrospective series of 42 aneurysms in 34 patients. Ann Vasc Surg 2004; 18: 695–703.

3.2.6   Arteriovenous malformations and other vascular malformations
Thomas Frieling

3.2.6.1   Clinical picture

Hepatic hemangiomas

Some 13% of hepatic lesions that are initially unclear when observed on ultrasound are hepatic hemangiomas. In the differential diagnosis, hepatic metastases are seen in 32% of cases, nonreproducible lesions in 19%, small hepatic cysts in 14%, abscesses in 11%, hepatocellular carcinoma in 5%, adenoma in 2%, and cholangiocarcinoma in around 1%.

The etiology of hepatic hemangiomas is unclear. Genetic factors may play a role. An autosomal-recessive inheritance pattern is present in hereditary telangiectasia (Osler-Weber-Rendu disease).

There are no definitive data on the incidence of angiodysplasias because they are asymptomatic in most cases. According to research studies, the incidence is approximately 1% in healthy individuals, 3% in patients without hemorrhage, and 6% in patients with hemorrhage. Older patients in the seventh and eighth decades of life are often affected.

Angiodysplasias in the gastrointestinal tract

Angiodysplasias are responsible for approximately 6% of cases of lower gastrointestinal bleeding and for 1.2–8% of cases of upper gastrointestinal bleeding. Small-bowel dysplasia is responsible for 30–40% of cases of bleeding of unclear origin (Fig. 3.2-53). The angiodysplasias are most often located in the cecum and ascending colon (54–100%). However, angiodysplasias may also be located in up to 46% of cases distal to the right colic flexure, or in the left-sided colon (21%), transverse colon (24%), or rectum (34%). Multiple lesions (40–75%) and multiple locations (17–60%), as well as concomitant small-bowel angiodysplasias (30%), are frequent. Angiodysplasias in the upper gastrointestinal tract are most often located in the stomach and duodenum. Intestinal angiodysplasias represent ectasia of previously normal submucosal vessels (not neovascularization) and superficial capillaries. The surrounding mucosa is intact.

The causes are unclear. It is suspected that angiodysplasias arise in the course of degenerative processes or are caused by low-grade obstruction in submucosal vessels at the points at which they penetrate the muscle layers. During the course of vascular ectasia, this leads to loss of the precapillary sphincter function and to the development of arteriovenous connections. It is suspected that many angiodysplasias have a congenital pathogenesis. There is no confirmed link to von Willebrand disease. Associations between angiodysplasia and aortic stenosis (Heyde syndrome), hepatic cirrhosis, and chronic pulmonary disease have also not been confirmed. Gastrointestinal angiodysplasias are frequently found in patients with hereditary telangiectasia (Osler-Weber-Rendu disease) (Fig. 3.2-53) and in those with collagen vascular disease (CREST syndrome: *c*alcinosis, *R*aynaud phenomenon, *e*sophageal motility disorders, *s*clerodactyly, and *t*elangiectasia).

Rare findings include what is known as watermelon stomach or gastric antral vascular ectasia (GAVE) syndrome. GAVE syndrome often occurs in combination with portal hypertension (Fig. 3.2-54). An association with autoimmune inflammation of various organs (e.g., of the thyroid, liver, and stomach) has been reported.

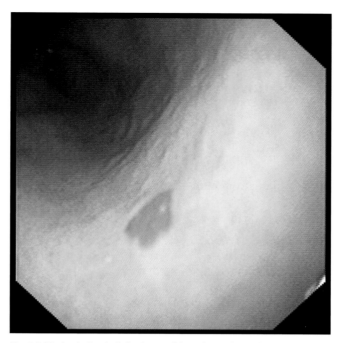

Fig. 3.2-53 Angiodysplasia in the small bowel in Osler-Webber-Rendu disease.

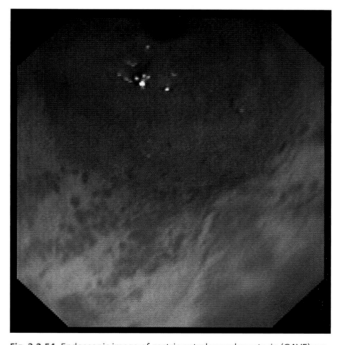

Fig. 3.2-54 Endoscopic image of gastric antral vascular ectasia (GAVE) syndrome (watermelon stomach), showing the typical striated angiectasias in the gastric antrum.

3.2.6.2   Clinical findings

Hemangiomas are usually asymptomatic and are incidental findings. During pregnancy, large hemangiomas may lead to high-output cardiac insufficiency. For this reason, large hemangiomas—e.g., in the context of Osler-Weber-Rendu disease—represent a contraindication for pregnancy.

Angiodysplasias and GAVE syndrome are also usually asymptomatic. Symptomatic patients have rectal bleeding (0–60%), melena

(0–26%), Hemoccult-positive feces (4–47%), and iron-deficiency anemia (0–51%).

Recurrent bleeding is usually seen (50% within 36 months). There are no parameters or events that have any predictive value for bleeding. Risk factors for bleeding from angiodysplasias include congestive heart failure, hypertension, renal insufficiency, collagen vascular disease, and coagulation disturbances. Mechanical factors associated with feces probably play only a subordinate role. Portal hypertension is a risk factor for bleeding in GAVE syndrome.

3.2.6.3   Diagnosis and differential diagnosis

Hepatic hemangioma

Typical hyperechoic, smooth-contoured structures are seen on ultrasonography, sometimes with detectable afferent and efferent vessels. On contrast ultrasonography, the early phase shows nodular enhancement with subsequent centripetal progression (iris diaphragm phenomenon). Multiple hemangiomas are seen in 10% of cases; the differential diagnosis needs to include all types of focal hepatic lesion that may have a hyperechoic appearance on ultrasound. These are primary hepatic tumors such as hepatocellular carcinoma and cholangiocellular carcinoma, or hepatic metastases. Dynamic computed tomography shows a characteristic triad, with a hypodense focus on noncontrast imaging, fast contrast enrichment on the periphery of the focus (known as the iris diaphragmatic phenomenon), and subsequent isodense complete filling of the focus over at least 30 min. In late-phase images (30–60 min), the initial hyperdensity typically declines.

Magnetic resonance imaging also shows small hemangiomas. A signal-rich T2 image is typical. More sensitive imaging is possible with contrast media containing ferrous oxide, as hemangiomas, focal nodular hyperplasia, and adenomas take up the iron particles due to the reticuloendothelial system.

Blood pool scintigraphy is the best method of distinguishing hepatic hemangiomas from other types of lesion. Strong enrichment of the hemangiomas is typical. Late-phase images using single-photon emission computed tomography (SPECT) provide better resolution.

Angiodysplasias

Colonoscopy, gastroscopy, small-intestinal endoscopy, capsule endoscopy, and angiography are the diagnostic methods of choice. Because angiodysplasias are small and do not cause any mucosal lesions, contrast enemas and laparoscopy are of no diagnostic relevance.

On endoscopy, angiodysplasias appear as shallow or slightly raised reddish lesions (2–10 mm in size) that are sharply demarcated from their surroundings (Fig. 3.2-55). Prominent hemangiomas are rarely found (Fig. 3.2-56). Only signs of hemorrhage (active bleeding, adherent coagulum) provide direct evidence of bleeding from angiodysplasias. The ability to detect angiodysplasias endoscopically may be impaired by severe anemia and by sedatives, which reduce the mucosal blood flow.

Colonoscopy is the primary method for clarifying bleeding from angiodysplasias, as the most frequent angiodysplasias are found in the colon. In addition to precise localization, simultaneous treatment of the angiodysplasias is possible. The sensitivity of colonos-

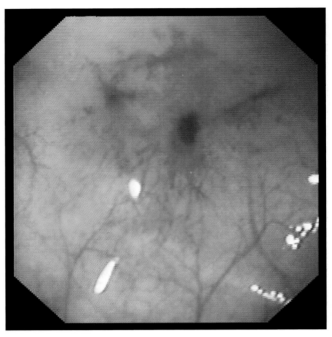

Fig. 3.2-55 Angiodysplasias in the duodenum.

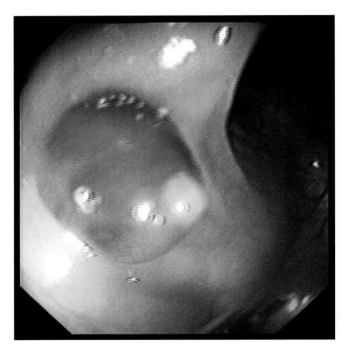

Fig. 3.2-56 Endoscopic image of a hemangioma in the colon.

copy for detecting angiodysplasias reported in the literature is up to 80%. The possibility of extracolic angiodysplasias should always be considered as well. Gastroscopy and small-intestinal endoscopy are indicated here.

Angiodysplasias in the small bowel are responsible for approximately 30–40% of cases of unclear bleeding. In up to half of the cases, the site of bleeding can be identified endoscopically. Intraoperative endoscopy has a sensitivity of 75–100%.

Angiography of the celiac trunk and superior and inferior mesenteric artery allows detection of angiodysplasias in the small bowel and colon (Fig. 3.2-57). Angiographic signs include vascular ectasia

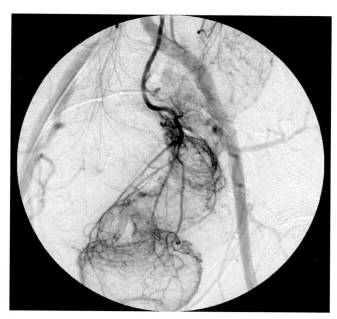

Fig. 3.2-57 Angiographic depiction of the inferior mesenteric artery. Angiodysplasias are seen in the descending colon and sigmoid (courtesy of Prof. V. Fiedler, Institute of Radiographic Diagnosis, HELIOS Hospital, Krefeld, Germany).

(70–75%) and early-filling veins (60–80%) or late-filling veins (85–90%). Only evidence of contrast in the lumen (6–20%) allows definitive localization of the bleeding source. Due to its low diagnostic value and the risk of inducing bleeding, biopsy of angiodysplasias is not recommended.

GAVE syndrome is characterized by its typical vascular ectasia, which appears on endoscopy as reddish stripes in the gastric antrum, resembling the pattern of a watermelon (Fig. 3.2-54).

3.2.6.4   Treatment

Hepatic hemangioma

Therapy is usually not needed, and there is no reduction in hepatic function or life expectancy. In large hemangiomas with clinical symptoms (e.g., high-output cardiac insufficiency), surgical resection may be indicated.

Angiodysplasias

Drug treatment

Although numerous uncontrolled and a few prospective studies have demonstrated reduced bleeding from angiodysplasias with estrogen treatment (0.5 mg ethinyl estradiol and 1.0 mg norethisterone), the mechanism of effect is unclear (e.g., with reduced bleeding time, stasis of microcirculation, stabilization of the endothelium). In some cases, patients with hereditary telangiectasia (Osler-Weber-Rendu disease) respond better to hormone therapy, as estrogen–progesterone receptors have been demonstrated in the affected tissue. A favorable effect with thalidomide, with inhibition of angiogenesis, has recently been reported.

Endoscopic treatment

Endoscopic treatment is usually easy to carry out. Local sclerotherapy procedures for angiodysplasia include monopolar electrocoagulation, polidocanol injection, thermocoagulation with contact probes (BICAP, gold probe, heater probe), Nd:YAG laser coagulation, and argon plasma coagulation. The injection technique, contact probes, and argon plasma coagulation (with a penetration depth of 1–2 mm) are currently preferred, as they are effective and simple procedures. As the wall of the right colon is very thin (50% thinner than the gastric wall), there is a high risk of perforation (2.4%). The risk is highest with monopolar electrocoagulation and Nd:YAG laser treatment. Repeated argon plasma coagulation therapy is a successful option in GAVE syndrome.

Surgical therapy

Surgical therapy is only indicated when bleeding cannot be managed with drug treatment or endoscopy, when there is a confirmed bleeding site and the angiodysplasias are located in one segment of the bowel. In GAVE syndrome, surgical antrectomy may be successful. The prognosis depends on hemostasis and the underlying diseases. The efficacy of endoscopic control of bleeding is 80–90%, and the rate of recurrent bleeding is 20–30%.

References

Biecker E, Heller J, Schmitz V, Lammert F, Sauerbruch T. Effiziente Diagnostik und Therapie oberer gastrointestinaler Blutungen (Diagnosis and Management of Upper Gastrointestinal Bleeding). Dtsch Arztebl 2008; 105 (5): 85–93. DOI: 10.3238/arztebl. 2008.0085.

Caselitz M, Wagner S, Chavan A, Gebel M, Bleck J, Wu A, Schlitt H, Galanski M, Manns M. Clinical outcome of transfemoral embolisation in patients with arteriovenous malformations of the liver in hereditary haemorrhagic telangiectasia (Weber-Rendu-Osler disease). Gut 1998 January; 42 (1): 123–6.

Foutch PG. Angiodysplasia of the gastrointestinal tract. Am J Gastroenterol 1993; 88: 807–18.

Kahl S, Kähler G, Dormann A. Interventionelle Endoskopie. Lehrbuch und Atlas. Elsevier, Urban & Fischer Verlag, München, Jena, 2006.

Schumacher B, Frieling T, Borchard F, Hengels KJ. Hereditary hemorrhagic telangiectasia associated with multiple pulmonary arteriovenous malformations and juvenile polyposis. Z Gastroenterol 1994 Feb; 32 (2): 105–8.

Zhi-Zheng Ge, Hui-Min Chen, Yun-Jie Gao, Wen-Zhong Lui, Chun-Hong Xu, Hong-Hong Tan, Hai-Ying Chen, Wei Wei, Jing-Yuan Fang, and Shu-Dong Xiao. Efficacy of thalidomide for refractory gastrointestinal bleeding from vascular malformation. Gastroenterology 2011; 141: 1629–37.

4 Diseases of the arteries of the extremities

4.1 Stenotic diseases of the proximal arteries of the upper extremity

Introduction and conservative treatment:
Thomas Zeller
Doppler/duplex ultrasonography: Tom Schilling
Conservative treatment: Thomas Zeller
Endovascular treatment: Thomas Zeller
Surgical treatment: Eric Lorenz

4.1.1 Anatomy of the proximal arteries in the upper extremities

See section A 2.1.1.

4.1.2 Clinical picture

Only 10% of all peripheral arterial vascular occlusions occur in the region of the upper extremities with approximately 25% of them located in the course of the shoulder arteries (the subclavian artery, brachiocephalic trunk, and axillary artery). Due to good collateralization, even occlusions of the subclavian and axillary arteries become symptomatic in only one-third of cases. A blood pressure difference of ≥ 20 mmHg present on repeated measures raises a suspicion of a subclavian artery lesion.

The causes of chronic occlusive disease in the proximal arteries of the upper extremity are:

- Atherosclerosis with an ostial or proximal location (more rarely distal) in the majority of cases.
- Local compression syndrome (thoracic outlet syndrome, TOS), usually caused by osseous malformations with compression in the costoclavicular space or a cervical rib. The chronic external compression leads to damage to the vascular wall, with intramural thrombosis, occlusion, or aneurysm.
- Inflammatory—e.g., Takayasu disease or Horton giant cell arteritis, mainly with an ostial location or other signs of generalized arteriosclerosis. This mainly affects women aged between 30 and 50 years.
- Thromboembolic—e.g., cardiac (atrial fibrillation, atrial myxoma) or from the aortic arch (plaque or dissection).
- Radiation vasculitis after tumor radiotherapy.

The causes of acute occlusions of the shoulder arteries are:

- Cardiac embolism with (intermittent) atrial fibrillation.
- Local thrombotic occlusion based on arteriosclerotic plaques that do not initially have hemodynamically stenotic effects.

- Chronic degenerative damage to the vascular wall due to external compression (TOS).
- Whiplash injury to the cervical spine can also lead to an acute compression syndrome or tearing of the intima, with subsequent thrombotic vascular occlusion.

Thoracic outlet syndrome (TOS) is described elsewhere in this book.

4.1.3 Clinical findings

The symptoms of *chronic occlusive diseases* of the proximal arteries in the upper extremities are characterized by underperfusion of the arm muscles and a cerebral steal effect.

- Subclavian steal syndrome or vertebral artery steal syndrome, with vertigo, nausea, transient pareses or paresthesias, visual disturbances, ataxia or syncope, which is usually triggered by manual activities, with arm movements leading to an increased perfusion demand. Only approximately 15% of patients with reverse flow or oscillating flow in the vertebral artery are symptomatic. Subclavian steal syndrome can only occur with stenoses or occlusions located proximal to the origin of the vertebral artery.
- Intermittent apraxia, occurring in compression syndromes usually during overhead work.
- Sensation of cold and pallor in the fingers.
- Recurrent finger embolism.

Acute occlusion of the subclavian or axillary arteries usually represents an emergency situation, with critical ischemia in the extremities. The principle symptoms are sudden resting pain in the hand affected, accompanied by weakness, pallor, a feeling of cold, and possibly paresthesias. Depending on the quality of the collateral network, the symptoms may either regress or progress and become life-threatening.

4.1.4 Diagnosis

A staged diagnostic workup, guided by the patient's history, is indicated in order to avoid unnecessary costs and radiation exposure.

- During inspection (at rest and after provocation—e.g., with repeated hand clenching), pallor in the affected hand is often noted, particularly after provocation. On palpation, the pulse in the brachial and radial arteries is either weak or not palpable.
- In stenoses of the subclavian artery or brachiocephalic trunk, a stenosal murmur can be auscultated in the supraclavicular fossa.
- Riva–Rocci blood pressure measurement (including provocation positions) confirms the suspected diagnosis if the blood pressure difference is > 20 mmHg.

- Arterial Doppler occlusive pressure measurement, like blood pressure measurement, is also used to confirm the diagnosis and provides information on the severity of the perfusion disturbance.
- Electronic segmental pulse volume recording of the upper and lower arm makes it possible to identify the level of the perfusion disturbance. Additional finger pulse volume recording (with cold and heat provocation if needed) can provide further information on embolic and functional perfusion disturbances in the finger arteries.
- Continuous-wave (CW) Doppler ultrasonography and color duplex sonography are used for precise assessment of the location and extent of the stenotic process and can provide evidence of any steal phenomena (in the vertebral artery and internal thoracic artery).
- X-ray of the chest skeleton is indicated if there is a suspicion of TOS.
- Capillary microscopy if there is suspected vasculitis.
- Intra-arterial angiography, magnetic resonance (MR) angiography, or computed tomography (CT) angiography are only indicated if there is also an indication for intervention.

4.1.4.1 Doppler/duplex ultrasonography

Examination technique in the proximal arteries of the upper extremity

The aortic arch is demonstrated, as well as the proximal **subclavian artery** and **brachiocephalic trunk** from supraclavicular and jugular, preferably with a 7.5-MHz microconvex probe; if that is not available, a low-frequency convex probe with adapted programming can be used, and further distally a (5.0)–7.5–(10.0)-MHz linear probe (*caution:* reverberation echoes with duplication of vascular images may occur at the cervical pleura).

When there is a suspicion of thoracic outlet syndrome, the relevant provocation tests can be carried out with duplex ultrasound imaging of the subclavian vein.

If there is flow obstruction in the proximal subclavian artery, an upper arm compression test can be carried out.

Differential diagnosis

- Arteriosclerosis:
  - Typical plaque morphology.
  - Classically located in proximal segments of the subclavian artery and in the brachiocephalic trunk.
- Embolism: hypoechoic to isoechoic occlusive material, potentially with a visible cervical pleura phenomenon—i.e., a convex configuration of the occlusive material toward the free lumen, with an otherwise unremarkable vascular system with no major atheromatosis.
- Arterial thrombosis: in addition to the hypoechoic occlusion, evidence of prior arteriosclerosis with echocomplex plaques and structures creating acoustic shadows, possibly "older" echogenic occlusive components.
- Large-vessel vasculitis:
  - Typically homogeneous and hypoechoic widened intima–media complex (macaroni sign).
  - Involvement of distal segments (e.g., axillary artery).

– *Caution:* there are often respiratory-modulated kinking stenoses in the subclavian artery, particularly on the left side; these regress on inspiration.

Specific findings

Subclavian artery

Stenotic findings in the subclavian artery:
- Increase in systolic peak frequency/maximum velocity (*caution:* respiratory-modulated kinking stenoses)
- Post-stenotic flow disturbances
- Loss of inverse early diastolic flow/DIP (*caution:* this may be mimicked if the insonation angle is too large)
- Post-stenotic drop in pressure
- Behavior of the vertebral artery and intracranial segments of the vertebrobasilar territory in resting conditions, as well as reactive hyperemia (in the upper arm compression test)
- If a prestenotic/intrastenotic/post-stenotic segment is well displayed: use of the peak velocity ratio (PVR; = V_{max} intrastenotic/ V_{max} prestenotic)

Low-grade stenosis (up to 50%). The clinical findings and CW/PW Doppler ultrasonography are unremarkable; direct duplex imaging of the reduced lumen, no significant difference in the occlusion pressure measured using Doppler ultrasound in the brachial artery or Riva–Rocci blood pressure findings (≤ 20 mmHg), PVR < 2.

Moderate stenosis (50–70%). At most only a slight difference in occlusion pressure in the brachial artery measured using Doppler ultrasound and in Riva–Rocci blood pressure (≥ 20 mmHg), possibly with auscultatory stenotic signal, slight increase in systolic peak frequency/maximum velocity, systolic turbulences, DIP reduction or loss (differential diagnosis: angle artefact), possibly with incipient systolic deceleration in the ipsilateral vertebral artery (subclavian steal effect I), PVR 2–3.

High-grade stenosis (70–99%). There is a clear difference in the occlusion pressure measured using Doppler ultrasound in the brachial artery and the Riva–Rocci blood pressure; auscultation shows a clear stenotic signal, with a marked increase in systolic peak frequency/ maximum velocity, distinct flow disturbances with a post-stenotically distorted systolic signal (sluggish increase in flow, widened spectrum, absent systolic window, retrograde flow components), DIP loss, subclavian steal effect II–IV, possible hyperperfusion of the afferent vessels supplying the ipsilateral vertebral artery, PVR 3 to ≥ 10.

Table 4.1-1 Duplex ultrasound grading of stenoses in the subclavian artery.

PVR	Stenosis grade
≥ 10	≥ 90%
5–9	Approx. 80–89%
5	Approx. 80%
3–4	Approx. 65–75%
2.5	Approx. 60%
2	Approx. 50%
1.5	Approx. 35%

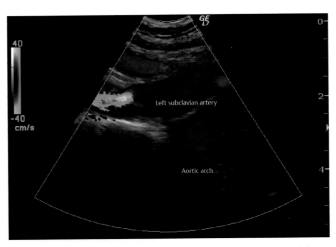

Fig. 4.1-1 Subclavian artery stenosis. The image shows the origin of the left subclavian artery from the aortic arch, with a typical color duplex signal showing higher-grade stenosis approximately 3 cm from the origin.

Occlusion. Steep pressure drop, no stenotic sounds on auscultation, no signal from the proximal subclavian artery, possible turbulent signal due to inflowing blood from collaterals with retrograde perfusion.

Variants of subclavian steal phenomenon

- Most frequently, supply to the ipsilateral vertebral artery via the contralateral vertebral artery → vertebra-vertebral steal
- Supply to the ipsilateral vertebral artery via the external carotid artery and its branches → externo-vertebral steal
- Supply to the basilar artery and ipsilateral vertebral artery via the internal carotid artery and circle of Willis → internobasilar steal
- Supply to the subclavian artery via external carotid branches and thyrocervical trunk or costocervical trunk → externocervical steal

Caution: the steal effect should not be equated with subclavian steal *syndrome* (which requires the associated symptoms).
Steal effects should be checked using an upper arm compression test. Procedure: ipsilateral hypersystolic block using an upper arm cuff for 20–30 s, with additional hand grips if appropriate, insonation of the ipsilateral vertebral artery, reactive hyperemia in the affected arm after rapid release of the cuff → reveals or intensifies corresponding steal effects in the vertebral artery.
Steal variants can be differentiated using a crossed upper arm compression test (as above, but with imaging of the contralateral vertebral artery or other afferent arteries).
When there are corresponding **cerebral symptoms** and hence a suspicion of subclavian steal *syndrome*, the upper arm compression test should be repeated with insonation of the basilar artery and additional segments of the arteries at the base of the brain if appropriate, in order to assess the extent of **intracranial steal effects**.

Brachiocephalic trunk

Stenotic findings in the brachiocephalic trunk:
- Difference in occlusion pressures measured using Doppler ultrasound in the brachial artery and Riva–Rocci blood pressure measurement, with lower pressures at the right side

- Stenotic sounds in the right infraclavicular region without definite direct Doppler/duplex ultrasound evidence of stenosis of the right subclavian artery
- Post-stenotic flow phenomena in the right common carotid artery and right subclavian artery
- Resulting in an **internosubclavian steal effect** → systolic decelerations or pendular flows in the common carotid artery and right internal carotid artery that occur or are intensified during the upper arm compression test
- CW/PW findings in the vertebral artery as in various degrees of subclavian steal effect

The information given in connection with the subclavian artery applies analogously in relation to an increase in systolic peak frequency, post-stenotic flow disturbances, and changes in the Doppler profile.

Axillary artery

Stenotic findings in the axillary artery:
- For the differential diagnosis of occlusive processes, see above; rarely with an arteriosclerotic pathogenesis; large-vessel vasculitis should be considered.
- Stenosis grading using the peak velocity ratio (PVR)

4.1.5   Differential Diagnosis

See Table 4.1-2.

4.1.6   Treatment

4.1.6.1   Conservative treatment

This is the most frequent form of therapy, as only 15–30% of patients are symptomatic. In patients with arteriosclerotic occlusion, it consists of secondary prophylactic administration of acetylsalicylic acid (ASA) 100 mg/d for long-term therapy and additional adjustment of known cardiovascular risk factors for prophylaxis against stroke and myocardial ischemia/infarction. In patients with asymptomatic vascular occlusion with no peripheral embolization caused by a compression syndrome, no further specific treatment is indicated. In those with functional stenosis, postural training is initially indicated, possibly along with a change in sleeping position if appropriate.

4.1.6.2   Endovascular treatment

Indications for percutaneous transluminal angioplasty (PTA)

- Symptomatic stenosis or occlusion of the subclavian artery (subclavian steal *syndrome*) affecting everyday life.
- Asymptomatic stenosis or occlusion of the subclavian artery (subclavian steal *phenomenon*), if the downstream internal mammary artery is needed or has already been used as a coronary bypass vessel.
- Bilateral asymptomatic stenosis or occlusion in patients with known arterial hypertension, to assure reliable blood pressure measurement and adjustment.
- Acute ischemia threatening the extremities.

Table 4.1-2 Differential diagnosis of subclavian artery lesions.

Symptom	Cause	Differential findings
Segmental paresthesias	Cervical nerve root compression syndrome	Palpable pulse No blood pressure difference
Segmental or complete paresthesias/dysesthesias in the arm	Bony nerve compression syndrome in the costoclavicular space	Palpable pulse Position-dependent symptoms No blood pressure difference
Intermittent apraxia with overhead movements	Thoracic outlet syndrome	Pulse not palpable in provocation position Blood pressure/Doppler pressure lowered in provocation position
Painful swelling in the arm	Thoracic inlet syndrome—e.g., bony compression syndrome, subclavian vein thrombosis	Livid, tense skin Edema Subcutaneous collateral veins Palpable pulse No Doppler pressure difference, but possibly a blood pressure difference
Recurrent painful paleness in individual fingers or all fingers	Primary or secondary Raynaud syndrome	Palpable pulse Symptoms inducible with cold
Recurrent vertigo or syncope	Neurocardial syncope Vertebral artery stenosis/occlusion	Palpable pulse Blood pressure and Doppler pressure similar on both sides
Pale, tense skin, acral lesions, contractures	Scleroderma	Palpable pulse Blood pressure and Doppler pressure similar on both sides Pathological capillary microscopy

Contraindications against PTA

- Asymptomatic stenosis/occlusion without the need for aorto-coronary bypass treatment
- Significant contraindications (e.g., hyperthyroidism, severe previous reaction to contrast administration, advanced renal insufficiency) for the use of iodine-containing radiographic contrast media, with no option for using alternative contrast media
- "Florid" vasculitis: in active vasculitis, immunosuppressive therapy should initially be started until inflammatory parameters have normalized. Exception: planned directional atherectomy (e.g., SilverHawk™, FoxHollow/ev3) to confirm the diagnosis

Patient preparation

- For elective procedures, the patient should receive information about the procedure and provide consent at least 1 day before the intervention.
- Fasting for at least 6 h before the intervention.

Medication

- Chronic premedication with ASA 100 mg/d or 500 mg ASA as an oral bolus before the intervention; clopidogrel 300 mg as a loading dose on the day before the procedure or on the day of the procedure.
- After placement of the sheath, a heparin bolus of 2500–5000 IU, depending on body weight and the time required for the procedure, is administered.

Access route

The femoral or brachial access routes are most often used or less often the radial access.

Femoral access

The femoral access route is the standard approach, except in untreated stenoses or occlusions of the infrarenal abdominal aorta or pelvic or femoral arteries (groin), marked tortuosity of the pelvic arteries, or an absent stump at the origin of the closed subclavian artery or brachiocephalic trunk. In these cases, the brachial access route can be selected instead. The intervention can be carried out either through a guiding catheter or a long sheath.

Guiding catheter technique (Fig. 4.1-2)

- After local anesthesia, placement of a 6–8F sheath (11 cm long) with a hemostatic valve in the common femoral artery. If there is tortuosity of the iliac arteries, using a 23-cm long sheath may be helpful.
- The guiding catheter (90 cm long)—a multipurpose "LIMA" or JR (Judkins right), depending on the anatomy—is used for selective probing of the origin of the left subclavian artery or brachiocephalic trunk.
- Alternatively, a 7–9F Vista BriteTip IG™ introducer sheath, 90 cm long, with a hemostatic valve can be used (a combination of a 90-cm long guiding catheter with a hemostatic valve; saves 1F in the sheath size).

Long sheath (Fig. 4.1-3)

- A straight 6F, 90-cm long sheath (e.g., Shuttle Sheath, Cook) is placed in the origin of the left subclavian artery or brachiocephalic trunk, either by slow withdrawal in the aortic arch or after probing using the telescope technique with a 6F JR-4 or IMA diagnostic catheter and a 0.035-inch Terumo J stiff wire.

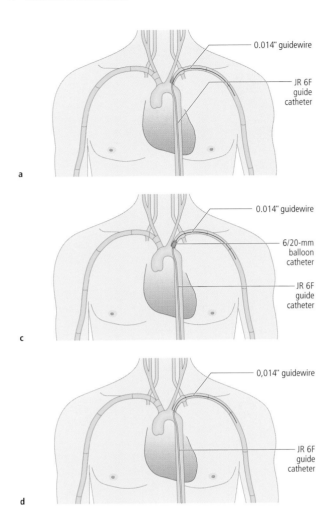

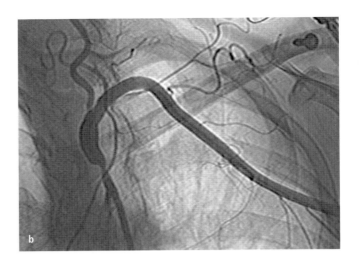

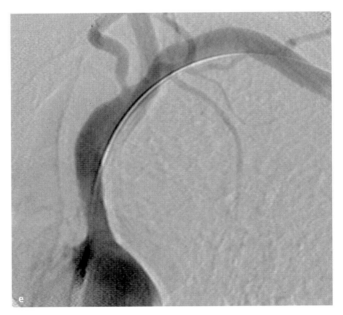

Fig. 4.1-2a–e (**a, b**) Stenosis near the origin of the subclavian artery on the left, demonstrated via a JR-4 guiding catheter. (**c**) 6-mm percutaneous transluminal angioplasty (PTA). (**d, e**) Check-up examination after 6-mm PTA in a 20° right anterior oblique (RAO) projection.

Brachial access route

A 5F or 6F sheath, 11 or 23 cm long, is placed retrograde in the brachial artery using the Seldinger technique. Retrograde brachial puncture is more difficult due to the usually nonpalpable brachial artery pulse, and can often only be achieved using CW Doppler or duplex ultrasonography. The lesion can then be crossed, using a 5F multipurpose or vertebral artery catheter for better guidance if appropriate, with a hydrophilic guidewire—e.g., a 0.035-inch Terumo stiff J wire. A disadvantage is that it is usually difficult to demonstrate the length of the target lesion via the retrograde access route.

Preinterventional angiography

The course of the proximal arteries in the upper extremities is not subject to any major anatomic variations; there are only variants in the origin, depending on the anatomy of the aortic arch. Several projections, and at least two levels—each 20–30° left anterior oblique (LAO) and right anterior oblique (RAO)—need to be used, depending on the configuration of the aortic arch, for precise localization of the origins of the vertebral artery and internal mammary artery (Fig. 4.1-2).

Intervention

Chronic perfusion disturbance

1. Stenosis (Figs. 4.1-2 and 4.1-3)
- With femoral access after selective probing of the subclavian artery or brachiocephalic trunk with a guiding catheter (6–8F) or guide sheath (JR 4, multipurpose, IMA), a guidable 0.014-inch, 0.018-inch, or 0.035-inch J guidewire is introduced, depending on the balloon catheter or stent system being used.
- Balloon dilation, usually with a PTA balloon catheter (usually 6–8 mm in diameter and 20 mm long) that can be traversed by a 0.014-inch or 0.018-inch guidewire. If primary stenting is planned, predilation should only be carried out with an undersized (2–3 mm) balloon catheter. This does not lead to normalization of the direction of flow in the vertebral artery and thus ensures natural protection against embolism during stent placement.
- If there is relevant residual stenosis or dissection, a stent (either balloon-expandable or self-expanding) is implanted. Most of the commonly used balloon-expandable stents up to a diameter of 7 mm can be introduced over a 6F guiding catheter. Stenting

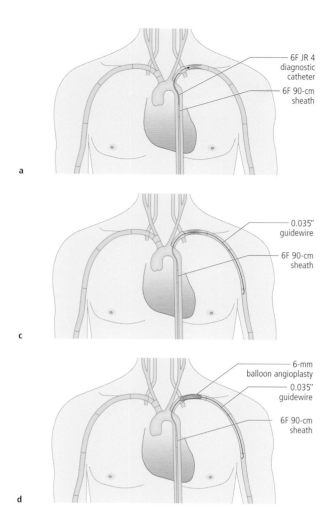

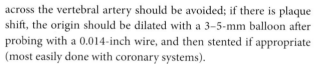

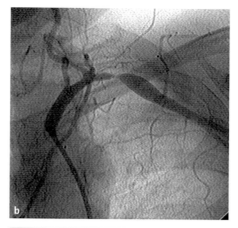

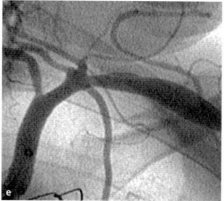

Fig. 4.1-3a–e (**a, b**) Stenosis in the middle left subclavian artery, demonstrated via a 90-cm straight 6F sheath. (**c**) Passage of the stenosis with a 0.035-inch wire (Terumo). (**d**) 6/40-mm percutaneous transluminal angioplasty (PTA). (**e**) The result after 6-mm PTA.

across the vertebral artery should be avoided; if there is plaque shift, the origin should be dilated with a 3–5-mm balloon after probing with a 0.014-inch wire, and then stented if appropriate (most easily done with coronary systems).

■ In stenoses of unclear etiology—e.g., in suspected vasculitis—a directional atherectomy (SilverHawk™, FoxHollow) can be helpful in obtaining tissue samples for histological processing (Fig. 4.1-8).

2. Occlusion (Fig. 4.1-4)

■ If there is a stump of the origin available or the occlusion is distal to the ostium, recanalization can be carried out transfemorally.

■ Stable positioning of the guiding catheter or long sheath is important so as to be able to penetrate the occlusion with a hydrophilic wire, best done with a 0.035-inch Terumo stiff J wire (260 cm long), stiffened with a 4F diagnostic catheter if appropriate. Alternatively, hydrophilic coronary 0.014-inch wires (e.g., Pilot™, Abbot Vascular; Crossit™, Terumo) or stiff recanalization wires (Confienza™, Boston Scientific; Crosswire™, Abbott Vascular), stabilized by using a coaxial technique if appropriate with a coronary 2-mm balloon catheter, can be used.

■ In chronic occlusions, wire recanalization often takes place subintimally. It is absolutely necessary to ensure that the guidewire becomes intraluminal again proximally to the level of the vertebral artery, as otherwise the vertebral artery will be occluded.

■ After passage of the occlusion with the guidewire, predilation can be carried out with a 5F balloon catheter with a diameter of 3–5 mm using a 0.035-inch guidewire (the shaft length must be at least 100 cm). With a 0.014-inch guidewire, monorail balloon catheters with a diameter of 2–7 mm can be used.

■ If it is necessary to implant a stent, either a self-expanding nitinol stent capable of traversing an 8F guiding catheter (6F sheath) can be placed, or—if the occlusion is severely calcified—a balloon-expandable stent premounted on a monorail catheter can be implanted over a 0.014-inch or 0.018-inch wire.

If antegrade recanalization is unsuccessful, a retrograde attempt can be made *transbrachially,* ideally during the same session or alternatively as a secondary procedure (Fig. 4.1-5). However, this involves a potential risk of aortic arch dissection if subintimal wire recanalization occurs.

Acute perfusion disturbance

The following treatment options are available for endovascular therapy for acute occlusion of the subclavian artery and axillary artery:

■ Local thrombolysis

■ Aspiration embolectomy (combined with local lysis if appropriate)

■ Rotation thrombectomy

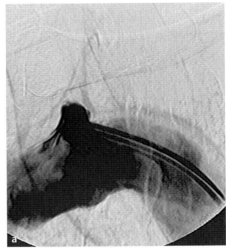

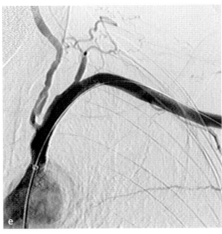

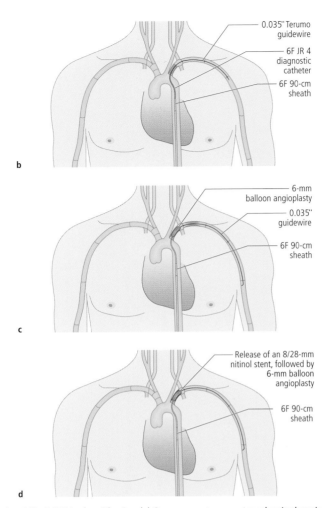

Fig. 4.1-4a–e (**a**) Occlusion of the left subclavian artery. (**b**) Passage using a hydrophilic 0.035-inch guidewire. (**c**) 6-mm percutaneous transluminal angioplasty (PTA). (**d**) Placement of a self-expanding nitinol stent and subsequent dilation. (**e**) Final result after recanalization.

Local thrombolysis

- A 5F or 6F sheath, 11 cm long, is positioned using a transfemoral access route.
- The origin of the subclavian artery or brachiocephalic trunk is probed using a diagnostic catheter (e.g., JR 4, vertebral artery) and diagnostic angiography is performed.
- The occlusion is traversed with a hydrophilic guidewire (e.g., 0.035-inch Terumo guidewire with a J-bend, 260 cm long).
- Placement of a side-hole lysis catheter (e.g., Cragg–McNamara™, Boston Scientific)
- Bolus administration of a lytic agent (e.g., Actilyse™ 5–10 mg) in combination with 5000 IU heparin, followed by a long-term infusion (e.g., Actilyse™ 0.5–2.0 mg/h in combination with heparin 600–800 IU/h) via the lysis catheter. The duration of local lysis treatment is guided by the success of the treatment, as documented clinically or with duplex ultrasonography.
- Angiographic checking of the findings may be needed after completion of lysis treatment if the duplex ultrasound findings are not sufficiently clear.

Caution: cerebral embolization must be excluded before the start of lysis treatment, as there is otherwise an increased risk of intracerebral hemorrhage.

Aspiration embolectomy

- Placement of either a 6–8F sheath, 11 cm long, or a 90 cm long 6–8F sheath with a removable hemostatic valve (Terumo).
- Probing of the origin of the subclavian artery or brachiocephalic trunk using a 5F or 6F diagnostic catheter (e.g., JR 4, vertebral artery) and performance of diagnostic angiography.
- Passage of the occlusion using a hydrophilic guidewire (e.g., 0.035-inch Terumo Glidewire with a J-bend, 180/260 cm long).
- When a short sheath is used, a 7F or 8F guiding catheter (multipurpose or JR 4) or a special aspiration catheter with an appropriate French size is advanced up to the start of the thrombotic occlusion. This is followed by removal of the guidewire and slow passage of the occlusion with the catheter, with continuous suction (e.g., via a 50-mL perfusion syringe). The advantages of using a guiding catheter for aspiration are the guidability of the catheter tip due to its curvature, its greater flexibility, and the wider internal lumen in comparison with the aspiration catheter, despite having the same French size.

If a long sheath with a removable hemostatic valve is used, the sheath itself can be used for aspiration. A potential disadvantage of this technique is that the whole sheath may have to be removed—for example, if an organized thrombus blocks the sheath.

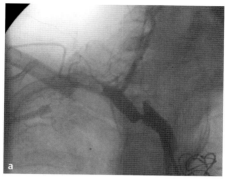

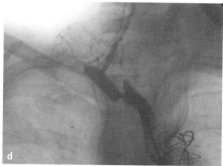

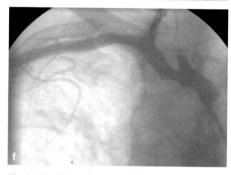

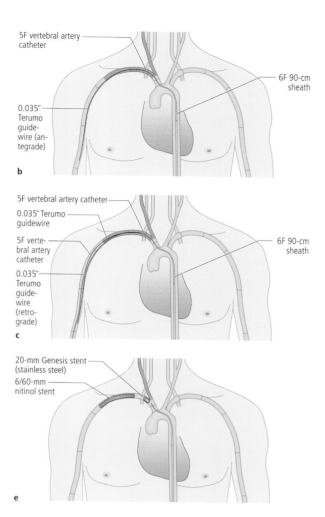

Fig. 4.1-5a–f Simultaneous bilateral recanalization of an occlusion of the right subclavian artery. (**a**) Occlusion of the right common carotid artery and stenosis at the origin of the right subclavian artery with downstream occlusion. (**b**) Subintimal 0.035-inch wire. (**c, d**) Bilateral access with one 5F vertebral artery diagnostic catheter each, after failed antegrade recanalization. (**e**) Placement of a 6/60-mm nitinol stent in the middle, plus a 6/20-mm stainless steel stent in the proximal subclavian artery. (**f**) Final result after placement of a balloon-expandable stent in the ostium and a self-expanding nitinol stent in the middle segment.

Rotation thrombectomy (Fig. 4.1-6)

- A 6F or 8F sheath is placed using transfemoral retrograde access.
- Probing of the origin of the subclavian artery or brachiocephalic trunk using a 5F or 6F diagnostic catheter (e.g. JR 4, vertebral artery) and performance of diagnostic angiography.
- Passage of the occlusion using a hydrophilic guidewire (e.g., 0.035-inch Terumo Glidewire with a J-bend, 180/260 cm long).
- Exchange of the 0.035-inch guidewire for a 300 cm long 0.018-inch wire (supplied in the Rotarex set) through a 4F diagnostic catheter.
- One to three passages either with a 6F (axillary artery) or 8F (subclavian artery) Rotarex™ catheter (Straub Medical).
- Switch back again to the diagnostic catheter for the final angiography.

Potential risks of the intervention

- Embolization in the vertebral artery or occlusion, with cerebellar insult (rare due to pre-interventional/peri-interventional retrograde flow and contralateral collateralization).

- Occasionally, transient neurological symptoms may arise peri-interventionally, probably due to the altered cerebral perfusion after the reversal of flow in the vertebral artery—with visual disturbances, vertigo, and tingling paresthesias in the ipsilateral half of the face.
- Contrast-induced nephropathy (the risk increases along with the degree of limitation of renal function, the amount of contrast administered, and in patients with diabetes).
- Incorrect stent placement.
- Local vascular complications at the puncture site, such as pseudoaneurysm, arteriovenous fistula, hematoma requiring transfusion, etc.

Postinterventional follow-up and medication

Long-term postinterventional therapy with ASA 100 mg/d; after stent implantation, in addition to 4 weeks clopidogrel 75 mg/d in addition.

- Bed rest for 6–12 h, depending on the size of the sheath in transfemoral access, or less when occlusion systems are used. Specialized neurological monitoring after the intervention is not necessary.

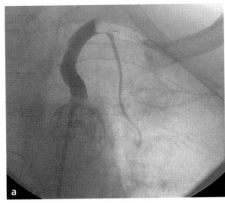

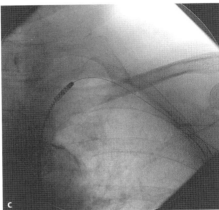

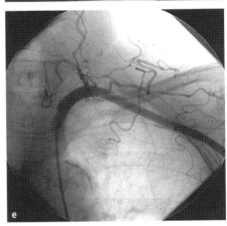

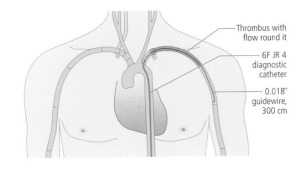

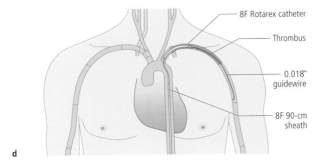

Fig. 4.1-6a–e (**a**) Cardioembolic occlusion of the left subclavian artery. (**b**) After passage with a 0.018-inch guidewire. (**c, d**) An 8F Rotarex catheter over a 0.018-inch guidewire. (**e**) Final result after Rotarex thrombectomy.

■ Before discharge, after 6 months and 12 months, and then at annual intervals: noninvasive angiologic check-up examinations, including segmental pulse volume recordings, arterial Doppler occlusion pressure measurement and color duplex sonography if there is a suspicion of residual stenosis (flow analysis in the vertebral artery). If the internal mammary artery has been used as a bypass artery, 6-monthly angiographic and cardiac check-ups are needed.

Course and prognosis

The prognosis depends on:
■ The duration and intensity of the ischemia (complete or incomplete)—i.e., the severity of the already existing ischemic tissue damage: → fixed muscular rigidity and completely eliminated sensation almost always require (primary) limb amputation

■ The underlying disease: atrial fibrillation (→ oral anticoagulation), aneurysm (→ covered stent, rib resection in thoracic outlet syndrome), (aortic) dissection, inflammatory, arteriosclerotic or traumatic vascular wall lesions

Prospects

Primary success rate: catheter revascularizations of subclavian artery and axillary artery stenoses can nowadays be carried out 100% successfully. However, recanalization, particularly of ostial occlusions, is limited—either due to the impossibility of penetrating the occlusion or due to failure to reconnect the false lumen distally to the true one in subintimal recanalization. Specialized recanalization systems such as the Frontrunner™ (Cordis) and the Crosser™ system (Bard), as well as the excimer laser (Spectranetics; Fig. 4.1-7), may make it easier

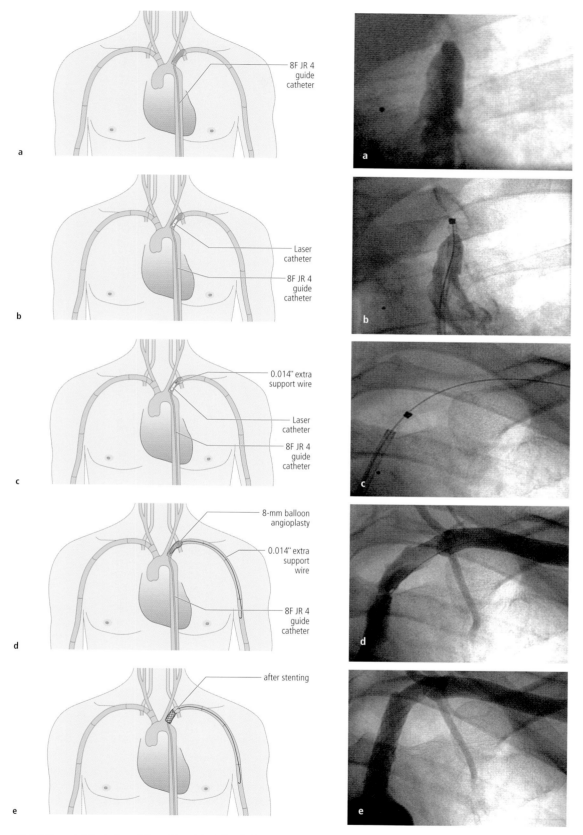

Fig. 4.1-7a–e (**a**) Occlusion of the origin of the left subclavian artery. (**b**) Penetration of the occlusion stump with a 2.0-mm excimer laser catheter. (**c**) 8F guiding catheter after passage of the occlusion with a wire. (**d**) Result after laser angioplasty and 7-mm balloon angioplasty. (**e**) Final result after implantation of a Palmaz–Schatz™ stent.

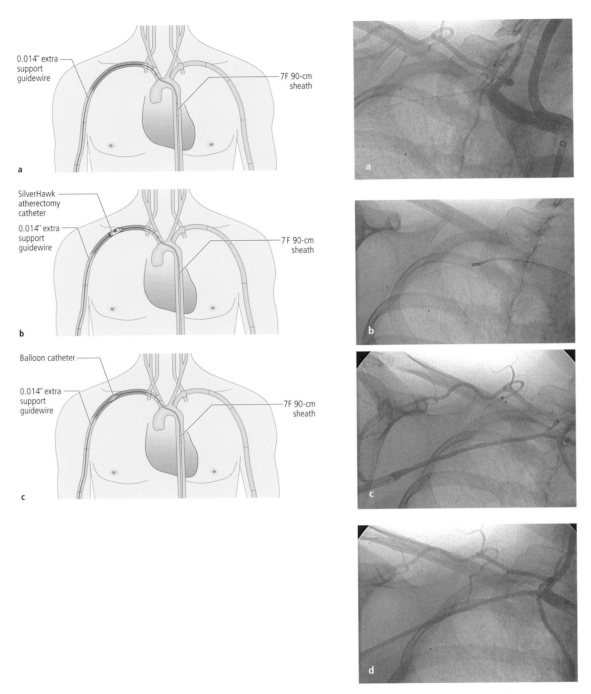

Fig. 4.1-8a–d (**a**) Functional occlusion of the right subclavian artery and axillary artery. (**b**) Directional SilverHawk™ atherectomy. (**c**) After SilverHawk™ atherectomy. (**d**) After additional 4-mm balloon angioplasty.

to pass hard occlusion stumps, or passage may only be possible at all with such systems. The same applies to specialized reentry systems such as Outback™ (Cordis) for subintimal recanalization.

Long-term technical success: One-year restenosis rates of approximately 30% are reported for both balloon dilation and stent implantation, although the results for PTA alone in recanalization procedures are probably poorer. In principle, the use of drug-eluting balloon-expandable stents is conceivable for these mainly focal lesions. However, manufacturers are not yet producing stent systems with the required diameters. The same applies to balloon catheters coated with paclitaxel (Taxol), which have thus far only been used successfully for femoropopliteal lesions.

Differential diagnosis: directional atherectomy (SilverHawk LS™, Covedian-ev3) allows both plaque material and vascular wall fragments to be removed from the lesion in sufficient quantity and quality for histological processing of the particles. This makes it possible to distinguish the basic cause underlying the occlusion process—e.g., differential diagnosis between a primary arteriosclerotic lesion and an inflammatory pathogenesis for the lesion in a chronic, serologically inactive state (Figs. 4.1-8–4.1-10). Controlled studies are needed in order to determine whether atherectomy can also achieve long-term patency rates similar to, or perhaps even better than, those achieved with stenting; but such studies are not currently being planned.

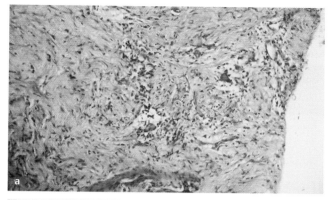

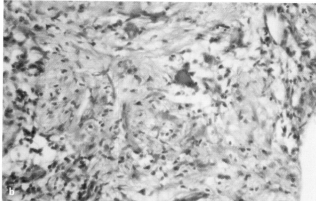

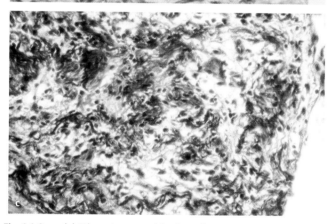

Fig. 4.1-9a–c (a) Atherectomy particles from the case illustrated in Fig. 4.1-8—enlarged detail showing the media with inflammatory changes, with dead granuloma cells and multinucleate giant cells. (**b**) High-resolution enlargement of granulomatous changes in the media and multinucleate giant cells. (**c**) Interrupted elastic fibers in the elastic media layer and multinucleate giant cells.

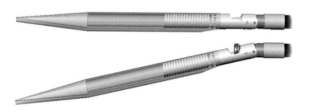

Fig. 4.1-10 A SilverHawk™ atherectomy catheter, extended in the inactivated state and deflected for directional atherectomy.

4.1.6.3 Surgical treatment

Chronic occlusive processes

Indication for surgery

In principle, the same guidelines for establishing the indication apply for surgery as for endovascular therapy. When the lesion location is unfavorable or if there is a symptomatic occlusion in the area of the proximal subclavian artery that cannot be passed interventionally, then vascular surgery is indicated. Due to collateral compensation in axillary or brachial occlusive processes, surgery is relatively rarely indicated—mainly in patients with intermittent apraxia that is handicapping them in working or other activities. Restoration of flow is always indicated if there is resting pain and distal necrosis.

Surgical procedure

There are basically three different surgical approaches that are available for treating occlusions near the origins of the branches of the aortic arch (Fig. 4.1-11a–c):
1. Vascular trunk transposition
2. Extra-anatomical and orthotopic bypass
3. Open local thromboendarterectomy and enlargement plasty and annular disobliteration

Due to the anatomic location of the proximal subclavian, orthotopic and local procedures often require sternotomy and therefore cause greater cardiopulmonary stress for the patients and are associated with a marked increase in the perioperative morbidity. Extra-anatomic bypass procedures are less burdensome. Largely unimpaired donor and recipient vessels are needed for the connection.

Reconstruction procedure

Subclavian–carotid transposition (Fig. 4.1-11a)

Surgical technique

The transposition operation is particularly suitable for the treatment of subclavian artery occlusions. The right or left subclavian artery is transposed to the ipsilateral common carotid artery and sutured end to side, without using an autologous or alloplastic vascular replacement. Access is obtained via a 4-cm long transverse incision above the sternoclavicular joint, with the insertions of the sternocleidomastoid and anterior scalene muscles being temporarily transected. The central vascular stump is closed blindly and the distal subclavian stump is positioned medially, in a cranial direction, to the common carotid artery. When there is substantial atherosclerosis in the donor or recipient vessel, it may in some cases also be necessary to carry out a local thromboendarterectomy or eversion endarterectomy in the subclavian artery.

Technical and clinical results

The good long-term results and low complication rates with the procedure make the subclavian–carotid transposition the surgical treatment of choice today for occlusions of the subclavian artery near its origin. The Düsseldorf research group reported in 1994 on the results in 116 patients with a mean age of 59 who all underwent this type of transposition operation. An ipsilateral thromboendar-

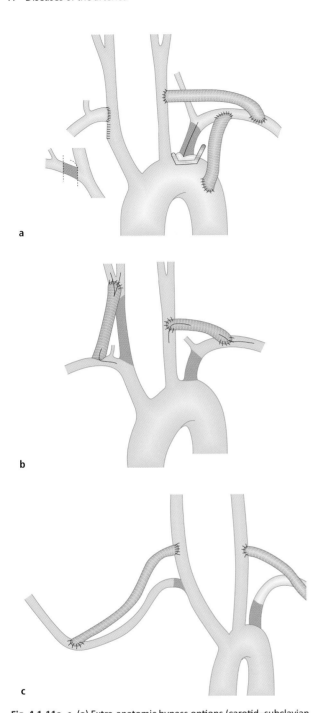

Fig. 4.1-11a–c (**a**) Extra-anatomic bypass options (carotid–subclavian bypass, aorta–subclavian bypass) and free transposition of the subclavian artery onto the common carotid artery. (**b**) Examples of carotid–subclavian and subclavian–carotid bypasses. (**c**) Positioning of bilateral carotid–subclavian bypasses.

Table 4.1-3 Results in 172 patients with isolated atherosclerotic lesions at the origin of the subclavian artery who were treated at the Center for Cardiovascular and Respiratory Sciences at the West Virginia University between 1993 and 2006.

	Carotid–subclavian bypass (PTFE) n = 51	Angioplasty n = 121
Mean follow-up	7.7 years	3.4 years
Primary technical success	100%	98%
Complications	5.9% — 2 phrenic nerve lesions — 1 myocardial infarction	5.9% — 4 emboli — 1 reperfusion edema — 1 false aneurysm — 1 cardiac insufficiency
Primary patency rates after 1, 3, and 5 years	100%, 98%, 96%	93%, 78%, 70%

tient had an occlusion. The results from the Division of Vascular Surgery at McMaster University in Hamilton, Ontario, where 27 transposition operations were carried out between 1990 and 2001, showed no stenoses or occlusions after 25 ± 21 months. Endarterectomy was carried out in the carotid artery in 12 patients, in the subclavian artery in seven, and in the vertebral arteries in six. The same group also reviewed the results for 516 patients who underwent carotid–subclavian bypass and 511 who received subclavian–carotid transplantation reported in the literature between 1966 and 2000. After a mean follow-up period of 59 ± 17 months, the patency rate was clearly superior for transposition (98%) in comparison with the bypass operation (84%).

Bypass procedures

Carotid–subclavian bypass (Fig. 4.1-11a, b)

Surgical technique

Placement of a bypass between the easily accessible common carotid artery and the supraclavicular or infraclavicular subclavian artery is a preferred reconstruction principle in single occlusive processes in the area of the origin of the subclavian artery. However, a prerequisite for this is the presence of a freely patent donor artery in the cervical or shoulder area. Clamping off the common carotid artery in particular is associated with an increased risk of stroke events. Prior atherosclerotic damage to the carotid artery therefore plays an important part in patient selection and in the surgical procedure. Stenoses or occlusions located distally or proximally that might have an unfavorable influence on the surgical result also need to be taken into account. In many patients, thromboendarterectomy of the common carotid artery or distal subclavian artery is therefore carried out in addition to creating the bypass. Autologous grafts (mainly from the great saphenous vein) or allogenic grafts can be used to bypass the occluded area. When the subclavian artery has a diameter of 5 mm or less, venous bypass is preferable to a vascular prosthesis made of Dacron or expanded polytetrafluoroethylene (ePTFE).

terectomy at the carotid bifurcation was also carried out in 33.6%, and an open thromboendarterectomy of the second segment of the subclavian artery and/or vertebral artery in 19%. Three patients died perioperatively (due to cardiac infarction or stroke), and early thrombotic occlusions occurred postoperatively in a further four patients, in three of whom patency was successfully restored again. In 70 patients who were followed up for a period of 59 ± 42 months, medium-grade stenoses were seen in two patients and a third pa-

Technical and clinical results

Comparison of angioplasty with surgical correction using a carotid–subclavian bypass is not entirely justified, since the two techniques have different indications, as mentioned earlier. However, interventional treatment should not be done at excessive risk, as the bypass operation has good long-term results with a comparatively low complication rate.

Endarterectomy procedures

Open thromboendarterectomy (TEA)

This requires exposure of the subclavian or axillary artery, with an osteotomy of the clavicle:

- After vascular control is established by placing atraumatic vascular clamps cranial and caudal to the occluded segment, the artery is opened longitudinally using a vascular scalpel or Potts scissors.
- This is followed by complete removal of the occlusive plaque using a vascular spatula under visual control. Any intimal edges at the distal removal point have to be avoided, due to the risk of dissection after flow is re-established, with subsequent thrombotic occlusion of the reconstructed vessel; edges may need to be tacked down using interrupted or continuous sutures.
- Closure of the longitudinal arteriotomy is carried out by suturing in a strip of autologous vein (usually from the distal great saphenous vein).
- After placement of Redon drains and re-approximation of the clavicle, the surgical wound is closed layer by layer.

Semi-closed TEA (annular endarterectomy)

The subclavian artery and axillary artery are exposed as described above:

- After vascular control is established (with vascular clamps on the subclavian, axillary, and thoracoacromial arteries), one longitudinal arteriotomy each, approximately 1.5–2.0 cm long, is made on the surface of the subclavian artery and axillary artery.
- The occlusive plaque is then detached and transected at its distal end (at the axillary artery) and threaded using a ring stripper with the correct luminal size. With slight pressure and spiral dissection, the occlusive plaque can now be removed through a suitable layer as far as the central arteriotomy, where it can be detached leaving a smooth edge.
- If a residual distal intimal edge remains, it may need to be tacked. As intimal flaps left in the area of the endarterectomized vascular segment can lead to recurrent occlusion (i.e., need to be removed), checking of the intravascular lumen (endoscopically or arteriographically) is critically important.
- Closure of the two arteriotomies is carried out by suturing in a venous patch (from the distal great saphenous vein). After placement of Redon drains, the surgical wounds are closed layer by layer.

Axilloaxillary bypass

Surgical technique

This procedure represents a technically simple extra-anatomic variant for correcting unilateral occlusions or stenoses of the subclavian artery. The donor and recipient arteries are located via an infraclavicular transverse incision, a side-to-end anastomosis is carried out, and the graft has a subfascial and prepectoral course. Allogenic prostheses are preferred as the bypass material, because of the better long-term results in comparison with a venous bypass.

Technical and clinical results

Extra-anatomic revascularization procedures are inferior to orthotopic reconstructions in the long term. There are therefore only very few current indications for this type of bypass—such as Takayasu aortitis with involvement of the proximal segments of the supra-aortic arteries. A follow-up study of 10 patients at Oxford University showed a patency rate of 75% after 12–24 months.

Acute occlusive processes

Indication for surgery

Surgery is indicated for practically all acute occlusions of the central arteries (subclavian, axillary, and brachial arteries), which are usually due to embolism. Exceptions include:

- Patients at high surgical risk, with reduced general operability and incomplete ischemia
- Patients with compensated occlusion and no impairment

As these are usually ill patients in poor general condition, the extent and duration of the surgical procedure need to be minimized.

Surgical procedure

The surgical procedure of choice is indirect embolectomy, with the patient in the dorsal decubitus position with the extremity to be operated on lying free on an arm table, with local anesthesia if possible.

Incision, preparation, and surgical procedure

Transcubital retrograde flow thrombectomy (brachial artery, axillary artery, subclavian artery) or antegrade flow thrombectomy (lower arm arteries) using Fogarty balloon catheters or with ring strippers of various sizes for thrombi that are adherent to the walls.

- Skin incision, 5–10 cm straight or S-shaped, in the area of the inside of the elbow, transection of the subcutaneous layer while protecting the veins that course there (the cephalic vein and basilic vein), and division of the tendon of the biceps muscle (*caution:* possible injury to the median nerve). The brachial artery is exposed, including its division into the lower arm arteries. Transverse arteriotomy of the brachial artery approximately 2 cm cranial to where it branches (or longitudinal arteriotomy if there are arteriosclerotic lesions).
- Retrograde thrombectomy of the central arteries (brachial artery, axillary artery, subclavian artery)—with digital compression of the common carotid artery on the right side to prevent embolization toward the brain—with appropriately sized balloon catheters until no more thrombus can be removed and strong pulsatile flow from the cranial side starts.

- After restoration of blood flow, checking of the inflow and out-flow is useful (with intra-arterial catheter angiography of the central arteries) to identify residual thrombi or iatrogenic vascular lesions (dissection, perforation, arteriovenous fistula) or a central aneurysm (as the cause of the embolism) and correct these in the same session.
- After a heparin–saline solution has been introduced into the thrombectomized arteries, closure of the transverse arteriotomy with a direct suture (with a longitudinal arteriotomy, a venous strip is sutured in) with a 6–0 monofilament thread.
- Acute central occlusions in the area of the axillary artery or subclavian artery that cannot be removed either with a balloon or a ring are an indication for graft reconstruction (e.g., carotid–subclavian bypass or carotid–axillary bypass). Distal embolization (aneurysm, dissection) is prevented by ligating the axillary artery before a bypass is carried out.

Risks and complications

The most frequent complication is recurrent occlusion, with an amputation rate of 4%. The causes include:

- Incomplete thrombectomy, with central or peripheral residual thrombi
- Untreated aneurysm
- Overlooked dissection
- Iatrogenic vascular lesion (mechanical damage to the endothelium, arterial spasm, perforation with subsequent arterial thrombosis)
- Absent run-off due to obstruction of the capillary bloodstream—e.g., in reperfusion damage with endothelial swelling or in compartment syndrome (for which immediate fasciotomy is required) after protracted ischemia
- Recurrent embolism
- Arterial thrombosis in a vessel with previous damage—e.g., in thoracic outlet syndrome (TOS) or in inflammatory or atherosclerotic wall lesions

By contrast, postoperative hemorrhage and local wound infections are rare events (in less than 1% of operated patients) and usually do not lead to any permanent damage if treated appropriately.

Postoperative follow-up

- Prevention of Haimovici–Legrain–Cormier syndrome (reperfusion damage with ischemic myopathy, myoglobulinuria, hyperkalemia, and acidosis) → checking and correction of any fluid-electrolyte imbalance, as well as renal and cardiac function.
- Prevention of recurrent occlusion → heparinization (low-molecular-weight heparin adjusted to weight, s.c.) immediately postoperatively, and possibly warfarin (Coumadin®) starting on the third postoperative day.

References

AbuRahma AF, Bates MC, Stone PA, Dyer B, Armistead L, Scott Dean L, Scott Lavigne P. Angioplasty and stenting versus carotid-subclavian bypass for the treatment of isolated subclavian artery disease. J Endovasc Ther 2007; 14: 698–704.

Baguneid M, Dodd D, Fulford P, Hadjilucas Y, Bukhari M, Griffiths G, Chalmers G, Walker M. Management of acute nontraumatic upper limb ischemia. Angiology 1999; 50: 715–20.

Cinà CS, Safar HA, Laganà A, Arena G, Clase CM. Subclavian carotid transposition and bypass grafting: consecutive cohort study and systematic review. J Vasc Surg 2002 Mar; 35: 422–9.

Duber C, Klose KJ, Kopp H, Schild H, Hake U. Angioplasty of the subclavian artery. The technique, early and late results. Dtsch Med Wochenschr 1989; 114: 496–502.

Halpin DP, Moran KT, Jewell ER. Arm ischemia secondary to giant cell arteritis. Ann Vasc Surg 1988; 2: 381–4.

Kniemeyer HW, Deich S, Grabitz K, Torsello G, Sandmann W. Subclavian-carotid transposition—experience in the treatment of arteriosclerotic lesions of the carotid artery near its origin. Zentralbl Chir 1994; 119: 109–14.

Kretschmer G, Teleky B, Mirosi L, Wagner O, Wunderlich M, Karnel F, Jantsch H, Schemper M, Polterauer P. Obliterations of the proximal subclavian artery: to bypass or to anastomose? J Cardiovasc Surg 1991; 32: 334–9.

Laperche T, Laurian C, Roudat R, Steg PG. Mobile thromboses of the aortic arch without aortic debris. A transesophageal echocardiographic finding associated with unexplained arterial embolism. Circulation 1997; 96: 288–94.

Mieno S, Horimoto H, Arishiro K, Negoro N, Hoshiga M, Ishihara T, Hanafusa T, Sasaki S. Axillo-axillary bypass for in-stent restenosis in Takayasu arteritis. Int J Cardiol 2004; 94: 131–2.

Nehler MR, Taylor LM, Moneta GL, Porter JM. Upper extremity ischemia from subclavian artery aneurysm caused by bony abnormalities of the thoracic outlet. Arch Surg 1997; 132: 527–32.

Perkins JM, Magee TR, Hands LJ, Collin J, Morris PJ. The long-term outcome after axillo-axillary bypass grafting for proximal subclavian artery disease. Eur J Vasc Endovasc Surg 2000; 19: 52–5.

Rosenthal D, Ellison RG, Clark MD, Lamis PA, Stanton PE, Codner MA, Daniel WW, Axilloaxillary bypass: is it worthwhile? J Cardiovasc Surg 1988; 29: 191–5.

Sixt S, Rastan A, Schwarzwälder U, Schwarz T, Frank U, Müller C, Pochert V, Bürgelin K, Gremmelmaier D, Branzan D, Hauswald K, Neumann FJ, Zeller T. Long term outcome after balloon angioplasty and stenting of subclavian artery obstruction: a single centre experience. VASA 2008; 37: 174–82.

Thompson RW, Petrinec D, Toursarkissian B. Surgical treatment of thoracic outlet compression syndromes. Supraclavicular exploration and vascular reconstruction. Ann Vasc Surg 1997; 11: 442–51.

Zeller T, Frank U, Bürgelin K, Sinn L, Horn B, Roskamm H. Treatment of an acute thrombotic occlusion of a subclavian artery with a new rotational thrombectomy device. J Endovasc Ther 2002; 9: 917–21.

Zeller T, Koch HK, Frank U, Bürgelin K, Schwarzwälder U, Müller C, Neumann FJ. Histological verification of non-specific aorta-arteritis (Takayasu's arteritis) using percutaneous transluminal atherectomy. VASA 2004; 33: 247–51.

4.2 Creation of dialysis fistulas and treatment of dialysis shunt insufficiency

Georg Nowak
Doppler/duplex ultrasonography: Tom Schilling
Endovascular therapy: Thomas Zeller

4.2.1 Introduction

The increased morbidity (such as diabetes and hypertension) associated with demographic changes has also led to a marked increase in the need for dialysis access operations. This is also reflected in the increasing numbers of publications on the topic. The expectations of all those involved—the patient, nephrologist, and surgeon—are high. The patient expects undisturbed long-term function; the nephrologist expects a high flow volume, with a puncture segment that is as long as possible; and the surgeon expects suitable vessels. Over time the need for frequent shunt revisions should be accepted. This becomes increasingly difficult, and revision procedures now make up the major proportion of everyday dialysis access surgery.

4.2.2 Shunt creation

Basically, the following types of dialysis access are normally used:

- Arteriovenous fistula (Brescia–Cimino)
- Arteriovenous bridging graft (with PTFE or biological materials)
- Catheters (Shaldon, Perm)
- Peritoneal dialysis

The first access is usually obtained with an arteriovenous fistula near the wrist or at the elbow. These autologous fistulas are certainly best with regard to their duration of function and susceptibility to complications. The primary patency rates after 2 years are 60–80%.

Since the 1970s, polytetrafluoroethylene (PTFE) bridging grafts have ensured that access is still possible when all of the veins have been exhausted as puncture segments. PTFE grafts have unlimited availability, but are second choice in view of their susceptibility to complications (e.g., with the risk of infection or shunt thrombosis). The patency rates after 2 years are approximately 30–40%.

Catheter-based access is unavoidable when dialysis is urgently indicated, but for long-term access they are limited to only a few indications, as central venous outflow obstructions often result (with reported frequencies of 2–29%).

Peritoneal dialysis (PD) can be used as a chronic outpatient method (continuous ambulatory peritoneal dialysis, CAPD) or as an automatic procedure (APD). PD represents some 5% of all dialysis procedures.

4.2.2.1 Preparation for surgery

Arterial inflow

The quality of inflow is tested using *Allen's test*. After the pulse has been suppressed near the wrist, the patient is asked to close the fist tightly several times. The hand becomes pale. One of the two arteries is then released, and the skin color is assessed. The test is then repeated with the other artery. When there is prompt arterial filling in both cases, the test result is "unremarkable"; otherwise, the result is described as "pathological" and prompts further diagnostic workup, initially with color duplex ultrasonography. The diameter of the radial artery should be more than 2 mm, as satisfactory shunt development is otherwise unlikely.

Contrast administration is contraindicated when there is residual renal function.

Venous outflow

The arm that has the more suitable veins should be selected as the shunt arm. Generally, the choice is the nondominant arm; however, if previous puncture procedures and indwelling cannulas have made the potential puncture segment unusable, the dominant arm is chosen.

The patient should be asked whether he or she has had any central indwelling catheters placed, as these may lead to central venous outflow obstructions.

The central venous segments are only partly visible with color duplex ultrasonography, so that if there are indirect signs of central flow obstruction, either magnetic resonance venography or conventional venography is indicated. It should be mentioned here that nephrogenic systemic fibrosis is a possible severe side effect if gadolinium is used in renal failure.

Anesthesia

A distinction needs to be made between anesthetic procedures used for initial placement and those used for shunt revisions. Initial placements at the wrist and elbow can be achieved without problems under local anesthesia. The site and extent of the procedure are familiar and usually hold no surprises.

Revision procedures are different. While local anesthesia is sufficient for thrombectomy and for any intraoperative dilation that may be required, general anesthesia is preferable if there have already been earlier revisions in the region or a possible "change of level" of intervention is required.

4.2.2.2 The arteriovenous fistula

Cimino fistula

The AV fistula is created near the wrist using a side-to-end anastomosis:

- As a radiocephalic fistula on the distal lower arm, or
- At the level of the elbow
- As a basilic vein transposition
- Additional variants: anatomic snuffbox fistula, ulnar fistula

Wrist

The incision runs slightly obliquely over the distal radius toward the radial styloid process; this allows exposure of sufficient lengths of both the cephalic vein and the radial artery. An adequate length of the cephalic vein is carefully mobilized, ligated distally, and transected. Instilling a blood–heparin–saline mixture provides information about possible outflow obstructions. With obstruction of the vein near the inside of the elbow, careful dilation can be carried out:

the use of a Fogarty catheter leads to serious and irreversible intimal lesions. Finally, a sufficient length of the radial artery is exposed, mobilized proximally and distally in the usual way, and occluded with soft bulldog clamps. The longitudinal incision is approximately 8–10 mm long. Here again, an injection with heparin–saline is carried out in both vascular limbs. Inflow can be tested again in the opened vessel. Instilling a heparin–saline solution via a glass flask syringe also gives an impression of the inflow quality.

The vein is now anastomosed side to end with the artery, using a monofilament nonresorbable double-reinforced 7–0 suture. Slight external rotation of the vein can prevent torsion near the anastomosis. Before the final tying of the sutures, blood flow is released by opening the individual clamps so that any thrombi present are rinsed out and the suture has an opportunity to expand. The venous limb is released last in order to prevent thrombi from passing into the vein. A palpable thrill above the shunt is a sign that the flow volume is good.

A pulsating shunt means there is an outflow problem, and the possible causes need to be identified:

- Thrombus
- Torsion
- Higher-level fibrotic segment

The primary patency rate with autologous fistulas is 60–80% after 2 years and 50% after 5 years.

Inside of the elbow

A side-to-end connection between the brachial artery and the cephalic vein is created. The anastomosis has to be smaller than that used at the wrist level (4–6 mm), as a steal phenomenon may arise as the shunt develops.

Basilic vein transposition

The vein is exposed above the medial epicondyle on the outstretched arm and an adequate length is also dissected distally, as the transposition to the ventral surface of the upper arm requires a sufficient surplus length of vein. Via a long skin incision along the medial upper arm, the vein is released from all of its branches, using ligatures, as far as the axillary confluence. Any fibers of the antebrachial cutaneous nerve that cross it must be protected. After distal transection, the vein is then led subcutaneously on the ventral side of the upper arm using a tunneling device at the free end, and is anastomosed to the artery without tension. Torsion and kinking must be avoided at all costs during this pull-through procedure.

In some centers, the basilic vein is left on the inner side of the upper arm after dissection. The transposition is only carried out over the fascia, which is then re-closed.

PTFE bridging graft

If the veins available for shunt surgery have been exhausted, PTFE is almost exclusively used as a substitute. Prostheses with normal walls and a diameter of 6–8 mm are used. Thin-walled prostheses are too easily damaged during the expected revisions (e.g., due to sutures cutting into them), and normal-walled prostheses are therefore preferable.

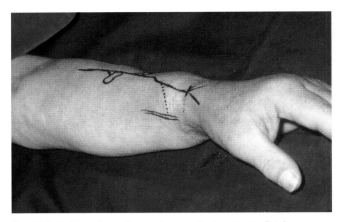

Fig. 4.2-1 Outlines drawn for creating a radioulnar Cimino fistula.

PTFE can be used in the lower arm as a straight or looped graft. Straight grafts are used for arterial inflow from the brachial artery to the preserved cephalic vein, which serves as the puncture segment. If both lower arm vessels are no longer usable, a PTFE loop with an anastomosis slightly above the inside elbow is used. One or two auxiliary incisions are needed on the distal lower arm on the inside of the elbow, through which the prosthesis is pulled. In the upper arm, a semi-loop can be created similarly between the brachial artery and the axillary vein. The puncture segment then runs along the ventral surface of the upper arm. If there is obesity in the upper arm, it should be ensured that the shunt is easily palpated, as the puncture procedure is more difficult if the course in the subcutaneous adipose tissue is too deep, and complications can be expected to result. When a revision is required, arterial inflow into the prosthesis limb is usually preserved, and an extension to the subclavian vein that is easily accessible on the ventral surface of the upper arm can be carried out.

A healing period of 14 days should be allowed before the first puncture.

Drug prophylaxis

There is evidence that administering acetylsalicylic acid has a favorable effect on the patency rate in arteriovenous fistulas and shunts. The dosages described in the relevant (Cochrane) meta-analysis are in the range of 160–500 mg/d.

4.2.3   Alternative dialysis procedures

4.2.3.1   Catheter dialysis

The principal indications for catheter placement are:
- Immediate need for dialysis
- As a bridging measure along with the first creation of a fistula
- When recovery of renal function is possible
- When there is borderline compensated cardiac insufficiency contraindicating the creation of a fistula

The following options are available:
- A single-lumen central venous catheter (Shaldon)
- An atrial catheter (Demers, Perm) with a tunneled subcutaneous course

Shaldon catheter

The two usual routes for placement of a Shaldon catheter are either via the internal jugular vein or via the subclavian vein. Access via the femoral vein is in most cases a route reserved for emergency indications. In sterile conditions and with local anesthesia, the catheter is introduced using the Seldinger technique. Positioning is carried out using fluoroscopic guidance. After puncture of the subclavian artery, a chest x-ray is obligatory in order to exclude pneumothorax. The puncture procedure itself may be easier with ultrasound assistance.

Demers catheter

In contrast to the Shaldon catheter, the atrial catheter has a plastic cuff that grows in when it is placed in the subcutaneous tissue near the catheter's exit point. The cuff provides resistance against ascending infections. The catheter can be introduced using the Seldinger technique or surgically.

In the surgical procedure, the relevant side of the neck is generously covered; boundaries formed by the earlobe, upper edge of the nipple, sternocleidomastoid muscle, and edge of the lower jaw should be visible. Local anesthesia is applied in the triangle between the insertions of the sternocleidomastoid muscle and the clavicle. A transverse skin incision 3–4 cm long between the two ends of the sternocleidomastoid muscle approximately 1–2 cm cranial to the clavicle provides adequate visualization of the internal jugular vein. An experienced surgeon can clamp the vein laterally or tunnel under it and snare it. A purse-string suture with a diameter of 5 mm is placed with a 5–0 monofilament thread. After a stab incision, the catheter can be introduced into the middle of the purse-string suture, in a proximal direction under radiographic guidance. The plastic sleeve is placed via the specially created tunnel in such a way that it can be easily released from the surrounding tissue under local anesthesia when the catheter is removed.

The tunnel should be created along the planned course of the catheter approximately 5–8 cm infraclavicularly, using a separate small incision. After correct placement in the atrium under fluoroscopic guidance, the catheter is filled with heparin, depending on its length and caliber, in accordance with the accompanying instructions. The heparin filling is withdrawn before dialysis.

4.2.3.2 Peritoneal dialysis (PD)

This alternative method is administered as a continuous ambulatory procedure (CAPD) or automated procedure (APD).
Indications:
- Patient's preference (for reasons of independence from the institution and quality of life)
- Cerebrovascular comorbidities
- Childhood dialysis
- Access problems due to surgical anatomy

Contraindications:
- Inflammatory bowel diseases
- Diverticular disease
- Abdominal adhesions
- Hernias
- Severe pulmonary diseases

Potential complications:
- Peritonitis
- Hernias (due to increased intra-abdominal pressure)

4.2.4 Dialysis shunt insufficiency

Frequent causes of shunt thrombosis and occlusion are:
- Stenoses near the anastomosis (myointimal hyperplasia usually occurs at venous anastomoses), with inadequate flow volume and increased recirculation
- Inadequate maturation after placement (unsuitable vessels, flow volume < 400 mL/min)
- Central venous stenoses after central venous catheter placement
- Stenosis or occlusion in the afferent arterial bloodstream
- Reduced blood pressure after major surgery

4.2.4.1 Diagnosis

A shunt that is still functional but is not providing adequate supply (a "failing shunt") can be identified with careful monitoring during the regular dialysis procedure before a sudden shunt occlusion develops. Simple monitoring measures include:
- Palpation and auscultation (thrill or only pulsation of the shunt; stenosal bruit)
- Observation of increased recirculation, increased venous outflow pressure

Color Duplex ultrasound allows simple noninvasive diagnosis of the location of the stenosis and precise planning of access for radiographic imaging in preparation for PTA.

Doppler/duplex ultrasonography

Examination technique

A 5.0–7.5 MHz (–10 MHz) sector scanner is used. If there is no definite local problem, the examination is carried out from the aortic origin of the afferent arteries up to the opening of the draining vein into the brachiocephalic vein. Optimally, the scanner should follow the path of the bloodstream → low application pressure with the scanner to avoid compressing the venous shunt segment. *Caution:* there are often septal stenoses that escape angiographic imaging → duplex ultrasonography has greater sensitivity here. The PRF has to be varied, as there are widely alternating flow velocities in various areas → imaging of the distal fistula arteries as well (obligatory if there is any suspicion of steal phenomenon with acral perfusion disturbances).

Specific findings

General characteristics

The shunt is a special form of arteriovenous fistula and has the corresponding classic duplex ultrasound characteristics:
- Continuous systolic–diastolic flow with high end-diastolic flow in the afferent fistula providing artery (sides should be compared).
- Perivascular tissue vibrations at the site of the fistula, particularly systolic (confetti phenomenon—the color display should be adjusted to high flow).

■ High flow and turbulence, with arterialization of the efferent vein, with wall fluttering in the inflow area.
■ Meanderings and dilations in the proximal fistula draining vein.

Measurement of shunt volume

V_{mean} × corresponding cross-sectional area × heart rate = shunt minute volume

Where and when to measure—what are the problems?
■ **Proximal fistula providing artery:**
  – If the distal fistula providing artery volume is disregarded:
    – Perfusion of the distal fistula providing artery may overestimate the volume.
    – Older secondary shunts may still be patent.
  – Or measuring the difference from the contralateral side:
    – Is the contralateral side regular? Are there any stenoses?
    – "Age" of a shunt that is still perfused on the contralateral side?
  – Or before/after fistula compression:
    – Completely compressed?
    – Postocclusive hyperemia?
■ **Difference between the proximal and distal fistula providing artery:**
  – Assessment is difficult due to turbulences near the anastomosis.
  – Not valid with steal phenomenon.
■ **Proximal fistula draining vein:**
  – Proximal the origin of side branches: occasional branches originating near anastomoses can make measurement more difficult.
  – In a straight segment with a normal caliber:
    – There are often huge lumen variations.
    – This can lead to a mismatch between the area and the assigned spectrum.
  – Outside of turbulences—laminar flow.
    – Occasionally difficult to observe due to the short anastomosis—luminal variation—side branch distance.
  – The optimal imaging point can therefore vary individually.
Measurement of V_{mean}: planimetry of the hemotachogram and integration of the Doppler spectrum (area under the curve) allows measurement of V_{mean} → must absolutely be carried out at the identical area measurement position, since otherwise values that do not correspond will be used for the calculation. Sample volumes should be adjusted to the shunt vessel diameter in order to include the entire spectrum → precise angle correction.
Measurement of the cross-sectional area:
1. By measuring the diameter and using the formula for the area of a circle, $A = \pi/4 \, d^2$
2. Using cross-sectional planimetry

Potential errors:
■ The venous cross-section is often not ideally circular.
■ Compression of the venous shunt segment.
■ Pulse-synchronous luminal variation, particularly in veins—planimetry should be carried out in mid-cycle in the veins.

Criteria for dialysis shunts (adapted from Thalhammer et al. 2007)

Preoperative requirements:
■ Absence of arteriovenous flow obstructions as far as the mediastinal area
■ Arterial diameter (radial artery) > 2.0 mm (shunt thrombosis rate 45% when < 1.5 mm)
■ Arterial inflow > 50 cm/s
■ Venous diameter (cephalic vein/basilar vein) and depth of the venous layer > 2.5 mm (< 2.5 mm reduces the rate of shunt development)
■ Venous diameter after stasis > 2.5 mm
■ Venous outflow shows respiratory/cardiac modulation

Shunt maturity:
■ Adequate dialysis is possible with a venous diameter of:
  – > 4 mm in 89% of cases
  – < 4 mm in only 44% of cases
■ Adequate dialysis is possible with flow volumes:
  – > 500 mL/min in 84% of cases
  – < 500 mL/min in only 43% of cases
■ Problems with insufficient shunt maturity usually involve:
  – Venous outflow obstruction (42%)
  – Anastomotic stenosis (34%)

Optimal shunt:
■ Flow volume approx. 600 mL/min
■ Vein a maximum of 6 mm under the skin surface
■ Minimum diameter of vein 6 mm
■ Latency for placement of the AV fistula > 6 months, with an AV graft > 6 weeks

Shunt volume:
■ Normal values:
  – Polytetrafluoroethylene (PTFE) fistulas: 614 ± 242 mL/min
  – Cimino–Brescia fistula: 464 ± 199 mL/min
  – Average shunt volume: 514 mL/min
■ Shunt insufficiency below 300 mL/min
■ Risk of shunt occlusion 40% at below 500 mL/min
■ Risk of shunt occlusion > 50% at below 300 mL/min

Shunt stenosis:
■ General:
  – Increased pulsatility in inflow
  – Reduced pulsatility in outflow
  – Reduced flow volume
  – B-mode image showing luminal reduction
  – Aliasing, acoustics
■ Arterial: PVR > 2
■ Anastomosis: PVR vs. prestenotic > 3 detects stenosis of more than 50%
■ Shunt prosthesis:
  – PVR 2.0–2.9: 50–74% stenosis
  – PVR > 3: > 75% stenosis
■ Venous:
  – PVR vs. prestenotic > 3
  – Collaterals

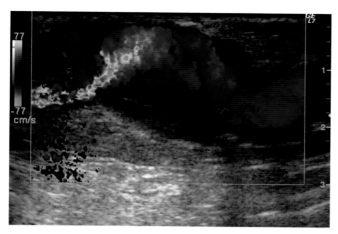

Fig. 4.2-2 Shunt stenosis: classic aliasing on color duplex ultrasound despite maximum PRF, with confetti phenomenon and inflow of the flow jet from the stenosis into an ectatic shunt segment with slight thrombosis at the margins.

Steal phenomenon:

- Occurs in up to 8% of cases
- Particularly in high-capacity upper arm shunts
- Criteria:
  - Typical clinical symptoms
  - + Retrograde arterial flow distal to the shunt (often asymptomatic)
  - + Regular arterial inflow
  - + Improved capillary filling and/or oscillography during shunt compression

Hypercapacity shunt:

- Shunt volume > 1000 mL/min in patients with cardiac disease
- Shunt volume > (1000–) 1500 mL/min or over 20–30% of heart minute volume, even in those with healthy hearts, leads to:
  - Left ventricular (LV) hypertrophy
  - LV dilation
  - Cardiac insufficiency

4.2.4.2   Shunt occlusion and shunt stenosis

In cases of occlusion, the cause of the shunt thrombosis cannot be diagnosed with primary imaging methods. There are then basically two approaches available:

- Lysis and subsequent percutaneous intervention (PTA/stent)
- Catheter thrombectomy with intraoperative angioplasty or immediate postoperative angioplasty.

Endovascular therapy

Local infiltration thrombolysis using a Cragg–McNamara side hole catheter that is introduced either proximally (arterial) or distally (venous). This is most safely done with ultrasound guidance. Infusion for a period of 1–2 h with:

- Streptokinase: 100,000 U/30 mL/30 min/30 cm, maximum dosage 250,000 U
- Urokinase: 50,000 units/300 mL NaCl/30 min/30 cm, maximum dosage 200,000 U

- Recombinant tissue plasminogen activator (rt-PA): 10 mg/10 mL solvent/10 min/30 cm, maximum dosage 20 mg (Brittinger method)

Contraindications

- Surgery < 10 days previously
- Gastrointestinal bleeding < 10 days previously
- Known coagulation disturbances
- History of cerebral bleeding

After thrombolysis, a venous stricture is usually revealed as the cause of the occlusion and has to be treated either endovascularly or surgically.

Alternatives to local thrombolysis include a mechanical thrombectomy catheter. In Europe, the catheters most often used are the Rotarex® (shunt prosthesis) and Aspirex® (venous dialysis fistula), while in the United States it is mainly the Angiojet® catheter that is used.

Use of a Cutting Balloon™ (Boston Scientific; Fig. 4.2.3a) has proved valuable in smaller single-center series in the treatment of shunt stenoses, which are usually scared and inelastic. The atherotomes attached to the balloon surface are used to cut through venous strictures, which often cannot be dilated using conventional balloon catheters, thereby reducing the vessel's resistance to dilation. This ensures both primary treatment success—i.e., the vessel becomes dilatable—as well as prevents early elastic recoil. Cutting Balloon angioplasty is also much less painful than dilation using traditional high-pressure balloon catheters. It is important to use a Cutting Balloon that is undersized by 1–2 mm (5–6 mm), in order to avoid perforating the vessel wall. In a second step, a balloon with an appropriate size for the vessel caliber can then be used for subsequent dilation. In centrally located stenoses, the use of self-expanding nitinol stents has proved valuable if the results of the initial dilation are inadequate (Fig. 4.2-3b, c). If recurrent stenoses develop in the stent, several stent-in-stent implantations can maintain shunt function, sometimes for several years (Fig. 4.2-3d, e).

The use of endoprostheses (Fluency®, Bard; Viabahn®, Gore) has proved to be more sustainable than balloon angioplasty alone. The endoprosthesis is used for extended coverage of both stenotic and ectatic shunt areas. The shunt can then be used for dialysis again immediately after the intervention; no major complications of needle puncture of the endoprostheses have so far been reported (Haskal et al. 2010).

Interventions using drug-coated balloon catheters (either as sole therapy or after previous Cutting Balloon angioplasty) and drug-eluting stents are still experimental.

Surgical treatment

As shunt occlusion is often only identified during preparation for dialysis, the time-frame for clinical treatment appears rather short. In our own practice, the surgical route, usually with local anesthesia, is therefore preferred.

Combined procedure

This requires radiographic equipment in the operating room allowing the road-map technique to be used.

The transverse incision must not be too close to the suspected location of the stenosis, as the segment available would not then be

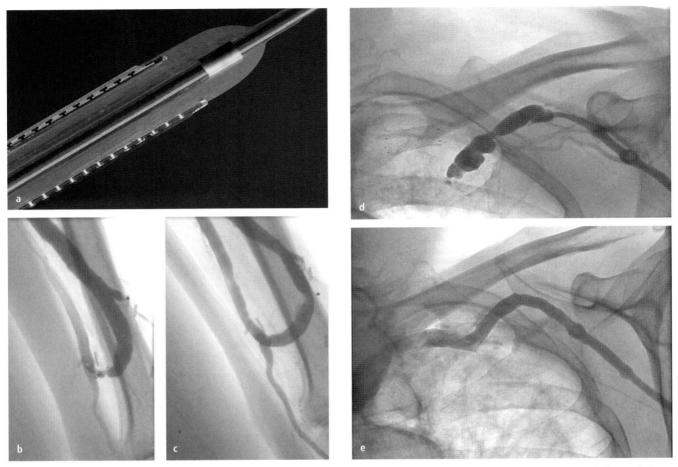

Fig. 4.2-3a–e (a) A Cutting Balloon with four longitudinally attached atherotomes. **(b, c)** A Cimino fistula stenosis near the anastomoses before and after Cutting Balloon™ angioplasty. **(d, e)** Occlusion of a shunt-draining basilic vein before and after stent angioplasty.

sufficient for good balloon placement. After thrombectomy with a Fogarty catheter, a 5F sheath can be introduced through the transverse incision. In short stenoses, a 6 mm/2 cm balloon can be used; in longer stenoses, balloons 4 cm long can be used. The inflation pressure is 8–25 atm (approx. 810–2533 kPa), and the duration of inflation is approximately 1 min. If the stenosis is not accessible to interventional therapy due to its morphology, the following surgical options are still possible:

- Lengthening of the venous outflow segment in a proximal direction (possibly with a prosthetic bridging graft)
- Anastomotic patch plasty (either autologous or alloplastic)

4.2.4.3 Central venous stenoses

These stenoses, caused by central venous catheters, cardiac pacemaker leads, or chronic shearing forces, particularly in the area of venous confluences, often remain initially unnoticed. It is only inadequate shunt function, associated with increasing swelling in the shunt arm and a visible collateral circulation that leads to the diagnosis (Figs. 4.2-4 and 4.2-5). It is usually the proximal segments of the subclavian vein, brachiocephalic trunk, and superior vena cava that are affected. If shunt function is maintained, anticoagulation measures can be administered while waiting to see whether adequate collateral outflow develops that would make further treatment steps initially unnecessary. If there is inadequate shunt perfor-

mance or occlusion, then PTA and stent placement, if needed, can be successfully carried out after thrombectomy. However, residual stenoses are frequent and regular checking of the proximal vessels is advisable.

Shunt ligation appears to be the simplest measure, accepting the loss of the shunt; however, this is a required treatment option in only a few cases.

If the external or internal jugular vein are accessible ipsilaterally, the stenosis or occlusion can be bypassed using a PTFE bridging graft. Surgical correction of a central venous obstruction is extremely challenging (e.g., with sternotomy and subclavioatrial diversion). The number of publications on surgical management is correspondingly small. Extra-anatomic diversions to the contralateral subclavian or ipsilateral external iliac vein are an alternative. Arterioarterial shunts (subclavian or femoral artery) have a smaller flow volume, but can be regarded as sufficiently functional for this indication.

4.2.4.4 Other dysfunctions

The following types of dysfunction can also be regarded as representing shunt insufficiency in the broader sense:

- Peripheral arterial ischemia (steal phenomenon)
- Shunt aneurysms
- Shunt infections
- Dysfunction due to central venous stenoses

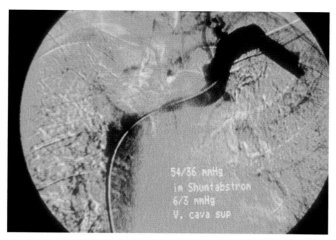

Fig. 4.2-4 Central venous stenosis in the left subclavian vein.

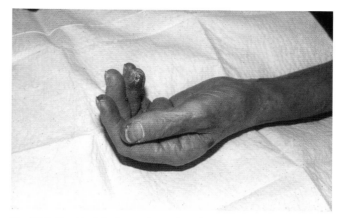

Fig. 4.2-6 Trophic disturbances in steal syndrome.

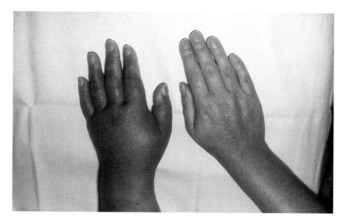

Fig. 4.2-5 Unilateral hand edema in a patient with central inflow congestion.

Steal phenomenon

Peripheral arterial insufficiency is also known as "steal." The term describes the effect of flow reversal in the artery distal to the anastomosis. If the collateral afferent vessels are not capable of compensating for the flow reversal, ischemic pain and trophic disturbances result. A distinction is made between steal phenomenon and the clinically manifest form, known as steal syndrome. Steal is often caused by the anastomosis being made too large, particularly in brachiocephalic anastomoses (Fig. 4.2-6).

The hemodynamic development of an arteriovenous fistula between the radial artery and the cephalic vein shows an increase in flow from 300 mL/min initially to approximately twice that amount after about 1 year. In elbow fistulas, the values are between 800 mL/min initially and approximately 1700–1800 mL/min after 1 year. In PTFE shunts, the progression is smaller; in these cases, there are higher flow rates to begin with and the increase is less marked.

Correction options

As an initial step, the radial artery can be ligated distal to the anastomosis. This changes the side-to-end anastomosis into a functional end-to-end anastomosis. However, this transfers the blood supply to the hand to the ulnar artery exclusively. Close follow-up monitoring is therefore necessary.

Another option is proximal transposition of the arterial anastomosis. This step reduces retrograde blood flow directed toward the anasto-

mosis. This proximal transposition can be carried out by accepting a shortening of the venous puncture segment available, or by implanting a PTFE bridging graft with a high anastomosis to the brachial artery. This eliminates or substantially reduces the "suction effect" of the anastomosis on the peripheral circulation that is threatened with ischemia. In ischemic complications caused by brachiocephalic fistulas with strong flow, it is also possible to interrupt the retrograde collateral flow by simple ligation of the brachial artery immediately distal to the anastomosis. This eliminates the retrograde flow, and an adequate blood supply to the hand is often provided via collaterals.

The distal revascularization and interval ligation (DRIL) procedure is more effective and safer, although it is also more elaborate. With ligation of the brachial artery distal to the anastomosis, a bridging bypass is placed from the central brachial artery to the trifurcation or one of the lower arm arteries. This maintains the shunt function and peripheral perfusion at the same time.

However, other authors consider that proximal transposition of the arterial inflow alone may also be able to relieve the steal problem.

4.2.5 Shunt aneurysms

Uniform distribution of the punctures along the entire course of the vein leads to a homogeneous volume increase along the course of the puncture segment used. Repeated punctures in the same area ("area punctures") can lead to aneurysm formation that may sometimes develop a grotesque appearance.

The presence of this type of dilation alone does not provide an indication for surgery; it is only when flow-obstructing thrombi form in the stagnant zones of the aneurysm and when the skin becomes thinner, with imminent erosion, that correction is indicated. Aneurysms of this type sometimes only form segment by segment. High-grade stenoses may sometimes develop in between, and these require surgical correction, as angioplasty is not successful.

Circumscribed sacculations can be corrected with excision and patch plasty. Extended aneurysms with the formation of stenotic kinks require circular exposure of their entire length. One option for maintaining the autologous shunt involves resective caliber reduction of the aneurysm along its whole length using a Hägar pin. The resection level is then closed with a continuous suture and covered with an external support. The external reinforcement consists of delicate wire netting that covers the entire vein but still allows puncture without difficulty (Biocompound®).

4.2.6 Shunt infection (Fig. 4.2-7)

Infection may become manifest immediately postoperatively or may appear as a consequence of shunt punctures. As dialysis patients are immunodeficient, infection always represents a serious complication, as severe complications (e.g., endocarditis, cerebral septic spread) can rapidly move centrally. Another feared complication is infection-related anastomotic rupture, with substantial blood loss.

If there is no clear evidence of the source of infection in a dialysis patient, it must be assumed that an apparently normal shunt or a catheter placed without irritation is the source—and even more so when a PTFE bridging graft is involved.

Autologous shunts are usually resistant to infections. Along with local measures to provide relief and antibiotic treatment (with vancomycin), tightly monitored efforts to maintain the shunt can be undertaken.

PTFE shunts are much more susceptible to infection. Circumscribed infections in one puncture area may be amenable to local surgical measures; otherwise, aseptic diversion and subsequent resection of the area are necessary.

If bleeding occurs in the context of an infection, shunt ligation is an adequate initial emergency measure. This controls the bleeding and avoids septic spread. If the infection involves the whole length of the bridging graft, prompt explantation is required. The arterial anastomosis is closed with a venous patch. Another shunt placement can only be undertaken once the infection has healed, after an interval of at least 4–6 weeks. In the meantime, catheter access needs to be used. Early shunt ligation must be considered in all cases as the initial option in order to prevent septic spread. Supplementary antibiotic treatment (with vancomycin) of the infection, which is usually caused by staphylococci, is carried out after each dialysis treatment for a period of 10–14 days.

4.2.7 Summary and prospects

It should be clear from this brief review that shunt surgery primarily means surgery for failing shunts. The greatest possible care in the planning and placement of shunts is a fundamental prerequisite for long-term functioning of these "lifelines." The shunt surgeon must be familiar with the wide range of possible variants and should always be thinking ahead to anticipate potential incorrect developments and ways of solving them.

The development of neointimal hyperplasia is a problem that has not yet been solved. Regular monitoring of shunt function must therefore be recommended in order to reduce the numbers of unexpected shunt thromboses. Implantation of endoprostheses has proved its value as the initial measure in the treatment of intima hyperplasia. Treatment approaches that are theoretically causal, such as drug-coated balloon angioplasty, are currently being tested in randomized studies and appear to have considerable potential for the future in the treatment of shunt stenoses.

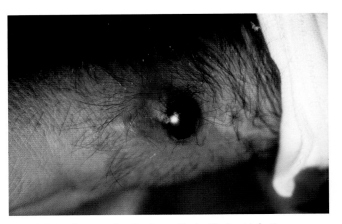

Fig. 4.2-7 Imminent perforation in a patient with shunt infection.

References

Brittinger W-D, Twittenhoff W-D. Anschlussverfahren an die künstliche Niere. Stuttgart, Georg Thieme Verlag, 2005.

Da Silva AF, Escofet X, Rutherford PA. Medical adjuvant treatment to increase patency of arteriovenous fistulae and grafts. Cochrane Database of Systematic Reviews 2003, Issue 2. Art. No.: CD002786. DOI:10.1002/14651858.CD002786.

European Best Practice Guidelines for Anaemia in Patients with Chronic Renal Failure. www.ndt-educational.org/guidelines.asp.

Haskal ZJ, Trerotola S, Dolmatch B, Schuman E, Altman S, Mietling S, Berman S, McLennan G, Trimmer C, Ross J, Vesely T. Stent graft versus balloon angioplasty for failing dialysis-access grafts. N Engl J Med 2010; 362: 494–503.

Haug M, Popescu M. Surgery of arteriovenous interposition grafts. European Surgery 2003 Dez; 35 (6).

Hepp W, Hegenscheid M. Dialyseshunts. Steinkopf-Verlag, 1998.

Kakkos SK, Andrzejewski T, Haddad JA, Haddad GK, Reddy DJ, Nypaver TJ, Scully MM, Schmid DL. Equivalent secondary patency rates of upper extremity Vectra Vascular Access Grafts and transposed brachial-basilic fistulas with aggressive access surveillance and endovascular treatment. Journal of vascular surgery: official publication, the Society for Vascular Surgery [and] International Society for Cardiovascular Surgery 2008; North American Chapter, Vol 47 (2): 407–14.

Krönung G, Kessler M, Klinkner J. Die CO2-Phlebographie vor Erstanlage des Dialysezugangs. Gefäßchirurgie 2007; 12: 179–83.

Maya ID, Weatherspoon J, Young CJ, Barker J, Allon M. Increased risk of infection associated with polyurethane dialysis grafts. Hemodialysis vascular access dysfunction from basic biology to clinical intervention. Seminars in Dialysis 2007; 20 (6): 616–20.

Mickley V. Zentralvenöse Obstruktionen beim Dialysepatienten. Gefäßchirurgie 2007; 12: 161–6.

Roy-Chaudhury P, Kelly BS, Narayana A, Desai P, Melhem M, Munda R, Duncan H, Heffelfinger SC. University of Cincinnati Medical Center, Cincinnati, OH, USA. Adv Ren Replace Ther 2002 Apr; 9 (2): 74–84.

Thalhammer C, Aschwanden M, Staub D, Dickenmann M, Jaeger KA. Duplex sonography of hemodialysis access. Ultraschall Med 2007 Oct; 28 (5):450–65.

Thermann F, Kornhuber M, Brauckhoff M. Dialysefistelassoziiertes Stealsyndrom – Ist ein Erhalt möglich? Gefäßchirurgie 2006; 11: 360–3.

Webb KM, Cull DL, Carsten CG 3rd, Johnson BL, Taylor SM. Outcome of the use of stent grafts to salvage failed arteriovenous accesses. Ann Vasc Surg 2010 Jan; 24 (1): 34–8.

Widmer MK, Uehlinger D, Do DD, Schmidli J. Shuntchirurgie bei Dialysepatienten. Gefäßchirurgie 2008; 13: 135–45.

4.3 Raynaud syndrome

Knut Kröger and Frans Santosa
Endovascular treatment: Christine Espinola-Klein

4.3.1 Introduction

Raynaud syndrome is named after the French physician Maurice Raynaud (1834–1881). In 1862, he described the phenomenon of local symmetrical ischemia in the extremities. Numerous synonyms for the condition are used in the literature, sometimes leading to confusion. Nowadays, it is therefore generally best to distinguish only between primary and secondary Raynaud syndrome.

In comparison with other regions, the circulatory system in the fingers has several peculiarities:

- Good vascular supply
- Variable blood pressure—e.g., during positional changes
- Variable perfusion—e.g., for thermoregulation

The finger arteries originate from the superficial and deep palmar arches. The superficial arch is larger and supplies the second to fifth fingers. According to the autopsy findings described by Coleman and Anson (1961), the superficial arch is fully formed in only 80% of cases, and there are seven different types of branching. The deep arch is complete in 97% of cases. The digital arteries on each side of a finger often have different calibers. In the thumb, index finger, and little finger, the dominant artery is usually on the medial side.

With good collateral circulation through the two palmar arches (superficial and deep) and the presence of double finger arteries, the vascular supply is disproportionately large. However, it is needed in order to protect the finger against circulatory disturbances in cold temperatures. In comparison with other arteries that have a similar caliber, the special characteristic of the finger arteries is that substantial changes in the vascular lumen can take place in these vessels in order to control perfusion. The finger arteries thus have a function similar to that of the precapillary arterioles. This is evident from the way in which the pressure differential between the wrist and the fingers, even with fully patent arteries, is strongly dependent on the current perfusion situation in response to cold and exercise.

The microcirculation in the skin of the fingers is mainly characterized by extensive arteriovenous anastomoses. These vascular bridges have a diameter of approximately $40\,\mu m$. Particularly in the nail bed, these hairpin anastomoses are easily visualized using reflective light microscopy. The mobility of the hand and its changing position relative to the heart lead to substantial variations in local perfusion pressure. These variations are much greater than hydrostatic pressure variations in the leg, since raising the hand above the level of the heart is accompanied by synchronous pressure reductions in the veins. The veins above the point of hydrostatic indifference (zero level) collapse. As a result of these pressure changes and the absence of circulatory autoregulation in the fingers, as well as thermoregulation, finger perfusion is subject to wide fluctuations even in healthy individuals. In the area of the finger pads, for example, it varies between 2 and $150\,mL$ per $100\,g$ of skin. In cold conditions, the finger circulation can be almost completely blocked by the hypothalamus in order to maintain thermoregulation. When it is cold, this mainly occurs through differences in sympathetic vasoconstrictor tone to the arteriovenous anastomoses and finger arteries, along with a si-

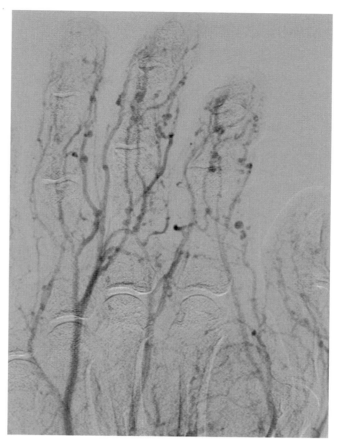

Fig. 4.3-1 Venous valves in the area of the finger veins.

multaneous local increase in the viscosity of the blood due to the cold. The viscosity is temperature-dependent. At 27–37°C, there is a linear relationship between blood temperature and viscosity. At lower temperatures, the viscosity increases proportionately with the declining temperature (Rand et al. 1964). Skin temperatures below 8°C activate pain receptors, and cold vasodilation caused by metabolic factors and axonal reflexes can occur in order to provide protection against frostbite.

The highly variable circulation in the fingers is normally well tolerated due to the relative insensitivity of the skin to ischemia. Venous valves are already present in the finger veins, and this is why blanching and whitening in the fingers is seen mainly after hand and finger movements when the Raynaud phenomenon occurs (Fig. 4.3-1). These movements shift the blood centripetally, with a simultaneous vasospastic arterial blockage.

There are many different causes of the disturbed finger circulation that is associated with Raynaud syndrome:

- Occlusions located proximal to the finger arteries—e.g., in the palmar arch or ulnar artery—lead to reduced perfusion pressure distal to the occlusion and thus promote vascular collapse even with minor external triggering factors.
- Medial or intimal hypertrophy produces an effect similar to that of an increased wall–lumen quotient. In accordance with the Laplace law, even minor vascular contractions are associated with substantial variations in the lumen. Medial or intimal hypertrophy may result from vibration trauma, hypertension, collagen vascular disease, or cold injury.

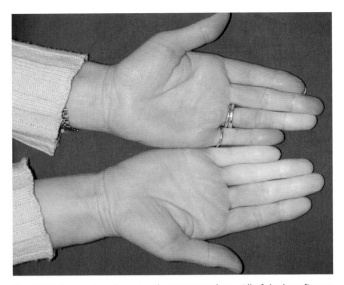

Fig. 4.3-2 Raynaud syndrome in the recovery phase. All of the long fingers of the right hand are still pale, but only the tip of D III on the left hand. The fingertips in D III and D V also appear hyperemic.

- Primary Raynaud syndrome is thought to be caused by increased vasoconstrictor activity. It may result from a compensatory increase in alpha constrictor tone due to low systemic blood pressure. In 1976, Thulesius showed that almost without exception, patients with primary Raynaud syndrome have low arterial systemic pressure. Low transmural pressure due to low systemic arterial pressure appears to be very important in Raynaud syndrome.

- Increased tissue pressure can theoretically lead to reduced transmural pressure, thereby impairing circulation in the fingers. This type of factor may also be important in scleroderma, but is unlikely to be the sole triggering factor. In 80% of the patients, the disease starts with vasospastic attacks even before fibrous changes become evident in the tissue.

- Rheological changes in the blood also play an important part in the genesis of disturbed finger circulation. Changes in hematocrit, plasma viscosity, platelet aggregation, blood cell aggregation, and erythrocyte deformability start to have pathological mechanical effects.

Primary Raynaud syndrome refers to a functional disturbance in which symmetrical blanching of the long fingers in both hands occurs, leaving the thumb unaffected (Fig. 4.3-2). It persists for several minutes and usually occurs as an effect of cold, although it can also be triggered by mental tension. The causes of primary Raynaud syndrome are not known. There are statistically significant associations with migraine (odds ratio 5.4; 95% confidence interval, 2.8 to 10.3) and nonspecific chest pain attacks (OR 4.4; 95% confidence interval, 2.4 to 9.3) in patients with primary Raynaud syndrome, so that it can be assumed that there is a systemic predisposition in the vascular system. The typical multiple-phase course, with paroxysmal pallor followed by reactive hyperemia with lividity and pain, is not always present. Many patients only report blanching of the fingers and a feeling of numbness. Trophic disturbances with distal necroses or poorly healing wounds exclude primary Raynaud syndrome.

Table 4.3-1 Possible causes of secondary Raynaud syndrome.

Neurovascular compression	Thoracic outlet syndrome
Arterial diseases	Thromboangiitis obliterans Embolism Atherosclerosis
Blood abnormalities	Monoclonal gammopathies Polycythemia
Occupational stress	Vibration injury Compressed-air injury Vinyl chloride
Drugs	Ergotamines β-blockers Triptans Chemotherapeutic agents
Connective tissue diseases	Systemic sclerosis Mixed connective tissue disease Rheumatoid arthritis Dermatomyositis, polymyositis
Other causes	Sympathetic reflex dystrophy Pheochromocytoma Pulmonary artery hypertension

Secondary Raynaud syndrome is a sequela of an organically manifest disease and is associated with a risk of tissue loss. It is mainly induced by cold and stress, and only rarely occurs with mental tension. Secondary Raynaud syndrome has a wide variety of causes (Table 4.3-1). These may affect the digital arteries themselves, the surrounding connective tissue, the flow characteristics of the blood, or the nerves supplying the hand. Secondary Raynaud syndrome with a paroxysmal onset and symptom-free intervals needs to be distinguished from acute acral ischemia with persistent pallor, cold, and pain in individual fingers. This type of ischemic syndrome against a background of acute arterial occlusion or distal embolism represents an acute emergency in relation to preserving tissue, and revascularization measures must be undertaken as quickly as possible.

Despite the simple definitions of primary and secondary Raynaud syndrome, it is often challenging for the physician to distinguish between them. As there is no evidence of the primary cause of Raynaud syndrome, the diagnosis can theoretically only be made after all possible secondary causes of the syndrome have been excluded. In addition, an assessment of the condition as "primary" is not conclusive, as there are several diseases that develop insidiously over several years before the full clinical picture becomes manifest. A systematic study of 112 patients with previously unclear Raynaud syndrome showed that primary Raynaud syndrome was diagnosed in 73 patients and secondary Raynaud syndrome in 39 at the first detailed workup. Further observation with regular 6-monthly examinations over 46 months showed that there was an annual conversion rate to secondary Raynaud syndrome of 1.4%.

Population-based data on the prevalence of Raynaud syndrome are scarce. The published data therefore always need to be interpreted in the light of the population studied and the definition of Raynaud syndrome used. Older publications reported a prevalence of 20–30% in populations in Britain and California. In more recent publications, the prevalence has been around 1–5%. Although the

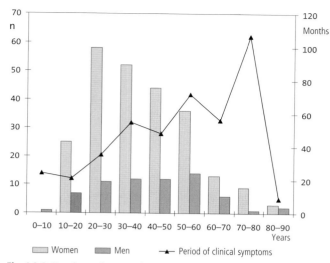

Fig. 4.3-3 Numbers of men and women, distributed by 10-year age groups, and the period of clinical symptoms in a population of 306 patients presenting for the first diagnostic examination.

female population is generally more often affected, data regarding the sex ratio also vary widely and the distinction between primary and secondary Raynaud syndrome is only rarely taken into account. Living conditions in various climatic zones appear to have an influence on the prevalence of Raynaud syndrome. An American–French study compared the prevalence of Raynaud syndrome in five different regions, taking migration movements into account. The majority of individuals affected by Raynaud syndrome in the colder climate zones had always lived in the colder zones. However, the majority of those with Raynaud syndrome in the warmer climate zones had moved there from colder zones.

In the clinical clarification of Raynaud syndrome, the prevalence in the general population is of lesser interest than the distribution within the population. Young women are the largest group presenting for diagnosis among our own patients (Fig. 4.3-3). Within this group, the diagnostic workup only leads to evidence of a secondary cause in a few cases. Although older women present more rarely, secondary Raynaud syndrome is more common in this group, since collagen vascular disease as a major cause of secondary Raynaud syndrome becomes manifest most often in the fifth and sixth decades of life. Men present less often than women in all age groups. The men affected mostly have manual occupations, and issues involving work-related traumatic arterial occlusions are therefore of immediate importance.

4.3.2 Diagnostic procedure

The following findings argue in favor of primary Raynaud syndrome:
- No organic cause identifiable
- Mainly symmetric manifestations
- Intermittent and brief (lasting only minutes)
- Thumb almost always spared

Despite these characteristics, primary Raynaud syndrome with the corresponding clinical findings can only be assumed indirectly after secondary Raynaud syndrome has been excluded. As the probability of primary or secondary Raynaud syndrome depends on sex, age,

comorbid conditions, and occupational stress, the strength of the evidence with which a secondary cause can be excluded varies widely. The structured approach described below can be recommended in order to make the diagnostic workup as efficient as possible.

4.3.2.1 History

In the patient history, the emphasis should be put on the distribution pattern of the Raynaud syndrome, general physical symptoms, and manual activities.

If all of the long fingers of both hands are affected, even if not equally severely, the picture fits primary Raynaud syndrome. If only the fingers on one hand or individual fingers are affected, a secondary Raynaud syndrome can be assumed initially. The time of the first appearance of the Raynaud syndrome should be established as precisely as possible. The patients have often had symptoms of primary Raynaud syndrome for several years. Raynaud syndromes that have a sudden onset tend to be secondary. Questions regarding the extent and duration of discoloration and the temporal sequence it shows (first pallor, then hyperemia, accompanied by pain) and provocation testing with iced water are not diagnostically helpful. This type of provocation procedure originally provided better information about the physiological sequences involved in Raynaud syndrome, but nowadays the tests are only useful for treatment check-ups in research conditions. A clinical distinction is made between Raynaud syndrome and acrocyanosis with paroxysmal or persistent cyanotic discoloring of the fingers. However, as acrocyanosis is only another type of digital perfusion disturbance, the diagnostic procedure is the same as that for Raynaud syndrome.

Details of general symptoms such as loss of appetite, weight loss, or a sudden lack of energy suggest a systemic cause such as collagen vascular disease, malignant hemopathy, or even myocarditis as a potential source of peripheral embolism. If general symptoms of this type are present, the emphasis in the further diagnostic workup must be placed on excluding them rather than on confirming Raynaud syndrome. Full details of the patient's medication history should be available if possible, and the patient should be asked about drugs taken for headache in particular. All of the ergotamines and ergotamine derivatives, as well as more recent migraine drugs such as the triptans, can trigger vascular spasm and thus cause Raynaud syndrome or aggravate an existing syndrome. Effects on the digital arteries have also been reported for many other preparations, but with the exception of chemotherapeutic agents they are rarely the sole cause of Raynaud syndrome.

The patient must always be asked about the temporal link between the first onset of Raynaud syndrome and manual exertion at work, at home, or during sporting activities. During the subsequent diagnostic workup involving blood tests and imaging procedures, the issue of whether there might be a chronic traumatic cause is never raised again—so that a potential causal connection will be overlooked if it is not explored and documented at the time the patient's history is taken.

4.3.2.2   Physical examination

The physical examination can be kept very organ-specific. The pulses over the radial and ulnar arteries on each side should be compared, so that even slight differences can be recognized. To exclude a clinically relevant thoracic outlet syndrome, a blood pressure measurement in the elevated and abducted arm is indicated. An Allen test (compression of the radial artery and ulnar artery for 30 seconds with fist clenching and evaluation of reactive hyperemia after opening of the two arteries) allows assessment of the arteries' areas of supply, but it has no diagnostic significance. In primary Raynaud syndrome, the Allen test should be unremarkable. In patients with well-compensated occlusion and Raynaud syndrome that only appears when working in cold conditions, the Allen test may also be negative. Although a positive Allen test suggests a secondary Raynaud syndrome, it does not help identify the cause. For example, if there is an absence of reperfusion after the ulnar artery is released, it may be due to a normal anatomic variant with primary absence of the ulnar artery, or the ulnar artery may have a traumatic or embolic occlusion.

Increased callosity or minor injuries in the hands suggest physical stress. This should be distinguished from trophic disturbances such as thickening of the cutis with an inability to form a fist, or cutaneous calcifications at the finger pads, or even rat-bite necrosis. Changes of this type are pathognomonic for collagen vascular disease. However, it is not always immediately possible to make the clinical distinction, and the diagnostic significance of the changes can only be recognized during the course of the disease due to failure to heal or episodic deterioration, with additional lesions. Changes in the feet as well as the hands should be inquired about, and the feet should be inspected. Thromboangiitis obliterans is an important differential diagnosis in young men and women. An inflammatory vascular disease, it occludes the medium-sized arteries in the arms and legs. If both the lower and the upper extremity are affected in a young patient with Raynaud syndrome, therefore, then thromboangiitis obliterans can be regarded as a possible cause. Simultaneous involvement of the feet in a primary Raynaud syndrome is rare.

4.3.2.3   Further diagnosis

In addition to measuring basic values such as erythrocyte sedimentation, the blood picture, and hepatic and renal values, evidence of autoantibodies is extremely important, as collagen vascular diseases and lupus erythematosus are the most frequent systemic diseases causing secondary Raynaud syndrome. Although both diseases become clinically evident more often with other organ manifestations, there are some patients who have only Raynaud syndrome for many years. A multicenter study including 761 patients with Raynaud syndrome found systemic sclerosis in 28.4%. Systemic lupus erythematosus was found in 6.8%, and rheumatoid arthritis in 5%. Other causes that may basically be associated with Raynaud syndrome—such as hypertension, Sjögren syndrome, mixed connective tissue disease, fibromyalgia, carpal tunnel syndrome, cryoglobulinemia, dermatopolymyositis, vasculitides, thoracic outlet syndrome, hypothyroidism, and diabetes mellitus—were together found in fewer than 5% of the patients. For target antibodies, it is sufficient to assess the antinuclear autoantibodies. Assessment of

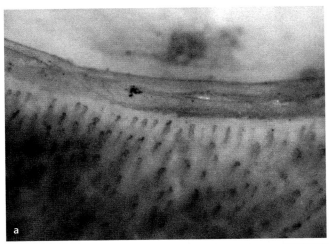

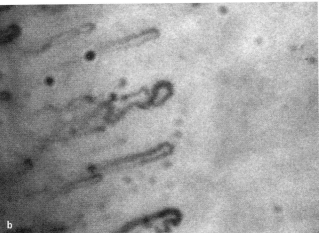

Fig. 4.3-4a, b The upper image (**a**) shows an overview of the capillaries. The capillaries in the last row clearly have a tilted course and are easily assessed. The lower image (**b**) is an enlarged one from a different patient. The slim capillaries with needle's-eye shapes are normal, whereas the larger, twisted capillaries are pathological.

other autoantibodies—such as extractable nuclear antigen (ENA), double-stranded DNA (dsDNA), and antineutrophilic cytoplasmic antibody (ANCA)—is useful when there is a relevant suspected diagnosis.

In capillary microscopy, the morphology of the capillaries in the nail fold can be assessed using light microscopy. The nail fold is useful for this examination, as the capillaries course obliquely in the skin and can be viewed from the side. Megacapillaries and avascular fields are the only pathological findings that constitute an almost pathognomonic criterion (Fig. 4.3-4). Evidence of megacapillaries also has prognostic significance for the development of collagenosis in patients with an otherwise unremarkable antibody status. All other changes in capillary density, length, visibility, and shape may be helpful in individual cases in interpreting the findings, but have no pathognomonic significance on their own.

Assessment of blood viscosity and cold agglutinins and cryoglobulins may be reserved for selected individual cases. Although earlier studies reported a high level of plasma viscosity in patients with primary Raynaud syndrome, the reason for this and the underlying cause have remained unclear, and the finding has no diagnostic significance. Cold agglutinins lead to reversible agglutination of erythrocytes at low temperatures. However, the agglutination does not lead to any intermittent pallor in the long fingers, but rather to underperfusion of all of the distal points (tip of the nose, auricle, fingers, and toes). If there are relevant titers of cold agglutinins that may have led to necroses at the distal points, the condition is known as cold hemagglutinin disease. When influenced by cold, cryoglobulins lead to the formation of immune complexes that are deposited on the basal membrane and therefore cause immune complex vasculitis with renal involvement. The early signs of this type of cryoglobulinemia are purpura-like skin changes, arthralgia, and neuropathy, and only rarely isolated Raynaud syndrome.

4.3.2.4   Functional tests

Distal volume pulse assessment and Doppler pressure measurement at the fingers can be used to identify digital artery occlusion or reduced pressure in the digital arteries. In volume pulse recording, the volume pulse is assessed qualitatively. Maintenance of dicrotism is an important diagnostic sign. Various procedures are available for measuring digital artery pressure. With simultaneous pressure measurement on various fingers, reproducible pressure differences of 15 mmHg between the fingers, or absolute pressure values of less than 70 mmHg, can be regarded as evidence of an arterial occlusion. However, a reduction in the volume pulse or digital arterial pressure can only be expected in secondary Raynaud syndromes with organic occlusion of the digital artery itself or a hemodynamically effective occlusion further up. In the great majority of patients with secondary Raynaud syndrome and all of those with primary Raynaud syndrome, these examinations do not provide any definitive evidence. Normal examination results obtained in resting conditions do not exclude compensated vascular occlusions. Functional examinations after cooling of the hand improve the yield of pathological findings, but are poorly reproducible and therefore unsuitable for clinical use.

4.3.2.5   Imaging procedures

Only vascular imaging is capable of determining whether there is an organic change present in the arterial system of the hand. Color duplex ultrasonography can be used to image the vessels in the shoulder girdle, upper arm, lower arm, and palmar arch. Individual variability in the digital circulatory system makes it difficult and sometimes impossible to assess the more distal vascular segments using ultrasound (Fig. 4.3-5). In addition, occluded digital arteries cannot be systematically imaged and delicate end branches are not capable of being assessed. Modern magnetic resonance (MR) angiography techniques are becoming increasingly important, but the required image resolution has not yet been achieved.

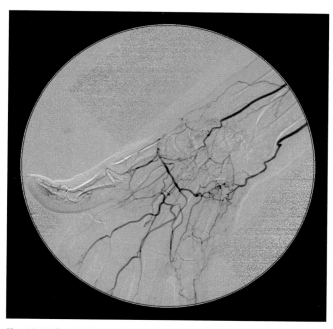

Fig. 4.3-5 The right hand of a 70-year-old patient with collagen vascular disease. Interestingly, the collateral vessels originate from the occluded lower arm arteries. This finding is repeatedly reported in patients with thromboangiitis obliterans, but is not pathognomonic of a palmar perfusion disturbance.

Optimal imaging of the vessels in the hand is only possible with angiography. Selective angiography is required, with catheter placement in the distal brachial artery and administration of a vasodilating agent such as tolazoline (Priscoline) or alprostadil (prostaglandin E_1).

4.3.2.6   Raynaud syndrome with a traumatic pathogenesis

Traumatic vascular changes in the area of the hands are not rare among people involved in manual work. They are thought to be present in up to 14% of all craftsmen and tradesmen. This type of occlusion is caused by stress due to mechanical vibrations, compressed air, and nonspecific use of the hand as a gripping, holding, or striking tool (Table 4.3-2). According to an estimate made in 1981, some 18% of employed individuals were subject to this type of mechanical vibration and approximately 0.5 million employees held vibration-causing devices in their hands for more than 2 hours per day. Preventive measures have not yet led to any marked reduction in this burden.

A distinction between types of damaging effect is made between vibration frequencies of around 50 Hz and those at around 1000 Hz. Changes in the area of the acromioclavicular joint or elbow joint, as

Table 4.3-2 The hand–arm system is subjected to a wide variety of different types of stress and demand in various types of work.

Physical stress from the tool	Physiology of effort conditions	Duration of exposure	Concomitant stress factors	Individual endogenous preconditions
Vibration characteristics	▪ Grasping strength of hand	▪ Daily	▪ Cold	▪ Constitution
▪ Amplitudes	▪ Arm pressure strength	▪ Annually	▪ Heat	▪ Disposition
▪ Frequencies	▪ Support effort	▪ At work	▪ Noise	▪ Congenital abnormality in the area of the hand/arm
▪ Rigidity	▪ Degree of practice	▪ Scheduled pauses		
▪ Vibration directions				

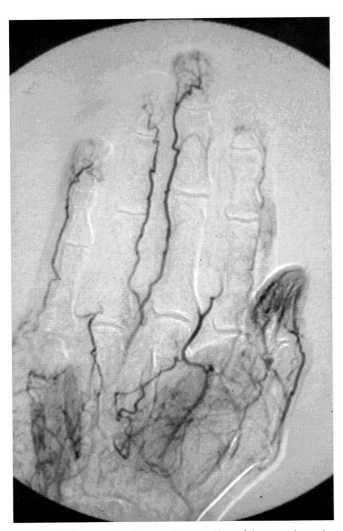

Fig. 4.3-6 Diffuse vascular changes with partial loss of the normal vascular anatomy are typical, but not diagnostic, for vibration injury. The thumb is less often affected.

Table 4.3-3 Stockholm classification of vibration-related vasospastic syndrome (adapted from Gemme 1987).

Stage	Characteristics/symptoms	Impairments
0	No blanching of the fingers	None
0T	Occasional tingling in the fingertips	No occupational disability
0N	Occasional sensation of numbness in the fingertips	No occupational disability
1	Blanching of one or more fingertips	No occupational disability
2	Blanching of one or more fingertips with numbness, but only during winter	Slight disability in the private and social field, no occupational disability
3	Comprehensive blanching of the fingers, usually in both hands. Frequent attacks in both winter and also summer	Severe impairment at work and in the private and social fields
4	Symptoms as in 3, but more severe and more frequent	Symptoms are not tolerated. Very severe impairment. Requires change of occupation

well as osteochondrosis dissecans, can be caused by 50-Hz vibration frequencies, and these are classified under no. 2103 among occupational diseases. Higher-frequency vibrations lead to aseptic necroses in the lunate bone or arthroses in the area of the wrist and are classified under no. 2104 (Fig. 4.3-6). These changes in the grasping apparatus are caused by vibration-induced vasomotor disturbances, which lead to underperfusion. If a vascular injury develops over the course of time, it becomes clinically evident with Raynaud syndrome. In addition to these vascular disturbances, nerve function disturbances can also occur (with reduced sensitivity at the fingertips), and this is referred to as vibration-related vasospastic syndrome. Raynaud syndrome and sensitivity disturbances occur independently of other changes and therefore have to be assessed separately (Table 4.3-3). Vibration sensitivity at the fingertips can be investigated using pallesthesiometry; in people occupationally exposed to vibrations, the vibration threshold values are increased threefold to fivefold in comparison with normal individuals. For occupational stress to be recognized as the cause of Raynaud syndrome, specific conditions need to be met (i.e., the patient concerned must have been working with vibration-causing devices for certain periods of time), and the theoretical daily assessed vibration

strength calculated by a technician must reach a given threshold value. The duration of the stress in particular is decisive. For example, a study including 1540 forest workers in Quebec, Canada, showed that there was a mean of 7.8 ± 5.6 years between the first use of a power saw and the appearance of Raynaud syndrome.

Raynaud syndrome in patients with no occupational exposure to vibration or pneumatic pressure stress, or which develop within brief periods of stress, are usually not recognized as having an occupational disease. Raynaud syndrome against a background of hypothenar hammer syndrome (Fig. 4.3-7) is an example of this. Hypothenar hammer syndrome is an occlusion or aneurysm formation with digital artery embolism as a form of direct traumatic injury in the area of the distal ulnar artery or superficial palmar arch. The hypothenar hammer syndrome occurs when the hypothenar eminence on the hand is used as a pushing or hitting instrument. It does not matter whether the stress occurs regularly or only once. The ways in which the hand can be used as a hitting or pushing tool are complex—ranging among our own group of patients from loosening of a vise to packaging work and laying tiles, or even baking activities. The triggering situation may be part of a routine activity. If the symptomatic picture is not paroxysmal with symptom-free intervals, then the symptoms should not be regarded as belonging to Raynaud syndrome. Depending on the extent of the vascular occlusion, a hypothenar hammer syndrome may also appear as acute ischemia with persistent pallor, cold, and pain. Acute ischemia in one or several fingers is very painful and represents an emergency situation that needs to be treated in order to preserve the tissue. Which particular patients are likely to develop a hypothenar hammer syndrome, and whether there are also individual predispositions for the condition in addition to external influences, is as yet unclear. An American study including 1300 patients with Raynaud syndrome identified a subgroup of 21 patients who had fibromuscular dysplasia in the area of the ulnar part of the palmar arch (Fig. 4.3-8). Surgery was performed in 19 of these 21 patients, with excision of the altered vascular segment and placement of a venous bridging graft. Evidence suggesting

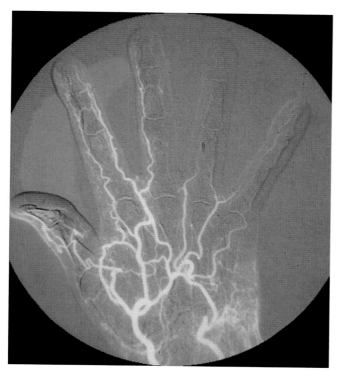

Fig. 4.3-7 This car mechanic who does bodywork had symptoms for about 2 months before the angiogram was taken. It shows an occlusion at the junction from the ulnar artery into the deep palmar arch—a classic sign of hypothenar hammer syndrome.

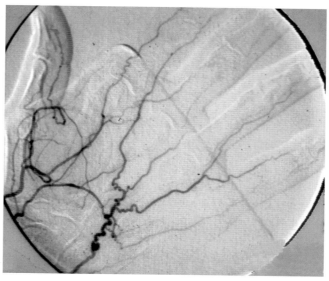

Fig. 4.3-8 The distal end of the ulnar artery has a sinuous course and aneurysmal dilation. The digital artery supplying the third and fourth ray is occluded by an embolism. This finding in a 23-year-old professional driver is consistent with the changes described in fibromuscular dysplasia.

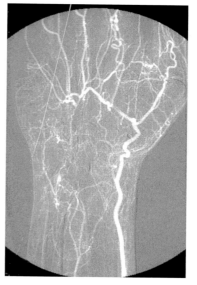

Fig. 4.3-9 In this 48-year-old lathe operator, there is a long occlusion in the ulnar artery. About 2 weeks after a blunt trauma from a rotating part, he noticed a feeling of coldness in the fingers. The accident was documented in his family physician's files. The occlusion was only confirmed 2 years later in connection with an acute heart attack. The trauma was not recognized by his trade association as being the cause, as the length of the occlusion led an assessor to regard diffuse atherosclerosis as the probable cause.

a predisposition resulting from fibromuscular dysplasia included the fact that 62% of the patients had the disease picture bilaterally and that the postoperative patency rate after 2 years, despite continued occupational exposure to the same stress, was more than 80%. It was unclear whether fibromuscular dysplasia was also present more frequently in these patients in other parts of the body, such as the renal and cerebral arteries, or whether fibromuscular transformation resulted from the chronic trauma.

4.3.2.7 Diagnostic differentiation of traumatic Raynaud syndromes

A suspected diagnosis of a traumatic cause always emerges only from the patient's history. As the patients themselves do not identify the causal link, it is the physician's task to inquire about manual activities, document them, and sum them up and assess them after all the examinations have been completed. Making the situation even more difficult is the fact that traumatized arteries often only occlude and become symptomatic after a latency period lasting hours to days.

As there is no evidence of a traumatic cause and patients can have other causes of Raynaud syndrome independently of their manual activities, the classic diagnostic workup has to be followed. Angiography is needed in order to obtain a definitive diagnosis and provide evidence for the relevant professional or trade association in relation to disability claims, with good depiction of both the afferent arteries in the lower arm and of the palmar arch, as well as the individual digital arteries right up to the terminal phalanges. On the other hand, the mechanism that may have led to traumatization of the hand arteries is not visible in an angiographic image. As-

sessment of such images can therefore only be carried out with full knowledge of all the findings. In some cases, direct abruption of the palmar arch in the ulnar area, with a residual stump or aneurysm formation, can be seen (Fig. 4.3-8). However, if there is ascending thrombosis in the ulnar artery, a long ulnar artery occlusion may also be present (Fig. 4.3-9). Differential diagnosis versus collagen vascular disease or thromboangiitis obliterans is also not possible with angiography.

4.3.3   Treatment

4.3.3.1   Conservative treatment

No specific therapy for primary Raynaud syndrome is available, as the cause is not known. Treatment of secondary Raynaud syndrome consists mainly of treatment for the underlying disease, along with all of the measures that are also indicated for primary Raynaud syndrome. Although Raynaud syndrome in itself has no influence on life expectancy, an early manifestation of Raynaud syndrome in patients with systemic scleroderma is a prognostically unfavorable sign (with a relative risk of death 1.30 over 10 years). Manifest digital ischemia does not represent Raynaud syndrome and needs to be treated as a case of ischemia of the extremities.

Basic measures

Symptomatic treatment is sufficient for the majority of young female patients with primary Raynaud syndrome. The course of the disease is benign, and the syndrome disappears as body weight increases during the third decade of life. Rigorous protection against cold can be recommended as a basic measure. In slim to anorectic patients who have problems with regulating body temperature, not only the affected extremities but also the entire body should be kept warm so that warmer blood reaches the fingers. Potentially vasoconstrictive drugs should be withdrawn. Drug therapy is rarely indicated. This is in contrast to secondary Raynaud syndrome, in which drug treatment is often necessary.

Calcium antagonists

It has often been recommended that Raynaud syndrome should be treated with calcium antagonists of the dihydropyridine type, in which the major effect is peripheral vasodilation and the cardiodepressive action is negligible (e.g., nifedipine 10–20 mg three times daily, felodipine or amlodipine 10 mg/d). In both primary and secondary Raynaud syndrome, the severity of the Raynaud attacks has been shown to improve with this type of treatment. However, the effect of calcium antagonists on the frequency of attacks (with a decline of 2.8–5.0 attacks per week) and their severity (with reductions by 33% or 35%) is fairly small in comparison with placebo. The patients' individual responses vary widely, and hypotension often limits the treatment, particularly in younger women with low blood-pressure values.

Prostacyclins and prostaglandins

Iloprost has been successfully used, particularly in patients with secondary Raynaud phenomenon against a background of systemic sclerosis. According to a Cochrane analysis, iloprost led to a reduction in the frequency and severity of Raynaud syndrome and to the healing of fingertip ulcers in 220 patients with systemic sclerosis. Interestingly, the positive effect persisted for up to 9 weeks after the end of the infusion treatments. The iloprost dosages used in the studies ranged from 0.5 to 2.0 ng/kg body weight/min for 6–8 h/d and the administration period from 3 to 21 days. Hypotension and flush symptoms can be expected as side effects. In this case, the concentration should be reduced and the duration of the infusion treatment should be increased. In older patients, attention should be given to deterioration in any existing form of cardiac insufficien-

cy, with increasing edema developing. There have only been case reports on the use of iloprost and alprostadil in primary Raynaud syndrome or in secondary Raynaud syndrome with a traumatic pathogenesis, for example.

Endothelin receptor antagonists

Administration of the endothelin receptor antagonist bosentan in patients with fingertip ulcers in systemic sclerosis appears to be a promising approach. In two randomized, prospective, placebo-controlled studies, the drug was found to be effective for prophylaxis against recurrent fingertip ulcers in patients with systemic sclerosis. This is an important aspect in high-risk patients after protracted healing of painful ulcers.

The *R*andomized *P*lacebo-Controlled *I*nvestigation of *D*igital Ulcers in *S*cleroderma (RAPIDS-1) study was a placebo-controlled clinical double-blind study in which the prevention of ischemic digital ulceration was investigated in 122 patients with systemic sclerosis (scleroderma) in 17 centers in Europe and North America. The study's design was specifically targeted at preventing ulcer development. During the course of treatment, patients who received bosentan in the study experienced a 48% reduction in the number of new digital ulcerations (1.4 vs. 2.7 new ulcerations; $P = 0.0083$). In addition, the treatment led to a significant improvement in the hand's functional capacity. This included the patients' ability to wash their hands, dress, and comb their hair.

The RAPIDS-2 study was conducted worldwide, with a total of 188 patients in 41 testing centers. Scleroderma patients with at least one digital ulceration were treated either with bosentan (62.5 mg twice daily for 4 weeks, followed by 125 mg twice daily for at least 20 and up to 32 weeks) or a placebo. The total number of new ulcerations over 24 weeks was 1.9 ± 0.2 in patients receiving bosentan treatment, in comparison with 2.7 ± 0.3 in patients receiving the placebo ($P = 0.035$). On the Scleroderma Health Assessment Questionnaire (SHAQ) scale, some improvements in the secondary end point of hand function were seen. Particularly with regard to hand functions associated with "dressing" ($P = 0.033$) and "eating" ($P = 0.098$), there were improvements after 24 weeks of treatment in the bosentan group in comparison with the placebo group. Pain scores, measured using the SHAQ visual analogue scale, improved after 12 weeks in the bosentan patients ($P = 0.034$).

Additional drugs

In small controlled studies comparing the agents with nifedipine, the AT_1 antagonist losartan and the selective serotonin reuptake inhibitor fluoxetine (20 mg/d) were reported to have similarly good effects, with a decrease in the frequency of attacks. The phosphodiesterase 5 inhibitor sildenafil (50 mg twice a day) also led to a significant reduction in the frequency and duration of Raynaud attacks in patients with secondary Raynaud syndrome. In a small pilot study including 19 patients with digital ulcers in systemic scleroderma, treatment with sildenafil for up to 6 months was found to have a positive effect on ulcer healing (49 ulcers at the start of the study, 17 at the end; $P < 0.001$).

The value of topically administered glycerol trinitrate or isosorbide nitrate ointment, oral acetylsalicylic acid, subcutaneous low-molecular-weight heparins, and oral pentoxifylline has not been confirmed. However, nitrate-containing ointments in particular are a valuable treatment approach. The ointment should be spread on the hands and lower arms and can help patients appreciate the importance of keeping the blood warm. A recent large study also showed that the angiotensin-converting enzyme (ACE) inhibitor quinapril has no effect. A randomized study investigated the effect of statins on the frequency of digital artery ulcers and noted a significant effect. Patients treated with 40 mg atorvastatin daily developed a mean of only 1.6 new ulcers within 4 months, in comparison with 2.5 in the placebo group.

4.3.3.2   Endovascular treatment

There is no endovascular treatment for primary Raynaud syndrome. In secondary Raynaud syndrome with vascular occlusions, weeks to months are unfortunately lost before the diagnosis is confirmed. This is because the causative trauma tends to be chronic or is part of the patient's occupational profile and does not prompt the patient to consult a physician immediately. Even in cases of acute trauma, it may be several days before the traumatic pain declines and the supervening Raynaud syndrome during stress and cold exposure comes to the fore.

There have been a few studies on the late use of fibrinolytic agents in the treatment of digital artery occlusions. The use of fibrinolytic agents in the retrograde venous perfusion technique is an interesting approach. In retrograde venous perfusion, a drug agent is injected into a vein following a "Bier blockade." In this procedure, arterial perfusion in one extremity is blocked using a blood-pressure cuff. The blood-pressure cuff is inflated to a suprasystolic pressure of approximately 50 mmHg. During the block, the desired drug is injected into a dorsal vein in the hand or foot. The block is maintained for about 20 min and then slowly released. This technique, which was developed in the anesthetic field, is used to administer antibiotics and vasodilators in patients with diabetic foot syndrome. It achieves a high local concentration of the agent while minimizing systemic side effects.

The use of the technique in patients with digital artery occlusion has been described in several studies. In most cases, these have been single case reports in which recombinant tissue plasminogen activator (rt-PA, alteplase) was used. In the reports, the fibrinolytic agent often has heparin, vasodilating agents such as prostanoids, and a local anesthetic added to it. Unfortunately, there have been no larger studies and there are no standard recommendations regarding the choice and dosage of the fibrinolytic agent. We can therefore only present our own experience here.

Our own experience is with a scheme developed by Pöhlmann and colleagues and modified by Schmiedel and von Flotow. In this procedure, a mixture of 5 µg alprostadil, 2500 IU heparin, 20 mL prilocaine 1%, and 10 mg alteplase with 0.9% NaCl is drawn up to a total volume of 45–50 mL. The medication is then injected slowly into a dorsal vein of the hand, with a suprasystolic pressure block, over about 10 min. The suprasystolic block is maintained for approximately 20 min and is then slowly released (over about 10 min). The total duration of the treatment is thus approximately 40 min. As the treatment can be very painful, particularly during the phase when the block is being released, adequate prophylactic pain therapy can be recommended—e.g., with an opiate. The treatment is repeated

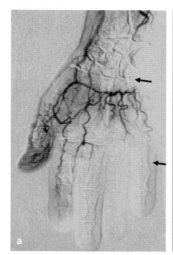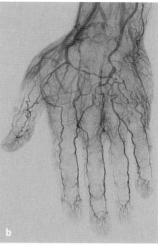

Fig. 4.3-10a, b A carpenter with occlusion of the ulnar artery and digital arteries of the third to fifth fingers on the right hand in hypothenar hammer syndrome. Before treatment (**a**) and after three 5-day cycles of retrograde venous lysis (**b**).

daily for 3–5 days. Clinical improvement in the symptoms is usually seen immediately after the infusion. It is possible to perform several treatment cycles; we leave an interval of 1–2 weeks between each cycle to allow decongestion of the hand or foot. In our experience, this method can also be successfully used to treat even older occlusions of the digital arteries—as shown in Fig. 4.3-10, for example. This was a 58-year-old patient with occlusion of the digital arteries and ulnar artery in hypothenar hammer syndrome. The patient only developed symptoms in the early winter months, although the acute event had been some 3 months before. Three cycles over 5 days each of retrograde venous lysis treatment in accordance with the scheme described above were administered in this patient. Minor bleeding problems, such as epistaxis, were only observed rarely when the treatment was being administered. Follow-up care depends on the cause of the digital artery occlusion; in most cases, we administer oral anticoagulation treatment with vitamin K antagonists for at least 6 months.

As retrograde venous lysis represents an "off-label" use and larger studies are not yet available, the patient should receive the appropriate information. However, in patients with digital artery occlusions, there are often very few treatment options remaining and there is often a risk of amputation. In the present author's view, retrograde venous lysis is therefore a suitable treatment method and one that usually leads to marked clinical improvement.

4.3.3.3   Surgical treatment options

Surgical procedures that may be considered in individual cases include sympathectomy (proximal cervical or peripheral digital), and—for occlusions in the area of the palmar arch—revascularization with vascular surgery.

Sympathectomy can be carried out temporarily with a CT-guided ganglion blockade, or permanently with a thoracoscopic sympathectomy at the T2–T4 level. However, this should only be considered when there is proven ischemia and an otherwise treatment-refractory disease course, associated with imminent amputation or uncontrollable resting pain. No systematic research has been conducted on the value of sympathectomy in patients with primary Raynaud syndrome. A problem deserving mention here is the potential for reinnervation to develop, which can even lead to post-sympathectomy syndrome.

In hypothenar hammer syndrome, surgical measures can be carried out to eliminate embolizing aneurysms and restore perfusion. Prophylactic surgery for aneurysms in the ulnar part of the palmar arch in particular is useful for prognostic reasons, as it can prevent peripheral embolism with obstruction of the digital terminal vessels.

As the digital arteries themselves are functional terminal arteries, revascularization measures in or at the digital arteries are not successful. In most cases, however, the digital arteries are not completely closed but are only constricted, either due to paroxysm or low perfusion pressure distal to the occluded palmar arch. After recanalization of the palmar arch, the perfusion of the digital arteries usually improves spontaneously. In inflammatory vascular changes in the context of collagen vascular disease or thromboangiitis obliterans, surgical correction is not promising.

References

Bier A. Über einen neuen Weg, Lokalanästhesie an den Gliedmaßen zu erzielen. Verh Dtsch Ges Chirur 1908; 37: 204.

Brand FN, Larson MG, Kannel WB, McGuirk JM. The occurrence of Raynaud's phenomenon in a general population: the Framingham Study. Vasc Med 1997; 2: 296–301.

Brueckner CS, Becker MO, Kroencke T, Huscher D, Scherer HU, Worm M, Burmester G, Riemekasten G. Effect of sildenafil on digital ulcers in systemic sclerosis: analysis from a single centre pilot study. Ann Rheum Dis 2010; 69: 1475–8.

Ferris BL, Taylor LM Jr, Oyama K, McLafferty RB, Edwards JM, Moneta GL, Porter JM. Hypothenar hammer syndrome: proposed etiology. J Vasc Surg 2000; 31: 104–13.

Gemme G, Pyykko I, Taylor W, Pelmear PL. The Stockholm Workshop scale for classification of cold-induced Raynaud's phenomenon in the hand-arm vibration syndrome. Scand J Work Environ Health 1987; 13: 275–8.

Gliddon AE, Doré CJ, Black CM, McHugh N, Moots R, Denton CP, Herrick A, Barnes T, Camilleri J, Chakravarty K, Emery P, Griffiths B, Hopkinson ND, Hickling P, Lanyon P, Laversuch C, Lawson T, Mallya R, Nisar M, Rhys-Dillon C, Sheeran T, Maddison PJ. Prevention of vascular damage in scleroderma and autoimmune Raynaud's phenomenon: a multicenter, randomized, double-blind, placebo-controlled trial of the angiotensin-converting enzyme inhibitor quinapril. Arthritis Rheum 2007; 56: 3837–46.

Grassi W, De Angelis R, Lapadula G, Leardini G, Scarpa R. Clinical diagnosis found in patients with Raynaud's phenomenon: a multicentre study. Rheumatol Int 1998; 18: 17–20.

Hirschl M, Kundi M. Initial prevalence and incidence of secondary Raynaud's phenomenon in patients with Raynaud's symptomatology. J Rheumatol 1996; 23: 302–9.

Ingegnoli F, Boracchi P, Gualtierotti R, Lubatti C, Meani L, Zahalkova L, Zeni S, Fantini F. Prognostic model based on nailfold capillaroscopy for identifying Raynaud's phenomenon patients at high risk for the development of a scleroderma spectrum disorder: PRINCE (prognostic index for nailfold capillaroscopic examination). Arthritis Rheum 2008; 58: 2174–82.

Kaminski M, Bourgine M, Zins M, Touranchet A, Verger C. Risk factors for Raynaud's phenomenon among workers in poultry slaughterhouses and canning factories. Int J Epidemiol 1997 Apr; 26 (2): 371–80.

Kommissari S. Dissertation: Die retrograde venöse Perfusion. Therapieoption der diabetischen Gangrän und anderer infizierter Läsionen der Extremitäten. 2002.

Kröger K, Billen T, Neuhaus G, Santosa F, Buss C, Kreuzfelder E, Henneberg-Quester KB. Relevance of low titers of cryoglobulins and cold-agglutinins in patients with isolated Raynaud phenomenon. Clin Hemor Microcirc 2001; 24: 167–74.

Letzel S, Kraus Th. Das Hypothenar-Hammer-Syndrom – eine Berufskrankheit? Arbeitsmed Sozialmed Umweltmed 1998; 33: 502–9.

Mannarino E, Pasqualini L, Fedeli F, Scricciolo V, Innocente S. Nailfod capillarscopy in the screening and diagnosis of Raynaud's phenomenon. Angiology 1994; 45: 37–42.

Maricq HR, Carpentier PH, Weinrich MC, Keil JE, Palesch Y, Biro C, Vionnet-Fuasset M, Jiguet M, Valter I. Geographic variation in the prevalence of Raynaud's phenomenon: a 5 region comparison. J Rheumatol 1997; 24: 879–89.

Maricq HR, Jennings JR, Valter I, Frederick M, Thompson B, Smith EA, Hill R. Raynaud's Treatment Study Investigators. Evaluation of treatment efficacy of Raynaud phenomenon by digital blood pressure response to cooling. Vasc Med 2000; 5: 135–40.

Martin M, Heimig T, Fiebach BJ, Magnus L, Riedel C. Lysis block treatment: a new form of local thrombolysis. Angiology 1994; 45: 143–8.

Monti G, Saccardo F, Pioltelli P, Rinaldi G. The natural history of cryoglobulinemia: symptoms at onset and during follow-up. A report by the Italian Group of the study of Cryoglobulinemias. Clin Experim Rheum 1995; 13: S129–S33.

O'Keeffe ST, Tsapatsaris NP, Beetham WP Jr. Increased prevalence of migraine and chest pain in patients with primary Raynaud disease. Ann Intern Med 1992; 116: 985–9.

Partsch H, Schoop W. Editorial: Biersche Sperre: neue Therapiemöglichkeit bei peripheren Extremitätenläsionen. Wien med Wschr 1993; 141: 143.

Pöhlmann G, Bär H, Siegmund R, Eidner G, Figulla HR. Verschluss der Fingerarterien nach Überstreckungstrauma. VASA 2002; 31: 122–4.

Seidel C, Buhler-Singer S, Richter UG, Hornstein OP. Regionale retrograd-venöse versus systemisch-venöse Infusion im therapeutischen Vergleich bei diabetischen Plantarulzerationen. Diabetes und Stoffwechsel 1994; 3: 343–7.

Theriault G, De Guire L, Gingras S, Laroche G. Raynaud's phenomenon in forestry workers in Quebec. Can Med Assoc J 1982; 126: 1404–8.

Tyndall AJ, Bannert B, Vonk M et al. Causes and risk factors for death in systemic sclerosis: a study from the EULAR Scleroderma Trials and Research (EUSTAR) database. Rheumatology (Oxford) 2010; 49: 583–7.

4.4 Stenoses and occlusive processes in the lower extremity

4.4.1 Clinical picture, clinical findings, diagnosis and differential diagnosis
Ernst Gröchenig, Thomas Zeller, Curt Diehm

Peripheral arterial occlusive disease (PAOD) is caused by atherosclerosis in 90% of cases. The prevalence of the disease is 3–10%; it increases with age and affects one in three individuals over the age of 75. The majority of these patients (two-thirds) does not develop any symptoms and thus do not become aware of their disease. Peripheral arterial occlusive disease is an important indicator for generalized atherosclerosis. Independently of whether the patients are symptomatic or asymptomatic, coronary or cerebral arterial occlusive disease is found in 40–60% of patients. Some 5–7% of the patients per year die as a result of cardiovascular events, and the incidence of nonfatal myocardial infarctions is 2–3% per year. The 5-year, 10-year, and 15-year morbidity and mortality rates for all cases are 30%, 50%, and 70%. Peripheral arterial occlusive disease is thus a very serious disease, not so much because of the risk to the leg, but rather as an indicator of generalized vascular disease from which two-thirds of the patients die.

4.4.1.1 Acute peripheral arterial occlusive disease

Clinical findings

Acute occlusion of the arteries of the extremities involves a sudden or rapidly developing complete cross-sectional blockage of an arterial conduit vessel. Depending on the location and the existing collateralization, the effects may range from a clinically silent occlusion (usually a local thrombotic one, with a preexisting stenosis) to an acute (embolic) ischemic syndrome that is an immediate threat to the extremity affected. In addition to the impending loss of the extremity, particularly in high-level thromboses, tourniquet syndrome after delayed recanalization of the occlusion may be life-threatening. The lower extremity is affected by acute occlusion in approximately 85% of cases and the upper extremity in roughly 15%. Some 70–85% of acute occlusions of the extremity arteries are caused by embolism, and approximately 15–30% involve local thrombosis. Other causes may be considered in 5–10% of cases (e.g., dissecting aneurysm, trauma, vasospasm, external compression). Some 80–90% of emboli have a cardioembolic pathogenesis (cardiac defects, atrial fibrillation, akinetic ventricular segment, or cardiac wall aneurysm following a myocardial infarction). Rarer sources of emboli include arterial aneurysms, atherosclerotic changes (arterioarterial embolism), compression syndrome in the upstream large arteries, and iatrogenic catheter-induced embolism. Other possibilities that also need to be considered include paradoxic venoarterial embolism in cases of open oval foramen, tumor embolism, foreign-body embolism, and fat embolism. In the typical case, the diagnosis can be made quite reliably on the basis of the patient history and physical findings, with Pratt's six Ps: pain, pallor, pulselessness, paralysis, paresthesia, prostration; only pulselessness occurs in all cases. To prevent unnecessary delays in the treatment of these acute emergencies, diagnostic imaging should be left as a matter of principle to the institution at which the final treatment will be given; after a clinically suspected diagnosis of "acute extremity artery occlusion," the patient should be transferred immediately, without any further diagnostic procedures, to a vascular center for in-patient admission.

Diagnosis

Patient history

If there is no existing collateralization, acute-onset, severe resting pain occurs in one extremity, typically "whiplash-like." If there is existing collateralization, there is frequently mild pain, which is often only perceived as dysesthesia, or rapid-onset intermittent claudication, or the condition may even be clinically completely silent. During the following hours, improvement is often seen—in favorable cases, this a sign of quickly developing collateralization, while in unfavorable ones it results from hypesthesia to anesthesia in very severe ischemia. Differential diagnosis: the differential diagnosis between embolism and thrombosis is also the most important aspect for follow-up (treatment of an embolism source, long-term anticoagulation treatment). Definitive clarification is not always possible.
Signs favoring embolism are:
- Adolescent age group or absence of arterial occlusive disease
- Atrial fibrillation, cardiac defects, cardiac wall aneurysm, reduced left-ventricular function
- Upstream arterial aneurysm

Signs favoring a local thrombotic occlusion are:
- Absence of the above criteria
- Prior arterial occlusive disease
- Previous local trauma
- Prior dilative arteriopathy at the occlusion site (popliteal artery)

Physical examination

Paleness in the extremity or livedo, along with pulselessness or weakening of the pulse distal to the occlusion, develop immediately; coldness in comparison with the contralateral side often only develops after a delay, depending on the outside temperature and the position of the extremity. Absent or reduced venous filling (which should be tested with the patient in the decubitus position with the leg elevated) reflects the severity of the ischemia. When there is a high occlusion in the area of the aortic bifurcation, paraplegic syndromes are possible (with involvement of the lumbar arteries). Ischemic rigidity of the muscles, paralysis, and sensory loss are signs of very severe ischemia with rapidly imminent loss of the extremity. In higher-level occlusions, the situation is life-threatening (with a mortality rate of up to 30%) due to impending circulatory shock and acute renal failure (crush kidney), and urgent action is needed.

Imaging examination

Color duplex ultrasonography makes it possible to locate the occlusion very quickly and assess its length so that the treatment approach can be planned (surgery or catheter intervention). If the extremity is not acutely threatened (in incomplete ischemia syndrome), other noninvasive methods such as ankle arterial pressure measurement and segmental pulse volume recordings, as well as diagnostic angiography, can be used. After successful reperfusion therapy, the cause should be clarified:

■ Search for the source of the embolism: electrocardiography, chest x-ray, abdominal ultrasound, computed tomography, magnetic resonance imaging

■ In acute popliteal artery occlusion: ultrasound to exclude a thrombotic aneurysm (including the contralateral side), cystic degeneration of the adventitia, or muscular entrapment syndrome

■ If there is a suspicion of dissecting aneurysm: chest x-ray, transesophageal echocardiography, computed tomography, magnetic resonance imaging, duplex ultrasonography of the abdominal aorta and pelvic arteries.

Treatment

For differentiated descriptions of the treatment, see also the specialized sections below for the different levels. *Immediate measures to be initiated by the first treating physician:*

■ 5000–10,000 IU unfractionated heparin intravenously for immediate anticoagulation

■ Pain treatment (not intramuscular!)

■ Moderately lower positioning of the legs and cotton-wool protective dressing

■ Oxygen administration

■ Referral to hospital accompanied by the emergency physician

Intramuscular injections, raising of the legs and exogenous warming are contraindicated.

General measures: continuation of heparin treatment, guided by the partial thromboplastin time (PTT), and oxygen administration. In prolonged ischemia with extensive muscle necroses, the patient requires intensive care. The correct balance of fluids and electrolytes is decisive for preventing crush kidney and multiple-organ failure. In cases of renal failure, hemofiltration treatment or hemodialysis is necessary. Cardiac rhythm problems and cardiac insufficiency must be expected, particularly after successful reperfusion of prolonged ischemia. Timely fasciotomy to prevent compartment syndrome must be considered. Measuring intramuscular pressure can be helpful here.

Vascular reconstruction: In principle, this can be done either surgically (embolectomy, thrombectomy, thromboendarterectomy, and bypass placement) or by catheter intervention; systemic fibrinolytic treatment is now obsolete. In the lower extremity, occlusions of the pelvic circulation as far as the femoral artery bifurcation carry a particularly high risk of life-threatening complications, in view of the large thrombus burden and the large mass of tissue affected by the ischemia, and such occlusions are usually treated acutely with surgery. However, new rotation thrombectomy catheters and self-expanding stents now also allow rapid catheter-based vascular recanalization. Infrainguinal occlusions are usually recanalized with catheter procedures, but vascular surgery methods are a possible alternative. The classical methods of aspiration embolectomy are available, often in combination with local catheter lysis (with urokinase or rt-PA) and supplementary percutaneous transluminal angioplasty for existing arteriosclerotic changes.

Primary amputation: Although preserving the extremity is normally the goal of treatment, primary amputation of the affected extremity may be the most useful and life-saving measure in individual cases—particularly in patients with extremely severe multimorbidity and when treatment has been delayed for severely advanced ischemia with resultant incipient necroses.

Follow-up and prophylaxis against recurrence

■ Elimination of the source of the embolism (e.g., regularization of atrial fibrillation, oral anticoagulation treatment, surgical elimination of aneurysms).

■ Anticoagulant treatment: if the source of embolism is not treatable or if an embolism is probable but the source has not been found (20–30% of cases), long-term anticoagulation treatment should be for the goal.

■ Antiplatelet medication: platelet inhibitors (ASA 100 mg, or alternatively ticlopidine 2 × 250 mg or clopidogrel 75 mg) are indicated after TEA, bypass surgery with plastic prostheses, and in generalized arteriosclerosis.

4.4.1.2   Chronic peripheral arterial occlusive disease

Symptoms

Typical symptoms include cramp-like pain in the legs during exercise (intermittent claudication). The pain is reproducible and occurs after a certain walking distance or after a defined effort. The location of the pain depends on the location of the flow obstruction. For example, patients with a stenosis or occlusion in the superficial femoral artery report calf pain, while patients with pelvic vessel problems describe pain in the upper and lower leg. A typical finding is rapid relief of the pain after a short rest.

It is only in advanced cases that a feeling of cold and resting pain occur, which often force the patient to let the leg hang downward. On the basis of the clinical findings, peripheral arterial occlusive disease is divided into four stages using the Fontaine classification in continental Europe (Table 4.4-1), while in English-speaking countries it is mainly the more precise Rutherford–Becker classification that is used (Table 4.4-2).

Table 4.4-1 Fontaine staging system (as adapted by Bollinger).

Stage	Symptoms
I	No clinical symptoms despite confirmed atherosclerotic changes or flow obstructions
II	Exercise-dependent pain in post-stenotic muscle groups, which is reversible (intermittent claudication)
IIa	Pain-free walking distance > 200 m
IIb	Pain-free walking distance < 200 m
(IIc)	Lesion with no evidence of a critical perfusion situation
III	Resting pain
IV	Resting pain with necroses or gangrene, with critical perfusion (post-stenotic pressure less than 50 mmHg)

Table 4.4-2 Rutherford–Becker classification.

Stage	Symptoms, test results
0	Asymptomatic arterial occlusive disease. Normal treadmill test
1	Slight claudication symptoms, with no relevant restriction to activities of daily living. Treadmill test > 250 m, ankle pressure after exercise < 50 mmHg but > 25 mmHg
2	Moderate claudication symptoms, rarely restricting activities of daily living. Treadmill test not completed (100–250 m)
3	Claudication symptoms restricting activities of daily living. On the treadmill test, walking distance less than 100 m, ankle pressure after exercise < 50 mmHg
4	Resting pain. Resting ankle pressure < 60 mmHg, toe pressure < 40 mmHg, shallow Doppler curve
5	Circumscribed tissue defects, return to normal possible with adequate wound care. Resting ankle pressure < 40 mmHg, toe pressure < 30 mmHg, shallow Doppler curve
6	Advanced hypoxic tissue damage, amputation unavoidable, resting ankle pressure < 40 mmHg, toe pressure < 30 mmHg, shallow Doppler curve

Depending on the location of the circulatory obstruction, various types are distinguished.

Pelvic type (aortoiliac type)

Circulatory obstructions in the infrarenal aorta and in the pelvic arteries mainly occur in chronic smokers, in whom some 60% of the lesions are found in this area. Typical findings include claudication symptoms in the area of the thigh and calf musculature, as well as in the buttocks area. Erectile dysfunction is often found if the internal iliac artery is affected bilaterally.

Leriche syndrome is a special form involving an occlusion of the aortic bifurcation. Abdominal pain and an iliofemoral steal phenomenon over the Riolan arcades may appear as the leading symptoms.

Thigh type

In the thigh type, claudication in the area of the calf is the most frequent major symptom. The superficial femoral artery and popliteal artery are most often affected in occlusions. Good collateral circulation may develop via the deep femoral artery, so that clinical symptoms may only appear at a late stage particularly in patients who are not very mobile. In this case, what is known as a "walk-through phenomenon" is also possible, in which the patient continues walking despite sudden pain, which subsequently resolves.

Lower leg type

In patients with diabetes mellitus, this segment is affected disproportionately often, in 50% of cases. All three lower leg arteries can be affected in principle. The typical locations for pain are the calf and foot. However, as there is often concomitant polyneuropathy, the clinical findings are unreliable. In diabetic patients, for example, there may be critical ischemia threatening the leg without any of the typical symptoms being present.

Distal type

In this form, the vascular supply is ensured as far as the lower leg, but often only collaterals can be identified distally. The symptoms mainly appear in the area of the foot, and in the toes in particular (e.g., in Winiwarter–Buerger disease).

Diagnosis

In most cases, the patient history and clinical examination provide certainty regarding the presence of peripheral arterial occlusive disease. The suspicion is then confirmed using noninvasive methods, and the location of the circulatory obstruction is narrowed down to one or more levels. The further diagnosis then depends on the extent of the disease. However, imaging methods going beyond duplex ultrasound are only justified if the results can be expected to have implications for treatment.

Clinical examination

The clinical examination of patients with peripheral arterial occlusive disease follows the usual rules: inspection, palpation, and auscultation.

Inspection

Peripheral arterial occlusive disease can sometimes be diagnosed at a glance, as Figs. 4.4-1 and 4.4-2 show. On inspection, particularly in advanced chronic stages, trophic disturbances such as reduced hair growth on the legs, slow nail growth, livedo, and thinning of the skin are noticed.

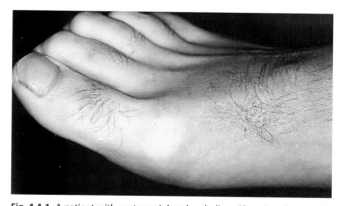

Fig. 4.4-1 A patient with acute peripheral embolism. There is paleness of the foot, and a clear temperature difference is evident on palpation. The source of the embolism in this case was a large infrarenal aortic aneurysm.

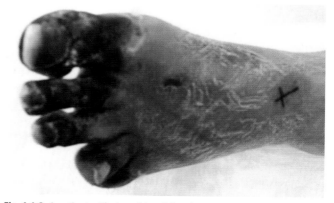

Fig. 4.4-2 A patient with stage IV peripheral arterial occlusive disease.

Ratschow's leg-position test: The patient lies on the back. Both legs are raised vertically upward, and rolling movements of the foot on the ankle joint are carried out for 2 min. The patient then sits up, with the legs hanging down from the examination couch. Any unilateral circulatory disturbance then becomes evident through an initially underperfused pale extremity; reactive hyperemia begins after a delay (> 15 s), as does venous filling (> 20 s). The reactive hyperemia lasts much longer than it does in the healthy extremity.

Palpation

All of the pulse sites are examined. The pulse in the upper extremity is palpated initially (radial, ulnar, and brachial arteries), then the carotid pulse bilaterally, and then the femoral pulse, popliteal pulse, and the pulse in the anterior tibial artery and dorsalis pedis artery. This makes it possible to narrow down a pathological process to one segment. For example, if the femoral pulse is easily palpated in one leg but the popliteal pulse and foot pulse are no longer palpable, the circulatory obstruction must be located in the area of thigh.

Auscultation

Auscultatory examination of the arteries starts with the heart. Any pathological heart murmur must be identified and included in the evaluation. The vascular circulation is auscultated with the stethoscope—i.e., the abdomen, course of the pelvic arteries, inner side of the thigh, and back of the knee. It is quite common to hear a flow noise that indicates a stenosis. The higher the frequency of the sound, the higher the grade of stenosis. If there are no flow noises and the pulse is absent distally, then there is a clinical suspicion of occlusion.

Noninvasive imaging diagnosis

Treadmill

Using a treadmill (gradient 12%, speed 3.2 km/h or 2 mph, Bruce protocol) allows objective testing of the distance the patient can walk without pain. Measurement of the ankle–brachial index (ABI) or tibiobrachial index (TBI) before and after exercise also provides objective evidence of the extent of the disease.

At our own institution, however, we no longer carry out these measurements routinely, as we believe the decisive element is the extent of impairment of the patient's quality of life and individual situation.

Arterial Doppler pressure measurement

The patient must have no exertion for 10–15 min before the measurement. The procedure is conducted with the patient supine, at a constant room temperature. Pressures in the upper arms are measured first, and then the pressures at the ankle arteries. Applying pressure with the Doppler probe should be avoided, and the Doppler probe should be held at an angle of around 60° to the vessel axis (Fig. 4.4-3). The measurement provides two values: the arm–ankle gradient and the ABI.

The arm–ankle gradient is calculated from the arm pressure minus the ankle artery pressure. Values from 0 to –20 are normal, while with values from –20 to –40 there is a suspicion of falsely high values—for example, due to marked medial sclerosis (in diabetics or dialysis patients). Positive pressure values greater than 5 are evi-

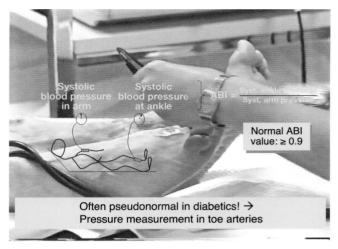

Fig. 4.4-3 Arterial blood pressure measurement in the legs.

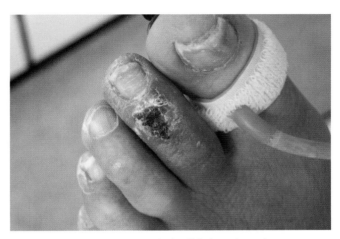

Fig. 4.4-4 Pressure measurement in the digital arteries at the toes.

dence of peripheral arterial occlusive disease. The ABI value is obtained by dividing the highest blood-pressure value measured in the lower extremity by the higher value in the upper extremity. A value greater than 0.97 is normal; 0.8–0.97 represents well-compensated PAOD; at 0.6–0.8 there is poor compensation or a multiple-level problem. Values below 0.6 indicate critical ischemia. Falsely low values occur when one carries out the measurement too soon after exercise or with multiple measurements, after pulse volume recording, or when the temperature is too low. Compression of the artery due to increased pressure from the probe also produces false low values. False high values are obtained when there is medial calcinosis. Signs of this include an ABI of more than 40, or an ankle artery pressure over 300 mmHg. In this case, measuring the toe pressure may allow one to objectify the findings (Fig. 4.4-4). Edema is another cause of false high values. ABI values are also falsely high when there is bilateral stenosis of the subclavian artery.

ABI measurement makes it possible to determine with a high degree of certainty whether PAOD is present, and it provides evidence of the severity of the disease. In addition, the ABI value also makes it possible to assess the prognosis for the patient, which is poorer the lower the ABI value.

Toe artery pressure measurement (toe brachial index, TBI)

This can be measured either with a strain gauge manometer, a laser Doppler, or photoplethysmography. TBI values greater than 0.6 are normal.

Segmental pulse oscillography

Each heartbeat pumps out a stroke volume that produces a pressure wave. This leads to variations in the caliber of the vessels and to volume variations in the perivascular tissue, both of which can be measured either mechanically or electronically. Pulse volume recording is now typically done electronically. However, the method is not capable of definitively excluding or confirming arterial occlusive disease. Side-to-side differences and the level of the circulatory obstruction can be evaluated. For example, an amplitude reduction and a delayed peak in one segment indicate an obstruction proximal to the cuff.

Color duplex ultrasonography

Color duplex ultrasonography is now the most important noninvasive examination method. It allows almost all vascular regions to be visualized and is just as reliable for treatment planning as the much more expensive method of magnetic resonance angiography. Duplex ultrasound provides a clear morphological image of the arteries and shows aneurysmal areas and the quality and composition of plaques, dissections, stenoses, and occlusions (Figs. 4.4-5 and 4.4-6). The size of thrombosed aneurysms can be measured and perivascular structures can be assessed (tumors, Baker cysts, cystic adventitial degeneration, etc.).

MR angiography

This is as good as duplex ultrasonography for treatment planning, although it is much more expensive. It has become indispensable for the planning of complex procedures. MR angiography allows three-dimensional imaging of vessels at any level. One problem with it is that it overestimates stenoses, while in addition the signal is obliterated when implants such as stents or joint prostheses are present. Calcified structures are not identified. Patients with defibrillators, spinal cord stimulators, intracerebral shunts, cochlea implants, etc., cannot be examined due to the strength of the magnetic fields.

CT angiography

Sixty-four–slice CT angiography provides very good three-dimensional imaging of the vessels. However, its disadvantages include the high level of radiation exposure, the need to use large amounts of contrast, and difficulty in distinguishing between a calcified, occluded lumen and a perfused lumen in the area of the lower leg arteries.

Intra-arterial angiography

This is now only indicated in exceptional cases for purely diagnostic purposes. Intra-arterial angiography can usually be combined with a therapeutic intervention. However, it is still regarded as the gold standard for imaging. As an invasive procedure, it is associated with potential complications such as arterial dissection, embolism, pseudoaneurysms, contrast-related renal failure, and contrast intolerance.

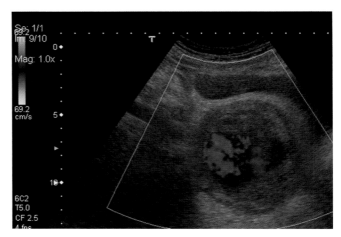

Fig. 4.4-5 A pelvic artery aneurysm as the source of an embolism in a patient with acute peripheral embolic arterial occlusions.

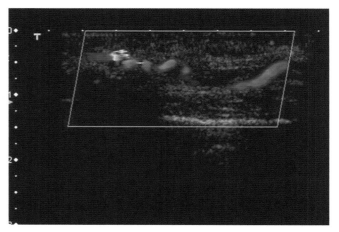

Fig. 4.4-6 Corkscrew-like arterial deformations in a patient with thromboangiitis obliterans (Winiwarter–Buerger disease).

Differential diagnosis

Neurogenic claudication

This is the most frequent differential diagnosis, and is caused by degenerative changes in the spine, or a herniated disk. Typical findings include pain radiating to the corresponding dermatomes and neurological abnormalities (such as reduced muscular proprioceptive reflexes and sensory deficits). Pain when walking down a slope or after prolonged standing is also typical of neurogenic claudication. Certain postures in which the affected nerves are relieved, such as bending of the hips, lead to symptomatic improvement. The pulse status and Ratschow test are usually unremarkable.

Arthropathies

Acute or chronic joint diseases, particularly coxarthrosis and gonarthrosis, can also lead to movement-dependent leg pain. With a precise patient history and clinical examination, it is usually possible to distinguish these from peripheral arterial occlusive disease.

Venous claudication

Patients with leg pain caused by venous conditions usually have a feeling of heaviness and a tendency to develop swelling in the legs, or pain after prolonged standing. Clinically, there are signs of chronic venous insufficiency. The patients are often free of symptoms in the morning, with the leg pain increasing during the course of the day.

Polyneuropathy

In the distal symmetrical polyneuropathy that is seen in most cases, patients usually report leg pain that begins when they are at rest, or often is triggered by the warmth of the bed during the night. The pain forces the patients to get up and walk about, after which the symptoms decline or disappear again. Typically, there is an absence of exercise-dependent pain. Clinically, there is often a sock-shaped sensory deficit, reduced muscular proprioceptive reflexes, reduced sensitivity to temperature, or a pathological neurofilament test.

References

Gröchenig E. Gefäßmedizin. Berlin: ABW Wissenschaftsverlag, 2002.

Jäger K, et al. Schweizer Richtlinien zum Management der PAVK-Patienten durch den Facharzt. Kardiovaskuläre Medizin 2007; 10: 403–11.

Kröger K, Gröchenig E (eds.). Nicht invasive Diagnostik angiologischer Krankheitsbilder. Berlin: ABW Wissenschaftsverlag, 2007.

Norgren L, et al. on behalf of the TASC II working group. Inter-Society Consensus for the management of peripheral arterial disease (TASC II). Eur J Vasc Endovasc Surg 2007; 33 (Suppl 1): S1–S75.

Ouriel K. Peripheral arterial disease. Lancet 2001; 358: 1257–64.

4.4.2   Prevention and management of cardiovascular risk factors

Thomas Cissarek

Cardiovascular diseases are the most frequent cause of early invalidity and death. High-risk patients have to be identified at an early stage in order to prevent cardiovascular deaths and diseases.

Who is at increased risk for vascular diseases?

- Patients with atherosclerotic vascular disease or diabetes mellitus have such a high rate of cardiovascular events that the best possible adjustment of all risk factors should be provided; risk stratification is not needed in these cases.
- First-degree relatives of patients with vascular disease.
- Individuals in the family of a patient with vascular disease.
- Individuals with very strong risk factors.

Risk stratification needs to be carried out in order to identify groups of people who do not have vascular disease or diabetes in whom there is an above-average probability of cardiovascular events.

4.4.2.1   Risk factors

The association between specific patient characteristics and the occurrence of atherothrombotic events has been examined in numerous epidemiological studies. A distinction is made here between *risk factors,* in which there is a confirmed causal link with atherothrombosis, and *risk markers,* in which although there is a clear association with ischemic events, the causal relationship has not (yet) been confirmed. Some risk factors and risk markers, such as physical inactivity, obesity, poor nutrition, and psychosocial factors are considered to be predisposing—i.e., they come into effect at least partly through other factors that in turn have a direct effect (e.g., obesity increases the blood pressure, blood glucose, etc.).

The following causal factors cannot be influenced:

- Age
- Sex
- Family history of vascular disease

The following causal factors can be influenced:

- Smoking
- Arterial hypertension
- Diabetes mellitus
- Cholesterol (LDL cholesterol $\uparrow$, HDL cholesterol $\downarrow$)
- Excess weight status/obesity
- Physical inactivity
- Poor nutrition
- Earlier ischemic events

4.4.2.2   Risk markers

- C-reactive protein
- Coagulation factors—e.g., plasminogen activator inhibitor type 1 (PAI-1), fibrinogen
- Psychosocial factors (e.g., depression, stress, etc.)
- Low socioeconomic status
- Triglycerides $\uparrow$
- Small LDL $\uparrow$
- Lipoprotein Lp(a) $\uparrow$
- CD 40L $\uparrow$

Risk stratification should be carried out in all patients who have more than one risk factor.

4.4.2.3   Risk-adjusted prevention, primary and secondary prevention

After an initial cardiovascular event, optimal action to influence all of the risk factors must be carried out in every case. However, even patients who have not yet had an event may have a similarly high risk for cardiovascular events. These patients can be recognized using risk stratification and can then receive appropriate treatment. It is not the individual risk factors that matter, but rather the overall risk as an effect of the sum of the individual risk factors and everyday habits. The overall risk can be assessed using risk algorithms. Two algorithms are commonly used in Germany:

- ESC-SCORE for Germany
- PROCAM score (www.chd-Taskforce.de)

(The Framingham Risk Score usually overestimates the event rate for European countries and is therefore not discussed here.)

The cardiovascular risk can be estimated reliably and quite individually for each patient using these scores. A 10-year risk of > 10% represents a very high level of cardiovascular risk; a 10-year risk of 5–10% represents a high risk level; and 1–5% represents a moderate risk level.

Differences between the scoring systems

The *European Society for Cardiology Systemic Coronary Risk Evaluation* (ESC-SCORE) and the *Prospective Cardiovascular Münster* (PROCAM) algorithms evaluate risk factors in slightly different ways. Only the ESC-SCORE assesses the risk of severe hypertension-dependent (fatal) events such as stroke, aortic rupture, and death, while the PROCAM algorithm better reflects the risk of cholesterol-dependent events such as heart attack. Calculation using both systems may be useful, depending on each patient's risk profile characteristics.

ESC-SCORE

The new risk charts published by the European Society for Cardiology (ESC) have been adjusted to conditions in Germany and estimate the risk of fatal cardiovascular events on the basis of heart attack, stroke, and peripheral vascular disease for the next 10 years. Factors such as sex, age, smoking status, blood pressure, and total cholesterol or the ratio of total/HDL cholesterol are used.

CARRISMA

(www.carrisma-pocket-ll.de)

In the *Cardiovascular Risk Management* (CARRISMA) algorithm, based on the scores mentioned above, the additional significance of lifestyle factors is also taken into account:

- Physical activity
- Number of cigarettes smoked
- Body mass index (BMI)

CARRISMA is not an independent system, but is based on the scores mentioned above and represents the score results with or without taking account of the additional lifestyle parameters that are also used in CARRISMA. In comparison with PROCAM and the ESC-SCORE, higher BMI and heavier cigarette consumption may double the overall risk. Depending on its intensity, regular physical activity can reduce the initial risk by up to 40%.

Calcium score

The calcium score (coronary calcium measurement using cardio-CT), which has been incorporated into the European Society for Cardiology's prevention guidelines, can allow further stratification, particularly in medium-risk patients. Patients with a medium risk (PROCAM 10–20%) are identified as high-risk patients if the coronary calcium score (e.g., the Agatston score) is above the age-related and sex-related 75th percentile. However, measurement of the calcium score is device-dependent. The radiation exposure resulting from calcium score measurement is at the level of 1 mSv and thus within the range permitted for pregnant women by recent radiation regulations, or a range equivalent to two transatlantic flights.

Evidence of coronary calcium must not be confused with the presence of coronary stenoses; a positive calcium score alone (without evidence of ischemia) is not an indication for a cardiac catheter examination.

Caution: None of the scoring systems is capable of predicting the future. Assessing the overall risk using risk stratification serves to enhance awareness on the part of the patient and physician that there is a potentially raised level of overall risk, thereby increasing motivation to change lifestyle or start medication treatment. The emphasis should be on the idea of using (side effect–free) improvements in lifestyle as an opportunity to prevent serious disease. The greater the overall risk of cardiovascular disease, the greater the absolute benefit resulting from effective prevention. The greater the overall risk, the more intensive the preventive measures should be.

4.4.2.4 Smoking

Approximately one-third of the population in Germany (about 20 million men and women) smokes. Smoking leads to a marked acceleration of the aging process. Consuming up to 20 cigarettes per day results in a 50-year-old man having the same level of cardiovascular risk as a 60-year-old. The risk of early death is increased 2.8-fold, and with more than 20 cigarettes per day it is increased 4.2-fold.

By their 60th year of life, smokers consuming 20 cigarettes per day lose 15 years of life in comparison with nonsmokers (British Doctors' Study). Measured in terms of tobacco consumption, smoking a pipe or cigars/cigarillos has similar cardiovascular effects to those of cigarette smoking. The cancer risks are distributed differently. Smoking only a few cigarettes per day or small amounts of tobacco is also damaging.

Smoking is the most important risk factor for PAOD and its extent correlates with the severity of PAOD, the amputation rate, and the bypass occlusion rate.

Independently of the patient's cardiovascular disease status, smoking should be discussed by the physician with every smoker every time he or she visits, and smokers should be encouraged to stop with a few friendly words relating to their current reason for presentation.

Aims of treatment

Experience shows that only stopping smoking completely is successful in the longer term. When smoking is completely stopped, the rate of cardiovascular events can be expected to be halved in comparison with persistent smoking.

Recommendations

- A clear recommendation should be given to the patient to stop smoking completely, with the patient's partner or family sharing involvement if possible.
- A date for stopping smoking should be set together with the patient.
- Psychosocial support or behavioral therapy can be used.
- Concomitant pharmacotherapy.

Pharmacotherapy

Nicotine replacement therapy

Nicotine replacement is administered for 8–12 weeks in various forms (e.g., chewing gum, plaster, tablets, nasal spray). This covers the receptor-linked nicotine addiction. Abstaining from the habitual daily self-reward activity of smoking a cigarette leads to a readjustment to a "nonsmoking personality type." As soon as this step has been reached, the nicotine replacement can be reduced or stopped. Nicotine chewing gum (2 mg and 4 mg), nicotine lozenge tablets (2 mg and 4 mg), and sublingual tablets are compounds that are sold without a prescription. Nicotine nasal sprays are only available with prescription and are currently only available from international pharmacies. For basic coverage, a nicotine plaster is applied in the morning and, depending on daily needs, can be supplemented with chewing gum and lozenges. For severely addicted smokers, the nicotine spray makes the nicotine available within seconds in the usual way.

Advantages:

- Pure nicotine, without the harmful substances contained in smoke
- Dosage can be adjusted
- Reduces withdrawal effects (nervousness, irritability, craving)

Contraindications:

- Postinfarction period (2 weeks)
- Unstable angina pectoris
- Severe disturbances of cardiac rhythm

Bupropion (Zyban®, Wellbutrin®)

Bupropion is an antidepressive agent with similar efficacy to that of individual nicotine replacement preparations. Patients report that their desire to smoke is reduced even with a gradually increasing introductory dosage before tobacco consumption has been stopped. Bupropion is a prescription drug.

- Inhibition of reuptake of dopamine and norepinephrine
- Reduction of:
  - Withdrawal symptoms
  - Craving
  - Weight increase
- Gradually increased dosage at 150 mg for 7 days
- 2 × 150 mg for 6–8 weeks

Varenicline (Champix®)

Varenicline is a partial nicotine receptor agonist (α_4-β_2-nicotine receptor) and thus stimulates the release of dopamine (a nicotine-like effect to reduce the withdrawal symptom). This blocks the effect of nicotine during smoking (antagonist). The agent is intended to be used for 12 weeks. The introductory dosage is initially 2 × 0.5 mg/d. The regular dosage is 2 × 1 mg/d. Varenicline is a prescription drug.

Side effects:

- Moderate nausea (25% 1 h after ingestion), vomiting, headache, flatulence
- Sleep disturbance, abnormal dreams, gustatory changes
- Evidence of suicidal ideation

Cardiovascular diseases are not a contraindication. Individual observations have shown that there is an increase in aggressive or depressive behavior and in suicidal tendency.

When smoking is stopped and the diet remains unchanged, a 5–7% increase in weight above the starting weight can be expected. When nicotine replacement and bupropion are used, this effect appears to be smaller. Increasing the amount of exercise during this period, along with medication support, can help reduce the weight increase effect. The patient should be prepared to expect an increase in weight and should be willing to accept it for a period of approximately 12 months. Applying weight reduction simultaneously is liable to be excessively demanding.

E-cigarette

An electronic cigarette, also known as an electric cigarette, e-cigarette, or smokeless cigarette, is a product in which an evaporated liquid is inhaled. The inhaled steam is similar to tobacco smoke in its consistency and the sensory impression created, but in contrast to smoking there is no combustion. The liquid is evaporated, rather than burned. The liquid may also contain nicotine. In contrast to smokers of traditional cigarettes, consumers do not inhale any carbon monoxide, formaldehyde, acrolein, hydrocyanic acid (prussic acid), arsenic, or carcinogenic polycyclic aromatic hydrocarbons.

However, the Food and Drug Administration (FDA) and public health experts have warned against electronic cigarettes and announced that a laboratory analysis of electronic cigarettes found samples containing carcinogenic and toxic chemicals such as diethylene glycol, an ingredient used in antifreeze.

Nicotine-containing liquids—i.e., capsules and cartridges containing nicotine as an inhalant—are subject to the federal drug law and therefore require licensing. In Germany, infringements may be subject to penalties of up to 1 year's imprisonment or a fine under legislation on the manufacture and distribution of medicines. Products with which drugs may be administered (e.g., an applicator) may only be sold with CE labeling (under the law on medical products). Under drug legislation, infringements are also subject to penalties of imprisonment for up to 1 year or a fine.

In summary, the e-cigarette can therefore currently not be recommended to assist patients in withdrawing from smoking.

4.4.2.5 Physical inactivity

An inactive lifestyle is a typical characteristic of modern cultures. The benefits of physical activity as a measure for primary prevention have been demonstrated by numerous studies. All adults should include a period of at least 30 min of physical activity daily at a moderate exercise level in their everyday routine. Daily training should take the form of dynamic endurance training. However, strengthening exercises are also useful and can be done for up to 20% of the planned time. The intended metabolic effect of the exercise (fat reduction, increased HDL level, improvement of endothelial function) is achieved by more prolonged exercise at a moderate level, and short phases at a high level increase the body's maximum performance capacity. Healthy individuals can reach their maximum cardiac frequency for short periods without risk. In patients with cardiovascular diseases, the intensity and duration of exercise need to be adjusted to the relevant guidelines.

4.4.2.6   Hyperlipidemia

Epidemiology and pathology

Independent risk factors for the occurrence of PAOD include raised total cholesterol concentrations, a raised LDL cholesterol level, and increased triglycerides and lipoprotein Lp(a). Primary genetic disturbances of lipid metabolism (e.g., a defective LDL receptor) lead to particularly severe hypercholesterolemia, with a high risk of infarction. Most disturbances of lipid metabolism are multifactorial, however, and only become clinically manifest as a result of environmental factors (e.g., diet, excess weight, lack of exercise).

Identifying high-risk patients

These include patients with coronary heart disease (CHD) or CHD-equivalent risk factors such as cardiac manifestations of atherosclerosis (PAOD, abdominal aortic aneurysm, symptomatic carotid stenosis) and manifest diabetes mellitus.

Risk stratification for non–high-risk patients

Risk stratification using PROCAM, ESC-SCORE, and CARRISMA as well if appropriate should be carried out in these patients in order to assess the 10-year risk level.

Treatment goals

The newly published European guideline (ESC/EAS) now sets out even stricter target values.
- In patients who are at moderate risk (with scores of 1–5%), an LDL cholesterol level of < 115 mg/dL should be aimed for.
- In those with a risk score between 5% and 10%, and those with prominent individual risk factors (e.g., familial hypercholesterolemia, marked hypertension), the LDL cholesterol value should be < 100 mg/dL.
- In patients with manifest coronary heart disease, peripheral arterial occlusive disease, type 2 diabetics, type 1 diabetics with end-organ damage, patients with chronic renal insufficiency and those with a risk score > 10% (very high cardiovascular risk), the LDL cholesterol level should be < 70 mg/L, or a reduction in LDL cholesterol of at least 50% should be aimed for.

However, these target values are very ambitious.

Aims of treatment

In order to prevent cardiovascular events, the priority in all patients with myocardial infarction and high-risk patients must be to achieve LDL cholesterol concentrations well below 100 mg/dL (2.58 mmol/L) after acute coronary syndrome, and if possible below 70 mg/dL (1.81 mmol/L) in those with CHD and concomitant metabolic syndrome or diabetes mellitus. Risk stratification is necessary in all patients who are not at high risk. Treatment is indicated when there is a 10-year risk of myocardial infarction greater than 20% or a risk of cardiovascular death greater than 5%.

Treatment management for lipid metabolism disturbances

In non–high-risk patients, the full potential for lifestyle changes should be initially exploited. There is clear evidence that reducing cholesterol levels using statins has a favorable prognostic effect in high-risk patients. The effect is very largely due to the reduction in LDL cholesterol.

A number of other drugs are also available for lipid-reducing treatment. Lipid-reducing drugs can also be administered in combination. In more severe forms of hypercholesterolemia, a combination of a resorption inhibitor and a statin can be effective, as well as administration of nicotinic acid.

Caution is advisable when fibric acids are combined with statins, due to the risk of myopathy and rhabdomyolysis. In patients receiving combination therapy, the serum activity of the muscle enzymes needs to be checked once every 3 months, or when there is any clinical suspicion of muscle symptoms. In 2011, the FDA advised against readjustment with high-dose statins (80 mg), as the SEARCH study showed that there was a severe increase in the risk of myopathy. However, patients who have taken 80 mg simvastatin for 1 year without any muscle problems can continue the treatment. (When there is co-medication with amiodarone, verapamil, or diltiazem, the maximum simvastatin dosage is 10 mg; when the patient is receiving co-medication with amlodipine or ranolazine, the threshold value is 20 mg/day). According to more recent studies, the clinical benefit of fibric acids in hypertriglyceridemia and diabetes mellitus is a matter of controversy in relation to hard clinical end points.

Importance of the HDL hypothesis

Ever since it was recognized that there is a strong inverse correlation between HDL cholesterol values and the risk of cardiovascular diseases, one of the goals of preventative treatment has been to increase HDL cholesterol levels.
- Physical activity leads to an increase in the HDL level.
- Nicotinic acid (niacin), which also increases HDL, has been found to reduce femoral atherothrombosis and to delay coronary atherothrombosis in patients with PAOD (2009 PAOD guideline: recommendation grade 0, class 2 evidence). However, a general recommendation can still not yet be given. The AIM-HIGH study (Atherothrombosis Intervention in Metabolic Syndrome with Low HDL Cholesterol/High Triglyceride and Impact on Global Health Outcomes) was abandoned after 18 months in May 2011 due to inefficacy and evidence of an increased rate of stroke. However, the first results from another large study (HPS2-THRIVE) will only become available in 2013.
- The cholesteryl ester transfer protein (CETP) inhibitor torcetrapib increases HDL cholesterol values, but has not been found to have any influence on the progression of atherosclerosis (as measured by atheroma volume on intravascular ultrasound). The cardiovascular mortality actually increased (probably in a molecule-specific fashion, due to an increase in blood pressure, serum aldosterone, and electrolyte disturbances). In addition, increased noncardiovascular mortality was also observed, mainly as a result of cancer diseases and infections. It is speculated that the immunological function of HDL was altered by torcetrapib treatment.

4.4.2.7   Arterial hypertension

Increased blood-pressure values are associated with a doubling of the risk of PAOD developing. Treatment for arterial hypertension in patients with PAOD has been shown to reduce the cardiovascular mortality rate.

Arterial hypertension is regarded as being confirmed if several measurements (three measurements on three different days) of systolic and/or diastolic blood pressure at the physician's office *reach* or *exceed* the threshold value.

Staging of hypertension (Hochdruckliga [Hypertension League] 2008)

- Optimal blood pressure: < 120 / < 80 mmHg
- Normal normotension: 120/80 to 129/84 mmHg
- High normal normotension: 130/85 to 139/89 mmHg
- Grade 1 hypertension: 140/90 to 159/99 mmHg
- Grade 2 hypertension: 160/100 to 179/109 mmHg
- Grade 3 hypertension: > 180/110 mmHg
- Isolated systolic hypertension: from systolic 140 mmHg with diastolic values < 90 mmHg
- Isolated diastolic hypertension: from diastolic 90 mmHg with systolic values < 140 mmHg.

The overall cardiovascular risk in patients with hypertension can be assessed using the familiar scores. The European Society of Hypertension (ESH) and the German Hypertension League (*Deutsche Hochdruckliga,* DHL) have included metabolic syndrome, diabetes mellitus, and end-organ damage as additional criteria in their *risk stratification:*

- Left ventricular myocardial hypertrophy
- Intima–media thickening
- Microalbuminuria
- Incipient restriction of renal function: creatinine clearance < 60 mL/min or estimated glomerular filtration rate (eGFR) < 60 mL/min/1.73 m^2

Lifestyle changes are regarded as providing the basis for every other effort. The lower the patient's cardiovascular risk, the longer the lifestyle changes can be implemented before drug therapy begins. In those at high risk or with blood pressure values below 180 mmHg systolic or 110 mmHg diastolic, immediate drug treatment is recommended alongside lifestyle changes (Table 4.4-3).

Table 4.4-3 Threshold values in various procedures for measuring blood pressure.

Measurement in physician's office	140/90 mmHg
Self-measurement of blood pressure	135/85 mmHg
24-h measurement	Daytime average: 135/85 mmHg Nocturnal average: 120/75 mmHg 24-h average: 130/80 mmHg

Aims of treatment

There have been a number of discoveries and publications in recent years with implications for treatment decision-making. Ideas and recommendations for target blood pressure in the treatment of hypertension have changed.

- The aim of antihypertensive treatment is to achieve normalization of the blood pressure *below 140/90 mmHg* in all patients, independently of age.
- For individuals who are at particularly high risk and patients with diabetes mellitus or nephropathy, blood pressure should be reduced to *below 130/80 mmHg.*
- There is currently insufficient evidence for a target blood pressure < 130 mmHg systolic in patients with diabetes mellitus. Blood-pressure values < 120/70 mmHg should not be aimed for.
- There appears to be an increased risk of cardiovascular events with excessively low blood-pressure values only in patients with coronary heart disease when diastolic blood pressure falls below a critical value (< 74 mmHg).
- In patients with renal insufficiency, a target blood pressure of < 130/80 mmHg appears to be beneficial to protect the kidneys, and when there is simultaneous proteinuria ≥ 1 g/day, the target value should be ≥ 125/75 mmHg.
- If treatment decisions are based on the patient's self-measurements at home or 24-h blood pressure measurements, the values should be a mean of 5–15 mmHg lower for systolic blood pressure and 5–10 mmHg lower for diastolic blood pressure.

Nondrug measures

Nondrug measures are based on lifestyle changes, which lead to a direct reduction in blood pressure and a reduction in the increased cardiovascular risk. In order of importance, these include the following *lifestyle changes:*

- Increased physical activity, particularly with endurance training
- Reduction or normalization of increased body weight
- Reduction of salt consumption to a maximum of 6 g/d and increased consumption of vegetables and fish
- Restriction of alcohol consumption (less than 30 g/d in men and 20 g/d in women)
- Reduction of stress and noise exposure

Successful implementation of such measures, particularly the first three, is as effective as any single-drug therapy.

Self-help groups such as those supported by the German Hypertension League provide support for long-term care in patients with hypertension.

Drug treatment

Drug treatment can be started with monotherapy or immediately with low-dose dual therapy. If the blood-pressure adjustment is insufficient, the dosage of the previous therapy can be increased, or a switch can be made to triple therapy. Low-dose combination therapy is recommended, as blood pressure can be adjusted in this way with fewer side effects than with high-dose monotherapy. The first choice of an antihypertensive agent is made in accordance with pathophysiological considerations, tolerability, and concomitant diseases. On the basis of the data provided by the HOPE Study, long-acting angiotensin-converting enzyme (ACE) inhibitors may be recommended in patients with PAOD and hypertension. β-Blockers are not contraindicated in PAOD, but instead reduce cardiac events. α_1-Blockers and central antihypertensive agents are now regarded as drugs of second choice for combination treatment.

Treatment monitoring is best carried out by having patients measure their blood pressure themselves, or with 24-h long-term measurement. Laboratory testing of serum potassium and serum creatinine is recommended.

4.4.2.8 Diabetes mellitus

Current data have demonstrated the importance of diabetes mellitus in the development of PAOD. Each 1% increase in hemoglobin A_{1c} increases the risk of PAOD by 28%. Diabetes mellitus increases the PAOD risk by a factor of three to four. After smoking, diabetes mellitus is the most important risk factor for the progression of PAOD.

Effective antihyperglycemic treatment is associated with a significant reduction in the risk of macrovascular events.

The prevalence of diabetes mellitus in Germany is approximately 8%, and it increases with advancing age. Between the 40th and 60th years of life, more men than women are affected, while after the age of 60 the proportions are reversed. Abnormal fasting glucose and impaired glucose tolerance are regarded as early stages of diabetes mellitus.

Diabetes mellitus:

- $HbA_{1c} \geq 6.5\%$ (48 mmol/L)
- Incidental plasma glucose value ≥ 200 mg/dL (≥ 11.1 mmol/L)
- Fasting plasma glucose ≥ 126 mg/dL (≥ 7.0 mmol/L)
- Oral glucose tolerance test (OGGT) 2-h value in venous plasma ≥ 200 mg/dL (≥ 11.1 mmol/L)

Impaired fasting glucose (IFG):

- Fasting glucose level of 100–125 mg/dL (5.6–6.9 mmol/L) in venous plasma

Impaired glucose tolerance (IGT):

- IGT for a 2-h plasma glucose level in an OGTT in the range of 140–199 mg/dL (7.8–11.0 mmol/L), with fasting glucose values < 126 mg/dL (< 7.0 mmol/L)

Aims of treatment

- Lifestyle changes (increased physical activity, weight reduction)
- Structured patient training for diabetics
- Self-monitoring of blood sugar
- Near-normoglycemic metabolic control ($HbA_{1c} < 7\%$)

Pharmacotherapy

- In addition to non-pharmacological treatment measures, antihyperglycemic drug treatment should be administered in most cases, depending on the pathophysiological stage involved. Data for cardiovascular end points are available for the following agents: metformin, glibenclamide, insulin, pioglitazone, and rosiglitazone.

- When there is additional arterial hypertension, antihypertensive agents should also be used that have organ-protective properties (on the brain, heart, kidney, and peripheral vessels) and counteract the development of manifest diabetes. The target blood pressure should be 130–140/80–85 mmHg. Even in patients with a high normal blood pressure level and simultaneous evidence of microalbuminuria, angiotensin-converting enzyme (ACE) inhibitors and angiotensin II type 1 (AT_1) antagonists should preferably be administered. These are the agents of choice for preventing progression of renal insufficiency in patients with diabetic nephropathy.

4.4.2.9 Value of hormone replacement therapy

Coronary heart disease and cardiovascular diseases are the most frequent causes of death in postmenopausal women. However, women substantially underestimate the risk of these diseases. In randomized studies in women with and without CHD, however, *no* favorable effect of hormone replacement therapy on the prognosis (e.g., the repeat infarction rate or stroke rate) was observed.

Recommendations

Due to its lack of positive effects despite simultaneous risks, hormone replacement therapy for prophylaxis against cardiovascular diseases cannot be recommended either in healthy women or in women with coronary heart disease or after stroke.

Hormone replacement therapy is only justified as a form of *treatment for severe menopausal symptoms*, after other contraindications have been checked and a careful risk–benefit analysis has been carried out.

Contraindications include breast cancer, a history including thromboembolism, congenital coagulation disturbances, cardiovascular diseases such as myocardial infarction, and status post stroke.

Women who are currently receiving hormone replacement therapy without severe menopausal symptoms should gradually discontinue it.

4.4.2.10 Importance of treatment for hyperhomocysteinemia

It is a matter of controversy whether drug treatment should be offered in order to reduce the homocysteine level and thus the cardiovascular risk. While observational studies have found that high plasma homocysteine levels were associated with increased cardiovascular events, clinical studies raised the question of whether hyperhomocysteinemia is a risk factor or a factor that is not involved in the pathological processes. Several large randomized studies showed that reducing homocysteine values with folic acid therapy did not reduce the numbers of cardiovascular events and that combined therapy with folic acid and vitamin B complex even actually increased the cardiovascular risk.

References

Baigent C, Keech A, Kearney PM, et al. Efficacy and safety of cholesterol-lowering treatment: prospective meta-analysis of data from 90,056 participants in 14 randomised trials of statins. Lancet 2005; 366: 1267–78.

Bönner G, Gysan DB, Sauer G. Prävention der Atherosklerose. Stellenwert der Behandlung der arteriellen Hypertonie. Z Kardiol 2005; 94 (Suppl 3): III/56–III/65.

Bonaa, KH, Njolstad I, Ueland PM, Schirmer H, Tverdal A, Steigen T, Wang H, Nordrhaug JE, Arnesen E, Rasmussen K. Homocysteine lowering and cardiovascular events after acute myocardial infarction (2-NORVIT-Trial). N Eng J Med 2006; 354: 1578–88.

Cooper-DeHoff RM, Gong Y, Handberg EM et al. Tight blood pressure control and cardiovascular outcomes among hypertensive patients with diabetes and coronary artery disease. J Amer Med Ass 2010; 304: 61–8.

De Backer G, Ambrosioni E, Borch-Johnsen K, et al. European guidelines on cardiovascular disease prevention in clinical practice. Third Joint Task Force of European and other Societies on Cardiovascular Disease Prevention in Clinical Practice. Eur Heart J 2003; 24.

Deutsche Gesellschaft für Angiologie, Gesellschaft für Gefäßmedizin, Arbeitsgemeinschaft der Wissenschaftlichen Medizinischen Fachgesellschaften (AWMF). Leitlinien zur Diagnostik und Therapie der peripheren arteriellen Verschlusskrankheit (PAVK), http://www.awmf-online.de, http://leitlinien.net/ (Stand 03/2009 – gültig bis 05/2012).

Deutsche Hochdruckliga e.V. DHL® – Deutsche Hypertonie Gesellschaft. Leitlinien zur Behandlung der arteriellen Hypertonie. 2011, online auf der Homepage der Hochdruckliga: http://www.hochdruckliga.de/tl_files/content/dhl/downloads/DHL-Leitlinien-2011.pdf.

Doll R, Peto R, Boreham J, Sutherland I. Mortality in relation to smoking: 50 years' observations on male British doctors. BMJ 2004; 328: 1529–33.

Eckert S, Tschöpe D. Der herzkranke Diabetiker – Stiftung in der Deutschen Diabetes Stiftung. Glukosestoffwechsel. Z Kardiol 2005; 94 (Suppl 3): III/88–III/91.

Empfehlungen zur Therapie der Tabakabhängigkeit. Arzneimittelkommission der deutschen Ärzteschaft, Arzneiverordnung in der Praxis, Sonderheft 1, 05/2001.

ESC/EAS Guidelines for the management of dyslipidaemias: the Task Force for the management of dyslipidaemias of the European Society of Cardiology (ESC) and the European Atherosclerosis Society (EAS). Eur Heart J 2011 Jul; 32 (14): 1769–818. Epub 2011 Jun 28.

ESC Guidelines on the diagnosis and treatment of peripheral artery diseases: Document covering atherosclerotic disease of extracranial carotid and vertebral, mesenteric, renal, upper and lower extremity arteries: the Task Force on the Diagnosis and Treatment of Peripheral Artery Diseases of the European Society of Cardiology (ESC). Eur Heart J 2011 Nov; 32 (22): 2851–906. Epub 2011 Aug 26.

Gohlke H. Das Gesamtrisiko für kardiovaskuläre Erkrankungen; ab wann ist eine medikamentöse Prophylaxe sinnvoll? Z Kardiol 2004; 93 (Suppl 2): 1–7.

Gohlke H. Ernährung. Z Kardiol 2005; 94 (Suppl 3): III/15–III/21.

Gohlke H, Schuler G (Hrsg.). Primärprävention kardiovaskulärer Erkrankungen. Z Kardiol 2005; 94 (Suppl 3): 1–115.

Gohlke H, et al. (Hrsg.). Leitlinie Risikoadjustierte Prävention von Herz- und Kreislauferkrankungen 2007 (online: http://leitlinien.dgk.org/images/pdf/leitlinien_volltext/2007-10_Risikoadjustierte.pdf).

Gohlke-Bärwolf C, von Schacky C. Stellenwert der Hormonersatztherapie zur Prävention der koronaren Herzerkrankung bei Frauen. Z Kardiol 2005; 94 (Suppl 3): III/74–III/78.

Grundy SM, Cleeman JI, Bairey Merz CN, et al. Implications of recent clinical trials for the National Cholesterol Education Program Adult Treatment Panel III Guidelines. Circulation 2004; 110: 227–39.

Hauner H, Buchholz G, Hamann A, et al. Evidenz-basierte Leitlinie: Prävention und Therapie der Adipositas. Endversion 2007 (www.adipositasgesellschaft.de/daten/Adipositas-Leitlinie-2007.pdf).

Heitzer T, Meinertz T. Rauchen und koronare Herzkrankheit. Z Kardiol 2005; 94 (Suppl 3): III/30–III/42.

Hering, T. Moderne medikamentöse Unterstützung der Tabakentwöhnung. Internist 2009; 50: 95–100.

Iestra JA, Kromhout D, van der Schouw YT, Grobbee DE, Boshuizen HC, van Staveren WA. Effect size estimates of lifestyle and dietary changes on all-cause mortality in coronary artery disease patients: a systematic review. Circulation 2005; 112: 924–34.

Kerner W, Brückel J. Definition, Klassifikation und Diagnostik des Diabetes mellitus. Diabetologie 2011; 6: 107–10.

Lichtenstein AH, Appel LJ, Brands M, et al. Diet and lifestyle recommendations revision 2006: a scientific statement from the American Heart Association Nutrition Committee. Circulation 2006; 114: 82–96.

Lonn E, Yusuf S, Arnold MJ, Sheridan P, Pogue J, Micks M, McQueen MJ, Probstfied J, Fodor G, Held C, et al. Homocysteine lowering with folic acid and B vitamins in vascular disease. N Eng J Med 2006; 354: 1567–77.

Mancia G, De Baker G, Dominiczak A, et al. 2007 Guidelines for the management of arterial hypertension: The task force for the Management of arterial Hypertension of the European Society of Hypertension (ESH) and of the European Society of Cardiology (ESC). Eur Heart J 2007; 28: 1462–1536.

Marcus BH, Williams DM, Dubbert PM, et al. Physical activity intervention studies: what we know and what we need to know: a scientific statement from the American Heart Association Council on Nutrition, Physical Activity, and Metabolism (Subcommittee on Physical Activity); Council on Cardiovascular Disease in the Young; and the Interdisciplinary Working Group on Quality of Care and Outcomes Research. Circulation 2006; 114: 2739–52.

Matthaei S et al. Medikamentöse antihyperglykämische Therapie des Diabetes mellitus Typ 2. Update der Evidenzbasierten Leitlinie der Deutschen Diabetes-Gesellschaft. Diabetologie 2009; 4: 32–64.

Nissen SE, Wolski K. Effect of rosiglitazone on the risk of myocardial infarction and death from cardiovascular causes. N Eng J Med 2007; 356: 2457–71.

Nissen SE, et al. Effect of torcetrapib on the progression of coronary atherosclerosis. N Eng J Med 2007; 356: 1304–16.

Pate RR, Davis MG, Robinson TN, Stone EJ, McKenzie TL, Young JC. Promoting physical activity in children and youth: a leadership role for schools: a scientific statement from the American Heart Association Council on Nutrition, Physical Activity, and Metabolism (Physical Activity Committee) in collaboration with the Councils on Cardiovascular Disease in the Young and Cardiovascular Nursing. Circulation 2006; 114: 1214–24.

Polosa R, Caponnetto P, Morjaria JB, Papale G, Campagna D, Russo C. Effect of an electronic nicotine delivery device (e-Cigarette) on smoking reduction and cessation: a prospective 6-month pilot study. BMC Public Health 2011; 11: 786.

Raupach T, Schäfer K, Konstantinides S, Andreas S. Secondhand smoke as an acute threat for the cardiovascular system: a change in paradigm. Eur Heart J 2006; 27: 386–92.

Schuler G. Körperliche Aktivität. Z Kardiol 2005; 94 (Suppl 3): III/11–III/14.

Stettler C, Allemann S, Jüni P et al. Glycemic control and macrovascular disease in types 1 and 2 diabetes mellitus: Meta-analysis of randomized trials. Am Heart J 2006; 152: 27–38.

Study of the Effectiveness of Additional Reductions in Cholesterol and Homocysteine (SEARCH) Collaborative Group, Armitage J, Bowman L, Wallendszus K, Bulbulia R, Rahimi K, Haynes R, Parish S, Peto R, Collins R. Intensive lowering of LDL cholesterol with 80 mg versus 20 mg simvastatin daily in 12,064 survivors of myocardial infarction: a double-blind randomised trial. Lancet. 2010 Nov 13; 376 (9753): 1658–69. Epub 2010 Nov 8. Erratum in: Lancet 2011 Jan 8; 377 (9760): 126.

Smith SC Jr, Allen J, Blair SN, et al. AHA/ACC guidelines for secondary prevention for patients with coronary and other atherosclerotic vascular disease: 2006 update: endorsed by the National Heart, Lung, and Blood Institute. Circulation 2006; 113: 2363–72 (Aktuelle Revision der AHA/ACC-Leitlinien zur Sekundärprävention; 40 Literaturhinweise).

Tabakbedingte Störungen – „Leitlinie Tabakentwöhnung" DG Sucht DGPPN 2004 (www.uni-duesseldorf.de/awmf/ll/076-006.htm).

Teo KK, Ounpuu S, Hawken S, et al. Tobacco use and risk of myocardial infarction in 52 countries in the INTERHEART study: a case-control study. Lancet 2006; 368: 647–58.

Völzke H, Neuhauser H, Moebus S, et al. Rauchen: Regionale Unterschiede in Deutschland. Dtsch Ärztebl 2006; 103: A2784–90.

Wirth A, Gohlke H. Rolle des Körpergewichts für die Prävention der koronaren Herzkrankheit. Z Kardiol 2005; 94 (Suppl 3): III/22–III/29.

4.4.3 Conservative treatment for chronic peripheral arterial occlusive disease

Jens Achenbach
Thomas Cissarek

4.4.3.1 Introduction

The aims of treatment in PAOD are to reduce the risk of all vascular complications in stages I–IV; to improve walking ability, mobility, and quality of life in stage II; and to preserve the extremities, reduce pain, and maintain quality of life in stages III and IV (2009 S3 guideline on PAOD).

The basic form of conservative treatment includes *control and treatment of the major cardiovascular risk factors for atherothrombosis* (see section 4.4.2 above).

Walking training is a particularly important part of a multimodal approach to treatment. *Drug therapy* is a further option. Drug treatment for chronic ischemia in the extremities can be divided into three types:

- Drugs that have a direct influence on the walking distance
- Drugs intended to prevent the progression of the disease itself (including prophylaxis against recurrence)
- Drugs for treating concomitant diseases and risk factors for PAOD (see section 4.4.2)

4.4.3.2 Walking training

Improving the walking distance means greater mobility and an improvement in quality of life for the patient. For older patients with a poor walking distance, limited mobility leads to increasing social isolation.

Physical activity is therefore particularly important in the treatment of PAOD. Structured walking training is the most important form of nondrug treatment, alongside consistent treatment of cardiovas-

cular risk factors. Studies have documented a significant improvement in walking distance (200% after 12 weeks) and a reduction in symptoms (such as claudication) with guided exercise (e.g., in a vascular exercise group), when interval training for 60 min with exercise periods of 5–15 min was carried out three times weekly for 3 months. The intensity of the exercise should extend up to the pain threshold. Unmonitored training is not as effective in comparison. Favorable prognostic factors include:

- History shorter than 1 year
- Occlusion of the superior femoral artery
- Good cardiopulmonary status

Unfavorable prognostic factors include:

- Pelvic artery stenoses and occlusions.
- Additional stenotic or occlusive processes in the deep femoral artery.
- Smoking, which leads to a poorer ability to undertake exercise treatment.
- Concomitant orthopedic and/or neurological diseases that are often present may make participation in exercise treatment impossible in some cases.

4.4.3.3 Drug therapy for improving walking distance

Vasoactive agents are preparations in which the pharmacological properties improve the blood's flow characteristics and thus improve arterial perfusion. It has not been precisely shown how the mechanism leads to improved perfusion, and it is still unclear whether it is due to vascular dilation and/or improved viscosity of the blood. Additional effects of many of the drugs include platelet inhibition and inhibited proliferation of smooth muscle cells (Table 4.4-5). At the stage of claudication, vasoactive agents should only be administered in a targeted fashion when the patient's quality of life is substantially restricted, the walking distance is less than 200 m, and walking training is not possible or limited (consensus recommendation in the 2009 PAOD guideline). Various medical societies (such as the ACC/AHA, TASC II) recommend only cilostazol, or naftidrofuryl with some restrictions.

Cilostazol (Pletal®)

Cilostazol is approved for the treatment of stage II PAOD, and it improves the walking distance through a mechanism of action that has not yet been precisely explained. Pharmacologically, cilostazol is a phosphodiesterase inhibitor (type III). In addition to platelet inhibition, it also has peripheral vasodilatory effects. As it has not been shown that the mechanisms of platelet inhibition and vasodilation lead to an increase in walking distance, the mechanism of action of many preparations that act in this way is unclear.

Cilostazol has been shown to lead to a significant improvement in walking distance in controlled studies. The increase in the walking distance may only become noticeable after several weeks. A time frame of 16–24 weeks has been reported.

Side effects can be expected, particularly at the start of treatment (the dosage should therefore be introduced gradually). The side effects include cephalgia, palpitations, and diffuse gastrointestinal symptoms. They usually decline during the course of treatment.

Contraindications: Cilostazol must not be combined with drugs that are metabolized via cytochrome P3A4. These include cimetidine, diltiazem, erythromycin, ketoconazole, lansoprazole, and omeprazole. Patients with manifest cardiac insufficiency should not receive cilostazol. However, the grade of cardiac insufficiency is not yet sufficiently clear. Simultaneous treatment with ASA and clopidogrel can be administered. Studies have not reported any increased risk of bleeding with this form of triple therapy.

Dosage: Cilostazol should be introduced gradually and should be administered with a maximum daily dosage of 2 × 100 mg p.o.

Naftidrofuryl

Naftidrofuryl is approved in Europe for the treatment of stage II PAOD with adequate circulatory reserve. It probably alters peripheral perfusion by improving the blood's flow characteristics. In addition to having a direct vasodilative effect and reducing the viscosity of the blood, platelet inhibition also takes place. Naftidrofuryl is a serotonin receptor blocker and an antagonist against serotonin's vasoconstrictive action.

Side effects include palpitations, transient hypertension, and gastrointestinal symptoms such as diarrhea, nausea, vomiting and loss of appetite.

Contraindications: Naftidrofuryl must not be administered in patients with acute myocardial infarction, severe cardiac insufficiency, recent hemorrhage, or cardiac dysrhythmia. Adequate hydration of the patient should also be ensured at the start of treatment.

Dosage: 600 mg p.o. is administered per day.

In addition to drug treatment with cilostazol or naftidrofuryl, the patient should be encouraged to undertake physical exercise and regular walking training.

The agents listed below do not provide adequate benefit in the treatment of patients with claudication symptoms.

Propionyl-L-carnitine (L-carnitine)

L-Carnitine is an agent shown in some studies to lead to an improved walking distance. It acts on muscle cell metabolism, where it influences the muscle cells' lipid metabolism. It is postulated that the improved muscle performance leads to an increase in the walking distance. However, the benefits reported in the initial studies have not been confirmed in everyday clinical practice. In recent years, the substance has also become available from many sources without prescription as a lifestyle drug for losing weight. L-Carnitine is a vitamin-like substance that is not only supplied in adequate amounts by a balanced diet, but is also produced by the body itself. As with many vitamins, additional amounts in excess of daily requirements are eliminated via the urine.

Side effects in overdosage include nausea, vomiting, and diarrhea. L-Carnitine can therefore only be recommended with qualifications.

Dosage: maximum daily treatment up to 2 g.

Pentoxifylline (Trental®, Pentohexal®, Pentoxy®, etc.)

Pentoxifylline is an agent with a mechanism of action that leads to an increased walking distance both by improving the blood's flow characteristics and also by producing an endothelial increase in prostacyclin (prostaglandin I_2, PGI_2), with platelet inhibition. However, only slight increases in the walking distance have been achieved in various studies. The clinical effect continues to be a subject of controversy, and the agent can therefore only be recommended with qualifications.

Contraindications include glaucoma and hypocoagulability.

Dosage: daily treatment 300–1000 mg/d p.o.

Buflomedil (Bufedil®, Buflohexal®, Buflomedil-CT®)

The drug probably acts by blocking the peripheral alpha receptors, but the precise mechanism of action is not known. It is assumed that buflomedil acts to improve oxygen utilization by optimizing the cell mechanism. Platelet disaggregation has also been discussed. In addition, improvements in flow characteristics and viscosity are thought to result. The clinical data for buflomedil are limited, and it can therefore only be recommended with qualifications.

Contraindications include high-grade cardiac insufficiency (New York Heart Association grade III), recent myocardial infarction, and a recent cerebral insult.

Side effects that can be expected are gastrointestinal symptoms and headache.

Dosage: Buflomedil is administered at a daily dosage of 150–300 mg p.o.

4.4.3.4   Drug treatment for critical ischemia in the extremities

Administering prostanoids in Fontaine stage II is not recommended in the TASC II document, but it is recommended for Fontaine stages III and IV, particularly when revascularization procedures cannot be used. Positive effects include:

- Improved wound healing
- Pain reduction
- A reduced amputation rate
- Reduced cardiovascular mortality

Iloprost (Ilomedin®)

This is a prostacyclin derivative that has a vasodilative effect and in addition to platelet inhibition also increases the blood's fibrinolytic activity. Iloprost is approved for the treatment of thromboangiitis obliterans, but is also used in PAOD in Fontaine stages III and IV and in chronic critical ischemia in the extremities. It is also used in secondary Raynaud syndrome.

Both a reduction in the amputation rate and an improved healing tendency in peripheral lesions have been reported in controlled studies using iloprost treatment.

Side effects include gastrointestinal symptoms such as nausea and vomiting, as well as flushing, headache, and rubescence at the injection site.

Dosage: It is administered intravenously at a dosage of about 20 µg.

Alprostadil—prostaglandin E₁ (Caverject®, Prostavasin®)

This is a form of prostaglandin E_1, administered intravenously and intra-arterially, that is a tried, tested and approved treatment for Fontaine stages III and IV. In addition to its vasodilative properties, the proliferation of smooth muscle cells is inhibited, as in many drugs of this type. It is already metabolized on first passage through the lungs and the metabolite is active.

In addition to the improved circulatory situation, with the associated improvement in healing in stages III and IV, it has been shown that analgetic requirements decline during treatment with alprostadil. It is not approved for use at the stage of intermittent claudication.

Side effects include gastrointestinal symptoms such as nausea and vomiting, as well as flushing, headache, and rubescence at the injection site.

Dosage: Alprostadil is administered parenterally at a dosage of 2×40 µg, or 1×60 µg i.v., or 20 µg intra-arterially. Treatment duration of 2 weeks with intravenous administration or 1 week with intra-arterial administration is recommended.

4.4.3.5 Antithrombotic treatment

The clinical value of platelet inhibition in the treatment of atherothrombotic vascular disease is undisputed. However, no convincing large studies have yet been published to confirm that it delays the onset of manifest PAOD or inhibits the progression of peripheral atherothrombosis. In patients with PAOD, the research data do not provide convincing results on secondary prevention of cardiac and cerebrovascular events, although there are insufficient data on primary prevention of peripheral vascular events. However, the value of platelet inhibition in reducing peripheral vascular events has been confirmed with invasive therapy. In patients with PAOD and confirmed CHD or cerebrovascular lesions, lifelong administration of platelet inhibition is obviously needed and is supported by good evidence. Administration of platelet inhibitors (ASA, clopidogrel) is also recommended in the treatment of patients with asymptomatic peripheral stenotic and occlusive processes, to reduce the risk of cardiac and cerebrovascular events. Acetylsalicylic acid (75–300 mg/d) and clopidogrel (75 mg/d) may be mentioned. Due to its side effects (neutropenia and thrombopenia), ticlopidine has been replaced with clopidogrel, and dipyridamole is not indicated in PAOD (Table 4.4-4).

Cyclooxygenase inhibitors

The most frequently used selective cyclooxygenase-1 inhibitor is acetylsalicylic acid (ASA). Its effect is based on irreversible inhibition of cyclooxygenase through acetylation of serine-529 and inhibition of thromboxane synthase (TXA_2). As a result of this irreversibility, thrombocyte aggregation is only possible with newly formed thrombocytes. Adequate antithrombotic treatment is already possible even at low dosages. It has not been demonstrated that ASA

prevents the progression of atherosclerosis. However, it is assumed that in combination with other drugs there is a reduction in the formation of neointima. This is an argument for using ASA as early as possible, while weighing up the risks. A positive effect has only been confirmed in PAOD patients who also had coronary heart disease and/or cerebral arteriovenous disease as well. ASA is not approved as a sole treatment for PAOD.

The gastrointestinal *side effects* are dose-dependent. The bleeding time is prolonged with ASA, so that there is a higher bleeding risk. An adenosine diphosphate (ADP) inhibitor is recommended if ASA is not tolerated.

Dosage: There are no precise dosage recommendations for platelet inhibition; 50–300 mg/d is reported in the literature. The established dosage in Germany is 100 mg/d.

Adenosine diphosphate (ADP) inhibitors

This class of drugs, including the agents clopidogrel, ticlopidine, and more recently prasugrel, irreversibly and selectively inhibits the binding of ADP to platelets. This inhibits ADP-induced platelet aggregation. Ticlopidine is an agent related to clopidogrel, with a similar mechanism of action. The agents, administered as prodrugs, are activated via cytochrome P450. Inhibitors of CYP3A4 such as erythromycin and cimetidine may therefore reduce the effect of clopidogrel. The delayed onset of action of the agents, administered as prodrugs, makes saturation necessary. Significant platelet inhibition only appears dose-dependently after 4 h at the earliest (after a loading dose of 600 mg; later at lower dosages).

Due to the *side effects* of ticlopidine, with leukopenia, thrombopenia, and high-risk thrombotic thrombocytopenic purpura, clopidogrel is nowadays used. Ticlopidine may be used if there is resistance to clopidogrel, as the metabolization pathways of the two agents differ.

Dosage: clopidogrel is approved at a dosage of 75 mg/d for the treatment of PAOD, and ticlopidine is administered at a dosage of 2×250 mg/d.

Dual platelet inhibition

Combination therapy with ASA and clopidogrel in high-risk patients with several risk factors and atherothrombotic signs (including PAOD) leads to an increased bleeding risk without conferring any advantages. Dual platelet inhibition with ASA (100 mg/d) and clopidogrel (75 mg/d) is decisively important in postinterventional coronary stent treatment, particularly after implantation of drug-eluting stents (DESs). A similar procedure is generally followed after peripheral arterial interventions with stent implantation. As

Table 4.4-4 Oral platelet inhibitors.

Drug	Site of action	Indication	Side effect(s)	Dosage
ASA	Cyclooxygenase-1	Secondary prophylaxis against CHD, cerebral perfusion disturbance	GIT complications (bleeding), dose-dependent	75–300 mg/d
Clopidogrel	ADP receptor	Secondary prophylaxis against PAOD and CHD, and in CHD after coronary intervention	Prolongs bleeding time	75 mg/d
Ticlopidine	ADP receptor	Secondary prophylaxis after TIA and ischemic insult, ASA intolerance	Changes blood count, thrombotic thrombocytopenic purpura	2×250 mg/d

ADP, adenosine diphosphate; ASA, acetylsalicylic acid; CHD, coronary heart disease; GIT, gastrointestinal tract; PAOD, peripheral arterial occlusive disease; TIA, transient ischemic attack.

DESs are rarely used in peripheral treatment at present, dual platelet inhibition is currently limited to 4 weeks after the intervention in patients with PAOD. It should be noted that clopidogrel is not approved for the prevention of stent thrombosis. The term "off-label use" refers to prescription of an agent outside the range of approved applications. However, clopidogrel is approved for the treatment of PAOD. Additional administration of ASA, although it is regularly done, is outside the range of approved uses here. The term "off–off-label use" can be used for a case in which a drug is used to treat a clinical picture for which it is has not been approved, while an alternative drug is available and has been approved. All of this applies to ASA and clopidogrel. ASA is not approved for PAOD, but clopidogrel certainly is.

Resistance to platelet inhibitors

Resistance to the effects of platelet inhibitors is becoming increasingly important. A lack of response to platelet inhibition is currently being investigated in several studies. Metabolic mechanisms and interactions with other substances are being discussed, on the one hand, while on the other inadequate patient compliance has been reported. It can be assumed that the causes of genuine pharmacological resistance would be quite complex.

In addition, there are clinical pictures that are associated with increased platelet function per se.

Diabetes mellitus is thought to be associated with what is known as "diabetic thrombocytopathy," with a tendency toward increased platelet aggregation. Inadequate platelet aggregation with ASA 100 treatment can be expected in one in five diabetic patients.

In general, the term "ASA resistance" is not consistently defined. There is a lack of standardized test procedures. Various authors distinguish between low responders and nonresponders. The group of low responders can be treated by increasing the dosage of platelet inhibitors, while that of the nonresponders can be treated by changing the drug group.

The pharmacological mechanism underlying this type of resistance is not known. In combination with platelet aggregation tests, an increase in the ASA dosage in low responders leads to complete inhibition again in vitro.

Resistance to the platelet inhibitor clopidogrel has also been reported. Various studies have estimated the rate at around 20%. Here again, metabolization and compliance are very important. The implications of genuine resistance could also be severe for PAOD patients after an intervention.

There are at present several laboratory methods of monitoring platelet inhibition. In everyday clinical work, pre-analysis is a particular problem. The blood should be obtained in as gentle a way as possible, and the time frame for analysis should be as short as possible. The test procedures determine platelet function, not a specific concentration. The PFA-100 is a test for measuring the "in vitro bleeding time"; this method has already been used to identify ASA nonresponders for some time. It is not possible to monitor platelet function during clopidogrel treatment using the PFA-100 test.

Monitoring of clopidogrel treatment is possible using impedance aggregometry, for example. The quality of platelet inhibition is determined here by assessing changes in resistance with the addition of ADP. The method can also be used to determine ASA resistance (in low responders) with the help of arachidonic acid.

Monitoring of platelet function has become increasingly important for diagnosis, and this has led to new analytic procedures being developed in recent years. Preanalytic conditions are extremely important for measuring platelet function, to prevent medical errors. The most frequent sources of error and distortion in the preanalytic assessment are:

- Patients in stress
- Veins too long and too strongly blocked during blood sampling
- Blood tube not inverted after the sample has been drawn
- Blood tube not filled sufficiently
- Tubes have been cooled and shaken during transport

The blood should therefore be drawn in the morning when the patient is well rested, without application of a tourniquet or after brief tourniquet blockage of the vein. The tube should then be gently inverted two or three times and transferred carefully to the coagulation laboratory at room temperature within 4 h.

Point-of-care (POC) procedures allow prompt analysis of platelet function even without extensive laboratory medicine experience and can be carried out without complex preanalytic procedures. In these procedures, an attempt is made to assess hemostasis satisfactorily, but in vitro test methods conducted with cell-free plasma do not adequately reflect in vivo processes. With POC test systems, the procedures are carried out close to the patient, outside of a classic laboratory setting, on the ward or in the operating room or catheter laboratory. The major advantage of POC analysis is that the assessment parameters are available rapidly.

Unfortunately, it is still unclear which of the available platelet function test systems is best for assessing the effect of platelet inhibition in order to predict thrombotic events or bleeding. It is questionable whether these in vitro laboratory methods actually reflect the in vivo effect of platelet inhibitors. With modern POC methods, it is already possible to quantify the effect of platelet inhibitors. However, the tests need to be standardized.

Glycoprotein (GP) IIb/IIIa receptor antagonists

This relatively new class of substances inhibits the GP IIb/IIIa receptors located on the platelets, independently of thromboxane and ADP. Three groups of agents have so far been used—abciximab (ReoPro®), eptifibatide (Integrilin®), and tirofiban (Aggrastat®). These drugs have favorable effects in percutaneous coronary interventions and acute coronary syndrome. The extent to which they have positive results during and after complex peripheral procedures has not yet been conclusively demonstrated. The RIO study (*ReoPro and Peripheral Arterial Intervention to Improve Clinical Outcome in Patients with Peripheral Arterial Disease*; results not yet published) has provided the first evidence of a lower rate of recurrent stenosis after femoral artery recanalizations. However, this powerful group of drugs is not yet approved for treatment of PAOD.

4.4.3.6   Anticoagulation in PAOD treatment

Oral anticoagulation

Oral anticoagulants such as coumarin (phenprocoumon, Marcoumar®) and warfarin (Coumadin®) have an established place in prophylactic treatment against cardiac thromboembolic events. The value of oral anticoagulation treatment alone to prevent thromboembolic events in PAOD has not currently been proven. According to more recent research, the administration of a coumarin preparation only has minor advantages in addition to existing platelet inhibition, and the advantages are canceled out by increased bleeding complications.

Vitamin K antagonists (coumarins)

Coumarin is a substance discovered in Canada during the 1920s that is produced in sweet clover and proved fatal for local cattle there, with many animals dying due to severe hypocoagulability. The agent's mechanism of action involves direct anticoagulation through inhibition of vitamin K. Carboxylation processes are inhibited via clotting factors II, VII, IX, and X and proteins C and S. Two substances are in use: phenprocoumon and warfarin. The main difference between them is their half-lives—150 h with phenprocoumon and 40 h with warfarin. While phenprocoumon is initially administered at a higher dosage than the subsequent daily dosage, the maintenance dosage can be started straight away with warfarin, due to its short half-life. The measurement range is given as the International Normalized Ratio (INR, formerly known as the Quick value), and it is dependent on the indication. In PAOD, coumarins are used for secondary prophylaxis after femorodistal bypass surgery, with the main indication being venous bypasses. In patients with plastic prostheses, treatment is usually only with ASA or with dual platelet inhibition with clopidogrel added (BOA study), independently of the location.

It is important to note the well-known drug interactions with vitamin K antagonists (Table 4.4-5).

Rivaroxaban (Xarelto®)

Rivaroxaban is a direct factor Xa inhibitor that is available as an orally administered coagulation inhibitor for prophylaxis against thrombosis during hip and knee joint operations. Since the end of December 2011, this factor Xa inhibitor has also been approved for prevention of stroke in high-risk patients with nonvalvular atrial fibrillation and for the treatment of deep vein thrombosis (DVT) in the legs and prophylaxis against recurrent DVT or pulmonary embolism.

Rivaroxaban acts independently of antithrombin, and treatment monitoring is not usually required. It has a half-life of 7–10 hours, and two-thirds is excreted via the kidneys.

However, rivaroxaban—even at prophylactic dosages—may influence many coagulation analyses (1–4 hours after administration/peak level). The results are not suitable for recording any overdosage or underdosage. Laboratory effects of rivaroxaban may include misleadingly low Quick and raised international normalized ratio (INR) results. The activated partial thromboplastin time (aPTT) may also be prolonged, although to a lesser extent. Antithrombin results are falsely raised when factor Xa–based tests are used. Lupus anticoagulant may also show a false-positive increase. Blood samples for coagulation diagnosis should therefore be taken after treatment has stopped or at trough level (immediately before the next dose).

In addition, providing details of the agent, dosage, and time of last ingestion of a drug that may influence coagulation generally seems sensible in screening examinations.

Table 4.4-5 Vitamin K antagonists and their interactions.

Inactivation	Potentiating
Amiodarone	Barbiturates
Allopurinol	Phenytoin
Cimetidine	Carbamazepine
ASA (high-dose)	Ethanol
Cephalosporins	Estrogens
Ciprofloxacin	Hypericum
Metronidazole/sulfonamides	Sulfonylureas
Thyroid hormones	Foods containing vitamin K
Fluvastatin/fibrates	Rifampicin

ASA, acetylsalicylic acid.

Dosage recommendation for prophylaxis against thrombosis

Rivaroxaban 10 mg is taken once a day. The first dose should be administered 6–10 hours after the surgical procedure and after checking of local hemostasis. Rivaroxaban can be taken at the 10-mg dosage with or without food. Prophylaxis against thrombosis should be continued on an individual basis for as long as there is a risk of thromboembolism. If it is noted that administration at the right time point has been forgotten, the omitted dose should be taken immediately and once-daily administration should continue the next day as usual.

No dose adjustment is necessary in patients with mild impairment of renal function (creatinine clearance 50–80 mL/min). In patients with moderately impaired renal function (creatinine clearance 30–49 mL/min), dose adjustment is also not required, except in patients who are simultaneously receiving other drugs that can lead to raised plasma rivaroxaban levels; rivaroxaban should be used with caution in such cases. In patients with severe renal insufficiency (creatinine clearance 15–29 mL/min) and those with renal insufficiency requiring dialysis (creatinine clearance < 15 mL/min), rivaroxaban should not be used. Rivaroxaban is contraindicated in all patients with hepatic disease and coagulopathy, as the risk of bleeding is increased in these cases. The agent must also not be used in pregnant patients or during lactation.

Dosage recommendation for thrombosis treatment

Rivaroxaban is initially administered at 15 mg twice daily for 3 weeks, followed by 20 mg once daily. In contrast to the 10-mg dosage, the 15-mg and 20-mg tablets should be taken at meals. According to the manufacturer, this type of intake improves the agent's bioavailability.

In patients with moderate (creatinine clearance 30–49 mL/min) and severe (creatinine clearance 15–29 mL/min) impairment of renal function, the dosage is 15 mg twice daily during the first 3 weeks, followed by 15 mg once daily. The recommended dosage of rivaroxaban in patients with simultaneous atrial fibrillation is 20 mg per day during long-term treatment. If anticoagulation treatment is switched from a vitamin K antagonist to rivaroxaban, it can be started in patients receiving thrombosis therapy and prophylaxis against recurrence from an INR of < 2.5, or in patients with atrial fibrillation at < 3.0. After withdrawal of the vitamin K antagonist, and depending on the half-life of the coumarin agent, rivaroxaban can usually be started at the maintenance dosage after 2 days. If a switch is made from rivaroxaban to a coumarin agent, overlapping administration is needed with INR measurements for 2–3 days.

One of the advantages claimed for this new anticoagulant is the fact that it can be administered without regular monitoring (such as regular INR checks). Despite this, however, events are conceivable for which optional monitoring would be desirable—for example, in cases of bleeding, or preoperatively following trauma. No tests are currently available, but they are apparently being developed.

Interactions between rivaroxaban and other drugs

Agents that inhibit excretory pathways via CYP3A4 and/or P-glycoprotein (P-gp) potentially increase the plasma concentration of rivaroxaban. Clarithromycin, a strong CYP3A4 inhibitor but a moderate P-gp inhibitor (500 mg twice daily) leads to a 1.5-fold increase in the mean steady-state area under the curve (AUC). Erythromycin, a moderate CYP3A4 and P-gp inhibitor (500 mg thrice daily) leads to a 1.3-fold increase in the mean steady-state AUC. These increases are within the range of normal variability and are therefore not regarded as being clinically relevant. Strong CYP3A4 inductors such as phenytoin and other anticonvulsants allow the mean AUC to be reduced by 50%. These also include St. John's wort and rifampicin. Administration of rivaroxaban is not recommended with strong inhibitors of CYP3A4 and P-gp such as azoles (e.g., ketonidazole) and HIV drugs such as ritonavir.

Note: analgesia

Patients with chronic and also critical ischemia of the extremities have constant pain that tends to become chronic. Effective analgesia is an important pillar in efforts to improve the patients' quality of life. Significant increases in walking distance cannot be achieved in this way. Constant analgesia treatment is often also needed for patients in the complicated Fontaine stage IIb. Administering painkillers only on demand should be avoided. The treatment recommendations issued by the specialist societies and/or the World Health Organization recommendations should be observed.

4.4.3.7 Concomitant medication in PAOD treatment

Concomitant medication in patients with PAOD depends on the patient's individual risk profile. As most patients have arterial hypertension, which represents one of the major risk factors for cardiovascular mortality, adequate antihypertensive treatment is indispensable. The mortality can be reduced by around 30% with targeted antihypertensive therapy (Hypertension Optimal Treatment [HOT] Study).

Independently of the cholesterol level, statin therapy is recommended in patients with hypercholesterolemia, as they frequently have comorbid conditions such as CHD and cerebral arteriovenous disease. Cholesterol reduction is not directly associated with an increased walking distance, but it has been shown that even with normal cholesterol values, patients have lower rates of myocardial infarction, cerebrovascular events, and peripheral vascular complications (Heart Protection Study, HPS). Statin therapy is therefore also recommended in high-risk patients with PAOD.

Recommended drug groups for patients with PAOD are discussed in detail below.

Angiotensin-converting enzyme (ACE) inhibitors

In these antihypertensive agents, the formation of angiotensin II, one of the strongest substances that act to increase blood pressure, is suppressed by inhibition of angiotensin-converting enzyme. Peripheral resistance in the vessels is also reduced. Lipid metabolism on the vascular wall is also thought to be positively influenced by ACE inhibitors. Many ultrasound studies have shown that the intima–media thickness is reduced during ACE inhibitor treatment, but in some of the studies the benefit was below the minimum level capable of being physically demonstrated with ultrasound. The studies are therefore not uncontroversial, particularly with regard to interobserver differences. However, ACE inhibitor treatment is generally recommended even in PAOD patients.

β-Receptor blockers (β-blockers)

β-Receptor antagonists inhibit the positive inotropic and chronotropic effects of catecholamines in the heart by blocking the β_1 receptors (cardioselectively). However, the selectivity is relative, as they occur not only in the heart but also in other organs. β_1-selective β-blockers are preferable to other nonselective ones if possible in patients with disturbed glucose tolerance and diabetes. They influence the carbohydrate metabolism less than nonselective ones. Administration of a β-blocker to treat hypertension in patients with PAOD is not contraindicated, as the benefits relative to cardiac mortality are greater.

The risk of a PAOD patient dying of the effects of a cardiac event is greater than the risk of suffering amputation during the course of the disease.

Statins (CSE inhibitors)

Low-density lipoprotein (LDL) is particularly important in the pathogenesis of arteriosclerosis. LDL can penetrate the vessel wall and can lead to the formation of atherosclerotic plaques on it, via metabolic pathways involving macrophages and foam cells.

Several studies have demonstrated that cholesterol synthase enzyme (CSE) inhibitors have a positive effect on the morbidity and mortality due to cardiac events. A direct effect on PAOD has not yet been confirmed. As some CSE inhibitors are metabolized via CYP3A4, interactions are possible; cilostazol may be mentioned, for example. There is an increased risk of rhabdomyolysis with these agents, which have low bioavailability. CSE inhibitors that are metabolized via CYP2C9 may influence (and increase) the anticoagulant effect of coumarins.

Fibrates

Fibrates increase the activity of lipoprotein lipase, with more very low-density lipoproteins (VLDLs) being transformed into LDLs. In addition, the level of high-density lipoproteins (HDLs) is also increased. The mechanism of effect involved has not been precisely explained. It is known that fibrates have a wide variety of effects.

They have also been reported to influence the nuclear transcription of peroxisome proliferator–activated receptor (PPAR) α-receptors, which are used in the treatment of diabetes mellitus. The glitazones act here to reduce blood sugar. Above all, fibrates reduce the triglycerides. They are thought to have a protective influence on atherosclerosis. However, fibrates also tend to have marked *interactions* not only with oral antidiabetic agents, but also with coumarins. Like statins, fibrates tend to cause muscular symptoms, which may even include rhabdomyolysis. This led to gemfibrozil and cerivastatin (Lipobay®) being withdrawn from the market.

Example drug treatment in a PAOD patient with intermittent claudication

Platelet inhibition:
- Clopidogrel/acetylsalicylic acid

Antihypertensive agents:
- ACE inhibitors
- β-blockers

Antilipemic agents:
- Statins/fibrates

Vasoactive substances:
- Cilostazol (first choice) or naftidrofuryl

Depending on the individual risk profile, the patient can be weaned from smoking using drug therapy.

References

Antithrombotic Trialists' Collaboration. Collaborative meta-analysis of randomised trials of antiplatelet therapy for prevention of death, myocardial infarction, and stroke in high risk patients. BMJ 2002; 324: 71–86.

Arzeimittelbrief 1997, 31, 13a Clopidogrel versus Azetylsalizylsäure in der Sekundärprophylaxe ischämischer Ereignisse.

Boccalon H, Lehert P, Mosnier M. Effect of naftidrofuryl on physiological walking distance in patients with claudication. Ann Cardiol Angéiol 2001; 50: 175–82 APIEC-STUDY.

CAPRIE Steering Committee C. A randomised, blinded, trial of clopidogrel versus aspirin in patients at risk of ischaemic events (CAPRIE). Lancet 1996; 348: 1329–39.

Creuzig A, Caspary L, Radeke U, Specht S, Ranke C, Alexander K. Prospektive randomisierte Doppelblindstudie zur Wirksamkeit von PGE1 bei schwerer Claudicatio intermittens. In: Heidrich H. Prostaglandin E1-Wirkungen und therapeutische Wirksamkeit. Berlin, Heidelberg, New York: Springer, 1998, 95–102.

Deutsche Gesellschaft für Angiologie, Gesellschaft für Gefäßmedizin, Arbeitsgemeinschaft der Wissenschaftlichen Medizinischen Fachgesellschaften (AWMF). Leitlinien zur Diagnostik und Therapie der peripheren arteriellen Verschlusskrankheit (PAVK). http://www.awmf-online.de, http://leitlinien.net/ (Stand 13.03.2009).

Die Einflüsse von Antikoagulanzien auf Routine- und Spezialdiagnostik im Gerinnungslabor. In Zusammenarbeit mit Fr. Prof. Dr. E. Lindhoff-Last und Herrn PD Dr. D. Peetz. 2010 Roche Diagnostics Xarelto® Fachinformation 2011.

Francis GS. ACE inhibition in cardiovascular disease. N Engl J Med 2000; 342: 201.

Grundy SM. Statin trials and goals of cholesterol-lowering therapy. Circulation 1998; 97: 1436–9.

Hansson L, et al. Effects of intensive blood-pressure lowering and low-dose aspirin in patients with hypertension: principal results of the hypertension optimal treatment (HOT) randomised trial. Lancet 1998; 351: 1755.

Heart Protection Study of cholesterol lowering with simvastatin in 20,536 high-risk individuals: a randomised placebo-controlled trial. Lancet 2002 Jul 6; 360 (9326): 7–22.

Herbert PR, Gaziano JM, Chan KS. Cholesterol lowering with statin drugs, risk of stroke and total mortality. JAMA 1997; 287: 313–21.

Mani H, Lindhoff-Last E. Aspirin- und Clopidogrel-Resistenz – kritische Bewertung. Vasomed 2007; 19. Jg. 3.

Mutschler E, Geisslinger G, Kroemer HK, Ruth P, Schäfer-Korting M. Arzneimittelwirkung – Lehrbuch der Pharmakologie und Toxikologie. Wissenschaftliche Verlagsgesellschaft mbH Stuttgart, 9. Auflage, 2008.

Norgren L et al. TASC II Guidelines for PAD. Eur J Vasc Endovasc Surg 2007 ; Vol 33 (Suppl 1).

Patel MR, et al. ROCKET-AF-Studie: Rivaroxaban versus Warfarin in Nonvalvular Atrial Fibrillation. N Engl J Med 2011; 365: 883–91.

Positionspapier der DGK (Deutsche Gesellschaft für Kardiologie) zur Vermeidung von Tod und lebensbedrohlichen Komplikationen nach koronarer Stentimplantation durch die zusätzliche Gabe von Clopidogrel. 2006.

Rudofsky G. Peripheral Arterial Disease: Chronic Ischemic Syndromes. In: Lanzer P, Topol EJ. Panvascular Medicine. Berlin, Heidelberg, New York, Springer, 2002.

The EINSTEIN Investigators. Oral Rivaroxaban for Symptomatic Venous Thromboembolism. N Engl J Med 2010; 363: 2499–510.

The ESPRIT Study Group. Aspirin plus dipyridamole versus aspirin alone after cerebral ischaemia of arterial origin (ESPRIT): Randomised controlled trial. Lancet 2006 May 20; 367: 1665–73.

United Kingdom Severe Limb Ischemia Study Group. Treatment of limb threatening ischemia with intravenous Iloprost: a randomised double-blind placebo controlled study. Eur J Vasc Surg 1992; 5: 511–6.

4.4.4   Conservative treatment of chronic ischemic wounds

Shanti Naskar

4.4.4.1   Introduction to the problem

Circulatory disturbances are one of the most important causes of chronic wounds. Lesions in Raynaud disease, thromboangiitis obliterans, and the condition known as trash foot represent special forms. Even in the presence of isolated peripheral AOD with critical ischemia in the extremity, regular wound healing is extremely difficult, particularly when adequate revascularization is not possible. However, PAOD is also associated with other diseases that limit healing processes (diabetes mellitus, chronic venous insufficiency, etc.).

In these patients, who often have multimorbid conditions, the wound therapist's task is difficult and a multimodal aggressive approach is required.

It should be clearly stated from the outset that revascularization is the only genuinely definitive treatment for ischemic ulceration. In addition to angiographic diagnosis, an attempt at revascularization should therefore always be made (Inter-Society Consensus 2007).

Even if a revascularization procedure does not initially appear possible or has been inadequate, options for interventional or surgical reopening of circulation, drug therapy, and more recently cell therapy or gene therapy, need to be checked again to improve local perfusion if the wound is not healing or is stagnating.

To avoid amputation, patients with a stable wound and pain situation should receive conservative multidisciplinary treatment in accordance with the TASC II recommendations (Inter-Society Consensus 2007). A study including 142 patients in whom revascularization was not possible showed that successful wound treatment is possible in some 30–40% of cases, although it is often protracted (Marston et al. 2006). The guidelines of the German Society for Angiology and Vascular Surgery also state that it is appropriate to treat patients with stage III or IV PAOD in specialized centers.

4.4.4.2 Definition and diagnosis

In the context of critical ischemia of the extremities, the wound is characterized by disturbed perfusion of the vascular bed in the wound area, the cause of which may be either microangiopathic or macroangiopathic.

In the current S3 guideline in Germany on "Local treatment for chronic wounds in patients at risk with chronic venous insufficiency, peripheral arterial occlusive disease, and diabetes mellitus," a chronic wound is defined as loss of the integrity of the skin and one or more underlying structures with failure to heal within 8 weeks.

Doppler pressure values are reported (depending on different authors) to fall to less than 50–70 mmHg at the ankle and less than 30 mmHg in the toes. In diabetic patients, and particularly when the disease continues for a prolonged period, occlusive pressure measurement and assessment of the ankle/brachial index (ABI) is only possible to a limited extent, due to incorrectly high values with medial calcinosis.

Assessing transcutaneous oxygen pressure (tcPo$_2$) is superior to measuring segmental occlusive pressure (Padberg et al. 1996) when assessing the grade of ischemia and the prognosis for wound healing in PAOD. An oxygen tension value of 30 mmHg indicates ischemia and a poor tendency to heal, although measurement variability of 10 mmHg is tolerable. When tcPo$_2$ is below 20 mmHg, no healing of the ulceration can be expected (Ubbink et al. 1994). A low Po$_2$ correlates significantly with reduced cell proliferation and increasing wound size (Coerper et al. 1999). Transcutaneous oxygen measurement is of subordinate clinical importance in diabetic foot syndrome (DFS), however. Even other techniques for examining the microcirculation, such as laser Doppler flowmetry and video capillary microscopy, appear to be unsuitable for more detailed quantification of the grade of ischemia in DFS (Lawall et al. 2000). In every chronic wound with evidence of an ischemic pathogenesis, therefore, digital subtraction angiography (DSA) of the pelvic and leg arteries, including imaging of the vascular supply of the foot, forms part of the standard diagnostic work-up in addition to color duplex ultrasonography.

Pathogenesis of foot ulcerations

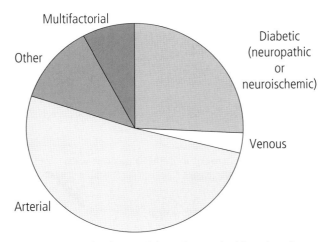

Fig. 4.4-7 Average distribution of the pathogenesis of foot ulcerations (adapted from Moulik et al. 2007).

4.4.4.3 Pathophysiology of the chronic ischemic wound

Normal wound healing is a delicately coordinated process that is temporally and spatially organized and in which the components of cells (leukocytes, thrombocytes, endothelia, keratinocytes and fibroblasts) and various hormonal factors (cytokines, chemokines, proteases) have to be present and capable of functioning at the right time in the right place.

The hormonal factors are formed by blood and tissue cells in order to control wound healing processes such as cellular proliferation and the synthesis of matrix components. Their secretion is usually precisely controlled by control circuits, with the appropriate inhibiting and activating factors.

The stages of wound healing (inflammation, granulation, and epithelialization/repair) basically proceed in the same way in ischemic processes as in wounds of other types. However, substantial differences are seen in the clinical course. The patient often does not remember an initial, usually (trivial) trauma. If the ischemia is sufficiently advanced, atraumatic tissue necrosis may even occur, usually in the toes. There may initially be no extensive exudation, with the first clinical sign apart from necrosis being pain.

1. The *first stage of healing (inflammation)* may have a comparatively rapid course. Deep necrosis or even gangrene develops after only hours or days. Secretion of tissue-active substances (prostaglandins, cytokines, etc.) leads to local edema due to increased capillary permeability. Inflammatory cells (initially thrombocytes and leukocytes, and later macrophages) are "lured" into the area of injury, although to a much lesser extent than normal or in subcritically perfused wounds, due to the circulatory disturbance. These cells ensure initial wound closure and begin phagocytosis of the necrotic tissue. These processes require large amounts of oxygen, and the surrounding tissue becomes hypoxic, as the terminal circulation is not capable of meeting the additional oxygen demand. Local necrosis develops. The tissue edema causes compression of the capillaries and can therefore lead to further deterioration of perfusion and of venous drainage.

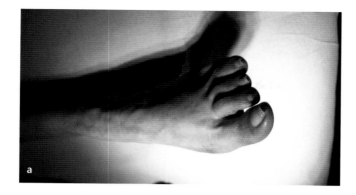

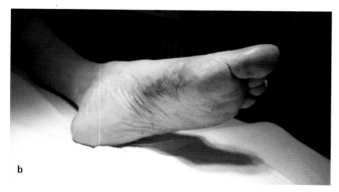

Fig. 4.4-8a, b Nail matrix infection in the large toe, with subsequent acute forefoot ischemia in a patient with severe arterial occlusive disease in the lower leg.

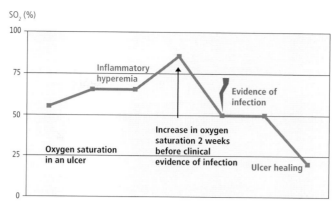

Fig. 4.4-9 The increase in local oxygen saturation 2 weeks before infection of a (nonischemic) wound. During infection, there is a severe drop in saturation, as a sign of an increased demand for oxygen. When the ulcer is healing, there is a gradual fall in saturation along with a decline in inflammatory hyperemia (measured with Micro-Light Guide O2C; adapted from Beckert et al. 2004).

The inflammatory cells in the area of the wound, which are undernourished, fail to overcome the initially low bacterial colonization and die, leaving cell detritus. From bacterial colonization, this quickly gives rise to manifest infection with all of the clinical signs of inflammation, constantly increasing the oxygen demand. The first phase of wound healing is inadequate, wound cleaning cannot be achieved in ischemic conditions, and instead the various inflammatory processes draw oxygen from the surrounding tissue and consequently lead to an even larger area of tissue necrosis (see Fig. 4.4-8). If this is followed by demarcation of the necrosis or it is possible to control the local infection with adequate wound therapy, the subsequent course is characterized by the wound remaining in stage 1 (chronic inflammation), independently of the extent of the ischemia.

2. The course of *stage 2 (granulation)* is also delayed. Usually, a chronic ischemic wound requires several weeks or sometimes even months until granulation tissue—usually sparse—begins to form from the edge of the wound. By contrast, the base of the wound often remains slow to heal unless other measures are carried out.

3. The course of *stage 3 (epithelialization/repair)* is also delayed. The scar tissue is often thin and remains more vulnerable than normally perfused skin.

Special case in ischemic wounds: diabetic foot syndrome

Only approximately half of foot lesions among diabetic patients have exclusively neuropathic causes; instead, neuropathy and circulatory disturbances are often present in combination.

In diabetic patients, most foot lesions are primarily neuropathic. However, the healing process and course are usually seriously lim-

ited by the degree of ischemia. Vascular changes in diabetes are extremely complex. Depending on other risk factors, the extent of neuropathy and the metabolic state, circulatory disturbances that have both macroangiopathic and microangiopathic causes are usually seen simultaneously.

It used to be thought that there is a diabetes-specific form of macroangiopathy involving obliterative or occlusive atherosclerosis, but this has so far *not* been demonstrated histopathologically. Instead, it is currently thought that the condition involves a progressive, severe form of "normal" atherosclerosis that particularly affects the crural arteries, often with coexistent mediasclerosis. The development of the media sclerosis is explained in part by neuropathic changes in the vasa vasorum.

The following pathophysiological aspects are distinguished:

- **Neuropathic development of cutaneous arteriovenous shunts** with steal phenomena in favor of the circulation in deeper tissue layers.
- **Hemostatic changes**, particularly hyperviscosity of the blood due to hyperglycemia and infection-related hyperfibrinogenemia, favoring microembolization and thrombosis of the arterial capillary system.
- **Complex glyceration processes:** prolonged hyperglycemia leads to irreversible formation of glycosylation end products (advanced glycosylation end products, AGEs) made up of glucose and matrix proteins, which cause complex changes particularly in the basal membrane. LDL particles are more easily deposited and a mainly macrophage-associated inflammatory reaction in the vessel wall is initiated, and this promotes atheroma formation (Brownlee et al. 1988).
- **Endothelial dysfunction:** in all secondary vascular diseases, particularly diabetes mellitus, this is a potent factor for atherogenesis. Nitric oxide (NO), known to be the most important mediator of endothelial vasodilation, also has inhibitory effects on the aggregation and migration of thrombocytes and leukocytes on the vessel wall, and it inhibits the binding of adhesion molecules.

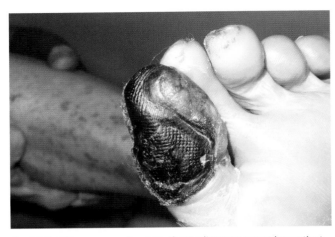

Fig. 4.4-10 D1 gangrene a few days after podiatry treatment in a patient with extremely severe multiple-level arterial occlusive disease in whom revascularization was not possible.

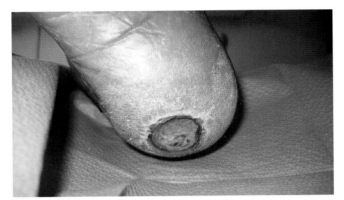

Fig. 4.4-11 Chronic ulceration of the heel, with a bradytrophic wound base.

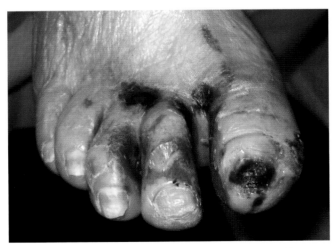

Fig. 4.4-12 Severe forefoot ischemia, with acral necroses caused by microembolism in a patient with severe arterial occlusive disease in the lower leg and long-standing diabetes mellitus.

Hyperglycemia causes inactivation of NO activity, mainly due to the formation of free O_2 radicals (Tesfamariam et al. 1992). In addition, cyclooxygenase-dependent vasoconstrictors are formed. The effects include increased adhesion of macrophages and thrombocytes, and impairment of the endothelium's fibrinolytic activity, with subse-

quent hypercoagulability due to increased thrombin activity and increased activation of thrombocytes.

These complex processes in the vascular system, combined with limited or even absent pain perception due to neuropathy, give rise to the more rapid progression of the wound that is often observed in DFS. Despite every therapeutic effort, angioneuropathic wounds have a poorer prognosis for healing and even today are associated with a much higher amputation rate (Heller et al. 2004).

4.4.4.4   Treatment

1. General measures:
- Near-normal values should be ensured: adjustment of blood sugar in diabetes mellitus
- Treatment of any disturbances of lipid metabolism
- Platelet inhibition
- Prophylaxis against thrombosis with low-molecular-weight heparin and adequate avoidance of hypothermia in the extremity (possibly by washing with warm water)
- Rigorous pressure avoidance (e.g., immobilization, cushioned dressings, ankle relief splints, alternating-pressure mattresses with a 30° tilt)
- Skin care
- Measures for protection against cold in Raynaud disease, nicotine abstinence, etc.
- Treatment of underlying internal medicine conditions:
  - Treatment of cardiac insufficiency. Caution: avoidance of hypotension, adjustment of systolic blood pressure to values in the range of 140–160 mmHg
  - Improvement in nephropathy
  - Improvement of protein deficiency
  - Treatment of anemia
  - Optimizing diet
- Monitoring of microbes to allow early antibiotic treatment

Intermittent manual compression may improve arterial perfusion and venous drainage. It involves repeatedly compressing the calf muscles while the patient is in a sitting position. Positive effects have been demonstrated by ultrasound measurements of the popliteal artery and laser Doppler flowmetry. This procedure, which is often used in the English-speaking countries, was found to be associated with improved wound healing in small groups of patients.

2. Drug treatment:

The established therapy is with prostaglandins, *alprostadil* (Caverject®, Prostavasin®).

Dosage: Once or twice daily 40–50 µg alprostadil, dissolved in 50–250 mL physiological saline, with an infusion over 2–3 h.

No other drugs that improve perfusion have so far been adequately evaluated. In patients with higher-grade ischemia and persistent disturbance of wound healing in whom the extremity is at risk, the following agents may be an option.

Low-dose urokinase lysis: Initial positive reports on this form of treatment were reported in the field of diabetology in 2000. A nonrandomized single-center study published in 2006 is now available that included 77 DFS patients with critical ischemia of the extremity and nonhealing wounds in whom revascularization was not possible. A dosage of 500,000–1 million IU, adjusted to the fibrinogen level, was administered as a short infusion over 30 min for 21 days. Sixty-one patients were ultimately available for analysis. After 12 months, the healing rate was 71%; 31% of the patients had no major amputation or ulcer. The amputation rate was 19% and the mortality rate was reported as 9%. Eighty-five percent of the patients survived. Only one case of severe bleeding occurred. Although there is still a lack of randomized studies, low-dose urokinase lysis represents a promising treatment option, particularly in DFS.

Administration of *sildenafil* (Revatio®) appears to improve wound healing in distal lesions in a setting of secondary Raynaud syndrome—e.g., in progressive systemic scleroderma (Friedrichson et al. 2007). Sildenafil is an inhibitor of type 5 phosphodiesterase and mediates NO-dependent vasodilation. Sildenafil can currently only be used "off label" (dosage 2×20 mg).

Cilostazol (Pletal®) is a selective phosphodiesterase-3 inhibitor with complex effects on the endothelium and on platelet aggregation. Treatment can be attempted for ulcers in the context of thromboangiitis obliterans, as well as in other lesions with microcirculatory causes.

3. Other as yet unevaluated forms of treatment:

Electrostimulation or similar forms of physical wound treatment, as well as tissue engineering with human fibroblasts, can be tried in individual cases, but have no major advantages over mechanical wound debridement.

Therapeutic angiogenesis using autologous bone-marrow cells is currently undergoing clinical testing, and the results of the current phase III study (BONMOT-CLI) are awaited. It might in the future offer an alternative form of treatment in patients with severe arterial occlusive disease (Amann et al. 2008).

Hyperbaric oxygen therapy and treatment with local growth factors have so far not shown any significant therapeutic success and should not be used.

4. Local wound therapy:
- Antiseptic local therapy
- Local debridement
- Wound dressings
- Vacuum therapy
- Pinch graft (Reverdin graft), split-thickness graft (Thiersch graft), mesh graft, flap plasty, etc. (see review by Kremer et al. 2008)

Local antiseptic treatment

The chronic ischemic wound must be regarded as potentially infected. This is due on the one hand to the local factors mentioned above, and on the other to the disturbed immunocompetence resulting from poor nutritive supply. Colonization, with slight microbial contamination, is found in practically all wounds. The progression of infection can take a very rapid course here, leading to sepsis. In addition, wound infection also causes persistent disturbance of the already weakened wound healing process. In the initial few days, therefore, even if there are only minor signs of clinical infection or if such signs are absent, local antiseptic treatment should be given. This applies especially to healing secondary wounds. For this reason, all ischemic wounds also receive additional systemic antibiotic treatment as a matter of principle. The aim is to achieve rapid elimination of pathogens and thus to reduce the oxygen demand in the tissue.

What is required, in addition to a safe microbicidal effect against possible pathogens, is a rapid onset of effect and adequate tolerability without relevant side effects (Kramer et al. 2004). Whenever possible, this treatment should be supported by previous wound debridement (see below). Alternatively (in cases of severe pain), the relevant solution can be rubbed in using "wiping debridement" with a gauze compress.

Appropriate *antiseptic agents:*
- Octenidine hydrochloride (Octenisept®). This has a microbicidal effect on Gram-positive and Gram-negative bacteria and fungi, as well as certain viruses, and has a sporicidal and protozoacidal effect. Carcinogenic or teratogenic effects are not known, and there is no relevant resorption and no toxic effect. It can be used as an undiluted rinse or can be applied moistly with sterile gauze compresses. It has a short application time of 1–2 min and is therefore the agent of choice for wound lavage. It can also be used for long-term application in special compresses with 24-h moistening (e.g., TenderWet®), which are changed daily.
- Polyhexanide. This has a microbicidal effect but is neither virucidal nor sporicidal. It has concentration-dependent effects in vitro, with an onset of effect of 5–20 min (a disadvantage in comparison with Octenisept®). It can be applied as a rinse or on a moistened gauze compress. No major resorption is known of, it has little interaction with human cell membranes and good tissue compatibility, and it can be used without pain. It must not be applied to hyaline cartilage or for joint rinsing because cartilage toxicity will occur.
- Prontosan®: combination of polyhexanide and undecylenamidopropyl betaine as a surfactant.
- Lavasept®: contains biguanide polyhexanide (PHMB) as the active agent, in an aqueous solution, and according to the manufacturer is only available as a concentrate for dilution to the desired concentration for application, with appropriate solutions such as Ringer's without lactate, or physiological saline. The concentration for application in aqueous solutions is (0.1–0.2% Lavasept concentrate corresponding to 0.02–0.04% polyhexanide); similar dosage recommendations apply to ointments, pastes, and gels. Preparation as a gel on the basis of hydroxyethyl cellulose has the advantage, in addition to the relatively low cost, that it can be combined with various wound dressings. This leads to longer contact time with the wound. The wound dressing must always be changed daily to begin with, so that maceration can be recognized early enough. As a result of the promotion of wound healing that has been observed, polyhexanide is suitable for use in combination with modern wound dressings (particularly with alginates and hydrofibers), according to the 2004 consensus recommendations on the choice of antiseptic agents. It can also be used under semiocclusive or occlusive dressings (Bruck et al. 2000). Polyhexanide is thus the agent of first choice for poorly healing chronic wounds.

Other suitable methods of eradicating bacteria include the use of fly maggots and the now-established application of silver-impregnated wound dressings (Atrauman® Ag, Actisorb® Silver 220, Aquacel® Ag, Contreet® H, Prisma®, Urgotül® Silver). These are discussed separately. Due to their cytotoxicity, the following (selected) agents are inappropriate or obsolete in the treatment of ischemic wounds: any form of topical antibiotic administration (Refobacin®, Leukase®, etc.), cytotoxic antiseptics such as chlorhexidine, ethanol, ethacridine lactate (Rivanol®), various dyes, organic mercury compounds (Mercurochrome®), and hydrogen peroxide. Povidone–iodine compounds (Betadine®) are contraindicated.

Wound cleaning by showering or with a foot bath, as recommended by some authors, sometimes with specially prepared drinking water, is contraindicated due to the possibility of introducing bacteria.

Local debridement

Due to the danger of the wound becoming larger, the indication for *mechanical debridement* with a scalpel and sharp spoon is very narrow in ischemic wounds. However, removal of nonvital tissue and fibrin coating is a prerequisite for healing (Steed et al. 1997). By contrast, when there is extensive infection, the focus is on generous opening to ensure wound drainage and prevent abscess formation. When debridement is used in chronic wounds, the aim is to reduce bacteria and promote granulation. In most cases, at least partial debridement is possible.

Care should be taken to ensure adequate analgesia. Pretreatment with local anesthetics alone (Emla® or a gauze compress soaked in 1–2% lidocaine solution) is only adequate for superficial wounds. The onset of action is approximately 20 min.

In deeper lesions, additional systemic analgesia with intravenous opioids or conscious sedation (with appropriate monitoring) has proved successful. Local injection into an underperfused or ischemic area to administer nerve blocks is contraindicated because of the risk of causing additional tissue damage.

If there is no success and the wound is extensive, there is an indication for surgical wound debridement or (after the perfusion situation has been clearly established) border zone amputation.

For wounds with refractory fibrin coating (biofilm) or necroses that are difficult to remove or are incompletely removed with a scalpel or sharp spoon, *biosurgery with fly maggots* is an important, if rather more elaborate treatment option. Sterile-bred maggots of the species *Phaenicia sericata* are applied to the wound in a controlled fashion and are able to perform highly targeted necrosectomy. As a result of saliva enzymes and protease secretion, necroses and fibrin are partially digested and broken down. A clean, bacteria-free wound base results (Prete 1997).

Application: After cleaning with Ringer's solution, the maggots are applied at a density of 5–10 per cm³ (approximately 50 for a moderately sized wound). If there has been previous antiseptic therapy, then only treatment with a lightly moistened Ringer's compress should be carried out for at least 24 h before application, as the larvae can be expected to die off more rapidly otherwise. After rinsing the wound with Ringer's solution, the maggots are applied under a loose dressing of gauze that serves as a cage; the edge of the wound is sealed well with a plaster (e.g., Fixomull®). Alternatively, a closed system using a "biobag" is possible; this makes it easier to create the dressing, but it is more expensive. The dressing is visually checked daily and removed after 2–5 days, depending on the size of the maggots and the wound surface. A second treatment cycle is sometimes necessary. The great advantage of this treatment is that it usually allows complete removal of bacteria, including problem bacteria such as multidrug-resistant *Staphylococcus aureus* (MRSA) and *Pseudomonas* spp.

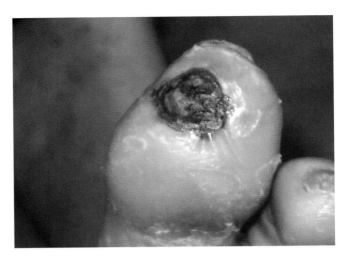

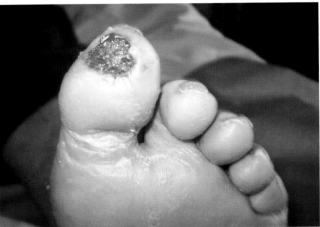

Fig. 4.4-13 and 4.4-14 D1 ischemic necrosis before and after appropriate debridement.

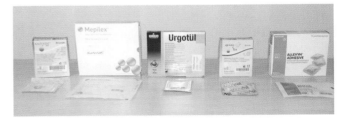

Fig. 4.4-15 A selection of the various wound dressings available.

With few exceptions, *enzymatic wound cleaning* with ointment preparations such as Iruxol® and Varidase® is obsolete in wound treatment, as it is ineffective.

Wound dressings

A vast number of different wound dressings are now commercially available, with constantly new approaches to treatment. Although "scientific" studies are often cited as part of the marketing strategy, there is as yet no research-based (randomized and blinded) evidence in comparison with moist gauze compresses. The selection presented here makes no claim to completeness, but the products listed are usually recommended in German wound centers and in the relevant wound manuals. Polypharmacy in the choice of wound dressing is not useful; standardization should be aimed for in each treatment center, with only a few preparations per indication. This not only makes economic sense, but also leads to a much wider base of experience with each dressing than a random choice from many different ones.

The principles involved in choosing a wound dressing are as follows. A wound dressing should in principle always be administered in accordance with each wound healing stage (i.e., adapted to the phase) and in accordance with the current extent of secretion.

In contrast to the wound compress, the more complex modern wound dressings basically carry out several tasks at the same time:

- Uptake and release of fluid (providing a moist wound environment)
- Promotion of granulation and epithelialization
- Antimicrobial effect (with silver compounds)
- Modulation of the wound secretion (protease binding, protection of growth factors)

Due to the high potential for microbial recolonization of chronic ischemic wounds, *excessively moist* wound treatment should be avoided. Moist agents such as hydrogels or hydrocolloid bandages can only be recommended here with qualifications due to their potential for maceration, and a strict indication for them is always required.

However, if a wound becomes too dry, its capacity for granulation—which is in any case poor—will cease altogether. A crust may form, which needs to be removed. The real difficulty for the therapist lies in recognizing the current situation and the secretion behavior of the wound and selecting a suitable dressing or changing it appropriately, as needed. In general, an ischemic wound needs more frequent changes of dressing. Due to the potential for deterioration, even in a stable wound situation, and in order to control the degree of infection, a maximum of 2–3 days must be set, even though this may contradict several published principles of treatment for wounds with other pathogeneses.

In *wound healing stage 1,* simple standard *sterile compresses* are still extremely important for initial treatment. During the first few days, they are used to absorb wound secretions and are extremely good for assessing the amount secreted. As described above, they are moistened with an antiseptic and placed over the wound if there are any important signs of infection. Their major disadvantage is that they dry out rapidly, so that moistening has to be carried out every 4–6 h.

Removing them when changing the dressing may be painful even after prior rinsing with Ringer's solution. Additional application of a *coated gauze* to the wound counteracts adhesion, leads to reduced evaporation of the antiseptic, and does not prevent rapid elimination of secretion. Suitable products include Urgotül® (a sterile lipidocolloid wound dressing made of polyester fibers with hydrocolloid particles, impregnated with Vaseline) and Atrauman® (a lattice mesh material made of hydrophobic polyester fibers, impregnated with an ointment containing no medical substances). Adaptic® may also be recommended with some qualifications, but not when there are large amounts of secretion (smooth-surfaced viscose fibers with a neutral oil-in-water emulsion).

Absorbent compresses are available for stronger levels of secretion (e.g., Surgipad®, Zetuvit®). It has been found that Sorbion plus® and Vliwasorb® (both with water-storing polymers known as "super-absorbers") barely adhere to the wound, although Sorbion sana®, which has a three-dimensional wound contact layer and has been commercially available since 2009, has proved particularly valuable for pain-sensitive wounds.

In cases of high levels of secretion with simultaneous infection, *activated carbon dressings* can also be used temporarily (e.g., Actisorb® Silver 220). These bind large amounts of secretion, are bactericidal, and absorb endotoxins, although the dressings themselves have no major granulation-promoting or wound-healing effects. An advantage is that they absorb unpleasant odors. They are applied directly, or with a coated gauze if there is a tendency for adhesion to develop, attached with compresses, and should be exchanged daily.

In practically *all three stages of wound healing, closed-pore foam materials* (e.g., Mepilex®, Biatain®, Urgocell®, Alleveyn®, and Tielle®) form a major pillar of treatment. They usually consist of a polyurethane foam and, as in Mepilex®, are coated with silicone or thermally smoothed.

They can absorb limited amounts of secretion and promote granulation and epithelialization. In addition, they have cushioning and thus pain-reducing characteristics, which are particularly useful for interdigital toe lesions. They are cut and applied to the wound with overlaps of approximately 1 cm. Wound adhesions are rare even in dry wound conditions, and changing the dressings is usually painless. In the first stage of wound healing, they can be combined with antiseptics (Lavasept or Prontosan gel; see above). In Biatain Ag® and Urgocell® Silver, silver is already incorporated into the foam texture, so that it is not necessary to apply an antiseptic when there is low-grade infection. *Alginates* and *hydrofibers* are used to maintain a moist wound environment in moderately to severely secreting wounds. They represent an important form of treatment in both the *inflammatory stage* and the *granulation stage.*

Alginates are obtained from brown algae and are available as wound compresses or wound tamponades in the form of fibrous calcium or calcium–sodium alginate. Their mode of action is based on ion exchange: calcium ions, high concentrations of which are incorporated into the alginate, are replaced by sodium ions that are present in the wound secretion. Alginates have a high capacity for absorption, and on absorbing the wound secretion they form a viscous gel with a stable shape that keeps the wound moist. They bind bacteria and tissue components and are therefore suitable for use in infected wounds, as well as fissured deep wounds.

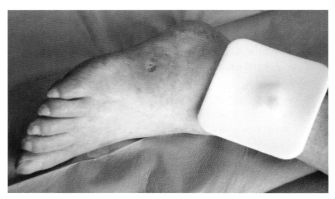

Fig. 4.4-16 Application of polyurethane foam (Mepilex®) in a patient with a superficial ischemic lesion.

Preparations available include Sorbalgon®, Suprasorb®, Algoster-il®, and Trionic®. In the inflammatory stage, they should always be moistened with polyhexanide, and they also need a secondary dressing—preferably with gauze or absorptive compresses, depending on the secretion. As the only calcium–sodium alginate available, Kaltostat® has also proved to have good granulation-promoting characteristics.

Hydrofibers (e.g., Aquacel®) consist of macromolecular sodium carboxymethylcellulose. This has a high absorptive capacity and beneficial management of exudate, as liquids are mainly absorbed vertically and are stored in the hydrofibers. The dressing should therefore be placed on the wound surface in such a way that it overlaps the wound by at least 1 cm on all sides; a secondary dressing should be placed in order to drain excess secretion. The dressing also changes into a shape-stable gel. As with the alginates, *targeted* moistening should be carried out in dry wounds. The dressing should be changed every 2 days, or a maximum of 3 days if the wound's grade of secretion and infection is known. A combination with silver (Aquacel® Ag) has proved useful for ischemic wounds.

If none of the wound treatments described above produce any progress, various *methods of promoting granulation* can be used. Although in traditional wound therapy these are all only recommended as a fall-back measure, due to their only slight advantages over conventional wound dressings and their higher cost, they may be a treatment option in critical ischemia of the extremities:

- Hyalofill® (hyaluronic acid 65% esterified with benzyl alcohol). This fibrous fleece material is moistened with Ringer's solution or polyhexanide, depending on the grade of secretion, until a gel-like matrix forms. The pieces of fleece are covered with compresses or with a foam as a secondary dressing.
- Hyalogran® (hyaluronic acid 100% esterified with benzyl alcohol in combination with sodium alginate). This powdery material can remain in the wound for up to 3 days or longer and has to be moistened with Ringer's solution until it forms a gel. It requires a semi-occlusive dressing—e.g., Tegaderm®—or alternatively foam.

Collagen-containing products: Collagen plays an important role in wound closure as a structural component and as an element required for cell migration, particularly of keratinocytes, which play a decisive role in epithelialization.

- Catrix® is a sterile collagen powder for the treatment of chronic wounds. It is compatible both with gauze dressings and with dressings designed for moist wound treatment.
- Promogran® (55% bovine collagen combined with 45% regenerated oxidized cellulose) is a wound fleece and is intended to produce a granulation-promoting effect by binding proteases and protecting growth factors. Depending on the secretion, moistening with Ringer's solution or polyhexanide is necessary. When it is combined with silver (Prisma®), antiseptic treatment is usually not necessary. Several studies have suggested that Promogran treatment reduces protease activity in the fluid present in chronic wounds, thereby providing protection against the degradation of growth factors such as platelet-derived growth factor (PDGF). Growth factors are intended to be temporarily stored in the matrix and released in an active form after resorption of the wound covering. In addition, a stimulatory effect on chemotaxis and proliferation of fibroblasts has been reported. This was dem-

onstrated for peptides that are produced during the degradation of collagen and for other degradation products of the extracellular matrix such as laminin, fibronectin, and elastin (Geesin et al. 1996).

Other products in the group of granulation-promoting materials include Dermax® and Suprasorb C.

In stage 3 (epithelialization/remodeling), open-pored *foam materials* or alternatively *coated gauzes* can again be used—e.g., Urgotül® or Adaptic® (see above). These products prevent adhesion to the wound and allow a slightly moist wound environment with a good air supply.

In this stage, the greatest danger is that the highly sensitive epithelium may dry out or undergo mechanical damage. Good cushioning (e.g., with wound compresses and surgical cotton) should therefore be ensured.

Vacuum suction treatment

The use of local negative pressure therapy (Vacuum-Assisted Closure, VAC®) has become increasingly accepted in recent years for the treatment of chronic wounds. In addition to the long-established KCI system, Smith & Nephew have since 2009 been supplying a comparable system (Renasys®), as has the Hartmann company. Both systems have proved practicable and effective in practical usage.

The therapeutic principle is based on a noninvasive wound closure system that produces controlled negative pressure limited to the local area and thereby accelerates the healing process in acute and chronic wounds. A sterile, open-pored foam dressing is placed in the wound defect, the surface is sealed with an adhesive foil, and controlled negative pressure of between 75 and 150 mmHg (40–120 mmHg in the Renasys® system) is then produced over the wound. Depending on the wound type and treatment goal, treatment can be carried out continuously or intermittently (e.g., 5 minutes on, 2 minutes off). The surplus wound secretion is sucked out of the wound and captured in a container. This procedure is therefore an important treatment option particularly in deep and superinfected wounds.

Granulation and neovascularization are promoted in comparison with treatment using moist dressings (Joseph et al. 2000). This may explain why treatment is successful even in cases of higher-grade ischemia of the extremities.

In addition, the wound base is ideally prepared for coverage with split skin, for example. This treatment procedure is now established in various fields of medicine—e.g., in DFS treatment, traumatology, abdominal surgery, and vascular surgery (Armstrong and Lavery 2005). In smaller wounds and those in acral locations, however, vacuum therapy is very restricted and often technically impossible. Other disadvantages include the still quite high cost of the procedure and the substantially increased amount of nursing care required. The development of small, portable pump systems—which are available from both manufacturers—has led to this form of treatment spreading to outpatient wound care as well in recent years. However, the use of the miniature pumps that have recently become available in the outpatient field is not advisable for the treatment of ischemic wounds, as the drainage lines are sometimes quite thin and the pump force is lower.

Table 4.4-6 Stage-adjusted drug administration for wound treatment and procedures.

Wound healing stage	Aim	Procedure	Preferred wound agent	Specialized treatment
WH 1 (inflammation)	Wound cleaning/eradication of bacteria	Mechanical debridement and necrosectomy VAC® therapy Biosurgery with maggots	Local antiseptics (polyhexanide) combined with: ■ Open-pored foam or alginates/hydrofibers, poss. combined with silver	Systemic antibiotics Analgesia
WH 2 (granulation)	Promoting granulation	VAC® therapy, poss. debridement	■ Open-pored foam ■ Alginates/hydrofibers ■ Poss. granulation-promoting agents	In case of stagnation, drug treatment, poss. use of as yet un-evaluated procedures (see text)
WH 3 (epithelialization)	Acceleration of epithelialization and wound closure	Moist wound care Cushioning	Open-pored foam Coated gauze Collagen-containing wound dressings	In case of stagnation, drug treatment, poss. use of as yet un-evaluated procedures (see text) In all stages: checking options for revascularization

VAC, vacuum assisted closure.

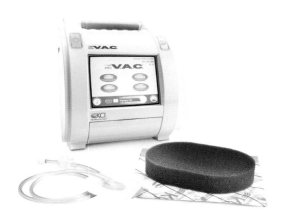

Fig. 4.4-17 Vacuum system (KCI®; manufacturer's photo).

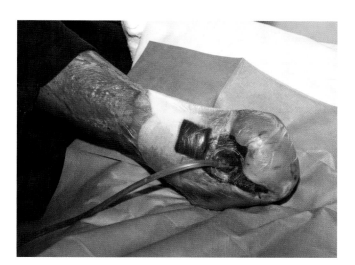

Table 4.4-6 provides an overview of the stage-adjusted application of the various agents and materials available for treating wounds and the procedures used.

References

Amann B, Lüdemann C, Rückert R, Lawall H, Liesenfeld B, Schneider M, Schmidt-Lucke J. Design and rationale of a randomized, double-blind, placebo-controlled phase III study for autologous bone marrow cell transplantation in critical limb ischemia: the BONe Marrow Outcomes Trial in Critical Limb Ischemia (BONMOT-CLI). VASA 2008; 37: 319–25.

Armstrong DG, Lavery LA. Negative pressure wound therapy after partial diabetic foot amputation: a multicentre, randomised controlled trial. The Lancet 2005 (12); 366 (9498): 1704–10.

Beckert S, WitteMB, Königsrainer A, Coerper S. The impact of the Micro-Lightguide O2C for the quantification of tissue ischemia in diabetic foot ulcers. Diabetes Care 2004; 27: 2863–7.

Brownlee M, Cerami A, Vlassara H. Advanced glycosylation end products in tissue and the biochemical basis of diabetic complications. N Engl J Med 1988; 318: 1315–22.

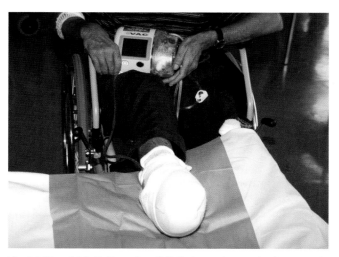

Fig. 4.4-18 and 4.4-19 Examples of VAC® therapy in a nonhealing wound after several failed attempts to create a bypass, with persistent ischemia and status post forefoot amputation.

Bruck JC, Koch S, Kramer A. Klinische und histologische Untersuchungen zur Wirksamkeit von Lavasept auf granulierenden bzw. epithelisierenden Wunden. Hyg Med Suppl 2000; 1: 46.

Coerper S, Wagner S, Witte M, Schaffer M, Becker HD. Temporary expression pattern in wound secretion and peripheral wound biopsies. Zentralbl Chir 1999; 124: 78–80.

Friedrichson E, Rehberger P, Fuhrmann JT, Walz F, Meurer M, Pfeiffer C. Rasche Abheilung von akralen Ulzera bei systemischer Sklerodermie unter Sildenafil. Der Hautarzt 2008; 59 (3): 230–3.

Geesin JC, Brown LJ, Liu Z, Berg RA. Development of a skin model based on insoluble fibrillar collagen. J Biomed Mater Res 1996; 33: 1–8.

Heller G, Günster, C, Schellschmidt H. Wie häufig sind Diabetes-bedingte Amputationen unterer Extremitäten in Deutschland? Dtsch Med Wochenschr 2004; 129: 429–33.

Inter-Society Consensus for the management of peripheral arterial disease (TASC II). Eur J Vasc Endovasc Surg 2007; Supplement 1: 40–1.

Joseph E, Hamori CA, Bergman S, Roaf E, Swann NF, Anastasi CW. A prospective randomized trial of vacuum-assisted closure versus standard therapy of chronic nonhealing wounds. Wounds 2000; 12 (3): 60–7.

Kammerlander G. Lokaltherapeutische Standards für chronische Hautwunden. Springer Verlag, 2005, S. 111ff.

Kramer A, Heeg P, Harke HP, Rudolph H, Koch S, Jülich WD, Hingst V, Merka V, Lippert H. Wundantiseptik. In: Klinische Antiseptik 1993: 163–91 (aus: Konsensempfehlung zur Auswahl von Wirkstoffen für die Wundantiseptik 2004: 4).

Kremer T, Germann G, Riedel K, Giessler GA. Plastisch-rekonstruktive Verfahren in der interdisziplinären Therapie chronischer Wunden. Chirurg 2008; 79: 546–54.

Lawall H, Amann B, Rottmann M, Angelkort B. The role of microcirculatory techniques in patients with diabetic foot syndrome. VASA 2000; 29: 191–7.

Marston WA, Davies SW, Armstrong B, Farber MA, Mendes RC, Fulton JJ, Keagy BA. Natural history of limbs with arterial insufficiency and chronic ulceration treated without revascularization. J Vasc Surg 2006; 44 (1): 108–14.

Moulik PK, Mtonga R, Gill GV. Amputation and mortality in new-onset diabetic foot ulcers stratified by etiology. Diabetes Care 2003; 26 (2): 491–494.

Padberg JFT, Back TL, Thompson PN, Hobson RW. Transcutaneous oxygen (TcPO2) estimates probability of healing in the ischemic extremity. J Surg Res 1996; 60 (2): 365–9.

Prete PE. Growth effects of phaeniciaserata larval extracts on fibroblasts: mechanism for wound healing by maggot therapy. Life Science 1997; 60: 505–10.

Steed DL, Donohoe D, Webster MW, Lindsley L. Effect of extensive debridement and treatment on the healing of diabetic foot ulcer. J Am Coll Surg 1997; 138: 61–4.

Tesfamariam B, Cohen RA. Free radicals mediate endothelial cell dysfunction caused by elevated glucose. Am J Physiol 1992; 263: H321–3.

Ubbink DT, Jacobs MJ, Tangelder GJ, Slaaf DW, Reneman RS. The usefulness of capillary microscopy, transcutaneous oximetry and laser Doppler fluxmetry in the assessment of the severity of lower limb ischaemia. Int J Microcirc Clin 1994; 14 (1–2): 34–44.

4.4.5 Regenerative treatment for peripheral arterial occlusive disease

Sigrid Nikol

4.4.5.1 Clinical background

A substantial proportion of patients with an advanced stage of peripheral arterial occlusive disease (PAOD) have diffuse coronary and peripheral disease in which all the available venous material for bypasses has been used. Typically, they also have disease of the small distal vessels and comorbid conditions in which interventional treatment, particularly bypass surgery, is contraindicated or associated with excessive risk, despite the advances that have been made in bypass surgery and peripheral vascular interventions in recent years. Due to the increasing age of the population and the rising prevalence of diabetes, a much higher incidence of advanced PAOD is expected in the coming years, with patients in whom conventional revascularization methods are no longer possible due to their poor general condition. In addition, there are also patients with thromboangiitis obliterans, in which interventional and surgical treatment is difficult.

For these reasons, it is necessary to develop new forms of treatment that can also be carried out on an adjuvant basis in addition to the traditional revascularization procedures. Local proangiogenetic therapy might represent a new noninvasive treatment option for such patients and even in what are known as "no-option" patients it might offer a possible way of achieving revascularization with comparatively low risk (Fig. 4.4-20).

In principle, several treatment options for these purposes have been developed in recent years, including the use of human growth factors in the form of biologically active proteins or their genes, and cell therapy. While protein therapy has not proved successful, angiogenetic gene therapy has overcome all obstacles after nearly 20 years of research and is currently being tested in phase 3 approval studies. Cell therapy, on the other hand, is a comparatively new field in which there are many open questions and no data from randomized studies are available.

4.4.5.2 Angiogenetic gene therapy

Angiogenesis is a complex process that depends on growth factor and involves a large number of steps before the final formation of mature new vessels from the preexisting vascular network (Fig. 4.4-21). In atherosclerotic vascular diseases, a lack of angiogenesis and inadequate formation of collateral vessels are a major problem. Cardiovascular risk factors such as diabetes mellitus and advanced age also limit the angiogenic response of the resident endothelial cells, as has been shown in animal studies using rabbits and mice. Collateral formation through angiogenesis is limited when there is peripheral ischemia in older and diabetic animals. The mechanisms responsible for this include gradually developing endothelial dysfunction and reduced expression of vascular endothelial growth factor (VEGF). However, greater age in the animals did not hinder collateral formation after administration of exogenous recombinant VEGF.

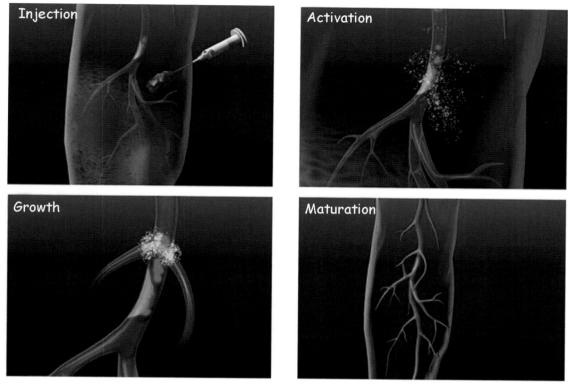

Fig. 4.4-20 Formation of new vessels in the extremity region during therapeutic angiogenesis.

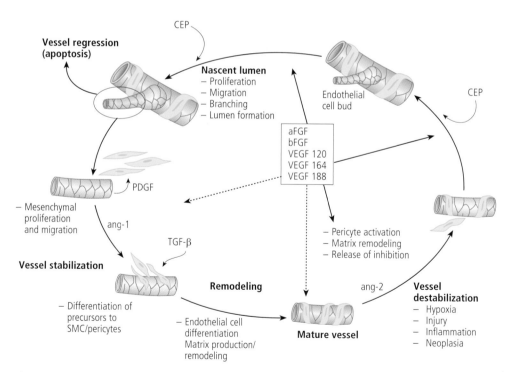

Fig. 4.4-21 Formation of a stable new vessel—a complex process. Increased local expression of angiogenetic factors such as fibroblast growth factor (FGF) and vascular endothelial growth factor (VEGF) during angiopoiesis destabilizes part of the existing vessels (usually a venule). This destabilization is associated with increased angiopoietin-2 (ang-2) expression and with pericyte activation, as well as matrix remodeling, induction of pericytes, and migration and proliferation of endothelial cells (ECs). Newly formed vessels may be dependent for their survival on exogenous factors before they have been transformed into completely mature structures. This transformation process includes the recruitment by the ECs of precursors from pericytes/smooth muscle cells (SMCs) via endothelial-derived platelet-derived growth factor (ED-PDGF). As soon as the wall precursor cell comes into contact with the vessel, transforming growth factor-β (TGF-β) is activated, which in turn down-regulates proliferation and migration and induces differentiation into SMCs/pericytes. In addition to TGF-β, ang-1—produced by the SMCs/pericytes—is also involved in the stabilization and maintenance of stable mature vessels. (Adapted from Ng and D'Amore 2001). aFGF, acidic fibroblast growth factor; bFGF, basic fibroblast growth factor; CEP, circulating endothelial precursor.

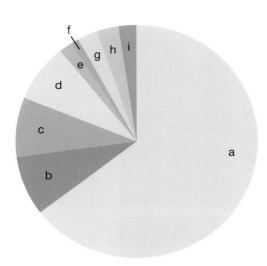

a Cancer diseases 64.5% (n = 1098)

b Cardiovascular diseases 8.5% (n = 144)

c Monogenic diseases 8.3% (n = 141)

d Infectious diseases (8%) (n = 137)

e Neurological diseases 1.8% (n = 30)

f Ocular diseases 1.2% (n = 20)

g Other diseases 2.5% (n = 43)

h Gene marking 2.9% (n = 50)

i Healthy volunteers 2.3% (n = 40)

Fig. 4.4-22 Indications in gene therapy studies to date (reproduced with permission from the Wiley website, accessed March 2011).

Table 4.4-7 Completed phase 2 studies on angiogenetic gene therapy in patients with peripheral arterial occlusive disease: efficacy.

Study	Growth factor	Vector	Route of administration	Patients (n)	Primary end point	Results	Reference
VEGF PVD	$VEGF_{165}$	Adenovirus Plasmid Liposomes	Local catheter support	54	Improved vascularization	Positive	Makinen et al. 2002
RAVE	$VEGF_{121}$	Adenovirus	Intramuscular	105	Maximum walking distance	Negative	Rajagopalan et al. 2003
Groningen Trial	$VEGF_{165}$	Plasmid	Intramuscular	54	Reduction in amputation rate	Negative	Kusumato et al. 2006
TALISMAN 201	FGF-1	Plasmid	Intramuscular	125	Complete ulcer healing	Negative (positive for amputation)	Nikol et al. 2008
WALK	(HIF)1-α/VP16	Adenovirus	Intramuscular	300	Maximum walking distance	Negative	US NIH 2010; Creager 2009
HGF-STAT	HGF	Plasmid	Intramuscular	104	TcPO2	Positive	Powell et al. 2010
HGF-CLI	HGF	Plasmid	Intramuscular	40	Resting pain, ulcer size	Positive	Shigematsu et al. 2010
DELTA-1	Del-1 (with poloxamer 188)	Plasmid	Intramuscular	105	Maximum walking distance	Negative	Conte et al. 2006

FGF, fibroblast growth factor; HGF, hepatocyte growth factor; RAVE, Regional Angiogenesis with Vascular Endothelial Growth Factor Trial; TALISMAN, Therapeutic Angiogenesis Leg Ischemia Study for the Management of Arteriopathy and Nonhealing ulcer; VEGF, vascular endothelial growth factor; VEGF PVD, VEGF for Peripheral Vascular Disease.

In various phase 1 and phase 2 studies, the value of therapeutic angiogenesis has also been demonstrated using a number of experimental agents, particularly VEGFs, fibroblast growth factors (FGFs) and hepatocyte growth factors (HGFs), administered in the form of protein or as plasmid DNA or an adenoviral gene construct. These agents are currently also being tested in phase 3 approval studies. Notable aspects in treatments conducted so far have been that gene constructs were regularly superior to the use of proteins—most probably due to their different half-life, with a sustained effect over weeks and sometimes even months; and lower rates of side effects such as hypertension (with VEGF) and nephrotoxicity (with basic FGF). For these reasons, there are currently high expectations from the development of angiogenetic gene therapy.

There were particularly high hopes after the identification of the gene that can be switched on by tissue hypoxia, known as hypoxia-inducible factor-1α (HIF-1α). HIF-1α is a transcription factor that regulates a large number of factors involved in the process of angiogenesis. The use of adenoviral HIF-1α in patients with intermittent claudication has now been evaluated in the randomized, double-blind, and placebo-controlled phase II Walk Study.

A total of 176 angiogenesis gene therapy studies throughout the world are currently registered (Fig. 4.4-22), including an estimated 3000–3500 patients (Wiley web page 2011). Table 4.4-7 summarizes all of the published phase 2 angiogenetic gene therapy studies on PAOD published from 2002 to 2011.

Efficacy results to date from clinical phase 2 angiogenetic gene therapy studies

The aims of the phase 2 study on VEGF in peripheral vascular disease by Ylä-Herttuala et al. (2002) were to evaluate the safety of the angiographic and hemodynamic effects of local catheter administration of the VEGF gene in ischemic legs immediately after percutaneous transluminal angioplasty (PTA). In the study, 18 patients received the adenoviral VEGF construct (VEGF-Ad), 17 received plasmid–liposome complexes of VEGF (VEGF-P/L), and 19 control patients received Ringer's lactate in each dilated area. On digital subtraction angiography (DSA), improved vascularization was seen in the VEGF-treated groups distal to each gene transfer area and in the VEGF-Ad group in the region with the clinically most severe ischemia. In the VEGF-Ad group and VEGF-P/L group, there was significant improvement in the Rutherford class and ankle–brachial index, but similar improvements were also seen in the control group. The angiographic end point is open to criticism in this study, since according to a consensus paper on suitable examination methods and end points in therapeutic angiogenesis, angiographically assessed vascularization in particular is an unreliable end point and cannot be recommended.

The Regional Angiogenesis with Vascular Endothelial Growth Factor (RAVE) study (2003) was a double-blind, placebo-controlled phase 2 study intended to evaluate the safety and efficacy of intramuscular administration of adenoviral VEGF (AdVEGF121) in the legs of patients with unilateral peripheral arterial occlusive disease (Rajagopalan et al. 2003). A total of 105 patients with unilateral exercise-limiting intermittent claudication were included after completing two treadmill ergometry tests with maximum walking distances of 1–10 min. The patients were randomly assigned to high-dose AdVEGF121, low-dose ADVEGF121, or a placebo, administered in the form of 20 intramuscular injections into the index leg during a single session. There were no differences between the groups with regard to the primary efficacy end point (i.e., the change in the maximum walking distance after 12 weeks). Secondary end points such as the ankle–brachial index, the interval to the start of claudication, and quality of life were similar after 12 and 26 weeks. However, administration of adenoviral VEGF121 was associated with more peripheral edema.

The double-blind, placebo-controlled Groningen study (Kusumanto et al. 2006) assessed the efficacy of intramuscular administration of nonviral phVEGF165 in patients with critical limb ischemia in comparison with a placebo. In 54 adult diabetic patients, 27 received the placebo and 27 received phVEGF165. After 100 days, six amputations were noted in the placebo group in comparison with three amputations in the treatment group (not significant), with a total of three responders versus 14 ($P = 0.003$). No severe adverse effects were observed. The authors concluded that this small randomized gene therapy study did not meet the primary end point of a significant reduction in the amputation rate, although it did show significant major improvement in the patients who received the VEGF165 plasmid.

It is important to note that the amputation rate in the gene therapy group in this study was only half that in the placebo group. Like many studies on angiogenetic gene therapy, the Groningen study was too small in terms of the number of patients included to identify any superiority for angiogenetic gene therapy relative to the hard end point of amputation. This is contrast to the following study,

which also showed a halving of the amputation rate and—with twice the number of patients included—also provided a statistically significant result.

In the WALK study, the safety and efficacy of Ad2/hypoxia-inducible factor (HIF)-1α/VP16 was investigated in patients with bilateral intermittent claudication (Creager 2009). In this randomized, double-blind, and placebo-controlled phase II study, it was tested whether an intramuscular injection of Ad2/HIF-1α/VP16 at various dosages into the ischemic leg was well tolerated and capable of improving the maximum walking distance on standardized treadmill ergometry. It was planned to include 75 patients with severe claudication per patient group (three groups with Ad2/HIF-1α/VP16 gene transfer at various dosages and one placebo group), with a total of 300 patients, but in fact 283 patients were recruited. Each patient received 20 injections (each 100 µL) per leg of gene construct or a placebo in one session, a total of 40 injections. However, the study's results showed no improvements in the maximum walking distance, onset of claudication, or ankle–arm index.

The HGF-STAT study was a phase II clinical trial in which hepatocyte growth factor (HGF) gene plasmid was investigated. This was also a randomized, double-blind, and placebo-controlled study with intramuscular injections of the HGF plasmid in patients with critical ischemia (Powell et al. 2010). The study included patients with critical ischemia in whom traditional revascularization was not indicated for anatomical reasons or due to unsuitable veins or comorbidities. After randomization, they received three treatment cycles each with eight injections on days 1, 14, and 28. The total dosages of HGF plasmid in each group were 0 mg (placebo), 1.2 mg (low dose), 8 mg (medium dose), and 12 mg (high dose). With regard to efficacy, no significant improvement was observed in the overall group, and transcutaneous oxygen pressure ($tcPO_2$) in the foot only increased significantly in the high-dose subgroup in comparison with the placebo. Six months after the treatment, $tcPO_2$ was higher than 30 mmHg in 39% of the placebo group, 57% of the low-dose group, 67% of the medium-dose group, and 80% of the high-dose group. With regard to ulcer healing, only a nonsignificant improvement was observed in the HGF treatment groups in comparison with the placebo. The safety of the treatment was good and did not differ among the groups. There are therefore at least some signs of possible benefit from intramuscular injections of HGF plasmid in relation to improved perfusion.

Intramuscular injections of naked HGF plasmid were also carried out in another randomized, double-blind, and placebo-controlled multicenter study in patients with critical limb ischemia (Shigematsu et al. 2010). Randomization was carried out with a plasmid:placebo ratio of 2:1. The injection sites were determined by the angiographic results. The placebo or plasmid was injected on days 1 and 28, and the follow-up period was 12 weeks. The primary end points were improvement in resting pain in patients without ulcers (Rutherford class 4) and a reduction in ulcer size in patients with ulcers (Rutherford class 5). Forty-five patients were treated, 40 of whom were examined in an interim analysis. Significant improvement with regard to the primary end point was observed in 70.4% of the patients (19/27) in the HGF group and 30.8% of patients (4/13) in the placebo group ($P = 0.014$). A significantly higher improvement rate after HGF therapy was seen in Rutherford class 5 patients (100%, 11/11) in comparison with the placebo group (40%, two of five; $P = 0.018$). There were no safety problems.

In the DELTA-1 study, VLTS-589 (a plasmid with the gene for the angiomatrix protein Del-1 in combination with poloxamer 188) in patients with intermittent claudication was compared with patients in a poloxamer 188 control group (Conte et al. 2006). Patients with bilateral intermittent claudication and a maximum walking distance of 1–10 min were included. The patients received VLTS-589 or the poloxamer 188 control, administered in the form of 21 intramuscular injections into each lower extremity (42 mL into each leg). The safety and tolerability of the treatment were assessed, as well as its efficacy in comparison with the control group and baseline values: a change in the maximum walking distance after 90 days (primary end point), and changes in the onset of claudication, in the ankle–arm index, and quality of life. Overall, 105 patients underwent randomization and were treated. After 30, 90, and 180 days of follow-up, all three clinical parameters had improved significantly in comparison with the baseline values, but without any difference between the treatment groups for any of the primary or secondary end points. The same applied to quality of life. There were no severe treatment-associated side effects, and the numbers of events were similar in both groups.

The Therapeutic Angiogenesis Leg Ischemia Study for the Management of Arteriopathy and Nonhealing Ulcer (TALISMAN 201) phase 2 study (Nikol et al. 2008) was a multinational 52-week study in which 125 patients with critical leg ischemia and nonhealing ulcers, with no options for conventional revascularization, were randomized 1:1 between eight intramuscular injections of nonviral FGF-1 (NV1F-GF) or a placebo on days 1, 15, 30, and 45. In this study, NV1FGF significantly reduced the risk of and time up to all amputations, including major amputations, in comparison with the placebo. In addition, there was a trend toward a reduced risk of mortality with nonviral FGF-1 (a synonym for acidic FGF). By contrast, the ulcer healing rate was similar with NV1FGF (19.6%) and placebo (14.3%; $P = 0.514$). The incidence of adverse effects was similarly high in the two groups, but far fewer severe events occurred in the gene therapy group.

Although the study did not succeed in reaching the primary end point of complete ulcer healing, it nevertheless represents a milestone, as it for the first time demonstrated a significant effect on a hard end point such as major amputation. It is probably difficult in the framework of angiogenesis studies to reach significant results with regard to ulcer healing, as there are extremely wide differences in the standards used in wound treatment between individual centers and individual countries, and the size of the ulcers in the patients included in the studies may also be extremely variable. In addition, a reduction in the amputation rate and an improvement in the amputation-free survival are clinically much more relevant than ulcer healing for the patients affected.

For this reason, a worldwide phase 3 approval study including 525 patients has been initiated in order to confirm the benefit of nonviral FGF-1 relative to the delay in the time to amputation and death in patients with critical limb ischemia with no options for revascularization (Therapeutic Angiogenesis for the Management of Arteriopathy in a Randomized International Study, TAMARIS).

Results of the largest phase III angiogenesis gene therapy study on PAOD worldwide

In a phase II approval study, the randomized, double-blind, and placebo-controlled TAMARIS study investigated whether viral FGF (NV1FGF) might improve the amputation-free survival in patients with critical limb ischemia (Belch et al. 2011). The study included a total of 525 patients with critical limb ischemia with no option for revascularization, from 171 institutions in 30 different countries. The patients all had ulcers in the lower extremity, with ankle pressures < 70 mmHg and/or toe pressures < 50 mmHg, or transcutaneous oxygen pressures < 30 mmHg in the leg being treated. After double-blind randomization, the patients received eight intramuscular injections of NV1FGF in the index leg or a placebo on days 1, 15, 29, and 43. The primary end point was a reduction in the rates of major amputation or death after 1 year. The patients' mean age was 70 ± 10 years; 70% were men, 53% were diabetic, and 45% had a medical history including coronary heart disease.

The results showed that there was no benefit either in relation to the primary end point or in relation to the individual components of the primary end point—major amputation or death—in the 86 patients (33%) in the placebo group and 96 patients (37%) in the active group: hazard ratio (95% CI) = 1.11 (0.83, 1.49); $P = 0.48$. There were no significant safety concerns. The TAMARIS study thus did not find any evidence of the efficacy of NV1FGF in relation to reducing the rate of amputation or death in patients with critical limb ischemia, although there was a good safety profile.

This shows that only a phase III study with a sufficient number of patients will be able to provide evidence as to whether a new treatment really offers any benefit; a phase II study is insufficiently powered for the purpose, even if there is a highly significant result. One possible explanation for the negative result of this large study might be that the patients affected were already too ill to obtain any benefit from the angiogenesis therapy. It is also conceivable that certain therapeutic agents might have different effects in different ethnic groups in a worldwide study of this type.

Safety profile of angiogenetic gene therapy

Altogether, more than 3000 patients with coronary and peripheral arterial occlusive disease have so far undergone angiogenetic gene therapy, and this form of treatment appears to be much safer than was originally thought. In comparison with placebo, there have in particular been no increases in the tumor incidence rate, and no negative influence on retinopathy, renal failure, or cardiovascular side effects such as unstable angina pectoris, myocardial infarction, stroke, or cardiac death. Excess vascular structures such as angiomas that have been observed in some cases have been shown to be reversible in animal experiments after a decline in VEGF expression. Cases of severe edema were observed in association with adenoviral VEGF121 treatment in the RAVE study and with the use of nonviral VEGF. Treatment for the edema was usually limited to oral diuretics, and the condition remained without lasting effects. Mild transient fever and the development of anti-adenoviral antibodies were observed after intra-arterial administration of adenoviral vectors, but these appear to be of minor clinical significance. It is now generally accepted that local intramuscular injection is better than other routes of administration, particularly intra-arterial injection, with regard to the distribution of the gene construct in the tissue, its retention, and the expression of the desired gene product in relation to safety and efficacy.

4.4.5.3 Angiogenetic cell therapy

Cell types used

The cell types so far best investigated in relation to their angiogenetic potential are precursor cells from the bone marrow. Bone marrow consists of various cell populations, including endothelial progenitor cells (EPCs), which can in turn differentiate into endothelial cells and can release various angiogenic growth factors (Asahara et al. 1997; Rafii and Lyden 2003). Clinical studies have so far used either au-

tologous bone marrow or mononuclear cells from the bone marrow, including the subgroup of EPCs and precursor cells from peripheral blood. In addition, there is also evidence here that mesenchymal stem cells (MSCs) and precursor cells from adipose tissue (adipose-derived stem cells, ADSCs) might be suitable for treating PAOD.

Clinical studies using stem cells

All of the clinical studies are listed in Table 4.4-8a, b.

Table 4.4-8a Published studies on angiogenesis in the lower extremity using mononuclear cells from bone marrow or peripheral blood, 2002–2010 (adapted from Lawall et al. 2010).

Study class	Indication	Cell type	Patients (n)	Ankle–arm index	Transcutaneous oxygen pressure measurement	Pain	Amputation	Overall benefit	Reference
1a	CLI	BMMNC	40	–		↓	→	→	Walter et al. 2011
1b	PAOD	BMMNC	45	↑	↑	↓	↓	+	Tateishi-Yuyama et al. 2002
1b	TAO	BMMNC	28	↑	↑	↓	↓	+	Durdu et al. 2006
2	CLI	PBMNC	28	↑	↑	↓	↓	+	Huang et al. 2005
2	PAOD	BMMNC	74	↑	↑	↓		+	Huang et al. 2007
2	PAOD	PBMNC	76	↑	↑	↓		+	Huang et al. 2007
4	CLI	BMMNC	8			↓	↓	+	Wester et al. 2008
4	PAOD, TAO	BMMNC	8	↑		↓	↓	+	Esato et al. 2002
4	PAOD	BMMNC	8	↑	↑	↓	↓	+	Saigawa et al. 2004
4	PAOD	BMMNC	8	↑	↑	↓	↓	+	Higashi et al. 2004
4	PAOD, CLI	BMMNC	12	↑		↓		+	Miyamoto et al. 2004
4	PAOD	PBMNC	5	→	↑	↓		+	Huang et al. 2004
4	TAO, CLI	BMMNC	10	↑	↑	↓	↓	+	Nizankowski et al. 2005
4	PAOD, CLI	PBMNC	30	↑	↑	↓	↓	+	Kawamura et al. 2005
4	CLI	PBMNC	7	↑	↑	↓		+	Lenk et al. 2005
4	TAO	PBMNC	6	↑	↑	↓		+	Ishida et al. 2005
4	PAOD, CLI	BMMNC	10	↑	↑			+	Bartsch 2006
4	TAO, CLI	BMMNC	8			↓		+	Miyamoto et al. 2006
4	CLI, TAO	BMMNC	7	→	(↑)	↓		+/–	Kajiiguchi et al. 2007
4	PAOD	BMMNC	12	↑	↑	↓	↓	+	Hernandez et al. 2007
4	PAOD, CLI	BMMNC	16	↑	↑	↓	↓	+	Gu et al. 2008
4	PAOD, CLI	BMMNC	28	↑	↑	↓	↓	+	Chocola et al. 2008
4	PAOD	BMMNC	27	↑	↑	↓		+	Van Tongeren et al. 2008
4	PAOD	BMMNC	16	→	↑	↓		+/–	De Vriese et al. 2008
4	CLI	BMMNC	51	↑	↑	↓	↓	+	Amann et al. 1009
4	CLI	BMMNC	37	↑	↑	↓		+	Prohazka et al. 2009
4	CLI	PBMNC	75	↑	↑	↓	↓	+	Kawamura et al. 2006
4	CLI	BMMNC	17	↑	↑	↓	↓	+	Kawamoto et al. 2009

Study classes: 1a, double-blind; 1b, randomized, unblinded controlled study; 2, controlled study; 3, cohort study/historical controls; 4, patient series/uncontrolled studies; BMMNC, bone marrow mononuclear cells; CLI, critical limb ischemia; PAOD, peripheral arterial occlusive disease; PBMNC, peripheral blood mononuclear cells; TAO, thromboangiitis obliterans.

Table 4.4-8b Angiogenesis studies on the use of precursor cells in the lower extremity that are not yet published or are currently in progress.

Indication	Comparison	Phase	Sponsor/institution
CLI	CD34$^+$ vs. placebo (ACT34-CLI study, 75 patients)	I/II	Baxter Health Corporation, USA
CLI	Concentrated autologous BMCs vs. placebo (BONMOT study, 90 patients)	II/III	Franziskus Hospital, Berlin, Germany
CLI	Autologous BMMNCs vs. placebo (ABC study, 108 patients)	II/III	Leiden University Medical Center, Netherlands
CLI	Cultured mesenchymal stem cells vs. placebo	II/III	Military Hospital, Chongqing, China
CLI	BMMNC vs. placebo (JUVENTAS study, 110–160 patients)	I/II	Utrecht University Medical Center, Netherlands
CLI	I.m. injection vs. i.m. injection and i.a. infusion of autologous BMMNCs	I/II	Harvest Technologies, India
CLI	G-CSF-mobilized PBMNCs vs. standard therapy	I/II	Beike Biotech, India
CLI	In vitro-expanded autologous bone marrow cells vs. placebo (RESTORE-CLI study, 150 patients)	II	Aastrom Biosciences, USA
CLI	Autologous CD133$^+$ cells vs. placebo	I	University of Wisconsin/Madison, USA
CLI	Autologous BMMNCs vs. placebo (48 patients)	II	Harvest Technologies, USA
CLI	Implantation of BMMNCs (BALI study, 110 patients)		Centre Hospitalier Universitaire de Reims, France
CLI	Intramuscular stem cell mixture (MESENDO study, 30 patients)	II	TCA Cellular Therapy, USA

BMC, bone marrow cell; BMMNC, bone marrow mononuclear cell; CLI, critical limb ischemia; G-CSF, granulocyte colony-stimulating factor; PBMNC, peripheral blood mononuclear cell.

A report by Matsui et al. (2003) was encouraging for the use of bone marrow cells or isolated mononuclear cells from bone marrow. Serum concentrations of macrophage colony-stimulating factor (M-CSF) were found to be higher in patients with PAOD than in control patients. Patients with thromboangiitis obliterans also had higher growth factor levels, although not quite as high as in patients with atherosclerotic PAOD. These observations thus pointed to physiological regenerative activities based on mobilized cells, which it might be possible to exploit therapeutically. Promising results from various preclinical studies then led relatively quickly to the initiation of clinical studies using bone marrow cells either alone or in combination with prior treatment with granulocyte colony-stimulating factor (G-CSF).

The first publication reporting the use of mononuclear cells from bone marrow was by Tateishi-Yuyama et al. (2002). The study essentially showed that mononuclear precursor cells from peripheral blood were superior. On angiography, increased collaterals were found in 27 of the 45 patients. The authors concluded that treatment with autologous bone marrow mononuclear cells is safe and that therapeutic angiogenesis with these cells was effective because bone marrow cells not only comprise EPCs but can also release angiogenic growth factors (Figs. 4.4-23 and 4.4.24).

This was followed by numerous mainly uncontrolled studies, often only patient series with in most cases small numbers of patients, ranging from five to 76. The patient groups involved were also inhomogeneous, with combinations of patients with thromboangiitis obliterans and atherosclerosis, as well as patients in various stages of PAOD. Mononuclear bone marrow cells were mostly used, but also peripheral mononuclear cells and circulating progenitor cells. In most of the studies, the cells were used without prior treatment with growth factors, although in some cases pretreatment with G-CSF was carried out at dosages of 300–600 mg/day or 5–10 mg/kg per day. There were also substantial variations in the numbers of cells used. While several publications gave no details of cell numbers, the others reported a minimum of $39 \pm 24 \times 10^6$ up to 2.8×10^9 cells being administered. The routes of administration also varied, with intramuscular and intra-arterial administration.

It is notable that all of these publications only report positive results, suggesting that negative pilot studies may not have been published at all. The variety of different protocols used also makes these pilot studies difficult to compare, even when the same end point is used. However, the end points also varied substantially, with evaluation of the pain-free walking distance, ulcer healing, amputation rate, pain reduction, angiographic collateralization, blood flow response to acetylcholine, ankle–arm index, flow-dependent dilation, transcutaneous oxygen pressure measurement, etc. (Table 4.4-8a).

Cell therapy showed a very good safety profile in all of the studies, if it was investigated. Reservations were only raised in connection with prior treatment with G-CSF or GM-CSF to mobilize mononuclear cells in the bone marrow or endothelial progenitor cells. There is some evidence here that G-CSF may trigger angina pectoris (Fukumoto et al. 1997) or acute arterial thromboses (Kawachi et al. 1996). This might be caused by leukocytosis and/or hypercoagulability caused by the mobilization. In particular, patients with previous coronary heart disease or cerebrovascular ischemia may be particularly susceptible to ischemic events after pretreatment with

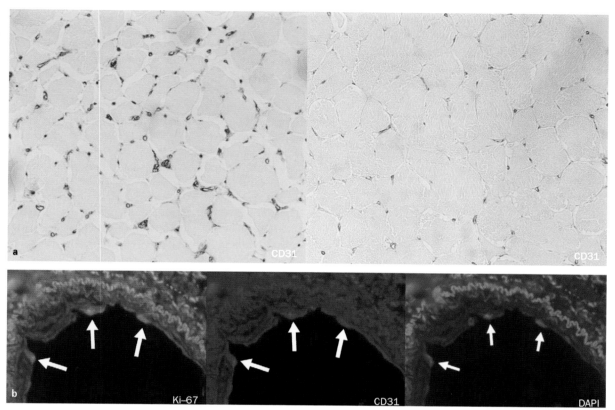

Fig. 4.4-23a, b Immunohistochemistry in new proliferating vessels in a patient treated with bone-marrow cells (BMCs). (**a**) There are markedly increased CD31-positive vessels (brown) in the leg after BMC therapy in comparison with the NaCl control (original magnification × 200). (**b**) The arrows mark endothelial cells that are positive for Ki-67, CD31, and 4,6-diamino-2-phenylindole (DAPI) (original magnification × 200). (From: Tateishi-Yuyama et al. 2002, reproduced with permission from Elsevier.)

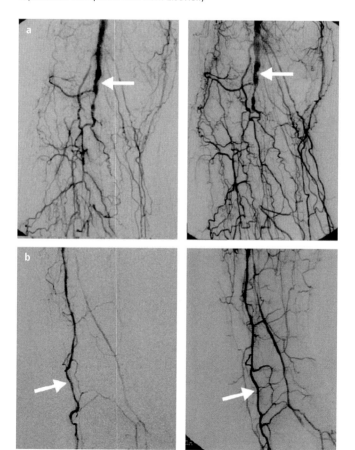

Fig. 4.4-24a, b Angiographic evidence of the formation of collateral branches in patients who received bone-marrow cells (BMCs). Clearly increased formation of collateral branches in the area of the knee and upper tibia (**a**) and in the lower tibia, ankle joint, and foot (**b**) before and 24 h after bone-marrow transplantation. The contrast densities in the femoral, posterior tibial, and dorsalis pedis artery (arrows) are similar before and after implantation. (From: Tateishi-Yuyama et al. 2002, reproduced with permission from Elsevier.)

G-CSF or GM-CSF. In view of the fact that hardly any data have so far been published from double-blind and placebo-controlled cell therapy studies on angiogenesis in PAOD and that unblinded controlled studies have also so far only been carried out rarely and even then with only small numbers of patients, large clinical studies with appropriate control groups and adequate follow-up periods of 12 months or more are needed in order to confirm any real benefit from cell therapy over the long-term course. Studies that are currently in progress or have not yet been published are listed in Table 4.4-8b.

In patients who have received preliminary treatment with growth factors such as G-CSF, M-CSF, or GM-CSF to mobilize EPCs, it will also need to be clarified whether even if there is any benefit, it might actually be due to direct effects of the growth factor in the preliminary treatment (Kuhlmann and Nikol 2007). Kuhlmann et al. (2006) found evidence of increased expression of the M-CSF receptor as a sign of sensitization of vascular cells in ischemic conditions, suggesting direct effects of these growth factors.

Even if it were possible to successfully optimize cell therapy using autologous cells to the extent that they could finally be clinically used effectively and safely, a major limitation of the treatment might be the limited availability of such cells in those patients who need this form of treatment most. Hill et al. (2003) noted that the number of EPCs was indirectly proportional to the cardiovascular risk assessed using the Framingham risk factor score. It was also found that in patients who were at high risk of cardiovascular events, EPCs showed higher aging rates in vitro than cells from patients who were at low risk. EPC levels might therefore represent biological markers for vascular function and cumulative cardiovascular risk.

4.4.5.4 Future prospects for cell therapy

A potential therapeutic effect has been demonstrated experimentally for mononuclear cells from bone marrow, including the subpopulation of EPCs, as well as for EPCs from peripheral blood and ADSCs. Almost all of these cell types have already been used clinically, but there has so far not been a single double-blind and placebo-controlled study including a sufficiently large number of patients and with a long enough follow-up period to confirm the clinical benefit of cell therapy in patients with peripheral arterial occlusive disease. While it was initially thought that precursor cells were incorporated into the new vessels (Asahara et al. 1997), it is now in most cases assumed that growth factors are released from the transplanted cells. A combination of cell therapy with growth factor therapy or angiogenesis gene therapy might therefore be useful in order to further enhance the potential clinical benefit. It has been shown, for example, that the combination of simultaneous expression of vascular endothelial growth factor (VEGF) and Ang-1 from a bicistronic vector in transduced skeletal myoblasts increased functional neovascularization.

The history of angiogenesis gene therapy can currently provide valuable guidance for the further development of cell therapy for peripheral arterial occlusive disease. In angiogenesis gene therapy, there was also initially a large number of positive pilot studies that only led to a few published double-blind and placebo-controlled phase II studies, of which in turn only a few were positive in relation to various end points (Nikol 2011). The decisive element here, still with relatively moderate numbers of patients in the phase II studies, was the fact that the placebo effect was usually underestimated. In addition, the follow-up intervals of only 3 months were too short, and there were end points that were of little clinical relevance or easily error-prone, such as transcutaneous oxygen pressure meas-

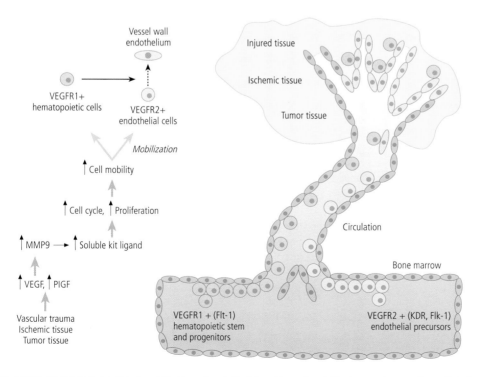

Fig. 4.4-25 Chemokine-mediated mobilization of endothelial and hematopoietic stem and progenitor cells (adapted from Rabbany et al. 2003).

urement and angiographic evidence of collaterals. The recommendations made by an expert committee for angiogenesis studies regarding the design of angiogenesis cell therapy studies should be taken into account here (Simons et al. 2000). The results of the largest worldwide phase III angiogenesis gene therapy approval study, TAMARIS, including 525 patients, are currently surprisingly sobering: the findings were negative for the primary end point and all of the secondary end points (Belch et al. 2011). This result shows that even when there are highly significant positive results in a phase II study—in this case the TALISMAN-201 study—confirmation with a large approval study is required before any clinical benefit can be safely assumed. This same is of course also true for angiogenesis cell therapy.

References

Amann B, Luedemann C, Ratei R, Schmidt-Lucke JA. Autologous bone marrow cell transplantation increases leg perfusion and reduces amputations in patients with advanced critical limb ischemia due to peripheral artery disease. Cell Transplant 2009; 18: 371–80.

Asahara T, Murohara T, Sullivan A, Silver M, van der Zee R, Li T, Witzenbichler B, Schatteman G, Isner JM. Isolation of putative progenitor endothelial cells for angiogenesis. Science 1997; 275: 964–7.

Bartsch T, Falke T, Brehm M, Zeus T, Kögler G, Wernet P, Strauer BE. Transplantation of autologous adult bone marrow stem cells in patients with severe peripheral arterial occlusion disease. Med Klin (Munich) 2006; 101 (Suppl 1): 195–7.

Belch JJF, Hiatt WR, Baumgartner I, Driver V, Nikol S, Norgren L, Van Belle E. Fibroblast growth factor NV1FGF does not prevent amputation or death, a randomised placebo-controlled trial of gene therapy in critical limb ischaemia. Lancet 2011; 377 (9781): 1929–37.

Chochola M, Pytlík R, Kobylka P, Skalická L, Kideryová L, Beran S, Varejka P, Jirát S, Køivánek J, Aschermann M, Linhart A. Autologous intra-arterial infusion of bone marrow mononuclear cells in patients with critical leg ischemia. Int Angiol 2008; 27: 281–90.

Conte MS, Bandyk DF, Clowes AW, Moneta GL, Seely L, Lorenz TJ. Results of PREVENT III: a multicenter, randomized trial of edifoligide for the prevention of vein graft failure in lower extremity bypass surgery. J Vasc Surg 2006; 43: 742–51.

Creager M. Study of Study of Ad2/Hypoxia Inducible Factor. (HIF)-1α/VP16 in Patients with Intermittent Claudication. directnews.americanheart.org/extras/pdfs/creager_accslides.pdf, 27 Mar 2009 http://directnews.americanheart.org/extras/pdfs/creager_accslides.pdf.

De Vriese AS, Billiet J, Van Droogenbroeck J, Ghekiere J, De Letter JA. Autologous transplantation of bone marrow mononuclear cells for limb ischemia in a Caucasian population with atherosclerosis obliterans. J Intern Med 2008; 263: 395–403.

Durdu S, Akar AR, Arat M, Sancak T, Eren NT, Ozyurda U. Autologous bone-marrow mononuclear cell implantation for patients with Rutherford grade II–III thromboangiitis obliterans. J Vasc Surg 2006; 44: 732–9.

Esato K, Hamano K, Li TS, Furutani A, Seyama A, Takenaka H, Zempo N. Neovascularization induced by autologous bone marrow cell implantation in peripheral arterial disease. Cell Transplant 2002; 11: 747–52.

Fukumoto Y, Miyamoto T, Okamura T, Gondo H, Iwasaki H, Horiuchi T, Yoshizawa S, Inaba S, Harada M, Niho Y. Angina pectoris occurring during granulocyte colony-stimulating factor-combined preparatory regimen for autologous peripheral blood stem cell transplantation in a patient with acute myelogenous leukaemia. Br J Haematol 1997; 97 (3): 666–8.

Gu YQ, Zhang J, Guo LR, Qi LX, Zhang SW, Xu J, Li JX, Luo T, Ji BX, Li XF, Yu HX, Cui SJ, Wang ZG. Transplantation of autologous bone marrow mononuclear cells for patients with lower limb ischemia. Chin Med J (Engl) 2008; 121: 963–7.

Higashi Y, Kimura M, Hara K, Noma K, Jitsuiki D, Nakagawa K, Oshima D, Chayama K, Sueda T, Goto C, Matsubara H, Murohara T, Yoshizumi M. Autologous bone-marrow mononuclear cell implantation improves endothelium-dependent vasodilation in patients with limb ischemia. Circulation 2004; 109: 1215–8.

Hernández P, Cortina L, Artaza H, Pol N, Lam RM, Dorticós E, Macías C, Hernández C, del Valle L, Blanco A, Martínez A, Díaz F. Autologous bone-marrow mononuclear cell implantation in patients with severe lower limb ischaemia: a comparison of using blood cell separator and Ficoll density gradient centrifugation. Atherosclerosis 2007; 194: e52–6.

Hill JM, Zalos G, Halcox JP, Schenke WH, Waclawiw MA, Quyyumi AA, Finkel T. Circulating Endothelial Progenitor Cells, Vascular Function, and Cardiovascular Risk. N Engl J Med 2003; 348: 593–600.

Huang PP, Li SZ, Han MZ, Xiao ZJ, Yang RC, Qiu LG, Han ZC. Autologous transplantation of peripheral blood stem cells as an effective therapeutic approach for severe arteriosclerosis obliterans of lower extremities. Thromb Haemost 2004; 91: 606–9.

Huang P, Li S, Han M, Xiao Z, Yang R, Han ZC. Autologous transplantation of granulocyte colony stimulating factor-mobilized peripheral blood mononuclear cells improves critical limb ischemia in diabetes. Diabetes Care 2005; 28: 2155–60.

Huang PP, Yang XF, Li SZ, Wen JC, Zhang Y, Han ZC. Randomised comparison of G-CSF-mobilized peripheral blood mononuclear cells versus bone marrow-mononuclear cells for the treatment of patients with lower limb arteriosclerosis obliterans. Thromb Haemost 2007; 98: 1335–42.

Ishida A, Ohya Y, Sakuda H, Ohshiro K, Higashiuesato Y, Nakaema M, Matsubara S, Yakabi S, Kakihana A, Ueda M, Miyagi C, Yamane N, Koja K, Komori K, Takishita S. Autologous peripheral blood mononuclear cell implantation for patients with peripheral arterial disease improves limb ischemia. Circ J 2005; 69: 1260–5.

Isner JM, Pieczek A, Schainfeld R, Blair R, Haley L, Asahara T, Rosenfield K, Razvi S, Walsh K, Symes JF. Clinical evidence of angiogenesis after arterial gene transfer of phVEGF165 in patient with ischaemic limb. Lancet 1996; 348: 370–4.

Kajiguchi M, Kondo T, Izawa H, Kobayashi M, Yamamoto K, Shintani S, Numaguchi Y, Naoe T, Takamatsu J, Komori K, Murohara T. Safety and efficacy of autologous progenitor cell transplantation for therapeutic angiogenesis in patients with critical limb ischemia. Circ J 2007; 71: 196–201.

Kawachi Y, Watanabe A, Uchida T, Yoshizawa K, Kurooka N, Setsu K. Acute arterial thrombosis due to platelet aggregation in a patient receiving granulocyte colony-stimulating factor. Br J Haematol 1996; 94 (2): 413–6.

Kawamoto A, Katayama M, Handa N, Kinoshita M, Takano H, Horii M, Sadamoto K, Yokoyama A, Yamanaka T, Onodera R, Kuroda A, Baba R, Kaneko Y, Tsukie T, Kurimoto Y, Okada Y, Kihara Y, Morioka S, Fukushima M, Asahara T. Intramuscular transplantation of G-CSF-mobilized CD34(+) cells in patients with critical limb ischemia: a phase I/IIa, multicenter, single-blinded, dose-escalation clinical trial. Stem Cells 2009; 27: 2857–64.

Kawamura A, Horie T, Tsuda I, Ikeda A, Egawa H, Imamura E, Iida J, Sakata H, Tamaki T, Kukita K, Meguro J, Yonekawa M, Kasai M. Prevention of limb amputation in patients with limbs ulcers by autologous peripheral blood mononuclear cell implantation. Ther Apher Dial 2005; 9: 59–63.

Kawamura A, Horie T, Tsuda I, Abe Y, Yamada M, Egawa H, Iida J, Sakata H, Onodera K, Tamaki T, Furui H, Kukita K, Meguro J, Yonekawa M, Tanaka S. Clinical study of therapeutic angiogenesis by autologous peripheral blood stem cell (PBSC) transplantation in 92 patients with critically ischemic limbs. J Artif Organs 2006; 9: 226–33.

Kuhlmann MT, Nikol S. Therapeutic angiogenesis for peripheral artery disease—Cytokine therapy. VASA 2007; 36: 253–60.

Kuhlmann MT, Kirchhof P, Klocke R, Hasib L, Stypmann J, Fabritz L, Stelljes M, Tian W, Zwiener M, Mueller M, Kienast J, Breithardt G, Nikol S. G-CSF/SCF reduces inducible arrythmias in the infarcted heart potentially via increased connexin43 expression and arteriogenesis. J Exp Med 2006; 203: 87–97.

Kusumanto YH, van Weel V, Mulder NH, Smit AJ, van den Dungen JJ, Hooymans JM, Sluiter WJ, Tio RA, Quax PH, Gans RO, Dullaart RP, Hospers GA. Treatment with intramuscular vascular endothelial growth factor gene compared with placebo for patients with diabetes mellitus and critical limb ischemia: a double-blind randomized trial. Hum Gene Ther 2006; 17: 683–91.

Lawall H, Bramlage P, Amann B. Stem cell and progenitor cell therapy in peripheral artery disease—a critical appraisal. Thromb Haemost 2010; 103: 696–709.

Lenk K, Adams V, Lurz P, Erbs S, Linke A, Gielen S, Schmidt A, Scheinert D, Biamino G, Emmrich F, Schuler G, Hambrecht R. Therapeutic potential of blood-derived progenitor cells in patients with peripheral arterial occlusive disease and critical limb ischaemia. Eur Heart J 2005; 26:1903–9.

Makinen K, Manninen H, Hedman M, Matsi P, Mussalo H, Alhava E, Yla-Herttuala S. Increased vascularity detected by digital subtraction angiography after VEGF gene transfer to human lower limb artery: a randomized, placebo-controlled, double-blinded phase II study. Mol Ther 2002; 6: 127–33.

Matsui K, Yoshioka T, Murakami Y, Takahashi M, Shimada K, Ikeda U. Serum concentrations of vascular endothelial growth factor and monocyte-colony stimulating factor in peripheral arterial disease. Circ J 2003; 67: 660–2.

Miyamoto M, Yasutake M, Takano H, Takagi H, Takagi K, Mizuno H, Kumita S, Takano T. Therapeutic angiogenesis by autologous bone marrow cell implantation for refractory chronic peripheral arterial disease using assessment of neovascularization by 99mTc-tetrofosmin (TF) perfusion scintigraphy. Cell Transplant 2004; 13: 429–37.

Miyamoto K, Nishigami K, Nagaya N, Akutsu K, Chiku M, Kamei M, Soma T, Miyata S, Higashi M, Tanaka R, Nakatani T, Nonogi H, Takeshita S. Unblinded pilot study of autologous transplantation of bone marrow mononuclear cells in patients with thromboangiitis obliterans. Circulation 2006; 114: 2679–84.

Ng YS, D'Amore PA. Therapeutic angiogenesis for cardiovascular disease. Curr Control Trials Cardiovasc Med 2001; 2: 278–85.

Nikol S, VanBelle E, Diehm C, Visona A, Capogrossi M, Ferreira-Maldent N, Gallino A, Pham E, Grek V, Coleman M, Meyer F, et al. Therapeutic angiogenesis with intramuscular NV1FGF improves amputation-free survival in patients with critical limb ischemia. Mol Ther 2008; 16: 972–8.

Nikol S. Therapeutische Angiogenese mittels Gen- und Stammzellentherapie bei der peripheren arteriellen Verschlusskrankheit. Deutsche Med Wochenschrift 2011; 136 (14):672–4.

Nizankowski R, Petriczek T, Skotnicki A, Szczeklik A. The treatment of advanced chronic lower limb ischaemia with marrow stem cell autotransplantation. Kardiol Pol 2005; 63: 351–60.

Powell RJ, Goodney P, Mendelsohn FO, Moen EK, Annex BH; HGF-0205 Trial Investigators. Safety and efficacy of patient specific intramuscular injection of HGF plasmid gene therapy on limb perfusion and wound healing in patients with ischemic lower extremity ulceration: results of the HGF-0205 trial. J Vasc Surg 2010; 52: 1525–30.

Procházka V, Gumulec J, Chmelová J, Klement P, Klement GL, Jonszta T, Czerný D, Krajca J. Autologous bone marrow stem cell transplantation in patients with end-stage chronical critical limb ischemia and diabetic foot. Vnitr Lek 2009; 55: 173–8.

Rabbany SY, Heissig B, Hattori K, Rafii S. Molecular pathways regulating mobilization of marrow-derived stem cells for tissue revascularization. Trends Mol Med 2003; 9: 109–17.

Rafii S, Lyden D. Therapeutic stem and progenitor cell transplantation for organ vascularization and regeneration. Nat Med 2003; 9: 702–12.

Rajagopalan S, Mohler ER, 3rd, Lederman RJ, Mendelsohn FO, Saucedo JF, Goldman CK, Blebea J, Macko J, Kessler PD, Rasmussen HS, Annex BH. Regional angiogenesis with vascular endothelial growth factor in peripheral arterial disease: a phase II randomized, double-blind, controlled study of adenoviral delivery of vascular endothelial growth factor 121 in patients with disabling intermittent claudication. Circulation 2003; 108: 1933–8.

Simons M, Bonow RO, Chronos NA, Cohen DJ, Giordano FJ, Hammond HK, Laham RJ, Li W, Pike M, Sellke FW, Stegman TJ, Udelson JE, Rosengart TK. Clinical trials in coronary angiogenesis: issues, problems, consensus: An expert panel summary. Circulation 2000; 102: E73–86.

Saigawa T, Kato K, Ozawa T, Toba K, Makiyama Y, Minagawa S, Hashimoto S, Furukawa T, Hanawa H, Kodama M, Yoshimura N, Fujiwara H, Namura O, Sogawa M, Hayashi J, Aizawa Y. Clinical application of bone marrow implantation in patients with arteriosclerosis obliterans, and the association between efficacy and the number of implanted bone marrow cells. Circ J 2004; 68: 1189–93.

Shigematsu H, Yasuda K, Iwai T, Sasajima T, Ishimaru S, Ohashi Y, Yamaguchi T, Ogihara T, Morishita R. Randomized, double-blind, placebo-controlled clinical trial of hepatocyte growth factor plasmid for critical limb ischemia. Gene Ther 2010; 17: 1152–61.

Tateishi-Yuyama E, Matsubara H, Murohara T, Ikeda U, Shintani S, Masaki H, Amano K, Kishimoto Y, Yoshimoto K, Akashi H, Shimada K, Iwasaka T, Imaizumi T. Therapeutic angiogenesis for patients with limb ischaemia by autologous transplantation of bone-marrow cells: a pilot study and a randomised controlled trial. Lancet 2002; 360: 427–35.

US National Institutes of Health. A Phase 2, Randomized, Double-blind, Placebo-controlled, Parallel-group, Multicenter, Dose-Selection Study of Ad2/Hypoxia inducible Factor (HIF)-1α/VP16 in Patients With Intermittent Claudication http://www.clinicaltrials.gov/ct2/search. Last access, 2010 http://clinicaltrials.gov/ct2/show/NCT00117650?term=WALK+HIF-1+alpha&rank=1.

Walter DH, Krankenberg H, Balzer JO, Kalka C, Baumgartner I, Schlüter M, Tonn T, Seeger F, Dimmeler S, Lindhoff-Last E, Zeiher AM; PROVASA Investigators. Intraarterial administration of bone marrow mononuclear cells in patients with critical limb ischemia: a randomized-start, placebo-controlled pilot trial (PROVASA). Circ Cardiovasc Interv 2011; 4: 26–37.

Wester T, Jørgensen JJ, Stranden E, Sandbaek G, Tjønnfjord G, Bay D, Kollerøs D, Kroese AJ, Brinchmann JE. Treatment with autologous bone marrow mononuclear cells in patients with critical lower limb ischaemia. A pilot study. Scand J Surg 2008; 97: 56–62.

Van Tongeren RB, Hamming JF, Fibbe WE, Van Weel V, Frerichs SJ, Stiggelbout AM, Van Bockel JH, Lindeman JH. Intramuscular or combined intramuscular/intra-arterial administration of bone marrow mononuclear cells: a clinical trial in patients with advanced limb ischemia. J Cardiovasc Surg 2008; 49: 51–8.

Wiley Website http://www.wiley.com/legacy/wileychi/genmed/clinical/ letzter Zugriff 23.06.2011.

4.4.6 Rehabilitation in peripheral arterial occlusive disease

Arndt Dohmen

The three pillars of treatment for PAOD are conservative treatment, interventional methods, and vascular surgery.

Conservative treatment has many different facets. This section focuses on the elements of treatment representing angiologic rehabilitation: in PAOD stage Fontaine II, structured vascular training and prosthesis training after amputations; and at all stages, secondary prevention through providing training in ways of dealing with cardiovascular risk factors.

Training therapy is the oldest method of treatment in angiology. Its origins go back to pioneers of the discipline such as Max Ratschow and Werner Schoop (Ratschow 1939; Köhler and Schoop 1973). From the 1960s to the 1980s, a number of scientific studies were published that clarified several of the pathophysiological mechanisms of effect, and the efficacy of treatment methods was also demonstrated in various studies (Dahllof et al. 1976; Womack et al. 1997; Larsen 1973). On the basis of these studies, the effects of vascular training can be described as follows:

- Development of an effective collateral circulation
- Redistribution of blood flow
- Metabolic adjustment of the muscles to a reduced oxygen supply (with an increase in mitochondria in the cells)
- Improvement of walking technique (providing equivalent performance with less oxygen consumption)
- Improvement in heart and lung function
- Improvement in joint function
- Pain "management" (developing realistic expectations)

The current national treatment guidelines for PAOD in Germany (S3-Leitlinie 2009) and international guidelines (Hirsch et al. 2006) classify conservative therapy—involving supervised structured vascular training in accordance with evidence-based medicine (EBM) criteria—as a class IA recommendation for patients with claudication. The guidelines partly go so far as to make the indication for vascular interventions and bypass surgery dependent on an inadequate response to a previous training phase with instruction for at least 6–12 weeks. The elements of a supervised structured training program are described in detail in the American Heart Association (AHA)/American College of Cardiology (ACC) guideline in particular. In contrast, a physician's recommendation to do walking exercises and independent training by the patient are ineffective and are therefore not recommended in the guidelines.

Unfortunately, the studies on which the evidence for the effectiveness of training therapy is based are already several decades old, and the same also applies to studies on the success of conservative therapy in comparison with catheter interventions (Creasy et al. 1990). It is all the more welcome that a national research project has been in progress in Switzerland since 2011 in which the results of training treatment are being checked in today's conditions in a multicenter study.

4.4.6.1 Statutory background

Medical rehabilitation is the statutory framework within which treatment measures are carried out that do not meet the German Appropriateness Evaluation Protocol (G-AEP) criteria for the necessity of acute in-hospital treatment, in accordance with the agreement reached between health-insurance companies and the German Hospital Association (Hansis 2003). This applies in particular to conservative treatment at the stage of claudication, but also to a number of other situations in which patients are faced, at the end of treatment for an acute condition, with resulting problems that they are unable to overcome without medical assistance—e.g., following minor or major amputation. In contrast to the acute treatment, rehabilitation measures have to be approved by the health-funding body in advance. The health-funding body for rehabilitation in patients who are in employment is usually the pension insurance fund, while for retirees it is the health-insurance company. Private insurance companies do not usually accept the costs of rehabilitation, with the exception of follow-up treatment with a specific rehabilitation program immediately after acute in-hospital therapy if the patient is not yet able to return to his or her previous environment. The follow-up treatment is intended to enable the patient to return to his or her private or occupational living conditions. This special form of rehabilitation is applied for by the acute hospital and has to start at the latest 14 days after discharge from the hospital.

When issuing approval for a rehabilitation program, the health-funding body also specifies the clinic in which the rehabilitation measures are to be carried out. However, patients have the right to choose a clinic themselves, provided that it meets the structural prerequisites for carrying out rehabilitation treatment. The health-funding body is obliged to accept the patient's preference and any refusal of it has to be justified to the patient in detail (German Social Code, Book V, para. 20).

4.4.6.2 Conceptual basis for rehabilitation

The concept of medical rehabilitation has substantially changed in recent years. The aim is not to cure a disease during the treatment—with chronic diseases, this cannot be achieved even in acute medicine—but rather to alleviate the symptoms and enable the patient to integrate into his or her environment again and cope with everyday life with little or no outside assistance, by providing information, training measures and practice in lifestyle changes, and to stop the progression of disabling sequelae of the disease.

To meet these treatment goals, the field of rehabilitation has implemented a biopsychosocial health model widely diverging from that used in acute medicine—one that focuses on limitations in personal activities and the resulting extent to which the patient is able to participate in society. Rehabilitation-specific interventions are intended to improve the range of activities possible and thus restore the patient's limited participation in the personal and occupational fields as far as possible. On the basis of this biopsychosocial approach, a new classification system, the International Classification of Functioning, Disability, and Health (ICF)—comparable to the International Classification of Diseases (ICD) in the field of acute medicine—has been established. Figure 4.4-26 gives an overview of the most important concepts in the two disease models (WHO 2001).

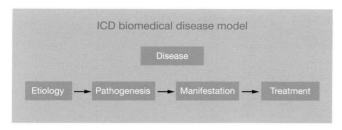

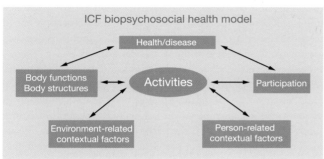

Fig. 4.4-26 The disease models underlying the International Classification of Diseases (ICD) and International Classification of Functioning, Disability and Health (ICF).

Table 4.4-9 Meaning of International Classification of Functioning, Disability and Health (ICF) terms as applied to angiologic rehabilitation.

ICF term	Meaning
Structural injuries	Stenosis/occlusion of an artery by arteriosclerotic plaques
Functional disturbance	Reduced circulation in the affected extremity
Activity restriction	Pain-related limitation of ability to walk
Restricted participation	Restriction of ability to cope with occupational requirements due to impaired mobility Restriction of ability to lead an independent private life due to impaired mobility
Contextual factors	Influences in the patient's personality and environment that have a positive/negative significance for his or her reintegration into the previous living environment

Although the concepts involved in the ICF system may at first seem unfamiliar, it is nevertheless important to understand what they mean, since even at the point when an application for a rehabilitation measure is being made, the health-funding bodies require a description of the patient's state of health using the relevant ICF categories. The planning and implementation of rehabilitation measures are nowadays also based on the ICF health model, in the ways in which the goals of treatment are defined for achieving specific gains in activities and participation options.

4.4.6.3　Indications for rehabilitation

At Fontaine stage II, the first treatment task in accordance with the guideline recommendations is to carry out structured vascular exercise training. Rehabilitation is therefore always indicated if the patient's mobility is restricted to the extent that he or she is no lon-

ger able to cope with the requirements of everyday life. However, a prerequisite for successful training treatment is previous angiologic diagnosis, with evidence of unobstructed circulation in the collateral vascular network that is most important for the treatment. For example, providing training in relation to occlusions of the superficial femoral artery, the most frequent type of occlusion (> 40% of all patients with PAOD) only makes sense if an upstream pelvic artery stenosis has been eliminated interventionally or with vascular surgery. Training treatment is indicated even when the imaging diagnosis does not offer any target for intervention or grounds for bypass surgery. With training and improvement of collateral vessel formation, a significant increase in the pain-free walking distance can be achieved even in these cases.

In cases of multiple-level disease, it is useful to combine several treatment procedures: after bypass surgery or interventions, for example, there is an indication for follow-on rehabilitation in order to train the collateral network in the downstream vascular region and thus further improve the patient's walking distance.

At Fontaine stage III, there is initially no indication for rehabilitation. It is only when all of the available revascularization options have been exhausted and after prostanoid infusion treatment for resting pain that subsequent training treatment as part of follow-up therapy will be able to improve the treatment success and sustainably extend the pain-free walking distance.

In Fontaine stage IV as well, the focus is on the acute medical treatment; training treatment here may even be counterproductive due to possible steal effects. Sequelae such as minor or major amputation then again become a challenge for rehabilitation in enabling the patient to cope with the radical consequences of the procedures in the framework of follow-up treatment and become sufficiently mobile once again despite the resulting disablement. This can be achieved through the patient learning how to walk safely with prosthesis, manage a wheelchair independently, and also through learning the required movement sequences for transferring from bed to wheelchair so that in the future nursing care will be possible in the patient's own social environment. The same also applies to patients with manifestations of PAOD in the upper extremities. The focus in rehabilitation treatment here is on functional training for the hands, including practicing how to use the appropriate aids.

4.4.6.4　Contraindications against rehabilitation

Rehabilitation is basically not indicated whenever (taking the patient's individual circumstances into account) a realistically achievable goal, improving the patient's ability to take part in occupational or social life, is not identifiable. In terms of the statutory requirements, this means specifically that patients whose inability to work or need for nursing care are insurmountable have no entitlement to receive rehabilitation treatment.

Additional diseases may represent a contraindication against angiologic rehabilitation if they are restricting the patient to a greater extent than the PAOD. This applies in particular to New York Heart Association (NYHA) III and IV heart failure, chronic obstructive pulmonary disease (COPD) in Global Initiative for Chronic Obstructive Lung Disease (GOLD) stages III and IV, and for disabling mobility restrictions in patients with arthrosis. In these situations, the first step is to compensate the cardiac insufficiency or COPD using drug treatment to such an extent that active participation in the treatment measures involved in structured vascular training becomes possible. Severe arthrosis may initially require a surgical joint replacement in order to make angiologic training therapy possible at all.

In special conditions, rehabilitation may also be at least relatively contraindicated independently of additional diseases when Fontaine stage II PAOD is the underlying condition. This may be the case if there is a hemodynamically significant stenosis in the arterial inflow in a patient with a peripheral vascular occlusion—most often at the level of the thigh or lower leg—that is impairing compensation reserves in the collateral network important for the training treatment. Before a decision is taken to carry out angiologic rehabilitation due to claudication symptoms, sophisticated imaging diagnosis must always be carried out so that corresponding upstream obstructions can be eliminated in cases of multiple-level disease using interventional or surgical treatment. It is only after this that the training treatment will make sense.

Vascular training should also not be carried out if coronary heart disease (CHD) or COPD is still limiting the patient's mobility, due to angina pectoris or dyspnea, at the same time as claudication pain, even after all the treatment options for those conditions have been exhausted. Improving exercise tolerance in relation to PAOD would make the risk of cardiac or pulmonary decompensation greater. As CHD symptoms are often unmasked by successful vascular training, it is important to recognize the change in symptoms in a timely fashion, interrupting the rehabilitation therapy and referring the patient for invasive cardiologic diagnosis and treatment if appropriate. The same precautions also apply to prosthesis training following major amputations. Cardiac symptoms can even be expected to develop more often in these patients, who are at a more advanced stage of PAOD in which simultaneous CHD is more likely and because walking with a prosthesis requires greater physical effort.

4.4.6.5 The rehabilitation process

Modern angiologic rehabilitation is only possible with an interdisciplinary team including the following professional groups:

- Physician specializing in internal medicine/angiology with additional qualification in the rehabilitation system or social medicine
- Physical therapist
- Sports therapist with additional training in vascular exercise groups
- Medical masseur with experience in connective-tissue massage and manual lymph drainage
- Social education worker

- Ergotherapist
- Nutrition consultant
- Psychologist
- Nurse with additional training in wound treatment
- Orthopedics technician
- Orthopedic footwear maker

The physician's task is to be responsible for heading the interdisciplinary rehabilitation team and guiding the rehabilitation process. The team should meet weekly in order to:

- Assess the rehabilitation progress made by each patient
- Recognize deviations from the course of rehabilitation relative to the goals that have been set
- If necessary, to adapt the goals to the patient's resources at a point when they have been better recognized, or to change the treatment previously administered

The rehabilitation process consists of the following interlocking stages.

Rehabilitation diagnosis

On the basis of an angiologic diagnosis of PAOD, information is collected that allows:

- Qualitative and quantitative assessment of the extent of the activity lost
- Recognition of the resulting restrictions in the ability to take part in occupational and private life that are relevant from the patient's point of view
- Description and evaluation of the major factors involved in the personal and social context of the patient's future living situation, in the light of whether they are beneficial for integrating the patient into the previous environment or are obstructing this goal

Defining the goals of rehabilitation

With the help of this comprehensive information, specific rehabilitation goals can then be defined and discussed with the patient. In Fontaine stage II PAOD, it is initially a matter of quantifying a realistically achievable improvement in walking distance and identifying the associated occupational and private participation goals. Clear goals also need to be defined in relation to contextual factors—which may include, for example, changes in lifestyle that should be practiced and then permanently established during the rehabilitation process in order to reduce the patient's cardiovascular risk and improve the long-term prognosis.

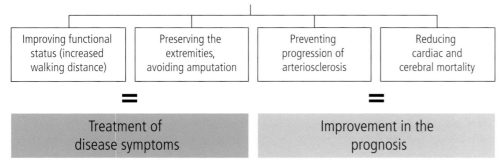

Fig. 4.4-27 Treatment goals for long-term care in patients with PAOD.

Course of rehabilitation

The individual treatment modules are then compiled into a treatment plan in accordance with the patient's special needs.

In Fontaine stage II PAOD, the focus is on structured vascular training. This consists of functional exercises in which the muscle groups distal to the occluded vascular level are specially activated. The same principle is followed in the choice of an appropriate training method: patients with pelvic artery occlusions benefit most from ergometer training, while those with occlusions at the thigh level should do more training in interval walking. Patients included in treatment groups should not have performance levels that diverge too widely, since otherwise the patients with the shortest walking distance would lose motivation and those with the longest ones would not be sufficiently stretched. For the same reason, patients with specific additional co-morbid conditions often need individual treatment. Motivating patients while at the same time not asking too much of them is the most important psychological task for the physical therapist, who in addition needs to recognize possible false habitual movements in the patient's gait resulting from several years of claudication symptoms and counteract them with individualized exercise treatment. Movement exercises in water can be helpful particularly in this type of situation, as patients are able to learn new movement patterns more easily in the reduced-gravity setting.

Additional treatment approaches include hot and cold foot baths, in which the temperature stimuli improve elasticity particularly in the peripheral vessels, and connective-tissue massage, which can lead to dilation of peripheral resistance vessels through responses via Head's zones (Hüter-Becker and Dölken 2004).

The structure of an exercise unit in movement training has been precisely described in the PAOD guidelines published by the AHA and ACC on the basis of an analysis of various studies (Table 4.4-10).

Additional specific tasks for rehabilitation therapy often arise in follow-up treatment after vascular surgery:

- After bypass surgery, particularly at the femoropopliteal and crural levels, postoperative lymphedema is often an obstacle to mobilization for the patients during the initial phase. This effect of surgery can usually be quickly resolved with manual lymph drainage, which is best combined with a compression bandage if there are adequate Doppler pressure values (over 80 mmHg).

- Complete or incomplete peroneal paralysis as a result of ischemia, or due to technical surgical causes, may substantially restrict the treatment options available in vascular training. Individualized physical therapy needs to be started here in a timely fashion, including use of a peroneal splint when there is marked disablement.

- Following vascular surgery with laparotomy, the treatment plan needs to take this special situation into account with temporary protection and subsequent cautious training of the abdominal muscles.

The rehabilitation process involved in follow-up treatment after amputations is a special type of problem. The patients come to the treatment after a surgical procedure that has radically changed their lives. Months of exhausting pain have often preceded this, hopes for healing after unsuccessful efforts to save the leg have been disappointed, and the patients are in an extreme psychological situation following this fruitless struggle. This usually leads to an extremely depressive general mood—not a favorable starting-point for the

Table 4.4-10 Key criteria for conservative vascular training in patients with PAOD (adapted from ACC/AHA 2005)

Key criteria for conservative vascular training in patients with PAOD
Warm-up and finishing phases of 5–10 min each with every exercise unit
Treadmill and walking training on a walking track are the most effective exercise methods
Isometric training is effective with other forms of cardiovascular disease and contributes to general fitness
The initial exertion level should be selected so that claudication occurs after 3–5 min
Patients should exercise until moderate claudication starts, followed by a short pause and then exercise until moderate claudication again
The exercise phases should start at a total of 35 min and should be increased by 5 min per exercise unit up to a total of 50 min
Three to five exercise units per week for at least 4–8 weeks, or preferably 3–6 months, have proved particularly effective

challenges that need to be faced in the rehabilitation treatment that follows. A high degree of psychological skill is therefore required from everyone involved in the therapy in order to avoid overstraining the patients, while at the same time encouraging them to contribute actively to the treatment process facing them and succeed with it despite the loss of physical integrity that they have suffered. The following points need to be clarified for rehabilitation diagnosis:

- Whether the patient will be in a position to cope successfully with a prosthesis, despite the presence of additional diseases (e.g., arthrosis, paralysis resulting from previous strokes, limited exercise capacity due to advanced stages of COPD or CHC, balance difficulties due to polyneuropathy in the remaining foot, compliance problems due to chronic alcohol dependency, insufficient mobility reserves in extreme obesity, lack of treatment motivation due to marked depression).

- If prosthesis is possible, whether it should be used only at home or elsewhere as well, and to what extent.

- If prosthesis is not realistic, whether wheelchair mobilization can be planned or nursing care is unavoidable—possibly made easier by giving the patient training in how to transfer from bed to wheelchair. Even success in mastering this transfer process alone may be decisive in determining whether a patient who has just undergone amputation can be cared for at home or whether long-term accommodation in a nursing home is unavoidable.

Once the mobility goal has been agreed with the patient in this way, treatment with conditioning of the amputation stump starts if prosthesis is planned, in order to prepare the stump for the future pressure load. Regular manual lymph drainage and additional compression therapy reduces the postoperative swelling of the stump in particular, creating the conditions for a well-fitting prosthesis. At the same time, balance exercises should be carried out during this phase to enable the patient to stand on the prosthesis safely later on. The subsequent prosthesis training itself can only start after the interim prosthesis has been made. Following initial standing exercises, walking exercises at graded stages of difficulty can start—progressing toward climbing stairs, which is particularly difficult with

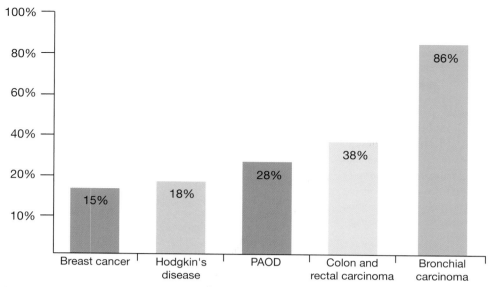

Fig. 4.4-28 Five-year mortality rates (adapted from Diehm et al. 2004).

a prosthesis. The patient also needs to be trained in independently putting the prosthesis on correctly, regularly inspecting the stump for pressure points, and ensuring correct and hygienically satisfactory skin care on the stump.

The most frequent reason for delays in the rehabilitation process is a prosthesis that has been fitted at the wrong time point.

In the course of rehabilitation and preparing patients for reintegration into their previous environment, social medicine considerations play a special role, and this needs to be analyzed during rehabilitation diagnosis and prepared in parallel with the training treatment. Depending on the work previously done, it can in some cases be predicted even at the start of rehabilitation that a return to the previous job will no longer be possible. For example, a machine fitter who previously had to climb ladders or scaffolding to carry out maintenance or repair of large machines will not be able to do the same job after amputation and prosthesis fitting. An immediate application for a disablement pass and—with the patient's consent—contact with the employer even during the rehabilitation process, when appropriate, are required in order to clarify where the patient may be able to work in the future. If it is foreseen that the patient will not be able to move about at home without a wheelchair, it needs to be clarified during rehabilitation what alterations need to be made in the house before the patient returns, so that they can be carried out as quickly as possible.

Probably the most difficult challenge in angiologic rehabilitation is the effort to influence cardiovascular risk factors that is required at all stages of PAOD. In addition to providing structured training to give the patient better information about the medical context, this also serves to motivate the affected individual—despite disease-related depression and often simultaneous loss of social contacts—to change living habits permanently, particularly in the areas in which unhealthy habits may have been established for decades: smoking, incorrect diet, and lack of exercise. Training methods, no matter how sophisticated, cannot solve this underlying problem. Despite this, all the energies of the whole rehabilitation team need to be used to achieve this treatment goal in particular. The fact that successful intervention is needed in order to reduce the cardiovascular risk profile is shown by the alarmingly high mortality rate particularly in

patients with PAOD (Diehm et al. 2004). For this reason, the same target values apply for the treatment of hypertension, hypercholesterolemia, and diabetes mellitus as after cardiovascular or cerebrovascular events.

As the patients' unhealthy lifestyle usually affects all three of these areas, the first task is to define goals that are realistically achievable for the patient. This involves initially selecting only the most important area for intervention from among the changes in lifestyle actually needed, but without losing sight of the others for the future. Failure is therefore usually inevitable if the physician asks an obese smoker to stop decades of nicotine abuse during a 3-week rehabilitation program while at the same time meeting a quantifiable weight reduction target. The task of the whole rehabilitation team is to recognize potentially excess demands on the patient in a timely fashion, instituting supportive measures when appropriate (e.g., additional, more intensive psychological care), or adapting the goal of the intervention to the patient's real capacities. Particularly in the area of lifestyle changes, a treatment goal that has not been achieved should not simply be blamed on the patient, but should always lead to critical questioning of the way in which the rehabilitation process is being managed, since patients who have a sense of failure and frustration will be even more difficult to motivate during the subsequent treatment course to face their individual responsibility for dealing with the disease.

4.4.6.6   Completion of rehabilitation

At the final examination, the patient and physician need to take stock:
- To what extent have the rehabilitation goals been achieved or missed?
- After partial success at the end of the treatment, what needs to be done to enable the goals still to be achieved?
- What level of activities and participation will be possible after the rehabilitation process?
- Depending on the individual demands involved in specific jobs, the patient's ability to work basically depends on the pain-free walking distance achieved. Another important aspect from the

social medicine point of view, particularly with PAOD, is the time that the patient takes to walk 500 meters at the end of the rehabilitation process, independently of the pauses required. If more than 20 minutes are needed for the distance, a PAOD patient is regarded as unfit for work.

- What measures are needed after the end of rehabilitation to maintain the results achieved for the longer term?
- Unfortunately, there are usually few suitable services available for patients with PAOD, except in a few of the large cities, to enable them to maintain or further extend the increased mobility they have achieved by making using of outpatient follow-up in the form of rehabilitation exercise. Experience with attempts to include PAOD patients in cardiac exercise groups has been poor, as the exercise levels appropriate for participants in cardiac exercise groups and claudication patients are too divergent.

4.4.6.7 New developments in rehabilitation for PAOD

Several new trends in rehabilitation have been emerging in recent years, and their implications for the treatment of PAOD patients are outlined below.

Increasing outpatient rehabilitation measures

Health-funding bodies are showing an increasing preference for outpatient rehabilitation services for almost every type of indication. Since those requiring rehabilitation with a diagnosis of PAOD only represent a small group of patients, appropriate treatment services for this indication are rarely available in outpatient rehabilitation institutions—particularly since the requirement for an acceptable distance from the patient's home means that the catchment area for this type of outpatient rehabilitation service is limited. It can therefore be expected that for administrative reasons, the assignment of the patient to a treatment group will no longer be carried out purely on the basis of disease-specific medical considerations. To ensure successful treatment, however, no compromises should be made here.

In relation to the interventions needed in order to achieve lifestyle changes, the chances of success are lower in an outpatient setting, since the patient returns every day at the end of the treatment to precisely the social environment that has played a major role in enabling unhealthy behavior to become chronic.

Medical-occupational guidance

The pension insurance funds—as the health-funding bodies responsible for patients' rehabilitation and return to work—are initiating and increasingly promoting the incorporation of elements of occupational rehabilitation into the process of medical rehabilitation. The aim is to combine these two aspects of the patient's reintegration into occupational life into a comprehensive process. From the point of view of the ICF biopsychosocial model of health, this development is a logical one. The problematic aspect, however, is that this extra rehabilitation task is supposed to take place within the same time frame, although several measures involved in medical-occupational guidance shorten the time available for training treatment. Since the reduction of the rehabilitation period to 21 days already runs counter to the EBM-based guideline recommendation for training therapy for PAOD, this further reduction of the time available for medical rehabilitation can be expected to lead to deterioration in the treatment results.

Making the rehabilitation period more flexible

With the pressure of rising costs to which all of the health-funding bodies are exposed, demands are being heard increasingly often for the period of rehabilitation measures to be further shortened by making it flexible on an individualized basis. With the exception of special cases in which after the initial examination it is found that there is no indication for angiologic rehabilitation or the patient shows no compliance with active participation in the therapy offered, there are no defensible grounds for shortening the course of treatment for patients with PAOD even further below the time frame set out in the guideline recommendations. For follow-up treatment after amputation, the time available for prosthesis training is even in principle too short already, and making it more flexible would place these patients, who are usually older and have multimorbid conditions, under unacceptable pressure.

Impediments in the application procedure for rehabilitation

The marked increase in the bureaucratic impediments that are appearing in the application procedure for rehabilitation treatment, particularly with the statutory health-insurance companies, is no longer merely a trend but has already been a reality for some time. A two-stage procedure has been established in which an initial application (Form No. 60) is needed in order apply for the actual application form (Form No. 61). After this, a four-page form has to be filled out, and only physicians who have completed a special training course are entitled to do this.

The rate of rejection of these applications by the Medical Service of the Health Insurance Companies (*Medizinischer Dienst der Krankenversicherung*, MDK) is high, partly because the complicated application forms are not filled out meticulously enough. This development is having far-reaching consequences for the care of patients with PAOD:

- The available statistical data are very imprecise (no specific diagnosis-related statistics are available for rehabilitation treatments carried out for the statutory health-insurance companies), but when the prevalence of PAOD in the population is taken into account, there are 1,570,000 PAOD patients who require treatment, according to data from the Federal Office of Statistics in Germany, in contrast to a total of 7174 rehabilitation treatments carried out per year.
- Rehabilitation treatments carried out specifically for ICD I70.20 and ICD I70.21 declined by 14% in the period from 2003 to 2009.

4.4.6.8 Prospects

Rehabilitation measures in vascular medicine will continue to be extremely important in the future, in view of the increasing prevalence of the disease. As revascularization measures become more and more effective, vascular interventions will increasingly tend to be combined with subsequent vascular training.

References

ACC/AHA. Practical Guidelines for PAD. 2005.

Creasy TS, McMillan PJ, Fletcher EW, Collin J, Morris PJ. Is percutaneous transluminal angioplasty better than exercise for claudication? Preliminary results from a prospective randomised trial. Eur J Vasc Surg 1990; 4: 135–40.

Dahllof AG, Holm J, Schersten T, Sivertsson R. Peripheral arterial insufficiency, effect of physical training on walking tolerance, calf blood flow, and blood flow resistance. Scand J Rehabil Med 1976; 8: 640–3.

Diehm C et al. Epidemiology of peripheral arterial disease. VASA 2004; 33: 183–9.

Hansis M. G-AEP Entwicklungsbericht. Essen, G-AEP_Bericht_703. doc-22.08.2003-53.

Hirsch AT et al. ACC/AHA Guidelines for the Management of Patients with Peripheral Arterial Disease (lower extremity, renal, mesenteric, and abdominal aortic): a collaborative report from the American Associations for Vascular Surgery/Society for Vascular Surgery, Society for Cardiovascular Angiography and Interventions, Society for Vascular Medicine and Biology, Society of Interventional Radiology, and the ACC/AHA Task Force on Practice Guidelines (writing committee to develop guidelines for the management of patients with peripheral arterial disease)—summary of recommendations. Circulation 2006 Mar 21; 113 (11): e463–654.

Hüter-Becker A, Dölken M. Physiotherapie in der Inneren Medizin, Thieme, 2004.

Köhler M, Schoop W (Hrsg.). Metabolische und hämodynamische Trainingseffekte bei normaler und gestörter Muskeldurchblutung. Bern, Huber, 1973.

Larsen OA. Effect of training on the circulation in ischemic muscle tissue. In: Köhler M, Schoop W (Hrsg.). Metabolische und hämodynamische Trainingseffekte bei normaler und gestörter Muskeldurchblutung. Bern, Huber, 1973, 50–6.

Ratschow M. Die peripheren Durchblutungsstörungen. Medizinische Praxis: Sammlung für ärztliche Fortbildung. Bd. 27, Dresden, Steinkopff Verlag, 1939.

S3-Leitlinie: Diagnostik und Therapie der peripheren arteriellen Verschlusskrankheit (pAVK), AWMF-Registernummer 065/003 (online: Volltext), Stand 03/2009.

WHO. International Classification of Functioning, Disability and Health. 2001.

Womack CJ, Sieminski DJ, Katzel LI, Yataco A, Gardner AW. Improved walking economy in patients with peripheral arterial occlusive disease. Med Sci Sports Exerc 1997; 29: 1286–90.

4.4.7 Endovascular and surgical treatment in the pelvic arteries—technique, clinical results, prospects

Pelvic arteries: Reinhard Putz
Clinical findings: Jörn O. Balzer
Diagnosis: Jörn O. Balzer
Doppler/duplex ultrasonography: Tom Schilling
Endovascular treatment: Jörn O. Balzer
Surgical treatment: Walther Schmiedt

4.4.7.1 Pelvic arteries

At the level of the fourth vertebra, the abdominal aorta divides at the aortic bifurcation into its two large branches, the right and left common iliac arteries, which—each lying on the associated common iliac vein—pass along on the inner side of the psoas major muscle (Fig. 4.4-29). Just above the bifurcation, the thin median sacral artery arises from the posterior wall of the aorta and passes over the promontory to the anterior surface of the sacrum.

At the level of the sacroiliac joint, the internal iliac artery (hypogastric artery) branches off into the lesser pelvis, while the external iliac artery continues the course of the trunk vessel along the pelvic inlet, lying close to the fascia of the iliopsoas muscle, until it passes through the vascular space of the retroinguinal compartment (lacuna vasorum) on the thigh. Along this route, it is crossed by the ureter and by the obliquely descending ovarian or testicular vessels. Before passing under the inguinal ligament, the external iliac artery gives off the inferior epigastric artery to the anterior abdominal wall, the deep circumflex iliac artery to the iliac crest, and small branches to the symphysis (Fig. 4.4-30). There is a small anastomosis between these branches and the obturator artery, but it may sometimes be so large that the obturator artery appears to arise from the external iliac artery.

The branches of the internal iliac artery form firstly a parietal group (Fig. 4.4-31). The first in this group, the iliolumbar artery, courses under the large iliac vessels in the depth of the ala of the ilium toward the iliacus and quadratus lumborum muscles. The obturator artery descends steeply and passes with the obturator nerve through the narrow obturator canal to the inner side of the thigh. The two gluteal arteries turn dorsally. The superior gluteal artery leaves the pelvis through the suprapiriform foramen and branches in the depths of the gluteal muscles. Along with the sciatic nerve and internal pudendal artery from the internal iliac artery, it passes through the infrapiriform foramen and supplies the gluteus maximus and deeper external rotation muscles.

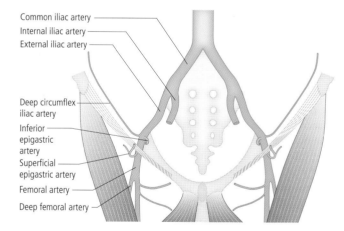

Common iliac artery
Internal iliac artery
External iliac artery

Deep circumflex iliac artery

Inferior epigastric artery

Superficial epigastric artery

Femoral artery

Deep femoral artery

Fig. 4.4-29 Division of the common iliac arteries.

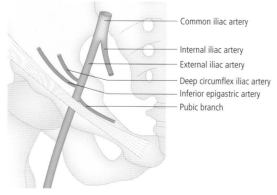

Common iliac artery

Internal iliac artery

External iliac artery

Deep circumflex iliac artery

Inferior epigastric artery

Pubic branch

Fig. 4.4.30 Branches of the external iliac artery.

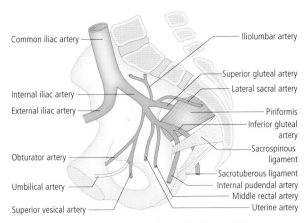

Fig. 4.4-31 Parietal and visceral branches of the internal iliac artery.

The second group of branches from the internal iliac artery, the visceral group, supplies the pelvic viscera (Fig. 4.4-31). These include the umbilical artery, the longer segment of which regresses after birth to form the cord of the umbilical artery. The inferior vesical artery passes to the base of the bladder and the middle rectal artery to the middle part of the rectum. In women, there is a uterine artery which in the base of the broad ligament of the uterus reaches the cervix from a lateral direction, crossing the ureter, and from there winds upwards along the body of the uterus. Small branches emerge from this artery to the ovary, to the uterine tube, and also to the vaginal fornix. Finally, the internal pudendal artery leaves the lesser pelvis along with the inferior gluteal artery and the sciatic nerve through the infrapiriform foramen and passes, winding closely along the ischial spine, into the pudendal canal (Alcock canal) on the inner side of the body of the ischium.

4.4.7.2   Clinical picture

In stage II, aortoiliac arterial occlusive disease often creates a diagnostic enigma. The patients do not necessarily have the calf claudication typically expected in vascular patients, and instead—particularly with this location for vascular disease—have hip and thigh claudication. These symptoms usually lead to a diagnostic odyssey for orthopedists and various other specialists and may even lead to pointless operations such as surgery for slipped disk, inguinal hernia, spinal canal stenosis, or even hip replacement—before a physician finally tries to palpate the inguinal pulse, fails to find it, and thus opens the way to the correct diagnosis. The typical patient is a "normal" atherosclerosis patient—i.e., a smoker, with hypertension, possibly combined with hyperlipidemia, and usually male. However, women are also affected, particularly those who are heavy smokers in their late 40s and those who have undergone radiotherapy at the pelvic level due to gynecological tumors.

4.4.7.3   Diagnosis

During examination of the patient, a weakened or absent pulse in the inguinal region and a reduced ankle–brachial index (ABI) on Doppler occlusive pressure measurement are often noted. Duplex ultrasound diagnosis is indicated for the relevant clinical picture; this can distinguish higher-grade stenosis and shows either a peak

systolic velocity ratio (PVR) $\geq$ 3.4 or a monophasic curve shape distal to the stenosis. Contrast-enhanced magnetic resonance angiography (MRA) or computed-tomographic angiography (CTA) can be used for noninvasive evaluation of the pelvic circulation before any intervention (Fig. 4.4-33a, b). Although angiographic clarification of a lesion in the area of the pelvic circulation using intra-arterial digital subtraction angiography (DSA) has the advantage that treatment can be carried out at the same time, it is now no longer used as a purely diagnostic procedure in advance of a planned intervention.

Doppler/duplex ultrasonography

Examination technique

Aortoiliac examination is usually carried out with a 3.5–5.0 MHz sector scanner. Due to the poor Doppler angle, the color setting should be adjusted fairly sensitively with a low pulse repetition frequency (PRF). The application pressure with the scanner should be strong enough to compress bowel contents etc. and improve the imaging quality. *Caution:* there are often septal stenoses that may escape angiographic imaging → duplex ultrasound is more sensitive here.

Differential diagnosis

Classic arteriosclerosis: classic plaque morphology—see the specific findings with femoropopliteal processes for ways of assessing the degree of stenosis and plaque morphology.
Large-vessel vasculitis: typically homogeneous and hypoechoic widened intima–media complex (macaroni sign).
Dissections: these are typically seen after interventions or after intra-arterial digital subtraction angiography (DSA); the floating dissection membrane should be demonstrated along with the partial lumens. If the B-mode image is unclear, the color mode can be used to display different color and flow patterns in the partial lumens. Hemodynamics in the lumens should be checked (for occlusions or stenoses).
Thrombosed aneurysms: there may be evidence of a preexisting aneurysm in a hypoechoic, occluded area.
Embolic processes: hypoechoic to isoechoic occlusive material is seen, and a dome phenomenon may be visible—i.e., a convex shape in the occlusive material towards the free lumen. Typical occlusion sites, multilocular processes, and an otherwise unremarkable vascular system with no major atheromatosis. In upstream arterial areas or structures that appear potentially emboligenic on echocardiography, there may be partly thrombosed or thrombosed aneurysms.
Arterial thrombosis: there is no evidence for the criteria that are suspicious for embolism mentioned above. In addition to the occlusion, there may be signs of prior arteriosclerosis, with echocomplex plaques and structures that create acoustic shadows → possibly "older" echogenic occlusive components in patients with a history of PAOD or status post interventional or surgical procedures.

Specific findings

For stenoses and occlusive processes in the lower extremity and femoropopliteal area, see the specific findings described in section A 4.4.8.

4.4.7.4 Endovascular treatment

Percutaneous transluminal angioplasty (PTA) with or without stent placement now plays an indispensable role in the treatment of peripheral arterial occlusive disease (PAOD). Since the first dilation of a vascular stenosis using a balloon in the 1970s, the percutaneous technique has developed to become a standard form of treatment for PAOD. Particularly in the area of the pelvic arteries, percutaneous intervention has become a safe and successful alternative to vascular surgery for a large number of patients. In comparison with the more invasive methods used in vascular surgery and the associated surgery-related complications, percutaneous interventions have much lower risks of morbidity and mortality.

Initially, percutaneous treatment in the pelvic arteries was largely limited to therapy for short stenoses. Even today, several authors consider that more complex lesions in the pelvic arterial circulation are only partly suitable for percutaneous recanalization, due to poor success rates and patency rates. Vascular surgery is therefore still regarded as the primary treatment method for specific lesions, multiple long stenoses and occlusions, particularly those longer than 5 cm, generally graded by the Trans-Atlantic Inter-Society Consensus (TASC) group as TASC II C and D (Table 4.4-11, Fig. 4.4-32).

In this classification, TASC A includes lesions in which endovascular treatment with very good long-term results is possible.

TASC B covers all lesions that can be treated using endovascular procedures with adequate long-term results provided there are no other lesions in the same area that require vascular surgery.

TASC C includes all lesions for which better long-term results are possible with vascular surgery unless surgery is contraindicated in the patient concerned.

TASC D includes all lesions for which satisfactory long-term results were not reported with endovascular treatment prior to the publication of the TASC II classification.

Recommendation 36 in the TASC II guidelines classifies the preferred treatment strategies in lesions of the aortoiliac circulation on the basis of publications on the treatment of aortoiliac vascular le-

Table 4.4-11 TASC II classification of pelvic artery lesions (2007).

TASC II classification	Description
Type A lesion	Unilateral or bilateral stenosis of the CIA Unilateral or bilateral single short (≤ 3 cm) stenosis in the EIA
Type B lesion	Short (≤ 3 cm) stenosis in the infrarenal aorta Unilateral occlusion of the CIA Single or multiple stenoses up to a maximum of 10 cm long with no involvement of the CFA Unilateral occlusion of the EIA with no involvement of the origins of the IIA or CFA
Type C lesion	Bilateral occlusion of the CIA Bilateral stenoses of the EIA up to 10 cm in length with no involvement of the CFA Unilateral stenoses of the EIA with involvement of the CFA Unilateral occlusions of the EIA with involvement of the origins of the IIA or CFA Severely calcified unilateral occlusion of the EIA with/without involvement of the origins of the IIA or CFA
Type D lesion	Infrarenal aortoiliac occlusion Diffuse lesions in the aorta and both iliac arteries, requiring treatment Diffuse multiple lesions of the unilateral CIA up to the CFA Unilateral occlusion of the common and external iliac arteries Bilateral occlusion of the EIA Stenoses of the iliac arteries in patients with abdominal aortic aneurysms requiring treatment in which stent grafting is not suitable, or other lesions in the aorta or iliac arteries that require open vascular surgery

CFA, common femoral artery; CIA, common iliac artery; EIA, external iliac artery; IIA, internal iliac artery; TASC, Trans-Atlantic Inter-Society Consensus.

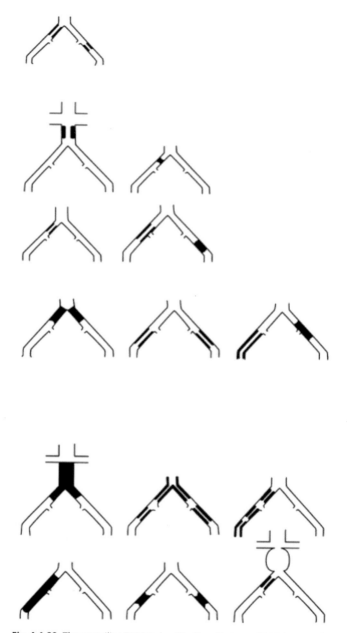

Fig. 4.4-32 The aortoiliac TASC II classification. First row: TASC A; second and third rows: TASC B; fourth row: TASC C; fifth and sixth rows: TASC D.

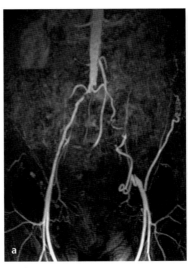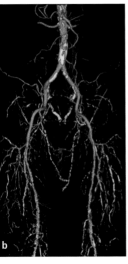

Fig. 4.4-33a, b Noninvasive vascular imaging of the pelvic arteries.
(**a**) Contrast magnetic resonance angiography, showing high-grade stenosis of the right common iliac artery and occlusion of the left common and external iliac arteries. (**b**) Computed tomographic angiography of the pelvic circulation, documenting calcified plaques in the area of the common iliac arteries bilaterally (right more than left) and internal iliac artery bilaterally.

Table 4.4-12 Treatment recommendations in accordance with TASC II Recommendation 36.

TASC classification	Primary treatment strategy
TASC A	Endovascular therapy
TASC B	Endovascular therapy
TASC C	Vascular surgery in operable patients; otherwise endovascular therapy
TASC D	Vascular surgery

TASC, Trans-Atlantic Inter-Society Consensus.

sions up to 2006 (Table 4.4-12). This classification is mainly based on older studies. However, due to improved technology and materials, good success rates and long-term patency rates can now be achieved in interventional treatment for multiple lesions and more complex lesions. There is also now a trend toward endovascular treatment even for TASC D lesions in experienced centers, due to the higher morbidity and mortality associated with surgical treatment.

Indications

The indication for interventional therapy is usually a reduced resting ABI, a deterioration in walking distance, with the corresponding pelvic or thigh-type claudication limiting everyday activities, or a wound healing disturbance.

Technique

For recanalization of lesions in the aortoiliac circulation, the following materials should be available: sheaths of various sizes and lengths (5–8F, 10–45 cm long), guidewires (0.035-inch, 180–260 cm long, hydrophilic, uncoated, stiff, soft, curved or straight), and diagnostic catheters and selective catheters of various sizes and shapes. Table 4.4-13 provides an overview of the interventional materials most commonly used.

Table 4.4.-13 Overview of materials used in the treatment of the aortoiliac circulatory pathway (selected).

Materials	Sizes
Sheath	Size: 6–8F Length: 10, 25, 45 cm Transbrachial: 80–90 cm
Guidewires	0.035 inch: e.g., Terumo soft and stiff, bent; Amplatz, Supracore 0.018 inch: e.g., Boston V18
PTA catheter	Diameter: 6–12 mm Length: 20–100 mm
Balloon-expandable stents	Diameter: 6–12 mm Length: 20–80 mm
Self-expanding stents	Diameter: 6–12 mm Length: 20–100 mm
Debulking catheter	Excimer laser catheter SilverHawk Straub Rotarex thrombectomy catheter system
Other	Cutting Balloon catheter Occlusion systems
Emergency materials	Introducer sheaths: 10–14F PTA catheters, diameter: 12, 18, 20 mm Stent grafts, diameter: 6–12 mm; length: 20–80 mm

PTA, percutaneous transluminal angioplasty.

Types of access route

The recanalization technique used (balloon angioplasty, stent implantation, etc.) initially depends on the type of lesion (stenosis or occlusion) and its length (short or long), and on the location—the common iliac artery or external iliac artery.

The interventional access route is usually via the common femoral artery, with local anesthesia. The most important advantage of this, apart from the vicinity of the lesion, is the ability to compress the vessel against the branch of the hip bone or the head of the femur for hemostasis at the end of the examination. The optimal puncture site is approximately 2 cm distal to the inguinal ligament (the line between the anterior superior iliac spine and the pubic symphysis)—i.e., slightly above the center of the head of the femur. Additional sedation or conscious sedation of the patient is usually not indicated and is only required in exceptional cases. Monitoring of circulatory parameters (pulse, blood pressure, oxygen saturation) is recommended and is obligatory in sedated patients. The main access route is via retrograde puncture of the common femoral artery. Depending on the type and location of the lesion in the area of the aortoiliac circulation, bilateral puncture of the common femoral artery or combined access via the brachial artery may be necessary.

For treatment of stenoses in the area of the common iliac artery and proximal external iliac artery, access to the lesion is obtained by retrograde puncture of the common femoral artery in the ipsilateral extremity. If the stenosis is located in the area of the distal common iliac artery or external iliac artery, crossover access is used, after puncturing the contralateral common femoral artery and navigating the guidewire through the iliac bifurcation (Fig. 4.4-34).

Recanalization of an occlusion in the common or external iliac artery should initially be attempted using an antegrade technique, so

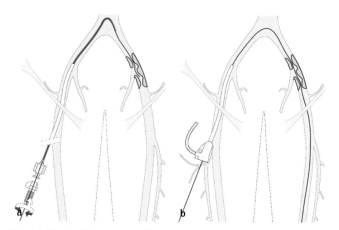

Fig. 4.4-34a, b Wire passage of a stenosis in the left common/external iliac artery using crossover access.

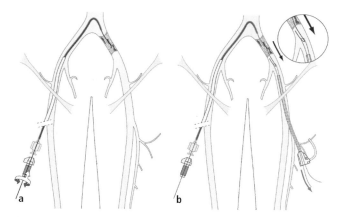

Fig. 4.4-35a, b Wire passage of an occlusion of the left common iliac artery using crossover access and subsequent recanalization via retrograde access.

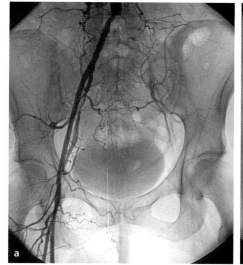
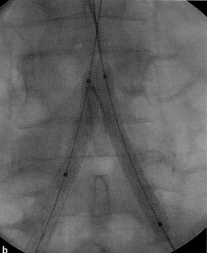
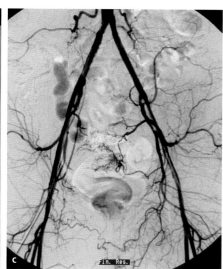

Fig. 4.4-36a–c Recanalization of an occlusion of the left common/external iliac artery and right common iliac artery using the kissing balloon technique.

that dissection of the abdominal aorta can be avoided if subintimal recanalization occurs. This initially requires retrograde puncture of the contralateral common femoral artery. After the wire has been successfully passed through the occlusion, the ipsilateral common femoral artery is also punctured and the guidewire is captured and brought out through it (Fig. 4.4-35). All of the other recanalization steps are then carried out in retrograde fashion over the wire on the ipsilateral side. If it is not possible to pass the wire using the crossover technique, an additional transbrachial access route with a long sheath can be used to achieve successful recanalization of the occlusion.

Primary bilateral puncture of the common femoral artery is used for recanalization of ostial lesions in the common iliac artery (with the kissing-balloon or stent techniques; Fig. 4.4-36). Alternatively, unilateral common femoral artery puncture can also be combined with transbrachial access here.

Recanalization techniques

The aim of the percutaneous intervention is not only to reopen the vessel but also to achieve long-term or permanent patency in it. It is not easy to compare the long-term patency rates reported in the published literature, since the same standards of definition are not used in all of the studies. For example, the post-interventional course may be assessed using either the Fontaine classification or the Rutherford system. The patency rate may also be defined in different ways—e.g., using these classification criteria, or by assessing the tibiobrachial index (TBI), the pain-free walking distance, or a recurrent lesion. For recanalization of pelvic artery stenoses or occlusions, primary or secondary stent implantation and ablation procedures (e.g., with an atherectomy catheter or laser angioplasty) are used. Sheath sizes of 6F 7F, or 8F are usually required for the intervention, depending on the materials that need to be used. The individual techniques are presented briefly below.

Balloon angioplasty

Percutaneous transluminal angioplasty (PTA), also known as balloon dilation angioplasty, is nowadays an important part of PAOD treatment. It is associated with lower risk in comparison with surgical treatment. The current indications for PTA in the pelvic arteries are short stenoses and occlusions that are less than 5 cm long (Fig. 4.4-37).

In PTA, a catheter is introduced over a guidewire into the area to be treated, where a balloon is inflated that dilates the stenosis and the affected vascular segment. Both the diameter and the length of the PTA catheter are adjusted relative to the diameter of the vessel being treated. The diameter of the PTA catheter used is adjusted to the

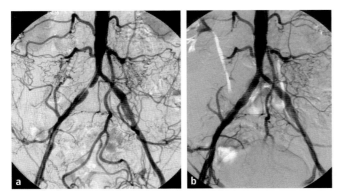

Fig. 4.4-37a, b Treatment of a stenosis of the right common iliac artery using balloon angioplasty.

length of the lesion being treated and is usually 2–6 mm. Over-the-wire catheter systems in combination with a 0.035-inch guidewire are normally used. In rarer cases, 0.018-inch guidewires are used (e.g., PTA with a Cutting Balloon system).

In higher-grade stenoses, predilation with a smaller or thinner PTA catheter may be necessary. For balloon inflation, it is best to use a manometer. Inflation pressures are usually in the range of 4–10 atm (approx. 405–1013 kPa). However, the relationship between the balloon diameter and the vessel diameter, and the patient's response to dilation with pain, are more important than the absolute pressure value. Balloon inflation should only be done up to the point at which the patient responds with a pain sensation, in order to prevent perforation of the vessel. There are no standard recommendations regarding the duration of dilation; periods of 1–2 min are usual.

Stent implantation

Stent implantation has proved its value in cases of substantial residual stenosis, recoiling (elastic rebound in the vessel) and dissection after PTA. It was in 1969 that Dotter first recommended the use of metal spiral endoprostheses to stabilize vessel lumina. Since that time, various endovascular stents have been developed. The first balloon-expandable stent (Palmaz®, Cordis Endovascular, Langenfeld, Germany) was developed in 1985 by J.C. Palmaz. It consists

of a stainless-steel mesh that is mounted on a balloon catheter in an unexpanded state. After correct placement, the stent is pressed into the vessel wall by inflation of the balloon. The Palmaz stent has a high radial force and is therefore well suited to use in severely calcified vessels. Precise placement using the balloon and the stent's freely selectable opening is advantageous. There is also only very slight shortening of the stent after dilation. The disadvantage with all stents of this type is that the length is limited to that of the balloon, so that these stents are not available with lengths sufficient to treat longer lesions. These balloon-expandable stents are nowadays usually made of a cobalt–chrome alloy.

Self-expanding nitinol stents are highly flexible and consist of a nickel–titanium alloy. They have a capacity for thermal memory. This means that the stents are able to preserve a previously set shape in "memory." When cooled, they become malleable and flexible and can therefore be easily introduced into a vessel. In the bloodstream, their temperature increases and the vascular wall support resumes its "memorized shape" again. Modern nitinol stents have more or less the same radial strength as those made of stainless steel or cobalt–chrome, but with a reduced tendency to shorten as compared to first generation devices (Fig. 4.4-38).

Both nitinol stents and steel stents that are coated with various graft materials can be used as stent grafts (or covered stents). Classic coating materials are polyethylene terephthalate (PET), expanded polytetrafluoroethylene (ePTFE), and polyurethane polycarbonate. This type of stent is indicated in aneurysms, arteriovenous fistulas, and ruptures. Recently, balloon-expandable stent grafts covered with ePTFE (Advanta™ V12, Atrium) are also recommended for the treatment of complex TASC C and D lesions. The COBEST study, which compared balloon-expandable stents with V12 stent grafts, reported higher patency rates for complex lesions after stent graft implantation than with traditional stents.

As mentioned earlier, stent implantation can prevent recoiling and remodeling in the vessel, so that the major remaining cause of residual stenosis after stent implantation is neointimal hyperplasia. It is hoped that new developments with coated stents covered with immunosuppressive or antiproliferative drug agents (drug-eluting stents, DESs) may prevent recurrent stenosis after PTA as a result of reduced neointimal hyperplasia.

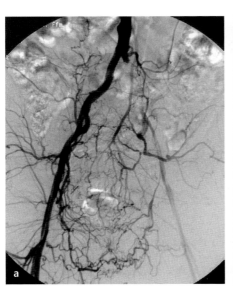
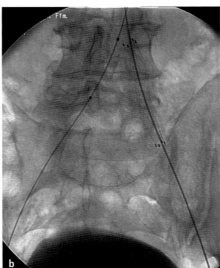
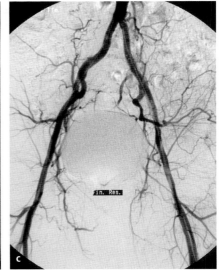

Fig. 4.4-38a–c Recanalization of an occlusion of the left common iliac artery using percutaneous transluminal angioplasty and nitinol stent implantation.

Atherectomy and thrombectomy systems

Atherectomy removes plaques through mechanical fragmentation and ablation of the atherosclerotic material using an endoluminal endarterectomy device that can be introduced over a guidewire. Several types of atherectomy system are available, and the SilverHawk® catheter (ev3, Inc., Plymouth, Minnesota) is the one most widely used. The catheter has a rotating blade inside its metal housing and a small collecting container in the catheter tip that stores the removed material for periodic emptying (see also section 4.1 above).

The Straub Rotarex® catheter (Straub Medical, Wangs, Switzerland) is used in a vasodilative procedure for acute and subacute occlusions. This thrombectomy system combines two basic mechanisms: mechanical thrombus fragmentation on the one hand, and removal of the thrombus particles on the other. The two processes are made possible by a rotating steel spiral. The rotation movement creates negative pressure, which in turns transports the fragmented material to the exterior. Distal embolization due to released particulates can thus be avoided. Although there is a risk of perforation, the reported long-term success rates range from 32% to 86%, depending on the type of occlusion being treated (see also section 4.1 above).

The oldest plaque removal technique is laser angioplasty (photoablation). Percutaneous transluminal laser angioplasty (PTLA) makes it possible to recanalize very long occlusions in which conventional methods of dilation treatment have not been successful. Only the excimer laser is currently used for PTLA. The excimer laser system is a pulsed high-pressure gas discharge laser that emits light in the ultraviolet wavelength range. It is able to photoablate atherosclerotic material without producing heat. As in the PTA technique, the laser is introduced over a guidewire, positioned at the lesion, and activated (Fig. 4.4-39). Laser angioplasty is used in addition to PTA and is indicated when the guidewire is unable to pass the occlusion (in the step-by-step technique), as it is the only atherectomy procedure that can be carried out without first placing a wire through the occlusion.

Pre-, peri-, and postinterventional medication

Peri-interventionally, 2500–10,000 IU of high-molecular-weight heparin is administered (weight-adjusted: 100 IU heparin/kg body weight).

In the longer term, all patients should receive platelet inhibitors after successful PTA, as these have favorable effects on the patency rate. ASA, clopidogrel, and other agents with antithrombotic effects can be used here. With PTA alone, only ASA 100 mg/d is usually administered; with stent implantations, clopidogrel 75 mg/d for 4 weeks is added. Drug treatment after percutaneous transluminal angioplasty is intended not only to prevent early thrombotic occlusions, but also to reduce the rate of slowly developing recurrent stenoses. Various pathophysiological mechanisms are responsible for the development of recurrent stenoses. Early elastic recoil, late vessel remodeling, and neointimal hyperplasia after interventions lead to an increase in late lumen loss. The recurrence rate depends on the location, length, and type of lesion involved.

Postinterventional follow-up

Technical success of the intervention is defined as successful recanalization with a residual stenosis grade of less than 30% and restoration of antegrade perfusion by the vascular segment treated, as evidenced by the arterial blood pressure gradients over the segment concerned.

All patients should be followed up for a set period, and the follow-up intervals given in the literature are (1 month), 3, 6, 12 months after the intervention, and thereafter annually. The follow-up examinations include a clinical examination, TBI measurement, and duplex ultrasonography. The American Heart Association (AHA) classification should be used for assessing the clinical success of the intervention (Table 4.4-14).

Clinical results

The reported technical success rates with PTA for pelvic artery stenosis are generally over 90%, or with focal stenoses up to 100%. The technical success rates for treatment of pelvic artery occlusions re-

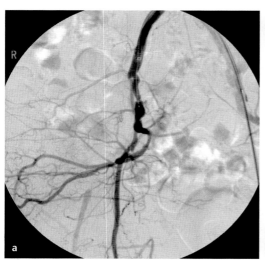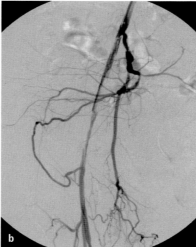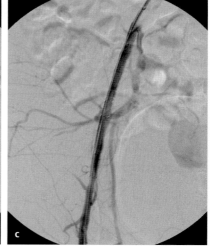

Fig. 4.4-39a–c Recanalization of an occlusion of the right external iliac artery using laser angioplasty and stent implantation with the crossover technique. (**a**) Occlusion of the right external iliac artery. (**b**) Imaging of the lumen after passing it with a 2.5-mm laser catheter three times. (**c**) Final result after stent implantation (nitinol stent, 7 × 80 mm).

Table 4.4-14 Guidelines of the American Heart Association (AHA) for symptomatic improvements in the disease after interventions.

Grade	Clinical description
3	Marked improvement: TBI > 0.9
2	Moderate improvement: TBI increase > 0.1, but not normal values, improvement by one class
1	Slight improvement: TBI increase > 0.1, but not normal values or no improvement by one class
0	No change
−1	Slight deterioration: no deterioration in class, but TBI < 0.1 poorer
−2	Deterioration by one class or unexpected minor amputation
−3	Deterioration by more than one class or unexpected major amputation

TBI, tibiobrachial index.

ported in the literature are 80–85%; among patients at our own institution, the rate is over 95%. The 5-year patency rates are 70–75%. Murphy et al. (2004) report an 8-year patency rate of 74% after stent implantation. Factors with a negative influence on patency include the quality of the outflow pathway, the severity of the ischemia, and the length of the diseased vascular segment. In the area of the external iliac artery, female sex also appears to be associated with a greater probability of recurrent stenosis after stent angioplasty. Although the interventional results with recanalization of the pelvic arteries are better than those with infrainguinal recanalization, both the indication in some groups of patients and the lesion morphology are currently matters of controversy. This particularly affects diabetic patients, females, lesions in the external iliac artery, and long occlusions.

Diabetics vs. nondiabetics

In a study in which they compared PAOD in the aortoiliac and femoropopliteal circulation in diabetics and nondiabetics, Jude et al. (2001) confirmed that severe forms of PAOD develop in diabetics. Significantly higher rates of amputation and mortality were observed in the group of diabetic patients with PAOD. Despite these observations, no significant differences in the success and patency rates were evident between diabetics and nondiabetics undergoing recanalization of the pelvic arteries. A possible reason for this is that there were no significant differences between the two groups with regard to the run-off conditions, degree of stenosis, or length of the lesions.

Lesion location and sex

Another matter of controversy is the issue of whether female sex and the location of the lesion in the external iliac artery have unfavorable effects on the long-term results after PTA. There are statistical trends in the evidence, but the data are not yet conclusively clear. Uher et al. (2002) reported one early recurrent stenosis and 16 recurrent stenoses an average of 27 months after recanalization of 76 occlusions. The locations of the occlusions treated were the common iliac artery in 33 cases and the external iliac artery in 34

cases, with both vessels being involved in nine patients. The mean occlusion length was 7 cm. Occlusions longer than 5 cm and stenoses longer than 10 cm have less favorable patency rates after PTA and have therefore so far been regarded as belonging to the field of vascular surgery. Müller-Leisse et al. reported a primary technical success rate of 100% in the treatment of 23 long pelvic artery occlusions (mean occlusion length 12 cm). During a follow-up period of 30 months, there were four early occlusions and five late occlusions, giving a primary patency rate of 61.0%. After successful repeat interventions in seven cases, there was a secondary patency rate of 91.3%. In 19 of the 23 interventions (82.6%), only the external iliac artery was affected or at least involved. Lower success rates and patency rates are reported for occlusions of the external iliac artery in nearly all of the studies. Johnston (1993) showed that PTA in the external iliac artery led to poorer long-term patency rates in comparison with PTA in the common iliac artery. He achieved a primary patency rate of 70.9% 3 years after PTA for common iliac artery stenoses, and primary patency rates of 57.0% in men and 34.0% in women after PTA for external iliac artery stenoses, despite similar success rates of 97.1% with the procedures. Timaran et al. (2001) also described both involvement of the external iliac artery and female sex as being two of the major factors associated with low patency rates. Suggested reasons for this were the smaller diameter of the external iliac artery and the usually slower flow velocity in it in comparison with the common iliac artery. Our own group of patients included 25 women (28.1%) and seven occlusions of the external iliac artery (36.8%). However, only three of the seven patients with external iliac artery occlusions were women (42.9%)—explaining the better primary and secondary patency rates of 89.9% and 95.5%, respectively, observed after a mean of 25 months in comparison with the data reported by Müller-Leisse and Johnston.

Length of the lesion

The data for clinical success rates published in recent years, as assessed using the AHA criteria, are in the range of 87.7–100%, depending on the morphology and location of the lesions treated. While Scheinert et al. reported a clinical success rate of 87.7% in the recanalization of long occlusions (average length 8.9 cm) in their study published in 2001, their 1999 study had reported a 100% clinical success rate in the treatment of 25 stenoses and 23 occlusions. Murphy et al. also noted clinical success in 95.0% of their patients after treatment of 505 lesions (82.6% stenoses and 17.4% occlusions). The few studies published to date that classify treated lesions using the TASC system, such as Timaran et al. 2001 and 2003, reported clinical success rates of 93.0% and 97.0% after interventions in patients mostly in TASC B and C grades, respectively (Fig. 4.4-40). The 129 lesions treated in our own group of patients included 24 of types which, in the view of other authors, lead to poor success rates and patency rates—such as stenoses more than 10 cm long, occlusions longer than 5 cm, and occlusions of the external iliac artery. Despite this, we achieved an outstanding technical success rate of 96.9%. There were no statistically significant differences between this result and the success rate in treating shorter lesions or occlusions of the common iliac artery. These results were confirmed by Sixt et al. (2008), who found no significant differences in the acute success and patency rates between TASC III A and B lesions versus C and D lesions.

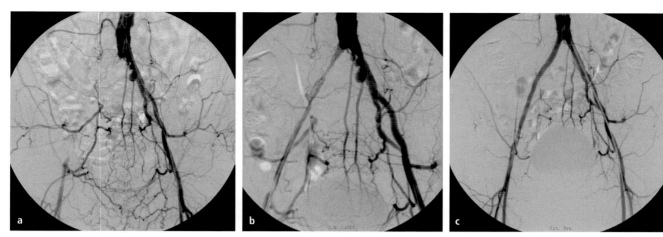

Fig. 4.4-40a–c Recanalization of an occlusion of the right common and external iliac artery using laser angioplasty and stent implantation. (**a**) Occlusion of the right common and external iliac artery, with ulcerated plaque in the left common iliac artery. (**b**) Imaging of the lumen on the right after passing it with a 2.5-mm laser catheter four times. (**c**) Final result after bilateral stent implantation (nitinol stent 9/60 and 7 × 80 mm right, with a balloon-expandable stainless steel stent 8/38 in the left common iliac artery).

The principal challenge in recanalizing long lesions lies in complication-free navigation of the guidewire through the vascular constriction. Some authors consider that the success of this maneuver is strictly correlated with the length of the segment. Colapinto et al. (1985) observed that the success rate in recanalizing occlusions declines along with increasing length. If the occlusions were longer than 5 cm, only 70% could be successfully passed, in comparison with a 92% success rate with shorter occlusions.

A possible explanation for the good technical results of 95.9% and 97.5% (in TASC C and TASC D, respectively) observed in our own group and by Sixt et al., despite the treatment of complex lesions, might be improvements in the materials used for the interventions.

Run-off

In more than half (15 of 24) of these complex lesions, unrestricted run-off distal to the vascular segment that was treated is a factor strongly influencing the long-term success of the intervention, in the view of several authors. Timaran et al. also showed that after stent placement in iliac occlusions in TASC categories B and C, restricted distal blood run-off can be regarded as the most important predictive factor for poor interventional results. Although the success rates observed in our own group showed a trend toward better results when there was good run-off (100% vs. 83.3%), the difference was not significant, in contrast to the other studies mentioned. The primary and secondary patency rates observed in our own group (89.9% and 95.5%, respectively) after a mean of 24 months are well above the previously published data on PTA for iliac stenoses and occlusions. In their analysis of the then-available literature, Kandarpa et al. (2001) reported 2-year patency rates of 76–84% and 60–67% after the treatment of iliac stenosis or occlusions, respectively, with PTA and stent placement. The lesions treated in the studies were focal stenoses of the common iliac artery and/or external iliac artery with lengths less than 10 cm, and unilateral occlusions of the common iliac artery. In the TASC classification, the lesions were classed as TASC B.

Another prognostically unfavorable factor, as mentioned earlier, is restricted blood flow through areas affected by arteriosclerosis in downstream vessels. There was no restriction in downstream blood flow in 58.4% (n = 52) of the patients in our own group. When there is an increased flow velocity in the treated segment, good distal run-off reduces platelet aggregation and thus reduces the risk of reocclusion. Lesions in the infrainguinal circulation should therefore always be treated at the same time, or at least shortly afterward in a second intervention.

Stent implantation

There are as yet no data from randomized studies comparing primary stent implantation in the area of the pelvic arteries with balloon angioplasty (PTA). A prospective randomized multicenter study compared primary stent implantation with "provisional stenting"—i.e., when stent implantation is only carried out if the results of the primary PTA are unsatisfactory. The 2-year reintervention rates were comparable in the two arms of the study (7% for PTA and stenting when needed, 4% for primary stenting). After a mean follow-up period of 5.6 ± 1.3 years, there were still no differences (target lesion revascularization 18% and 20%, respectively).

Harnek et al. compared the development of intimal hyperplasia after placement of a self-expanding nitinol stent with and without prior PTA in nine healthy swine, and reported a lower rate of intimal hyperplasia with primary stenting. The arteries treated with PTA and a selective stent had a significantly thicker intima (10.24 mm^2 vs. 2.69 mm^2 in the group in which a stent was placed primarily) and a higher intima–media ratio (1.95 vs. 0.56). The recurrent stenosis index for the group treated with selective stent placement was 2.63 in comparison with 1.35 after primary stent placement. The results published by Harnek et al. suggest that the intimal hyperplasia that ultimately leads to recurrent stenoses occurs less often with primary stent placement.

In our own group of patients, we achieved a primary patency rate of approximately 90.0% in both the TASC C and TASC D groups, with no significant differences between the groups and with no significant differences between stenoses and occlusions or complex and noncomplex lesions. Several recently published studies have confirmed these observations. Kim et al. (1999) carried out primary placement of a self-expanding spiral stent for 36 occlusions in 34 patients and achieved an outstanding technical success rate of 100%, with clinical improvement in 94% of cases. After a mean follow-up period of 11.9 months (6–35 months), the authors only observed two reocclusions.

Postinterventionally, the patients we treated also received optimal long-term anticoagulation treatment, or had their existing long-term medication adjusted to the progression of their PAOD. ASA was administered for long-term medication in 46.1% of the patients, clopidogrel in 40.4%, and a combination of the two in 7.9%. According to the CAPRIE study, clopidogrel has a slight advantage over ASA with regard to the range of side effects and risk reduction. However, the high cost of clopidogrel is still a disadvantage. Before the intervention, 2.2% of the patients were already receiving phenprocoumon (Marcoumar®), and this was left unchanged postinterventionally. In view of the cardiovascular risk and increased mortality in PAOD patients mentioned earlier, both pharmacological risk therapy and also uninterrupted follow-up care are an important part of secondary prophylaxis against atherosclerotic vascular changes.

Complications

An overall complication rate of 5.62% was observed in our own group. Although lesions were treated for which primary PTA is not the recommended form of therapy, this is a relatively low percentage. Matsi et al. (1998) reported an overall complication rate of 10.5% after PTA treatment for 410 occlusions. In their group, 66% of the stenoses treated were in the femoropopliteal region, but this was regarded as a negligible factor, as the authors found that it was not the location of the lesion but rather the grade of stenosis that was the decisive factor relative to the complication rate. The findings published by Gardiner et al. (1986) support this view. In their study, there were complication rates of 3% for iliac PTA and 3% for femoropopliteal PTA. However, significantly more complications were associated with occlusions and fewer with stenoses (18% vs. 7%).

The most frequent incidents during PTA are hemorrhage, pseudoaneurysms, hematomas, and arteriovenous fistulas at the puncture site, or more rarely thromboembolism and perforations (Fig. 4.4-41). Matsi et al. (1998) evaluated the complications that occurred in

410 interventions using 5F sheaths (both stenoses and occlusions) in 295 patients, and reported 22 hematomas, two arteriovenous fistulas, five pseudoaneurysms at the puncture site, two retroperitoneal hematomas, and 12 thromboembolic complications. Despite the larger sheath systems (6–8F) used in our own group, the complication rate was much lower (10.5% vs. 5.62%).

There are also other patient-related factors that contribute to increased complication rates, such as obesity, coagulation disturbances, and concomitant cardiac and renal diseases.

Prospects

The results of recently published studies show that percutaneous recanalization of lesions in the aortoiliac circulation can be carried out in both TASC A or B and also C or D lesions with high technical and clinical success rates and low complication rates. The primary and secondary patency rates achieved with these interventions are comparable with those obtained after the treatment of short (< 10 cm) focal stenoses. Interventional therapy can therefore certainly also be recommended as a method of treating TASC C and D lesions, and it is likely to play an increasingly important role in the future in more complex lesions as well.

4.4.7.5 Surgical treatment

As aortoiliac occlusive disease has now become a field for interventional therapy, these procedures are being performed less often in routine vascular surgery. However, the poor durability of the interventions and early recurrent stenoses (after 3 months in this region) and stent thromboses lead to renewed presentation for vascular surgery and definitive surgical care. Vascular surgery in this region is thus required when occlusive disease is progressing rapidly or interventional measures have failed.

Indications for surgery

The recommendations given in the Trans-Atlantic Inter-Society Consensus (TASC) document on the management of peripheral arterial disease, published in 2000, and its 2007 amendment can be used for guidance on the type of therapy required.

Brewster (2005) distinguishes three types of aortoiliac occlusive disease:

- Type I, approximately 10%, TASC A and B lesions, is limited to the aortic bifurcation and common iliac arteries, only leads to claudication, and is usually treated interventionally.
- Type II, approximately 25%, TASC A, B, and C lesions, affects the distal aorta and pelvic arteries up to the inguinal ligament and causes stages II–III arterial occlusive disease. This type can be treated interventionally or surgically, or both.
- Type III, approximately 65%, TASC C and D lesions, is always extended to the distal aorta, pelvic arteries, femoral and calf arteries, and is the most frequent type. The majority of lesions are in stages II–IV, and they can be treated with hybrid procedures (i.e., with combined surgical and interventional measures) or surgically.

When establishing the indication, it should be borne in mind that the usual imaging procedures, particularly MRA, often give the impression of a better vascular situation than is then actually encountered intraoperatively. This also means that the preoperative

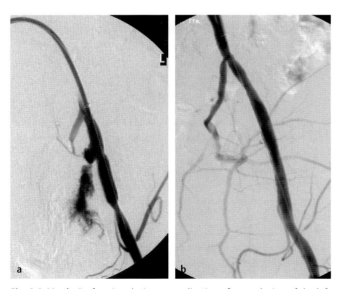

Fig. 4.4-41a, b Perforation during recanalization of an occlusion of the left external iliac artery. (**a**) Perforation after dilation of the left external iliac artery with a 7/40-mm percutaneous transluminal angioplasty catheter. (**b**) No further evidence of a perforation after implantation of a covered stent.

Table 4.4-15 Differences in results: comparison of published data.

Authors	Year	Patients (n)	Lesions (n)	Occlusions (n)	Stenoses (n)	CIA	EIA	CIA/EIA	Technical success (%)	PPR (%, months)			SPR (%, months)			Complications (%)
										12	24	36	12	24	26	
Kim et al.	1999	34	36	36	0	13	12	11	100	94.1	n.a.	n.a.	100	n.a.	n.a.	2.9
Önal et al.	1998	19	22	0	22	19	2	0	95	94.7	n.a.	n.a.	n.a.	n.a.	n.a.	0.0
Matsi et al.	1998	295	552	180	372	n.a.	n.a.	n.a.	88	n.a.	n.a.	n.a.	n.a.	n.a.	n.a.	10.5
Scheinert et al.	1999	48	48	23	25	22	0	26	100	97.2	86.8	n.a.	100	100	n.a.	6.2
Scheinert et al.	2001	212	212	212	0	67	74	71	90	84	81	78	88	88	86	8.0
Tetteroo et al.	1998	279	356	29	327	245	111	0	84/88	n.a.	71	n.a.	n.a.	n.a.	n.a.	5.7
Murphy et al.	2004	365	505	88	417	n.a.	n.a.	n.a.	98	89	86	83	95	93	91	7.0
Funovisc et al.	2002	78	80	80	0	52	29	9	96	78.1	74.5	n.a.	88.8	88.8	n.a.	9.0
Müller-Leisse et al.	2001	23	23	23	0	3	12	8	100	82.6	n.a.	60.9	91.3	n.a.	91.3	43.5
Orr et al.	2002	84	104	29	75	n.a.	n.a.	n.a.	100	n.a.	58.7	n.a.	n.a.	90.3	n.a.	3.0

CIA, common iliac artery; EIA, external iliac artery; n.a., not available; PPR, primary patency rate; SPR, secondary patency rate.

diagnostic findings may tempt one into carrying out interventional procedures that are hardly capable of leading to long-term success, as the arteriosclerosis proves to be far too advanced (e.g., due to underestimated inflow or outflow problems).

Surgical technique

Surgical treatment is performed in patients in whom interventional therapy does not appear possible, or is possible only with limited success; those with in-stent stenoses or occlusion that do not appear to be treatable interventionally; and those with TASC C and D lesions. The choice of surgical procedure depends on the stage of the disease, the extent of the morphological changes, and comorbid conditions. Fontaine stage III, with resting pain, and stage IV, with ulcers and gangrene, have to be treated; stage II may be treated, but the risks involved in the comorbid conditions need to be weighed. A wide range of treatment procedures are available, as detailed below.

Retroperitoneal or transperitoneal access

- Direct thromboendarterectomy (TEA) and patch plasty
- Vollmar semi-closed ring stripper disobliteration
- Unilateral and bilateral aortofemoral/iliacofemoral bypass, Y prosthesis
- Iliacofemoral crossover bypass
- Laparoscopic aortofemoral/iliacofemoral bypass

Superficial subcutaneous/subfascial access (without opening body cavities)

- Femorofemoral crossover bypass
- Axillofemoral bypass
- Combinations with iliac–PTA/stenting from the femoral direction

Standard surgical access routes

Left-sided retroperitoneal access (Rob; Fig. 4.4-43)

The patient is placed in the dorsal decubitus position, with the left half of the chest slightly raised.

An oblique skin incision is made lateral to the rectus sheath in the center, between the symphysis and umbilicus, starting toward the costal arch in the direction of rib XI.

This is followed by transection of the aponeurosis of the external oblique muscle and transection of the internal oblique and transversus abdominis muscles and the transversalis fascia, and careful release of the peritoneum from the fascia.

Blunt pushing of the peritoneal sac in the medial direction follows. The left kidney and ureter may also be pushed medially here or can be left in a retroperitoneal position, depending on requirements. For ease of exposure, a frame of lockable hooks (i.e., a self-retaining system such as the Omnitract retainers) is very useful. In this way, the whole of the infrarenal aorta, the origin of the inferior mesenteric artery, all of the left common, internal, and external iliac arteries, and the beginning of the right common iliac artery can be demonstrated. If exposure of the right iliac bifurcation or right external iliac artery is also necessary, it can also be done retroperitoneally via a smaller contralateral incision parallel to the right inguinal ligament.

The peritoneal sac must be retracted to the right; the infrarenal aorta with the origin of the inferior mesenteric artery, origin of the right external iliac artery, and common, internal, and external iliac artery are well demonstrated. The ureter remains in its retroperitoneal bed; alternatively, in the retrorenal variant of this approach used to expose the suprarenal aorta as well, the ureter can be repositioned medially along with the left kidney.

Right-sided retroperitoneal access

To demonstrate the right iliac bifurcation and aortic bifurcation, the approach described above can also be used on the right side. However, access to the infrarenal aorta from the right is more difficult, as the small-bowel mesentery and ascending colon also have to be mobilized.

Transperitoneal access

Inguinal vessels: To keep the cooling caused by the laparotomy as brief as possible, particularly when prolonged dissection of the inguinal vessels is expected (e.g., when there is a distal connection to the deep femoral artery with profundoplasty) the inguinal vessels are demonstrated first.

The femoral bifurcation is demonstrated with an incision coursing in the inguinal crease, with the incision direction gradually becoming more vertical, and careful pushing of the lymphatic and fatty tissue from lateral to medial. If there is occlusion of the superficial femoral artery and prolonged dissection of the deep femoral artery is expected, a skin incision lateral to the inguinal vessels is recommended, as this makes the distal dissection of the deep artery easier.

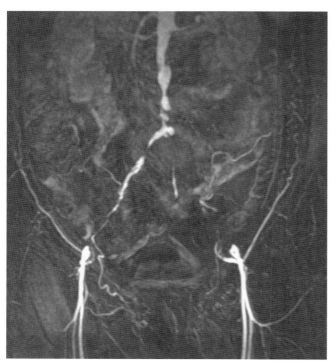

Fig. 4.4-42 Leriche syndrome, Brewster type III. Magnetic resonance angiography: severe aortoiliac arterial occlusive disease on the right side, clinically representing Fontaine stage IV.

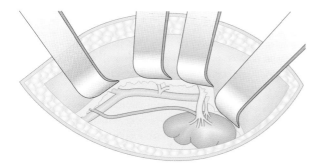

Fig. 4.4-43 Retroperitoneal access (Rob approach). The peritoneal sac is retracted to the right, and the infrarenal aorta with the origin of the inferior mesenteric artery and the origins of the right common, internal, and external iliac arteries on the left are well demonstrated. The ureter is left in its retroperitoneal bed, or—in the retrorenal variant of this access route for additional exposure of the suprarenal aorta—is transposed medially along with the left kidney.

In preparation for the peripheral connection—e.g., when there is stenosis at the origin of the deep femoral artery—TEA of the common femoral artery and deep femoral artery has to be carried out here. If there is a long area of plaque formation, the exploration has to continue beyond the first or second/third lateral branch in the form of a profundoplasty. The patch plasty that is then needed is best made with endarterectomized superficial femoral artery or another biological material such as a strip of bovine pericardium. This material is soft and smooth and is easier to suture to the extremely delicate wall of the deep artery, which is also thin after TEA, than a relatively rigid Dacron prosthesis or a long tongue of the Dacron prosthesis limb used as a patch. It is important to be aware of the femoral nerve, which courses lateral to the vessels. Careful and superficial use of the wound spreader makes it possible to avoid nerve lesions, pareses, and pain syndromes.

Aorta: The median laparotomy from the xiphoid process to the umbilicus, or passing around it on the left, then follows. This ensures adequate exposure of the infrarenal aorta. There is then just sufficient space between the origin of the renal arteries and the inferior mesenteric artery, which may be patent and therefore important, for the end-to-side anastomosis with the vascular prosthesis that is usually carried out. If any fibers from the right lateral hypogastric plexus and passing around the origin of the inferior mesenteric artery are visible, they should be protected as much as possible in order to avoid potency problems. Before the anastomosis is done, local thromboendarterectomy is often necessary, particularly when there is a thrombotic occlusion of the aorta immediately distal to the origin of the renal arteries; suprarenal clamping may be necessary here in some circumstances. The greatest care needs to be taken when pulling the prosthesis limb through the pelvis in order to protect the ureters, veins, and lymph vessels.

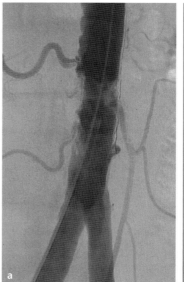
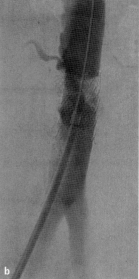

Fig. 4.4-44a, b Special form of aortoiliac arterial occlusive disease in a 48-year-old patient. There is a coral-reef aorta in the infrarenal segment. High-grade in-stent stenosis with severe calcification and recurrent claudication. Pressure gradient 20 mmHg. Thromboendarterectomy with explantation of the stent and patch plasty via a retroperitoneal access route was needed in this case.

Thromboendarterectomy (TEA) and patch plasty

Isolated occlusive processes that are limited to the infrarenal aorta and the initial part of the common iliac artery can be managed using a direct local TEA and direct suturing or patch plasty. This avoids the need to introduce large amounts of plastic material and thus largely excludes the risk of prosthesis infection or ureteral problems—e.g., erosion by the Dacron prosthesis with the resulting deleterious effects.

Stenoses of the infrarenal aorta or ostia of the common iliac artery in particular are often so calcified that they cannot be adequately dilated with balloon catheters, or cannot be kept permanently patent. The left retroperitoneal access route (see above) is useful here. With this approach, the aorta can be clamped at a suitable point, and the external and internal iliac arteries and lumbar arteries can be controlled with slight mobilization of the aorta. Through a longitudinal incision from the aorta into the internal iliac artery, a balloon catheter is placed in the contralateral right internal iliac artery to block the reverse flow.

In what is known as *open* endarterectomy, the aorta/artery is incised longitudinally over the whole occlusion segment, and a suitable layer in the media or internal/external elastic membrane is then sought with the dissector, so that a complete endarterectomy is carried out. The vascular wall is then reconstructed using a direct suture if there is sufficient residual volume, or by suturing in patch material as an enlargement plasty.

In isolated stenoses of the aortic bifurcation, a TEA and patch plasty to form a "Mercedes star plasty" are possible, again with a left retroperitoneal or transperitoneal approach, if the plaques extend far into the right common iliac artery.

In stenoses and occlusions of the aortoiliac and femoral axis, *semiclosed* endarterectomy may be suitable, using the Vollmar method with a ring stripper. The common and external iliac arteries do not have to be completely incised longitudinally to do this. Via several short transverse incisions when the artery has a sufficient caliber, or longitudinal incisions (which can later be managed with a patch plasty) in decisive positions (i.e., the common femoral artery, above the origin of the internal iliac artery, and at the aortic bifurcation) intimal atheroma can be dissected and isolated with the ring stripper and then removed with the dissector, so that a normal lumen is created. The ostium of the internal iliac artery (*caution:* possible vascular erectile dysfunction) is also easily accessed for endarterectomy in this way. If the lumen diameter is not sufficient for direct suturing, each incision has to be closed with a patch plasty, preferably of biological material such as a bovine pericardium patch. If the common iliac artery and aortic bifurcation are involved in the occlusive process, this procedure is elaborate and it may be difficult to control bleeding from the opened vessels. Ring stripper endarterectomy is ideal for occlusions that are limited to the external iliac artery and common femoral artery.

Unilateral aortoiliacofemoral bypass

This operation is probably the most frequently used surgical technique in the whole range of aortoiliac reconstructions, as it is the simplest and fastest and is also very effective. Access is normally retroperitoneal (see above), so that the procedure is also more sparing and can be carried out bilaterally. Numerous types of bypass can be used, depending on the type of occlusion—aortoiliac, aortofemoral, iliacofemoral or iliacoprofundal, and also transverse (see below). The retroperitoneal access route allows occlusive processes in the internal iliac artery to be specifically considered. Patients with this type of occlusion often report erectile dysfunction, with vascular causes, which can also be elegantly treated at the same time as this operation. With an incision over the origin of the internal iliac artery, an endarterectomy can be carried out in that vessel at the same time as the other measures for the aortofemoral/iliacofemoral bypass. However, with this access route, special attention has to be given to the fibers of the hypogastric plexus that course over the common iliac artery, at least in patients who are still sexually active, as injury to the fibers can result in retrograde ejaculation.

Extra-anatomic surgical technique with crossover bypass

If the intention is to perform the operation as sparingly as possible in patients with multimorbid conditions (i.e., avoiding a laparotomy) extra-anatomic procedures are available for long unilateral external/common iliac artery occlusions, such as the femorofemoral or iliacofemoral crossover bypass. After exposure of the femoral arteries (see above), a prosthesis is anastomosed end to side to the donor artery against the direction of flow, pulled through subcutaneously above the symphysis to the contralateral side, and anastomosed there again end to side, so that the prosthesis is moved in a C shape. To ensure stability against kinking and to prevent needle track bleeding, a warp-knit Dacron prosthesis with a diameter of 7 or 8 mm is preferable to an ePTFE prosthesis. For prophylaxis against the theoretically greater risk of infection in the inguinal region, it is best to impregnate the Dacron prosthesis with rifampicin—although rifampicin only binds to collagen-coated (presealed) vascular prostheses. Silver-impregnated Dacron prostheses also appear to have a bactericidal effect that is sustained for weeks or months. When there is a clearly increased risk of infection or an already contaminated inguinal region, the great saphenous vein or alternative veins should be used as the bypass material.

If there is also an iliac stenosis in the donor artery, an iliacofemoral crossover bypass can also be created. However, this requires a slightly more invasive procedure, with exposure of the external iliac artery via a—limited—retroperitoneal access site 5 cm above the inguinal ligament. The vascular prosthesis is either anastomosed directly onto the iliac stenosis, thereby simultaneously producing an enlargement plasty, or if the stenosis is cranial to the anastomosis, it is dilated through the prosthesis or kept patent with a stent. Another option is later percutaneous PTA/stenting via the surgically untouched inguinal region.

Axillobifemoral bypass

If the aorta shows extreme circular calcification and is therefore not capable of being clamped (the extreme example being coral-reef aorta), and/or if the patient is at very high surgical risk (e.g., with severe obstructive pulmonary disease) revascularization of the lower half of the body by creating an axillobifemoral (or actually subclavian bifemoral) bypass is a good solution. The subclavian artery, preferably on the right side (subclavian artery stenoses more often occur on the left side than the right), is demonstrated under the clavicle after transection of the pectoralis major muscle in the

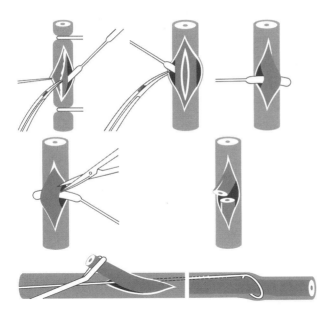

Fig. 4.4-45 Principle of ring stripper endarterectomy. An intimal cylinder is obtained by dissection between the intima and media/adventitia.

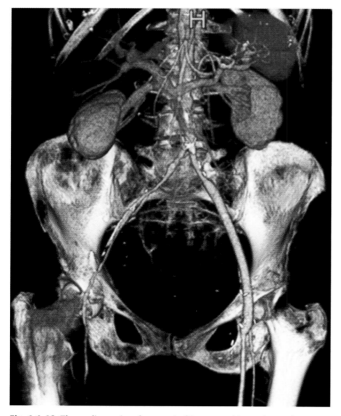

Fig. 4.4-46 Three-dimensional computed tomographic angiography. Severe arterial occlusive disease with a rarefied aortoiliac vascular system and still-adequate perfusion on the right. On the left, there is an iliaco-femoral (Dacron) bypass and a femoropopliteal venous bypass.

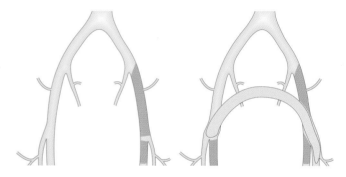

Fig. 4.4-47 A crossover bypass from the right common femoral artery to the left side in a patient with unilateral pelvic occlusion—in this case to the deep femoral artery, due to the occluded superficial femoral artery.

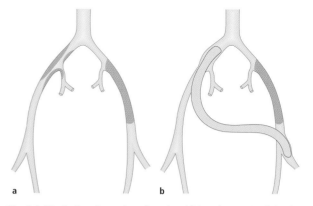

Fig. 4.4-48a, b A variant when there is additional stenosis of the donor artery. Thromboendarterectomy of the iliac bifurcation, with an iliaco-femoral bypass on the right and a femoral crossover bypass on the left.

course subcutaneously, with dressing forceps via auxiliary incisions in the costal arch and in the lower abdomen, and the prosthesis limbs are each anastomosed end to side onto the femoral arteries. This procedure is now rarely used, but may be justified in certain cases; in view of the not infrequent complications (with a great deal of foreign material being used and the risk of prosthesis infection), it must be regarded rather as a palliative procedure.

Thoracofemoral bypass may be mentioned as an exotic variant. In this procedure for revascularizing the lower half of the body (e.g., in patients with Leriche syndrome or coral-reef aorta) the ascending aorta via a sternotomy or the descending aorta via open or endoscopic exposure of the descending aorta is anastomosed, and the vascular prosthesis is pulled through subfascially and preperitoneally to one or both of the common iliac arteries or common femoral arteries and anastomosed. This is rarely useful or necessary.

Y prosthesis, aortobifemoral bypass

With the development of vascular prostheses made of plastic in the 1960s, it became much easier to bridge an aortoiliac occlusion in comparison with endarterectomy procedures. After demonstration of the aorta retroperitoneally or transperitoneally, as described above, the vascular prosthesis, which is usually a presealed collagen-coated warp-knit Dacron prosthesis, is anastomosed proximally end to end or end to side.

If there is residual perfusion of the internal iliac artery circulation, an end-to-side anastomosis is carried out in order to maintain the

direction of the fibers dorsocranial to the subclavian artery over a length of 3 cm. A presealed axillobifemoral Dacron prosthesis (e.g., $10 \times 8 \times 8$ mm with circular reinforcement with a flow divider, similar to a Y prosthesis) is anastomosed end to side to the subclavian artery and then pulled through subpectorally, and in the subsequent

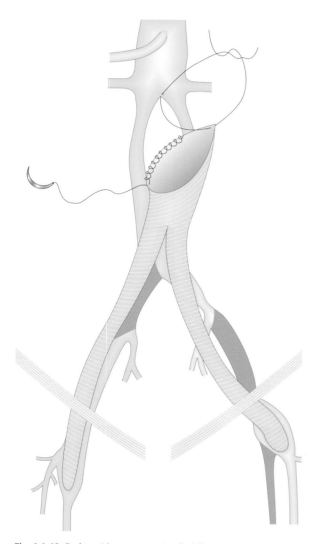

Fig. 4.4-49 End-to-side anastomosis of a bifurcation prosthesis to the infrarenal aorta.

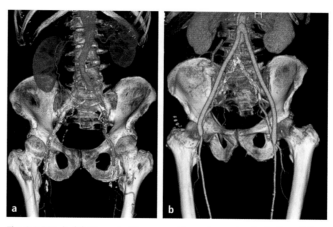

Fig. 4.4-50a, b (**a**) Computed tomographic angiography. Occlusion of the aortic bifurcation, with substantial calcification and small-caliber external iliac arteries in Fontaine stage IIb. (**b**) A bifurcation prosthesis with central and peripheral end-to-side anastomoses, providing retrograde perfusion of the internal iliac region.

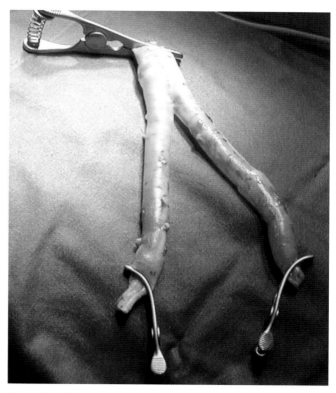

Fig. 4.4-51 A Y prosthesis constructed from the deep femoral vein.

perfusion there and also that of a still patent inferior mesenteric artery. The aortic wall should be semicircularly excised here to avoid creating an anastomosis aneurysm.

If the aortic bifurcation is already occluded, the hemodynamically more favorable end-to-end anastomosis can be created. Immediate contact between the vascular prosthesis and the duodenum must be avoided. As a late complication, erosion of the duodenum by the vascular prosthesis can trigger infection of the aortic anastomosis, with the development of an aortoduodenal fistula and potentially massive intestinal bleeding. If there is insufficient retroperitoneal fatty tissue available for interposition between the duodenum and the vascular prosthesis, part of the greater omentum should be dissected as a pedicle, pulled through a slit in the mesentery, and attached to the aortic anastomosis.

The prosthesis limbs are then moved retroperitoneally, and depending on the pattern of the occlusion it needs to be ensured that there is sufficient retrograde perfusion of the internal iliac artery regions at the femoral connection. If this is not ensured, the aim should be to achieve a side-to-side anastomosis above the origin of the internal iliac artery on the way to the common femoral artery (possibly with simultaneous ostial TEA in the internal iliac artery).

Special forms

Younger patients under the age of 55, and among these women in particular who have what is known as premature atherosclerosis (synonyms for which include hypoplastic aortoiliac syndrome, and young woman's disease) are probably able to benefit to a decisive extent from the vascular replacement material selected. It has been shown in these young patients that plastic prostheses, Dacron, and PTFE often lead to excessive intimal hyperplasia and rapid development of anastomotic stenoses and consequently prosthesis limb thromboses. The use of autologous material is therefore definitely preferable in order to improve the long-term prognosis (Fig. 4.4-51)—e.g., the femoral vein, which is very good for the purpose owing to its caliber (6–12 mm). A length of up to 24 cm of the femoral vein can be removed between the adductor canal and the junction of the deep femoral vein with no risk of deep venous thromboses. However, most vascular surgeons are not familiar with dissection of unilateral or bilateral femoral veins, and it makes the operating time 1–2 h longer. If an additional occlusion of the superficial femoral artery is found during dissection, all collaterals to the popliteal artery and lower leg arteries must be scrupulously protected. Accidental ligation of the collaterals could restrict compensation at the occluded thigh levels and lead to critical ischemia and then possible emergency revascularization at a more distal level.

Specialized surgical procedures

Laparoscopic creation of an iliacofemoral or aortofemoral (unifemoral or bifemoral) bypass is attracting increasing interest in Canada and various European countries such as France, although less so in Germany. In this procedure, five to seven transabdominal or retroperitoneal trocars are instrumented and the aortoiliac segment is usually exposed retroperitoneally and also retrorenally. This minimally invasive procedure requires previous laparoscopic experience, of course, and involves long operating times during the learning curve, but on the other hand the patient's recovery after the abdominal intervention is faster. The procedure is mainly intended for high-risk patients, who must be carefully selected in relation to the feasibility of the operation.

Acute embolism/thrombosis in the aortoiliac segment

Most aortoiliac occlusive processes are chronic and can be treated electively; however, there are also cases of acute arterial embolism or thrombosis in the aorta and iliac artery in patients with existing arterial occlusive disease and severe ischemia in the lower extremity in which immediate action is needed. If the inguinal pulse is absent, CT angiography or MR angiography can provide additional information about the extent of the occlusion or existing arterial occlusive disease. In patients with severe ischemia, immediate exposure of the common femoral artery is also sometimes indicated, with intraoperative balloon catheter thrombectomy, angiography, local TEA, and intraoperative transluminal angioplasty (ITA) or stenting at the pelvic level if needed. It may be possible to carry out this type of intervention with local anesthesia. If recanalization is not possible, a crossover bypass from the contralateral side, which is hopefully patent, or even an (aorto-)iliacofemoral bypass may be created on an emergency basis. Fasciotomy may be necessary in addition in cases of imminent compartment syndrome.

Clinical results

Surgical aortoiliac reconstruction with TEA or bypass procedures was the most frequent vascular surgery intervention in the 1970s and 1980s. Valid results are mainly available for the standard procedure with the aortobifemoral Y prosthesis and are presented in the study by Reed et al. (2003), a meta-analysis by de Vries et al. (1997), and TASC II (Norgren et al. 2007). The perioperative mortality has declined from the 4.6% figure reported in pre-1975 studies to 3.3% after 1975, and is nowadays in the range of 1–3%.

The patency rates in the first few years after the procedure are outstanding at 90–100% (Table 4.4-16), and were found in the meta-

Table 4.4-16 Patency rates with various treatment procedures for aortoiliac arterial occlusive disease.

Patency rate (%)	1 year	5 years	10 years	References
PTA/stent	86 (81–94)	71 (64–75)	?	TASC II
Direct endarterectomy		60–94		Brewster
Semiclosed ring stripper disobliteration	94	83		Van den Dungen
Y prosthesis for claudication	> 90	85–91	86.8	TASC II de Vries
Y prosthesis for critical ischemia	> 90	80–87	81.8	TASC II de Vries
Unilateral aortoiliacofemoral	> 90			TASC II
Femorofemoral crossover bypass	> 90	75 (55–92)		TASC II
Axillobifemoral	> 90	71 (50–76)		TASC II

PTA, percutaneous angioplasty; TASC, Trans-Atlantic Inter-Society Consensus.

Table 4.4-17 Relationship of patency rates to patient age, according to Reed.

5-year patency rates for Y prostheses by age group (%)	Primary patency (%)	Secondary patency (%)
< 50 years	66 ± 8	79 ± 7
50–59 years	87 ± 5	91 ± 4
> 60 years	98 ± 2	98 ± 2

analysis to be higher for claudication (85–91%) than for critical ischemia (80–87%). No stage-dependent differences were found in the study by Reed et al. (2003), but there was a significant difference in the patency rates in different age groups (Table 4.4-17). In the under-50 age group, for example, transplant failure occurred much earlier and more often than in the 50–59 age group, in which it was also more frequent than in those aged over 60. This is thought to be due to a more aggressive form of atherosclerosis in younger patients, the smaller diameter of the aorta and pelvic arteries with the resulting smaller diameter of the vascular prostheses used, and more frequent involvement of multiple levels—e.g., with simultaneous superficial femoral artery occlusion. No advantages with the hemodynamically more favorable central end-to-end anastomosis in comparison with an end-to-side anastomosis have been confirmed.

Late complications

Prosthesis limb thrombosis: Prosthesis limb thrombosis, which is usually unilateral, is the most frequent late complication after aortofemoral bypass, at 5–10% over 5 years. It is due to progression of the atherosclerosis, particularly at the distal anastomosis. This complication can usually be resolved with a prosthesis thrombectomy and anastomosis patch plasty, although this often needs to be performed in emergency conditions with critical ischemia.

Anastomotic aneurysm: Aneurysms of the anastomosis or suture are rare, at 1–5% for the whole working life of an aortofemoral by-pass, but they are potentially a threat to the extremity due to thrombosis and peripheral embolization. Aneurysms usually cause local symptoms, pain and nerve lesions, and timely treatment is therefore possible. Rupture of this type of aneurysm is rare. Treatment consists of replacement of a short length of the vessel connecting to the bridging prosthesis limb with a vascular prostheses or venous segment (femoral vein, if there is a risk of prosthesis infection).

Prosthesis infection: Infections of vascular prostheses may be non-specifically symptomatic and smolder away for many years, kept reasonably in check with antibiotic therapy, or they may lead to acute to septic clinical pictures that require speedy action. Both of the above complications—prosthesis thrombosis and aneurysms—may be caused by infection. Most infections originate in the inguinal region, as a result of the inevitable bacterial colonization.

However, the immediate vicinity of the aorta or vascular prosthesis can lead to erosion of the sensitive duodenum, which then causes infection of the prosthesis and anastomosis, with a potentially catastrophic aortoenteric fistula and massive gastrointestinal bleeding. This may require complete replacement of the prosthesis material with plastic prostheses with anti-infectious silver coating or soaked in antibiotic. The safest way of providing protection against recurrent infection is to use autologous material—e.g., the femoral vein (see above)—as is done in our own institution.

Ureteral complications: The immediate vicinity of the ureter to the iliac artery or a vascular prosthesis positioned parallel to it can lead to urinary stasis due to scar formation. This can usually be temporarily relieved by placing a ureteral catheter (double J). In rare cases, it can lead to erosion and necrosis of the ureter, with urosepsis and prosthesis infection, which then require nephrectomy and replacement of the vascular prosthesis.

Prospects

The indication for surgery in aortoiliac occlusive disease depends on the stage and morphological extent of the disease and the extent of the patient's usually severe comorbid or multimorbid conditions. The most sparing method can be selected depending on the intended effect—i.e., treatment either for critical ischemia or only for claudication. Particularly at the aortoiliac level, interventional procedures are preferable initially, and then the combined hybrid procedure; a unilateral or bifemoral replacement with retroperitoneal access, which is still a sparing procedure, or transperitoneal access, is only selected when these procedures appear impossible. If the patient is at very high surgical risk, the extra-anatomic procedures of femoral or iliacofemoral crossover bypass, or finally axillobifemoral bypass, may be considered. Total laparoscopic aortofemoral or iliacofemoral bypass, which are also sparing procedures, has so far only been carried out in a few centers in Germany. Although it is minimally invasive, with only small incisions, it requires a much longer operating time. Despite all the advances that have been made in interventional and minimally invasive treatment options, the use of open surgical therapy is likely to continue, not least due to the outstanding long-term results it provides.

References

Antiplatelet Trialists' Collaboration. Secondary prevention of vascular disease by prolonged antiplatelet treatment. BMJ (Clin Res Ed) 1988; 296: 320–31.

Balzer JO, Gastinger V, Ritter R, Herzog C, Mack MG, Schmitz-Rixen T, Vogl TJ. Percutaneous interventional reconstruction of the iliac arteries: primary and long-term success rate in selected TASC C and D lesions. Eur Radiol 2006, 16: 124–31.

Balzer JO, Gastinger V, Thalhammer A, Ritter RG, Lindhoff-Last E, Schmitz-Rixen T, Vogl TJ. Percutaneous laser assisted recanalization of long chronic iliac artery occlusions: primary and mid-term results. Eur Radiol 2006, 16: 381–90.

Barbera L, Geier B, Kemen M, Mumme A. Klinische Erfahrungen mit 43 laparoskopischen Rekonstruktionen an der aortoiliakalen Etage. Eine Analyse hinsichtlich Morbidität, Effektivität und Behandlungskomfort. Zentralbl Chir 2001; 126: 134–7.

Bosch JL, Hunik MG. Meta-analysis of the results of percutaneous transluminal angioplasty and stent placement for aortoiliac occlusive disease. Radiology 1997; 204 (1): 87–96.

Brewster DC. Direct reconstruction for aortoiliac occlusive disease. In: Rutherford RB (ed.). Vascular Surgery. Philadelphia, Pennsylvania: Elsevier, 2005.

CAPRIE Steering Committee. A randomized, blinded, trial of clopidogrel versus aspirin in patients at risk of ischaemic events (CAPRIE). Lancet 1997; 348: 1329–39.

Colapinto RF, Stronell RD, Johnston WK. Transluminal angioplasty of complete iliac obstruction. AJR 1985; 146: 859–62.

Comerota A. Endovascular and surgical revascularization for patients with intermittent claudication. Am J Cardiology 2001; 87 (Suppl): 34D–43D.

de Vries SO, Hunink MGM. Results of aortic bifurcation grafts for aortoiliac occlusive disease: a meta-analysis. J Vasc Surg 1997; 26: 558–69.

Di Centa I, Coggia M, Cerceau P, Javerliat I, Alfonsi P, Beauchet A, Goëau-Brissonnière. Total laparoscopic aortobifemoral bypass: short- and middle-term results. Ann Vasc Surg 2008; 22: 227–32.

Dotter CT. Transluminally-placed coilspring endarterial tube grafts. Long-term patency in canine popliteal artery. Invest Radiol 1969; 4 (5): 329–32.

Duda S, Heller S, Wiesinger B, Tepe G. Modifizierte Stents für die interventionelle Therapie der pAVK. VASA 2004; 33 (S64): 55–8.

Duda SH, Wiskirchen J, Tepe G, Bitzer M, Kaulich TW, Stoeckel D, Claussen CD. Physical properties of endovascular stents: An experimental comparison. J Vasc Interv Radiol 2000; 11: 645–54.

Funovics MA, Lackner B, Cejna M, Peloschek P, Sailer J, Philipp MO, Maca T, Ahmadi A, Minar E, Lammer J. Predictors of long-term results after treatment of iliac artery obliteration by transluminal angioplasty and stent deployment. Cardiovasc Intervent Radiol 2002; 25: 397–402.

Gardiner GA, Meyerovitz MF, Stokes KR, Clouse ME, Harrington DP, Bettmann MA. Complications of transluminal angioplasty. Radiology 1986; 158: 201–8.

Goldhaber SZ, Manson JE, Stampfer MJ, LaMotte F, Rosner B, Buring JE. Low-dose aspirin and subsequent peripheral arterial surgery in the physicians' health study. Lancet 1992; 340: 143–5.

Harnek J, Zoucas E, Stenram U, Cwikiel W. Insertion of self-expandable nitinol stents without previous balloon angioplasty reduces restenosis compared with PTA prior to stenting. Cardiovasc Intervent Radiol 2002; 25: 430–6.

Jackson MR, Ali AT, Bell C, Modrall JG, Welborn MB 3rd, Scoggins E, Valentine RJ, D'Addio VJ, Clagett GP. Aortofemoral bypass in young patients with premature atherosclerosis: is superficial femoral vein superior to Dacron? J Vasc Surg 2004; 40 (1): 17–23.

Johnston KW. Iliac arteries: reanalysis of results of balloon angioplasty. Radiology 1993; 186: 207–12.

Jude EB, Chalmers N, Oyibo SO, Boulton AJM. Peripheral arterial disease in diabetic and nondiabetic patients. Diabetes Care 2001; 24: 1433–7.

Kandarpa K, Becker GJ, Hunink M, McNamara TO, Rundback JH, Trost DW, Sos TA, Poplausky MR, Semba CP, Landow WJ. Transcatheter interventions for the treatment of peripheral atherosclerotic lesions: Part I. J Vasc Interv Radiol 2001; 12: 683–95.

Kim JK, Kim YH, Chung SY, et al. Primary stent placement for recanalization of iliac artery occlusions: using a self-expanding spiral stent. Cardiovasc Intervent Radiol 1999; 22: 278–81.

Klein WM, van der Graaf Y, Segers J, Moll FL, Mali WP. Longterm cardiovascular morbidity, mortality, and reintervention after endovascular treatment in patients with iliac artery disease: The Dutch Iliac Stent Trial Study. Radiology 2004; 232 (2): 491–8.

Kröger K. Postinterventionelle Behandlung nach peripheren Interventionen. VASA 2004; 33 (S64): 73–9.

Lee ES, Coleman Steenson C, Trimble KE, Caldwell MP, Kuskowski MA, Santilli SM. Comparing patency rates between external iliac and common iliac artery stents. J Vasc Surg 2000; 31: 889–94.

Liermann D, Kirchner J. Punktionstechniken. In: Angiographische Diagnostik und Therapie. Stuttgart: Thieme, 1997: 30–8.

Mahler F, Do DD, Baumgartner I, Triller J, Zeller T. Techniques of catheter aspiration and local thrombolysis. The Paris course on revascularization 2004: 461–70.

Matsi PJ, Manninen HI. Complications of lower-limb percutaneous transluminal angioplasty: a prospective analysis of 410 procedures on 295 consecutive patients. Cardiovasc Intervent Radiol 1998; 21: 361–6.

Müller-Leisse C, Janßen R, Hajeck KL, Korsten F, Kippels A, Kamphausen U. Perkutane Therapie langstreckiger Beckenarterienverschlüsse: Technische Durchführbarkeit, kurz- und mittelfristige Ergebnisse. Fortschr Röntgenstr 2001; 173: 1079–85.

Murphy TP, Ariaratnam NS, Carney WI, Marcaccio EJ, Slaiby JM, Soares GM, Kim HM. Aortoiliac insufficiency: long-term experience with stent placement for treatment. Radiology 2004; 231: 243–9.

Mwipatayi BP, Thomas S, Wong J, Temple SE, Vijayan V, Jackson M, Burrows SA; Covered Versus Balloon Expandable Stent Trial (COBEST) Co-investigators. A comparison of covered vs bare expandable stents for the treatment of aortoiliac occlusive disease. J Vasc Surg 2011 Dec; 54 (6): 1561–70. e1. Epub 2011 Sep 9.

Norgren L, on behalf of the TASC Working Group. The TransAtlantic Inter-Society Consensus (TASC II) document on management of peripheral arterial disease. Eur J Vasc Endovasc Surg 2007; 33 (Suppl 1): S1–S70.

Önal B, Ilgit ET, Yücel C, et al. Primary stenting for complex atherosclerotic plaques in aortic and iliac stenoses. Cardiovasc Intervent Radiol 1998; 21: 386–92.

Orr JD, Leeper NJ, Funaki B, Leef Jeffrey, Gewertz BL, Desai TR. Gender does not influence outcomes after iliac angioplasty. Ann Vasc Surg 2002; 16: 55–60.

Palmaz CJ, Sibbitt RR, Reuter SR, Tio FO, Rice WJ. Expandable intraluminal graft: a preliminary study. Work in progress. Radiology 1985; 156 (1): 73–7.

Reed AB, Conte MS, Donaldson MC, Mannick JA, Whittemore AD, Belkin M. The impact of patient age and aortic size on the results of aortobifemoral bypass grafting. J Vasc Surg 2003; 37: 1219–25.

Rutherford RB, Baker D, Ernst C, Johnston KW, Porter JM, Ahn S, Jones DN. Recommended standards for reports dealing with lower extremity ischemia: revised version. J Vasc Surg 1997; 26: 517–38.

Scheinert D, Laird JR, Schröder M, Steinkamp H, Balzer JO, Biamino G. Excimer Laser-assisted recanalization of long, chronic superficial femoral artery occlusions. J Endovasc Ther 2001; 8 (2): 156–66.

Scheinert D, Schröder M, Balzer JO, et al. Stent-supported reconstruction of the aortoiliac bifurcation with the kissing balloon technique. Circulation 1999; 100 (Suppl II): II-295–II-300.

Scheinert D, Schröder M, Ludwig J, et al. Stent-supported recanalization of chronic iliac artery occlusions. The American Journal of Medicine 2001; 110: 708–15.

Schulte KL. Interventionelle endovaskuläre Therapie bei Patienten mit der peripheren arteriellen Verschlusskrankheit – Ballonangioplastie. VASA 2004; 33 (S64): 5–7.

Sixt S, Alawied AK, Rastan A, Schwarzwälder U, Noory E, Schwarz T, Frank U, Müller C, Hauk M, Beschorner U, Nazary T, Bürgelin K, Hauswald K, Leppänen O, Neumann FJ, Zeller T. Acute and long-term outcome of endovascular therapy for aortoiliac occlusive lesions stratified according to the TASC Classification: A single-centre experience. J Endovasc Ther 2008; 15: 408–16.

Tetteroo E, van der Graaf Y, Bosch JL, van Engelen AD, Hunink MG, Eikelboom BC, Mali WP. Randomised comparison of primary stent placement versus primary angioplasty followed by selective stent placement in patients with iliac-artery occlusive disease. Dutch Iliac Stent Trial Study Group. Lancet 1998 Apr 18; 351 (9110): 1153–9.

Timaran CH, Prault TL, Stevens SL, et al. Iliac artery stenting versus surgical reconstruction for TASC type B and type C iliac lesions. J Vasc Surg 2003; 38: 272–8.

Timaran CH, Stevens SL, Freeman MB, et al. External iliac and common iliac artery angioplasty and stenting in men and women. J Vasc Surg 2001; 34: 440–6.

Timaran CH, Stevens SL, Freeman MB, Goldman MH. Predictors for adverse outcome after iliac angioplasty and stenting for limb-threatening ischemia. J Vasc Surg 2002; 36: 507–13.

Tsetis D, Raman U. Quality improvement guidelines for endovascular treatment of iliac artery occlusive disease. Cardiovasc Intervent Radiol 2008; 31: 238–45.

Uher P, Nyman U, Lindh M, Lindblad B, Ivancev K. Long-term results of stenting chronic iliac artery occlusions. J Endovasc Ther 2002; 9: 67–75.

Van den Dungen JJAM, Boontje AH, Kropfeld A. Unilateral iliofemoral occlusive disease: long-term results of the semiclosed endarterectomy with the ringstripper. J Vasc Surg 1991; 14: 673–7.

Vorwerk D, Schürmann K. Endoluminale Gefäßprothesen. Fortschr Röntgenstr 2000; 172 (6): 493–9.

Wissgott C, Steinkamp HJ. Perkutane Transluminale Laserangioplastie zur Behandlung der pAVK. VASA 2004; 33 (S64): 18–23.

Zeller T, Frank U, Bürgelin K, Schwarzwälder U, Flügel PC, Neumann FJ. Initial clinical experience with percutaneous atherectomy in the infragenicular arteries. J Endovasc Ther 2003; 10: 987–93.

Zeller T, Frank U, Müller C, Bürgelin KH, Sinn L, Horn B, Roskamm H. Erste Erfahrungen mit einem 6F kompatiblen selbstexpandierenden Nitinol-Stent. Fortschr Röntgenstr 2002; 174: 93–8.

Zeller T. Rekanalisation thrombotischer Verschlüsse Becken-Beinversorgender Arterien und Bypässe durch Rotationsthrombektomieverfahren unter besonderer Berücksichtigung des Straub-Rotarex-Katheters. VASA 2004; 33 (S64): 32–7.

4.4.8   Conservative, endovascular, and surgical treatment for femoropopliteal lesions

Basic anatomy: Reinhard Putz
Epidemiology and etiology: Thomas Zeller
Clinical findings: Thomas Zeller
Diagnosis: Thomas Zeller
Doppler/duplex ultrasonography: Tom Schilling
Differential diagnosis: Thomas Zeller
Conservative treatment: Thomas Zeller
Endovascular treatment: Thomas Zeller
Brachytherapy: Erich Minar
Surgical treatment: Achim Neufang

4.4.8.1   Basic anatomy

Thigh arteries

After passing through the vascular space of the retroinguinal compartment (lacuna vasorum) under the inguinal ligament, the external iliac artery changes its name and becomes the common femoral artery. At this point, it lies just distal to the ligament in the saphenous opening, covered with fascia lata, which is slightly loosened here (Fig. 4.4-52). Medial to it, the femoral vein is closely adjacent, and the femoral nerve courses lateral to the artery, slightly deeper in the fascia of the iliopsoas.

The following arteries branch off from the common femoral artery in this region: the superficial circumflex iliac artery to the iliac crest, the external pudendal arteries to the pubic region, and the superficial epigastric artery, which takes a retrograde course to the abdominal wall. The terminal branches of these arteries enter into small anastomoses with branches of the iliac arteries, which may develop into collateral circulatory pathways.

A few centimeters distal to the inguinal ligament, the deep femoral artery (Arteria profunda femoris, APF), which is similarly quite thick, arises from the (superficial) femoral artery (SFA, Arteria femoralis superficialis). The two branches of the deep femoral artery, the anterior and posterior circumflex femoral branches, span the neck of the femur and the proximal part of the femoral shaft, and branch into the upper parts of the adductors and flexors and the articular capsule of the hip joint. Further distally, the three perforating arteries branch off to the adductors and to the dorsal muscles

of the thigh (Fig. 4.4-52). Anatomic variants occur in up to 20% of cases and mainly involve separate origins of the deep femoral artery (main trunk) and one of its side branches. The lateral and/or medial circumflex femoral arteries may also originate not from the main trunk, but from one of the side branches of the deep femoral artery. If there is obstruction of the superficial femoral artery, both the main trunk of the deep femoral artery and also its side branches may serve as collaterals. In approximately 5% of cases, the deep femoral artery arises from the (superficial) femoral artery immediately or just after the transition to the external iliac artery under the inguinal ligament (high femoral bifurcation). This anatomic variant needs to be taken into account during antegrade puncture.

In its course in the iliopectineal fossa distally in the groove between the vastus medialis and the adductor longus muscles, the superficial femoral artery continues to be covered with fascia lata and passes, at approximately the level of the mid-thigh, under the firm vastoadductor membrane into the adductor canal. Along the course of the canal, the superficial femoral artery turns dorsally and passes, as the popliteal artery, through the adductor hiatus between the two heads of the adductor magnus muscle into the popliteal fossa. While still in the canal, it gives off the descending genicular artery. The transition from the superficial femoral artery into the popliteal artery is defined radiographically on an anteroposterior projection as the intersection of the artery with the femur.

In the popliteal fossa, three pairs of arteries, each with a medial and lateral branch, are given off in tiers to the knee joint and calf (Fig. 4.4-53). These arteries together form the genicular anastomosis, a complex network of delicate arteries all round the knee joint. Unfortunately, the volume of this network is not sufficient for a relevant collateral circulation to develop if the popliteal artery is occluded.

The popliteal artery continues as far as its division into the infrapopliteal arteries, which is usually located approximately 5 cm below the knee joint space. It is divided into three segments: P1, from the distal end of the femur to the upper margin of the patella; P2, from the upper margin of the patella to the knee joint space; and P3, from the knee joint space to the division of the infrapopliteal arteries. A high infrapopliteal bifurcation at the level of the lower margin of the patella may be present as an anatomic variant in approximately 5% of cases.

4.4.8.2   Epidemiology and etiology

In arterial occlusive disease, more than 50% of lesions are located in the femoropopliteal segment. Occlusions are predominant here by a factor of three in comparison with other segments of the vasculature. For pathoanatomic reasons, the occlusions are mostly long and form part of a multiple-level disease. When the femoropopliteal segment alone is affected, the patients may be either asymptomatic if the deep femoral circulation is intact, or restricted by intermittent claudication; when several levels are involved, critical ischemia of the extremity may also be present. The femoropopliteal segment is usually affected in older patients with a diffuse form of arteriosclerosis. There is a high correlation with coronary heart disease and stenoses of the extracranial cervical vessels. The major risk factors are nicotine abuse and diabetes mellitus.

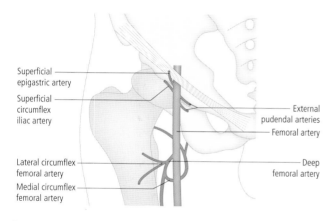

Superficial epigastric artery
Superficial circumflex iliac artery
External pudendal arteries
Femoral artery
Lateral circumflex femoral artery
Medial circumflex femoral artery
Deep femoral artery

Fig. 4.4-52 Branching of the femoral artery in the saphenous opening.

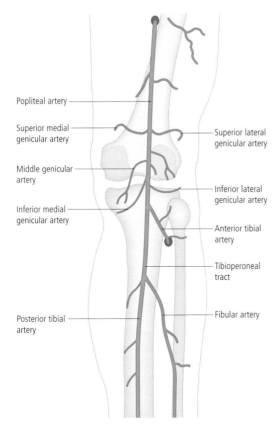

Popliteal artery

Superior medial
genicular artery

Middle genicular
artery

Inferior medial
genicular artery

Posterior tibial
artery

Superior lateral
genicular artery

Inferior lateral
genicular artery

Anterior tibial
artery

Tibioperoneal
tract

Fibular artery

Fig. 4.4-53 Branches of the popliteal artery.

4.4.8.3   Clinical findings

Intermittent claudication is the typical clinical sign. The walking distance to the point at which calf pain starts is the "relative walking distance." The definition of the "absolute walking distance" is the distance after which the pain forces the patient to stop, which depends on walking speed, the gradient of the walking distance, and collateralization. After a few minutes' rest, the symptoms decline and the patient is able to walk a certain distance again without pain. Resting pain or nonhealing lesions are rare when only the femoropopliteal vascular axis is involved and are usually a sign of disease at several levels.

The causes of acute femoropopliteal occlusions are either local thrombosis, usually originating in the adductor canal, or embolism, with the embolus becoming caught in a preexisting stenosis and not being washed as far as the bifurcation of the lower leg arteries. Acute and subacute thromboembolic and local thrombotic occlusions in the arteries supplying the lower extremities are still the most frequent reason for amputation.

4.4.8.4   Diagnosis

■ The physical examination, with inspection (including Ratschow test), palpation (for pulse status), and auscultation at rest and after exercise (for flow murmurs) usually make it possible to identify the level of the perfusion disturbance, along with the patient's history.

■ Pulse volume recording documents the segmental distribution of the perfusion disturbance.

■ Arterial Doppler occlusive pressure measurement at rest and after exercise makes it possible to assess the severity of the perfusion disturbances (with the exception of cases of medial calcinosis).

■ Using a standardized exercise test (with a defined walking distance on a flat surface or on the treadmill—e.g., Bruce protocol: speed 3.3 km/h and 12% gradient) can be used to assess the restriction of everyday activities.

■ Color duplex ultrasonography is used to identify the precise location and extent of the lesion. The morphological assessment of the occlusion can be used to assist in decision-making on whether catheter intervention can be used (and if so which type), and which access route to the occlusion should be selected (antegrade or crossover).

Doppler/duplex ultrasonography

Examination technique

A (5)–7.5 MHz scanner should be used starting the examination at the iliacofemoral transition; in extremely obese thighs, a 3.5-MHz sector scanner can also be used here. The examination has to be adjusted to more difficult ultrasound conditions along the course, particularly in the adductor canal (PRF, gain, insonation direction). Alternatively, insonation from the dorsal direction is possible, often with a better imaging quality. In patients with suspected entrapment syndrome, the popliteal artery should also be examined with active and passive dorsal and plantar flexion.

Differential diagnosis

Classic arteriosclerosis: classic plaque morphology—see under special findings.

Compression syndrome: entrapment syndrome: compression effects on the distal popliteal artery. Evidence of stenosis or occlusion on active and passive dorsal/plantar flexion—best detected actively with the patient standing.

Large-vessel vasculitis: typical intima–media complex with homogeneous hypoechoic widening (halo sign, macaroni sign).

Cystic adventitial degeneration: typically, an hourglass-shaped stenosis of the popliteal artery, thickened hypoechoic wall, with no signs of atherosclerosis and possibly varying degrees of stenosis.

Dissections: typically postinterventional; the floating dissection membrane and partial lumina should be imaged. If necessary when B-mode imaging and color mode are unclear, the color M-mode can be used to demonstrate different color and flow patterns in the partial lumina. The hemodynamics of the lumina should be checked (for possible occlusions and stenoses).

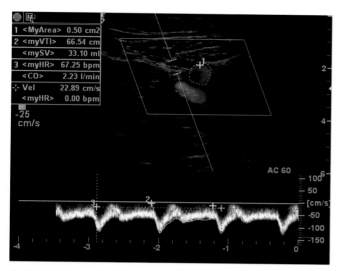

Fig.4.4-54 Flow profile in the common femoral artery, with typically increased diastolic flow as a sign of reduced peripheral outflow resistance in a patient with a (post-traumatic) arteriovenous fistula—measurement of flow volume (for details, see the section on "measurement of shunt volume" in section A 4.2).

Thrombosed aneurysms: there may be evidence of a preexistent aneurysm in a hypoechoic occluded area.

Arteriovenous shunts: A high fistula volume may lead to critical peripheral perfusion in the distal fistula providing artery, with typical pulsatility differences and monophasic flow in the proximal fistula providing artery (Fig. 4.4-54).

Embolic processes: hypoechoic to isoechoic occlusive material, possibly with imaging of a dome phenomenon—i.e., a convex configuration toward the free lumen in the occlusive material. Typical occlusion sites, multilocular processes, otherwise an unremarkable vascular system with no major atheromatosis. There may potentially be emboligenic structures and partly thrombosed or thrombosed aneurysms in the area of the upstream arteries.

Arterial thrombosis: There is no evidence of the criteria suspicious for embolism mentioned above. In addition to the occlusion, there may be evidence of prior arteriosclerosis with echocomplex plaques and structures creating acoustic shadows, possibly with "older" echogenic occlusive components, history of previous PAOD, history of interventional or surgical procedures.

Specific findings

Normal findings

CW/PW Doppler: Regular triphasic flow profile, with a clean acoustic signal with no flow disturbances, steep systolic signal increase, short acceleration time, regular systolic peak frequency or velocity; the systolic peak is sharp, not rounded; regular DIP, free systolic window.

B-mode image: narrow double-line pattern, anechoic vascular lumen, normal vascular diameter.

Color duplex mode: whole lumen filled with color, imaging of the physiological color change (triphasic), no aliasing (with adjusted PRF), no intraluminal jets, demonstration of maximum flow velocities in the central jet.

Early atheromatosis

CW/PW Doppler: normal findings.

B-mode image: widened intima–media complex, possible shallow plaque formation with no relevant lumen reduction; the femoral bifurcation is a site of predilection.

Color duplex mode: still largely normal findings, with the possible exception of a slightly irregular lumen boundary, no relevant flow disturbances.

Mediasclerosis

CW/PW Doppler: normal findings are seen here if the patient has isolated media sclerosis; *caution:* Doppler pressure measurements are not valid. In patients with the polyneuropathy with autosympathectomy that often accompanies the condition, there is a monophasic hemotachogram due to peripheral vasodilation. Differential diagnosis: versus post-stenotic signal showing monophasic distortion, identified above all by noting the acceleration time (short, in contrast to post-stenotic flow) and curve shape.

B-mode image: in patients with mediasclerosis, the vascular lumen is unremarkable, but intramurally there are very echodense (bright), beadlike, nodular structures that create acoustic shadows. If the condition is severe, particularly in the infrapopliteal region, assessment of the lumen behind may be very difficult.

Color duplex mode: the color image may be "disrupted" by color voids when acoustic shadows form, otherwise unremarkable in cases of isolated media sclerosis.

Stenoses

In principle, identical criteria apply for grading stenotic processes using Cw/Pw Doppler, B-mode image, and color duplex ultrasonography in all sections of the arterial pathways in the pelvis and legs.

Low-grade stenosis (< 50%)

CW/PW Doppler:

Prestenotic: the triphasic flow profile is still regular.

Intrastenotic: higher-frequency acoustic signal, increasing systolic peak frequency or velocity, use of the peak velocity ratio (PVR) on the basis of the continuity equation: with a 50% stenosis, there is approximate doubling of V_{max} and the pressure gradient over the stenosis can be estimated using a simplified Bernoulli equation.

Poststenotic: triphasic flow profile still regular, still with a steep systolic signal increase and short acceleration time, shape of the systolic peak still sharp, not rounded; possibly a reduced DIP.

B-mode image: there is usually a widened double-line pattern and plaques of varying morphology at the site of the stenosis, with a luminal reduction of around 50% that can be detected using planimetry. Only the ultrasound morphology of the plaques should be described, with no use of histological criteria such as calcium plaque, cholesterol plaque, fat plaque, etc.

The following are assessed:

- Plaque location and extent: longitudinal and cross-sectional diameters, relationship to the lumen (mural, shallow, semicircular, circular, concentric, eccentric), pulse-synchronous plaque deformation (consistency) and/or longitudinal pulsation (shearing forces), degree of lumen reduction.

Table 4.4-18 Age-dependent and sex-dependent normal values for the double-line pattern (intima–media thickness, IMT) in the common femoral artery (CFA), superficial femoral artery (SFA), and popliteal artery. Data are given as means, standard deviation, and 95% confidence intervals (Temelkova-Kurktschiev et al. 2001) (all data in mm).

	Men 40–54 y	Men 55–70 y	Women 40–54 y	Women 55–70 y
IMT – CFA	0.55 ± 0.11 (0.50–0.61)	0.63 ± 0.14 (0.55–0.71)	0.44 ± 0.10 (0.38–0.49)	0.49 ± 0.08 (0.43–0.54)
IMT – SFA	0.45 ± 0.07 (0.41–0.48)	0.49 ± 0.07 (0.45–0.53)	0.38 ± 0.05 (0.35–0.40)	0.43 ± 0.05 (0.39–0.47)
IMT – Popliteal artery	0.55 ± 0.09 (0.49–0.60)	0.66 ± 0.09 (0.60–0.71)	0.49 ± 0.07 (0.45–0.52)	0.51 ± 0.05 (0.47–0.55)

Table 4.4-19 Duplex ultrasound grading of stenoses, based on the peak velocity ratio (PVR).

PVR	Degree of stenosis
≥ 10	≥ 90%
5–9	approx. 80–89%
5	approx. 80%
3–4	approx. 65–75%
2.5	approx. 60%
2	approx. 50%
1.5	approx. 35%

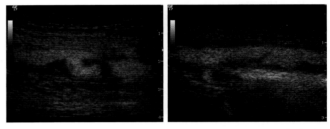

Fig. 4.4-55 Special types of plaque morphology that may be overlooked by angiographic imaging are often found in the superficial femoral artery. Left: undermined, "ulcerated" plaque as a source of peripheral/acral emboli; right: septal plaque.

- Internal plaque echoes: isoechoic with the flowing blood—hypoechoic/hyperechoic, homogeneous/inhomogeneous, coarse/delicate pattern in the internal echo, distribution of various echo qualities, structures creating acoustic shadows (Fig. 4.4-55).
- Plaque surface: smooth/irregular contour, interrupted or continuous border lamella, niches or "ulcerated" segments, floating structures (Fig. 4.4-55).
- Plaque dynamics: changes in the parameters described above during the course of follow-up examinations.

When ultrasound conditions are good and in the absence of major signal voids, cross-sectional planimetry can already be carried out on the B-mode image for guidance, although this needs to be supplemented with color Doppler mode assessment.

Color duplex mode: the lumen is incompletely filled with color; gaps in the lumen are caused by plaques. The contours of the plaques and free lumen are well imaged, particularly with power mode. The lumen reduction that can be quantified in cross-section is around 50%; in the longitudinal section only the diameter reduction can be quantified. Precise cross-sectional planimetry requires painstaking adjustment of the various color imaging parameters (color enhancement, PRF, etc.) in order to avoid either exaggeration of the free lumen or underestimation. The intraluminal jet should be imaged, with an increase in the intrastenotic Doppler frequency/flow velocity and typical turbulence phenomena.

Moderate stenosis (50–70%)

CW/PW Doppler:

Prestenotic: there may be increased pulsatility.

Intrastenotic: Very high-frequency acoustic signal, strongly increasing systolic peak frequency or velocity. The peak velocity ratio (PVR) should be used on the basis of the continuity equation—with stenosis of around 70%, there is an approximate tripling or quadrupling of the V_{max}. The pressure gradient over the stenosis can be estimated using a simplified Bernoulli equation.

Poststenotic: Monophasic flow profile, rather sluggish systolic signal increase and prolonged acceleration time, rounded profile at the systolic peak, clear turbulences. With purely segmental, noncontinuous CW Doppler ultrasound, the level of the primary finding of these post-stenotic flow curves provides evidence of the location of the hemodynamically relevant process.

B-mode image: Widened double-line pattern, plaques of various morphology at the site of the stenosis, with a lumen reduction on planimetry of approximately 70%.

Color duplex mode: the lumen is incompletely filled with color, on the cross-section there is a quantifiable lumen reduction of approximately 70%; in the longitudinal section, only the diameter reduction can be quantified. Imaging of an intraluminal jet with an increase in the intrastenotic Doppler frequency/flow velocity, with clear turbulence phenomena (Fig. 4.4-56).

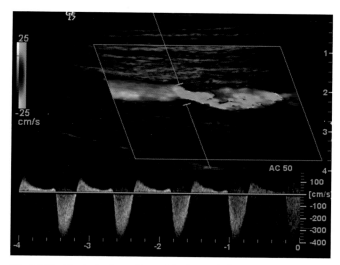

Fig. 4.4-56 A typical color pattern with aliasing (color coding with variance optimizes visualization of hemodynamic effects).

High-grade stenosis (> 70%)

CW/PW Doppler:

Prestenotic: increased pulsatility, or in cases of poor distal collateralization with maximum vasodilation, there may also already be a flow signal with monophasic deformation.

Intrastenotic: Very high-frequency acoustic signal, strongly increasing systolic peak frequency or velocity. The peak velocity ratio (PVR) should be used on the basis of the continuity equation—with stenosis of around 80%, there is an approximately fivefold increase in the V_{max}. The pressure gradient over the stenosis can be estimated using a simplified Bernoulli equation.

Poststenotic: there is a marked monophasic flow profile, with a rather sluggish systolic signal increase and prolonged acceleration time; rounded profile at the systolic peak, marked turbulences.

B-mode image: Widened double-line pattern, plaques of various morphology at the site of the stenosis (see above), with a lumen reduction on planimetry of more than 80%.

Color duplex mode: the color-filled lumen is massively reduced at the site of the stenosis (Fig. 4.4-57), with a high-grade lumen reduction on cross-section. Imaging of an intraluminal jet with an increase in the intrastenotic Doppler frequency/flow velocity, with clear turbulence phenomena and perivascular color artefacts caused by vessel wall vibrations: confetti effect.

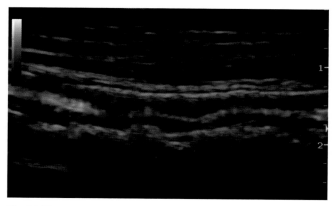

Fig. 4.4-57 A stent in situ, with hypoechoic concentric intimal hyperplasia and a filiform residual lumen (color B-flow).

Occlusion

CW/PW Doppler:

Preocclusive: increased pulsatility, or in cases of poor distal collateralization with maximum vasodilation, there may also already be a flow signal with monophasic deformation.

Occlusion: No signal in the vascular lumen.

Postocclusive: there is a marked monophasic flow profile, with a sluggish systolic signal increase and prolonged acceleration time depending on the degree of collateralization; rounded profile at the systolic peak, possibly marked turbulences due to inflow from hyperperfused collaterals.

B-mode image: Plaques of widely varying morphology in the entire lumen; in cases of fresh occlusion by an arterial embolus or thrombosis, there may be occlusive material that is isoechoic with the flowing blood. In cases of arterial embolus, there may be a dome phenomenon (a convex boundary on the occlusion toward the free lumen). In cases of arterial thrombosis, there tend to be signs of previous atherosclerosis.

Color duplex mode: No color signal at the site of the occlusion. Using a low adjustment of the PRF (or power mode, as appropriate), differentiation from filiform stenoses/pseudo-occlusions and precise assessment of the length of the occlusion are carried out (overestimation is possible with incorrect device settings). Attention should be given to retrograde postocclusive refilling from collaterals that enter distally.

Serial stenotic and occlusive processes

There is an increasing reduction in flow velocity, so that despite higher-grade local stenosis the typical Doppler phenomena may be missed. In these cases, the peak velocity ratio, diameter reduction, and cross-sectional planimetry should be used as tools for grading the stenosis.

Bypass stenosis

In cases of critical stenosis in the proximal or distal anastomosis, or along the course of the bypass, the risk of re-occlusion increases; Table 4.4-20 sums up the duplex ultrasound criteria.

Table 4.4-20 Duplex ultrasound criteria for the risk of occlusion in bypass stenoses (adapted from Mofidi et al. 2007).

Occlusion risk	PSV (cm/s)	PVR	PSV in graft (cm/s)
Low	< 200	< 2	> 45
Moderate	200–350	> 2	> 45
High	> 350	> 3.5	> 40

PSV, peak systolic velocity; PVR, peak velocity ratio.

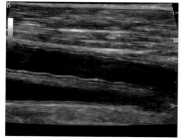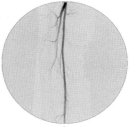

Fig. 4.4-58 "Standing wave" phenomenon in thromboangiitis obliterans, caused by segmental vasospasms. Right: the corresponding angiographic findings.

- Magnetic resonance angiography or computed tomographic angiography can be used to allow better treatment planning when the disease involves several levels, but these can usually be dispensed with.
- The same applies to intra-arterial angiography—because of its inadequate image quality, digital subtraction angiography (DSA) is now obsolete. We perform angiography at the same time as the intervention, and the patient does not usually have to undergo invasive diagnostic procedures before that.

4.4.8.5 Differential diagnosis

See Table 4.4-21.

Table 4.4-21 Differential diagnosis of intermittent claudication.

Symptoms	Diagnosis	Differential findings
Usually symmetrical walking distance-dependent pain stretching from the feet over the calves up to the thigh	Neurogenic claudication with a narrow vertebral canal	No pulse deficit Normal pulse volume recordings and Doppler occlusive pressure
Starting pain in the thigh or calf, with improvement after a longer walking distance	Coxarthrosis and/or gonarthrosis	No pulse deficit Normal pulse volume recordings and Doppler occlusive pressure
Pain during walking, radiating from the buttocks to the outer thigh, calf to back of the foot	Sciatica in lumbar intervertebral disk prolapse	No pulse deficit Normal pulse volume recordings and Doppler occlusive pressure
Pain in the foot and calf after prolonged standing, tendency to improve during walking	Flatfoot	No pulse deficit Normal pulse volume recordings and Doppler occlusive pressure
Typical intermittent claudication	Venous claudication after leg vein thrombosis at several levels, with involvement of the pelvic veins	History of thrombosis Difference in leg circumferences No pulse deficit Normal pulse volume recordings and Doppler occlusive pressure

4.4.8.6 Treatment

Conservative treatment

1. Structured walking training using the Schoop method is indicated for attempted treatment if:
- The collateral circulation areas are sufficient—i.e., there is no stenosis and the first segment of the popliteal artery is free.
- There are no upstream obstructions to the circulatory inflow.

- There are no concomitant diseases that might impede walking training.
- There are no serious occupational limitations or restrictions in private everyday life.

2. Drug therapy:
- The focus here is on adjusting cardiovascular risk factors to ensure secondary prophylaxis against cardiocerebral events. The standard treatment is administration of a platelet inhibitor, usually acetylsalicylic acid (ASA) 100 mg/d; in diabetics, particularly those requiring insulin, the CAPRIE study showed that clopidogrel 75 mg/d has an advantage. In addition, administration of a cholesterol synthesis inhibitor (CSE) and—if there is arterial hypertension with or without renal insufficiency—an angiotensin-converting enzyme (ACE) inhibitor, particularly ramipril, is indicated (ESC Guidelines 2011).
- Vasoactive agents: the only adequately validated data available from randomized studies are for cilostazol (Pletal®), showing a significant improvement in walking distance with a daily dosage of 2 × 100 mg/d. This drug has therefore been included in the guideline recommendations published by the German Society for Angiology.

Endovascular treatment

Indications for endovascular treatment of chronic femoropopliteal lesions

- Decompensation of stable compensated arterial occlusive disease—e.g., due to progressive lower artery lesions in a patient with critical ischemia of the extremity (Fontaine stages III and IV, Rutherford 4–6). The aims of the intervention are to improve arterial inflow into the lower leg, as well as additional percutaneous transluminal angiography (PTA)/recanalization of lower leg artery lesions, as this may also improve the prognosis with the femoral intervention.
- Complicated Fontaine stage II (Rutherford 1–3)—e.g., neuropathic ulcer in diabetes mellitus, mixed arteriovenous ulcer, venous ulcer, requiring compression therapy.
- Intermittent claudication restricting activities of daily life, usually in stage IIb, but occasionally also Fontaine IIa (Rutherford 1–3).

When there are relevant contraindications against contrast media for ionizing radiation (e.g., manifest hyperthyroidosis, borderline renal insufficiency, etc.), a catheter intervention with CO_2 or gadodiamide (Omniscan®, if GFR > 30 mL/min) can be used as an alternative method of contrast imaging with the DSA technique.

Contraindications against PTA

- Asymptomatic occlusive disease (Fontaine stage I, Rutherford 0)
- Massive long calcifications in the occlusive segment are a relative contraindication if alternative options for vascular surgical treatment are available.

Absence of stump of the origin of the superficial femoral artery is *not* a contraindication, as occlusions of the lower leg arteries can also be recanalized.

Patient preparation

- The patient should receive information, including mention of the relatively high risk of recurrence and repeat intervention, and should provide consent on the day before the procedure at the latest.
- Fasting for 6 h beforehand.
- Adequate preinterventional hydration for prophylaxis against contrast-induced nephropathy in high-risk patients.
- Metformin administration should be interrupted at least 24 h before the intervention, particularly in patients with chronic renal insufficiency (due to the risk of lactate acidosis).

Preinterventional and peri-interventional medication

- Chronic prior treatment with ASA 100 mg/d or 500 mg ASA as a bolus before the intervention. This is the accepted standard, despite the lack of data. Clopidogrel 600 mg as a loading dose on the day before the intervention or on the same day is increasingly being recommended, adapted from the procedure with coronary interventions, particularly when stent implantation is planned. However, the necessity for this measure has not been documented by any research studies.
- In patients with a high risk of developing contrast-induced nephropathy, such as those with manifest renal insufficiency or diabetes mellitus, administration of acetylcysteine 2 × 600 mg/d orally on the day before and the day of the intervention.
- After catheter placement, administration of a heparin bolus of 5000 IU. Depending on the duration of the intervention, repeated doses of 2500 IU can be administered. Routine measurement of activated clotting time (ACT) to monitor the peri-interventional anticoagulation status has not yet become an established practice.
- Peri-interventional administration of a glycoprotein IIb/IIIa receptor antagonist during recanalization of chronic femoropopliteal occlusions is associated with a better patency rate, although there is no reduction in peri-interventional embolic events or subacute recurrent occlusions (RIO Study; abciximab, ReoPro®).

Access routes

- Transfemoral antegrade (Fig. 4.4-59) or alternatively via the distal superficial femoral artery (the patient does not need to be turned to the prone position for this, Fig. 4.4-62) if the occlusions are located distal to the femoral bifurcation; retrograde crossover from the contralateral side (Fig. 4.4-60) in occlusions of the origin of the superficial femoral artery or if the patient is substantially obese.
- Transpopliteal retrograde (Fig. 4.4-61) in occlusions of the origin of the superficial femoral artery with no stump at the origin, or when an attempted antegrade recanalization has failed.
- The retrograde transtibial access route via the posterior tibial artery or dorsalis pedis artery is only used in exceptional cases, when there is complete occlusion of the popliteal artery (see section 4.4.9).

Familiarity with the anatomy and ultrasound morphology of the occlusion is essential for planning the correct access route and selecting an appropriate recanalization technique (primary balloon angioplasty, laser angioplasty, local lysis and thrombectomy, etc.)

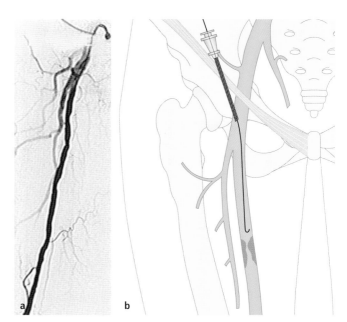

Fig. 4.4-59a, b Antegrade transfemoral access.

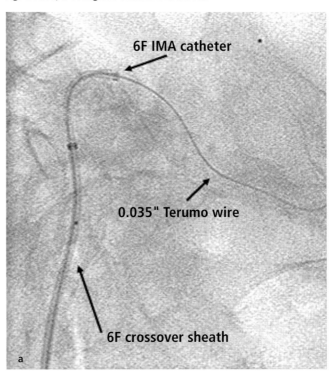

Fig. 4.4-60a–c Retrograde transfemoral crossover access.

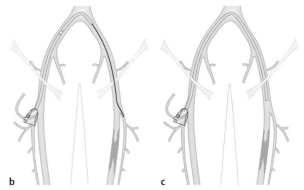

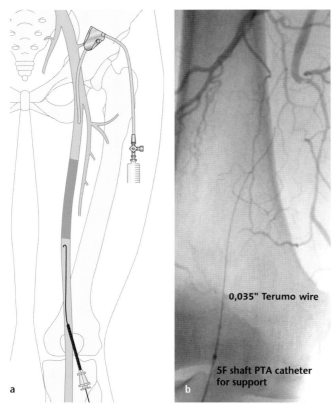

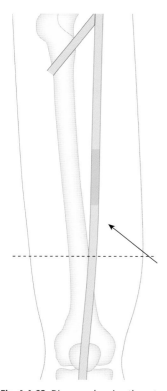

0,035" Terumo wire

**5F shaft PTA catheter
for support**

Fig. 4.4-61a, b Transpopliteal retrograde access (the femoral sheath shown in the graphic should be placed antegrade).

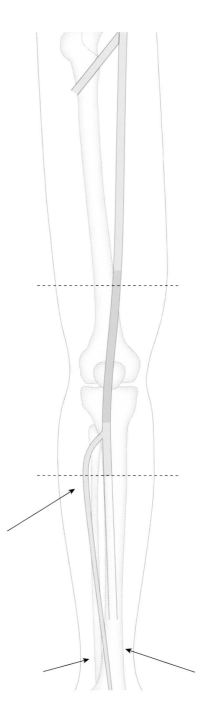

Fig. 4.4-63 Alternative retrograde transtibial access routes when there is occlusion of the distal superficial femoral artery or popliteal artery.

Fig. 4.4-62 Diagram showing the retrograde transfemoral access route proximal to the upper margin of the patella.

Femoral access

3. The *antegrade* femoral access route is the standard approach for occlusions of the superficial femoral artery or popliteal artery that start at least 5 cm distal to the origin, if the anatomic situation permits (e.g., due to obesity or a high femoral bifurcation; Fig. 4.4-59). The argument often raised against the antegrade access route, that the sheath compromises the inflow or that there is compression after removal of the sheath, has not yet been proved. However, the risk of complications, and particularly retroperitoneal bleeding, is increased particularly in patients over the age of 75 in comparison with the retrograde access route. The advantages of the antegrade access route in comparison with contralateral access are that the wires and catheter materials are easier to guide and that there is better contrast in the peripheral vessels due to the selective placement of the sheath tip in the superficial femoral artery. Vascular puncture should be carried out in the common femoral artery distal to the inguinal ligament, but proximal to the femoral bifurcation. It is important to puncture at the level of the head of the femur so that the latter can be used to support compression after removal of the sheath. It is useful to outline the fluoroscopically identified head of the femur on the skin with a waterproof pen before the patient is draped. Local anesthesia and the skin incision can then be carried out approximately 5 cm proximal to the center of the femoral head. Use of an 11 cm long sheath is recommended; the sheath diameter depends on the recanalization technique chosen (5–8F).

4. For the *retrograde crossover intervention* (Fig. 4.4-60), use of a 35–45 cm long crossover sheath (Cook, Terumo, etc.) has proved valuable. After puncture of the common femoral artery under local anesthesia, a 180 cm long stiff 0.035-inch Terumo J wire is advanced under fluoroscopic guidance as far as the abdominal aorta, and the sheath is positioned over the wire at the level of the aortic bifurcation. After removal of the dilator, a pelvic scout angiography is initially done. The actual crossover maneuver is then started. It has proved useful to probe the origin of the contralateral common iliac artery using a 6F LIMA diagnostic catheter (or alternatively Cobra 1, Sidewinder, SOS Soft VU, Sheppard–Hook, etc.), and then to advance the guidewire (e.g., stiff Glidewire, Terumo) into the contralateral femoral bifurcation (Fig. 4.4-60a). In the next step, a 6F or 7F sheath is used to advance the LIMA catheter into the common femoral artery, with the sheath following it in a telescopic technique. The diagnostic catheter is then removed. If an 8F sheath is used, the 6F diagnostic catheter has to be exchanged for the dilator after placement of the Terumo wire in the deep femoral artery, as the size difference between the 6F diagnostic catheter and the 8F sheath is too large (with a risk of plaque rupture or dissection in the contralateral common iliac artery near the origin). If necessary, a switch may need to be made to an extra support wire (Amplatz super-stiff or similar) in order to introduce the stiff 8F sheath.

Popliteal access

Basically, there is experience with three different puncture techniques.

1. Initially, antegrade (or alternatively retrograde) transfemoral placement of a 4F sheath (puncture site: common femoral artery; sheath tip in the deep femoral artery), with good fixation and a long contrast line via the side port of the hemostatic valve. The patient is then placed in the prone position and sterile draping of the popliteal fossa is carried out. Injecting contrast through the femoral sheath allows the course of the popliteal artery to be identified if there is no calcification present. Targeted local anesthesia then follows, and the popliteal artery should be capable of being punctured in the P2 segment. After a repeated contrast injection with fluoroscopy, targeted puncture of the contrast-filled artery is carried out (with a 5F or 6F sheath).

2. The patient is initially placed in the prone position, and the course of the popliteal artery is marked using duplex ultrasonography before sterile draping (this is not as precise as the angiographic method).

3. As in 2, but before the ultrasound marking, fluoroscopy of the popliteal fossa is briefly done to search for any calcification in the popliteal artery. If calcification can be identified, the artery is punctured with continuing fluoroscopy (*caution:* radiation protection for the examiner's hand is required).

Preinterventional angiography

This is used to locate the occlusion precisely and to document the preinterventional lower leg outflow (in case a peri-interventional embolization is needed). It is helpful to use a radiopaque tape measure for later guidance. Imaging should be carried out with a lateral 20–30° projection, so that the femoral bifurcation can be freely rotated. Saving a working image (with overlay or road-map imaging) allows better orientation and reduces the contrast and radiation dosage.

Intervention

Controlled comparative data are only available for treatment of the superficial femoral artery, but not for the common or deep femoral arteries or popliteal artery. This section therefore mainly focuses on treatment of the superficial femoral artery and concludes with a few technical recommendations for treatment of the other vascular areas.

Treatment of chronic lesions of the femoropopliteal circulation

Conventional balloon angioplasty (PTA, uncoated or drug-coated)

Various balloon systems can be used to treat *stenoses,* and can be introduced either over a 0.018-inch or 0.035-inch wire. The standard procedure uses a Glidewire® (standard or stiff, Terumo) with a curved tip. For outpatient procedures, 0.018-inch wire-guided systems are preferable, as a 4F or 5F sheath is sufficient. Only the relevant stenosis of the vessel should be dilated, in order to avoid injury to areas of the vessel wall that are not significantly diseased. The established dilation time is 2 min, although there have been no comparative studies on the optimal PTA technique (to investigate dilation times, the balloon-to-vessel diameter ratio, and dilation pressure).

For recanalization of *occlusions,* a 0.035" antifriction J wire (Glidewire®, Terumo), or a 0.018-inch wire also with hydrophilic coating at the tip (e.g., V-18 Control Wire®, Boston Scientific, Natick, Massachusetts), is used.

In principle, there are two possible techniques for recanalizing occlusions—intraluminal and subintimal wire passage.

In *intraluminal passage,* an attempt is made to pass the whole length of the occlusion intraluminally. However, particularly in chronic occlusions in which the vascular diameter has already narrowed due to fibrotic transformation, this may be almost impossible. Using splinting with a catheter—a special hydrophilic-coated support catheter (e.g., Quickcross®, Spectranetics, Colorado Springs, Colorado); or a straight or angled (vertebral, multipurpose) 4F or 5F diagnostic catheter; or simply a balloon catheter adapted to the guidewire diameter—the occlusion is probed with a straight or curved hydrophilic-coated wire, with gradual advancement of the support catheter after it. An attempt is made to bore an intraluminal channel with the hydrophilic-coated wire tip with the help of a torquer. Specially developed catheter systems (e.g., Frontrunner® XP, Cordis, Crosser®, C. R. Bard) were designed to increase the success rate for passage through intraluminal occlusions. However, no advantage in comparison with the use of a hydrophilic-coated wire has been demonstrated for any of these systems—not even for the excimer laser (Spectranetics). The principal argument in favor of intraluminal passage of occlusions is that it makes it possible to use mechanical catheter systems such as atherectomy and thrombectomy catheters. A new wire system (Enabler®, EndoCross), basically consisting of a compliant balloon, a pressure control unit and a straight uncoated 0.035" wire, has for the first time made it possible to pass even hard femoropopliteal occlusions intraluminally, with a success rate of more than 80% (Zeller et al. 2012). The system cannot be used for occlusions at vascular orifices. The system is based on the principle of placing a balloon catheter approximately 1–2 cm proximal to the occlusion and creating a block there. The straight guidewire is directly placed at the cap of the occlusion and pressure in the balloon is then intermittently increased via the pressure control unit by 2 atm. This expands the tip of the balloon axially to distal and shifts the wire a few millimeters into the occlusion. The pressure is then reduced, and the balloon releases the wire and becomes shorter again. This process is repeated automatically until the occlusion has been passed. Advancement of the wire can also be supported manually (Figs. 4.4-64, 4.4-65, and 4.4-66).

PTA with embolic protection represents a new balloon approach: the Proteus™ catheter (Angioslide) combines the characteristics of a normal PTA balloon (with a balloon length of up to 30 cm) with a protection system. After dilation of the vessel, the balloon pressure is reduced to 2 atm and the distal 50% of the balloon catheter is rolled inwards (invaginated) using a handle at the distal end of the catheter (Fig. 4.4-68). The balloon catheter is then completely deflated. The invagination of the balloon catheter creates a vacuum that is intended to suck any potentially emboligenic material into the balloon. A multicenter study showed that it was possible to remove plaque particles with every balloon catheter, with particle sizes > 2 mm long in 25% of cases. However, the clinical relevance of this angioplasty technique is as yet unclear.

The technique of *subintimal vascular recanalization* (Fig. 4.4-67) allows the wire to be placed in the subintimal vascular wall layer using an angled catheter, with the occlusion being completely passed at the subintimal level (the Bolia technique). This is usually achieved with a loop of a hydrophilic-coated wire. Reentry into the true lumen may be problematic, particularly when there are severely calcified wall layers in the postocclusive vascular area. Reentry is achieved either using continuous advancement of the catheter loop, the spring force of which leads to penetration of the intima and consequently intraluminal positioning of the wire (*caution:* compromise of deep collaterals must be avoided in the distal segment of the superficial femoral artery); or with targeted navigation of the re-straightened recanalization wire, possibly guided with a curved 4F or 5F diagnostic catheter (e.g., vertebral artery, Bernstein, or Judkins right). Re-

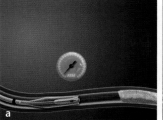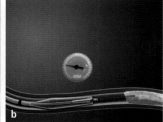

Fig. 4.4-65a, b With increasing balloon pressure, the balloon tip expands distally and pushes the wire into the occlusion.

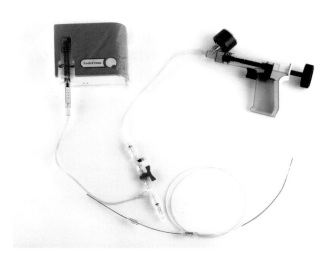

Fig. 4.4-64 The Enabler recanalization system, consisting of a balloon catheter, inflator/deflator, and pressure control unit.

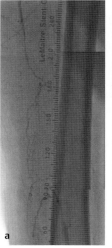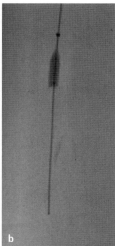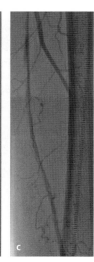

Fig. 4.4-66a–c Example case of a medium-length occlusion in the left superficial femoral artery before and after passage with the Enabler.

canalization success rates of over 90% have been reported with this technique. Using what are known as reentry systems (Outback®, Cordis J&J, Fig. 4.4-69; Pioneer®, Medtronic), the primary success rate can be increased to nearly 100%. The rationale behind primary subintimal vascular recanalization is to create a new smooth lumen free of thrombi and atheromas, thereby reducing the risk of embolism and avoiding the need for stent implantation. Factors limiting the technique include severely calcified plaques in the closed true lumen, which compress the newly created false lumen to such an extent that stent implantation is unavoidable.

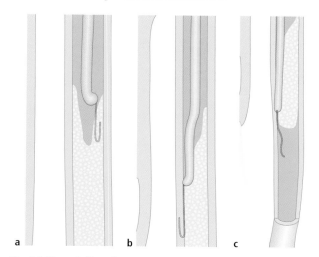

Fig. 4.4-67a–c Bolia technique for subintimal passage of an occlusion. (a) Penetration of the intima with a curved 4F or 5F diagnostic catheter and a hydrophilic wire proximal to the occlusion. (b) Subintimal passage of the occlusion with a small loop of the wire. (c) Reentry of the wire (either spontaneously or guided with a curved support catheter) into the true lumen distal to the occlusion.

After successful passage of the occlusion with the guidewire, the occlusion is dilated from distal to proximal in overlapping steps with the balloon catheter (2 min per segment; the inflation pressure depends on the rigidity of the occlusion and the size ratio of the balloon to the vascular diameter—usually 2 atm above the pressure needed to completely expand the balloon). Balloon lengths of up to 30 cm are now available that substantially reduce dilation times for longer occlusions and show better angiographic acute results (Admiral® extreme, Medtronic-Invatec; Proteus®, Angioslide).

Depending on the results of the primary dilation (the aim being to achieve a residual stenosis of ≤ 30%), a second dilation may be carried out in which thrombi are aspirated, or more rarely local lysis is carried out, or stenting if there is imminent re-occlusion (or dissection).

When recanalization of the femoropopliteal circulation has been completed, angiogram of the infrapopliteal circulation is obligatory (to exclude emboli or wire-induced dissection).

A promising and easily implemented approach is to apply a drug with antiproliferative effects to the vascular wall during balloon dilation. Four randomized studies and an Italian registry study (THUNDER, FEMPAC, LEVANT 1, PACIFIER) on paclitaxel-coated balloon catheters, which release the drug in the vessel wall during balloon dilation, have in the meantime shown that there is a highly significant reduction in the rate of restenosis in comparison with conventional PTA. In the THUNDER study, these results were sustained for up to 5 years after the treatment. Interestingly, dissections after drug-coated balloon angioplasty do not appear to have a negative effect on patency rates; on the contrary, in significant but not flow-limiting dissections it was found that positive remodeling occurred. Coated balloon catheters from various manufacturers (Medtronic-Invatec, Medrad, Eurocor, Bard-Lutonix etc.) have been approved for femoropopliteal procedures since May 2009.

Step 1: angioplasty

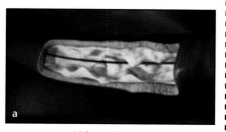

Wire passage

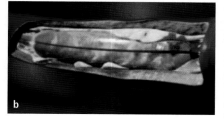

Balloon inflation 8 atm

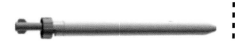

Step 2: Removal of embolic particles

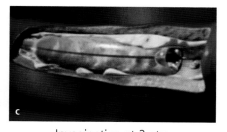

Invagination at 2 atm

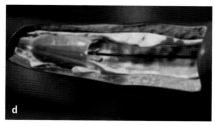

Creating negative pressure

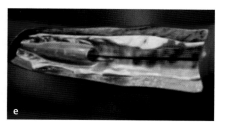

Suctioning particles

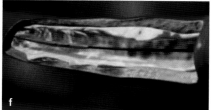

Balloon deflation & withdrawal

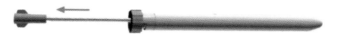

Fig. 4.4-68a–f The principle of Proteus-angioplasty.

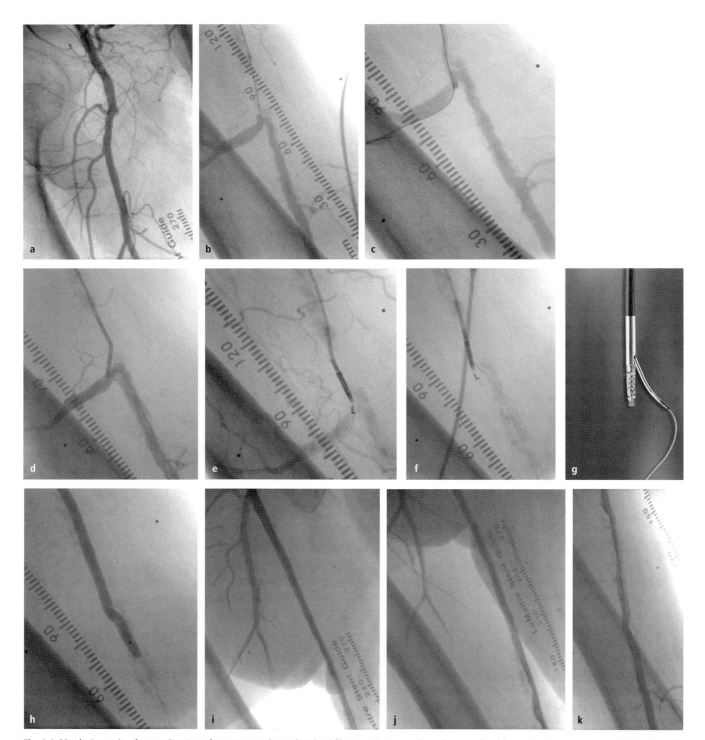

Fig. 4.4-69a–k Example of an application of a reentry catheter (Outback®). An occlusion in the right superficial femoral artery is passed subintimally with the Glidewire®, which can only be placed in a deep collateral. The true lumen is punctured with the Outback® catheter, and the final result after percutaneous transluminal angioplasty and distal stent implantation is shown.

Stent angioplasty (uncoated and drug eluting)

With the exception of one study, the FAST study, in which a first-generation self-expanding nitinol stent (Luminexx™) was used, all controlled studies comparing primary stenting and "provisional" stenting after unsatisfactory PTA results with balloon angioplasty alone ended with significantly better patency rates for the stent groups, independently of the stent type used (Fig. 4.4-71). The advantage of stenting becomes all the greater the longer the lesions being treated are.

On the basis of the available data, balloon-expandable stents should today only be used in severely calcified lesions in which nitinol stents would be compressed. In this type of lesion, the results with balloon-expandable stents are comparable with those for nitinol stents in lesions with minor calcification. Alternatively, specially woven nitinol stents with a closed cell design such as the Supera™ stent (IDEV) and Samba™ stent (NovoStent) can be used even with severely calcified lesions, since in their fully expanded state they have a compression resistance up to four times that of traditional slotted tube laser-cut nitinol stents. In addition, both stent types have the advantage of excellent flexibility, preventing kinking of the vessel at the edges of the stent (kink stenosis, Figs. 4.4-72 and 4.4-73).

In general, it is not yet clear whether there are relevant differences between the various nitinol stents available on the market with regard to patency rates. The first-generation nitinol stents (e.g., Luminexx™ and Smart™) showed a remarkably high rate of fracture—although in contrast to initial assumptions, no direct connection was found between the stent fracture rate and the recurrent stenosis rate (Table 4.4-22).

TASC 2000: Morphological stratification and treatment of femoropopliteal lesisons (adapted from J Vasc Surg 2000; 31 [1Pt 2]: S104, Recommendation 34/35; crit. issue 14)		TASC II 2007: TASC classification and treatment of femoral popliteal lesions (adapted from Europ J Vasc Endovasc Surg 2007; 33 [Suppl 1]: S58–S59; Recommendation 37)	
TASC type A lesions: *Endovascular treatment of choice*		**TASC type A lesions:** *Endovascular therapy is the treatment of choice*	
1. Single stenosis up to 3 cm in length, not at the origin of the superficial femoral artery or the distal popliteal artery	4 cm	1. Single stenosis ≤ 10 cm in length 2. Single occlusion ≤ 5 cm in length	
TASC type B lesions: *Currently, endovascular treatment is more often used but insufficient evidence to make recommendation*		**TASC type B lesions:** *Endovascular treatment is the preferred treatment*	
2. Single stenosis or occlusions 3–5 cm long, not involving the distal popliteal artery 3. Heavily calcified stenoses up to 3 cm in length 4. Multiple lesions, each less than 3 cm (stenoses or occlusions) 5. Single or multiple lesions in the absence of continuous tibial runoff to improve inflow for distal surgical bypass	5–6 cm 4 cm 4 cm	3. Multiple lesions, each ≤ 5 cm (stenoses or occlusions) 4. Single stenosis or occlusion ≤ 15 cm, not involving the infrageniculate popliteal artery 5. Single or multiple lesions in the absence of continuous tibial vessels to improve inflow for a distal bypass 6. Heavily calcified occlusions ≤ 5 cm in length 7. Single popliteal stenosis	
TASC type C lesions: *Currently, surgical treatment is more often used but insufficient evidence to make recommendation*	3–5 cm	**TASC type C lesions:** *Surgery is the preferred treatment for good-risk patients*	
6. Single stenosis or occlusion longer than 5 cm 7. Multiple stenoses or occlusions, each 3–5 cm, with or without heavy calcification	4–5 cm 4–5 cm	8. Multiple stenoses or occlusions, totalling > 15 cm, with or without heavy calcification 9. Recurrent stenoses or occlusions that need treatment after two endovascular interventions	
TASC type D lesions: *Surgical treatment of choice*		**TASC type D lesions:** *Surgery is the treatment of choice*	
8. Complete common femoral artery or superficial artery occlusions or complete popliteal and proximal trifurcation occlusions	> 5 cm	10. Chronic total occlusion of the CFA or SFA (> 20 cm, involving the popliteal artery) 11. Chronic total occlusion of popliteal artery and proximal trifurcation vessels CFA, common femoral artery; SFA, superficial femoral artery.	

Fig. 4.4-70 TASC I (2000) versus TASC II (2007) recommendations on the treatment of femoropopliteal lesions.

Table 4.4-22 Stent fracture rate and restenosis rate with various types of nitinol stent.

Study	Fracture rate	Restenosis rate
Vienna (Dynalink & Absolute)	1% (6 months)	25% (6 months)
FAST (Luminexx)	12% (6 months)	21% with fracture (6 months) 28% without fracture (6 months)
SIROCCO (Smart)	9% and 18% (6 months)	18% and 0% (6 months)
RESILIANT	3.1% (12 months)	18.7% (12 months)
ZILVER randomized	0.9% (12 months)	27% (BMS, 12 months)

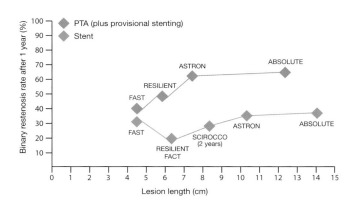

Fig. 4.4-71 Randomized and controlled studies comparing nitinol stenting with balloon angioplasty for femoropopliteal lesions.

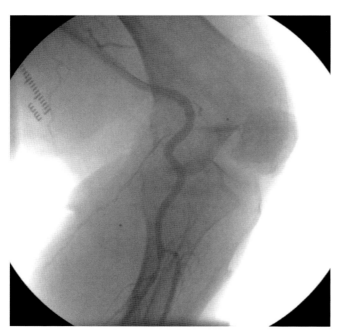

Fig. 4.4-72 The popliteal artery after recanalization and overlapping implantation of two Supera stents as far as the tibioperoneal tract, with 90° knee flexion.

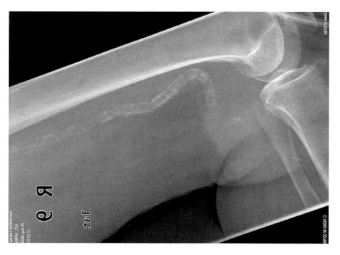

Fig. 4.4-73 A Hyperion stent (the predecessor of the Samba™ stent) in the middle popliteal artery, with the knee in 90° flexion.

More recent stents (e.g., LifeStent™, C.R. Bard; Ever-Flex™, ev3, Inc.; Supera™, IDEV) are more fracture-resistant and more flexible, although they have not been shown to provide better patency rates. The main problem with stent fracture, in addition to the potential injury to the vessel (with pseudoaneurysm), is blocking of the vessel lumen by dislocated stent fragments, which can make a repeat intervention impossible.

The first two studies on drug releasing nitinol stents (drug eluting stents, DES) produced sobering results. The SIROCCO study found no benefit with sirolimus release for a maximum of 30 days in relation to the 1-year and 2-year patency rates, although the 2-year restenosis rate was remarkably low at 25% both for the uncoated and drug eluting Smart™ stent. The STRIDES study, which used a stent releasing everolimus, found a lower restenosis rate after 6 months than had been observed in the historical control group in the Vi-

enna ABSOLUTE study, but after 1 year no further difference was noted. By contrast, the polymer-free paclitaxel-coated Zilver™ PTX stent (Cook Medical) documented a significantly better patency rate for up to 2 years both in comparison with PTA and also in comparison with implantation of the identical uncoated Zilver™ stents (Fig. 4.4-74).

The results of the stent studies have led to further liberalization of the TASC II recommendations (Fig. 4.4-70). Intervention is now regarded as being indicated in TASC B lesions up to 15 cm long.

Endoprosthesis implantation

Balloon-expandable and self-expanding endoprostheses (covered stents) are available for peripheral use. While the balloon-expandable systems (e.g., Jostent™ graft, Abbott Vascular) are mainly used to treat complications such as perforations, it is hoped that the use of self-expanding stent prostheses may lead to improved long-term patency rates, as they have fewer components that can lead to recurrent stenosis due to neointimal hyperproliferation. A randomized study is currently in progress comparing the Viabahn™ endoprosthesis (W.L. Gore) with nitinol stents in the follow-up phase, a registry study on the treatment of long superficial femoral artery lesions treated with up to two 25-cm long endoprostheses; it was still recruiting patients up to August 2012. Potential disadvantages of using self-expanding endoprostheses include the sheath size needed for these large-caliber systems (≥ 7F or 8F), the occlusion of side branches, a nonspecific systemic febrile reaction to the graft resembling Dressler syndrome, and their high cost. Due to the relatively low radial force of the endoprostheses, particularly when used in recurrent stenoses and occlusions, it is important to create an adequate lumen to allow the prosthesis to be introduced and expanded. Particularly in cases of in-stent recurrent occlusion, atherectomy or thrombectomy if appropriate can be recommended before implantation of the endoprosthesis. Endoprostheses up to 15 cm long are available.

Atherectomy

Photoablation (excimer laser): contact laser is the oldest technique for removing atheromas. No clear advantage has yet been demonstrated with the use of lasers for femoropopliteal occlusions. The randomized PELA study (comparing PTA with laser in occlusions of the superficial femoral artery < 10 cm long) only showed a reduced stenting rate in the laser group. Technological advances such as the Turbo Elite™ and Turbo-Booster™ (Fig. 4.4-75a) may potentially be able to increase the effectiveness of laser atherectomy, but have not yet been tested in controlled studies.

Technique of laser atherectomy (with the over-the-wire system):

- Placement of a hydrophilic-coated 0.018-inch or 0.035-inch guidewire and the excimer laser catheter (2.2 mm, 7F or 2.5 mm, 8F) over the occlusive stump.
- Attempted penetration of the occlusion with the guidewire using splinting with the laser catheter. If this is not successful, the laser catheter can be placed without wire guidance on the cap of the occlusion and a laser series can be applied without pressure. This penetrates the fibrous cap of the occlusion, and the guidewire can then usually be advanced without effort into the occlusion. In the step-by-step technique, the occlusion is probed with the guidewire for a few centimeters, and the laser catheter follows it

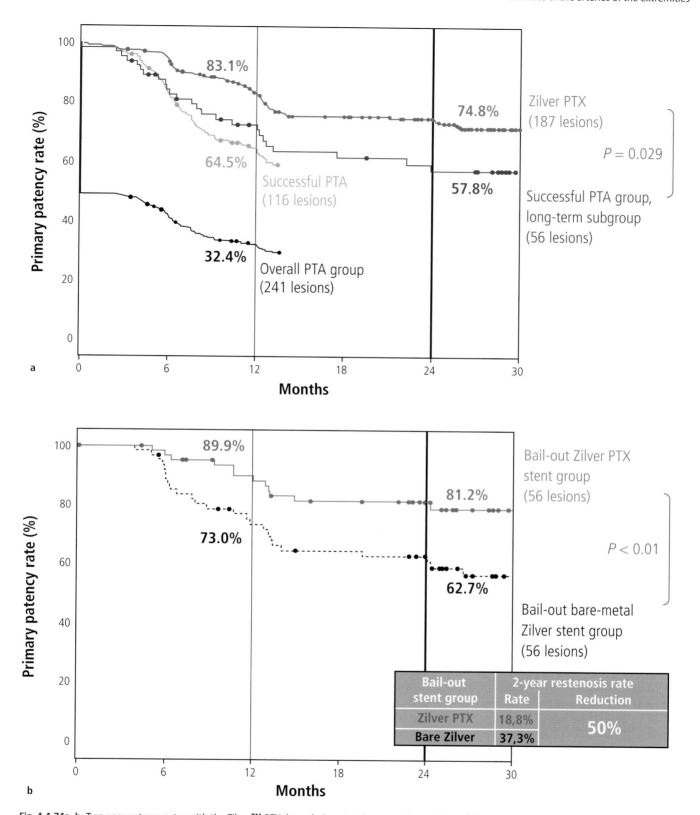

Fig. 4.4-74a, b Two-year patency rates with the Zilver™ PTX drug-eluting stent in comparison with PTA (**a**) and in comparison with an uncoated Zilver™ stent (**b**).

with energy being applied (with a pushing speed of 1 mm/s). The procedure is repeated until the occlusion has been completely passed. After this, the occlusion can be passed once again with the laser catheter if needed, although a saline rinse through the guidewire lumen is then needed.

- Once a pilot channel has been established, the occlusion is passed once again with the Turbo-Booster™ catheter at least four times rotating in quadrants or until the desired final results have been achieved.

Directional atherectomy: The SilverHawk™ catheter (ev3, Inc.; Fig. 4.4-75b) is a 0.014-inch guidewire-controlled (monorail) atherectomy catheter with an eccentrically placed cutting device that also allows eccentric atheromas to be removed. Due to its limited reservoir capacity, the system has to be regularly cleansed of excised atheroma material during the intervention. A further development of the catheter (the TurboHawk™) has also made it possible to treat calcified lesions, although a distal protection filter (e.g., Spider™, Covidien-ev3) should be used in all cases during the treatment of such lesions. However, severely calcified stenoses often have to be predilated, as the lesion first has to be passed with the catheter tip ("nose cone") before the cutter comes into contact with the atheroma. The results of our own registry study and of a larger American multicenter registry show high primary success rates even with occlusions; additional balloon dilations are needed in 10–20% of cases. The 1-year patency rates for short de novo lesions up to 5 cm long are over 80%. A multicenter registry study including 800 patients (DEFINITIVE LE) will be able to provide further information about differential indications for atherectomy. Ideal indications for this procedure are segments involved in movement (common femoral artery, femoral bifurcation, popliteal artery), as well as in-stent recurrent stenoses (this is an off-label use). Subgroup analyses of the registries mentioned indicated a particularly favorable effect in diabetics. Fresh thrombotic occlusions are rather unsuitable due to the potential risk of embolism, unless a protection system is used. Technique of SilverHawk atherectomy:

- Passage of the lesion either with a 0.014-inch guide catheter (e.g., Pilot™, Abbott Vascular; Galeo™ ES, Biotronik) in case of stenoses, or with a 0.035-inch hydrophilic-coated guidewire that is exchanged for a 0.014-inch wire after the occlusion has been passed.
- After the catheter has been introduced, at least 12 passages of the lesion with the atherectomy catheter should be carried out. Using a grid button, the catheter can be rotated in 10° steps, so that with a 30° rotation after each passage of the vessel lesion, one circumferential atherectomy is completed. Residual plaques can then be removed in a targeted fashion. The decisive aspects for avoiding potential embolism are that the catheter should only be moved forward when it is in the activated state and that atherectomized material should be regularly cleared.
- Additional procedures such as PTA or stenting are only necessary in occasional cases.

Rotation aspiration atherectomy (Fig. 4.4-75c): rotation aspiration atherectomy (Jetstream™, Pathway Medical Technologies, Redwood City, California) is the newest method of atherectomy. The catheter is led over a 0.014-inch guidewire, and the current version has 2.1-mm and 3.0-mm atherectomy in its single head. Continuous suc-

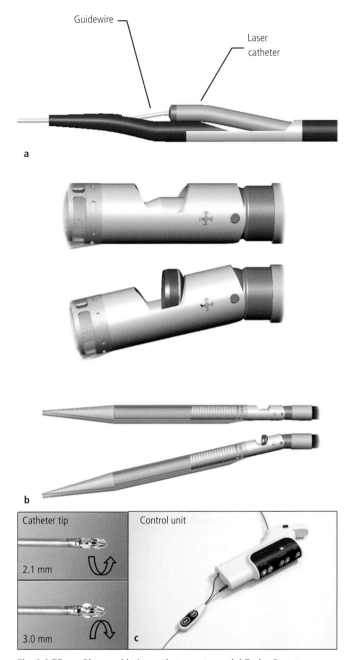

Fig. 4.4-75a–c Plaque-ablating catheter systems. (**a**) Turbo-Booster. (**b**) SilverHawk. (**c**) Jetstream.

tion irrigation allows continuous removal of the atherectomized material. Strict intraluminal use of the system is necessary, as otherwise there is a substantial risk of perforation. An initial multicenter study showed that the system can be well used in calcified lesions and that additional PTA is necessary with vascular diameters larger than 4.5 mm. A planned 4-mm atherectomy system is intended to allow effective treatment of vessels up to a nominal diameter of 6 mm. The system has been approved with certification since May 2009. Due to the continuous aspiration of the atherectomized material, the system is also suitable for treating subacute occlusions with a high thrombus burden—e.g., recurrent in-stent occlusions. As with directional atherectomy, diabetic patients can benefit from Jetstream atherectomy to the same extent as nondiabetics.

Technique of Jetstream atherectomy:

- Passage of the lesion either with a 0.014-inch guidewire (e.g., Pilot™ 300 cm long, Abbott Vascular; Extrasupport™, Abbott Vascular) in case of stenoses, or in occlusions with a 0.035-inch hydrophilic-coated guidewire that is exchanged for a 0.014-inch wire once the occlusion has been passed.

- As with the laser catheter, there is an initial passage of the lesion with the 2.1-mm head size (clockwise rotation), with an advancement speed of about 1 mm/s. If the rotation speed declines in spite of the slow advancement speed, the catheter should only be advanced further again once the rotation speed has returned to normal. Withdrawing the catheter in the activated state is not recommended. After the first complete passage, the catheter is positioned proximal to the lesion again, and it is passed a second time in the same way using the 3.0-mm head size (with counterclockwise rotation). If appropriate, further dilation can be carried out with a 5-mm or 6-mm balloon catheter.

Endovascular brachytherapy to prevent recurrences

This involves local intravascular application of ionizing radiation to prevent recurrent stenoses after endovascular revascularization. Despite the limited use of this form of treatment for logistic reasons, it is currently an effective method of avoiding recurrent stenosis and is therefore discussed here in detail.

Pathophysiological background: the treatment approach of irradiating the vascular wall for prophylaxis against recurrent stenosis is based on discoveries regarding the pathogenesis of recurrent stenosis. Recurrent stenosis is an excessive response by the vessel wall to the injury caused during the intervention. Excessive scar formation (keloids) has long been successfully treated using local radiation therapy. Increased cell growth in malignant diseases can also be prevented with radiation therapy. It was therefore an obvious step to attempt to influence the processes that lead to recurrent stenosis by carrying out brachytherapy immediately after PTA or stent implantation. The validity of the principle underlying this approach has been confirmed in animal experiments.

Foundations of radiation physics and dosimetry: in principle, either beta or gamma emitters can be used in intravascular brachytherapy:

- Beta emitters (electrons): these have a narrow depth of travel, and the beta emitters that used to be used for this indication for large-caliber peripheral vessels (diameter > 4 mm) were therefore not very suitable. However, this disadvantage has been overcome by the use of the fluid beta emitter rhenium-188, which is introduced into the target lesion via a special application set directly over a conventional PTA balloon. The main advantage of using a beta emitter is that the brachytherapy can be carried out immediately after the revascularization procedure in the catheter laboratory.

- Gamma emitters (photons): these have a longer range and are therefore also suitable for peripheral vessels. Iridium-192 is the main agent that has so far been used. The major disadvantage of using a gamma emitter is that local postprocedural radiotherapy cannot be carried out in the catheter laboratory; patients have to be transported to the radiotherapy department with the catheter in place. In addition, many hospitals do not have such a department. This is the main reason why this form of treatment has not ultimately come into widespread use, for logistic reasons.

Radiation dosage: this is defined as the energy absorbed per kilogram of matter; the unit is Gray (Gy), with 1 Gy = 1 J/kg. This is a very small amount of energy. However, as the energy is in the form of ionizing radiation, it has a powerful biological effect. The effective dose range for preventing recurrent stenosis is a single dose of approximately 15–20 Gy. The dosage details familiar from tumor therapy are usually higher, but they refer to the total dosage administered in fractionated single doses. Due to cellular recovery processes between applications, the biological effect of this total dosage on the target tissue is not directly comparable with a single dose.

The target cells in brachytherapy for prevention of recurrent stenosis are located in the area of the vascular wall media and adventitia. However, the luminal lining of endothelial cells needs to be protected as much as possible, particularly due to its antithrombogenic properties. To reach the outer layers of the vascular circumference with an effective dosage while at the same time sparing the endothelium as much as possible, as low as possible a radial dosage decline in the vessel wall is preferable. The problem with the radial dosage distribution is considerably exacerbated by the asymmetric plaque formations that are often present. This usually leads to varying distances between the geometric center of the lumen and the target volume. During brachytherapy planning, attention therefore needs to be given to achieving an adequate dosage in the area of the outer media and adventitia even when there is marked thickening of the vascular wall.

Terminology in intravascular brachytherapy (Fig. 4.4-76): a systematic and common terminology is needed for the planning and implementation of this form of treatment, as well as for comparing the results of different studies. Relevant recommendations have been published by the endovascular group of the European Society for Radiotherapy and Brachytherapy.

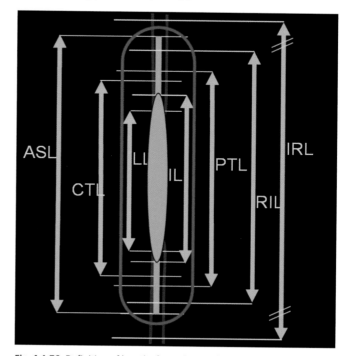

Fig. 4.4-76 Definition of lengths for endovascular brachytherapy in accordance with the recommendations of the European Society for Radiotherapy and Brachytherapy (adapted from Potter et al. 2001). ASL, Active Source Length; CTL, Clinical Target Length; IL, Interventional Length; IRL, Irradiated Length; LL, Lesion Length; PTL, Planning Target Length; RIL, Reference Isodose Length.

Intravascular brachytherapy procedure

Only systems currently available on the market are discussed here.

- *Application of a beta emitter (strontium-90) using an afterloader system,* in which a centering catheter is inflated using CO_2 (Novoste Corp.). The results of a study conducted with this system have unfortunately never been published. Our own long-term results in patients with (in-stent) recurrent stenoses were very promising for this group of patients, with a relatively low recurrence rate of around 30% after 3 years.

- *Application of a fluid beta emitter using a PTA balloon* (system manufactured by the itm FlowMedical company; it has been approved as a medical product in Europe since September 2008). The rhenium-188 that is used is eluted from a wolfram-188 generator and made available on the day of the planned procedure. The main advantages are the ability to apply the treatment directly in the catheter laboratory, on the one hand, and on the other precise centering with uniform irradiation of the target tissue. The target dose used in studies so far is 10 Gy at a tissue depth of 2 mm. The short half-life of approximately 17 hours allows for easy disposal.

- *Application of a gamma emitter using the afterloading procedure* (see Fig. 4.4-77): in the studies conducted to date on intravascular brachytherapy in the peripheral vascular area, it has mainly been a computer-controlled high dose-rate (HDR) afterloading device (Nucletron MicroSelectron) that has been used (as in brachytherapy for oncological diseases such as cervical carcinoma). The only radioactive source used has been iridium-192 (with activity of 5–10 Ci; active length 3.5 mm), and the afterloader allows movement of the radioactive source within the brachytherapy catheter in 5-mm steps. The treatment is administered in a special radiation therapy room with continuous audiovisual monitoring of the patient, and depending on the length needing to be treated, it takes 5–10 min.

Centering (Fig. 4.4-77): both uncentered and centered brachytherapy catheters are available for intravascular brachytherapy. The disadvantage of uncentered catheters is the potential for eccentric positioning of the source inside the vascular lumen, resulting in a possibly inhomogeneous dose distribution in the vessel wall—although eccentric positioning is less problematic with a gamma emitter than when a beta emitter is used.

Brachytherapy length: all of the positions used in balloon dilation (the intervention length) have to be precisely documented in order to establish the treatment length. The zones of marginal vascular wall trauma have to be included in the radiation field (Fig. 4.4-76). A safety margin of 5 mm at each end, both proximal and distal to the intervention length, is added. This margin is necessary because the traumatization to the vascular wall caused by the angioplasty usually extends beyond the documented balloon length. An additional 5 mm is added at both ends to take account of imprecise positioning of the treatment catheter. After successful recanalization, the radiotherapy catheter is positioned 15 mm distal to the last intervention, over the guidewire. A radiopaque marking wire and a marking strip attached to the skin are used to set the relevant parameters. The catheter is fixed to the sheath for patient transport to the brachytherapy department.

Brachytherapy planning: this is carried out on the planning computer with knowledge of the relevant parameters, based on the x-

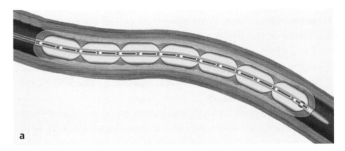

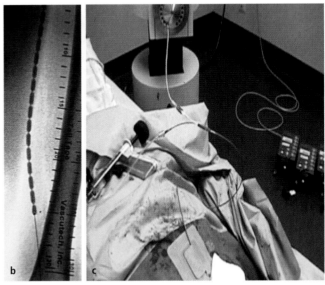

Fig. 4.4-77a–c Brachytherapy with a centering catheter. (**a**) Diagram of the segmented inflated balloon. (**b**) The balloon inside the vessel. (**c**) The catheter connected to the afterloader.

ray documentation. Calculations are carried out using the mean postinterventional vascular radius. The usual treatment approach is to administer the planned dosage within a set depth in the vessel wall. The recommended reference depth for peripheral vessels is 2 mm, and the reference point for the prescribed dosage is therefore $r + 2$ mm distance to the source axis.

Prerequisites for carrying out intravascular brachytherapy: the radiotherapy planning and quality assurance must meet the usual safety standards for clinical radiation therapy for malignant tumors, and there must be close collaboration with the radiotherapist and medical physicist. When a gamma emitter is used, there must be a department for brachytherapy in the vicinity (if possible in the same hospital), although this is not a requirement when a beta emitter is used. In addition, notification to the relevant authorities is required when this method is used.

Potential problems in using intravascular brachytherapy: appropriate radiation protection measures are required due to the radiation exposure for patient and staff (when a beta emitter is used, only direct contact is dangerous, while with a gamma emitter additional protection has to be ensured by using afterloading devices). In addition, ionizing rays are capable of giving rise to radiation-induced tumors. However, the likelihood of radiation-induced carcinogenesis in the context of intravascular brachytherapy is extremely low (small volumes, relatively insensitive tissue).

An arterial segment that has been injured during the interventional procedure but does not then receive the planned radiation dosage is known as a "geographic miss"—with incorrect positioning of the radiation source. This can be avoided by careful documentation of the length of the angioplasty and precise positioning of the radiation source.

A new stenosis that appears at the edge of the treatment zone is known as an "edge effect." This may be caused by incorrect positioning of the radiation source, with the lower dosage in the marginal area (every radiation source has a dose decline at its edge) inducing increased cell proliferation due to proinflammatory radiation effects. The effectiveness of brachytherapy with a beta emitter may be limited by metal stent struts or when there are severely calcified stenoses.

Results of intravascular brachytherapy (Table 4.4.-23)

1. **Brachytherapy after femoropopliteal PTA:** several studies conducted in the German-speaking countries—primarily with the gamma emitter iridium-92, while no randomized studies are available yet for the beta emitter rhenium-188 that has recently been used—have reported a positive effect of endovascular brachytherapy both for de novo and for recurrent stenoses, with significant and clinically relevant reductions in the recurrence rate within the first 6–12 months (Minar et al. 2000; Zehnder et al. 2003; Gallino et al. 2004; Wohlgemuth et al. 2010). However, the frequency of late recurrences after more than 12 months increased, so that—at least at the dosage used—brachytherapy ultimately does not lead to the elimination of recurrences, but only to a delay in their appearance (Diehm et al. 2005; Wolfram et al. 2006). This phenomenon is known as "regrowth delay" in experimental tumor biology. In a large study conducted in the USA, the PARIS study, no differences were observed after femoropopliteal angioplasty between the group receiving brachytherapy and the placebo group. Along with the logistic problems, this unpublished negative study has meant that endovascular radiotherapy for prophylaxis against recurrences after peripheral interventions has not become established in the USA.

2. **Brachytherapy after femoropopliteal stent implantation** (Fig. 4.4-78): in principle, this combination is capable of influencing both of the basic mechanisms underlying recurrent stenoses. Brachytherapy is intended to prevent neointimal hyperplasia, and stent implantation is meant to prevent negative remodeling. However, due to the markedly delayed endothelialization, there

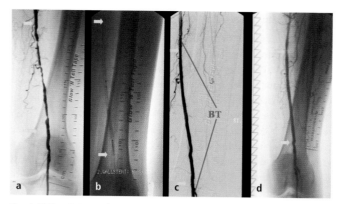

Fig. 4.4-78a–d Example case from a randomized study. (**a**) Multiple femoropopliteal stenoses before the intervention. (**b**) Long stent implantation (between the arrows). (**c**) Control angiography after stent implantation. (**d**) Control angiogram 7 months after stent implantation and endovascular brachytherapy.

is a relatively high risk of late thrombotic occlusions when secondary prophylaxis with aspirin alone is used. Optimizing the antithrombotic therapy (dual platelet inhibition treatment with aspirin and clopidogrel for at least 12 months) can be used to reduce this risk. In a randomized study, brachytherapy after peripheral stent implantation was ultimately found to offer no advantage in comparison with a group who did not undergo radiotherapy, due to the higher frequency of early and late thrombotic occlusions (Wolfram et al. 2005).

3. **Brachytherapy in femoropopliteal in-stent recurrent stenosis:** In the Frankfurt study (Böttcher et al. 1994)—the first clinical application of intravascular therapy anywhere in the world—a 5-year clinical patency rate of 82% was reported, although with only a relatively small group of patients. Our own results in Vienna with a beta emitter, taking account of the more recent high recurrence rates in the treatment of in-stent recurrent stenoses, are also very promising. The research group in Leipzig recently published a study (Werner et al. 2012) including 90 patients with long femoropopliteal in-stent restenoses, in which rhenium-188 was used as a beta emitter and a target dosage of 13 Gy at a tissue depth of 2 mm was used. The primary 12-month patency rate of 80% confirmed earlier results in a relatively large group of patients.

Table 4.4-23 Randomized studies on endovascular brachytherapy after femoropopliteal angioplasty.

Study	n	De novo (%)	Recurrent lesions (%)	Dosage (Gy) RD	Centering	Positive short-term effect of BT	Positive long-term effect of BT
Vienna-2	113	51	49	12-0	No	Yes: 12-month recurrence rates 36% vs. 65%	No: 60-month recurrence rates 72.5% vs. 72.5%
Vienna-3	134	78	22	18-2	Yes	Yes: 12-month recurrence rates 23% vs. 53%	Not known
Bern	100	–	100	12-2	No	Yes: 12-month recurrence rates 23% vs. 42%	Mixed group
Switzerland	335	100	–	12-2	No	Yes: 6-month recurrence rates 17% vs. 35%	32-month recurrence rates 36% vs. 53% (n.s.)
Cologne	30	100	–	14-2	Yes	Yes: 6-month recurrence rates 0% vs. 47%	Not known

BT, brachytherapy.

External brachytherapy

Several studies have been carried out in recent years on the use of external postinterventional brachytherapy after femoropopliteal angioplasty, with varying results.

This treatment approach avoids the decisive logistic disadvantages of using a gamma emitter, as the patients can, in principle, be treated in an external department after revascularization has been completed. A randomized study conducted in Canada in which one course of external administration of 14 Gy in the area of the angioplasty site was carried out 24 h after revascularization reported a reduction in the 1-year recurrence rate from 50% to 25% (Therasse et al. 2005).

Summary: brachytherapy

The validity of the concept of using endovascular radiotherapy to reduce the recurrence rate has been confirmed, particularly after femoropopliteal angioplasty. The absence of any long-term benefit as a result of increased numbers of late recurrences may possibly be attributed to the dosage used in the studies being too low. Endovascular therapy with a gamma emitter has not become established due to the associated logistic problems, and further research on ways of optimizing the treatment, particularly with regard to the optimal dosage, has not therefore been possible. External postinterventional radiotherapy with a gamma emitter, which is easier and more practicable to carry out, would need to be investigated in further studies before it can be recommended as a method of preventing recurrences. In contrast to gamma emitters, beta emitters can be applied directly in the catheter laboratory immediately after revascularization, and this of course makes this method much easier. At present, treatment for femoropopliteal in-stent restenoses is the most promising indication, particularly since there are only very few alternative treatment options available.

Endovascular treatment of acute femoropopliteal occlusions

1. **Local lysis.** Local lysis, either with an end-hole or side-hole catheter (e.g., Cragg–McNamara™, Boston Scientific), is still the most frequently used form of treatment—either alone or in combination with thrombus aspiration. In this procedure, the catheter is placed either proximal to the occlusion (end-hole) or, following complete passage with a hydrophilic-coated guidewire, within the thrombotically occluded vascular segment (side-hole catheter, with side holes over a length of 10–50 cm). A bolus of the lytic agent is then administered—e.g., urokinase 200,000–400,000 IU or recombinant tissue plasminogen activator (rt-PA) 1–10 mg. This is followed by continuous infusion of the lytic agent in combination with heparin (target partial thromboplastin time: 60–80 s) for a variable period of 6–24 h, depending on local hospital practices and the thrombus burden. Depending on the clinical course, an angiographic check on the result of the lysis procedure and additional therapy if needed, such as aspiration, PTA, or stent placement, then follows. With the need for intensive-care monitoring and a check-up angiography, local thrombolysis is time-consuming and costly, and it is associated with an increased risk of peripheral embolism and local or systemic bleeding. In addition, the underlying stenosis in

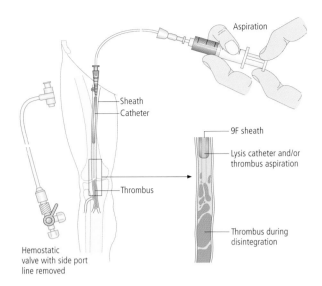

Fig. 4.4-79 Schematic depiction of a thrombus aspiration maneuver in the distal popliteal artery.

local thrombotic occlusions carries an increased risk of recurrent occlusion. The primary success rates with local lysis treatment can be substantially increased using additional thrombus aspiration and balloon angioplasty. The possibility of fatal hemorrhage as a complication of this form of treatment, particularly in long-term thrombolysis and in older patients, needs to be pointed out despite all the clinical success with the therapy.

2. **Aspiration embolectomy.** In aspiration embolectomy, either a special straight aspiration catheter (5–8F) with a stiff shaft that does not collapse during suction applications is used, or guide catheters, which have the advantage of a softer and less traumatic catheter tip and are available both as straight catheters and in various curved versions (e.g., Multipurpose). The latter allow targeted thrombus aspiration even in tortuous vascular segments or in areas where vessels divide. The easiest way of creating suction is to use a 50-mL (perfusion) syringe and a three-way stopcock (Fig. 4.4-79).

3. **Mechanical thrombectomy.** Various thrombectomy catheter systems for optimizing endovascular treatment have become commercially available in recent years. Most of these systems have various specific limitations—such as only being usable with fresh thromboses, only achieving incomplete thrombus removal, causing injury to the vascular wall, or involving elaborate and time-consuming application. Only a few systems have been approved or are suitable for use with femoropopliteal occlusions. The most commonly used systems and the way in which they are operated are briefly described below.

    –   *Straub Rotarex system:* this catheter system consists of three components (Fig. 4.4-80)—an electric control unit, a 40-W electric motor, and a 6F or 8F thrombectomy catheter that is connected to the electric motor via an electromagnetic coupling. The system is passed over a 0.018-inch guidewire. A coated steel helix rotates inside the catheter at a speed of 40,000 revolutions/min and thus produces a continuous vacuum with a suction force of around 43 mmHg. The catheter tip consists of two overlying cylinders, each with two side openings; the outer cylinder is connected to the rotating helix

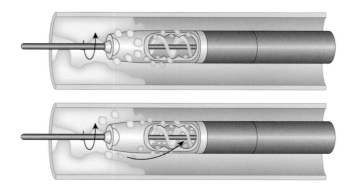

Fig. 4.4-80 Diagram showing the Straub Rotarex device. The external part of the catheter head is driven by the inner spiral at 40,000 rpm. The device removes and fragments thrombotic material, which is sucked into the side holes at a pressure of 36 bar and transported away.

and the inner one to the catheter shaft. The vacuum sucks soft and hard thrombus particles into the side holes, where they are fragmented and then transported via the rotating helix to the proximal part of the shaft, where the material is collected in a bag. After initial passage of the occlusion, usually with a hydrophilic-coated 0.035-inch wire, the 0.018-inch guidewire is exchanged via a 4F diagnostic catheter. The catheter is then slowly guided through the occlusion, with occasional withdrawal and rotating movements (fresh blood flowing in helps to cool the catheter). The advancement speed is approximately 1 cm/s. The occlusion is passed repeatedly (usually two or three times) until no further thrombi can be identified.

– *Hydrolyser catheter:* this is a 6F or 7F triple-lumen catheter with a narrow injection lumen, a larger outlet lumen, and a 0.020-inch guidewire lumen. The system is available with various lengths and is activated by a standard contrast injection pump filled with 0.9% saline. It is a rheolytic catheter that uses a Venturi effect and can be safely used in vessels with diameters of 3–8 mm without causing any significant vascular wall reactions. After initial passage of the occlusion, using a 0.035-inch wire if necessary, the inlet lumen is infused under high pressure with a saline jet in the retrograde direction. The jet is directed at the catheter's central outlet lumen. The fluid jet fragments and removes the thrombus.

– *AngioJet catheter:* The catheter consists of a guidewire–controlled 3.2–6.0F double-lumen tube enclosing a small injection lumen and a larger outlet lumen. Via multiple side holes at the catheter tip, saline is injected under high pressure into the outlet lumen, fragmenting and removing the thrombus. This requires a special pump that produces a pressure of 70,000–105,000 kPa.

– *PMT system:* this is a 6F double-lumen catheter, 120 cm long. A helix that fragments the thrombus rotates at the catheter tip. A second lumen is attached to a vacuum-producing capture system, through which the fragmented thrombus material is removed.

The efficacy of the Straub Rotarex rotation thrombectomy catheter system for treating acute and subacute occlusions of the femoropopliteal arteries has been confirmed in research studies. The major

application for the system is for local acute and subacute thrombotic occlusions, as well as thromboembolic occlusions in previously untreated arteries. Successful primary treatment of a high percentage of long intrastent occlusions is also possible. As with balloon angioplasty, however, the long-term course after recanalization of intrastent occlusions shows high rates of recurrent occlusion. The other thrombectomy catheters listed above are less effective for thrombectomy in comparison.

A common factor with all of the mechanical thrombectomy systems is a specific potential complication—vascular perforation. Safe intraluminal positioning of the wire has to be documented before the systems are operated. Comparison of the clinical results, in terms of amputation-free survival and recurrence of critical ischemia of the extremity, with the results of the STILE and TOPAS studies (both of which compared recanalization of thrombotically occluded vessels using surgical measures or local lysis in patients with acute ischemia of the extremities) shows that treatment with the Rotarex catheter is superior. In the TOPAS study, the 1-year amputation-free survival rate in the lysis group was 65%, in comparison with 69.9% in the surgical group. With comparable patient characteristics, the 1-year limb preservation rate in patients in our own study was 95%. In the STILE study, recurrent critical ischemia of the extremity was reported in 64% of the patients in the lysis group and 35% of those in the surgical group. In our own group of patients, the repeat intervention rate, as an indicator of recurrent relevant ischemia, was much lower at 41% than in the surgical group in the STILE study. The high repeat intervention rate was due to a relatively high number of recurrent stenoses or occlusions in bypass or in-stent occlusions. These groups of patients generally have a reduced long-term prognosis with regard to the postinterventional patency rate. While the amputation rate in the lysis group in the STILE study was 10% during the follow-up, in our own research group the rate was 0%.

No results for acute treatment have so far been published for the other catheter systems that are commercially available. Primary success rates of up to 82% have been reported for the Hydrolyser catheter in infrainguinal applications, with positive clinical results of 73% for previously untreated vessels and 53% for use in bypass occlusions. However, additional local lysis therapy was required in approximately 50% of the successful interventions. Peripheral embolizations are reported in up to 15% of cases. The limitation of the system is that vascular occlusions that are more than 14 days old usually have to undergo additional lysis treatment. The AngioJet thrombectomy system was investigated in a multicenter study. Use of the thrombectomy system alone was successful in 52% of the cases, and a 90% success rate was achieved after additional lysis or thrombus aspiration. Peripheral embolizations occurred in 2% of cases. The advantage of this catheter system is its small diameter of 6F, which means that the system can also be used for occlusions of the lower leg arteries. Its disadvantage is the relatively high proportion of additional treatment measures such as lysis and aspiration that are needed. The PMT system was investigated in a small single-center study. For infrainguinal applications, the system's primary technical success rate was 16%; with additional balloon angioplasty, stent implantation, and laser application, an interventional success rate of 92% was achieved.

Postinterventional medication and follow-up

- In chronic lesions and local thrombotic occlusions, long-term postinterventional therapy with ASA 100 mg/d for secondary cardiovascular prophylaxis is administered, plus 4 weeks clopidogrel 75 mg/d with stent implantation. If a DES is implanted, clopidogrel is administered for at least 6 months.
- In acute embolic occlusions, depending on the etiology, oral anticoagulation treatment with warfarin (Coumadin) with overlapping therapeutic heparinization with fractionated or unfractionated heparin or platelet inhibition is administered, as described above.
- Neither the recommendation for clopidogrel administration nor the occasionally recommended postinterventional follow-up treatment with fractionated, weight-adjusted heparin for 14 days has yet been confirmed by research results.
- Before discharge, postinterventional success should be documented by a clinical examination (including pulse status), segmental oscillography, arterial Doppler occlusion pressure measurement, and color duplex ultrasonography (including checking of the puncture site). Due to the high rate of recurrence of complex lesions, particularly during the first 6 months, outpatient angiographic follow-up examinations should be ensured after 3, 6, and 12 months so that focal recurrent stenosis can be recognized quickly and a repeat intervention can be carried out to prevent recurrent occlusion. Rigorous follow-up of the patients can achieve assisted and secondary patency rates similar to those achieved with bypasses.
- Attention should be given to ensure optimal secondary prophylaxis (see under conservative therapy above). Due to the high incidence of concomitant coronary heart disease, regular cardiac check-ups are indicated.

Potential risks of the intervention

- Peripheral embolization, with a need for thrombus aspiration and/or local lysis.
- Contrast-induced nephropathy, as with any use of contrast media (the risk increases in proportion to the restriction of renal function). Using CO_2 is an alternative if DSA facilities are available.
- Vascular wall dissection or perforation (of the target vessel or lower leg arteries). Treatment consists of several minutes of balloon dilation, and if this fails, implantation of a stent, which should covered in cases of perforation (e.g., Jostent™ graft, Abbott Vascular) and, if necessary, reversal of anticoagulation using protamine.
- Local vascular complications at the puncture site, such as pseudoaneurysm, arteriovenous fistulas, hematoma requiring transfusion, etc.

Course and prognosis with endovascular therapy

The patency rates (Table 4.4-24) depend on the length of the lesion, its degree of calcification, the type and length of stent, and the recanalization procedure used. In addition, there is evidence that the quality of the outflow is also very important for the prognosis, and we therefore also aim to achieve optimal revascularization of the lower leg arteries. The best prognosis with atherectomy procedures is seen when intraluminal recanalization is successful.

Table 4.4-24 Recurrent stenosis rates after femoropopliteal interventions relative to the treatment procedure.

	Lesions (n)	1-y recurrent stenosis rate	Lesion length
Balloon (FAST)	121	39%	4.5 ± 2.8 cm
Balloon (Absolute)	53	63%	9.2 ± 6.4 cm
Luminexx® stent (FAST)	123	32%	4.5 ± 2.8 cm
Conformexx® stent (FACT)	110	23%	5.9 ± 4.9 cm
Absolute® stent (Vienna-Absolute)	51	37%	10.1 ± 7.5 cm
Smart® stent (Scirocco, bare stent and DES)	90	25% (2 years)	8.5 ± 3.5 cm
LifeStent® (RESILIANT)	134	20%	7.9 ± 4.4 cm
Atherectomy for de novo lesion	45	16%	4.3 ± 5.4 cm
Atherectomy for recurrent stenosis	43	46%	10.5 ± 12.2 cm
Atherectomy for in-stent recurrent stenosis	43	46%	13.1 ± 11.1 cm
Paclitaxel-coated balloon (THUNDER)	48	24%	7.5 ± 6.2 cm
Paclitaxel-coated stent (Zilver PTX, randomized)	236	16.9%	6.5 ± 4.0 cm

DES, drug-eluting stent.

Prospects for endovascular therapy

Although the technical success rates are now very high, the limitation of this type of treatment lies in the still unsatisfactory long-term patency rates, particularly with long femoropopliteal occlusions. Studies currently in progress with drug-eluting balloons, either with or without atherectomy procedures (DEFINITIVE AR, PHOTOPAC), are raising hopes for a better long-term prognosis with endovascular treatment. Paclitaxel-coated stents already represent a good treatment option in short and medium-length lesions, including in-stent lesions.

Surgical therapy

Acute occlusive processes

Causes

Acute arterial occlusive processes in the lower extremity are mainly caused by embolism or thrombosis in an artery that already has severe arteriosclerotic damage. More rarely, severe acute ischemia can also be caused by emboli from a proximally-located aneurysm, with additional complete thrombotic occlusion of the aneurysm itself. In occasional cases, an acute surgical intervention may be necessary after a failed endovascular procedure. Vascular compression syndrome (entrapment of the popliteal artery) or cystic adventitial degeneration (CAD) can also very rarely cause acute ischemia. Trauma in the lower extremity, with luxation or fractures near the joints, as well as severe soft-tissue injuries, occasionally causes acute ischemia due to traumatic vascular occlusion.

Indication for surgery

Nearly all forms of acute limb ischemia represent emergency or urgent indications for surgery. In cases of complete acute ischemia with extreme pain symptoms in which loss of sensation and motor control has already occurred, immediate restoration of the circulation is essential, since with complete ischemia lasting more than 6 h, irreversible damage to the neural structures and skeletal musculature is certain to occur. However, if there is incomplete acute ischemia with residual sensorimotor function, time is available before the procedure for additional diagnostic procedures and preoperative optimization of the patient's general condition by regulating the fluid and electrolyte metabolism and treating any concomitant cardiac disease that may be present. The surgical procedure that is then selected must always be planned so as to include elimination of the cause of the acute vascular occlusion after the relevant diagnosis. This applies particularly to acute arterial thrombosis against a background of advanced arteriosclerosis or with a thrombosed peripheral aneurysm. The initial treatment after diagnosis should always consist of an intravenous bolus dose of 5000–10,000 IU heparin, to prevent further thrombosis in the peripheral vasculature. The extremity must be placed in a lowered position and protected against pressure and loss of temperature. In cases of arterial thrombosis, the indication for intra-arterial lysis should always be considered.

Surgical procedure

General preparations

The easiest way of removing an embolus or local thrombus is with direct or indirect thromboembolectomy. Intravenous access must be obtained to allow continuous administration of fluids and for intravenous administration of heparin and other drugs. Local anesthesia (e.g., with mepivacaine 1% 20–30 mL) is applied along the line of the planned incision in the inguinal area, with additional deep infiltration. The presence of an anesthetist to allow possible analgesia and sedation if necessary and for monitoring circulatory function is also recommended. It may also be necessary to switch to general anesthesia if the operation needs to be extended. Sterile preparation of the whole extremity that is to be operated on is carried out, followed by draping leaving the extremity mobile. If the treatment plan needs to include possible placement of a femorofemoral bypass in patients with concomitant arterial occlusive disease of the iliac arteries, the contralateral inguinal region should also undergo sterile preparation and draping. Systemic heparin (5000–10,000 IU, depending on body weight) is administered before clamping and incision of the artery.

Access routes

Transfemoral thromboembolectomy under local anesthesia. A 5(–10) cm slightly oblique skin incision is made, which should not cross the inguinal crease proximally if possible. The wound is held open with retractors. The femoral nerve must be protected. The femoral bifurcation is exposed from the lateral direction, protecting the lymph vessels and lymph nodes. The vessels are exposed spar-

ingly, and the common, superficial, and deep femoral artery and any side branches are snared with vessel loops.

Occlusion situation

Embolic occlusion of the femoral bifurcation. Palpation of the vessel, which is usually healthy, is carried out to identify any atherosclerotic changes in the wall. This is followed by clamping of the superficial and deep femoral arteries slightly distal to the bifurcation, and finally the common femoral artery proximal to the embolus. Transverse arteriotomy of the common femoral artery approximately 0.5 cm above the origin of the superficial femoral artery follows, with possible direct inspection of the origin of the deep femoral artery. In the simplest case, the embolus can be manually expressed or rinsed out of the lumen by carefully opening the vascular clamp. After an additional thrombectomy maneuver using a balloon catheter (Fogarty no. 4 or 5), a check is made that there is flow returning from the individual vessels. Heparin is instilled and the arteriotomy is closed using interrupted or continuous sutures (polypropylene 5.0 or 6.0). A Redon drain is placed, and the wound is closed layer by layer.

Thrombotic occlusion of the femoral bifurcation. The operation can basically also be carried out with local anesthesia. Dissection is carried out proximally and distally as far as the region of slight atherosclerotic change. If necessary, the inguinal ligament can be mobilized by releasing it from the fascia tangentially, with dissection of the transition from the external iliac artery to the common femoral artery. If there is severe stenotic alteration of the deep femoral artery, dissection is carried out distally as far as an area showing fewer changes, with transection of the ventrally crossing circumflex vein. After systemic heparinization and clamping, a longitudinal arteriotomy is carried out along the whole length of the occlusion. Apposition thrombi are removed locally. Thromboendarterectomy of the stenotic plaque causing the arterial thrombosis is then carried out, if necessary including the deep femoral artery and centrally as far as the distal external iliac artery. The atherosclerotic cylinder is transected and trimmed proximally. If necessary, a distal intimal step can be attached with a transmural interrupted tacking suture. All intimal flaps are removed and the arteriotomy is closed with a patch (Fig. 4.4-81b, c). If the caliber is large, continuous direct suturing of the arteriotomy is possible. This is preceded by a thrombectomy maneuver of the proximal and distal vessel with an embolectomy balloon catheter. Intraoperative PTA and stent implantation in an upstream or downstream stenosis may be necessary. A preexisting chronic occlusion of the superficial femoral artery can usually be left when inflow to the deep femoral artery is restored (Fig. 4.4-81d).

Arterial thrombosis of the femoropopliteal axis

It must be assumed that the atherosclerotic lesion is advanced. If the patient is in poor general condition (e.g., bedridden), simple local thrombus removal from the deep and superficial femoral artery may be sufficient to restore adequate resting perfusion. The procedure is analogous to that used for embolectomy from the femoral bifurcation. If necessary, the thrombectomy catheter can be advanced under fluoroscopic guidance over a guidewire placed in the peripheral vasculature. After removal of the thrombi, additional PTA of a higher-grade stenosis causing the condition may be necessary. In individual cases, it may also be necessary to implant a stent with an appropriate diameter into the underlying lesion as well. Finally,

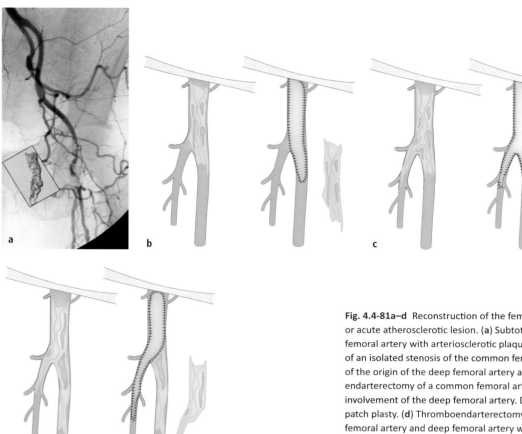

Fig. 4.4-81a–d Reconstruction of the femoral bifurcation in a chronic or acute atherosclerotic lesion. (**a**) Subtotal stenosis of the left common femoral artery with arteriosclerotic plaque. (**b**) Thromboendarterectomy of an isolated stenosis of the common femoral artery, with disobliteration of the origin of the deep femoral artery and patch plasty. (**c**) Thrombo-endarterectomy of a common femoral artery stenosis with simultaneous involvement of the deep femoral artery. Disobliteration and Y-shaped patch plasty. (**d**) Thromboendarterectomy of a stenosis of the common femoral artery and deep femoral artery with an occluded superficial femoral artery. Profundoplasty with a patch up to the second branching of the deep femoral artery.

intraoperative angiography is carried out to document the results. The arteriotomy can be closed either with direct suturing or with a patch plasty after local reconstruction.

Embolism in the popliteal trifurcation and lower leg and foot arteries

In principle, it is still possible to remove thrombi via the common femoral artery using an indirect embolectomy under local anesthesia. The entrance is made with a 4F Fogarty catheter in the distal direction, with careful removal of the embolus from the popliteal artery using slow withdrawal of the catheter, which is kept sufficiently blocked. The embolus is inspected for completeness. Restoration of the circulation is checked using intraoperative angiography. If complete indirect removal of the embolus is not possible, the popliteal trifurcation is exposed via a skin incision approximately 5–8 cm long parallel to the posterior edge of the tibia, with the patient under general anesthesia. The saphenous nerve and great saphenous vein must be protected. The lower leg fascia is opened and the popliteal artery, the origin of the anterior tibial artery, the tibioperoneal trunk and if necessary the posterior tibial artery and the peroneal artery are dissected free and controlled using vessel loops. Palpatory assessment of the popliteal artery is carried out to identify any atherosclerotic plaques that may be present. In principle, a transverse or slightly oblique arteriotomy opposite the origin of the anterior tibial artery may be used; otherwise, a longitudinal arteriotomy of the distal popliteal artery is carried out. The embolus is extracted through the arteriotomy. Thrombectomy maneuvers are performed centrally and peripherally with 4F or 2F Fogarty catheters to check on the in-

flow or backflow. Heparin is instilled locally and the arteriotomy is closed (using a venous patch for a longitudinal incision). The results of the operation are documented using intraoperative angiography.

Arterial thrombosis in the popliteal artery and lower leg and foot arteries

The procedure is analogous to embolectomy in the popliteal artery. The indication for additional intraoperative local lysis should be considered, and if appropriate, local administration of up to 100,000 IU (total dose) of urokinase into the individual crural arteries can be carried out. The thrombolytic agent should be administered via small-lumen catheters introduced into the individual vessels, and this must be done before closure of the arteriotomy. The intraoperative results are checked and documented using angiography of the peripheral vasculature. If necessary for very distal thrombi, the posterior tibial artery can also be exposed at the medial malleolus and the dorsalis pedis artery at the dorsum of the foot, and antegrade and retrograde thrombectomy can be carried out via a transverse or longitudinal arteriotomy. The transverse arteriotomy is closed using interrupted sutures (polypropylene 7–0 or 8–0), or the longitudinal arteriotomy is closed with a venous patch after local instillation of a heparin solution.

Differential diagnosis between embolus or thrombus material

After the material has been obtained, all of it is sent for histological examination along with a precise description of the location. This is because there may occasionally be evidence of a tumor (atrial myxoma or an embolizing carcinoma with invasive growth). The histological findings differentiate between thrombus and embolus and document the material actually removed, identifying the age of the thrombus by its degree of organization (the age of the thrombus may have legal significance in some situations).

Acute revascularization with vascular prosthesis or bypass procedure

In acute ischemia due to arterial thrombosis against a background of advanced peripheral arterial occlusive disease and unsuccessful thrombectomy, after failed endovascular therapy or lysis with severe acute ischemia, or in cases of acute thrombosis of a peripheral aneurysm with additional peripheral embolization, emergency placement of a peripheral bypass may be necessary (for details, see the sections on chronic occlusive processes in the femoropopliteal arteries and lower leg arteries).

Fasciotomy

This is always indicated if there is complete ischemia or severe incomplete ischemia preoperatively. The operation should be carried out under general anesthesia if the fasciotomy is anticipated. The most important muscle group is the extensors in the lower leg, as they have a relatively tight envelope of muscular fascia and there is a risk of early pressure damage to the fibular nerve. In cases of severe acute ischemia, the fascia of this muscle group is completely divided along its entire length. Carrying out the incision at the level of the fibula makes it possible to divide the superficial flexor group as well here, and also the deep flexors retrofibularly. *Caution:* damage to the proximal fibular nerve must be avoided. On the medial side of the lower leg, the surgical access route to the popliteal artery can be extended to include a fasciotomy. The contractility of the muscles should be checked (as a sign of vitality)—e.g., by tapping them with forceps.

If a fasciotomy is not carried out primarily, as the ischemia period has only been short, the patient should be monitored with clinical examinations repeated at short intervals to assess any incipient swelling of the operated extremity, with secondary loss of sensorimotor function. In this case, there is an indication for rapid secondary fasciotomy.

The muscles are covered with a moist compress dressing or a temporary skin replacement (e.g., Epigard®). Once the reperfusion edema has declined, the skin is closed with secondary sutures or the wound covered with a mesh graft.

Special case: acute ischemia due to pathology in the popliteal artery (entrapment syndrome or cystic adventitial degeneration)

If acute ischemia usually develops in young patients with previous atypical or unclear symptoms of claudication, the underlying lesion can be revealed using emergency thrombectomy or intra-arterial lysis during acute treatment. Additional tomographic diagnosis with CT or MRI using contrast is required in order to demonstrate local compressive structures. Acute surgical intervention may rarely be necessary. After diagnosis, the local cause is relieved by decompression of the popliteal artery, splitting the pathological muscle insertion, and local repair of the popliteal artery if necessary. The operation is carried out using general anesthesia with the patient in the prone position, via an S-shaped skin incision in the popliteal fossa. Gentle dissection of the popliteal artery is carried out, avoiding trauma of the tibial nerve. The pathological muscle origin is identi-

fied and completely split, and the artery is released. If necessary, the popliteal artery can be corrected with a venous patch plasty or vein graft. The wound is closed with a simple skin suture after placement of a drain.

Special case: acute ischemia due to concomitant arterial damage in the context of severe trauma to the lower extremity

This often results from severe open or closed trauma with fracture near a joint or luxation (the knee joint) in cases of massive violent injury. Diagnosis is possible with signs of severe ischemia even at the primary examination. There is an indication for emergency angiography, in the operating room if needed. The injury is treated in collaboration with a trauma specialist. Primary emergency stabilization of the fracture or luxation is carried out with a distraction–compression apparatus or intramedullary nailing. Then the angiographically identified lesion is dissected free. The vessels are snared and clamped after heparin administration. There is often initially no visible bleeding, even when there is laceration due to intimal involution. It is therefore often very difficult to identify the distal vascular stump in cases of laceration. The lesion can occasionally be managed with direct suturing after mobilization (e.g., lesions in the superficial femoral artery). Replacement or bypassing of the damaged vessel using autologous great saphenous vein is usually necessary (in emergencies, it can also be taken from the traumatized extremity). Careful local debridement is needed, as there is a significant risk of wound infection. The arterial reconstruction must always be covered with viable muscle tissue. Due to the often massive local tissue trauma, there is a generous indication for open fasciotomy and healing by secondary intention.

Postoperative follow-up

- *Systemic heparinization:* this starts immediately postoperatively with unfractionated heparin via infusion, or with low-molecular-weight heparin subcutaneously.
- *Monitoring the patient for possible reperfusion syndrome:* after prolonged complete ischemia of the leg or massive trauma, this is a highly likely complication. Repeated measurement of creatine kinase (CK), myoglobin, electrolytes, creatinine and if possible lactate, correction of electrolytes with continuous intravenous infusion therapy, stimulation of diuresis to eliminate muscle degradation products, and renal replacement treatment (hemofiltration) may be needed in an intensive care setting.
- *In cases of arterial embolism and confirmed cardiac rhythm disturbance:* overlapping oral long-term anticoagulation treatment.
- *After emergency placement of a peripheral bypass:* long-term oral anticoagulation (vein bypass) or long-term administration of a platelet inhibitor (prosthetic bypass).
- *Cardiac diagnosis:* echocardiography; targeted cardiac or cardiovascular surgical therapy.
- *Further vascular diagnosis:* if a cardiac source of embolism has been excluded, a targeted search should be conducted for another arterial cause (aortic or other aneurysm, intra-aortic thrombi, thrombotic endovascular implant) and treatment should be provided for the lesion responsible.
- *Coagulation diagnosis:* in individual cases, analysis of thrombophilia parameters; exclusion of a heparin-induced thrombocytopenia (HIT) syndrome.

Results

Surgical therapy for severe acute ischemia is associated with comparatively high mortality and general complication rates. This is because acute ischemia in older individuals is almost always the result of advanced disease of the entire cardiovascular system. Although restoration of circulation within 12 h can still lead to preservation of the leg in 93% of cases, the mortality rate may be as high as 19%. With prolonged ischemia of more than 12 h, the leg preservation rate declines to 78% and the mortality rises to more than 30%. In comparison, acute treatment with interventional methods, with a similarly high risk of amputation of 18% within 12 months, appears to be associated with a much lower mortality. In the final analysis, only rapid diagnosis and immediate treatment adapted to the specific cause in the individual case can improve the prognosis for this severe vascular emergency.

Chronic occlusive processes

Causes

Chronic occlusive processes in the lower extremity are mainly caused by advanced atherosclerosis, with the formation of single or multiple stenoses or long occlusions, sometimes at several vascular levels. In individual cases, chronically thrombosed peripheral aneurysms (popliteal aneurysms) or, very rarely, chronic arterial occlusion after local vascular trauma can lead to ischemia. In rare cases, a local pathological process may be present in the popliteal artery (entrapment of cystic adventitial degeneration), particularly in younger patients without typical risk factors for arteriosclerosis. Chronic inflammatory vascular occlusions may be encountered in young patients with severe nicotine abuse.

Indications for surgical treatment

The most common approaches include either local open or extended endarterectomy of the affected arterial segment, or bypass of the stenotic or occluded vascular segment (Table 4.4-25). Local replacement of the diseased vessel is usually only necessary in exceptional cases. The decision as to which approach is employed is based on the location and extent of the lesion. In stenoses or occlusions at a vascular bifurcation that is important for the collateral circulation, such as the femoral bifurcation, local endarterectomy with reconstruction of the vessel is the most appropriate option. By contrast, bypass procedures are more suitable for long lesions. According to the TASC II document, there is consensus that surgical procedures should be used for long occlusive processes in the femoropopliteal axis and at the trifurcation of the popliteal artery, or for multiple stenoses or multiple recurrences after endovascular therapy (TASC D and C lesions). The indication for the procedure of choice is based not only on the underlying occlusion pattern and the distal vessel that may need to be anastomosed, but also and primarily on the clinical symptoms and the general condition of the extremity or of the patient (Tables 4.4-25 and 4.4-26). The basic rule is that the more distal the anticipated anastomosis of the bypass, the smaller the caliber of the vessel. The more restrictive the indication—counterbalanced by a greater imminent risk of amputation, the more generous the indication for revascularization procedures. Thus, while a popliteal bypass may be indicated in Fontaine stage IIb with intermittent claudication in order to improve the walking distance, one should still usually refrain from a crural reconstruction. By contrast, infrapopliteal bypass procedures—i.e., crural or pedal bypasses—should always basically be considered when there is critical ischemia of the extremity with a long vascular occlusion (Table 4.4-25). If there is already very ad-

Table 4.4-25 Surgical treatment procedures for chronic occlusive processes in the lower extremity.

Procedure type	Indication	Materials	Advantages	Disadvantages
Thromboendarterectomy (TEA) in CFA with patch plasty (SFA still patent) or deep femoral artery plasty (SFA occluded)	PAOD II(a)/b, III, (IV)	Prosthetic patches (Dacron, PTFE), autologous vein, endarterectomized autologous artery, biological material (e.g., denatured bovine pericardium)	Locally limited procedure Restoration of original vessel Optimization of collateral supply Low risk of late occlusion	Aneurysmal degeneration possible in the late course Infection (risk in later puncture) Usually inadequate as a sole measure in stage IV
Ring stripper endarterectomy in SFA	PAOD IIb, III, IV	Closure of the arteriotomy in the inguinal region with prosthetic patch (Dacron, PTFE), autologous vein, or biological material (e.g., denatured bovine pericardium)	Locally limited procedure Restoration of original vessel Combination with endovascular procedures possible Bypass anastomosis possible	Risk of distal intimal step; residual arteriosclerotic material in the lumen Recurrent stenosis due to myointimal hyperplasia
Popliteal bypass	PAOD IIb, III, IV	Autologous vein Synthetic prosthesis (PTFE, Dacron) Biological prosthesis (collagen conduit, denaturized human umbilical vein (HUV)	Direct pulsatile inflow to the periphery Combination with central reconstruction possible Good patency rates	Bypass and anastomotic stenoses possible during the later course Progressive degeneration of outflow Risk of implant infection
Infrapopliteal bypass (crural or pedal anastomosis)	PAOD III, IV (IIb with minimal walking distance in selected individual cases)	Autologous vein Plastic (PTFE, Dacron) Biological prosthesis (collagen conduit, denaturized human umbilical vein (HUV)	Direct pulsatile inflow to the periphery Combination with central reconstruction possible Good patency rates Good limb salvage in critical ischemia	Bypass and anastomotic stenoses possible during the later course Progressive degeneration of outflow Risk of implant infection

Table 4.4-26 Indications and contraindications for crural and pedal bypass surgery.

Indications	Contraindications
Resting pain	Extensive gangrene up to the proximal third of the metatarsals
Distal gangrene	Combination of heel gangrene and forefoot gangrene in diabetic dialysis patients
Nonhealing ulcerations	Established fixed contracture of the knee joint
Rapidly progressive infection	Definitive confinement to bed
Heel necrosis	Very severe general sepsis with diabetic foot infection
Perforating ulcer of the foot with foot ischemia	
Nonhealing osteomyelitis	
Nonhealing minor amputation	

Table 4.4-27 General and specific preoperative diagnosis and preparatory measures.

Measures and diagnosis	Goal
Adjustment of nicotine consumption (surgery in stage II if possible only with credible permanent nicotine abstention)	Raising patient's awareness of the prognosis in his/her disease; controlling risk factors
ECG; possibly echocardiogram; cardiac consultation if previous cardiac damage or coronary heart disease (CHD) present	Recognition of high-risk patients and planning for possible perioperative intensive monitoring If appropriate, treatment for the cardiac disease (therapy for insufficiency or arrhythmia, PTCA, CABG)
Carotid Doppler imaging	Assessment of stroke risk
Pulmonary function (if specific history)	Adjustment of anesthetic procedure (surgery with peridural anesthesia)
β-blockers	Reducing the perioperative rate of myocardial ischemia
Platelet inhibition	Reducing cardiac risk
Statins	Reducing cardiac risk
Blood-pressure adjustment and targeted antibiotic treatment after microbiological smear in peripheral gangrene	Optimizing conditions for undisturbed wound healing Limiting infection and necrosis development
Immobilization and sparing local debridement in gangrene	Avoidance of additional necroses during exercise; controlling infection
Imaging diagnosis in arteries	Planning of arterial reconstruction; differential indication for PTA or surgical revascularization
Duplex ultrasonography of the peripheral veins Particularly when brachial vein harvesting is planned, no venous punctures	Precise planning for obtaining bypass material; avoidance of venous inflammation and unusability of veins

CABG, coronary artery bypass grafting; CHD, coronary heart disease; ECG, electrocardiography; PTA, percutaneous transluminal angioplasty; PTCA, percutaneous transluminal coronary angiography.

vanced necrosis or limited mobility in the extremity, vascular reconstructive procedures are no longer indicated (Table 4.4-26). Consideration also needs to be given to a primary major amputation here.

Preoperative examinations, surgical planning, and patient information

Permanent cessation of smoking in Fontaine stage IIb improves the overall prognosis. In Fontaine stages III or IV, the patient should of course be urgently reminded of the negative effects of smoking with regard to the further prognosis, particularly after surgery. However, the indication for surgery itself should not be made dependent on smoking behavior, as there is a very high level of discomfort in critical ischemia as well as a high risk of amputation.

Since generalized and potentially life-threatening vascular lesions (with CHD and cerebrovascular insufficiency) can be expected in all patients with advanced PAOD, the relevant preoperative diagnostic work-up should be initiated, particularly when surgery can be electively planned, including invasive therapy if necessary. ASA should not be withdrawn, except when the operation inevitably requires epidural spinal anesthesia (Table 4.4-27).

The operation can be performed with general anesthesia or regional anesthesia, with local reconstruction procedures (such as isolated femoral TEA) carried out with local anesthesia in occasional cases.

Preoperative patient information. The procedure should be described to the patient (bypass or local reconstruction) along with the expected implant material. General potential complications of surgery should be mentioned, such as wound infection, wound healing disturbances, thrombosis and embolism, hemorrhagic complications with the need for blood transfusions, and also hematoma development secondary to anticoagulation. The surgical strategy should always be clearly explained, and it should be assumed that the surgeon will basically make an effort to use the preferred method of grafting with the patient's own veins during the bypass procedure. The ipsilateral or contralateral great saphenous vein, arm veins, and small saphenous vein are typically used. Synthetic or biological vascular prostheses are used if vein is lacking, including bypasses that extend beyond the knee joint, and a combination of vein and prostheses may also be used. Potential paresthesias along the course of the saphenous vein (which usually slowly resolve spontaneously) should always be mentioned, as well as the risk of transient femoral nerve weakness, especially in recurrent procedures. Thrombotic occlusion of the reconstruction may result in a need for secondary procedures. Foreseeable amputations that may be required (e.g., toe amputation) when gangrene has already developed, as well as the risk of losing the limb if the operation fails, particularly in cases of critical ischemia. The patient should be informed about the reperfusion edema that may occur particularly after mobilization in the operated extremity, as in some cases it may persist for several weeks to months and may even require specific treatment with lymph drainage. The necessity for perioperative and long-term anticoagulation treatment should be explained, as well as the potential bleeding risks and the pharmacological manipulation (i.e., low-molecular-weight heparin) if the anticoagulant treatment needs to be interrupted in connection with other general surgical procedures, as well as the importance of specific follow-up care and any subsequent procedures that may be necessary (duplex ultrasound monitoring of the reconstruction, subsequent corrective/reconstructive procedures) to ensure durable perfusion. It is also useful to give this information not only to patients themselves, but also to any relatives who may be caring for them.

Role of the implant material

It is generally accepted that autologous vein with a suitable caliber is the preferable implant type for all infrainguinal bypass procedures, followed by the available synthetic and biological vascular prostheses. Autologous vein and artery material, as well as a number of synthetic or biological materials, are also available for patch angioplasties (Table 4.4-28).

- **Autologous greater saphenous vein.** When a venous bypass is reversed, the venous valves do not have to be destroyed, as the vein is implanted in the direction of flow. However, caliber mismatches may be a disadvantage, particularly in case of anastomosis to narrow-lumen crural and pedal vessels. Some authors therefore recommend using the vein in a non-reversed fashion. The greater saphenous vein is harvested either via a continuous skin incision, or with individual incisions leaving in place skin bridges that are as long as possible. Endoscopic harvesting is also possible. The side branches are ligated centrally with nonresorbable sutures (e.g., Mersilene or silk, 4–0) or—after careful dilation of the vein with heparinized blood or a cooled saline solution—with purse-string ligation using polypropylene (7–0 or 6–0). If the nonreversed method is chosen, careful destruction of the venous valves is carried out from central to peripheral with the retrograde Mills valvulotome or with Böhmig valve scissors during continuous filling of the vein with saline solution. While reversed and nonreversed venous bypasses require complete removal of the vein and ligation of the side branches, it is also possible to leave it largely in its vascular bed and simply ligate the larger side branches after atraumatic destruction of the venous valves using a special valvulotome. This technique is known as an in situ greater saphenous vein bypass. Due to the anatomic course of the great saphenous vein and the recipient artery, this method is particularly suitable for bypasses near the ankle, to the foot, or in the proximal crural area.
- **Alternative veins.** If the greater saphenous vein is not available, other autologous veins can also be used for bypass material, such as the superficial brachial veins (cephalic and basilic vein), the lesser saphenous vein, and occasionally also the superficial femoral vein. A venous bypass can also be put together from individual venous segments (spliced vein grafts) in order to achieve the required graft length. In this case, the individual venous segments are anastomosed with continuous polypropylene 7–0 suture after appropriate spatulation (45°).

Preoperative clinical assessment of autologous veins. The autologous vein material that is available must already be assessed at the time when the indication for a surgical reconstruction procedure is being established. The ipsilateral greater saphenous vein is inspected and palpated, preferably with the patient in a standing position. The residual length of the vein should be assessed if part of it has been removed previously during cardiac or vascular surgery. A search should be made for possible inflammatory or varicose changes. Varicose changes in the vein do not in principle preclude its use, as varicose segments can be resected or externally covered with synthetic prosthetic material. The lesser saphenous vein is assessed with the patient in the standing position. The cephalic and basilic veins are inspected and palpated after a tourniquet has been placed on the proximal upper arm. A search should be made in the cubital fossa for possible scarring or inflammatory changes. In principle, veins from both arms can also be used. If arm veins are to be used, then the patient and medical and nursing staff should be instructed that no further venous punctures or infusion treatments must be carried out on the arm preoperatively, in order to prevent damage to the veins. An appropriate mark can be made on the arm if necessary. If clinical assessment is difficult, a duplex ultrasound examination of the superficial venous system is helpful (known as venous mapping). The courses and diameters of the veins should be marked on the skin during this examination.

- **Synthetic and biological implants.** As autologous veins only provide suitable implant material in up to 80% of cases, even with alternative veins, the use of vascular prostheses in peripheral bypass surgery has in practice become indispensable. Narrow-lumen synthetic implants with a diameter of 6–8 mm are available, either made of Dacron (polyethylene terephthalate), which has been in use for a substantial period, or polytetrafluoroethylene (PTFE). Human umbilical vein (HUV) with an internal diameter of 5 or 6 mm, obtained from the umbilical cord, denatured using glutaraldehyde solution, and reinforced externally with a polyester coating, can also be used. However, this is at present no longer commercially available, so that the only biological vessel implant now commercially available is a biosynthetically manufactured narrow-lumen prosthesis consisting of a combination of ovine collagen and a polyester mesh integrated into the implant wall (Omniflow® II). Homologous vein and artery can, in principle, be used in peripheral artery bypass, but the logistic effort involved is high. Homografts are consequently not in widespread use, although for special indications such as infection of a synthetic prosthesis they do offer a potential alternative (Table 4.4-28).

Surgical reconstruction of the femoropopliteal segment

Depending on the extent of atherosclerotic changes, either the continuity of the diseased vessel can be restored using local procedures (thromboendarterectomy, TEA) or the diseased segment can be bypassed. Replacement of the diseased vessel is only necessary in exceptional cases with complete local destruction of the artery.

Table 4.4-28 Bypass and patch materials used in reconstructing arteries in the thigh and lower leg.

Type of material	Bypass suitability	Advantages	Disadvantages	Patch suitability	Advantages	Disadvantages
Autologous vascular replacements						
Greater saphenous vein	++	Adequate caliber Good patency rates	Limited availability	++	Availability Resistance to infection	Later usability of the vein for additional operations limited Possible degeneration and late formation of aneurysm
Lesser saphenous vein	+	Adequate caliber Good patency rates	Limited availability Insufficient length	+	Availability Resistance to infection	Caliber rather small
Arm veins (cephalic vein, basilic vein)	++	Adequate caliber Good patency rates	Limited availability Insufficient length	(+)	Availability	Wall rather thin Risk of patch rupture and aneurysmal degeneration
Superficial femoral vein	+	Good patency rates	Caliber mismatch (caliber rather large) Limited availability Insufficient length	(+)	Availability	Harvesting procedure rather invasive
Autologous artery	–		Not used routine in peripheral bypass surgery	+	Availability Resistance to infection Autologous patch material from occluded endarterectomized superficial femoral artery easily obtained	More extensive dissection
Synthetic vascular replacements						
Dacron (polyethylene terephthalate)	+	Good availability Acceptable patency in popliteal bypass above the knee	Risk of infection Poor patency rates in distal bypass	++	Availability Suitable for larger and middle-sized calibers	Not suitable for small calibers (crural and pedal arteries) Risk of infection Suture line aneurysm possible
PTFE (polytetrafluoro-ethylene)	+	Good availability Acceptable patency in popliteal bypass above the knee	Risk of infection Poor patency rates in distal bypass	++	Availability Suitable for larger and middle-sized calibers	Not suitable for small calibers (crural and pedal arteries) Needle-track bleeding Risk of infection Suture line aneurysm possible
Biological vascular replacements						
Denatured human umbilical vein (HUV)	+	Good availability (currently not commercially available) Good patency in popliteal bypass	Biodegeneration, risk of infection Moderate patency rates for distal bypass	–	–	Not suitable as patch material
Heterologous collagen conduits (ovine collagen prosthesis, Omniflow®)	+	Good availability Acceptable patency in popliteal bypass	Biodegeneration Moderate patency rates for distal bypass	–		Not intended as a patch material
Denatured bovine pericardium	–		Not intended as a vascular conduit	+	Good availability and handling qualities Infection resistance	Not suitable for the smallest calibers Patch aneurysm possible
Homologous veins and arteries	+	Adequate caliber Infection resistance	High logistic effort Poor patency rates	(+)	Infection resistance	Restricted availability Patch aneurysm possible

Reconstruction of the femoral artery with profundoplasty (Fig. 4.4-81a–d)

This is indicated in case of stenosis or occlusion of the femoral bifurcation (Fig. 4.4-81a). The subcutaneous fatty tissue is incised to the level of the fascia lateral to the neurovascular sheath. The lymphatic vessels and lymph nodes are carefully protected. The common femoral artery is exposed proximally until the vessel becomes soft and compressible. The side branches are controlled with vessel loops. If necessary, the inguinal ligament can be mobilized tangentially as far as the external iliac artery. The femoral bifurcation and deep femoral artery are dissected including the first bifurcation. The circumflex vein, which crosses ventrally, is transected and ligated.

After systemic administration of 5000–10,000 IU heparin i.v., the vessels are clamped in an area that shows as few pathologic changes as possible. A longitudinal arteriotomy is made for approximately 5–10 mm beyond each stenotic or occluded segment, and open thromboendarterectomy of the arteriosclerotic plaque is carried out in an appropriate layer of media. If necessary, it may be decided to carry out additional simultaneous ring stripper endarterectomy of the external iliac artery or balloon angioplasty and stenting of the external iliac artery. Ring endarterectomy must be carried out before completion of the patch plasty and PTA after it. If the superficial femoral artery is already completely occluded at its origin, the artery may be checked for its suitability for use as patch material. Removal and thromboendarterectomy of an appropriate segment follows, and the patch is then cut to size. *Caution:* this procedure means that it will no longer be possible to reopen the superficial femoral artery using endovascular techniques.

Otherwise, it has to be decided whether to use synthetic biological material or autologous vein for patching. The arteriotomy is then closed with an adequately sized patch, using a continuous suture (polypropylene 5-0 or 6-0), starting proximally. If there is an isolated stenosis in the common femoral artery or the deep femoral artery is also involved, endarterectomy and patch plasty up to the origin of the still patent superficial femoral artery is carried out (Fig. 4.4-81b). Thromboendarterectomy of the common femoral artery and deep femoral artery requires reconstruction of the deep femoral artery using a Y-shaped patch (Fig. 4.4-81c). If the superficial femoral artery is occluded, endarterectomy should include the initial part of the deep femoral artery as a profundoplasty as far as the second bifurcation of the artery (Fig. 4.4-81d). If simultaneous PTA and stenting of the iliac artery is planned, then once the patch has been completed, central puncture of the patch under pulsatile blood flow and endovascular treatment of the iliac artery are carried out. The puncture site in the patch is closed after the introducer sheath has been removed. A Redon drain is placed and the wound is closed layer by layer; the perivascular sheath should be restored. The drain is left in place for 2 days. The patient is mobilized starting on the third postoperative day.

Antegrade or retrograde endarterectomy of the superficial femoral artery. Endarterectomy of the superficial femoral artery in cases of multiple stenoses or long occlusions is a long-established procedure that has attracted fresh attention as a result of modern endovascular techniques. It combines limited surgical access with extended restoration of the diseased original vessel. The femoral bifurcation is exposed as described above. If endovascular fixation of the distal intimal step is to be carried out with a stent, a flexible guidewire now has to be advanced with fluoroscopic guidance through the diseased vascular segment into the popliteal artery. Retrograde endarterectomy, which is now hardly ever done, requires additional exposure of the popliteal artery through a skin incision in the distal thigh, along the distal course of the sartorius muscle. Systemic heparinization is carried out with 5000–10,000 IU heparin before clamping of the inguinal vessels and longitudinal arteriotomy of the common femoral artery as far as the initial part of the superficial femoral artery. The atherosclerotic plaque is identified and isolated, with central excision in the femoral bifurcation. The cylinder is threaded over the guidewire, if in place, onto a suitably sized ring stripper, which is slowly advanced peripherally with slow rotating movements and with slight pressure on the vessel wall until the occlusive plaque is completely freed in the distal lumen. The released plaque is then extracted centrally, and angiography is carried out to document the vessel lumen. Angioscopic control of the lumen for residual intimal flaps may occasionally be required. If necessary, a stent can be placed in the transitional zone to the popliteal artery to prevent a distal intimal step, followed by a final angiography. The central arteriotomy is closed with an appropriate patch. The wound is closed in the same way as in femoral TEA.

Femoropopliteal bypass (Figs. 4.4-82a, 4.4-83a, 4.4-84a, b). In the popliteal bypass, the location of the peripheral anastomosis is based on the preoperative angiographic findings and the intraoperative findings of the exposed popliteal artery (Fig. 4.4-82a). If the greater saphenous vein is used, a 7 cm long skin incision is first made along the course of the vein in the distal thigh at the level of the popliteal artery, if a connection to the first popliteal segment appears possible on angiography (Fig. 4.4-83a, b). If use of the vein is not initially intended—e.g., after stripping of the greater saphenous vein has been carried out—an incision is made before the anterior edge of the sartorius muscle directly over the course of the popliteal artery. The vein is exposed and its caliber is assessed; careful dilation of the lumen with a saline solution via a side branch can be carried out in case of doubt. The vein should have a caliber of at least 4 mm at the level of the distal anastomosis. At no time should peripheral transection of the vein be carried out at this point. The fascia is opened in front of the anterior edge of the sartorius muscle, with the saphenous nerve being protected. The popliteal artery is identified and exposed, with meticulous protection of all collaterals, as far as the popliteal fossa. The venous plexus around the artery should be protected. The extent of atherosclerosis and wall calcification in the artery is assessed. If there is still substantial calcification or thickening in the arterial wall, raising justifiable doubt regarding the durability of a bypass connection above the knee joint, the decision may be taken to explore the distal part of the popliteal artery. A 7 cm long skin incision is made approximately 1 cm parallel to the dorsal edge of the tibia. The greater saphenous vein is dissected free and assessed, without transecting it. The popliteal fascia is opened. The gastrocnemius muscle is retracted dorsally and the artery is dissected between the two accompanying veins. The popliteal artery usually shows only relatively few atherosclerotic changes here.

A 7–10 cm long skin incision along the course of the proximal greater saphenous vein is made, and the vein is exposed as far as its junction with the femoral vein. The incision can end below the inguinal crease. The vascular sheath is opened, and the femoral bifurcation is dissected with cranial retraction of the soft tissue far enough for any local TEA to be carried out if necessary.

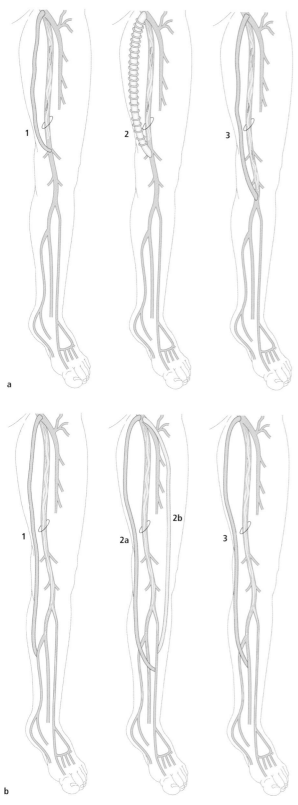

a

b

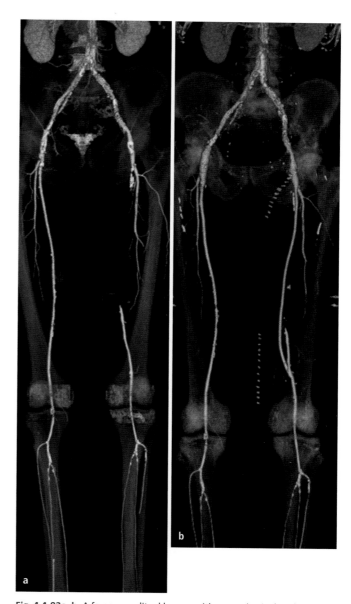

a

b

Fig. 4.4-83a, b A femoropopliteal bypass with a prosthesis that does not cross the knee joint. (**a**) An extended occlusion of the left superficial femoral artery, with inadequate collateralization and intermittent claudication limiting the walking distance. (**b**) A bypass to the popliteal artery above the knee joint, with a collagen prosthesis (Omniflow); the greater saphenous vein was not usable.

Fig. 4.4-82a, b Schematic depiction of occlusion types in the thigh and lower leg, with popliteal and crural bypasses. (**a**) An extended occlusion of the superficial femoral artery with a femoropopliteal venous (1) and prosthetic (2) bypass above, and a venous bypass below (3) the knee joint. (**b**) An extended occlusion of the superficial artery and popliteal artery with femorocrural bypass variants to the posterior tibial artery (1), anterior tibial artery with a medial and lateral (2) course, and the fibular artery (3).

Depending on the quality of the popliteal artery, a decision is taken as to whether the distal anastomosis should be placed above or below the knee joint. If the vein shows marked narrowing distally, implantation in the nonreversed position is carried out (Fig. 4.4-84a, b). If the in situ technique is selected to connect the third popliteal segment, the proximal anastomosis has to be created first. It is then best to tunnel the distal venous segment through the popliteal fossa after mobilization and then create the distal anastomosis after eliminating the venous valves. Systemic administration of 5000–10,000 IU heparin is carried out. Looping or careful clamping of the popliteal artery is then done using soft bulldog clamps, ensuring protection of all the collaterals, and a longitudinal arteriotomy 10–12 mm long is made in an area free of atherosclerosis. The vein is spatulated, and an end-to-side anastomosis is created using a continuous technique, starting with a parachute suture at the heel of the anastomosis (polypropylene 6–0). The double parachute technique, in which the sutures starting at the heel and tip of the anastomosis are each tied in the middle of the arteriotomy, may be helpful. Air is removed from the anastomosis and it is tested using a heparinized saline solution. If the distal connection is being made below the knee joint, the vein is tunneled through the popliteal space to the popliteal fossa above the knee joint through a tissue tunnel created digitally between the femoral condyles ventral to the vessels, and from there, bypassing the adductor canal, under the sartorius muscle subfascially to the groin. The inguinal vessels are clamped, a longitudinal arteriotomy 1.5–2.0 cm long is made in the femoral artery (this can be extended to allow for a TEA if necessary), and an end-to-side anastomosis is made between the vein and the artery (Fig. 4.4-85a). The central anastomosis can also be created on the initial part of the superficial femoral artery or deep femoral artery, if necessary after local TEA with or without a patch plasty (Fig. 4.4-85b). If the superficial femoral artery is already occluded directly at its origin from the femoral bifurcation, the central anastomosis can also be created as an oblique end-to-end anastomosis after separation of the superficial femoral artery. It is helpful here to leave a stump of the superficial femoral artery approximately 5–10 mm long, incising it longitudinally in a proximal direction in the common femoral artery and then trimming it after local TEA in such a way that a harmonious end-to-end anastomosis is established with the proximal end in the common femoral artery (6–0 or 5–0 polypropylene) (Fig. 4.4-85c).

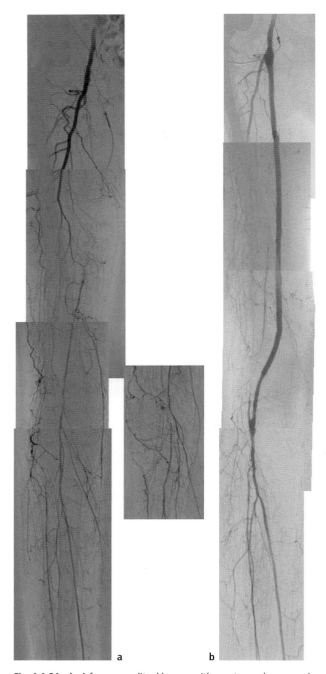

Fig. 4.4-84a, b A femoropopliteal bypass with greater saphenous vein, crossing the knee joint. (**a**) An extended occlusion of the superficial femoral artery, with additional high-grade stenosis of the popliteal artery at the level of the knee joint. (**b**) Bypass with nonreversed great saphenous vein, after destruction of the venous valves, to the distal popliteal artery below the knee joint. The marked changes in the popliteal artery at the level of the knee joint proximal to the anastomosis are well visualized.

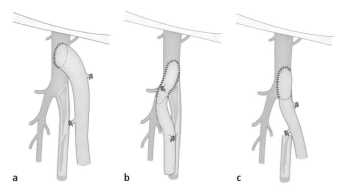

a   b   c

Fig. 4.4-85a–c Possible anastomotic configuration at the femoral bifurcation with femoral anastomosis of a popliteal or distal bypass. (**a**) End-to-side anastomosis between the bypass graft and the common femoral artery, leaving the occluded superficial femoral artery. (**b**) End-to-side anastomosis between the bypass graft and the transition from the common femoral artery to the deep femoral artery, with elimination of the stenosis at the origin of the deep femoral artery. (**c**) End-to-end anastomosis between the bypass graft and the origin of the occluded and centrally detached superficial femoral artery. The arteriotomy is extended into the common femoral artery and if necessary, local thromboendarterectomy of the origin of the deep and superficial femoral artery is carried out.

The procedure is analogous when a synthetic or biological vascular prosthesis is used, but if a PTFE prosthesis is used to cross the joint, a ring-reinforced prosthesis should always be used. When the popliteal artery is connected above the knee joint and the artery has a suitable caliber, an 8-mm Dacron or PTFE prosthesis may be useful instead of a 6-mm prosthesis. When a PTFE prosthesis is used, PTFE suture material can also be used.

Clinical results with surgical reconstruction of the femoropopliteal arteries

The femoropopliteal bypass is a method that was introduced into the repertoire of vascular surgery techniques at a very early stage, 60 years ago, and it has good long-term function. Despite this, the need to harvest and dissect the autologous vein has been regarded as a disadvantage by many surgeons, and the synthetic implants made of PTFE and Dacron that have been available since the mid-1970s, as well as biological implants such as denatured human umbilical vein, have been preferred both for primary bypass material and in order to shorten the operating time. It has also been argued that this procedure spares the autologous saphenous vein for later secondary interventions in case the prosthesis becomes occluded. Despite this, however, there appears to be growing recognition that the vein, particularly above the knee, provides better results in terms of long-term patency and less severe recurrent ischemia in case of later bypass occlusion, so that it should always be implanted if available.

Only autologous vein should be used primarily for all popliteal bypass operations that cross the knee joint; synthetic or biological vascular replacements should only be resorted to if autologous vein is not available. Patency rates of 70–80% after 5 years can be expected when autologous vein is used for bypasses to the above-knee and also below-knee popliteal segment. The patency rates with synthetic implants are much poorer, even though a statistically significant difference is not seen during the first 2 years after the operation. Although no significant difference was observed with regard to patency after 36 months with popliteal bypasses not crossing the knee joint, with rates of 57% for PTFE and 61% for Dacron, the 5-year patency rates with HUV reported by two randomized studies were significantly better at 76% and 53%, in comparison with 51% and 39% for PTFE. Good long-term results with supragenicular and infragenicular bypasses, with 5-year and 6-year patency rates of 76% and 67%, respectively, have been reported in single-center studies in which oral long-term anticoagulation treatment was administered. The long-term results with bovine collagen conduits also appear to be acceptable, with patency rates of 44–62%. Placement of a distal anastomosis using an end-to-end technique has no advantages in comparison with the end-to-side technique. A higher amputation rate can then be expected if bypass failure occurs.

Local reconstruction of the femoral artery using a patch plasty is usually a very durable method of reconstruction, with good improvement of the hemodynamics. This has been confirmed in two current studies, with very good long-term function in the common femoral artery reconstructed using a thromboendarterectomy. However, a patch aneurysm may develop during the long-term follow-up, with late infection or leading to suture disruption. Ring stripper endarterectomy is currently being used more frequently again, particularly in combination with endovascular methods, and initially encouraging results with 2-year patency rates of 86% have

been reported with the method—the principle of which can be regarded as less invasive. However, in prospective studies, the 5-year patency rates were only 44%, below the level of function expected for a bypass operation. Ring stripper endarterectomy can therefore not be regarded as the method of choice for surgical treatment of occlusions in the thigh arteries. The results of a current study in the Netherlands confirm similar results for antegrade endarterectomy with stent angioplasty and placement of an above-knee bypass with a PTFE prosthesis. However, the rate of bypass patency when an autologous vein was used was far superior to both procedures.

Prospects for surgical therapy

Occlusive disease in the femoropopliteal and crural vascular area is increasingly being regarded as a field for endovascular techniques, which have proved to be very useful for treating short vascular lesions and should be primarily used for these. Although TASC C and D lesions are considered to belong to the field of open surgical revascularization, it also has been suggested that long interventional recanalizations can be carried out for extended vascular occlusions, using endoluminal laser techniques or with multiple stents, sometimes even below the knee joint and at the level of the knee joint. Stents are also commonly implanted over very long distances in the crural arteries. Encouraging results have been reported with subintimal angioplasty in the femoropopliteal and crural axis.

With the increasing variety of methods and materials available, however, further systematic research on the value of these procedures is needed, and prospective randomized studies in particular are needed in order to compare them with the surgical bypass procedures. This is especially important in view of the fact that autologous venous bypass in this region still offers excellent long-term results that have not yet been improved on. However, a combination of endovascular therapy at the level of the thigh with placement of a distal-origin venous bypass to treat severe ischemia is also conceivable in the future. When prosthetic materials are used for bypass surgery, improvements can be expected to result from antithrombogenic coating of PTFE and Dacron grafts. Favorable 1-year and 2-year results with the use of heparin-coated PTFE prostheses in comparison with autologous vein in positions crossing the knee show that this implant is a possible alternative if a vein is not available.

Colonization of PTFE with autologous endothelium has also provided very encouraging results. Current research work has suggested the possibility of developing homologous or heterologous collagen scaffolds colonized with autologous cells in order to create new, partly autologous, vascular conduits. It may also be possible to slow the course of neointimal hyperplasia by impregnating the bypass graft with antiproliferative substances, or by using external reinforcement of the normal venous graft to reduce the mechanical irritation that stimulates the proliferation of smooth muscle cells in the vascular wall.

References

Aalders GJ, van Vroonhoven TJ. Polytetrafluoroethylene versus human umbilical vein in above-knee femoropopliteal bypass: six-year results of a randomized clinical trial. J Vasc Surg 1992; 16(6): 816–23.

Abbott WM, Green RM, Matsumoto T, Wheeler JR, Miller N, Veith FJ, et al. Prosthetic above-knee femoropopliteal bypass grafting: results of a multicenter randomized prospective trial. Above-Knee Femoropopliteal Study Group. J Vasc Surg 1997; 25 (1): 19–28.

Abbott WM, Maloney RD, McCabe CC, Lee CE, Wirthlin LS. Arterial embolism: a 44 year perspective. Am J Surg 1982; 143(4): 460–4.

Aune S, Laxdal E. Above-knee prosthetic femoropopliteal bypass for intermittent claudication. Results of the initial and secondary procedures. Eur J Vasc Endovasc Surg 2000; 19 (5): 476–80.

Ballotta E, Renon L, Toffano M, Da Giau G. Prospective randomized study on bilateral above-knee femoropopliteal revascularization: polytetrafluoroethylene graft versus reversed saphenous vein. J Vasc Surg 2003; 38 (5): 1051–5.

Ballotta E, Gruppo M, Mazzalai F, Da Giau G. Common femoral artery endarterectomy for occlusive disease: an 8-year single-center prospective study. Surgery 2010; 147 (2): 268–74.

Bausback Y, Botsios S, Flux J et al. Outback catheter for femoropopliteal occlusions: immediate and long-term results. J Endovasc Ther 2011 Feb; 18 (1): 13–21.

Berglund J, Bjorck M, Elfstrom J. Long-term results of above knee femoro-popliteal bypass depend on indication for surgery and graft-material. Eur J Vasc Endovasc Surg 2005; 29 (4): 412–8.

Beschorner U, Sixt S, Schwarzwälder U, Rastan A, Mayer C, Noory E, Macharzina R, Buergelin K, Bonvini R, Zeller T. Recanalization of Chronic Occlusions of the Superficial Femoral Artery Using the Outback™ Re-Entry Catheter: A Single Centre Experience. Cath Cardiovasc Intervent 2009, 74: 934–8.

Beschorner U, Rastan A, Zeller T. Recanalization of femoropopliteal occlusions using the crosser system. J Endovasc Ther 2009 Aug; 16 (4): 526–7.

Bolia A, Brennan J, Bell PR. Recanalisation of femoro-popliteal occlusions: improving success rate by subintimal recanalisation. Clin Radiol 1989; 40: 325–32.

Bosiers M, Deloose K, Verbist J, Schroe H, Lauwers G, Lansink W, et al. Heparin-bonded expanded polytetrafluoroethylene vascular graft for femoropopliteal and femorocrural bypass grafting: 1-year results. J Vasc Surg 2006; 43 (2): 313–8; discussion 318–9.

Bosiers M, Torsello G, Gißler H-M, Ruef J, Muller-Hulsbeck S, Jahnke T, Peeters P, Daenens K, Lammer J, Schroe H, Mathias K, Koppensteiner R, Vermassen F, Scheinert D. Nitinol stent implantation in long superficial femoral artery lesions: 12-month results of the DURABILITY I study. J Endovasc Ther 2009; 16: 261–9.

Burger DH, Kappetein AP, Van Bockel JH, Breslau PJ. A prospective randomized trial comparing vein with polytetrafluoroethylene in above-knee femoropopliteal bypass grafting. J Vasc Surg 2000; 32 (2): 278–83.

Capek P, McLean GK, Berkowitz HD. Femoropopliteal angioplasty: factors influencing long-term success. Circulation 1991; 83: 70–80.

Daenens K, Schepers S, Fourneau I, Houthoofd S, Nevelsteen A. Heparin-bonded ePTFE grafts compared with vein grafts in femoropopliteal and femorocrural bypasses: 1- and 2-year results. J Vasc Surg 2009; 49 (5): 1210–6.

Dake MD, Ansel GM, Jaff MR, Ohki T, Saxon RR, Smouse HB, Machan LS, Zeller T, Roubin GS, Burket MW, Khatib Y, Snyder SA, Ragheb AO, White JK, On behalf of the Zilver PTX Investigators. Paclitaxel-Eluting Stents Show Superiority to Balloon Angioplasty and Bare Metal Stents in Femoropopliteal Disease: 12-month Zilver PTX Randomized Study Results. Circulation Cardiovasc Intervent 2011; 4: 495–504.

Dake M, Bosiers M, Fanelli F, Kavteladze Z, Lottes A, Ragheb A, Ruhlman C, Scheinert D, Tepe G, Tessarek J, Zeller T. A Single-Arm Clinical Study of the Safety and Effectiveness of the Zilver® PTX® Drug-Eluting Peripheral Stent: Twelve-Month Results. JEVT 2011; 18: 613–23.

Dardik H, Wengerter K, Qin F, Pangilinan A, Silvestri F, Wolodiger F, et al. Comparative decades of experience with glutaraldehyde-tanned human umbilical cord vein graft for lower limb revascularization: an analysis of 1275 cases. J Vasc Surg 2002; 35 (1): 64–71.

Dave RM, Patlola R, Kollmeyer K, Bunch F, Weinstock BS, Dippel E, Jaff MR, Popma J, Weissman N; CELLO Investigators. Excimer laser recanalization of femoropopliteal lesions and 1-year patency: results of the CELLO registry. J Endovasc Ther 2009 Dec; 16 (6): 665–75.

Deutsch M, Meinhart J, Fischlein T, Preiss P, Zilla P. Clinical autologous in vitro endothelialization of infrainguinal ePTFE grafts in 100 patients: a 9-year experience. Surgery 1999; 126 (5): 847–55.

Dick P, Wallner H, Sabeti S, Loewe C, Mlekusch W, Lammer J, Koppensteiner R, Minar E, Schillinger M. Balloon angioplasty versus stenting with nitinol stents in intermediate length superficial femoral artery lesions. Catheter Cardiovasc Interv 2009 Dec 1; 74 (7): 1090–5.

Diehm N, Silvestro A, Do DD, et al. Endovascular brachytherapy after femoropopliteal balloon angioplasty fails to show robust clinical benefit over time. J Endovasc Ther 2005; 12: 723–30.

Duda SH, Bosiers M, Lammer J, Scheinert D, Zeller T, Oliva V, et al. Drug-eluting and bare nitinol stents for the treatment of atherosclerotic lesions in the superficial femoral artery. J Endovasc Ther 2006; 13: 701–10.

Efficacy of oral anticoagulants compared with aspirin after infrainguinal bypass surgery (The Dutch Bypass Oral Anticoagulants or Aspirin Study): a randomised trial. Lancet 2000 Jan 29; 355 (9201): 346–51.

Fischer M, Schwabe C, Schulte KL. Value of the Hemobahn/Viabahn endoprosthesis in the treatment of long chronic lesions of the superficial femoral artery: 6 years of experience. J Endovasc Ther 2006; 13: 281–90.

Freyhardt P, Zeller T, Kröncke TJ, Schwarzwaelder U, Schreiter NF, Stiepani H, Sixt S, Rastan A, Werk M. Plasma Levels Following Application of Paclitaxel-Coated Balloon Catheter in Patients with Stenotic, or Occluded Femoro-Popliteal Arteries. Röfo 2011; 183: 448–55.

Galland RB, Whiteley MS, Gibson M, Simmons MJ, Torrie EP, Magee TR. Remote superficial femoral artery endarterectomy: medium-term results. Eur J Vasc Endovasc Surg 2000 Mar; 19 (3): 278–82.

Gallino A, Do DD, Alerci M, et al. Effects of probucol versus aspirin and versus brachytherapy on restenosis after femoropopliteal angioplasty: the PAB randomized multicenter trial. J Endovasc Ther 2004; 11: 595–604.

Gisbertz SS, Ramzan M, Tutein Nolthenius RP, van der Laan L, Overtoom TT, Moll FL, et al. Short-term results of a randomized trial comparing remote endarterectomy and supragenicular bypass surgery for long occlusions of the superficial femoral artery [the REVAS trial]. Eur J Vasc Endovasc Surg 2009; 37 (1): 68–76.

Gray BH, Olin JW. Limitations of percutaneous transluminal angioplasty with stenting for femoropopliteal arterial occlusive disease. Semin Vasc Surg 1997; 10: 8–16.

Green RM, Abbott WM, Matsumoto T, Wheeler JR, Miller N, Veith FJ, et al. Prosthetic above-knee femoropopliteal bypass grafting: five-year results of a randomized trial. J Vasc Surg 2000; 31 (3): 417–25.

Heider P, Hofmann M, Maurer PC, von Sommoggy S. Semi-closed femoropopliteal thromboendarterectomy: a prospective study. Eur J Vasc Endovasc Surg 1999; 18 (1): 43–7.

Hirsch AT, Haskal ZJ, Hertzer NR, et al. ACC/AHA Guidelines for the Management of Patients with Peripheral Arterial Disease 2005 (Lower Extremity, Renal, Mesenteric, and Abdominal Aortic): executive summary. JACC 2006; 47: 1239–312.

Hunink MG, Donaldson MC, Meyerovitz MF, Polak JF, Whittemore AD, Kandarpa K, et al. Risks and benefits of femoropopliteal percutaneous balloon angioplasty. J Vasc Surg 1993; 17: 183–92.

Hunink MG, Wong JB, Donaldson MC, Meyerovitz MF, de Vries J, Harrington DP. Revascularization for femoropopliteal disease: a decision and cost-effectiveness analysis. JAMA 1995; 274: 165–71.

Johnson WC, Lee KK. A comparative evaluation of polytetrafluoroethylene, umbilical vein, and saphenous vein bypass grafts for femoral-popliteal above-knee revascularization: a prospective randomized Department of Veterans Affairs cooperative study. J Vasc Surg 2000; 32 (2): 268–77.

Kang JL, Patel VI, Conrad MF, Lamuraglia GM, Chung TK, Cambria RP. Common femoral artery occlusive disease: contemporary results following surgical endarterectomy. J Vasc Surg 2008; 48 (4): 872–7.

Klinkert P, Post PN, Breslau PJ, van Bockel JH. Saphenous vein versus PTFE for above-knee femoropopliteal bypass. A review of the literature. Eur J Vasc Endovasc Surg 2004; 27 (4): 357–62.

Klinkert P, Schepers A, Burger DH, van Bockel JH, Breslau PJ. Vein versus polytetrafluoroethylene in above-knee femoropopliteal bypass grafting: five-year results of a randomized controlled trial. J Vasc Surg 2003; 37 (1): 149–55.

Koch G, Gutschi S, Pascher O, Fruhwirth H, Glanzer H. Analysis of 274 Omniflow Vascular Prostheses implanted over an eight-year period. Aust N Z J Surg 1997; 67 (9): 637–9.

Krankenberg H, Schlüter M, Steinkamp HJ, Bürgelin K, Scheinert D, Schulte CL, Minar E, Peeters P, Bosiers M, Tepe G, Reimers B, Mahler F, Tübler T, Zeller T. Nitinol Stent Implantation vs. Percutaneous Transluminal Angioplasty in Superficial Femoral Artery Lesions up to 10 cm in Length: the Femoral Artery Stenting Trial (FAST). Circulation 2007; 116: 285–92.

Laird JR, Katzen BT, Scheinert D, Lammer J, Carpenter J, Buchbinder M, Dave R, Ansel G, Lansky A, Cristea E, Collins TJ, Goldstein J, Jaff MR; RESILIENT Investigators. Nitinol stent implantation versus balloon angioplasty for lesions in the superficial femoral artery and proximal popliteal artery: twelve-month results from the RESILIENT randomized trial. Circ Cardiovasc Interv 2010 Jun 1; 3 (3): 267–76.

Laird JR, Zeller T, Gray BH, Scheinert D, Vranic M, Reiser C, Biamino G, MD for the LACI Investigators. Limb salvage following laser-assisted angioplasty for critical limb ischemia: results of the LACI multicenter trial. J Endovasc Ther 2006; 13: 1–9.

Lammer J, Bosiers M, Zeller T, Schillinger M, Boone E, Zaugg MJ, Verta P, Schwartz LB. First clinical trial of nitinol self-expanding everolimus-eluting stent implantation for peripheral arterial occlusive disease. J Vasc Surg 2011; 54: 394–401.

Melliere D, Desgrange P, Allaire E, Becquemin JP. Long-term results of venous bypass for lower extremity arteries with selective short segment prosthetic reinforcement of varicose dilatations. Ann Vasc Surg 2007; 21 (1): 45–9.

Mofidi R, Kelman J, Berry O, Bennett S, Murie JA, Dawson AR. Significance of the early postoperative duplex result in infrainguinal vein bypass surveillance. Eur J Vasc Endovasc Surg 2007 Sep; 34 (3): 327–32. Epub 2007 May 22.

Moll FL, Ho GH. Endarterectomy of the superficial femoral artery [published erratum appears in Surg Clin North Am 2000 Feb; 80 (1): following table of contents]. Surg Clin North Am 1999; 79(3): 611–22.

Murray JG, Apthorp LA, Wilkins RA. Long-segment (>10 cm) femoropopliteal angioplasty: improved technical success and long-term patency. Radiology 1995; 195: 158–62.

Neufang A, Espinola-Klein C, Dorweiler B, Messow CM, Schmiedt W, Vahl CF. Femoropopliteal prosthetic bypass with glutaraldehyde stabilized human umbilical vein (HUV). J Vasc Surg 2007; 46 (2): 280–8.

Noory E, Rastan A, Schwarzwälder U, Sixt S, Beschorner U, Bürgelin K, Neumann FJ, Zeller T. Retrograde Trans-popliteal Recanalization of Chronic Superficial Femoral Artery Occlusion in Case of Failed Antegrade Attempt. J Endovasc Ther 2009; 16: 619–23.

Norgren L, et al. Inter-Society Consensus for Management of Peripheral Arterial Disease (TASC II). Eur J Vasc Endovasc Surg 2007; 33 (1 Suppl): S1–S75.

Ouriel K, Shortell CK, DeWeese JA, Green RM, Francis CW, Azodo MV, et al. A comparison of thrombolytic therapy with operative revascularization in the initial treatment of acute peripheral arterial ischemia. J Vasc Surg 1994; 19 (6): 1021–30.

Pötter T, Van Limbergen E, Dries W, Popowski Y, Coen V, Fellner C, Georg D, Kirsits C, Levendag P, Marijnissen H, Marsiglia H, Mazeron JJ, Pokrajac B, Scalliet P, Tamburini V; EVA (endovascular) GEC (Groupe Européen de Curiethérapie) ESTRO (European Society for Therapeutic Radiation Oncology) Working Group. Prescribing, recording, and reporting in endovascular brachytherapy. Quality assurance, equipment, personnel and education. Radiother Oncol 2001 Jun; 59 (3): 339–60. Erratum in: Radiother Oncol 2001 Sep; 60 (3): 337–8.

Pokrajac B, Kirisits C, Schmid R, Schillinger M, Berger D, Peer K, Tripuraneni P, Pötter R, Minar E. Beta endovascular brachytherapy using CO2-filled centering catheter for treatment of recurrent superficial femoropopliteal artery disease. Cardiovasc Revasc Med 2009 Jul–Sep; 10 (3): 162–5.

Rastan A, Sixt S, Schwarzwälder U, Kerker W, Bürgelin K, Frank U, Noory E, Gremmelmeier D, Branzan D, Hauswald K, Brantner R, Schwarz T, Zeller T. Initial Experience with Directed Laser Atherectomy: The Bias Sheath First in Man Study. JEVT 2007; 14: 365–73.

Robinson BI, Fletcher JP, Tomlinson P, Allen RD, Hazelton SJ, Richardson AJ, et al. A prospective randomized multicentre comparison of expanded polytetrafluoroethylene and gelatin-sealed knitted Dacron grafts for femoropopliteal bypass. Cardiovasc Surg 1999; 7 (2): 214–8.

Scheinert D, Biamino G. Access sites for peripheral interventions. In: Marco J, Serruys P, Biamino G, Fajadet J, de Feyter P, Morice M, et al. (eds). The Paris Course on Revascularization course book. Europa edition, Poitiers, France, 2003: 405–10.

Scheinert D, Grummt L, Piorkowski M, Sax J, Scheinert S, Ulrich M, Werner M, Bausback Y, Braunlich S, Schmidt A. A novel self-expanding interwoven nitinol stent for complex femoropopliteal lesions: 24-month results of the SUPERA SFA registry. J Endovasc Ther 2011 Dec; 18 (6): 745–52.

Scheinert D, Scheinert S, Sax J, Piorkowski C, Braunlich S, Ulrich M, et al. Prevalence and clinical impact of stent fractures after femoropopliteal stenting. J Am Coll Cardiol 2005; 45: 312–5.

Schillinger M, Minar E. Advances in vascular brachytherapy over the last 10 years: focus on femoropopliteal applications. J Endovasc Ther 2004; 11 (Suppl II): II-180–91.

Schillinger M, Sabeti S, Loewe C, Dick P, Amighi J, Mlekusch W, et al. Balloon angioplasty versus implantation of nitinol stents in the superficial femoral artery. N Engl J Med 2006; 354; 1879–88.

Schouten O, Hoedt MT, Wittens CH, Hop WC, van Sambeek MR, van Urk H. End-to-end versus end-to-side distal anastomosis in femoropopliteal bypasses; results of a randomized multicenter trial. Eur J Vasc Endovasc Surg 2005; 29 (5): 457–62.

Sixt S, Rastan A, Beschorner U, Noory E, Schwarzwälder U, Bürgelin K, Schwarz T, Müller C, Hauk M, Brantner R, Möhrle C, Linnemann B, Macharzina R, Neumann FJ, Zeller T. Acute and long-term outcome of Silverhawk assisted atherectomy for femoro-popliteal lesions according the TASC II classification: a single-center experience. Vasa 2010; 39: 229–36.

Sixt S, Scheinert D, Rastan A, Krankenberg H, Steinkamp H, Schmidt A, Sievert H, Minar E, Bosiers M, Peeters P, Balzer JO, Tübler T, Wissgott C, Nielsen C, Schwarzwälder U, Zeller T. One-Year outcome after percutaneous rotational and aspiration atherectomy in infrainguinal arteries in patient with and without diabetes mellitus type 2. Ann Vasc Surg 2011; 25: 520–9.

Sixt S, Rastan A, Scheinert D, Krankenberg H, Steinkamp H, Schmidt A, Sievert H, Minar E, Bosiers M, Peeters P, Balzer JO, Tübler T, Wissgott C, Nielsen C, Schwarzwälder U, Zeller T. The 1-Year Clinical Impact of Rotational Aspiration Atherectomy of Infrainguinal Lesions. Angiology 2011 May 8; [Epub ahead of print].

Temelkova-Kurktschiev T, Fischer S, Koehler C, Mennicken G, Henkel E, Hanefeld M. [Intima-media thickness in healthy probands without risk factors for arteriosclerosis]. Dtsch Med Wochenschr. 2001 Feb 23; 126 (8): 193–7. German.

Tendera M, Aboyans V, Bartelink ML, Baumgartner I, Clement D, Collet JF, Cremonesi A, De Carlo M, Erbel R, Fowkes FGR, Heras M, Kownator S, Minar E, Ostergren J, Poldermans D, Riambau V, Roffi M, Röther J, Sievert H, van Sambeek M, Zeller T. ESC Guidelines on the diagnosis and treatment of peripheral artery diseases: Document covering atherosclerotic disease of extracranial carotid and vertebral, mesenteric, renal, upper and lower extremity arteries. European Heart Journal 2011; 32: 2851–906, doi:10.1093/eurheartj/ehr211.

Tepe G, Zeller T, Albrecht T, Heller S, Schwarzwälder U, Beregi JP, Claussen CD, Oldenburg A, Scheller B, Speck U. Local taxane with short exposure for reduction of restenosis in distal arteries: THUNDER Trial. N Engl J Med 2008; 358: 689–99.

The TASC-working group. Management of peripheral arterial disease—the TransAtlantic Inter-Society Consensus (TASC). J Vasc Surg 2000; 31 (Suppl. 1).

Therasse E, Donath D, Lespérance J, et al. External beam radiation to prevent restenosis after superficial femoral artery balloon angioplasty. Circulation 2005; 111: 3310–5.

Werner M, Scheinert D, Henn M, Scheinert S, Bräunlich S, Bausback Y, Friedenberger J, Schuster J, Hertting K, Piorkowski M, Rosner C, Schmidt A, Ulrich M, Gutberlet M. Endovascular brachytherapy using liquid Beta-emitting rhenium-188 for the treatment of long-segment femoropopliteal in-stent stenosis. J Endovasc Ther 2012; 19 (4): 467–75.

Wolfram R, Budinsky A, Pokrajac B, et al. Endovascular brachytherapy for prophylaxis of restenosis after femoropopliteal angioplasty: five-year follow-up—prospective randomized study. Radiology 2006; 240: 878–84.

Wolfram R, Budinsky A, Pokrajac B, Pötter R, Minar E. Vascular brachytherapy with 192-Iridium after femoropopliteal stent implantation in high risk patients: twelve-month follow-up results from the Vienna-5 trial. Radiology 2005; 236: 343–51.

Wohlgemuth WA, Leissner G, Wengenmair H, Bohndorf K, Kirchhof K. Endovascular brachytherapy with (192)Ir and (188)Re to treat de novo and recurrent infrainguinal restenoses. J Cardiovasc Surg 2010; 51: 573–8.

Zeller T, Frank U, Bürgelin K, Schwarzwälder U, Horn B, Flügel PC, Neumann FJ. [Long-term results after recanalization of acute and subacute thrombotic occlusions of the infra-aortic arteries and bypass grafts using a rotational thrombectomy device.] article in German. Röfo – Fortschr Röntgenstr 2002; 174: 1559–65.

Zeller T, Krankenberg H, Rastan A, Sixt S, Schmidt A, Tübler T, Schwarz T, Frank U, Bürgelin K, Schwarzwälder U, Hauswald K, Kliem M, Pochert V, Neumann FJ, Scheinert D. Percutaneous rotational and aspiration atherectomy in infrainguinal peripheral arterial occlusive disease: a multi-centre pilot study. JEVT 2007; 14: 357–64.

Zeller T, Rastan A, Schwarzwälder U, Schwarz T, Frank U, Bürgelin K, Sixt S, Müller C, Rothenpieler U, Flügel PC, Tepe G, Neumann FJ. Long-term results after directional atherectomy of femoro-popliteal lesions. JACC 2006; 48 (8): 1573–8.

Zeller T, Tiefenbacher C, Steinkamp HJ, Langhoff R, Wittenberg G, Schlüter M, Rastan A, Krumsdorf U, Sixt S, Bürgelin K, Schulte K-L, Tübler T, Krankenberg H. Nitinol stent implantation in TASC A and B superficial femoral artery lesions: the femoral artery conformexx trial (FACT). J Endovasc Ther 2008; 15: 390–8.

Zeller, T, Bräunlich S, Waldo M, Cheng C, Macharzina R, Scheinert D, Rastan A. The NovoStent® SAMBA™ Stent—a novel alternating helix self-expanding nitinol stent design. Interventional Cardiology 2011; 3: 247–61.

Zeller T, Krankenberg H, Steinkamp HJ, Rastan A, Sixt S, Schmidt A, Sievert H, Minar E, Bosiers M, Peeters P, Balzer JO, Gray W, Tübler T, Wissgott C, Schwarzwälder U, Scheinert D. One-year outcome of percutaneous rotational and aspiration atherectomy in infrainguinal peripheral arterial occlusive disease: the multi-centre pathway PVD Trial. J Endovasc Ther 2009; 16: 653–62.

Zeller T, Kambara A, Samuel M, Atar E, Chulsky A, Sixt S, Tepe G, Rastan A, Buchbinder M. Recanalization of femoropopliteal chronic total occlusions using the ENABLER-P Catheter System. J Endovasc Ther 2012; in press.

4.4.9 Endovascular and surgical treatment in the infrapopliteal arteries: technique, clinical results, prospects

Anatomy of the arteries in the lower leg and foot: Reinhard Putz
Endovascular treatment: Andrej Schmidt and Dierk Scheinert
Doppler/duplex ultrasonography: Tom Schilling
Surgical treatment: Achim Neufang

4.4.9.1 Anatomy of the arteries in the lower leg and foot

The popliteal artery leaves the popliteal region distally under the tendinous arch of the soleus muscle and continues as the posterior tibial artery. The latter passes in a common connective-tissue neurovascular sheath in the depths of the calf muscles as far as the medial malleolar groove, and from there supplies the sole of the foot (Fig. 4.4-86).

Just after the emergence of the soleus below the tendinous arch, the anterior tibial artery branches off ventrally and passes through a gap in the interosseous membrane, lying distal to the tibiofibular joint, into the anterior lower leg compartment. In the extensor loge, it passes distally deeply embedded between the anterior tibial and extensor hallucis longus muscles. It crosses under the tendon at the level of the ankle and after giving off small branches to the malleolar network, it reaches the back of the foot as the dorsalis pedis artery (Fig. 4.4-87).

The next branch given off, also far proximally, is the fibular (peroneal) artery, which lies dorsal to the fibula and branches into the muscles of the fibular compartment. Its end branches also supply the malleolar network.

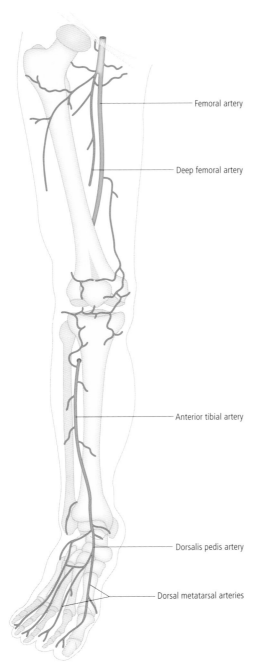

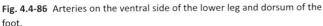

Fig. 4.4-86 Arteries on the ventral side of the lower leg and dorsum of the foot.

Labels on figure: Femoral artery / Deep femoral artery / Anterior tibial artery / Dorsalis pedis artery / Dorsal metatarsal arteries

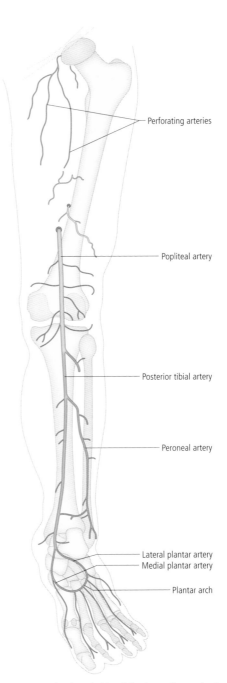

Fig. 4.4-87 Arteries on the dorsal side of the lower leg and sole of the foot.

Labels on figure: Perforating arteries / Popliteal artery / Posterior tibial artery / Peroneal artery / Lateral plantar artery / Medial plantar artery / Plantar arch

The malleolar network around the distal end of the lower leg, like the arterial network around the knee, is able to ensure an adequate supply to the foot if one of the two tibial arteries or the fibular artery is interrupted.

Covered by the aponeurosis that closes the tarsal sinus and from which the abductor hallucis muscle originates, the posterior tibial artery branches into the two plantar arteries. The medial plantar artery remains embedded between the abductor hallucis and the flexor digitorum brevis muscles on the medial side of the foot and gives off a deep branch toward the plantar arterial arch. The slightly thicker lateral plantar artery, lying on the quadratus plantae muscle, crosses under the thick belly of the flexor digitorum brevis muscle and passes laterally from there to the midfoot, where it supplies the deep plantar arch that lies on the metatarsal bone and interosseous muscles.

The dorsalis pedis artery becomes the arcuate artery at the level of the tarsometatarsal joint. The metatarsal arteries branch off from it and pass distally in the spaces between the metatarsal bones to supply the dorsal digital arteries of the toes. There are numerous anastomoses between the dorsal and plantar arteries of the foot via the perforating branches, which pass through the intermetatarsal spaces proximally.

4.4.9.2 Endovascular treatment in the infrapopliteal arteries

Introduction

Interventional treatment for arteriosclerotic lesions in the infrapopliteal region was still being administered with great caution only a few years ago. This was because on the one hand, there were hardly any endovascular materials available for this region, while on the other interventions in the area were regarded as potentially dangerous and unpromising due to high rates of failure and restenosis. The treatment recommendations for infrapopliteal obstructions (TASC-I 2000) were correspondingly cautious. An infrapopliteal occlusion more than 2 cm long was regarded as a clear indication for surgical revascularization. However, since an indication for infrapopliteal recanalization is mainly restricted to patients who are at the stage of critical ischemia, and these patients often have extended arteriosclerotic occlusions, there was only rarely any indication for endovascular therapy. There is currently a marked increase in interest in endovascular treatment in the lower leg, however, particularly since the increasing numbers of diabetic patients and patients of advanced age, with the corresponding increase in cases of critical ischemia, are associated with a high level of surgical risk due to comorbid conditions and a less invasive approach would be advantageous. The development of materials specifically designed for this region has also contributed to a shift in treatment toward endovascular therapy. This trend is also reflected in the revision of the TASC recommendations (TASC-II 2007). As the approach used is currently undergoing a process of change, no clear recommendations are given by TASC for selecting the treatment method in relation to the complexity of the lesions, and the physician involved therefore has greater freedom of choice. The recommendation given in the S3 guideline issued by the German Angiology Association is clearer, advocating endovascular therapy even for lesions > 10 cm long (Lawall et al. 2009). Several authors have already described endovascular therapy as the treatment of choice (Bosiers et al. 2006).

Indications for PTA in the lower leg arteries

Critical ischemia in Fontaine stages III and IV or Rutherford 4–6 represents the main indication for recanalization of obstructions in the lower leg. Treatment at the stage at which the walking distance is restricted is a controversial topic, as there is some doubt as to whether infrapopliteal obstructions are capable of causing intermittent claudication. However, several publications have shown that marked symptomatic improvement in this regard occurs after revascularization of the lower leg (Rastan et al. 2011). Treatment of the infrapopliteal arteries is indicated in order to improve outflow and also to improve the patency rate after revascularization at the thigh and/or popliteal level—e.g., after bypass placement (Lawall et al. 2009). Before any planned amputation, the option of recanalization in the infrapopliteal region should also be checked in order to improve wound healing in the stump area.

Contraindications against PTA in the lower leg arteries

Recanalization is not indicated in asymptomatic lower leg obstructions, as there is as yet no evidence of prognostic benefit. In patients with manifest hyperthyroidism, interventions can be carried out using gadolinium as the contrast agent.

Precise preinterventional diagnosis (e.g., with MR angiography) is extremely helpful here to ensure that the angiography is limited to the affected area and thus keeping within the recommended maximum dosage of 0.1 mmol gadolinium/kg body weight.
CO_2 angiography is another alternative and should be used in particular in patients with renal insufficiency. However, selective injection of CO_2 into the lower leg is sometimes found to be very uncomfortable or painful. An examination with the quality required can then only be carried out with the patient under general anesthesia. In patients who are in the active stage of thromboangiitis obliterans, angioplasty is generally carried out only with caution, particularly with the small arteries in the lower leg.

Preinterventional diagnosis and angiography

The noninvasive methods used to identify PAOD in the lower leg area are duplex ultrasonography, segmental plethysmography, and tibial occlusive pressure measurement with a Doppler probe, as well as occlusive pressure measurement and light plethysmography at the toes. The latter two methods are very important, due to the large numbers of patients who have medial calcinosis as a result of diabetes mellitus, in whom ankle occlusion pressure measurements are consequently unreliable. In the hands of an experienced examiner, duplex ultrasonography provides valuable additional information for establishing the indication for catheter angiography in readiness for an intervention.

Doppler/duplex ultrasonography

Examination technique

A (5)–7.5 MHz linear scanner is used, as the ultrasound conditions are often poor (particularly with slow post-stenotic flow and in cases of mediasclerosis). The examination is carried out with low-flow settings (low PRF, increased gain, or use of power mode or B-flow as appropriate). The examination is often easier from distal to proximal, and the origin of the anterior tibial artery is most easily identified from the anterolateral direction below the head of the fibula. When the patient has acral and foot symptoms, the arteries of the foot should be imaged (particularly the medial and lateral plantar arteries and metatarsal arteries), along with the arteries of the toes. Continuous imaging is often difficult (due to signal loss), but segmental imaging provides information about the extent to which the hemodynamics are generally compromised. In patients with diabetic foot (with autosympathectomy) and peripheral inflammation (and subsequent vasodilation), there is often a monophasic flow profile with no upstream flow compromise. The differential diagnosis is against a signal with post-stenotic and monophasic deformation, with particular attention to the acceleration time (short, in contrast to post-stenotic flow) and the shape of the curve.

Measurement of occlusion pressure (ankle–brachial index) using continuous-wave Doppler

Procedure

The patient should be supine, with an adequate resting phase. The blood-pressure cuff is then applied and the correct cuff width should be selected depending on the circumference of the extremities:
- Thigh and proximal lower leg 15–16 cm
- Arm and distal lower leg 13 cm
- Large toe 2 cm

The cuff is initially applied bilaterally in the upper arm area with assessment of each radial artery and measurement of the occlusion pressure in the brachial artery with a suprasystolic block and then a slow reduction in the cuff pressure. The cuff is then placed in the distal lower leg area with assessment of each posterior tibial artery and dorsalis pedis artery, and measurement of occlusion pressure in the dorsalis pedis and posterior tibial arteries using a slow release of the cuff pressure. When pressures in these infrapopliteal arteries are critically reduced, the peroneal artery can also be assessed.

N.B.: Measurement of occlusion pressures always captures the pressure at the level of the cuff and not at the level of the probe—and should be described as such (i.e., not pressure in the dorsalis pedis artery, but in the anterior tibial artery). Pressure can be measured in the toe arteries as an alternative or supplement (this is less error-prone in cases of mediasclerosis).

Evaluation

Occlusion pressures in the infrapopliteal arteries are normally approximately 10% higher than the occlusion pressure in the brachial artery.

The pressure difference $P_{upper\ arm} - P_{lower\ leg}$ is thus –10 mmHg to –20 mmHg; in pathological cases, it is a sign of compensation in patients with PAOD.

The pressure ratio (synonym: pressure index or ankle–brachial index, ABI), $P_{lower\ leg}/P_{brachial}$ is > 1. Values of 0.92–1 represent a gray area that requires further investigation, supplemented by curve analysis and spectral analysis of the signal. The normal value at rest does not safely exclude low to moderate PAOD.

To establish a **diagnosis** of PAOD and calculate the ABI, the lowest pressure in the infrapopliteal arteries is always used. The highest absolute value measured is used to estimate the degree of compensation in PAOD. *Caution:* new automatic measurement procedures do not provide adequate discrimination here.

Potential errors

Incorrectly high occlusion pressure:
- Mediasclerosis (pressure measurement in the toe arteries may be needed)
- Lower leg edema and/or sclerosis of the skin and subcutaneous tissue (repeat examination after edema has regressed)
- Cuff too narrow
- Hypersystolic block too long
- Upper part of the body raised

Incorrectly low occlusion pressure:
- Pressure cuff deflated too quickly
- Probe dislocated
- Resting period too short
- Measurements repeated too often

Incorrect measurement of brachial pressure:
- Only unilateral pressure measurement when in the presence of an upstream stenosis (e.g., subclavian artery stenosis)
- Bilateral upstream stenoses

Differential diagnosis

Classic arteriosclerosis: classic plaque morphology—see under specific findings.

Thromboangiitis obliterans: segmental involvement particularly of medium-sized and smaller arteries—thus in particular the lower leg arteries.

Functional compartment syndrome: pain symptoms in the anterior muscle compartment after heavy physical exercise, due to muscular edema (see under specific findings).

Specific findings

Arteriosclerotic stenoses and occlusions

The methods used to grade stenoses are identical with those used in the femoropopliteal region (see corresponding text) (Fig. 4.4-88).

Critical ischemia

Occlusion pressure in the infrapopliteal arteries < 50 mmHg and/or in the toe arteries < 30 mmHg. The acceleration time on the hemotachogram, measured as distally as possible, is > 180 ms, V_{max} usually < 30 cm/s.

Thromboangiitis obliterans

A specific but not pathognomonic finding is atypical collaterals that appear as "corkscrew collaterals" in the region of the infrapopliteal arteries, particularly the anterior tibial artery (meandering collaterals within the boundaries of the adventitia, Fig. 4.4-89). Another sign is an abrupt (cut-off) start in proximal occlusions, a terminal filum appearance in distal occlusions, vasospasms ("rippling,"

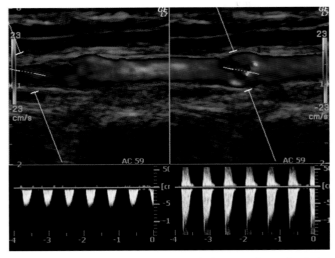

Fig. 4.4-88 Septal stenosis of the posterior tibial artery with a peak velocity ratio (PVR) of 3—corresponding to an approximately 60–70% stenosis, i.e., moderate stenosis.

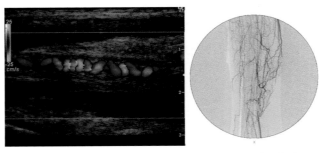

Fig. 4.4-89 Convoluted "corkscrew collaterals" coursing within the boundaries of the adventitia of the occluded infrapopliteal artery, as a classic sign of thromboangiitis obliterans; right: the corresponding angiogram.

"standing wave phenomenon"), and small vessels and collaterals with a convoluted course.

Functional compartment syndrome

There is increased pulsatility in the anterior tibial artery at its origin. On side-to-side comparison, there is a larger distance between the skin surface and the interosseous membrane in the symptomatic leg, as a sign of intrafascial edema.

Other diagnostic procedures

The clinical findings and evidence of relevant PAOD based on one of the above-mentioned diagnostic methods are sufficient to establish the indication for invasive angiographic imaging of the infrapopliteal arteries in readiness for percutaneous transluminal angioplasty (PTA). Angiography should be carried out selectively, either after the catheter has been advanced using a cross-over technique as far as the distal superficial femoral artery or directly via a sheath advanced antegrade into the distal superficial femoral artery, or preferably via a catheter positioned in the popliteal artery. When the beam direction is anteroposterior, the anterior tibial artery and peroneal artery are superimposed in the middle lower leg region, so that various angulations need to be used. It is indispensable to have complete pre-interventional imaging of the foot arteries at two levels as well, with an anteroposterior beam and approximately 30° cranial angulation, as well as a lateral beam (e.g., right foot, left anterior oblique 60–70°).

Noncontrast fluoroscopy provides information about the degree of sclerosis and any mediasclerosis that may be present that could serve for guidance during guidewire passage. Injection of contrast medium into the infrapopliteal arteries can be painful and can lead to vasospasm. Adequate dilution of the contrast medium with physiological saline and the use of low-osmolar nonionic contrast medium should be ensured. Intra-arterial administration of nitroglycerine solution should be considered if blood-pressure conditions are sufficient, particularly in younger patients.

Considerations when planning the intervention

The concept of the angiosome has been receiving increasing attention during the planning of these interventions. The idea is to consider which area of the foot is supplied by which artery and ought to be treated with priority relative to the location of the ischemic foot lesion. When there is ischemia in the area of the dorsal toe region, an attempt should therefore be made to recanalize the anterior tibial artery. Via its medial and lateral plantar branches, the posterior tibial artery supplies a large part of the sole of the foot and plantar toes, as well as the medial area of the heel. Recanalizing the peroneal artery can be helpful in healing ischemic lesions in the lateral area of the heel. Recognizable individual variants in the arterial system of the foot and the collateral supply must of course be taken into account. Retrospective analyses have shown that recanalization based on the angiosome concept leads to better clinical results than recanalization of an artery that does not directly supply the ischemic foot area (Alexandrescu et al. 2011). However, it should be remembered that the morphological conditions involved in arteriosclerotic obstruction in many cases prevent interventionalists from following the angiosome concept and they may need to be satisfied with opening an artery that does not directly supply the ischemic area. Other research groups have noted that the number of recanalized arteries is the only positive predictive factor for clinical success, and they prefer recanalization of as many arteries as possible, independently of the angiosome concept (Peregrin et al. 2011).

Endovascular treatment technique

Access routes

Antegrade access via the ipsilateral inguinal region is the most commonly used approach. Due to the miniaturization of the materials, a 4F or 5F sheath is usually sufficient, and these are also available with lengths of 35, 45, and 55 cm (Cordis, Cook), allowing direct access to the lesion (alternatively, a guide catheter 55 cm or 100 cm long can be used). Puncture of the superficial femoral artery should be avoided, as compression at the end of the procedure is more difficult, and bleeding and pseudoaneurysms may occur more frequently. However, antegrade puncture of the common femoral artery may be difficult in obese patients, and contralateral crossover access may be necessary. Puncture above the inguinal ligament must be absolutely avoided, as bleeding there can lead uncontrollably to a retroperitoneal hematoma. However—with the 90-cm sheaths currently available (Cook, Terumo, Cordis) and balloons (Amphirion Deep, with a working length of 150 cm, Invatec)—crossover access via retrograde puncture in the contralateral inguinal region can be used even to carry out angioplasty of the foot arteries. Marked tortuosity or severe calcification of the pelvic arteries may lead to a significant loss of maneuverability in the guidewire in the lower leg area, however, in which case ipsilateral antegrade access is preferable.

If an occlusion in an infrapopliteal artery cannot be passed with the guidewire, transpedal access and retrograde recanalization may be successful. Reconstitution of the dorsalis pedis artery or posterior tibial artery in the area of the upper ankle joint is a prerequisite for this. However, puncture of the peroneal artery in the dorsal area of the lower leg is also possible (Fig. 4.4-90a–j). The puncture should be carried out with a 21-gauge needle, with the assistance of the "roadmap" function or preferably with fluoroscopy with simultaneous contrast injection (Fig. 4.4-90c). If a sheath is used, it should be as small as possible (e.g., 4F Terumo sheath for a 0.025" guidewire). A 3F sheath is now available that has been specially developed for this type of access (Transpedal Set, Cook), over which a support catheter (CXI, Cook) or coronary balloon with a particularly low profile (e.g., the MiniTrek OTW balloon, Abbott) can be used. To minimize traumatization of the pedal artery, a guidewire can also be introduced directly over the puncture needle and a balloon or support catheter can be introduced over it directly into the vessel as a support catheter without using a sheath (Fig. 4.4-90f). After successful retrograde passage of the arterial occlusion, the guidewire is maneuvered—using a catheter (4–6F) introduced antegrade into the popliteal artery via a second access site—out of the inguinal sheath, so that the 300-cm guidewire can now be used as a rail for a balloon introduced from the antegrade direction. While the angioplasty is being carried out from the antegrade direction, the wire along with the guide catheter and balloon or sheath should be removed from the pedal artery in order to minimize the dwell time in the vessel. Compression by a second operator for a few minutes is usually sufficient to achieve hemostasis, even under anticoagulation. In puncture procedures above the ankle, a blood-pressure

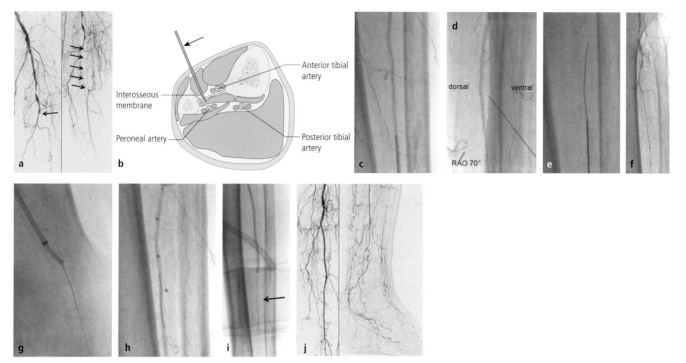

Fig. 4.4-90a–j (a) Occlusion of the middle peroneal artery on the left side (arrows). (b) Puncture of the peroneal artery requires a 7-cm long 21-gauge needle (arrow). The peroneal artery lies dorsal to the interosseous membrane, which has to be penetrated by the needle. (c) Puncture of the left peroneal artery; the C-arm is at a left anterior oblique (LAO) angle (approx. 30°), so that the needle forms a line with the peroneal artery. (d) The C-arm can be moved to right anterior oblique (RAO, approx. 70°) to allow estimation of the distance between the needle tip and the artery. (e) The LAO projection is then restored and after puncture of the peroneal artery a 0.018" guidewire (V18 Control, 300 cm, Boston Scientific) is introduced into the vessel. (f) After a support catheter has been introduced (QuickCross 0.018", 90 cm, Spectranetics), directly through the skin (without a sheath), the occlusion is passed from the retrograde direction. (g) After passage of the occlusion from the retrograde direction, the wire is maneuvered into a catheter that has been advanced from antegrade (Judkins R 5F) so that it can be led out of the proximal sheath. (h) After the wire has been pulled from the proximal sheath and a balloon has been introduced from antegrade, the wire is pulled and is now led in an antegrade direction distal to the balloon on the QuickCross catheter that is still in position in the peroneal artery. (i) Compression of the puncture site using a blood-pressure cuff for 10 minutes while the angioplasty of the lesion is carried out. (j) The final result, with an unremarkable appearance at the puncture site.

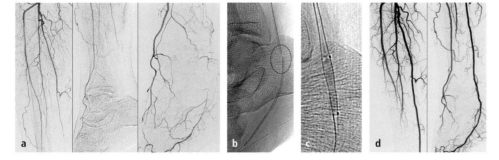

Fig. 4.4-91a–d (a) A long occlusion in the dominant posterior tibial artery, with clinical signs of dysesthesia particularly in the area of the heel sole of the foot. (b) Due to a fibrotic stenosis in the malleolus area, a normal balloon does not open completely even at 16 bar (broken circle). (c) Using a "scoring" balloon, which presses two wires (one attached to the outside of the balloon and the guidewire) into the plaque during inflation, reducing vessel wall rigidity, the residual stenosis is easily eliminated. (d) The result after balloon dilation.

cuff is raised to hypersystolic pressure for a few minutes over the puncture site (Fig. 4.4-90i); heparin antagonization with protamine should not be carried out. Using this technique, which is only indicated if an attempt at traditional antegrade recanalization has failed, a very high rate of success can be achieved (Montero-Baker et al. 2008).

There has also been increasing interest in interventional recanalization of arteries distal to the ankle, as well as the foot arteries. Using what is known as the "foot loop technique," an occlusion that can not be crossed from the antegrade direction is recanalized with a retrograde approach, with the plantar arch being used as the access route (Fig. 4.4-91a–d), or with recanalization of the plantar arch in order to reach an area that is not accessible from antegrade (Manzi et al. 2009)—following the angiosome concept. However, there is as yet little information about success and complication rates with this technique, and in particular about the restenosis rates.

Intervention

Balloon dilation is the standard technique. Alternatively, percutaneous atherectomy and stent implantation can also be performed.

Guidewires and support catheters

Whether a stenosis or an occlusion is present is the major factor involved in deciding on the choice of guidewire. Whereas shorter stenoses are best treated using coronary materials—i.e., a short guidewire and coronary monorail balloons, usually 20 mm long (Abbott Vascular, Medtronic, Cordis, etc.)—300-cm long wires that allow over-the-wire (OTW) balloons to be used are advantageous for passing longer occlusions. Guidewires with a diameter of 0.014" in particular are being increasingly used, as they allow very low-profile balloons to be used. Polymer-coated hydrophilic wires (e.g., PT2 or Journey™, Boston Scientific; Hydro ST, Cook Medical) are most often used. For severely calcified occlusions, a number of wires specifically developed for these difficult obstructions are now available (Winn 200 T, Abbott; CTO Approach 18g and 25g, Cook Medical). A 0.018" guidewire (V18 Control Wire, Boston Scientific) offers greater stability. More recent developments specifically for calcified lesions are 0.018" guidewires (Connect 250 T, Abbott; Astato 30g, Asahi Intecc). Finally, the rigid 0.035" Terumo wire with a straight tip is also used in occlusions that are difficult to pass, while accepting a high risk of perfusion and loss of the low profile.

Intraluminal passage of the wire is generally preferred in the area of the lower leg, although subintimal recanalization has also been reported to be successful using advancement of a Terumo wire loop (with a soft wire configuration or 0.035" Terumo half-stiff). However, maneuvering the wire back into the true lumen of the artery after passing the occlusion may be a difficult step. Long obstructions in particular require the guidewire to be stabilized with a support catheter (Quick-Cross™, Spectranetics; XCI, Cook; TrailBlazer, Covidien), but the balloon can also be used as a support catheter as an alternative.

Balloons

While coronary balloons using the monorail technique are often used for short stenoses, longer lesions are usually treated with an over-the-wire or coaxial technique. For successful passage of a total occlusion, it is best to use balloons with as small a profile as possible—e.g., balloons that can be guided over a 0.014-inch guidewire (Amphirion Deep™, Medtronic). The diameter of the balloon should not exceed 2.0 mm up to a maximum of 2.5 mm for the distal segment and 2.5–3.0 mm for the proximal area of the infrapopliteal arteries. Balloons with lengths of 120 mm and sometimes up to 220 mm (Amphirion Deep, Medtronic; Sleek, Cordis; Armada 14, Abbott; Coyote, Boston Scientific) are available. This technology also makes it possible to treat very lengthy lesions. Patients sometimes find the dilation process painful, but there is no risk of perforation as long as the balloon is not oversized. Pressures of 14–16 atm are maintained for a dilation time of up to 5 min.

Cutting balloons (Boston Scientific) are required in rare cases of severely calcified or fibrotic stenoses that cannot be dilated with a traditional balloon. The Angio-Sculpt™ PTA catheter (Angioscore, Biotronik), a balloon spirally wrapped with a nitinol wire, or the Vascutrak balloon (Bard) is based on a similar concept (Fig. 4.4-92a–d).

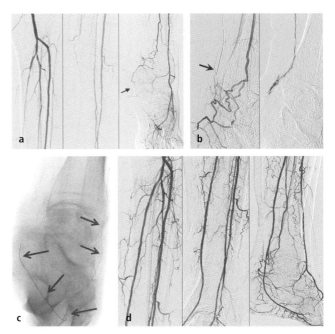

Fig. 4.4-92a–d (**a**) A patient with diabetes mellitus and mainly ischemic ulceration on the left heel, with no recognizable perfusion in the heel area (arrow). (**b**) A wire passage attempt through the occluded posterior tibial artery (arrow) is unsuccessful and leads to perforation. (**c**) However, wire passage is successful from the retrograde direction via the anterior tibial artery and plantar arch (arrows). (**d**) The result after balloon dilation.

No data are available comparing this with the traditional balloon angioplasty.

Cryoplasty (CryoBalloon™, Boston Scientific) uses fluid nitrogen oxide for balloon inflation. The phase transition from liquid to gas that occurs during inflow into the balloon leads to cooling of the arterial wall to –10°C. This system has also not yet been compared with traditional balloons in controlled studies.

Percutaneous catheter atherectomy

Although the efficacy of laser atherectomy in the treatment of critical ischemia has been confirmed in one single-center study and one multicenter registry study, it is now only carried out in a few centers. The laser can be helpful for passing severely calcified lesions, but the high purchasing price of the device is preventing its widespread use. The SilverHawk™ system and TurboHawk™ system (Covidien) are atherectomy catheters incorporating a rotating cutting blade that is available in various sizes for the arteries of the thigh and lower leg. This catheter allows resection and removal of obstructive material in *de novo* stenosis, recurrent stenosis, and in-stent restenosis. The TurboHawk™, a further development of the catheter, can now also be used in calcified lesions, although only with a filter system, due to the high risk of embolization with calcified lesions. A high rate of technical success was achieved with SilverHawk atherectomy in 36 patients with 49 infrapopliteal lesions, with remarkably high primary and secondary patency rates for infrapopliteal obstructions of 60% and 80% being achieved after 2 years (Zeller et al. 2007). More recent atherectomy systems such as the Jetstream system (Pathway Medical) and the Diamondback™ system (CSI) have proved effective in initial clinical studies, but are currently only available to a limited extent in Europe, if at all.

Stenting in the infrapopliteal arteries

A number of mainly self-expanding stents have been designed for use in the lower leg (e.g., Xpert™, Abbott; Maris Deep™, Medtronic; Astron Pulsar™, Biotronik; Sinus 18™, Optimed) that also make it possible to treat more extended lesions. Although the data on stents in the infrapopliteal region are much more sparse than those for the thigh region, systematic implantation of uncoated stents is not superior to balloon angioplasty in relation to patency rates or clinical end points, in contrast to the superficial femoral artery (Brodmann et al. 2011). The indications for stent implantation are therefore limited to unsatisfactory results after balloon angioplasty, such as flow-limiting dissection, significant residual stenosis, or significant recoil after PTA. A self-expanding stent should—if possible—be used at the transition from the popliteal artery to the infrapopliteal arteries, as it adapts better to different vascular diameters. This type of stent is also preferable in the distal infrapopliteal region, where there is a risk of stent compression by external forces.

Balloon-expandable stents are more suitable for reconstructing bifurcations, although there is a substantial restenosis rate with this application. Shortly after its origin, the anterior tibial artery passes through the interosseous membrane, where it is exposed to particular forces that may be the cause of the (rare) stent fractures in this area.

Systematic implantation of drug-eluting stents (DES) is a different matter. Three randomized studies, two of which have already been published (Rastan et al. 2011; Bosiers et al. 2011) have shown that coronary DES are clearly superior to uncoated stents for up to 1 year with regard to the restenosis rate. However, as DES are only available with a maximum length of 38 mm (although with approval for use in the peripheral arteries—e.g., Xience BTK, Abbott Vascular), only short lesions can be usefully treated with them.

Peri-interventional anticoagulation

The standard procedure is to administer 5000 IU unfractionated heparin during the intervention. Activated clotting time is not usually measured. Transpedal recanalizations have been carried out by one group using only additional administration of glycoprotein IIb/IIIa blockers, but sufficient data are not yet available to provide a basis for any recommendations. Anticoagulation therapy after balloon angioplasty consists of administration of 100 mg ASA daily, and after stent implantation additional administration of 75 mg/d clopidogrel for 4 weeks, or after implantation of DESs for at least 6 months.

Vasodilation during lower leg PTA

Intra-arterial administration of vasodilators plays an important role in lower leg recanalization. Particular in younger and female patients, there is an extremely strong tendency for vasospasm to develop during the dilation process, which is exacerbated by the injection of contrast.

Before or directly after balloon dilation or other recanalization techniques, administration of nitroglycerin 0.2–0.3 mg (1 mg nitroglycerin diluted in 10 mL NaCl, administration of 2–3 mL), 30–60 mg papaverine, calcium antagonists (e.g., up to 5 mg verapamil), or adenosine is carried out. The guidewire sometimes promotes spasm and consequently has to be withdrawn in order to assess the results of the PTA.

Detailed angiography is needed in order to distinguish between long or occult dissection and spasm.

Recanalization of acute infrapopliteal occlusions

Acute occlusions of the lower leg arteries are usually etiologically due to embolism. Spontaneous embolism is often cardiogenic, particularly in patients with atrial fibrillation, or may have arterioarterial causes—e.g., embolism from an aneurysm. In the latter case, a popliteal aneurysm always needs to be excluded. Angiography is not the method of choice, as it can only demonstrate the perfused lumen, but not the whole extent of an aneurysm that may be partly thrombosed. Duplex ultrasonography is the first-choice diagnostic method here. Iatrogenic emboli occur after recanalization of pelvic arteries, more frequently from occlusions of the superficial femoral artery or after arterial access via the common femoral artery—e.g., after coronary angiography.

Aspiration is the treatment of choice for occlusions that appear embolic. This requires a 6–8F end-hole guide catheter (e.g., Bard) for the distal popliteal artery and proximal lower leg arteries and a 5F catheter for distal emboli. Depending on the course of the artery, the catheters may be straight or curved (e.g., Multipurpose). As guide catheters are only available with lengths of 100 cm, crossover aspiration is often not possible and antegrade access is required. Thrombolysis (e.g., rt-PA 10 mg for 15 min) administered proximally at the thrombus, or after placement of a lysis catheter with multiple perforations into the occlusion (Cragg–McNamara, Micro Therapeutics), makes aspiration much easier. Aspiration is carried out with a 50-mL perfusion syringe, and the catheter is withdrawn slowly while maintaining aspiration. As the aspirate is sometimes lost at the sheath's hemostatic valve during catheter withdrawal, sheaths with removable valves are preferable (e.g., Destination, Terumo; Tuohy–Borst sheaths, Cook Medical). If complete aspiration is successful, local lysis via a side-hole lysis catheter for 12–24 h can follow.

Alternatively, various thrombectomy catheters (Rotarex, Straub Medical; Oasis, Boston Scientific; AngioJet, Possis Medical) can be used if the morphology of the occlusion is suitable. Laser treatment may also be successful, particularly after prior or simultaneous administration of a thrombolytic agent in acute occlusions. A coronary aspiration catheter (e.g., Diver-CE, Medtronic) may also be helpful in cases of acute distal embolization of thrombotic material. The main advantage of this system is that the guidewire (0.014") can be left in place and does not have to be removed for each aspiration.

Complications of infrapopliteal interventions

Complications of endovascular treatment in this region are generally rare. Peripheral embolization is a rarity. Guidewire perforations are rare, but are probably the most frequent complication, although they do not always make it necessary to stop the intervention and rarely require treatment. However, angiographically visible bleeding must always be stopped before the end of the intervention, as there is otherwise a substantial risk of compartment syndrome. If external compression—e.g., using a blood pressure cuff and/or heparin antagonization using protamine—is not sufficient, coil embolization or implantation of a stent graft (Graft-Master, Abbott Vascular) is available.

Results of infrapopliteal angioplasty

Although interventional therapy has not yet been compared with surgical treatment for infrapopliteal obstructions in randomized studies, a number of (partly prospective) registry studies have reported clinical results equivalent to those with surgery. In particular, even long occlusions affecting the entire course of the tibial arteries can be successfully treated with a high rate of technical and also clinical long-term success (Ferraresi et al. 2009). Since interventional treatment can be carried out with a very low complication rate and patients with critical ischemia represent a high-risk group for surgical procedures due to the frequent co-morbid conditions that are present, endovascular treatment is increasingly being regarded as the method of choice. In addition—in contrast to bypass surgery—the interventional procedure can be easily repeated in case of restenosis.

The restenosis rate after angioplasty for infrapopliteal lesions is inferior to the patency rates after bypass placement, but restenosis does not necessarily lead to clinical failure of the treatment. Nevertheless, it would be desirable to optimize endovascular treatment methods regarding restenosis rate. This seems worthwhile particularly in patients with intermittent claudication or resting pain, as it can be assumed that restenosis will necessarily also lead to recurrence of the symptoms in these cases. This is in contrast to ischemic ulcerations and gangrene. With these clinical findings, it is often assumed that optimizing the blood supply by carrying out recanalization is only required during the period of healing and less for maintaining tissue integrity over the long-term course. However, reducing the restenosis rate in these cases could also be beneficial, as several months often pass before ischemic lesions heal and restenosis during this period could have negative effects on the healing process.

Particularly for long lesions, a restenosis rate of nearly 70% only 3 months after PTA has been reported after angioplasty with traditional balloons (Fig. 4.4-93a–c), and clinical success can probably only be achieved with a high rate of repeat procedures (Schmidt et al. 2011).

As mentioned above, three randomized studies have now shown that patency rates of 80–85% after 1 year can be expected after DES treatment for short lesions (Rastan et al. 2011; Bosiers et al. 2011). In addition, registry studies have shown that restenoses can be expected mainly during the first year after implantation and that a stable result during the subsequent course can be expected (Werne et al. 2012).

Paclitaxel-coated balloons (drug-eluting balloons, DEB) lead to better results with long lesions. Initial studies using the first DEB to obtain approval (In.Pact Amphirion, Medtronic) showed a clear 60% reduction in the restenosis rate after 3 months following PTA for long infrapopliteal lesions, in comparison with traditional uncoated balloons (Schmidt et al. 2011) (Fig. 4.4-94a–c). However, randomized studies with clinical end points are still needed in order to confirm these positive results before DEB can enter everyday clinical work.

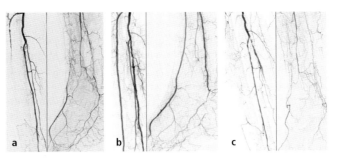

Fig. 4.4-93a–c (a) A long occlusion of the anterior tibial artery and stenosis of the posterior tibial artery in a patient with toe ulcerations on the right side. (b) After PTA in the anterior and posterior tibial arteries with traditional uncoated balloons. (c) Three months after PTA, the anterior and posterior tibial arteries once again appear occluded on angiography.

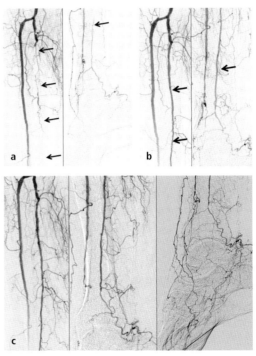

Fig. 4.4-94a–c (a) Occlusion of the distal anterior tibial artery and entire posterior tibial artery. Only the peroneal artery is filling small collaterals in the foot area, distal to a long occlusion (arrows: occlusion of the peroneal artery). (b) Results after angioplasty of the peroneal artery using two drug-eluting balloons (In.Pact Amphirion 2.5/120 mm, Medtronic) (arrows). (c) Despite the previous long occlusion, the small caliber of the vessel, and poor outflow, the peroneal artery is still without any significant restenosis even after 9 months.

Prospects

There has recently been a tremendous surge of interest in endovascular therapy for infrapopliteal obstructions. Even long occlusions do not currently present a technical obstacle, and endovascular therapy can therefore be used for almost every type of infrapopliteal obstruction. Using DES in short lesions and DEB in long lesions represents a solution for the high rates of restenosis, although the clinical superiority of DEB in comparison with uncoated standard balloons still needs to be confirmed. Angioplasty is feasible in very distal infrapopliteal and foot arteries, but the published data on this type of intervention are at present still sparse.

References

Alexandrescu V, Vincent G, Azdad K, Hubermont G, Ledent G, Ngongang C, Filimon A-N. A reliable approach to diabetic neuroischemic foot wounds: below-the-knee angiosome-oriented angioplasty. J Endovasc Ther 2011; 18: 376–87.

Bosiers M, Hart JP, Deloose K, Verbist J, Peeters P. Endovascular therapy as the primary approach for limb salvage in patients with critical limb ischemia: experience with 443 infrapopliteal procedures. Vascular 2006; 14: 63–9.

Bosiers M, Scheinert D, Peeters P, Torsello G, Zeller T, Deloose K, Schmidt A, Tessarek J, Vinck E, Schwartz LB. Randomized comparison of everolimus-eluting versus bare-metal stents in patients with critical limb ischemia and infrapopliteal arterial occlusive disease. J Vasc Surg 2011 Dec 12; [Epub ahead of print].

Brodmann M, Froelich H, Dorr A, Gary T, Portugaller RH, Deurschmann H, Pilger E. Percutaneous transluminal angioplasty versus primary stenting in infrapopliteal arteries in critical limb ischemia. Vasa 2011; 40: 482–90.

Ferraresi R, Centola M, Ferlini M, et al. Long-term outcomes after angioplasty of isolated, below-the-knee arteries in diabetic patients with critical limb ischemia. Eur J Vasc Endovasc Surg 2009; 37: 336–42.

Lawall H, Diehm C, Pittrow (Hrsg.). Deutsche Gesellschaft für Angiologie, Gesellschaft für Gefäßmedizin. Leitlinien zur Diagnostik und Therapie der peripheren arteriellen Verschlusskrankheit (PAVK). VASA 2009; 38 (Suppl 75): 1–72.

Manzi M, Fusaro M, Ceccacci T, Erente G, Dalla Paola L, Brocco E. Clinical results of below-the knee intervention using pedal-plantar loop technique for the revascularization of foot arteries. J Cardiovasc Surg (Torino) 2009; 50: 331–7.

Montero-Baker M, Schmidt A, Bräunlich S, et al. Retrograde approach for complex popliteal and tibioperoneal occlusions. J Endovasc Ther 2008; 15: 594–604.

Peregrin JH, Koznar B, Kovác J, et al. PTA of infrapopliteal arteries: long-term clinical follow-up and analysis of factors influencing clinical outcome. Cardiovasc Intervent Radiol 2010; 33: 720–5.

Rastan A, Tepe G, Krankenberg H, et al. Sirolimus-eluting stents vs. Bare-metal stents for treatment of focal lesions in infrapopliteal arteries: a double-blind, multicentre, randomized clinical trial. Eur Heart J 2011; 32: 2274–81.

Schmidt A, Ulrich M, Winkler B, et al. Angiographic patency and clinical outcome after balloon-angioplasty for extensive infrapopliteal arterial disease. Catheter Cardiovasc Interv 2010; 76: 1047–54.

Schmidt A, Piorkowski M, Werner M, et al. First experience with drug-eluting balloons in infrapopliteal arteries restenosis rate and clinical outcome. J Am Coll Cardiol 2011; 58: 1105–9.

Soder HK, Manninen HI, Jaakkola P, et al. Prospective trial of infrapopliteal artery balloon angioplasty for critical limb ischemia: angiographic and clinical results. J Vasc Interv Radiol 2000; 11: 1021–31.

TASC-I: Dormandy JA, Rutherford RB. Management of peripheral arterial disease (PAD). TASC Working Group. TransAtlantic Inter-Society Consensus (TASC). J Vasc Surg 2000 Jan; 31: S1–S296.

TASC-II: Norgren L, Hiatt WR, Dormandy JA, Nehler MR, Harris KA, Fowkes FG; on behalf of the TASC II Working Group. Inter-Society Consensus for the Management of Peripheral Arterial Disease (TASC II). Eur J Vasc Endovasc Surg 2007; 33 (Suppl 1): S1–S75.

Werner M, Schmidt A, Freyer M, Bausback Y, Bräunlich S, Friedenberger J, Schuster J, Botsios S, Scheinert D, Ulrich M. Sirolimus eluting stents for the treatment of infrapopliteal arteries in chronic limb ischemia: Clinical and angiographical long-term follow-up. J Endo Ther 2012; accepted.

Zeller T, Sixt S, Schwarzwälder U, et al. Two-years results after directional atherectomy of infrapopliteal arteries with the SilerHawk device. J Endovasc Ther 2007; 14: 232–40.

4.4.9.3 Surgical treatment in the lower leg arteries

Basic principles and general preparation

With the development of increasingly sophisticated diagnostic methods, the indication for bypass surgery has been extended more and more to the crural and pedal level during the last 30 or more years. The autologous venous bypass technique has dramatically improved the prognosis in critical ischemia and is now an indispensable component of peripheral surgical methods. In principle, all of the arteries in the course of the lower leg and foot can be considered for bypass anastomosis. The length and course of the required bypass depend entirely on the angiographic occlusion pattern present in the individual case (Figs. 4.4-82b, 4.4-95a–c) and on the materials available (Table 4.4-29).

In addition to cardiovascular evaluation, particularly in cases of critical ischemia in which gangrene is already established, general preparatory measures include initiating antibiogram-tested antibiotic therapy after a microbiological smear taken during primary local debridement, particularly in patients with ischemic diabetic foot syndrome. The affected limb should also be protected and adequate pain therapy should be provided in order to prevent further mechanical damage to the ischemic tissue. Complete angiographic imaging of the crural and pedal vessels is always required for surgical planning. Particularly in diabetic patients, if a patent femoropopliteal axis is visible with a distal type of occlusion (Fig. 4.4-96a and c), then the "distal origin" method is preferable—i.e., placement of the

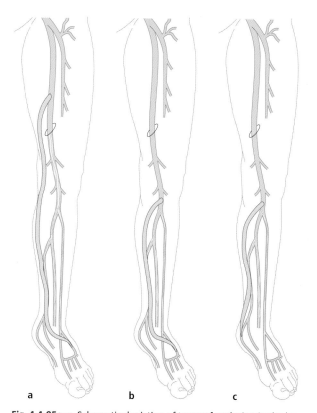

a b c

Fig. 4.4-95a–c Schematic depiction of types of occlusion in the lower leg, with pedal bypasses, including distal-origin bypass. Arterial occlusion in the lower leg with (**a**) and without (**b, c**) involvement of the popliteal artery. A long femoropedal venous bypass to the dorsalis pedis artery (**a**), and a popliteal distal-origin bypass to the dorsalis pedis artery (**b**) and to the plantar artery (**c**).

Table 4.4-29 Peripheral bypass types and anastomosis locations.

Bypass type	Central anastomosis	Peripheral anastomosis
Popliteal bypass	External iliac artery Common femoral artery Deep femoral artery Superficial femoral artery Popliteal artery	Popliteal artery above the knee joint (popliteal segment, above-knee bypass) Popliteal artery below knee joint before the trifurcation (third popliteal segment, below-knee bypass)
Crural bypass	Common femoral artery Deep femoral artery Superficial artery Popliteal artery	Tibioperoneal trunk Anterior tibial artery Posterior tibial artery Peroneal artery
Pedal bypass	Common femoral artery Deep femoral artery Superficial femoral artery Popliteal artery Proximal lower leg arteries	Dorsalis pedis artery Lateral tarsal artery Posterior tibial artery below the ankle joint Medial plantar artery Lateral plantar artery
Short distal bypass (distal-origin bypass)	Distal femoral artery Course of the popliteal artery Proximal lower leg arteries	Popliteal trifurcation Anterior tibial artery Posterior tibial artery Peroneal artery Dorsalis pedis artery Lateral tarsal artery Posterior tibial artery below the ankle joint Medial plantar artery Lateral plantar artery

proximal bypass anastomosis in the best possible distal donor vessel, often in the course of the popliteal artery (Fig. 7.4-96b and d).

If possible, a crural or pedal bypass should always consist entirely of autologous vein—ideally with the ipsilateral greater saphenous vein. As the autologous veins and potential recipient arterial vessels have adjoining courses, the in situ technique avoiding complete vein excision is a useful option in distal crural and pedal bypass surgery (Fig. 4.4-96d). If the greater saphenous vein is unsuitable or only partly usable, use of arm veins can also play an important role. If it is anticipated that the arm veins have to be used, the operation can be planned with two surgeons for simultaneous vein harvesting and exposure of the arteries. If the veins are being used in reversed or nonreversed manner, the distal anastomosis should be created first, if possible, in order to allow easier placement of the graft, but this is not absolutely necessary. When there are marked differences in vein caliber after harvesting and assessment of the greater saphenous vein for long femorodistal reconstructions, it is best to use the vein in a nonreversed direction after destruction of the venous valves (Fig. 4-4-96a). Caliber differences are less evident in short distal bypasses, and the vein can therefore also be implanted in the reversed position in these cases.

Surgical technique for crural and pedal reconstructions

A crural bypass anastomosis can be placed at the tibiofibular trunk (Fig. 4.4-97d) and along the complete course of the anterior tibial artery (Fig. 4.4-97a), posterior tibial artery (Fig. 4.4-97b), and peroneal artery (Fig. 4.4-97c, Table 4.4-29). In principle, the best possible crural vessel with unobstructed outflow to the foot should be selected for the distal anastomosis. When there are two vessels suitable for anastomosis, both peripheral vessels can also be included in what is known as a sequential bypass, if appropriate (Figs. 4.4-96e and f, 4.4-100a). The bypass graft is placed along the natural vascular course deep between the corresponding muscle groups (Fig. 4.4.-97c), or superficially in the subcutaneous tissue, particularly in patients who have previously undergone surgery (Fig. 4.4-97a, b, d). Subcutaneous placement of the bypass, particularly with spliced vein grafts (Fig. 4.4-97b and d), allows easier later bypass graft surveillance using duplex ultrasound. The ring-reinforced PTFE prosthesis bypass can also be easily placed in the subcutaneous position. In this case, the bypass is positioned using an atraumatic tunneling instrument with which the bypass graft can be gently passed through the tissue. Ideally, the course of the ipsilateral greater saphenous vein can be marked during the preoperative examination, so that possible incisions to expose the arterial donor and recipient vessels are already planned.

The artery is then carefully and sparingly dissected along a suitable-looking segment and is controlled with a thin vessel loop. After systemic anticoagulation with 5000–10,000 IU heparin, the crural and pedal anastomoses are created using a continuous technique with monofilament suture material (polypropylene 7–0 or 6–0), as thinly as possible. The parachute suturing technique and endoluminal control of backbleeding using thin probes, a blocking catheter, or putting slight tension on the vessel loops is recommended (Fig. 4.4-99). Clamping of these small vessels, which in diabetic patients sometimes have rigid walls due to significant sclerosis of the media layer, should be avoided at all costs in order to prevent development of early restenosis in the anastomotic region. Creation of the distal anastomosis in severely calcified vessels can be done in a bloodless field using a tourniquet for the same reason. Redon drains are placed during wound closure to prevent wound hematomas. The fascia is loosely adapted without constricting the bypass transit site. Loose subcutaneous suturing and skin closure with staples or interrupted sutures are recommended. Intracutaneous sutures should be avoided, particularly in patients requiring hemodialysis, as wound edge necrosis may occur with these. The skin suture material should be left in place for 2 weeks, or 3 weeks with pedal incisions.

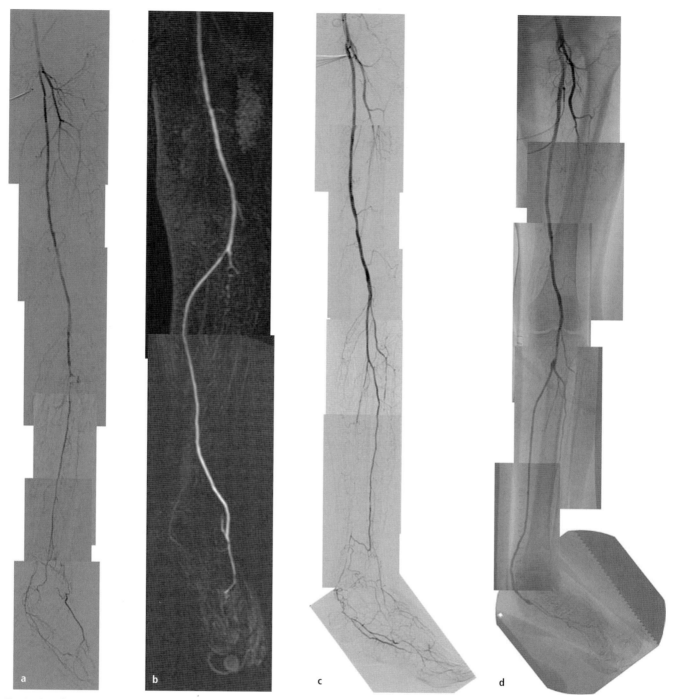

Fig. 4.4-96a–f Distal-origin bypass. (**a, b**) Typical appearance of lower leg arterial occlusion in a patient with diabetes mellitus with inadequate collateral-ization to the dorsalis pedis artery and severe infection of the foot with gangrene. A popliteopedal bypass was carried out from the popliteal artery above the knee joint to the dorsalis pedis artery. Magnetic resonance angiography 58 months postoperatively due to severe ischemia in the contralateral foot. (**c, d**) Arterial occlusion in the lower leg in a patient with diabetes mellitus with a preserved plantar artery and critical forefoot phlegmon with necroses. A popliteoplantar distal-origin in situ bypass was carried out using great saphenous vein to the plantar branching; forefoot amputation postoperatively.

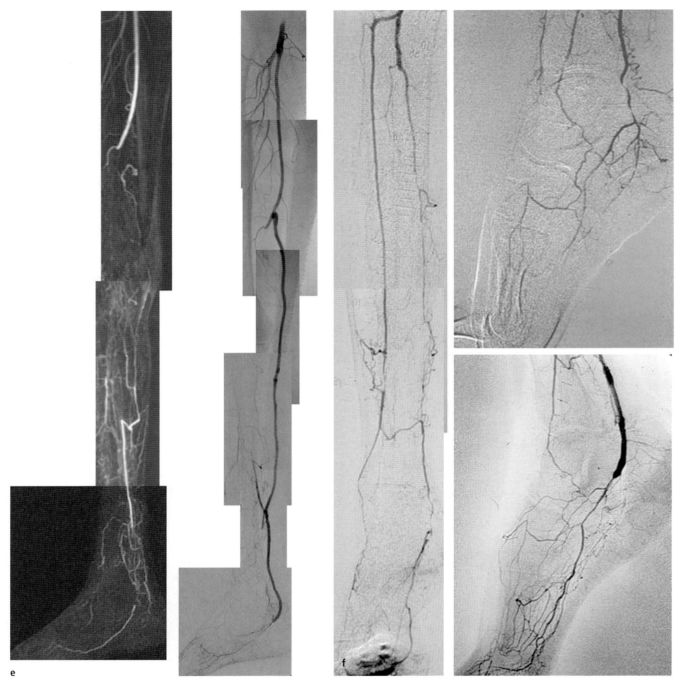

e

f

Fig. 4.4-96a–f Continuation. (**e**) A sequential distal-origin bypass with composite basilic vein and cephalic vein, from the distal superficial femoral artery to a segment of the posterior tibial artery and lateral plantar artery. (**f**) A sequential distal-origin bypass to the distal posterior tibial artery and medial plantar artery in a diabetic patient with an ulcer at the heel. Patent for 11.5 years.

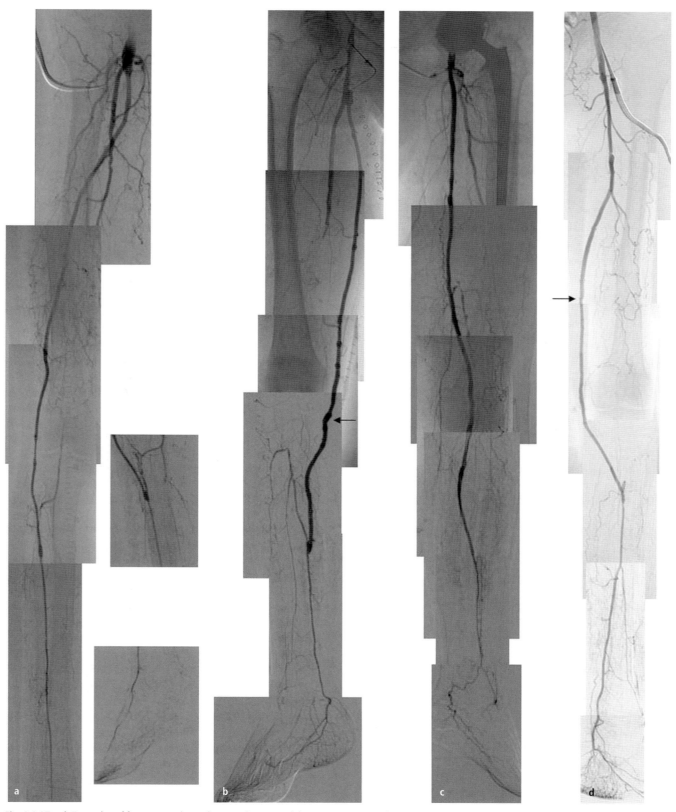

Fig. 4.4-97a–d Examples of femorocrural crural venous bypasses. (**a**) An extra-anatomic bypass to the proximal anterior tibial artery with nonreversed great saphenous vein. Course over the extensor side in the thigh. There are still marked changes in the proximal part of the anterior tibial artery in front of the anastomosis. (**b**) A femorocrural bypass from the proximal superficial femoral artery to the proximal posterior tibial artery, using composite great saphenous vein from both legs. The subcutaneous bypass course is well visualized, with a venovenostomy (arrow). (**c**) A femorocrural bypass from the transition between the middle and distal thirds of the peroneal artery with nonreversed great saphenous vein. The bypass vein has an anatomic course through the popliteal region. (**d**) A femorocrural bypass with brachial veins, from the deep femoral artery to the tibioperoneal trunk. Composite basilic vein and cephalic vein (arrow); a subcutaneous bypass course following several previous operations.

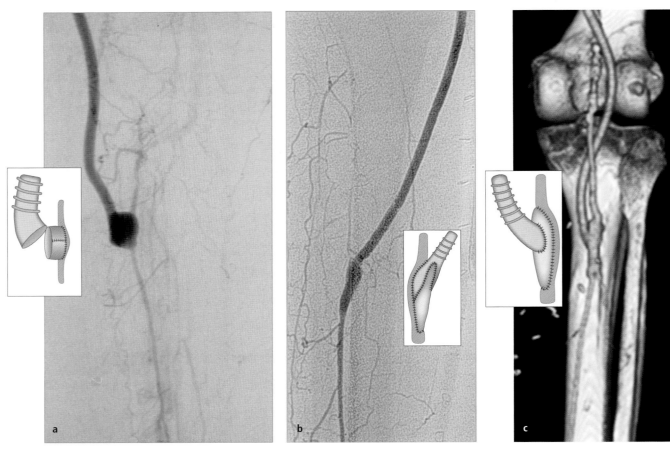

Fig. 4.4-98a–c Special anastomosis techniques for a distal prosthesis bypass. (**a**) Miller cuff: diagram and postoperative angiogram of an extra-anatomic bypass with a ring-reinforced 6-mm PTFE prosthesis to the proximal anterior tibial artery. (**b**) Taylor patch: diagram and postoperative angiogram of an extra-anatomic bypass with a 6-mm human umbilical vein prosthesis to the middle peroneal artery. (**c**) Linton patch: diagram and postoperative CT angiography of a bypass with a 6-mm Omniflow prosthesis to the tibioperoneal trunk.

In-situ technique

Initially, the proximal greater saphenous vein is exposed at the level of the proximal arterial donor vessel. The site for the central anastomosis can be selected at the femoral bifurcation, at the proximal superficial femoral artery, or anywhere along its whole course as far as the distal popliteal artery (Fig. 4.4-96d). Exposure of the distal recipient vessel and distal venous segment then follows as much as is necessary to allow tension-free passage of the vein to the site of planned anastomosis. Complete exposure of the vein is not necessary. If there is any doubt about the course of the vein, it can be checked by careful advancement of an unblocked Fogarty catheter. After heparinization, the vein is detached centrally, possibly with excision of a small cuff from the common femoral vein, with continuous suturing of the stump or of the femoral vein using 6–0 polypropylene. After this, the artery is clamped and the central arteriotomy is carried out. If tension-free mobilization of the proximal segment of the vein to reach the femoral bifurcation does not appear possible, the arteriotomy can initially be extended in the distal direction into the superficial femoral artery in order to expand it peripherally with a patch of prosthetic or biological material far enough to allow a tension-free anastomosis with the mobilized vein. Before this, the proximal segment of the vein is carefully everted, and the first venous valve is excised under direct vision. The vein is spatulated, and the central anastomosis is created with 6–0 polypropylene. Af-

ter completion of the anastomosis circulation into the peripheral vessel and the proximal vein the blood flow is restored. A flexible valvulotome (Le Maître Intervascular; In-Situ Cut, Braun Melsungen) is then introduced from the distal direction and advanced to the level of the proximal anastomosis. The valvulotome is slowly withdrawn during blood inflow, and all venous valves are carefully destroyed until distal pulsations can be felt. The distal anastomosis is created without tension using an end-to-side technique. Larger side branches of the greater saphenous vein are then located using a Doppler probe, flow measurement, or angiography, and are ligated or closed with vascular clips via small separate incisions.

Pedal bypass construction

Both the dorsalis pedis artery (Fig. 4.4-96a, b) with the lateral tarsal artery and also the distal posterior tibial artery (Fig. 4.4-96d) and its two terminal branches, the medial (Fig. 4.4.-96f) and lateral (Fig. 4.4-96e) plantar artery, can be used for a pedal bypass. The procedure can be done as a distal-origin bypass to bridge a lower leg arterial occlusion if the femoropopliteal axis is still intact, or as a long femoropedal bypass when there are additional occlusions at the thigh level. The indication is very often seen in patients with ischemic diabetic foot syndrome with gangrene already present in the toes and forefoot, or after nonhealing amputations if the underlying impaired perfusion has not been dealt with during a previous

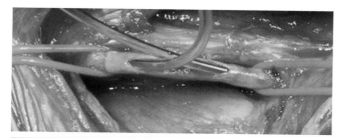

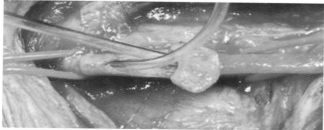

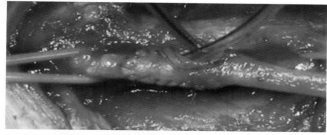

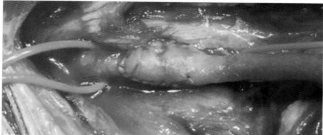

Fig. 4.4-99a–d Crural and pedal anastomosis technique without vascular clamping. (**a**) Looping of the artery using vessel loops, longitudinal arteriotomy and splinting of the lumen with fine probes, instillation of a heparin solution. (**b**) End-to-side anastomosis using a continuous double-parachute suture, starting at the heel of the anastomosis and continuing up to the middle of the arteriotomy, with polypropylene 7–0. (**c**) Completion of the anastomosis from the tip with a second suture, leaving the probes in place. The last sutures are placed loosely around the probes, which are left in position. (**d**) The last suture in the center of the anastomosis is tied after the probes have been removed. The anastomosis is complete.

surgical procedure. In these cases, it is imperative to optimize the blood flow to the ischemic tissue in order to ensure healing and to control the infection that is normally present after toe amputations, ray amputations, and forefoot amputations. The connection to the small-caliber pedal vessels, with a diameter of 2 mm, should always be done with autologous vein using the technique described above, with 7–0 Prolene. Wound closure at the ankle or on the dorsum of the foot is done with simple interrupted Prolene sutures of the skin, without placing drains. The skin sutures are left in place for about 3 weeks, as premature removal can lead to wound rupture, with the risk of a bypass infection.

Concept of the distal-origin bypass

The distal type of occlusion often seen in diabetic patients, with the femoropopliteal vascular axis often well preserved as far as the popliteal trifurcation, is particularly suitable for placement of a central bypass anastomosis to the distal superficial femoral artery (Fig. 4.4-96e) or along the course of the popliteal artery (Fig. 4.4-96b, d). It is mainly the infragenicular segment that is used. This distal origin for the bypass substantially reduces the length of the venous material required and makes it possible to use the in situ technique, particularly for the pedal anastomosis to the dorsalis pedis artery or distal posterior tibial artery. With these distal-origin bypasses, the nonreversed or reversed venous bypass can be placed subcutaneously (Fig. 4.4-96b).

Exposure and anastomosis of the crural and pedal arteries

Tibioperoneal trunk

The tibioperoneal trunk (TPT) is an arterial segment, usually 2–3 cm long, after the origin of the anterior tibial artery that divides into the posterior tibial artery and peroneal artery. It is surrounded by the converging lower leg veins, which fuse in this area to form the popliteal veins. After the tendinous arch of the soleus muscle has been released from the posterior edge of the tibia and the muscle has been retracted dorsally, the TPT is exposed from the medial direction. This may be necessary if a high-grade stenosis is found at the trifurcation when a connection to the distal popliteal artery is planned, for example. The stenosis can be resolved by extending the arteriotomy into the TPT. However, the TPT itself is often difficult to access and may be calcified. In these cases, it is recommended to expose the division into the posterior tibial artery and peroneal artery and to carry out the anastomosis to the less-altered vessel there. The bypass can pass to this region via the popliteal region, as well as subcutaneously. A particularly straight bypass course is possible here, especially when the in situ technique is used.

Anterior tibial artery

The anterior tibial artery is exposed at an angiographically suitable vascular segment using a skin incision 8–10 cm long over the extensor side of the lower leg approximately 3 cm lateral to the edge of the tibia. However, the first 1.5–2.0 cm of the artery can also be exposed from the medial direction starting at the popliteal fossa, possibly after incision of the proximal interosseous membrane. After a longitudinal incision in the lower leg fascia, the bellies of the anterior tibial muscle and extensor digitorum muscle are separated, and after placement of a wound retractor the artery and accompanying veins are dissected in the deep area. In its distal course above the ankle, the artery crosses under the tendon of the extensor hallucis longus. The positioning of the bypass anastomosis depends on the planned course of the bypass. The arteriotomy is made laterally when an extra-anatomic course is planned for the bypass, along the extensor side of the thigh. It can be placed anteriorly or even slightly medially if the bypass is to pass through the interosseous membrane. To do this, the interosseous membrane is cautiously exposed at the level of and above the selected anastomosis region, from the lateral side. This region is also exposed from the medial side after retraction of the posterior tibial muscle. Cruciform incision of the membrane and careful blunt tunneling of the bypass graft with a curved dressing forceps to the lower leg flexor side and to the popliteal area follow. When an extra-anatomic bypass course is planned, this can be done with an external ring-reinforced PTFE prosthesis over the thigh extensor side, for example, tunneling through the subcutaneous tissue above the fibula head lateral to the patella to the groin. However, it is also possible to place the greater saphenous vein here subcutaneously (Fig. 4.4-97a).

Posterior tibial artery

A skin incision 8–10 cm is made 2 cm dorsal to the medial edge of the tibia, protecting the great saphenous vein. The fascia of the soleus muscle is transected with the muscle at the tibia with a margin of 5–10 mm in the direction of the fibers, and the muscle is retracted dorsally. The artery with the accompanying vein lies embedded between the flexor digitorum muscle ventrally and the flexor hallucis longus dorsally. At the level of the ankle, the vascular bundle is also covered by the flexor retinaculum, which is transected for exposure. Due to its adjoining course, the greater saphenous vein is suitable for the in-situ technique in a bypass to the posterior tibial artery.

Peroneal artery

The access route is the same as for the posterior tibial artery. The vascular bundle is retracted ventrally or dorsally to expose the peroneal artery in the proximal part. Dissection is carried out in the depth between the flexor hallucis longus and tibialis posterior muscles. There is a thin layer of fascia separating the vessels. After an incision into the fascia, the veins—often relatively large—that surround the artery are exposed. It may sometimes be necessary to transect the communicating veins. The middle and distal thirds of the artery are exposed after dorsal retraction of the flexor hallucis longus muscle. In the distal third, exposure may be very difficult when there is strong musculature. Use of the lateral access route, in which the artery is exposed more superficially, may then be indicated. In individual cases, resection of a segment of the fibula may be necessary in order to demonstrate the vessel. This requires exposure of the fibula, which is circled and resected for several centimeters using a Gigli saw at the level of the selected segment. The peroneal artery can then be easily demonstrated from the lateral side after an incision into the medial periosteum. This access route is very suitable for repeat procedures.

Dorsalis pedis artery

The artery is exposed using a longitudinal incision over the course of the artery, which can be marked using Doppler ultrasound if needed, lateral to the tendon of the extensor hallucis muscle. The retinaculum is transected and the artery is carefully dissected, ensuring protection of the surrounding veins. If an anastomosis to the lateral tarsal artery is required, it is followed laterally after exposure of its origin from the dorsalis pedis artery. The bypass is passed distally under a skin bridge to the dorsum of the foot, no matter which technique is used to implant the vein. In individual cases, it may be necessary to make additional small relief incisions on the dorsum of the foot to ensure tension-free wound closure.

Distal posterior tibial artery and its terminal branches

The posterior tibial artery is exposed via a slightly curved skin incision approximately 2 cm behind the medial malleolus, with transection of the flexor retinaculum. The vessel divides into the medial plantar artery, which courses on the medial side towards the first ray, and the larger-caliber lateral plantar artery, which courses into the plantar arch. The latter can be followed further peripherally by retracting and incising the abductor hallucis and flexor digitorum muscles.

Special types of bypass and anastomotic techniques when using synthetic and biological vascular prostheses (Fig. 4.4-98a–c)

Direct anastomosis of a vascular prosthesis to a narrow-lumen artery often leads to early development of an anastomotic stenosis, due to neointimal hyperplasia resulting from its relative rigidity, particularly with synthetic prostheses, in comparison with the attached artery. In addition, blood flow in the crural arteries is often relatively low, and stagnation thrombosis in a synthetic implant may therefore develop. A number of techniques have therefore been developed either to delay the development of neointimal hyperplasia by incorporating the small amount of autologous venous material that may still be available into the crural anastomosis of a prosthesis bypass (as cuffs and patches), or to increase flow in the bypass by sequential anastomosis of the entire distal arterial bed that is still available or by diverting part of the flow volume into the venous system via an arteriovenous fistula. Venous material that is still available, although not long enough, can also be combined with a prosthesis in the form of a composite bypass. The distal anastomosis is then carried out using the conventional technique with the venous part. A sequential composite bypass incorporates several still available distal vessels into the structure with the venous bypass segment.

Miller cuff

After an arteriotomy approximately 2.0–2.5 cm long in the crural artery, a venous strip is sutured onto the artery using continuous sutures. The suturing is completed to form a venous cuff that is mounted on the crural artery like a chimney. The prosthesis is then anastomosed to the venous cuff using continuous sutures (Fig. 4.4-98a).

Taylor patch

An arteriotomy approximately 3 cm long is made in the crural artery, followed by anastomosis of the heel part of the prosthesis to the artery with continuous sutures up to half of the arteriotomy. A longitudinal incision is made in the anterior wall of the prosthesis from the tip to a point proximal to the prosthesis heel, with resection of a small wedge at each tip. This incision is closed with a continuously sutured diamond-shaped venous patch that fills out the anterior half of the incision (Fig. 4.4-98b).

Linton patch

After a 3-cm arteriotomy in the crural artery, an autologous venous patch is sutured into the arteriotomy with continuous sutures. After the patch has been completed, an incision is made in the proximal third of it and an S-beveled prosthesis is implanted into the patch (Fig. 4.4-98c).

Composite bypass

In the composite bypass, autologous venous material that is still available with a sufficient caliber but not sufficiently long is combined with a vascular prosthesis using a 45° beveled end-to-end anastomosis, in such a way that the part of the bypass that crosses the knee joint consists of vein (Fig. 4.4-100a–c). The anastomosis should not lie at the level of the knee joint space.

Sequential technique

If several potential distal recipient vessels are identified angiographically, they can be connected in the form of a sequential bypass both with autologous vein and with a composite bypass. The hope is that this will lead to increased bypass flow and optimization of the peripheral outflow (Figs. 4.4.96e, f, 4.4-100c).

Arteriovenous fistula

The technique most frequently used is known as the common ostium fistula, in which the crural artery and an accompanying vein are first dissected over 3 cm and incised longitudinally. A continuous anastomosis of the artery and vein is then made. The long anterior side of the arteriovenous fistula created in this way is then anastomosed with a correspondingly long incised prosthesis. However, it is also possible to use the composite technique to connect a side branch of an autologous venous segment with an accompanying vein in the anastomosed crural or pedal artery. The Linton patch technique can also be modified in such a way that the patch is initially implanted over the crural or pedal artery that is to be connected and over the corresponding accompanying artery, creating a common-ostium arteriovenous fistula, with the prosthesis bypass then being anastomosed to the patch.

Perioperative complications and risks

Systemic and local complications are distinguished. Local complications are caused by the type of surgical reconstruction used, while systemic complications are signs of the multiple comorbid conditions of a patient with progressive limb ischemia.

Local complications include acute thrombotic occlusion of the arterial reconstruction, with a frequency of 2–10%, depending on the type of implant used. Possible causes include:

- Technical errors at the anastomoses, with a lesion in the artery
- Defective venous material
- Thrombus formation in the bypass graft
- Low bypass flow, with stagnation thrombosis

Immediate revision with thrombectomy and elimination of the mechanical cause, if necessary with complete replacement of the bypass, is necessary.

Other local complications include:

- Postoperative bleeding; hematoma formation, in which surgical revisions are needed in up to 5% of cases. This does not usually lead to any impairment in the surgical results.
- Wound healing disturbances: rare with prosthetic implants, but up to 10% of cases when autologous vein is used; the long-term results are not affected.
- Bypass infection: this is a severe local complication that is rare at 0.5–1.0% with autologous vein, but up to 3% with vascular pros-

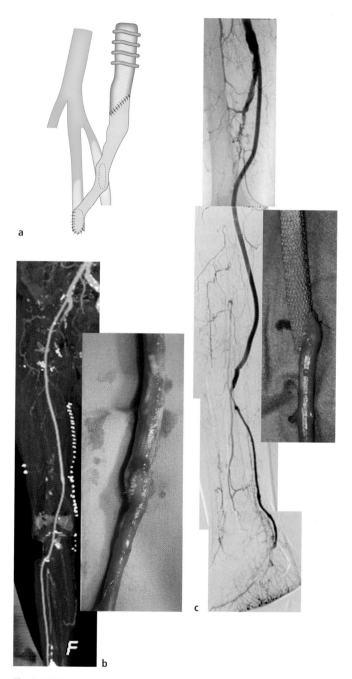

Fig. 4.4-100a–c Composite bypass. **(a)** Schematic depiction of a composite anastomosis between a synthetic prosthesis and an autologous vein. **(b)** A long iliacocrural composite bypass from the common iliac artery to the proximal anterior tibial artery via a medial access site, with a 6-mm Omniflow prosthesis and residual great saphenous vein. Composite anastomosis above the knee. **(c)** A femoropedal sequential composite bypass from the middle superficial femoral artery to the middle peroneal artery and to the plantar artery, using 6-mm human umbilical vein and residual great saphenous vein.

thesis. An infected synthetic implant bypass graft almost always has to be abandoned in this case. However, preservation of the bypass graft should always be considered and it can also be successfully achieved in individual cases with biological safeguarding and coverage with vital muscle.

- Major amputation: 0–5% (with severe critical ischemia).

Systemic complications are associated with mortality rates of 0–6% and are usually caused by myocardial infarction (very rare in intermittent claudication; high risk in dialysis-dependent patients with critical ischemia; intensive-care monitoring is useful here). Other complications that occur include:

- Other cardiac complications: up to 10% (including arrhythmia).
- Stroke: 1%.
- Pneumonia, respiratory insufficiency: up to 3%. This is a sign of poor general condition.

Postoperative treatment and quality control

Critical aspects for the long-term prognosis after surgical reconstruction include not only extremely good preoperative imaging diagnosis, but also already controlling the results intraoperatively with angiography, duplex ultrasound, or flowmetry. If there is any doubt about the findings, the anastomoses should be revised, any thrombi found should be removed, and mechanical errors should be corrected by redoing the anastomoses concerned, possibly with distal extension of the bypass to another arterial segment. Postoperative control of the whole reconstruction, with an additional duplex ultrasound examination and/or angiography, makes it possible to recognize stenoses, residual valves, or thrombi that have only developed later at residual valves, or wall changes due to unnoticed intraoperative lesions. Surgical revision or endovascular correction should then be carried out. It is important, although not always possible (in cases of pedal anastomoses with incisions near the malleolus), to measure and document the brachiopedal gradient before the patient is discharged.

Postoperative swelling (known as postoperative reperfusion edema) regularly occurs in the operated extremity, and this may be particularly marked with distal reconstructions for very severe ischemia. The limb should be elevated, with simultaneous physiotherapy exercises, and the patient should receive information about the cause of the swelling tendency and its good prognosis.

Drug therapy and follow-up

Systemic anticoagulation therapy is required perioperatively, with unfractionated or low-molecular-weight heparin. In autologous venous bypasses, the current research data show that long-term oral anticoagulation is beneficial, while administration of a platelet inhibitor is useful with prosthetic bypasses. According to the results of the CASPAR study, combined administration of acetylsalicylic acid (ASA) and clopidogrel in patients who have received bypasses crossing the knee in which a synthetic graft was used is superior to administering ASA alone, whereas there is no benefit here with regard to patency when autologous vein is used. Combined administration of vitamin K antagonists with a platelet inhibitor is also possible in individual cases. With autologous venous bypasses, duplex ultrasound monitoring of the reconstruction is useful. This should be done after 3, 6, 12, 18, and 24 months and thereafter annually. If evidence of a developing stenosis is found, prophylactic intervention to eliminate the stenosis using local patch plasty, partial bypass replacement, PTA of the bypass, PTA of the anastomosis, and repositioning of the bypass or distal extension of it have all proved beneficial. When biological bypass grafts are used, duplex ultrasound monitoring is useful, as aneurysmal graft degeneration can occur in some cases after the bypass has been functioning for a long period. However, with synthetic bypass grafts, the value of duplex ultrasound monitoring is a matter of controversy, as acute occlusion of the prosthesis can occur here even when the conditions are morphologically unremarkable.

Results of surgical reconstruction in the crural and pedal arteries

The long-term patency and limb salvage rates after placement of a crural or pedal venous bypass can be regarded as good (Table 4.4-30). For crural and venous bypasses, the 5-year patency rate is 60–70%. The limb salvage rate is 70–90%, as adequate residual circulation may be present even when a bypass occlusion develops (usually a slow process) and the distal anastomosed vessel is preserved after the original ischemic lesion has resolved. The long-term results with the pedal venous bypass to the dorsalis pedis artery are surprisingly good, with 5-year patency rates of more than 60% and even better limb salvage rates. By contrast, the historical results after placement of a crural bypass with a PTFE prosthesis in particular are much poorer, with patency rates of only 12–43% after 5 years. Improved bypass function with PTFE prostheses has mainly been achieved by using special anastomotic techniques (such as the Miller cuff and venous patch techniques). This puts the 5-year bypass patency rates in the range of 40–50%. The adjuvant arteriovenous fistula technique emphasized by some authors shows good function, particularly with biological prostheses, although more recent randomized studies have not demonstrated any advantage with it in comparison with the venous cuff when a PTFE prosthesis is used. Neville's research group has published a modification of the common-ostium arteriovenous fistula technique in combination with a distal venous patch using a PTFE implant, with a 2-year patency rate of 62% in high-risk patients with severely advanced occlusion patterns. The composite technique holds a moderate position with regard to function and limb salvage. Experienced centers have reported astonishingly good patency rates of 40–68% after 3 years with this method, with limb salvage rates of 60–88%, particularly with the sequential technique. The present author's experience with the use of biological implants and the sequential composite technique has also been very encouraging with regard to function and limb salvage.

Prospects

Occlusive disease in the femoropopliteal and crural vascular area in particular is increasingly becoming a field for endovascular techniques, which have proved to be very useful for treating short vascular lesions and should also be used for these primarily. Although TASC C and D lesions are regarded as being a domain for open surgical revascularization, long recanalizations of occluded long vessel segments using interventional methods with endoluminal laser techniques or the use of multiple stents are nevertheless being proposed. Implantation of stents over very long distances in the crural arteries is also common practice. Encouraging early results have also been reported with subintimal angioplasty of the crural arteries. Particularly in view of the increasing variety of methods and materials available, however, the value of these procedures still requires further systematic investigation in prospective randomized studies comparing them with surgical procedures—all the more so since autologous venous bypass in this region still offers unrivaled and excellent long-term results. A future combination of endovas-

Table 4.4-30 Overview of examples of long-term results in peripheral bypass surgery with crural and pedal venous bypasses.

First author	Year	Bypass	N	Special features	Patency (%)	Leg preservation (%)
Donaldson	1993	Popliteal/crural/pedal	585	Great saphenous vein and other veins	72 (5 y)	92 (5 y)
Gloviczki	1994	Pedal	100	None	69 (3 y)	79 (3 y)
Shah	1995	Crural/pedal	2058	Saphenous vein in situ	70 (10 y)	90 (10 y)
Darling	1995	Pedal	238	Dorsalis pedis artery	67 (5 y)	86 (5 y)
Gentile	1996	Popliteal/crural	702	Great saphenous vein	7582 (5 y)	8492 (5 y)
			187	Alternative veins	72 (5 y)	78 (5 y)
Eckstein	1996	Pedal	56	Also PTFE composites	62 (4 y)	66 (4 y)
Luther	1997	Pedal	109	None	72 (2 y)	72 (2 y)
Berceli	1999	Pedal	432	Dorsalis pedis artery	62 (5 y)	
Faries	2000	Popliteal/crural/pedal	520	Brachial vein	57 (5 y)	71 (5 y)
Connors	2000	Pedal	24	Pedal side branches	70 (2 y)	78 (2 y)
Wölfle	2000	Crural/pedal	130	Distal-origin vein	49 (7 y)	63 (7 y)
Chew	2001	Popliteal/crural/pedal	165	Spliced vein	65 (5 y)	81 (5 y)
Roddy	2001	Pedal	19	Plantar artery	74 (15 months)	74 (15 months)
Schmiedt	2003	Crural/pedal	140	Distal-origin vein	70 (5 y)	81 (5 y)
Neufang	2003	Pedal	84	In situ technique	75 (5 y)	78 (5 y)
Pomposelli	2003	Pedal	1032	Dorsalis pedis artery	62 (5 y)	78 (5 y)

PTFE, polytetrafluoroethylene.

cular therapy at the level of the thigh with placement of a distal-origin venous bypass might also be conceivable in the treatment of severe ischemia. When prosthetic materials are used for bypass surgery, improvements can be expected with the use of antithrombogenic coating on PTFE or Dacron grafts. Encouraging initial results with heparin-coated PTFE prostheses have already been published. Colonization of PTFE with autologous endothelium has also provided very encouraging results. Current research suggests that it may be possible to develop homologous or heterologous collagen scaffolds colonized with autologous cells, leading to a new type of partly autologous vascular conduit.

References

Abbott WM, Maloney RD, McCabe CC, Lee CE, Wirthlin LS. Arterial embolism: a 44 year perspective. Am J Surg 1982; 143 (4): 460–4.

Ascer E, Gennaro M, Pollina RM, Ivanov M, Yorkovich WR, Lorensen E. Complementary distal arteriovenous fistula and deep vein interposition: a five-year experience with a new technique to improve infrapopliteal prosthetic bypass patency. J Vasc Surg 1996; 24 (1): 134–43.

Belch JJ, Dormandy J, Biasi GM, Cairols M, Diehm C, Eikelboom B, et al. Results of the randomized, placebo-controlled clopidogrel and acetylsalicylic acid in bypass surgery for peripheral arterial disease (CASPAR) trial. J Vasc Surg 2010; 52 (4): 825–33, 833 e1–2.

Berceli SA, Chan AK, Pomposelli FB, Jr., Gibbons GW, Campbell DR, Akbari CM, et al. Efficacy of dorsal pedal artery bypass in limb salvage for ischemic heel ulcers. J Vasc Surg 1999; 30 (3): 499–508.

Bosiers M, Deloose K, Verbist J, Peeters P. Nitinol stenting for treatment of „below-the-knee" critical limb ischemia: 1-year angiographic outcome after Xpert stent implantation. J Cardiovascular Surg (Torino) 2007; 48: 455–61.

Connors JP, Walsh DB, Nelson PR, Powell RJ, Fillinger MF, Zwolak RM, et al. Pedal branch artery bypass: a viable limb salvage option. J Vasc Surg 2000; 32 (6): 1071–9.

Daenens K, Schepers S, Fourneau I, Houthoofd S, Nevelsteen A. Heparin-bonded ePTFE grafts compared with vein grafts in femoropopliteal and femorocrural bypasses: 1- and 2-year results. J Vasc Surg 2009; 49 (5): 1210-6.

Dardik H, Silvestri F, Alasio T, Berry S, Kahn M, Ibrahim IM, et al. Improved method to create the common ostium variant of the distal arteriovenous fistula for enhancing crural prosthetic graft patency. J Vasc Surg 1996; 24 (2): 240–8.

Darling RC, 3rd, Chang BB, Paty PS, Lloyd WE, Leather RP, Shah DM. Choice of peroneal or dorsalis pedis artery bypass for limb salvage. Am J Surg 1995; 170 (2): 109–12.

Deutsch M, Meinhart J, Howanietz N, Froschl A, Heine B, Moidl R, et al. The bridge graft: a new concept for infrapopliteal surgery. Eur J Vasc Endovasc Surg 2001; 21 (6): 508–12.

Dorros G, Jaff MR, Dorros AM, et al. Tibioperoneal (outflow lesion) angioplasty can be used as primary treatment in 235 patients with critical limb ischemia: five-year follow-up. Circulation 2001; 104: 2057–62.

Ducasse E, Chevalier J, Chevier E, Forzy G, Speziale F, Sbarigia E, et al. Patency and limb salvage after distal prosthetic bypass associated with vein cuff and arteriovenous fistula. Eur J Vasc Endovasc Surg 2004; 27 (4): 417–22.

Eckstein HH, Schumacher H, Maeder N, Post S, Hupp T, Allenberg JR. Pedal bypass for limb-threatening ischaemia: an 11-year review. Br J Surg 1996; 83 (11): 1554–7.

Faries PL, Arora S, Pomposelli FB, Jr., Pulling MC, Smakowski P, Rohan DI, et al. The use of arm vein in lower-extremity revascularization: results of 520 procedures performed in eight years. J Vasc Surg 2000; 31 (1 Pt 1): 50–9.

Gentile AT, Lee RW, Moneta GL, Taylor LM, Edwards JM, Porter JM. Results of bypass to the popliteal and tibial arteries with alternative sources of autogenous vein. J Vasc Surg 1996; 23 (2): 2729; discussion 279–80.

Gloviczki P, Bower TC, Toomey BJ, Mendonca C, Naessens JM, Schabauer AM, et al. Microscope-aided pedal bypass is an effective and low-risk operation to salvage the ischemic foot. Am J Surg 1994; 168 (2): 76–84.

Griffiths GD, Nagy J, Black D, Stonebridge PA. Randomized clinical trial of distal anastomotic interposition vein cuff in infrainguinal polytetrafluoroethylene bypass grafting. Br J Surg 2004; 91 (5): 560–2.

Krankenberg H, Sorge I, Zeller T, Tübler T. Percutaneous transluminal angioplasty of infrapopliteal arteries in patients with intermittent claudicatio: Acute and one-year results. Catheter Cardiovasc Interv 2005; 64: 12–7.

Kreienberg PB, Darling RC, 3rd, Chang BB, Paty PS, Lloyd WE, Shah DM. Adjunctive techniques to improve patency of distal prosthetic bypass grafts: Polytetrafluoroethylene with remote arteriovenous fistulae versus vein cuffs. J Vasc Surg 2000; 31 (4): 696–701.

Laird JR, Zeller T, Gray BH, et al. Limb salvage following laser-assisted angioplasty for critical limb ischemia: results of the LACI multicenter trial. J Endovasc Ther 2006; 13: 1–11.

Laurila K, Lepantalo M, Teittinen K, Kantonen I, Forssell C, Vilkko P, et al. Does an adjuvant AV-fistula improve the patency of a femorocrural PTFE bypass with distal vein cuff in critical leg ischaemia? A prospective randomised multicentre trial. Eur J Vasc Endovasc Surg 2004; 27 (2): 180–5.

Luther M, Lepantalo M. Arterial reconstruction to the foot arteries—a viable option? Eur J Surg 1997; 163 (9): 659–65.

Mahmood A, Garnham A, Sintler M, Smith SR, Vohra RK, Simms MH. Composite sequential grafts for femorocrural bypass reconstruction: experience with a modified technique. J Vasc Surg 2002; 36 (4): 772–8.

Melliere D, Desgrange P, Allaire E, Becquemin JP. Long-term results of venous bypass for lower extremity arteries with selective short segment prosthetic reinforcement of varicose dilatations. Ann Vasc Surg 2007; 21 (1): 45–9.

Mills JL, Gahtan V, Fujitani RM, Taylor SM, Bandyk DF. The utility and durability of vein bypass grafts originating from the popliteal artery for limb salvage. Am J Surg 1994; 168 (6): 646–50; discussion 650–1.

Neufang A, Dorweiler B, Espinola-Klein C, Reinstadler J, Kraus O, Schmiedt W, et al. [Limb salvage in diabetic foot syndrome with pedal bypass using the in-situ technique]. Zentralbl Chir 2003; 128 (9): 715–9.

Neufang A, Espinola-Klein C, Dorweiler B, Reinstadler J, Pitton M, Savvidis S, et al. Sequential femorodistal composite bypass with second generation glutaraldehyde stabilized human umbilical vein (HUV). Eur J Vasc Endovasc Surg 2005; 30 (2): 176–83.

Neville RF, Tempesta B, Sidway AN. Tibial bypass for limb salvage using polytetrafluoroethylene and a distal vein patch. J Vasc Surg 2001; 33 (2): 266–71; discussion 271–2.

Neville RF, Dy B, Singh N, DeZee KJ. Distal vein patch with an arteriovenous fistula: a viable option for the patient without autogenous conduit and severe distal occlusive disease. J Vasc Surg 2009; 50 (1): 83–8.

Parsons RE, Suggs WD, Veith FJ, Sanchez LA, Lyon RT, Marin ML, et al. Polytetrafluoroethylene bypasses to infrapopliteal arteries without cuffs or patches: a better option than amputation in patients without autologous vein. J Vasc Surg 1996; 23 (2): 347–54; discussion 355–6.

Pomposelli FB, Kansal N, Hamdan AD, Belfield A, Sheahan M, Campbell DR, et al. A decade of experience with dorsalis pedis artery bypass: analysis of outcome in more than 1000 cases. J Vasc Surg 2003; 37 (2): 307–15.

Roddy SP, Darling RC, 3rd, Chang BB, Kreienberg PB, Paty PS, Lloyd WE, et al. Outcomes with plantar bypass for limb-threatening ischemia. Ann Vasc Surg 2001 Jan; 15 (1): 79–83.

Scheinert D, Ulrich M, Scheinert S, et al. Comparison of sirolimus-eluting vs. bare-metal stents for the treatment of infrapopliteal obstructions. EuroIntervention 2006; 6: 169–74.

Schmiedt W, Neufang A, Dorweiler B, Espinola-Klein C, Reinstadler J, Kraus O, et al. [Short distal origin vein graft in diabetic foot syndrome]. Zentralbl Chir 2003; 128 (9): 720–5.

Schweiger H, Klein P, Lang W. Tibial bypass grafting for limb salvage with ringed polytetrafluoroethylene prostheses: results of primary and secondary procedures. J Vasc Surg 1993; 18 (5): 867–74.

Soder HK, Manninen HI, Jaakkola P, et al. Prospective trial of infrapopliteal artery balloon angioplasty for critical limb ischemia: angiographic and clinical results. J Vasc Interv Radiol 2000; 11: 1021–31.

Spinosa DJ, Harthun NL, Bissonette EA, et al. Subintimal arterial flossing with antegrade-retrograde intervention (SAFARI) for subintimal recanalization to treat chronic critical limb ischemia. J Vasc Interv Radiol 2005; 16: 37–44.

Stonebridge PA, Prescott RJ, Ruckley CV. Randomized trial comparing infrainguinal polytetrafluoroethylene bypass grafting with and without vein interposition cuff at the distal anastomosis. The Joint Vascular Research Group. J Vasc Surg 1997; 26 (4): 543–50.

Tartari S, Zattoni L, Rizzati R, et al. Subintimal angioplasty as the first-choice revascularization technique for infrainguinal arterial occlusions in patients with critical limb ischemia. Ann Vasc Surg 2007; 21: 819–28.

TASC I: Dormandy JA, Rutherford RB. Management of peripheral arterial disease (PAD). TASC Working Group. TransAtlantic Inter-Society Consensus (TASC). J Vasc Surg 2000 Jan; 31: S1–S296.

TASC II: Norgren L, Hiatt WR, Dormandy JA, Nehler MR, Harris KA, Fowkes FG; on behalf of the TASC II Working Group. Inter-Society Consensus for the Management of Peripheral Arterial Disease (TASC II). Eur J Vasc Endovasc Surg 2007; 33 (Suppl 1): S1–S75.

Veith FJ, Gupta SK, Wengerter KR, Goldsmith J, Rivers SP, Bakal CW, et al. Changing arteriosclerotic disease patterns and management strategies in lower-limb-threatening ischemia. Ann Surg 1990; 212 (4): 402–12; discussion 412–4.

Wolfle KD, Bruijnen H, Reeps C, Reutemann S, Wack C, Campbell P, et al. Tibioperoneal arterial lesions and critical foot ischaemia: successful management by the use of short vein grafts and percutaneous transluminal angioplasty. Vasa 2000; 29 (3): 207–14.

Zeller T, Sixt S, Schwarzwälder U, et al. Two-years results after directional atherectomy of infrapopliteal arteries with the SilverHawk device. J Endovasc Ther 2007; 14: 232–40.

4.5 Aneurysms in the arteries of the extremities

4.5.1 True aneurysm

Introduction and conservative treatment:
Franz Santosa, Elias Noory, and Sebastian Sixt
Doppler/color duplex ultrasonography:
Tom Schilling
Endovascular treatment: Thomas Zeller and
Franz Santosa
Surgical treatment: Jörg Heckenkamp and
Dietrich Koch

4.5.1.1 Clinical picture

Aneurysmal dilation can occur throughout the whole course of the peripheral arteries, but the iliac arteries and the popliteal segment are particularly affected. Some 20% of aneurysms are in extra-aortic locations. Nonaortic aneurysms also mainly have an atherosclerotic pathogenesis (in 85% of cases); other causes include infections, trauma, and arterial wall abnormalities. In the early 1900s, syphilis and tuberculosis also caused this type of aneurysm. Other infections with *Salmonella, Staphylococcus, Escherichia coli, Pseudomonas,* and *Klebsiella* have also been reported. Trauma is the major cause of pseudoaneurysms, but it can also occasionally cause true aneurysms. Rare causes include connective-tissue diseases, Marfan syndrome and Ehlers–Danlos syndrome, fibromuscular dysplasia, Takayasu arteritis, Behçet disease, and cystic medial necrosis. In addition to risk factors such as hypertension, there also appears to be an individual predisposition.

The clinically manifest signs of aneurysms are defined by their extent and location. Most aneurysms remain asymptomatic up to a certain size.

Peripheral aneurysms occasionally become symptomatic as pulsatile tumors, or are found incidentally on ultrasonography (in the femoral and popliteal areas), but the diagnosis is usually only made on the basis of complications. As in the aorta, aneurysms in the arteries of the extremities tend to develop mural thromboses, which can lead to embolism and more often to occlusion of the vessel. Aneurysmal dilation can cause nerve irritation and thromboses in the neighboring veins (popliteal). The risk of rupture increases in proportion to the diameter. However, the natural course is much less predictable with peripheral aneurysms than with aneurysms of the abdominal aorta. There is consequently little evidence for size criteria on which to base treatment indications. What is certain is that when an increase in size is documented, there is an increasing risk of rupture and occlusion with these aneurysms. The risk of embolism and acute occlusion is the main clinical problem in the area of the extremities. The popliteal artery is by far the most frequent site for aneurysms in the extremity arteries, at 30–60%, followed by the pelvic arteries (8–15%).

Aneurysms in the iliac arteries

The prevalence of iliac artery aneurysm is 0.6%; additional aneurysms in the femoral and popliteal artery are found in 50% of cases. The risk of rupture in iliac artery aneurysms is reported to be up to 33% (with an outer diameter > 2 cm). Aneurysms remain asymptomatic for many years during their growth phase before becoming symptomatic as a result of complications. Local symptoms can also occur as a result of increasing size, and the risk of rupture and thrombosis also increases (Fig. 4.5-1). Iliac artery aneurysms with a diameter of 3 cm or less expand at an average rate of 0.05–0.15 cm/year. Aneurysms with a diameter of more than 3 cm expand on average by 0.28 cm/year. The growth rate of iliac aneurysms that are larger than 5 cm is unclear, as most patients with aneurysms as large as this undergo emergency treatment. Internal iliac artery aneurysms are often found in connection with other aneurysms in the abdominal arteries, with a reported incidence of around 10%; isolated internal iliac artery aneurysms are rare. By definition, an aneurysm of the internal iliac artery is present if the diameter grows to double that of the upstream or downstream artery without an additional aneurysm in another location being present. The majority of patients with isolated aneurysms of the internal iliac artery are over the age of 65–70. On the other hand, clinical presentations have also been reported in patients aged 26–72, as well as in neonates. Aneurysms occur more frequently in men than in women, at a ratio of 6:1.

Aneurysms in the iliac arteries can lead to compression of surrounding structures such as the sacral plexus, colon, iliac veins, and ureter. Nerve irritations with pareses, ischialgia, tenesmus, and constipation are clinically prominent. Other patients may visit a urologist initially. However, patients may also have claudication or insidious leg ischemia. A ruptured iliac arterial aneurysm becomes symptomatic with severe lower abdominal pain or hip and flank pain. In rare cases, the aneurysm may also arrode the iliac vein, leading to an arteriovenous fistula with cardiac overload and swelling of the leg. Typical symptoms of internal iliac artery aneurysm also include abdominal pain, urinary symptoms, lumbosacral pain, and inguinal pain (Fig. 4.5-2). However, the majority of the aneurysms are asymptomatic at the time when they are diagnosed incidentally.

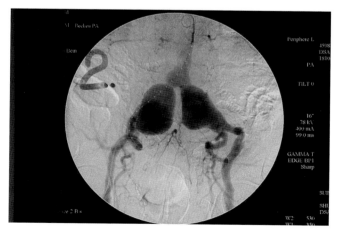

Fig. 4.5-1 A bilateral, previously asymptomatic aneurysm in the common iliac artery.

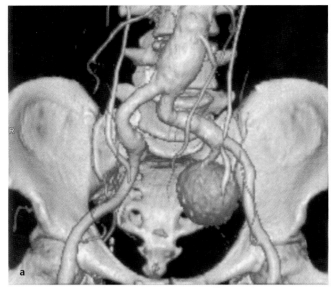

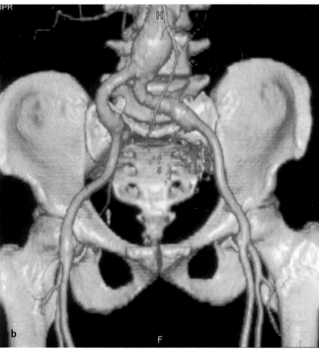

Fig. 4.5-2a, b An isolated aneurysm in the internal iliac artery that became symptomatic due to dysuria, before (**a**) and after (**b**) surgical exclusion.

Aneurysms in the femoral arteries

True aneurysms may affect the common, superficial, and deep femoral arteries, but they are generally rare. Femoral artery aneurysms tend to occur at an advanced age, in those older than 70. There is a clear male predominance, with a ratio of 15–20:1. Some 30–40% of patients are asymptomatic at the time of diagnosis. Approximately one-third have local symptoms with pain and a feeling of tension, and 10–65% of the patients present with complications such as local thrombosis, claudication, acute thrombosis, or rupture. Distal embolization is notably rare.

Aneurysms in the popliteal artery

Popliteal artery aneurysm needs to be included in the differential diagnosis in all occlusive syndromes distal to the popliteal regions. Popliteal artery aneurysms are the most frequent type of aneurysm in the peripheral arteries of the extremities, at around 85%. More than half of the aneurysms are bilateral, and 40–50% are also associated with aneurysmal changes in the infrarenal abdominal aorta. Conversely, up to 14% of patients with an abdominal aortic aneurysm also have popliteal aneurysms. A popliteal aneurysm is present when the diameter of the dilated segment is twice the vascular diameter of the upstream or downstream arterial segments. Some publications use the term "aneurysm" only when the diameter of the artery is more than 2 cm. The condition occurs almost exclusively among men (Fig. 4.5-3). The longitudinal extension of the aneurysm increases along with its size. Aneurysms with a diameter smaller than 2 cm have been reported in some studies to grow by 1.5 mm/year, and aneurysms with a diameter of 2–3 cm by 3.7 mm/year. In another study, popliteal aneurysms larger than 2 cm had a mean increase of 1.5 mm/year, while aneurysms smaller than 2 cm grew by 0.7 mm/year.

The popliteal artery has certain characteristics that predispose it to aneurysm development. The properties of the vessel wall resemble those of the central elastic arteries rather than those of the typical muscle arteries in the periphery. The major risk with popliteal artery aneurysms is thromboembolic complications (24% after 1 year, 74% after 5 years), which are associated with amputation in 20–50% of cases. Acute rupture is less frequent, with a rupture risk of only 2–7%. It is not clear why popliteal artery aneurysms become symptomatic with acute thrombosis much more frequently than with rupture. Regional differences in mechanical stress, particularly due to bending at the knee joint, have been suggested. An aneurysmal popliteal artery may lose its longitudinal elasticity, and knee-bending leads to pre-aneurysmal or postaneurysmal kinking, with interruption or reduction of the blood flow. Local stasis can then promote thrombus formation. Compression of the surrounding structures with irritation of the nerves and thrombus formation is also possible.

Aneurysms in the infrapopliteal arteries

Isolated aneurysms in the lower leg arteries are rare. The aneurysms described in case reports tend to affect the area of the trifurcation rather than individual lower leg arteries, and they usually have a post-traumatic pathogenesis.

The most extreme form of degenerative vascular wall dilation is represented by the aneurysmal form of atherosclerosis (atherosclerosis dilatans), in which whole segments of the iliac and femoral arteries are inhomogeneously dilated. Flow speeds are severely reduced in these arteries. Mural thrombus formation and embolism occur and may make long-term oral anticoagulation treatment necessary. Surgical vascular reconstruction is only an option when localized complications occur (such as acute occlusion or rupture), but is often not possible due to unfavorable anastomotic conditions.

The second most frequent cause of peripheral aneurysms is infection ("mycotic aneurysm"), with bacteria being the main cause (usually staphylococci or Gram-negative bacteria). An attempt should be made to identify the pathogen using blood culture. Up to 85% of mycotic aneurysms are located outside the aorta. Their sites

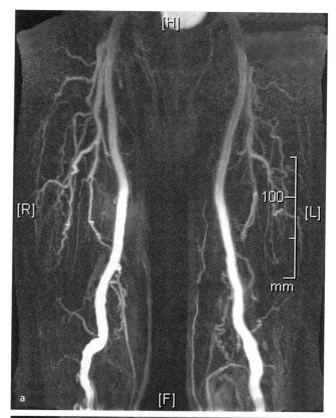

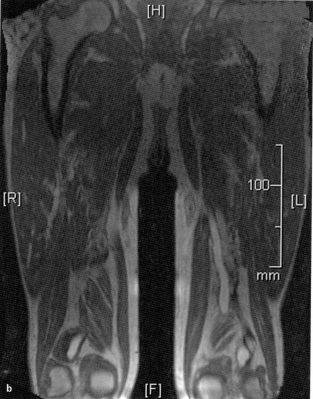

Fig. 4.5-3a, b An aneurysm in the right popliteal artery with general dilative angiopathy. The important aspect is that the aneurysm is not seen on pure angiography (**a**), as only the lumen is shown. On the coronary images, however, a 28-mm partly thrombosed aneurysm in the right popliteal artery is recognizable (**b**, arrows).

of predilection include medium-sized arteries (e.g., the iliac artery, mesenteric vessels, and also cerebral arteries). The patients are often immunocompromised (e.g., by diabetes mellitus, malignant diseases, or drug abuse). The disease can also be caused by conducted infections in the vicinity (e.g., paravertebral abscess) or septicemia. The major symptom is fever of unclear cause, and the disease needs to be included in the differential diagnosis of fever, with the appropriate ultrasound screening. In addition, mycotic aneurysm can also be revealed by local complications (e.g., urinary stasis with iliac artery aneurysm) or peripheral embolism. Death can be caused by aneurysmal rupture and septic complications. Only high-dose antibiotic therapy that is as pathogen-specific as possible, and with agents easily accessible to the tissues, is promising. The aneurysms are removed surgically. In-situ reconstructions after high-dose targeted antibiotic treatment are often possible, and this has markedly reduced the very high medium-term mortality rate seen before the development of such methods. Septic complications (such as cerebral abscess and endocarditis) should be excluded.

Involvement of the vessel wall in various types of inflammatory disease (such as panarteritis nodosa, Behçet disease, Kawasaki arteritis, etc.) can lead to the development of single or multiple peripheral aneurysms. However, they only represent a small proportion of such lesions, at around 1%. Treatment depends on the underlying disease.

4.5.1.2 Diagnosis

Peripheral aneurysms may be difficult to diagnose. They are often not recognizable during the physical examination. Calcification may occasionally be seen on the abdominal or popliteal x-rays as incidental findings and should suggest an aneurysm. As there are no definite clinical signs of an aneurysm with the exception of palpable vascular dilation, an underlying aneurysm should in principle be considered in every case of peripheral occlusion. The possibility of an upstream aneurysm also has to be considered with every peripheral embolism. In patients with peripheral perfusion disturbances, at least the most frequent locations in the area of the popliteal and iliac arteries should be routinely examined, in addition to the abdominal aorta.

Aneurysms are easily overlooked on angiography, as partial thrombosis often reduces the perfused lumen to a normal size (Fig. 4.5-4). Color duplex ultrasonography is the diagnostic method of choice. Its sensitivity depends of course on the extent to which ultrasound imaging is possible in the patient.

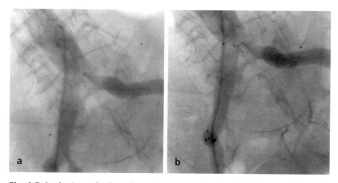

Fig. 4.5-4a, b A partly thrombosed aneurysm in the right common iliac artery before (**a**) and after (**b**) implantation of a Fluency® Plus 13.5/60-mm stent graft.

Doppler/color duplex ultrasonography

Examination technique

Depending on the region, a 3.5-MHz convex scanner (iliac region) or 5–7.5-MHz linear scanner (femoropopliteal region, lower leg, upper extremity) is used. Settings optimized for low flow or (color) B flow imaging should be used to demonstrate the freely perfused lumen and demarcate intravascular thrombi in the aneurysm.

Differential diagnosis

- True aneurysm: circumscribed luminal dilation up to > 1.5 times the size of the upstream and downstream vascular segments
- Pseudoaneurysm: perivascular hematoma communicating with the lumen, with typical hemodynamics
- Dilating arteriopathy: long or generalized vascular ectasia, with above-normal diameters
- Perivascular hematoma: hypoechoic perivascular structure with no sign of communication with the lumen and with no internal perfusion
- Dissecting aneurysm: dissection with a preexisting aneurysm

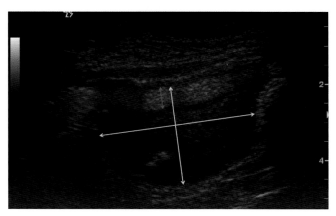

Fig. 4.5-5 An aneurysm in the common femoral artery. The free lumen of the common femoral artery had a regular appearance (on angiography). Duplex ultrasonography reveals an eccentric and largely thrombosed aneurysm, with simultaneous dilating arteriopathy.

- Dissection: classic primary separatation of the vascular wall, with a subsequent increase in the outer diameter of the vessel over a long distance

Specific findings

Issues for Doppler/duplex ultrasonography

- Location of the aneurysm.
- Type and shape of the aneurysm (true aneurysm, pseudoaneurysm, fusiform, sacciform, fusisacciform).
- Size of the aneurysm: length, transverse diameter, ventrodorsal diameter (always measured vertical to the vascular axis, rather than to the body axis, to avoid overestimation).
- Vascular diameter proximal and distal to the aneurysm (for treatment planning).
- Relationship to branches that are given off.
- Signs of impairment of neighboring structures (compression effects).
- Thromboses? (Extent, distribution, consistency, pulse-synchronous behavior).
- Signs of emboligenicity in endoluminal thrombi (floating structures, niches).
- Signs of distal embolizations.
- Width of the residual lumen—occlusion caused by thrombosis?
- Evidence of an inflammatory pathogenesis (wall structures with hypoechoic thickening).
- Signs of instability in the wall: flow around thrombi, hypoechoic vascular wall structures as signs of dissection, perivascular hypoechoic structures as signs of rupture, leakage.
- Signs of arteriovenous fistula formation in the area of the aneurysm or distal to it, with secondary aneurysmatic degeneration.
- Is there any evidence of dilating arteriopathy?
- Are any other aneurysms present? E.g., simultaneous popliteal and aortic aneurysms, as well as contralateral popliteal aneurysms.
- Differentiation between dissection and dissecting aneurysm.
- If dissections are present, imaging of the entry and reentry, length, thickness of the dissection membrane, hemodynamic effects, side branches originating from which lumen? Thromboses in a lumen? *Caution:* during a hurried examination, reverberation echoes may mimic thin dissection membranes.

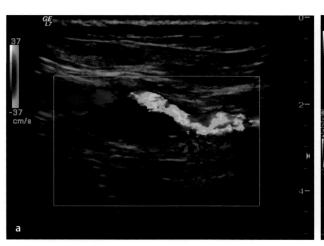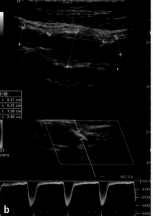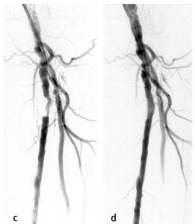

Fig. 4.5-6a–d An aneurysm of the superficial femoral artery. (**a, b**) High-grade stenosis of the superficial femoral artery in the F1 segment. The cause was a subtotally thrombosed aneurysm of the superficial femoral artery in a patient with dilating arteriopathy. (**c**) Angiography naturally only shows the stenosis and not the aneurysmatic structure. (**d**) The result after treatment, with a Viabahn® prosthesis that was indicated based on the pathogenesis.

Additional diagnostic procedures

Alternative procedures such as CT and MRI are reserved particularly for imaging of unclear duplex ultrasound findings in the iliac artery when there is severe tortuosity, and for specialized investigations. In addition to pure size measurements in the longitudinal and transverse directions, the extent of thrombosis and residual perfusion have to be assessed. As the disease mainly occurs with multiple and bilateral locations, it is obligatory to examine all of the vascular levels and also the contralateral side.

Segmental pulse volume recordings and arterial Doppler occlusive pressure measurement are obligatory for establishing the diagnosis, even when there are no symptoms, as this makes it possible to recognize clinically silent peripheral embolization during the subsequent course (as an indication for prophylactic surgery in popliteal artery aneurysms). Before surgery, imaging of the lower leg and foot arteries must be performed, either with intra-arterial DSA or MR angiography.

4.5.1.3   Treatment

Conservative treatment

Genuinely conservative treatment for peripheral aneurysms is not possible, as aneurysmal dilation is irreversible and the degenerative processes that lead to vascular dilation cannot be treated in a targeted way. Assuming that the cause is atherosclerotic, all patients should receive risk-reduction therapy. In peripheral aneurysms with diameters that do not yet make invasive treatment necessary, conservative therapy for iliac artery aneurysms consists of strict secondary prophylaxis with drug treatment to normalize arterial pressure, and administration of a platelet inhibitor. It is not yet clear whether administering a statin can prevent progression of the disease. The patient should be forbidden to lift heavy weights of more than 10 kg.

With femoral artery aneurysms, the same considerations apply in principle as for iliac artery aneurysms. However, the indication for surgery can be established more generously in this case, as the procedure is easier.

The situation with popliteal artery aneurysms is a special one, as these aneurysms only rarely rupture but often thrombose. The size of a popliteal aneurysm therefore does not represent a contraindication to antiplatelet therapy. It has even occasionally been discussed whether oral anticoagulation is indicated. A research group in Germany has recommended oral anticoagulation (INR 3.0) in patients with smaller popliteal aneurysms, in order to avoid acute thrombosis. The recommendation is based on follow-up data for 2.5 years in 36 patients with 46 aneurysms, 19 of whom received antiplatelet treatment while 16 had oral anticoagulation. The complication rates with regard to acute thrombosis and peripheral embolism were 14.3% and 0%, respectively. However, there is a lack of controlled studies on this treatment approach.

An absolute indication for invasive treatment only arises here when there are symptoms of acute ischemia or local compression syndrome in the neighboring anatomic structures.

Differential considerations on conservative treatment versus invasive/surgical therapy

Invasive treatment of an isolated iliac artery aneurysm is recommended in the following cases:

- If symptoms develop
- If the aneurysm is 3–4 cm in size (urgent treatment should be aimed for in aneurysms larger than 5 cm)
- If the aneurysm is growing rapidly: > 7 mm in 6 months or > 1 cm in 1 year

Although rupture occurs with increasing diameter in this type of aneurysm, it is a matter of controversy whether there is a direct connection between the size of the aneurysm and the risk of rupture. A survey by Dix et al. in 2005 showed that the median diameter of ruptured aneurysms was 7 cm (range 5–13 cm). By contrast, unruptured aneurysms were 6 cm in diameter (range 2–11 cm). As the risk of rupture is 14–33% starting with a diameter of 3 cm, conservative and expectant management should be limited to patients in whom the surgical risk is not acceptable and who have aneurysms smaller than 3 cm.

Prophylactic surgery for nonthrombosed femoral and popliteal aneurysms larger than 2 cm may be useful. There is a close correlation between the complication rate and the size of the aneurysm, and it is therefore recommended that all femoral artery aneurysms larger than 2.5 cm should be treated. The standard therapy so far has been aneurysmal resection (with a surgical mortality rate of 0–2%). When the vascular morphology is favorable, however, stent graft implantation is now a less invasive treatment option. In general, symptomatic aneurysms are an indication for primary treatment. When there is complete occlusion of a popliteal aneurysm, the treatment approach is based on the clinical situation, in which there is usually an acute threat to the extremity. Anticoagulation treatment is also possible as an alternative to vascular reconstruction in embolizing aneurysms < 2.0–2.5 cm.

Endovascular therapy

As an alternative to surgical procedures, percutaneous transarterial treatment can exclude aneurysms by bridging with a stent graft. The long-term results of this approach with regard to patency rates and possible embolic complications are still awaited, with the exception of popliteal artery aneurysms. Suitable treatment procedures include local lysis combined with thrombus aspiration, and rotation embolectomy with subsequent stent graft implantation in local thrombotic occlusions.

Iliac artery aneurysm

CT angiography of the aorta and pelvic arteries is necessary before endovascular treatment, in order to confirm the size and length of the proximal and distal neck and the length of the aneurysm, the degree of torsion of the iliac arteries, and the patency of the internal iliac artery. Examinations using three-dimensional reconstruction may be helpful in individual cases. Endovascular treatment for an isolated iliac artery aneurysm typically involves a combination of the actual aneurysm treatment with embolization or exclusion of side branches using occluders. The specific anatomy of the aneurysm has to be taken into account here, and adequate perfusion of

Table 4.5-1 Classifications of isolated iliac artery aneurysms relative to options for endovascular treatment (Fahrni et al. 2003 and Sakamoto et al. 2005).

Fahrni classification	Anatomy	Treatment approach	Sakamoto classification
Type Ia	CIA aneurysm with good proximal anchoring zone	Stent extending from the CIA to the EIA (possibly covering the IIA), embolization of the ipsilateral IIA	Type III
Type Ib	Bilateral aneurysm in the CIA or unilateral aneurysm in the CIA without suitable proximal anchoring zone	Embolization of the ipsilateral IIA and additionally either aortoiliac bifurcation prosthesis or uni-iliac prosthesis plus femorofemoral crossover bypass	Type IV
Type IIa	Aneurysm in the IIA with broad entrance (no proximal anchoring zone)	Embolization of the distal IIA, stent placement in the CIA with coverage of the hypogastric artery	Type I
Type IIb	Aneurysm in the IIA with a good proximal anchoring zone	Coil embolization of the afferent and efferent supply (no stent placement)	Type II
Type IIc	Aneurysm in the IIA with conical proximal neck Aneurysm in the CIA or IIA that develops after endovascular treatment for an infrarenal abdominal aortic aneurysm	Packing of the aneurysm with coils	Type V

CIA, common iliac artery; EIA, external iliac artery; IIA, internal iliac artery.

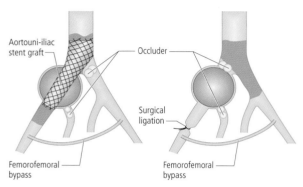

Fig. 4.5-7 An aneurysm in the common iliac artery without a proximal anchoring zone. To achieve the treatment goal of excluding the aneurysm, perfusion of a pelvic circulatory pathway has to be deliberately abandoned in these cases and replaced with a femorofemoral crossover bypass. There are two ways of doing this. Left: perfusion is preserved on the aneurysm side.

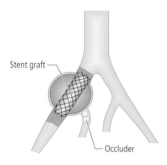

Fig. 4.5-8 An aneurysm in the common iliac artery with an adequate proximal anchoring zone. Embolization of the ipsilateral internal iliac artery is carried out first. The aneurysm is then excluded using a tube prosthesis.

the pelvic arteries needs to be maintained. The aneurysms are usually in the common iliac artery (Fig. 4.5-4); isolated aneurysms of the internal or external iliac artery are rarer. Sakamoto and Fahrni have developed slightly differing classifications of iliac artery aneurysms (Table 4.5-1). According to these systems, an aneurysm of the common iliac artery that is less than 2 cm away from the aortic bifurcation (Fahrni type 1B, Sakamoto type 4) can either undergo bifurcation-preserving treatment using a bifurcation prosthesis or can be treated with a tube prosthesis, excluding the bifurcation and placing a crossover bypass. The tube prosthesis can be placed via the aorta in the nonaneurysmal iliac artery segment, in which case the aneurysmal side needs to be occluded using coil embolization (Fig. 4.5-7). Alternatively, the tube prosthesis can also be placed in the aneurysmal side, in which case the nonaneurysmal side needs to be occluded using coil embolization or placement of an occluder. In both cases, however, the ipsilateral internal iliac artery has to be additionally occluded using coil embolization in order to exclude the possibility of retrograde filling of the aneurysm.

In contrast, a unilateral iliac artery aneurysm that includes the internal iliac artery but has a good proximal anchorage zone (Fahrni type 1A, Sakamoto type 3) can be bridged with a tube prosthesis (Fig. 4.5-8). The prosthesis should be anchored in the ipsilateral common iliac artery and external iliac artery, and the ipsilateral iliac artery again has to be excluded using coil embolization.

Technique of endovascular treatment

Common iliac artery. To exclude an isolated aneurysm of the common iliac artery using stent graft implantation, the following conditions need to be met:

- Adequate neck at the origin of the target vessel for anchoring an endoprosthesis (> 1 cm long)
- Adequate distal neck proximal to the iliac bifurcation if there is a contralateral occlusion of the internal iliac artery. If the contralateral internal iliac artery is patent, the vessel can be stented ipsilaterally.
- Angulation of the target vessel must be < 90%.

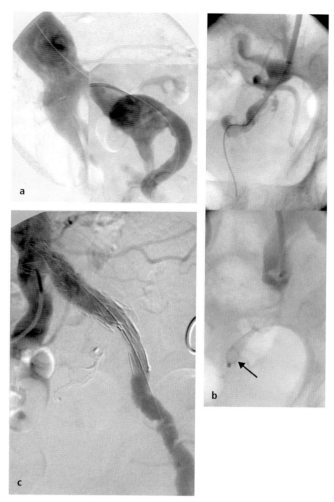

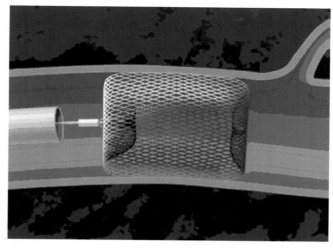

Fig. 4.5-10 The Amplatzer® Vascular Plug is a self-expanding nitinol wire mesh with a platinum marking at the proximal and distal ends. A diameter of around 30–50% larger than the vessel being occluded should be selected in order to achieve secure placement and occlusion.

Fig. 4.5-9a–c An aneurysm in the left common iliac artery involving the iliac bifurcation (**a**). Selective probing of the internal iliac artery (**b**), after occlusion of the internal iliac artery with an occluder (see also arrow in b) (**c**) and after implantation of two iliac Talent prosthesis limbs.

Interventional technique: ipsilateral retrograde transfemoral access, 8–12F depending on the diameter of the stent graft to be implanted (Viabahn®/Hemobahn®, Gore; Fluency® Plus, Bard; Wallgraft®, Boston Scientific). The limit of the usual stent grafts is a maximum diameter of 13.5 mm (Fluency® Plus). When there is an ectatic aneurysmal neck, an iliac limb or an extension of an aortic bifurcation stenosis has to be used (Fig. 4.5-9) (e.g., AneuRx®, Medtronic; Excluder, Gore). By contrast, balloon-expandable stent grafts (e.g., Jostent graft, Abbott Vascular) are usually only used in very circumscribed aneurysms or pseudoaneurysms, due to their limited length and rigidity. Precise selection of the stent graft size is essential, and the diameter of the graft should be at least 1 mm larger than the reference diameter. A landing zone at least 2 cm long at both ends is ideal in order to ensure safe exclusion of the aneurysm. When several stent grafts are placed in overlapping fashion, a 2-cm long overlap zone should also be ensured. After the endoprothesis has been released, the stent graft is subsequently dilated in the area of the landing zones using a balloon catheter adjusted to the vascular diameter.

If the iliac bifurcation is involved, the internal iliac artery has to be stented. Before this, however, the main trunk has to be closed with

an occluder (Amplatzer® Vascular Plug, AGA Medical; Fig. 4.5-10) to prevent retrograde perfusion of the aneurysm (Fig. 4.5-9).

Alternatively, the internal iliac artery can be occluded with coils. However, one should avoid occluding the terminal branches of the internal iliac artery using coil embolization. Coil embolization of the internal iliac artery can either be carried out as the initial measure, or should take place in parallel with endovascular exclusion of the aneurysm. In patients in whom the inferior mesenteric artery is occluded or an abdominal aortic aneurysm has been excluded during previous surgery, it should be confirmed that the superior mesenteric artery is patent in order to ensure perfusion of the bladder and colon. Embolization of the internal iliac artery can be carried out using stainless-steel coils with a diameter of 0.035" (Tornado, Cook), 0.035" platinum coils, or 0.018" platinum coils (Tornado Embolization Microcoils, Cook). In comparison with standard coils, the Amplatzer® Plug can be positioned more precisely in the artery and only a single catheter intervention is required in order to occlude the artery.

Normally, patients require long-term anticoagulation treatment after stent graft implantation. A few patients experience what is known as postimplantation syndrome in the first 10 days after placement. Fever over 38°C, leukocytosis, and raised C-reactive protein may occur. However, these changes should resolve within 3 days. Other potential complications include colon ischemia, thrombus embolization in the lower extremity, as well as graft thrombosis due to kinking and external compression, infection, and delayed aneurysmal rupture due to an endoleak.

Internal iliac artery. Aneurysms of the internal iliac artery are rarer; for anatomic reasons and if iliac tortuosity is not too marked, they are usually treated via contralateral transfemoral access (40–50-cm long crossover sheath; e.g., Cook, Terumo). After placement of the 6F sheath in the ipsilateral common iliac artery, the affected internal iliac artery can be selectively probed with a 4F or 5F diagnostic catheter. Via this catheter itself, or using a telescope technique with a microcatheter, the terminal branches of the internal iliac artery distal to the aneurysm are first occluded using coils (Tornado, Cook, or similar) in order to prevent retrograde perfusion of the aneurysm

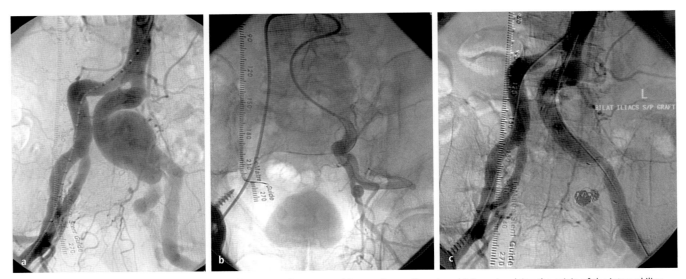

Fig. 4.5-11a–c Angiograms of an aneurysm in the left common iliac artery with a maximum diameter of 4.2 cm, involving the origin of the internal iliac artery. Steel coils were released in the left iliac artery via a 4F catheter. As the common iliac artery had an adequate landing zone of more than 2 cm, it was possible to cover the complete length of the aneurysm. (Reprinted with permission from John Wiley & Sons, Inc., from Bacharach and Slovut 2008.)

after occlusion of the proximal vascular neck. If the aneurysm has a proximal neck of at least 2 cm in front of it, it is closed with an occluder (Amplatzer® Vascular Plug, AGA Medical). If an adequate neck on which to anchor an occluder is not present, a stent graft (if necessary via an ipsilateral retrograde access site) is placed from the common iliac artery to extend as far as the proximal external iliac artery.

Late complications can include a typical form of buttock claudication (12–55%) and erectile dysfunction (1–13%). In individual cases, occlusions have also been reported with direct injection of fibrin glue as a technical variant.

Endoluminal stent placement is now an established method, and a combination of coil embolization and an endoprosthesis is therefore the method of choice (Fig. 4.5-11). This reduces the surgical burden, particularly for older patients. However, it should be pointed out that although the aneurysm can be excluded with this technique, reducing the risk of rupture, the local pressure symptoms that the aneurysm exerts on the surrounding organs are not immediately relieved or may be impossible to relieve. In cases in which local pressure symptoms of this type are clinically predominant, open surgical treatment is indicated if the surgical risk is acceptable.

Common femoral artery. Endovascular treatment for an aneurysm in the common femoral artery is only given when there is already an occlusion of either the superficial or deep femoral artery, as the aneurysm usually involves the femoral bifurcation or the neck proximal to the bifurcation is too short for a stent graft to be safely anchored. Invasive treatment for common femoral artery aneurysms is a field for vascular surgery.

Superficial femoral artery. True aneurysms are a rare finding, and post-traumatic or iatrogenic pseudoaneurysms are more frequent. In general, self-expanding stent grafts are preferable due to their flexibility (e.g., Viabahn®/Hemobahn®, Fluency® Plus, Wallgraft®). Depending on the patient's general condition and the diameter of the access artery, the prostheses can be placed using either an ipsilateral antegrade or a contralateral retrograde crossover technique via a femoral access site. The sheath size is based on the diameter of the stent graft selected. Due to the high level of mechanical stress on

the target vessel, the prosthesis has to overlap the aneurysm proximally and distally with at least 2 cm of "healthy" vessel in order to prevent stent graft dislocation during movement. The diameter should be 1–2 mm larger than the reference diameter of the target vessel. After release, the ends of the stent graft should be dilated in the area of the landing zones.

Popliteal artery. Endovascular treatment of an aneurysm in the popliteal artery is technically easier, although the special biological characteristics of the popliteal artery and the extreme angles of bending that can occur in the knee area make the long-term results poorer. The ideal prosthesis should be more flexible and should be able to absorb external compressions with a high degree of radial resistance in order to prevent mechanical occlusions and dislocations. In principle, the same technical considerations apply here as in aneurysms of the superficial femoral artery. A perfused popliteal artery aneurysm can thus be excluded from the circulation by implanting a stent graft if a sufficiently long landing zone of at least 2 cm is available, particularly distally, and the aneurysm is not more than 10 cm long (Fig. 4.5-12).

The Hemobahn endoprosthesis (Gore) is mainly used to treat popliteal aneurysms. This is a self-expanding nitinol prosthesis with an inner lining formed by an ultrathin PTFE tissue. With the smooth surface presented to the blood-perfused interior side, it is biocompatible. In addition, the special nitinol design has a reduced number of what are known as cross-links (the longitudinal struts linking the individual segments of the prosthesis). This provides greater flexibility while at the same time a high degree of radial rigidity, minimizing the risk of kinking. The endoprosthesis sizes needed for popliteal aneurysms are in the range of 6–13 mm, with lengths of 5–15 cm. The stent lengths and stent diameters to be used should be determined during intraoperative angiography. The diameter should be roughly 20% larger than the diameter of the proximal and distal artery. When selecting the length, it should be ensured that the landing zone does not lie in the area directly proximal to the knee joint space, which is where the maximum bending forces in the popliteal region occur. To avoid this zone, the endoprosthesis should always land at least 2–3 cm above the knee joint space.

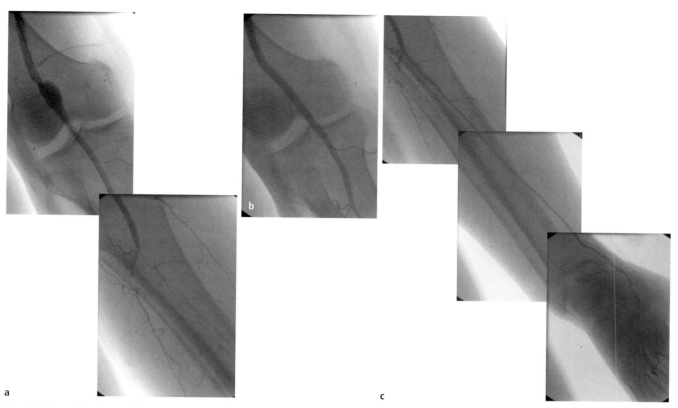

Fig. 4.5-12a–c (**a**) A circumscribed, partly thrombosed aneurysm in the right popliteal artery and chronic occlusion of the tibioperoneal trunk and anterior tibial artery. (**b**) Implantation of a 7/100-mm Viabahn® endoprosthesis. (**c**) Stent recanalization of the tibiofibular tract.

Endovascular treatment for longer aneurysms can only currently be recommended in individual cases (Fig. 4.5-13). It is not recommended in particular when the aneurysm diameter is more than 3 cm and there is severe vascular kinking. If multiple endoprostheses are needed to exclude a popliteal aneurysm, adequate overlapping (of approximately 3 cm) should be ensured.

Finally, the endoprosthesis should be documented radiographically with the leg outstretched so that the stent structures and possible later deformations can be demonstrated. In addition, an angiographic check with the knee bent by at least 90° should be done to confirm that there is no kinking. If kinking and stenoses of more than 50% occur, the results are not optimal for the longer term, and conversion of the procedure to a surgical aneurysm operation should be considered. After implantation of the endoprosthesis, dual platelet inhibition is indicated, probably indefinitely, as the endoprosthesis does not usually become completely endothelialized.

An acutely occluded aneurysm in the popliteal artery is initially recanalized either using rotation thrombectomy (8F Rotarex® system, Straub Medical) or local lysis. Ideally, the two forms of treatment can be combined, with rotation thrombectomy for rapid restoration of adequate lower leg perfusion and subsequent lysis to dissolve any peripheral emboli that may be present. Fixed stenoses or occlusions are revascularized conventionally with PTA and/or stent implantation (Fig. 4.5-12). After this, the aneurysm can either be treated during the same interventional session or in a second procedure, either with an endoprosthesis or using vascular surgery if the anatomy is unfavorable.

At follow-up examinations for popliteal aneurysms that have been treated endovascularly, the same complications are observed as for all of the aortic and pelvic artery aneurysms. Complications that have been reported include early thrombotic occlusion, stenosis and migration of the endoprostheses, development of endoleaks, and increases in the size of the excluded aneurysm. A feasibility study in 2007 reported on 73 popliteal artery aneurysms that had been treated from 1998 to 2007. Early thrombotic occlusions occurred in 18 endoprostheses, and nine migrations, three fractures, and two cases of stenosis of the endoprosthesis were observed. The primary patency rates after 3 and 5 years were 77% and 70%, and the secondary patency rates were 86% and 76%. In the period before the introduction of dual platelet inhibition, the occlusion rate was higher at 35% than it was after platelet inhibition was introduced (20%; $P = 0.22$). Another study has reported the 2-year results with 57 popliteal artery aneurysms that were treated with coated endografts. Twenty-one percent became occluded during that period, and the primary and secondary patency rates were 77% and 97%.

Surgical treatment

In addition to the endovascular options for excluding aneurysms, the open surgical procedure is still generally accepted, and good long-term results have been documented. However, treatment has to be planned on an individual basis.

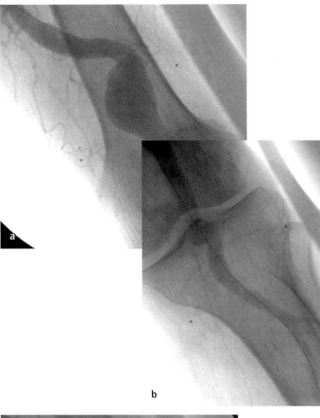

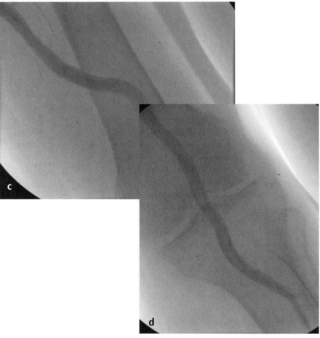

Fig. 4.5-13a–d (**a, b**) A long, partly thrombosed aneurysm in the left popliteal artery. (**c, d**) After implantation of a total of four Viabahn®/Hemobahn endoprostheses with diameters of 8 and 9 mm.

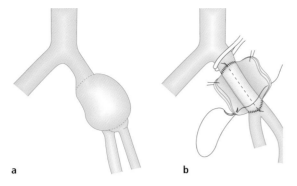

Fig. 4.5-14a, b A circumscribed aneurysm in the common iliac artery. For surgery, the healthy proximal and distal vascular segments are dissected and looped in order to stop the circulation intraoperatively. The aneurysmal sac is then opened, and the diseased segment is anastomosed end to end through a vascular prosthesis with the original vascular stumps.

Iliac artery aneurysm: standard surgical procedure

Isolated aneurysms of the iliac arteries are usually operated on via a retroperitoneal access route. The skin incision is along a line between the tip of the eleventh rib and the pubic tubercle. The abdominal wall muscles are opened, and the peritoneal sac with the attached ureter is retracted medially. After placement of a retractor system (ideally a self-retaining one), the distal aorta and iliac vessels can be well demonstrated. The basic surgical technique for excluding the aneurysm also corresponds to that for an abdominal aortic aneurysm. After dissection of the aneurysm and of a clampable proximal and distal vascular segment (Fig. 4.5-14), the aneurysm is clamped off after systemic heparin administration, and opened longitudinally. After the marginal thrombus that is often present has been cleared, vascular branches with potential backflow are sutured. The vessel is incised on its anterior wall proximally and distally to form door flaps. The posterior circumference of the original vessel is left as it is. A vascular prosthesis (usually 8 mm PTFE or Dacron) is then anastomosed end to end with the original vascular stumps using nonresorbable monofilament suture material (3–0, 4–0), with the posterior wall being sutured using the insertion technique. Careful protection of the pelvic veins should be ensured, particularly with aneurysms in the common iliac artery and external iliac artery. Due to the veins in the vicinity, no resection of the aneurysmal sac should be attempted. The sutures are tied using a continuous and over-and-over technique. Before the suturing of the anastomosis is completed, the arterial inflow and outflow are checked and the reconstruction is rinsed with a heparin–saline solution. When the anastomosis is completed and the blood flow has been restored, the aneurysm wall is sutured over the prosthesis. If the iliac bifurcation is included in the aneurysm, the distal anastomosis should be repositioned accordingly, and if necessary the internal iliac artery should be reinserted into the prosthesis. In any case, however, the anastomoses should lie outside of the dilated vascular area, as otherwise there is an increased risk of anastomotic aneurysm.

When there are bilateral iliac aneurysms, a transabdominal approach should be selected, as it is usually necessary to implant an aortobi-iliac prosthesis in these cases.

Isolated aneurysms in the internal iliac artery are rare, but the mortality rate is 30–60% if they rupture. In unilateral internal iliac aneurysms, the method of choice is ligation without reconstruction. To do this, the aneurysm is demonstrated via a retroperitoneal approach. As dissection is often difficult in this location, the distal vessels can be selectively blocked with Fogarty catheters and then grasped with endoluminal stitches. The vessel is ligated proximally near its origin. In bilateral internal iliac aneurysms, unilateral reconstruction of the internal iliac artery is often necessary in order to prevent ischemia in the pelvic organs, particularly the sigmoid colon. However, when a two-stage approach is used, it is possible that adequate collateral circulation may develop in the intervening period, and this should be clarified angiographically before the second procedure.

Common femoral artery aneurysm

True aneurysms are very rare in the femoral arteries. The aneurysms found here are usually iatrogenic aneurysms of the common femoral artery after puncture of the inguinal arteries (pseudoaneurysms), or more rarely suture aneurysms at the inguinal division after previous surgical procedures. Possible infectious components need to be taken into account during treatment planning.

Exposure is via a longitudinal incision below the inguinal ligament on a line connecting the anterior superior iliac spine and the inner knee joint space. The lymphatic vessels are lifted as a curtain and retracted medially. Exposure of the aneurysm and femoral bifurcation then follows and extended exposure of the deep femoral artery is often necessary. When there is proximal extension under the inguinal ligament, suprainguinal exposure of the external iliac artery either via an additional incision or via a balloon blockade is indicated. After the aneurysm has been clamped off, it is resected, and a vascular prosthesis is anastomosed end-to-end both proximally and distally using 8–10 mm Dacron or polytetrafluoroethylene (PTFE). In the inguinal region, particular attention should always be given to the deep femoral artery, as the vessel plays a critical role in collateral formation, so if the femoral bifurcation is involved in the dilation, careful reconstruction of the deep femoral artery is required. To do this, either the origin of the deep femoral artery is reinserted into the prosthesis after completion of the graft, or the deep femoral artery can be connected via an additional graft. As there is often already an older thrombotic occlusion in the superficial femoral artery, a femoral–deep femoral bridging graft alone is also possible.

Special case: standard surgical procedure with suture aneurysms

The surgical procedure with inguinal suture aneurysms mainly depends on the anatomic relationships of the aneurysm and the type of vascular surgery reconstruction previously carried out. After the aneurysm has been exposed, it needs to be decided whether a prosthesis graft is required or whether the aneurysm can be excluded using a direct reconstruction of the anastomosis (Fig. 4.5-15).

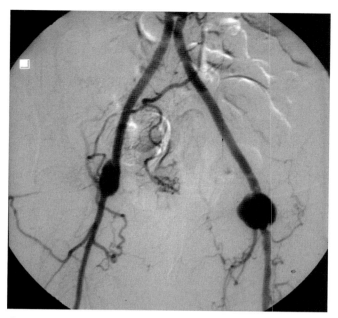

Fig. 4.5-15 Bilateral suture aneurysms in an aortobifemoral prosthetic bypass carried out 8 years before. Depending on the length of the vascular segment that needs to be replaced, the aneurysms can be excluded using a new direct suturing between the prosthesis and the vessel, or it may be necessary to extend the prosthesis with a short bridging graft.

Superficial femoral artery aneurysm

True aneurysms of the superficial femoral artery without the presence of dilative arteriopathy are a rarity. Surgical treatment usually consists of exclusion using a femoropopliteal bypass with a proximal anastomosis to the femoral bifurcation and distal connection of the bypass at the level of the supragenicular popliteal segment. The great saphenous vein should be used for bypass material if available. Although the major risk is of peripheral embolism, proximal as well as distal ligation of the artery bearing the aneurysm should be done to prevent later rupture.

Alternatively, the aneurysm can be excluded using a bridging graft. Aneurysms of the superficial femoral artery are exposed with a direct incision along the course of the artery. Superficial femoral artery aneurysms are often long. Exposure then follows from two separate incisions over the femoral bifurcation and over the lower segment of the femoral artery proximal to the knee. The aneurysm is ligated, and the artery is reconstructed with the bypass. Depending on the location, autologous material or an ePTFE or Dacron prosthesis can be used for the conduit. The two vessel stumps are beveled and then anastomosed end to end with the conduit using continuous over-and-over sutures (Fig. 4.5-16).

Popliteal artery aneurysm

As popliteal segments PI and PII are the main locations affected, exclusion using a femoropopliteal or popliteopopliteal venous bypass is usually possible. However, patency in the lower leg circulation is absolutely decisive for the later patency rate.

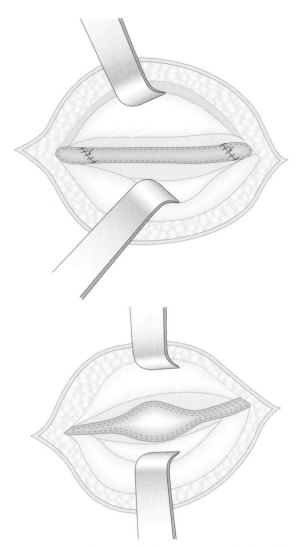

Fig. 4.5-16 Direct dissection of a short aneurysm in the femoral artery and implantation of a conduit of autologous venous material or ePTFE or Dacron prostheses.

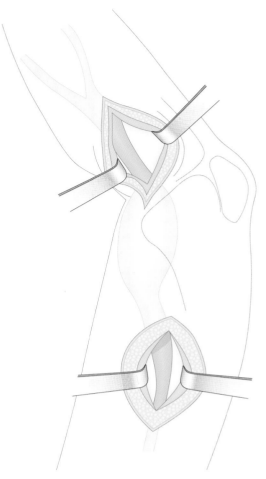

Fig. 4.5-17 Medial access to exclude popliteal aneurysms, with skin incisions in the medial distal thigh and medial proximal lower leg.

The medial access route is the one most often used for exclusion of popliteal aneurysms. Skin incisions are made on the medial distal thigh and on the medial proximal lower leg (Fig. 4.5-17). The subcutaneous great saphenous vein needs to be protected and should be used as a conduit if its caliber is adequate. On the thigh, after transection of the subcutaneous layer, the deep fascia is split and the neurovascular bundle is identified. The vein, which often courses in closely to the artery, has to be carefully dissected away, and the artery must be looped. This access route ensures exposure of the upper neck of the aneurysm. After transection of the subcutaneous fatty tissue, the deep fascia in the lower leg distal to the tibia has to be incised. There are no major vessel origins in the distal third of the popliteal artery. It has proved valuable to carry out early ligation of the upstream blood flow in order to prevent intraoperative embolizations. To avoid injury to structures in close vicinity to the aneurysm (such as the popliteal vein and tibial nerve), the aneurysm is usually not resected, except when compression-related symptoms are present. In these cases, the size of the aneurysmal sac can be reduced using a continuous gathering suture. Reconstruction of the popliteal artery is preferably done with autologous great saphenous vein, which can be pulled through in an anatomically reversed position. Both popliteal stumps are beveled and anastomosed to the vein end to end using continuous over-and-over sutures. With autologous graft material, a resorbable monofilament suture size 5–0 or 6–) can be used for stitching. If the patient does not have any suitable venous material, it is also possible to use ring-reinforced ePTFE or Dacron prostheses, and in this case nonresorbable suture material must be used. Before the anastomosis is completed, the blood flow must be checked and if any thromboembolic material is washed out, a Fogarty maneuver should be carried out. Intraoperative angiography can be used to document the surgical results if appropriate. Complete exclusion of the aneurysm is necessary in order to prevent later reperfusion (Fig. 4.5-18).

Minor aneurysms in the popliteal artery can also be approached from the dorsal direction. The patient must be placed in the prone position. To expose the vessel, the incision should be made from a top lateral point transversely across the popliteal region to a bottom medial point. After division of the posterior popliteal fascia, the popliteal fossa lies exposed. Crossing nerve branches must be carefully isolated and protected while the artery is being dissected free. The basic surgical strategy otherwise corresponds to the one also used with the medial access route.

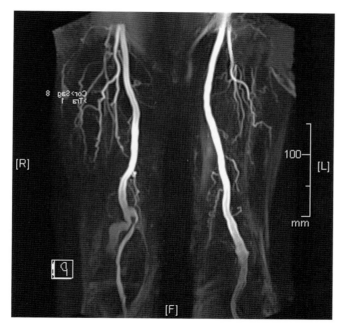

Fig. 4.5-18 Status post surgical exclusion of a popliteal artery aneurysm on the right side using proximal and distal ligation and implantation of an autologous venous bypass. The MR angiogram, 1 year after the operation, shows inflow into the patent bypass and contrast inflow into the previously excluded aneurysm.

Infrapopliteal artery aneurysms

True aneurysms of the infrapopliteal arteries are extremely rare. The aneurysms seen are usually post-traumatic or iatrogenic, following interventions and bypass operations. The aim of the operation is to exclude the aneurysm and reconstruct the artery.

Standard surgical procedure

The access route depends on the location and size of the aneurysm. The anterior tibial artery can be exposed starting from the lateral lower leg. After an incision along the cutis and division of the subcutaneous fatty tissue, the crural fascia, which is quite strong, is also opened longitudinally. The neurovascular bundle can be found between the tibialis anterior muscle and the extensor digitorum longus muscle (Fig. 4.5-19). Separation of the arterial trunk from the accompanying veins can be difficult due to the close positional relationship of all of the lower leg arteries. The posterior tibial artery courses mediocrurally along with the tibial nerve. The artery is exposed from the medial direction. The skin incision is made longitudinally, one or two fingerbreadths dorsal to the tibial edge. After splitting of the crural fascia, the soleus musculature is separated from the flexor digitorum longus muscle. This makes the neurovascular bundle accessible (Fig. 4.5-20).
The peroneal artery is embedded at the lowest position in the lower leg musculature. After its origin from the tibioperoneal trunk, it descends laterally. It courses very close to the fibula along the posterior tibial muscle. Exposure is usually from the medial direction, although lateral incisions have also been described. The skin should be opened at the posterior edge of the tibia. After opening of the fascia, dissection is carried out between the soleus musculature. The flexor digitorum longus muscle is then demonstrated, and af-

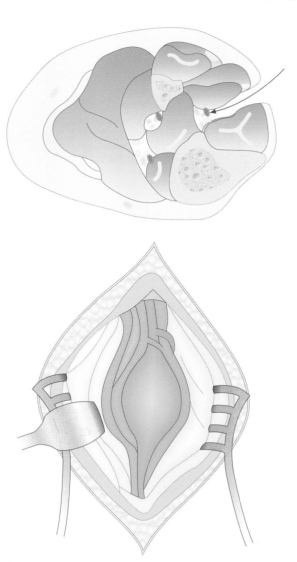

Fig. 4.5-19 Exposure of the anterior tibial artery from the lateral lower leg with a longitudinal incision into the cutis, subcutis, and crural fascia.

ter retraction of the posterior neurovascular bundle, dissection as far as the peroneal artery follows. It is also possible to demonstrate the artery (Fig. 4.5-21). After demonstration of each aneurysm and clamping or blocking of the artery with a Fogarty catheter, the aneurysm is opened and the artery is reconstructed with autologous vein as described above whenever possible. If the aneurysm is in an anatomically unfavorable location, proximal and distal ligation and use of a venous bridging graft are also possible, as in reconstruction for more proximal aneurysms.

Prospects

Implantation of multilayer stents represents a promising new treatment procedure. These two-layer or three-layer woven stents, made of a cobalt–chrome alloy (Fig. 4.5-22), are placed over the aneurysm with broad overlapping in the same way as stent grafts. Laminarization of blood flow in the multilayer stent leads to rapid thrombosis of the aneurysm. The flow changes also result in a reduction of pressure in the thrombosed aneurysmal sac and thus to reduced tension in the wall. Initial feasibility studies are in progress. This new treat-

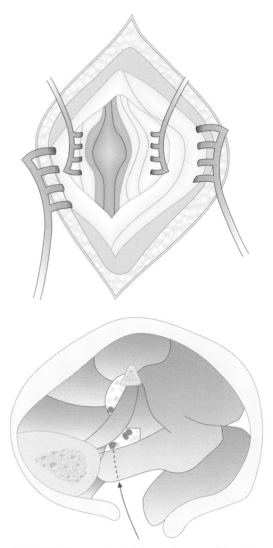

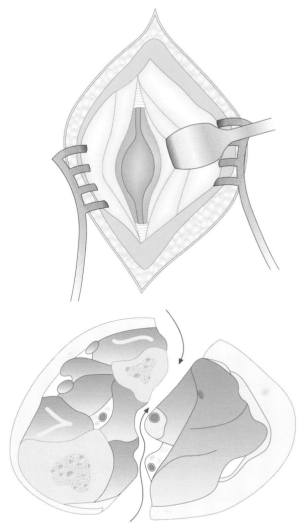

Fig. 4.5-20 The posterior tibial artery is exposed from the medial direction with a longitudinal incision approximately one to two fingerbreadths dorsal to the edge of the tibia, and the soleus musculature is dissected away from the flexor digitorum longus muscle.

Fig. 4.5-21 Exposure of the peroneal artery from the medial direction. After opening of the fascia, dissection is carried out between the soleus musculature, followed by demonstration of the flexor digitorum longus muscle. The posterior neurovascular bundle is held aside, and dissection then continues up to the peroneal artery.

ment approach can be expected to become established as an alternative to stent graft implantation—at least in the treatment of arterial aneurysms below the inguinal ligament in which the focus is on restoring the lumen and providing protection against distal emboli— since prolonged dual platelet inhibition treatment is not necessary, and particularly since side branches that are occluded by endoprostheses can be preserved using the multilayer technique. Randomized studies will be needed to investigate whether the technique is suitable for preventing life-threatening aneurysmal ruptures—e.g., in the iliac region.

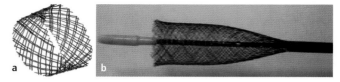

Fig. 4.5-22a, b The Cardiatis multilayer stent.

References

Antonello M, Frigatti P, Battocchio P, Lepidi S, Dall'Antonia A, Derui GP, Grego F. Endovascular treatment of symptomatic popliteal aneurysms: 8-year concurrent comparison with open repair. J Cardiovasc Surg 2007; 48: 267–74.

Bacharach JM, Slovut DP. State of the Art: Management of Iliac Artery Aneurysmal Disease. Cath Cardiovasc Intervent 2008; 71: 708–14.

Boules TN, Selzer F, Stanziale SF, Chomic A, Marone LK, Dillavou ED, Makaroun MS. Endovascular management of isolated iliac artery aneurysms. J Vasc Surg 2006; 44: 29–37.

Caronno R, Piffaretti G, Tozzi M, Lomazzi C, Rivolta N, Lagana D, Carrafiello G, Recaldini C, Castelli P. Endovascular treatment of isolated iliac artery aneurysms. Ann Vasc Surg 2006; 20: 496–501.

Casana R, Nano G, Dalainas I, Stegher S, Bianchi P, Tealdi DG. Midterm experience with the endovascular treatment of isolated iliac aneurysms. Int Angiol 2003; 22: 32–5.

Corriere MA, Guzman RJ. True and false aneurysms of the femoral artery. Semin Vasc Surg 2005; 18: 216–23.

Cronenwett JL, Rutherford RB. Decision Making in Vascular Surgery. St. Louis: W. B. Saunders Company, 2001: 132–46.

Dawson I, Bockel JH van, Brand R et al. Long-term follow-up of aneurysmal disease and results of surgical treatment. J Vasc Surg 1991; 13: 398–407.

Fahrni M, Lachat MM, Wildermuth S, Pfammatter T. Endovascular therapeutic options for isolated iliac aneurysms with a working classification. Cardiovasc Intervent Radiol 2003; 26: 443–7.

Ferrero E, Ferri M, Viazzo A, Robaldo A, Carbonatto P, Pecchio A, Chiecchio A, Nessi F. Visceral artery aneurysms, an experience on 32 cases in a single center: treatment from surgery to multilayer stent. Ann Vasc Surg 2011 Oct; 25 (7): 923–35.

Galland RB, Magee, TR. Management of popliteal aneurysm. Br J Surg 2002; 89: 1382–5.

Heberer G, van Dongen RJAM. Gefäßchirurgie. Berlin, Heidelberg, New York: Springer, 2004: 286–94.

Hepp W, Kogel H. Gefäßchirurgie. München: Urban & Fischer, 2001: 282–9.

Jarrett F, Makaroun MS, Rhee RY Bertges DJ. Superficial femoral artery aneurysms: An unusual entity? J Vasc Surg 2002; 36: 571–4.

Kalyanasundaram A, Elmore JR, Manazer JR, Golden A, Franklin DP, Galt SW, Zakhary EM, Carey DJ. Simvastatin suppresses experimental aortic aneurysm expansion. J Vasc Surg 2006; 43: 117–24.

Leon LR, Benn Psalms S, Stevensos S, Mills JL. Nontraumatic aneurysms affecting crural arteries. Vascular 2007; 15: 102–8.

Lozano F, Sánchez-Fernandez J, Gómez Alonso A. Ruptured aneurysm of the deep femoral artery. Case report and historical review. J Cardiovasc Surg (Torino) 2001; 42: 821–4.

Mahmood A, Salaman R, Sintler M, Smith SR, Simms MH, Vohra RK. Surgery of popliteal artery aneurysms. J Vasc Surg 2003; 37: 586–93.

Manouguian S, Mlynek-Kersjes ML. Spontaneous complete rupture of a thrombotic aneurysm of the tibiofibular trunk. Pathologe 2000; 21: 303–7.

Parsons RE, Marin ML, Veith FJ, Parsons RB, Hollier LH. Midterm results of endovascular stented grafts for the treatment of isolated iliac artery aneurysms. J Vasc Surg 1999; 30: 915–21.

Pittaluga P, Batt M, Hassen-Khodja R, et al. Revascularization of internal iliac arteries during aortoiliac surgery: a multicenter study. Ann Vasc Surg 1998; 12: 537.

Richardson JW, Greenfield LJ. Natural history and management of iliac aneurysms. J Vasc Surg 1988; 8: 165–71.

Roggo A, Hoffmann R, Duff C et al. Wie oft rupturiert das Aneurysma der A. poplitea? Helv Chir Acta 1993; 60: 145–8.

Sakamoto I, Sueyoshi E, Hazama S, Makino K, Nishida A, Yamaguchi T, Eishi K, Uetani M. Endovascular treatment of iliac artery aneurysms. RadioGraphics 2005; 25: S213–S227.

Sanchez LA, Patel AV, Ohki T, Suggs WD, Wain RA, Valladares J, Cynamon J, Rigg J, Veith FJ. Midterm experience with the endovascular treatment of isolated iliac aneurysms. J Vasc Surg 1999; 30: 907–13.

Sandhu RS, Pipinos II. Isolated iliac artery aneurysms. Semin Vasc Surg 2005; 18: 209–15.

Sapienza P, Mingoli A, Feldhaus RJ, et al. Femoral artery aneurysms: long-term follow-up and results of surgical treatment. Cardiovasc Surg 1996; 4: 181–4.

Schermerhorn ML, Cronenwett JL. Isolated iliac artery aneurysms. In: Rutherford RB (Hrsg.). Vascular Surgery. 6. Aufl., St. Louis: Elsevier Saunders, 2005: 1440–1.

Shortell CK, DeWeese JA, Quriel K et al. Popliteal artery aneurysms: A 25-year surgical experience. J Vasc Surg 1991; 14: 771–9.

Sixt S, Rastan A, Schwarzwälder U, Schwarz T, Frank U, Gremmelmaier D, Noory E, Bürgelin B, Zeller T. Coil Embolisation of an internal iliac artery aneurysm after surgical repair of an infrarenal aortic aneurysm. VASA 2007; 36: 138–42.

Stiegler H, Mendler G, Baumann G. Prospective study of 36 patients with 46 popliteal artery aneurysms with non-surgical treatment. Vasa 2002; 31: 43–6.

Strinemann P, Schwery S. Operationsindikation bei Poplitealaneurysma. Dtsch Med Wochenschr 1986; 108: 691–4.

Tielliu IF, Verhoeven EL, Zeebregts CJ, Prins TR, Oranen BI, van den Dungen. Endovascular treatment of iliac artery aneurysms with a tubular stent-graft: mid-term results. J Vasc Surg 2006; 43: 440–5.

Tielliu IF, Verhoeven EL, Zeebregts CJ, Prins TR, Bos WT, Van den Dungen JJ. Endovascular treatment of popliteal artery aneurysms: is the technique a valid alternative to open surgery? J Cardiovasc Surg (Torino). 2007; 48: 275–9.

Van Bockel JH, Hamming JF. Lower extremity Aneurysms. In: Rutherford RB (Hrsg.). Vascular Surgery. 6. Aufl., St. Louis: Elsevier Saunders, 2005: 1535–48.

4.5.2   Pseudoaneurysm

Introduction and conservative treatment:
Aljoscha Rastan
Endovascular treatment: Aljoscha Rastan
Surgical treatment: Wolfgang Peck

4.5.2.1   Clinical picture

Pseudoaneurysms arise due to interruption of the continuity of all three of an artery's wall layers, with subsequent bleeding into the perivascular space. The resulting hematoma and the surrounding tissue form the wall of the aneurysm. Pseudoaneurysms can arise:

- During diagnostic or interventional catheter examinations, at the arterial puncture sites after the sheath has been removed
- At bypass anastomoses (e.g., iliacofemoral, femoropopliteal, femorocrural) between the original vessel and synthetic bypass materials (e.g., Dacron, ePTFE)
- As a result of trauma
- As mycotic aneurysms, due to infection

This section focuses on the diagnosis and treatment of pseudoaneurysms that develop as a result of catheter examinations.
Pseudoaneurysm is one of the most frequent complications after arterial catheter examinations. The incidence after diagnostic procedures (e.g., angiography, coronary angiography) is in the range of 0.2–2.0%, and after therapeutic procedures 2–6%. Risk factors favoring pseudoaneurysm are:

- Female sex
- Age > 65
- Obesity
- Arterial hypertension
- Peripheral arterial occlusive disease
- End-stage renal disease
- Simultaneous venous and arterial puncture
- The sheath size used to carry out the intervention
- Complex, time-consuming interventions (e.g., with atherectomy)
- Platelet-inhibiting medication (e.g., aspirin, clopidogrel, ticlopidine)
- Peri-interventional treatment with glycoprotein IIb/IIIa receptor antagonists
- Lysis therapy (e.g., rt-PA, streptokinase)
- Inadequate compression (duration and/or location) at the puncture site after removal of the sheath

In arterial catheter examinations via the inguinal region, the preferable puncture site should always be the common femoral artery, as the head of the femur provides an ideal base for manual compression after the sheath is removed. A high puncture site (external iliac artery) or low puncture site (superficial or deep femoral artery) is therefore an additional risk factor for the development of pseudoaneurysm.

4.5.2.2   Clinical findings

The symptoms of pseudoaneurysms may result both from the defect in the artery and also from the space-occupying hematoma, with associated compression of tissue or vascular and neural pathways. Persistent pain at the puncture site is the principal symptom. Other possible symptoms include local hematoma, cutaneous necrosis, paresthesias, newly developing intermittent claudication and/or edematous swelling of the extremity (hematoma-related arterial perfusion disturbance and/or venous outflow obstruction). Severe complications are: critical ischemia in the affected extremity, progression in the size of the aneurysm with an increased risk of rupture from a diameter of 3 cm upwards, arterial thromboembolism, and infections with septic emboli.

4.5.2.3   Diagnosis and differential diagnosis

- Possible findings on inspection: painful (and possibly pulsatile) swelling, hematoma, skin necrosis, edema in the extremity affected, symptoms and findings seen in critical ischemia of the extremities.
- Auscultation: systolic–diastolic flow murmur at the puncture site.
- In principle, the presence of a pseudoaneurysm cannot be definitely excluded even without the clinical findings and examination findings mentioned. Every patient with pain at the arterial puncture site should therefore receive diagnostic clarification using color duplex ultrasonography.
- Color duplex ultrasonography (this is the gold standard, with a sensitivity of 95% and a specificity of 98%) with a 5–7-MHz linear probe. With a high puncture site (inguinal access), and/or a large hematoma, and/or obesity, a sector probe often provides better results. The typical finding here is usually a sacculation, located ventral to the artery, with single or multiple loculations and with a connection to the artery. On Doppler imaging, this afferent channel shows a typical inflow and outflow signal (Fig. 4.5-23b).

4.5.2.4   Treatment

Until the early 1990s, surgery was the only way of treating pseudoaneurysms. Other established noninvasive and invasive treatment procedures are described below.

Conservative treatment

On the basis of the current literature, an expectant attitude may be considered if the patient does not have any pain in the area of the puncture site and the maximum diameter of the pseudoaneurysm is less than 2 cm. Without anticoagulation or platelet-inhibiting medication, the spontaneous thrombosis rate is 60–90% during a follow-up period of 3–4 weeks. No data on the thrombosis rate with anticoagulation and/or platelet inhibition are available. In those cases, one of the following treatment measures should therefore be used.

Ultrasound-guided compression

First described by Fellmeth et al. in 1991, ultrasound-guided compression has a success rate of 80–98%. The ultrasound probe is pressed onto the pseudoaneurysm, so that both the aneurysm and the associated arterial supply channel to the aneurysm are compressed. The artery from which the supply channel arises (e.g., the common femoral artery) must not be compressed. After compression for 5–10 min, the degree of thrombosis in the aneurysm is checked. This cycle is then repeated until complete thrombosis can be documented. The size and position of the aneurysm (e.g., a deep location) and the number of aneurysm locules, as well as the patient's general physical condition (e.g., obesity) and anticoagulation status, may substantially reduce the success rate. Complications of this treatment procedure are: a vasovagal reaction (venous access and emergency medication are obligatory), rupture of the aneurysm, and with prolonged compression the development of deep venous thromboses and cutaneous necroses. Without anticoagulation treatment, the treatment time is between 10 and 15 minutes. In patients who are receiving anticoagulation treatment, much longer treatment periods can be expected, and the number of patients in whom the treatment fails is considerably increased. Ultrasound-guided compression is time consuming involving qualified staff and a reduces patient comfort due to compression-related pain (local anesthesia is obligatory) and immobilization for several hours (Fig. 4.5-23a–c).

In principle, *non*–ultrasound-guided manual or device compression (e.g., with FemoStop®) is possible. However, this does not en-

Table 4.5-2 Differential diagnosis of pseudoaneurysm.

Symptoms	Cause	Differential findings
Pain, swelling of the extremity, varicosis, intermittent claudication	Arteriovenous (AV) fistula	Auscultation: high-frequency systolic–diastolic flow murmur Duplex ultrasonography: evidence of AV fistula
Pain, swelling of the extremity, varicosis, intermittent claudication	Thrombosis	Also occurs as a complication of mechanical or manual compression Compression ultrasonography: evidence of thrombosis
Pain, restlessness	Hemorrhage	Hypertension/shock, duplex ultrasonography, CT angiography Angiography: evidence of bleeding
Pain, fever, emboli	Mycotic aneurysm	Local redness/excess warmth; rising infection parameters Duplex ultrasonography: evidence of aneurysm; septic emboli

sure selective compression of the aneurysm and arterial connecting channel. This leads to a lower success rate while at the same time involving a longer treatment time and thus a greater risk of the above complications developing.

Ultrasound-guided thrombin injection

Transcutaneous thrombin injection to treat pseudoaneurysms was first reported by Cope and Zeit in 1986. The procedure was later modified to include ultrasound-guided puncture of the aneurysm. The principle is to induce thrombin-mediated conversion of fibrinogen into fibrin. In comparison with ultrasound-guided compres-

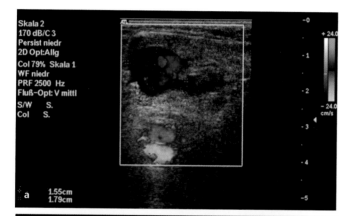

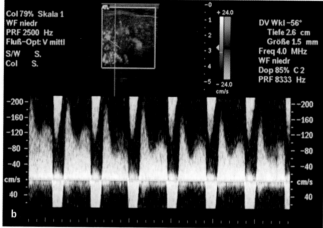

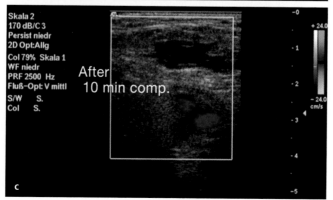

Fig. 4.5-23a–c (a) Color duplex ultrasonography of a pseudoaneurysm in the common femoral artery (cross-section). (b) The Doppler signal in the afferent channel of the aneurysm. (c) After ultrasound-guided compression, with complete thrombosis of the aneurysm.

sion, complete thrombosis of the aneurysm occurs within seconds of the thrombin injection. In addition, the patient can be mobilized immediately without the need for a compression bandage. Independently of the patient's coagulation status and platelet-inhibiting medication, success rates with this form of treatment are in the range of 91–100%. However, this is qualified by the fact that this treatment is not an officially approved area of application for standard commercially available thrombin (i.e., it is an off-label use). The complication rate is 0.5–1.3%. The complications observed include: venous/arterial thromboembolism, venous/arterial occlusion (caused by dislocation of the puncture needle), infection, and allergic reactions. The patient must therefore receive detailed information (with a written informed consent) beforehand.

Technique of ultrasound-guided thrombin injection:

The following materials are required:

- Sterile surgical gown
- 2 × sterile surgical gloves
- Sterile drape
- Sterile fenestrated drape
- Sterile gauze compresses (12)
- 2 × 10-mL syringes with screw caps
- 2 × no. 1 cannulas
- 10 mL NaCl 0.9%
- Three-way stopcock
- Infusion line
- 5 mL thrombin (e.g., bovine thrombin, Vascular Solutions, Inc.)
- Puncture needle
- Emergency medication
- 5–10 mL Xylocaine 1–2% (optional)

After venous access has been obtained and after duplex ultrasound imaging of the pseudoaneurysm, sterile draping of the puncture site is carried out. In sterile conditions, a short infusion line, a 10-mL (NaCl 0.9%) syringe, and the thrombin dissolved in the second 10-mL syringe are connected to the three-way stopcock. The puncture needle is connected to the other end of the infusion line. Puncture of the pseudoaneurysm follows (after optional local anesthesia), with duplex ultrasound guidance. The location of the puncture needle in the pseudoaneurysm is initially confirmed by the emergence of arterial blood from the distal end of the infusion line and then, after a substantial injection of NaCl 0.9% (with a 10-mL syringe), by turbulences appearing in the aneurysm on the (B-mode) ultrasound image. The three-way stopcock is then readjusted so that the thrombin injection (with a mean of 1.5–2.0 mL = 1500–2000 U thrombin) can be carried out via the infusion line. Complete thrombosis of the aneurysm can be observed within seconds on duplex ultrasonography. Puncture of the connecting channel between the artery and the pseudoaneurysm should be avoided here, due to much higher complication rates. After the thrombin injection, both the arterial and local venous status of the extremity involved should be documented (Fig. 4.5-24a–c). The disadvantage of this method of treatment, in addition to its high cost (ca. € 150–250 per treatment), is the workload—consenting the patient information, treatment in sterile conditions, and at least two staff members being required.

Contraindications for ultrasound-guided thrombin injection include mycotic aneurysm, anastomotic aneurysm (e.g., between synthetic bypass material and the artery), a pseudoaneurysm causing displacement, which may lead to the development of cutaneous

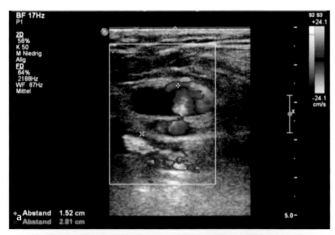

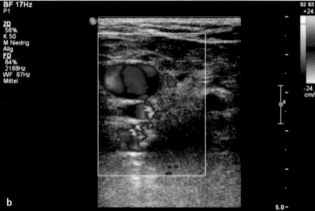

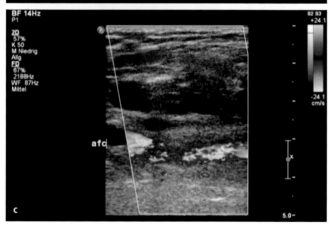

Fig. 4.5-24a–c (a) A multilocular pseudoaneurysm in the common femoral artery (longitudinal section). (b) A multilocular pseudoaneurysm in the common femoral artery (cross-section). (c) Complete thrombosis of the aneurysm after thrombin injection.

necrosis or compression of nerves and/or vessels. Surgical treatment is preferable in these cases.

Endovascular therapy

The most important options for interventional treatment for pseudoaneurysm include prolonged balloon dilation, coil embolization, and endoprosthesis implantation. The procedures are only rarely used. They are mainly indicated when the conservative measures described above are contraindicated or have failed. Before coil em-

bolization (Fig. 4.5-25a–c) or endoprosthesis implantation (Fig. 4.5-26a–c), balloon-supported interruption of perfusion to the pseudoaneurysm should be attempted first in interventional treatment. A balloon is placed and dilated in the affected artery in such a way that perfusion of the connecting channel to the aneurysm is interrupted. The balloon remains in this position for 5–10 min. This can often achieve complete occlusion of the aneurysm.

Patient preparation

- Patient information and consent
- Fasting for at least 4 hours before the intervention

Medication

- When endoprosthesis implantation is planned, a loading dose of 300 mg clopidogrel is given on the day before the intervention or on the same day.
- After placement of the sheath, a heparin bolus of 2500–5000 IU is administered, depending on the patient's body weight and the duration of the intervention.

Catheter technique in coil embolization

- After local anesthesia, a 5F or 6F crossover sheath (e.g., Cook, Terumo) with a hemostatic valve is placed in the contralateral common femoral artery.
- A crossover maneuver is then performed, usually with a 5F IMA or SOS or "SIM" catheter and a 0.035" Terumo J wire.
- In cases of kinking and/or occlusion of the contralateral pelvic arteries, the intervention can alternatively be carried out via the brachial access route.
- After local anesthesia, a 6F 90-cm sheath (e.g., Shuttle Sheath, Cook) with a hemostatic valve is placed in the left brachial artery.
- Using the telescope technique with a 6F IMA diagnostic catheter and a 0.035" Terumo J stiff wire, the sheath is advanced into the distal segment of the abdominal aorta and if possible to the corresponding pelvic arteries.

Preinterventional angiography

For precise assessment of the femoral artery bifurcation (deep femoral artery/superficial femoral artery) and localization of the pseudoaneurysm or its afferent channel, the femoral arteries are imaged with a 30° right anterior oblique view. Additional projections are necessary if any anatomic variants are present.

Intervention in coil embolization

The connecting channel between the artery and the pseudoaneurysm is probed with a guidable 0.014", 0.018", or 0.035" J guidewire and a suitable guide catheter, usually a 5F IMA or vertebral artery catheter. After successful probing, the guidewire is removed and the coil (e.g., Tornado 0.035", Cook) is introduced into the catheter.
The coil is advanced into the aneurysm with the guidewire (Fig. 4.5-25a).

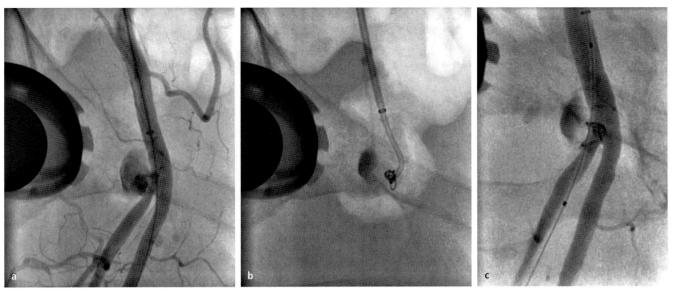

Fig. 4.5-25a–c (a) Angiographic imaging of a pseudoaneurysm in the right common femoral artery. (b) Probing of the aneurysm (with an IMA catheter) and coil embolization. (c) The completely thrombosed aneurysm after coil embolization (with contrast left in the pseudoaneurysm sac after coil application).

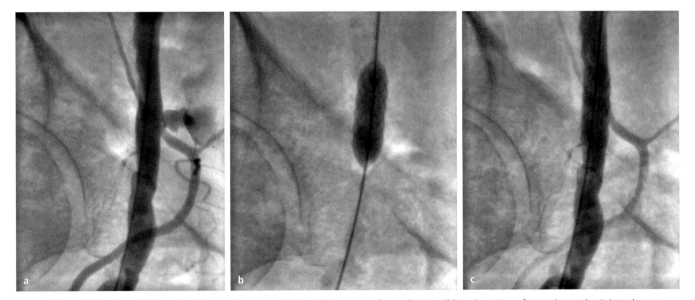

Fig. 4.5-26a–c (a) Angiographic imaging of a pseudoaneurysm in the right common femoral artery. (b) Implantation of an endoprosthesis into the common femoral artery (17-mm Jostent® graft). (c) Complete exclusion of the aneurysm after implantation of the endoprosthesis.

Catheter technique in endoprosthesis implantation

- After local anesthesia, a 7–9F crossover sheath (e.g., Cook, Terumo), depending on the diameter of the endoprosthesis required (4–9 mm Jostent® graft, Abbott Vascular; 6 mm and 7 mm Viabahn®, Gore) with a hemostatic valve is placed in the contralateral common femoral artery.
- The crossover maneuver is performed, depending on the anatomy of the pelvic arteries, with the 5F IMA or SOS-Omni catheter and a 0.035" hydrophilic-coated J wire (Terumo). The sheath must only be placed or advanced over the corresponding dilator.
- Due to the increased risk of complications, the indication for the intervention via the brachial access route with a sheath ≥ 7F needs to be established cautiously.

Preinterventional angiography

Preinterventional angiography is the same as described in the section on coil embolization above.

Intervention with endoprosthesis implantation

- A 0.035" wire is advanced into the affected artery—e.g., the common femoral artery.
- The balloon-expandable endoprosthesis (e.g., Jostent® graft) or self-expanding endoprosthesis (e.g., Viabahn®) is placed in the arterial segment supplying the pseudoaneurysm. It is important for the endoprosthesis to be large enough (at least 1 mm oversized), as it may otherwise dislodge distally when the vascular surface is smooth.

■ Further dilation in the endoprosthesis is carried out using a suitably sized balloon for better adaptation to the vessel wall (recommended in self-expanding endoprostheses; Fig. 4.5-26a–c).

Postinterventional follow-up and medication

Special medication such as platelet inhibition is not recommended after coil embolization. After endoprosthesis implantation, combined platelet inhibition with ASA 100 mg/d and clopidogrel 75 mg/d should be continued for at least 3 months.

■ 6–8 hour bed rest, depending on the sheath size used for transfemoral access, or 2–4 hours, if occlusion systems are used.

■ Check-up angiographic examinations with color duplex ultrasonography should be carried out before discharge and 6 and 12 months later.

Surgical treatment

Indication

Even today, surgical treatment is still an important treatment option for pseudoaneurysms. Due to the size of the aneurysm, compression of neighboring structures can occur in rare cases, leading to neuropathy, skin necrosis, thrombosis, or critical leg ischemia. In these cases, a surgical approach with removal of the hematoma and suturing of the artery is unavoidable. Additional indications for surgical therapy include failure of noninvasive treatment measures, bypass aneurysm, and mycotic aneurysm.

Disadvantages and potential complications with this form of treatment include a longer hospital stay, postoperative infection or neuralgia, perioperative bleeding, myocardial infarction, and rarely death.

When assessing the urgency of surgical intervention, priority must be given to establishing whether it is an acute pseudoaneurysm, less than 3 days old, or a chronic one. Chronic forms include pseudoaneurysms that develop after placement of a prosthesis–arterial anastomosis (anastomotic aneurysm) and local thromboendarterectomy (TEA), disobliteration aneurysm. Both in prosthesis–arterial aneurysms and those developing after TEA, pseudoaneurysm formation is often caused by technical errors: lack of caliber adaptation between the prosthesis and vessel leads to later ectasias, and when disobliteration is too radical, often in combination with patch dilation, the stability of the vessel wall is weakened.

The inguinal region is a site of predilection, as traction, shearing, and vibration forces all occur there. Suture aneurysms arise due to suture leaks and are functionally equivalent to pseudoaneurysms after persistent puncture defects (Fig. 4.5-15). These mainly require surgical revision and improvement.

Mycotic aneurysms arise as a result of inflammatory bacterial processes (rarely fungal) that infiltrate and destroy the vessel wall. In formal pathogenetic terms, two different routes of infection can be distinguished:

■ Hematogenous: internal. In this case, either septic microembolizations with scattered foci in the vasa vasorum lead to local vasculitis with necrosis and thinning of the wall, or septic macroemboli (e.g., in valvular endocarditis) obliterate a peripheral vascular lumen, resulting in local abscess formation with inflammatory wall damage.

■ Continuous: external. In this case, paravascular inflammatory processes that spread to the vascular wall, either in continuity or via lymph vessels, lead to necrotizing vasculitis with destruction of the wall texture (e.g., abscess-forming lymphadenitis; abscess-forming pulmonary processes penetrating the parietal pleura; or infected Angio-Seal anchors).

Inflammatory disintegration of the vessel wall promotes early rupture and rapid size growth in mycotic pseudo-aneurysms and requires rapid surgical intervention when the diagnosis is established.

Vascular surgery treatment

Surgical treatment for pseudoaneurysm may be limited to direct demonstration and suturing of the puncture defect, but may also lead to complete prosthetic replacement of the vessel (e.g., in vessels with high-grade calcification or in cases of stent perforation).

The surgical procedure for pseudoaneurysm in the common femoral may be used as an example here, as it is the one that occurs most frequently. Depending on the intensity of bleeding, manual compression of the bleeding site by an assistant is urgently continued. At least one large-lumen venous access is placed, electrocardiography and arterial blood-pressure monitoring are instituted, and intubation anesthesia (due to the high risk of aspiration in these patients, who are usually no longer in a fasting state), surgical disinfection, and draping follow. If there is severe bleeding and hemorrhagic shock, non–cross-matched blood must be requested.

This is followed by rapid exposure of the pseudoaneurysm with demonstration of the proximal neck of the aneurysm, and then heparinization (100 U/kg body weight) and clamping off of the vessel central to the pseudoaneurysm, opening of the aneurysm, and demonstration and direct suturing of the puncture defect. Distal (i.e., segmental) clamping of the punctured artery is not necessary in most cases, as bleeding is easily stopped using the fingers. After the skin incision, experienced vascular surgeons prefer blunt digital spreading of the subcutaneous tissue and aneurysmal sac, and direct digital sealing of the wall defect, which is often only 2–3 mm in size, once the bleeding source has been found. After this, broad forceps can be used to control bleeding by pressing the adventitia together, and the defect can be directly sutured. Alternatively, the vessel wall defect can be clamped off tangentially using a Cooley or Satinsky vascular clamp. Routine exploration of the posterior wall can be dispensed with if there is no further bleeding after the primary defect has been sutured, as double wall puncture with aneurysm formation is rare. If there is bleeding from the posterior wall, a search needs to be made for an iatrogenic arteriovenous fistula, and if necessary the venous puncture site will also have to be sutured. After hemostasis, the hematoma is aspirated or evacuated digitally, so far as this is possible without causing additional damage to the musculature. Finally, a large-caliber (16F) Redon drain is placed in the hematoma cavity.

A skin wound in the inguinal region is always closed using interrupted sutures (Allgöwer vertical mattress sutures). Deep sutures in the subcutis should be avoided because of possible damage to the femoral nerve or superficial cutaneous nerve, or to the centrally confluent lymphatic vessels here (the inguinal lymph collectors). Frequent complications (3–8%) of emergency surgical procedures in the inguinal region include wound healing disturbances and persistent lymphatic fistulas/seromas. Postoperative duplex ultrasonography is recommended in order to exclude stenosis of the afferent artery caused by the vascular suture.

Mycotic aneurysm always requires generous segmental resection of the infected vessel. A large-caliber venous segment should be used for the vascular bridging graft whenever possible. If no more usable saphenous vein is available, the femoral vein can be used as an alternative, preferably harvested from the distal third of the thigh. With the good collateralization that is usually present, swelling of the dependent lower leg due to stasis only occurs in exceptional cases. Silver-impregnated (commercially available) Dacron prostheses can also be used as replacements, but stable impregnation should be ensured.

4.5.2.5   Prospects

As has already been recommended in the international literature, it can be expected that thrombin injection will become the treatment method of choice, in view of the high success rate and low risk of the intervention, both depending on the patient's anticoagulation status, and as it is also much more comfortable for the patient.

References

Cope C, Zeit R. Coagulation of aneurysms by direct percutaneous thrombin injection. American Journal of Roentgenology 1986; 147: 383–7.

Coughlin BF, Paushter DM. Peripheral pseudoaneurysms: evaluation with duplex ultrasound. Radiology 1988; 168: 339–42.

Doyle BJ, Ting HH, Bell MR, Lennon RJ, Mathew V, Singh M, Holmes DR, Rihal CS. Major femoral bleeding complications after percutaneous coronary intervention: Incidence, predictors, and impact on long-term survival among 17,901 patients treated at the Mayo Clinic from 1994 to 2005. JACC Cardiovasc Interv 2008; 1: 202–9.

Fellmeth BD, Roberts AC, Bookstein JJ, Freischlag JA, Forsythe JR, Buckner NK, Hye RJ. Postangiographic femoral artery injuries: non-surgical repair with US-guided compression. Radiology 1991; 178: 671–5.

Gabriel M, Pawlaczyk K, Waliszewski K, Krasinski Z, Majewski W. Location of femoral artery puncture site and the risk of postcatheterization pseudoaneurysm formation. Int J Cardiol 2007; 120: 167–71.

Katzenschlager R, Uguruoglu A, Ahmandi A, Hulsmann M, Koppensteiner R, Larch E, Maca T, Minar E, Stumpflen A, Ehringer H. Incidence of pseudoaneurysm after diagnostic and therapeutic angiography. Radiology 1995; 195: 463–6.

Kobeiter H, Lapeyre M, Becquemin JP, Mathieu D, Melliere D, Desgranges P. Percutaneous coil embolization of postcatheterization arterial femoral pseudaneurysms. Journal of Vascular Surgery 2002; 36: 127–31.

Kresowik TF, Khoury MD, Miller BV, Winniford MD, Shamma AR, Sharp WJ, Blecha MB, Corson JD. A prospective study of the incidence and natural history of femoral vascular complications after percutaneous transluminal coronary angioplasty. Journal of Vascular Surgery 1991; 134: 328–36.

La Perna L, Olin JW, Goines D, Childs MB, Ouriel K. Ultrasound-guided thrombin injection for the treatment of postcatheterization pseudoaneurysms. Circulation 2000; 102: 2391–5.

Muller DWM, Shamir KJH, Ellis SG, Topol EJ. Peripheral vascular complications after conventional and complex percutaneous coronary interventional procedures. American Journal of Cardiology 1992; 69: 63–8.

Popma JJ, Satler LF, Pichard AD, Kent KM, Campbell A, Chuang YC, Clark C, Merritt AJ, Bucher TA, Leon MB. Vascular complications after balloon and new device angioplasty. Circulation 1993; 88: 1569–78.

Sridevi R. Pitta, Abhiram Prasad, Gautam Kumar, Ryan Lennon, Charanjit S. Rihal, David Holmes. Location of Femoral Artery Access and Correlation with Vascular Complications. Catheterization and Cardiovascular Interventions 2011; 78: 294–9.

Thalhammer C, Kirchherr AS, Uhlich F, Waigand J, Gross CM. Postcatheterization pseudoaneurysms and arteriovenous fistulas: repair with percutaneous implantation of endovsascular covered stents. Radiology 2000; 214: 127–31.

Webber WG, Jang J, Gustavson S, Olin JW. Contemporary management of postcatheterization pseudoaneurysms. Circulation 2007; 115: 2666–74.

4.6   Arteriovenous fistula

Sebastian Sixt and Thomas Zeller

4.6.1   Clinical picture

Local peri-interventional complications after inguinal puncture include inguinal hematomas, active bleeding, pseudoaneurysms, and arteriovenous fistulas (AVFs). An AVF can develop if the femoral artery and vein or their side branches are punctured simultaneously. These arteriovenous fistulas are usually narrow and of no hemodynamic relevance. They represent approximately 12% of all complications in the inguinal region. In a retrospective study after coronary catheter interventions, an incidence of associated AVFs in the range of 0.006–0.140% was observed, although the analysis only included cases that were treated surgically. The most comprehensive analysis so far conducted, by Kelm et al. (2002), included 10,271 consecutive patients who were followed up for 3 years; not unexpectedly, the incidence was higher at 0.86%. In addition, slightly more arteriovenous fistulas were found after catheter interventions than after purely diagnostic angiographies (1.1% vs. 0.75%; $P = 0.12$). Arterial hypertension and female sex were independent, patient-related risk factors for inguinal complications. Degenerative changes in the vessel wall and a need for several punctures appear to have some influence on the development of arteriovenous fistulas here.

In addition, risk factors associated with the catheter intervention and a correlation with the intensity of anticoagulation treatment was also observed. Puncture in the left groin, which is comparatively unusual for access, was associated with more than twice the risk of arteriovenous fistula. High heparin dosages and warfarin (Coumadin) treatment increased the risk twofold. Intensive anticoagulation treatment thus makes it easier for arteriovenous fistulas to develop, as has already been demonstrated for the development of postinterventional pseudoaneurysms and hemorrhage. Patient-associated factors influencing the development of AVFs included age and overweight status. The sheath size and the number of sheaths used had no influence on the frequency of iatrogenic AVFs. Manual compression to remove the sheath after peripheral intervention, particularly after antegrade puncture in combination with local ly-

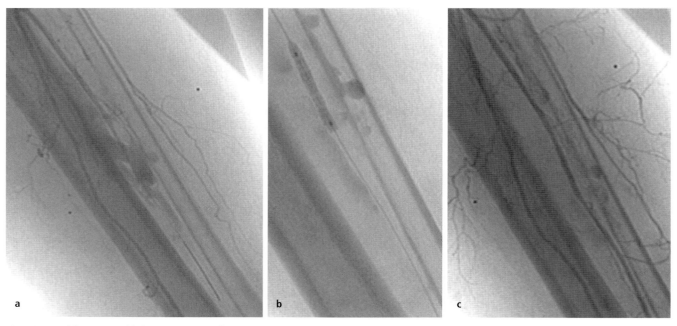

Fig. 4.6-1a–c (a) Iatrogenic fibular arteriovenous fistula and pseudoaneurysm following Fogarty embolectomy. (b) Introduction of a covered stent (Graftmaster™). (c) Results after elimination of the arteriovenous fistula.

sis therapy, is considered to be problematic. There is an increased risk of an iatrogenic AVF occurring during puncture of the popliteal artery (rarely required), as the popliteal vein lies ventral to the artery here and the puncture procedure often penetrates through it. During the subsequent withdrawal of the sheath with manual compression, relevant AV fistulas can occur that are sometimes hemodynamically relevant.

A less well known but typical complication is an AV fistula in the lower leg following a Fogarty maneuver (Fig. 4.6-1).

4.6.2 Clinical findings

The clinical signs of an arteriovenous fistula are sometimes subtle, and auscultation of the puncture site is needed in order to document a newly developed clear, holosystolic–diastolic flow murmur. Opinions differ widely regarding the potential sequelae of persistent AVF. In a group of 88 patients with a follow-up period of 3 years, neither clinical symptoms such as edema development, reduced walking distance, abnormal pulse status, local pain, cold sensation in the affected extremity, nor any signs of cardiac insufficiency were observed (Ruebben et al. 1998). Alternatively, there have been reports of cardiac insufficiency due to high-output cardiac failure, as well as evidence of aneurysmal degeneration at the puncture site and leg edema as a consequence of AVFs (Fig. 4.6-2). An arteriovenous fistula can become potentially clinically significant due to a hemodynamically relevant left–right shunt with subsequent reduced blood flow in the periphery, as well as increased volume loading with signs of cardiac insufficiency. However, shunt flow measurements only showed variations of only 160–510 mL/min. This was low in comparison with larger cardiac left–right shunts and even much lower than the level seen in hemodialysis shunts; the authors therefore concluded that the hemodynamic relevance of AVFs appears to be extremely questionable.

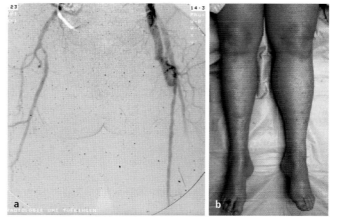

Fig. 4.6-2a, b A femoral arteriovenous fistula (a), leading to swelling of the left leg (b).

4.6.3 Differential diagnosis and diagnosis

A newly developing flow murmur or pulsatile resistance after arterial puncture always requires diagnosis. The principal differential diagnosis is pseudoaneurysm. An important aspect of the differential diagnosis is an initial clinical approach with palpation and auscultation, and imaging with color duplex ultrasonography is always finally required, which is safe and cost-effective here. Typical findings, as seen in Fig. 4.6-3, include severely turbulent flow directed out of the artery, with high peripheral resistance into the vein, with low peripheral resistance. Imaging should always be carried out with a high repetition rate, as this is the best way of narrowing down and classifying the shunt flow. In pathognomic terms, there is a loss of three-phase arterial flow proximal to the fistula and reduced arterial flow distal to it, as well as markedly increased pulsatile flow (Fig. 4.6-4) proximal to the fistula in the affected vein. Occasionally, high-speed pulsatile flow can transfer vibrations to the surrounding tissue, so that

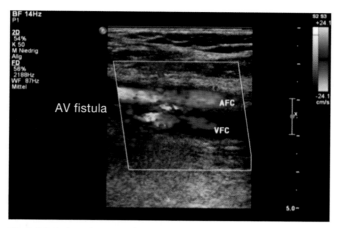

Fig. 4.6-3 A shunt between the common femoral artery (AFC) and common femoral vein (VFC).

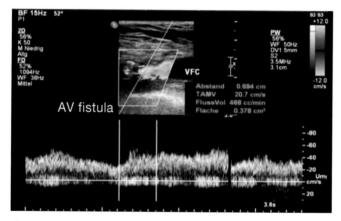

Fig. 4.6-4 Arterialized, turbulent flow in the common femoral vein (VFC) with a shunt volume calculated at approximately 450–500 mL/min.

precise ultrasound localization may be difficult. It should be noted that the typical flow changes only occur with arteriovenous fistulas of the large vessels; if smaller side branches are affected, such changes may be absent and it may be more difficult to confirm the diagnosis. There have been rare cases in which a pseudoaneurysm also had a connection to the accompanying vein, so that a pseudoaneurysm with an accompanying AVF was present at the arterial puncture site.

4.6.4 Prevention

Many efforts have been made to make catheter interventions safer, but inguinal complications after cardiac and peripheral interventions are still the most frequent. Use of an occlusion system to control hemostasis after arterial puncture and allow early mobilization of the patient appears to be promising. Ways of shortening the hospitalization period involved are attracting attention, with increasing numbers of catheter interventions being conducted on an outpatient basis.

4.6.5 Treatment

Three different treatment strategies are available for symptomatic AVFs: ultrasound-guided compression, surgical inguinal revision, and implantation of a covered stent. Although the success rate with compression is relatively low, it is recommended as the treatment of choice due to its noninvasiveness. There are differing views on the spontaneous occlusion rate, which varies from one-third of all AVFs within 1 year to 81% within 1 month. There is also controversy regarding the prospects for success with ultrasound-guided compression, which patients often find extremely painful. For example, successful occlusion was not achieved in one report even after repeated compression for 20–40 min—although these compression times may perhaps be too short, as a success rate of one in three was observed with a longer period (up to 80 min). As an alternative to manual compression, prolonged compression of the inguinal region by placing a compression dressing for several days has been carried out, without compromising arterial perfusion, with local pressure relief for 45 min each during daily duplex ultrasound check-ups and dressing replacement. In a group of 16 patients, occlusion was observed with this approach after periods of 4–46 days. However, complications developing during treatment included two skin ulcerations in the inguinal region and an asymptomatic thrombosis of the femoral vein, and this method can therefore not be recommended.

Administration of a platelet inhibitor or oral anticoagulation makes spontaneous occlusion substantially more difficult and reduces the likelihood that manual compression will succeed.

Use of percutaneous intervention with implantation of a covered stent or stent grafts was for a long time limited to case reports, but has now become a noteworthy alternative treatment strategy, including coil embolization (Fig. 4.6-3). However, a limiting factor is the unknown rate of recurrent in-stent occlusions and thromboses during the long-term course. For this reason, stents should be used with some caution in younger patients. Stent angioplasty near the bifurcation should also be avoided.

The recommendation for surgical revision of iatrogenic AVFs is based on observations of relevant congenital and traumatic fistulas. However, this treatment approach is associated with an appreciable rate of perioperative complications. It is generally recommended that the indications for surgical revision should be kept narrow and that it should only be done in exceptional situations. These may include cardiac insufficiency, leg ischemia, and varicosis. Relevant complications of surgical revision include bleeding, wound healing disturbances, and secondary lymphedema; the cosmetic disturbance represented by the scar should also be mentioned.

References

Igidbashian VN, Mitchell DG, Middleton WD, Schwartz RA, Goldberg BB. Iatrogenic femoral arteriovenous fistula: diagnosis with color Doppler imaging. Radiology 1989; 170 (3 Pt 1): 749–52.

Kelm M, Perings SM, Jax T, Lauer T, Schoebel FC, Heintzen MP, Perings C, Strauer BE. Incidence and clinical outcome of iatrogenic femoral arteriovenous fistulas: implications for risk stratification and treatment. J Am Coll Cardiol 2002; 40 (2): 291–7.

Messina LM, Brothers TE, Wakefield TW, Zelenock GB, Lindenauer SM, Greenfield LJ, Jacobs LA, Fellows EP, Grube SV, Stanley JC. Clinical characteristics and surgical management of vascular complications in patients undergoing cardiac catheterization: interventional versus diagnostic procedures. J Vasc Surg 1991; 13 (5): 593–600.

Paulson EK, Kliewer MA, Hertzberg BS, Tcheng JE, McCann RL, Bowie JD, Carroll BA. Ultrasonographically guided manual compression of femoral artery injuries. J Ultrasound Med 1995; 14 (9): 653–9.

Paulson EK, Kliewer MA, Hertzberg BS, O'Malley CM, Washington R, Carroll BA. Color Doppler sonography of groin complications following femoral artery catheterization. AJR Am J Roentgenol 1995; 165 (2): 439–44.

Ruebben A, Tettoni S, Muratore P, Rossato D, Savio D, Rabbia C. Arteriovenous fistulas induced by femoral arterial catheterization: percutaneous treatment. Radiology 1998; 209 (3): 729–34.

Schaub F, Theiss W, Heinz M, Zagel M, Schomig A. New aspects in ultrasound-guided compression repair of postcatheterization femoral artery injuries. Circulation 1994; 90 (4): 1861–5.

Thalhammer C, Kirchherr AS, Uhlich F, Waigand J, Gross CM. Postcatheterization pseudoaneurysms and arteriovenous fistulas: repair with percutaneous implantation of endovascular covered stents. Radiology 2000; 214 (1): 127–31.

Toursarkissian B, Allen BT, Petrinec D, Thompson RW, Rubin BG, Reilly JM, Anderson CB, Flye MW, Sicard GA. Spontaneous closure of selected iatrogenic pseudoaneurysms and arteriovenous fistulae. J Vasc Surg 1997; 25 (5): 803–8.

Waigand J, Uhlich F, Gross CM, Thalhammer C, Dietz R. Percutaneous treatment of pseudoaneurysms and arteriovenous fistulas after invasive vascular procedures. Catheter Cardiovasc Interv 1999; 47 (2): 157–64.

Waksman R, King SB, 3rd, Douglas JS, Shen Y, Ewing H, Mueller L, Ghazzal ZM, Weintraub WS. Predictors of groin complications after balloon and new-device coronary intervention. Am J Cardiol 1995; 75 (14): 886–9.

Zhou T, Liu ZJ, Zhou SH, Shen XQ, Liu QM, Fang ZF, Hu XQ, Li J, Lu XL. Treatment of postcatheterization femoral arteriovenous fistulas with simple prolonged bandaging. Chin Med J 2007; 120 (11): 952–5.

4.7   Compression syndromes in the extremities

Thomas Cissarek

4.7.1   Thoracic outlet syndrome (TOS)

TOS is a generic term for several syndromes in the area of the superior thoracic outlet that are associated with compression of vessels and nerves (neurovascular compression syndrome) and which are impossible (or difficult) to differentiate from one another diagnostically:

- Costoclavicular syndrome
- Hyperabduction syndrome
- Scalenus syndrome
- Scalenus minimus syndrome
- Cervical rib syndrome
- Pectoralis minor syndrome
- Paget–von Schroetter syndrome

If only the subclavian vein is compressed, the condition can be described as thoracic inlet syndrome (TIS), although there is concomitant arterial involvement in 66% of cases and neurological involvement in 57%.

4.7.1.1   Epidemiology

It is not possible to give precise details on the frequency of TOS. There are large numbers of unreported cases, and the diagnosis is usually only made at a late stage. It particularly affects younger, asthenic individuals, and women more frequently than men at a ratio of 3:2 (probably due to the deeper position of the sternum, resulting in an increase in constrictive areas further up). Men who are affected are often muscular and athletic (and involved in weight training and body-building). The peak age is between 20 and 40 (when there is physiological lowering of the pectoral girdle). The brachial plexus is involved in 97% of cases, mainly arterial compression occurs in 24%, and mainly venous compression in 36%. Cervical rib is found to be the cause in > 10%; patients with a subclavian artery aneurysm have cervical ribs in 21% of cases.

4.7.1.2   Etiology

Compression of vessels and nerves may occur intermittently, but it can also be chronic. It is caused by:

- Constitutional bony and fibromuscular anomalies. Roos distinguishes nine different types of band anomaly.
- Post-traumatic changes—e.g., cicatricial muscular contraction after crushing, tissue lacerations, and muscle hematomas, and excessive callus formation after clavicular fractures. Some two-thirds of patients have a history including a corresponding trauma.

Sequelae include vessel wall injuries (local intimal lesions due to the action of shearing forces) and pressure lesions in the brachial plexus. Compression and strain lead to microhematomas in the perineural tissue, which develop fibrous healing and lead to cicatricial contraction. The plexus lesions may be reversible.

4.7.1.3   Clinical findings

Major symptoms

The major symptoms are:

- Movement-dependent shoulder–arm pain
- Nocturnal tingling paresthesias
- Weakness and a feeling of heaviness in the arm
- Increased perspiration tendency in the affected arm

The major symptoms in an advanced course are:

- Disturbance of fine motor skills in the fingers
- Atrophy of the small muscles of the hand

When there are vascular complications, the major symptoms are:

- Claudication-like pain (intermittent apraxia)
- Pallor and coldness in the hand
- Punctate skin necroses
- Swollen, livid arm

The symptoms mainly depend on whether neural or vascular structures are affected. In most cases, veins, arteries, and plexus are compressed, although to varying degrees. Detailed neurological examinations show involvement of the plexus in as many as 97% of cases. The symptomatic picture may vary extremely widely among individuals, but remains largely the same in each individual over long periods.

Pain

- Lateral and dorsal headache, pain in the shoulder and lateral upper arm when there is injury/compression in the upper plexus (C5–7)
- Pain in the area of the hand and fingers, particularly in the area of the ulnar distribution (D IV and V), and medial shoulder–arm pain when the lower plexus is affected (C8/T1)
- Feeling of heaviness and tension in the entire arm with venous outflow disturbances

The neurological and vascular symptoms are typically exacerbated when the arms are raised (with overhead work) and resolve with physical rest.

Paresthesias and motor disturbances

- Disturbances in the distribution area of the damaged plexus parts—e.g., a feeling of numbness in the elevated arm
- Rapid fatigability in the upper extremity during hyperabduction
- Tingling paresthesias on elevation and abduction
- Increasing clumsiness with prolonged manual work (dropping objects from the hand)
- Nocturnal pain after overexertion or prolonged overhead work
- Moist, cold hands, caused by compression of sympathetic fibers

Circulatory disturbances

- Claudication-like symptoms when there is mainly arterial compression
- Multiple occlusions of the hand and digital arteries, with exercise pain and pain on exposure to cold. Seventy-five percent of TOS patients who undergo surgery have angiographic evidence of digital artery occlusions
- Cyanosis and bulging protrusion of the brachial veins, with swelling during overhead work, in patients with venous compression
- Increased extent and consistency, with increased venous markings, in acute subclavian vein thrombosis
- Increased venous markings at the shoulder and anterior chest wall, with increased extent in the affected arm, in patients with post-thrombotic syndrome in the upper extremity

Skin changes

- Punctate skin necroses and trophic disturbances at the fingertips when there are arterioarterial emboli from mural or parietal thrombi:
  - From a vessel wall lesion resulting from chronic, repetitive trauma
  - From aneurysms resulting from post-stenotic dilations
- Edema and (massive) swelling in the hand and lower arm when there is deep vein thrombosis in the axillary–subclavian region (with chronic and also intermittent compression) due to the venous outflow disturbances (not found in scalenus syndrome, as the subclavian vein does not penetrate the scalene fissure)

- Increased perspiration and feeling of cold, changes in skin color (neural) when there is irritation of the sympathetic neural supply to the brachial plexus
- Pallor:
  - In acute ischemia with an embolic arterial occlusion
  - Due to vasospasm (with subsequent reactive hyperemia) in secondary Raynaud phenomenon

4.7.1.4 Diagnosis

History

A precise and careful patient history is an absolute necessity. Most patients have usually undergone many years of orthopedic, chiropractic, rheumatologic, hand-surgery, psychotherapeutic, and psychiatric treatment before the diagnosis is established. Establishing the diagnosis takes an average of 4.5 years, with an average of 6.3 physicians being consulted. Many patients have previously undergone surgical treatment—for carpal tunnel syndrome, ulnar sulcus syndrome, radial or ulnar epicondylitis, etc.

The patients often have occupations involving heavy labor. They are often actively involved in high-performance sports such as tennis, table tennis, sailing, hang-gliding, surfing, and body-building. Hyperabduction pain occurs with overhead work. Nocturnal symptoms include tingling paresthesias when sleeping in the prone position and when the arms are raised. Loss of skill and coordination capacity in finger movements is noted, with unexpected dropping of objects and difficulty in writing and working on the computer or in playing a musical instrument. When there is venous compression, the arm is swollen and shows livid discoloring in the mornings.

Inspection and palpation

Inspection and palpation include the following items:

- Examination of the patient in the standing position: evidence of postural anomalies
- Skin color:
  - Pallor (in embolic occlusion, vasospasm in Raynaud phenomenon)
  - Livid discoloration (in venous compression)
  - Punctate skin necroses (emboli)
- Skin temperature (cold with arterial symptoms)
- Perspiration (secondary Raynaud phenomenon)
- Increased extent and venous markings in the upper and lower arm in comparison with the contralateral side
- Checking grip and pinch strength
- Signs of muscular atrophy
- Sensitivity of neural pressure points (brachial plexus in the axilla and supraclavicular area)
- Mobility in the shoulder joint and cervical spine
- Cervical rib possibly palpable: springy resistance in the supraclavicular area
- Pulse status (axillary artery, brachial artery, radial artery, ulnar artery)
- Characteristically, tension in the trapezius muscle and pressure pain at the upper edge of the trapezius

Clinical examination—provocation tests

The multitude of tests that have been described (the Eden test, Adson test, Wright test, etc.) have proved to be unnecessary since the comparative studies conducted by Roos. Disappearance of the radial pulse on elevation and abduction of the arm with simultaneous rotation of the head to the affected side, as well as dorsal flexion of the head and deep inspiration, only provide hints. However, this examination provides no evidence of disease in the absence of clinical symptoms, as 30% of the normal population also has disappearance of the radial pulse on elevation and abduction.

By contrast, the abduction, elevation, and external rotation test, known in the English-language literature as the elevated arm stress test (EAST), is extremely useful. During the test, both arms are abducted by about 90°. With the hands externally rotated, the patient carries out slow and strong fist-forming exercises for 3 min. This test can usually trigger all of the symptoms that are typical in these patients:

- Tingling paresthesias
- Numbness
- Feeling of heaviness
- Pain
- Prolonged pallor
- Bulging protrusion of the veins in the hand and lower arm
- Blue livid discoloration, etc.
- In severe cases, patients are unable to tolerate the 3-min test time.

A positive EAST is practically pathognomonic for TOS. The test is negative in carpal tunnel syndrome, ulnar sulcus syndrome, and cervical syndrome.

Diagnostic imaging

Basic examinations

- Duplex ultrasonography
- X-ray of the cervical spine at four levels
- Special imaging of the superior thoracic outlet
- Digital subtraction angiography to demonstrate the subclavian artery and vein in a sitting position
- Neurological diagnosis

Doppler duplex ultrasonography

With a provocation test:
- Direct imaging of hemodynamically effective compression phenomena on color duplex
- Compression ultrasonography and color duplex to confirm/exclude thrombosis
- Imaging of local vessel wall changes such as aneurysms, plaque, and stenoses
- Typical local stenosis signal in the supraclavicular area in scalenus syndrome or in the infraclavicular region in hyperabduction syndrome, with typical aliasing and cessation of flow in some cases
- Imaging of the distal "post-stenotic" flow changes on continuous-wave Doppler

- Monophasic flow signal or cessation of flow in the lower arm arteries during the provocation

X-ray

- Imaging of the cervical spine at four levels to exclude or confirm degenerative changes in the cervical spine, or a cervical rib if present.
- Special imaging of the superior thoracic outlet (lordosis imaging) to confirm cervical rib or other congenital or acquired bony anomalies at the superior thoracic outlet (e.g., excessive callus formation after clavicular fracture).
- To confirm vascular lesions (stenosis, aneurysm, peripheral embolization), intra-arterial digital subtraction angiography is done (with readiness to perform percutaneous transluminal angioplasty if needed).
- It is difficult to confirm compression (without a vascular lesion) with angiography (in the supine position). Arteriography or phlebography in the supine position is meaningless if the findings are negative. This provides no information about anatomic structures that might lead to compression. Alternatively, intravenous DSA can be used to image the subclavian artery and vein in the normal position with the arm held horizontally and in elevation and abduction. This examination has to be done with the patient seated or standing.
- To confirm anatomic structures (bony or muscle structures, fibrous bands) that represent the extent of vascular compression, CT and MRI can be carried out in combination with CT angiography or MR angiography. However, even with high-resolution MRI, evidence of fibrous bands is difficult to obtain and unreliable. As the tomographic examinations are carried out with the patient in the supine position, there is a very high rate of false-negative findings. Assessment of the venous circulation is also unsatisfactory.

Neurological consultation (electrophysiology)

Proximal nerve conduction velocity (NCV) in the ulnar and median nerves:
- Delayed NCV confirms compression of the plexus, but normal findings do not exclude TOS.
- A long NCV delay in combination with atrophy of the small muscles of the hand suggests plexus damage, with a poor prognosis.

Caution: even if symptoms are only present on one side, the contralateral side always has to be assessed as well.

4.7.1.5 Differential diagnosis

Pain (shoulder and arm)

See Table 4.7-1.

Paresthesias and motor disturbances

See Table 4.7-2.

Table 4.7-1 Pain (shoulder and arm).

Major symptoms	Minor symptoms	Suspected diagnosis	Diagnosis
Symptomatic (more severe on raising arm), intermittent, in the ulnar distribution area	Paresthesias, motor disturbances, weakening of the radial pulse on raising the arm	Thoracic outlet syndrome	Chest x-ray
Differential diagnoses			
Constant, often on the radial side, limited to specific dermatomes	Restricted movement in the cervical spine	Radiculopathy with constriction of the intervertebral foramina (disk prolapse/protrusion, bony degenerative changes in the cervical spine)	Cervical spine x-ray at four levels Computed tomography (CT) Magnetic resonance imaging (MRI)
Neck pain	Restricted movement in the cervical spine, muscle rigidity	Functional segmental disturbances in the cervical spine (e.g., blockages, muscle rigidity)	Manual examination
Shoulder pain	Restricted mobility in the shoulder	Wear at the glenohumeral joint (omarthrosis), acromioclavicular arthrosis	Shoulder x-ray at two levels
Ubiquitous pain possible	Functional restriction in the arm	Scapulohumeral periarthritis and subforms (impingement syndrome, calcific tendinitis, subacromial bursitis)	Orthopedic consultation Clinical examination Shoulder x-ray at two levels Ultrasound MRI
Appearing suddenly after around 1 week	Persistent paralysis of the shoulder musculature	Neuralgic shoulder amyotrophy/ plexus neuritis	Surveillance Neurologic consultation (electromyography)
Ubiquitous pain possible	Malpositioning of the extremities Signs of external injury	Trauma Luxation Subluxation	Clinical examination X-ray
Severe shoulder pain (usually lower plexus)	Swelling of the hand (lymphostasis and outflow obstruction in the subclavian vein), Horner syndrome, loss of perspiration	Pancoast tumor	Chest x-ray (arrosion of first rib) Chest CT Neurological consultation
Dull, aching pain in a radicular distribution area	Group of segmentally arranged blisters	Herpes zoster	Clinical examination
Aching pain in the arm together with a feeling of retrosternal pressure	Radiating into the jaw, dyspnea	Coronary heart disease	History Electrocardiography Ergometry

Circulatory disturbances

In the differential diagnosis, the vascular complications that are possible in TOS have to be distinguished from complications of other underlying diseases.

4.7.1.6 Treatment

Conservative treatment

Conservative measures lead to decisive improvement in approximately two-thirds of the patients. Among 2013 TOS patients, 852 underwent transaxillary disarticulation of the first rib (Gruss et al. 1980). All minor and moderate cases undergo primary conservative treatment:

- Avoidance of overhead work
- Local heat application (hot packs, warm air)
- Massage to loosen muscle tension
- Adjuvant drug therapy to relax muscle tension is initially useful—e.g., tetrazepam (Musaril) $1–4 \times 50$ mg
- Physiotherapeutic exercises to strengthen the shoulder–arm musculature and improve posture in patients with postural anomalies, particularly cervical spine position in those with poor cervical posture

Treatment of symptoms with venous causes

Acute subclavian vein thrombosis is currently *no longer* treated with surgical thrombectomy or systemic lysis. There is controversy over the indication for local lysis treatment for brachial vein thrombosis (only a few studies, some of them 10–20 years old, have shown trends in favor of fibrinolytic treatment).

Table 4.7-2 Paresthesias and motor disturbances.

Major symptoms	Minor symptoms	Suspected diagnosis	Diagnosis
Tingling paresthesias with arm raised (mainly ulnar)	Motor weakness	Thoracic outlet syndrome	Nerve conduction velocity (NCV)
Differential diagnoses			
Burning paresthesias in the middle finger and flexor side of the first three fingers (median nerve distribution)	Hypotrophy of the thenar musculature, reduced perspiration (median nerve)	Carpal tunnel syndrome	NCV
Sensory disturbances on the ulnar side of the hand, on the fifth and half of the fourth finger		Ulnar sulcus syndrome	Pathological sulcus NCV implies damage at the level of the elbow joint
Persistent paralysis of the shoulder muscles	Sudden-onset shoulder pain for approx. 1 week initially	Neuralgic shoulder amyotrophy/plexus neuritis	Surveillance Electromyography
Dissociated sensory disturbances	Trophic disturbances caused by lesions	Syringomyelia	Myelography Computed tomography Magnetic resonance imaging
Arm hangs down limply and cannot be raised (upper plexus C5–6) Paresis of small hand muscles, disturbed ulnar sensory function (lower plexus, C8–T1)		Pressure lesion on plexus	History (carrying heavy loads—e.g., rucksack paralysis)
Restricted movement (e.g., elevation no longer possible)	Initial pain	Rotator cuff injury	Clinical examination Ultrasonography

Table 4.7-3 Circulatory disturbances.

Major symptoms	Suspected diagnosis	Underlying disease	Diagnosis
Cold, pale, pulseless arm	Arterial embolism	Atrial fibrillation Paradoxical embolism with atrial septal defect	Electrocardiography, transesophageal echocardiography
Tricolor phenomenon, usually in both hands (pale, cold fingers alternating with reactive hyperemia)	Primary or secondary Raynaud phenomenon	Collagenosis and vasculitides	Continuous-wave Doppler, capillary microscopy, laboratory tests
Persistently pale, cold fingers, skin necroses	Digital artery occlusions	Endangiitis obliterans in a setting of collagenosis and vasculitis, traumatic, hyperviscosity syndrome, cryoglobulinemia	Continuous-wave Doppler, intra-arterial angiography, capillary microscopy, laboratory tests
Acute unilateral arm swelling	Subclavian or brachiocephalic thromboses	Effort-induced, in tumor diseases (paraneoplastic or due to tumor compression)	Compression ultrasonography, phlebography if appropriate Chest computed tomography

Decision-making criteria for lysis treatment for deep shoulder–arm venous thrombosis:

- *Extent of thrombosis:* central site with centrally directed growth and no available collateralization, with involvement of the jugular vein
- *Age of thrombosis:* 6–10 days old
- *Individual circumstances:* above-average requirements for arm usability

After reopening of the vein, phlebographic evidence of the underlying compression is indispensable. When there is positive evidence of compression, transaxillary disarticulation of the first rib is carried out within the next 24 hours.

In Germany, untreated subclavian thrombosis and subclavian thrombosis that is only treated with heparin lead to clinically and medicolegally relevant post-thrombotic syndrome in the upper extremity in 13% of cases.

Alternative: appropriate treatment with low-molecular-weight heparin (LMWH), oral anticoagulation, and compression treatment.

Endovascular therapy

Reference may be made here to section A 4.1 above, on stenotic diseases of the proximal arteries of the upper extremity. Although stenoses and short occlusions in the arterial circulation may appear to be accessible for treatment using catheter interventions, the aim should be to achieve causal therapy with resection of the compressive structure and removal of aneurysms as a source of embolism.

Surgical treatment

The success rate is 80–90%. The indications for surgery and the optimal timing are:

- Filiform compression of the subclavian vein on elevation and abduction
- Documented compression of the subclavian vein after catheter lysis of an acute subclavian thrombosis
- Post-thrombotic syndrome in the upper extremity, with confirmed compression of the recanalized subclavian vein and compression of the collaterals
- Morphological changes in the subclavian vein, mural thrombi, dilation, aneurysms
- Peripheral macroembolization or microembolization
- Delayed ulnar nerve and/or median nerve conduction velocities

Surgical procedure

The aim is to achieve complete decompression of the neurovascular bundle by expanding the superior thoracic outlet.

Position

Lateral recumbent position: sterile packing of the arm, which is held by an assistant in abduction (110°); slight pulling may provide a better overview (*caution:* prolonged traction must be avoided).

Incision (transaxillary access)

A curved skin incision is made at the lower margin of the axillary hair, coursing from the posterior edge of the pectoralis major muscle to the anterior edge of the latissimus dorsi ("smiling incision").

Dissection and surgical procedure

Ensuring protection of the intercostobrachial nerve, the fatty, glandular and lymphatic tissue in the axilla is retracted cranially and the anterior and posterior scalene hiatus are demonstrated to provide a clear view. The insertions of the subclavian muscle tendons and of the scalenus anterior and scalenus medius muscles are transected. The intercostal musculature is separated from the first rib, and further free dissection is carried out, releasing the cervical pleura. Fibrous anomalies now become visible and can be removed. The first rib is now completely free and can be transected ventrally and dorsally and removed.

Complete disarticulation of the dorsal costal stump is then carried out (*caution:* there should be no traction on the arm, because of the risk of a plexus lesion; the pleura is accidentally opened during disarticulation in approximately one-third of cases, and Bülau drainage is then required). The ventral costal stump is shortened as far as the cartilage at the manubrium of the sternum. If a cervical rib is also being removed, the connection to the first rib should be left in place, as traction at the first rib allows better manipulation of the cervical rib.

In cases of aneurysm and acute or subacute occlusions, arterial reconstruction can also be carried out with:

- Resection of subclavian aneurysms with grafting of a great saphenous vein segment or a PTFE prosthesis
- Embolectomy

Thoracic sympathectomy is carried out by resecting the sympathetic ganglia at T2–T3/4; this influences the neuropeptides neuropeptide Y, substance P, and calcitonin gene–related peptide that act in the vessel walls, and leads to improved peripheral circulation and positive effects on inflammatory reactions and pain stimuli. When there are venous complications, it may be necessary to remove callused cicatricial tissue around the subclavian vein and to do a patch plasty for a cicatricial stenosis after transaxillary disarticulation of the first rib.

Risks and complications

Bleeding complications arise as a result of sharp dissection of the subclavian artery and vein; hematomas in the axilla are resorbed, but lead to fibroses that can cause recurrent pain symptoms. *Neurological deficits* can be caused by nerve injuries—e.g.:

- Sensory disturbances (intercostobrachial nerve)
- Winged scapula (long thoracic nerve)
- Elevation of the diaphragm (phrenic nerve)
- Horner syndrome (cervicothoracic ganglion)
- Overrotation of the brachial plexus
- Peripheral ulnar and median neuropathy (claw hand deformity, atrophy of the forearm and hand with loss of function, permanent numbness, pain)

Injury to the thoracic duct (lymphatic fistula) is possible with the supraclavicular access route that is used for persistent or recurrent TOS. *Caution:* due to the potential complications and the low prevalence of the disease, appropriate treatment should only be carried out in specialized centers.

Postoperative follow-up

- Chest x-ray immediately postoperatively (in case of pneumothorax)
- Removal of Bülau drain after 24 or 48 hours (one-third of TOS operations)
- Patients are usually symptom-free after a few days (with discharge between the seventh and tenth days postoperatively) and should protect the arm for 8 weeks (with no physiotherapy during this period)
- If there was reduced nerve conduction velocity preoperatively, a check-up should be done 4 weeks postoperatively.
- Heavy physical work and overhead work should be avoided during the first 3–4 months.

4.7.1.7 Prognosis and course

Without treatment, the pain symptoms lead to a relieving posture with subsequent muscle atrophy and painful shoulder stiffness. In rare, advanced cases, paresis of the affected muscles occurs (e.g., in the area of the hand, with disturbance of fine motor skills). Arterial complications include fingertip necroses, amputations of the fingers, hand, and lower arm; post-thrombotic syndrome in the upper extremity is a venous complication.

Results in surgical centers: after the first procedure,

- 85% of patients are completely free of symptoms.
- 12% have decisive improvement.
- 3% have a similar or poorer condition.

Persistent compression syndromes develop in the immediate postoperative period, with:

- Insufficient rib resection (only partial resections) or incorrect disarticulation of the dorsal costal stumps
- Previous plexus lesions
- Overlooking compressive bands, tendons, and muscles

Recurrent compression syndromes are:
- Unfavorable scar formation (e.g., with an inadequately blood-free surgical field at the first operation, or when physiotherapy exercises are started too early)
- Rib regeneration

It is important to carry out a high-standard repeat operation with careful neurolysis of the brachial plexus, removal of cicatricial tissue, scalenectomy, resection of dorsal costal stumps or osseous regeneration, using the neurostimulator. Apical pleurectomy.

After a secondary procedure, only approximately 50% of the patients become symptom-free; 30% have decisive improvement, and 20% remain unchanged.

4.7.2 Compression syndrome in the brachial artery

This involves compression of the brachial artery by a musculotendinous anomaly in the biceps brachii muscle. A distinction needs to be made between:
- Third biceps head syndrome
- Lacertus fibrosus syndrome

4.7.2.1 Anatomy

In the third biceps head syndrome, there is an accessory third biceps head that is too long, arising from the distal upper arm and crossing the neurovascular bundle towards the ulna.

In the *lacertus fibrosus syndrome*, the brachial artery crosses at the elbow underneath the lacertus fibrosus (bicipital aponeurosis), an aponeurosis-like extension of the biceps tendon. Very rarely, there is a supracondylar insertion of the pronator teres muscle. In addition, a ligament of Struthers and abnormal lower arm muscle may be seen.

4.7.2.2 Epidemiology

This is an extremely rare syndrome. A short third head of the biceps is seen in 10% of the population in Europe, but the variant is common in South Africa.
- Women and children in particular have slight hyperextensibility of the elbow joint.
- Muscular men are particularly affected (heavy laborers and body-builders).
- There are patients who have a pathological absence of the physiological inhibition of extension, with elbow joint luxations and fractures.

4.7.2.3 Pathophysiology

- Movement-dependent compression of the brachial artery occurs.
- Venous obstruction does not occur, as unobstructed venous outflow is possible extrafascially.

4.7.2.4 Clinical findings

The clinical symptoms correspond to those in arterial occlusive disease, with:
- Signs of fatigue
- Sensory disturbances

Due to the possible damage to the vessel wall, peripheral embolisms can occur in the digital arteries.

4.7.2.5 Differential diagnosis

- Chronic occlusion on the basis of an arteriosclerotic pathogenesis
- Acute occlusion in embolisms with a cardiac pathogenesis (e.g., atrial fibrillation)
- Digital artery occlusion with other pathogeneses

4.7.2.6 Diagnosis

History

- Young (male) patients who do not have a vascular risk profile
- Involvement of the movement-dominant arm
- Exclusion of a traumatic pathogenesis

Clinical examination

A provocation maneuver is carried out with hyperextension at the elbow joint, in order to achieve weakening and elimination of the radial pulse.

Ultrasound diagnosis

The arm is hyperextended and direct duplex ultrasound imaging of the occlusion is carried out, followed by Doppler ultrasound detection of compromising peripheral flow until the signal is interrupted, and then detection of any distal embolic occlusions.

X-ray

An x-ray is made of the elbow joint to exclude atypical bone and a CT (or MRI) to clarify the anatomy (e.g., with a musculotendinous apparatus surrounding the brachial artery).

4.7.2.7 Treatment

Vascular surgery

The *surgical procedure* consists of division of the lacertus fibrosus, the compressive biceps head, and any abnormally coursing muscles and tendons. Thrombectomy is carried out if there is an acute vascular occlusion.

- *Anesthesia:* plexus anesthesia in the outstretched arm.
- *Risks and complications:* after extended manipulation, vascular spasms with peripheral circulatory disturbances may result. Intraoperative and postoperative intravenous heparin are given.
- *Follow-up and prognosis:* postoperatively, the arm is placed in a slightly flexed position on a cushioned splint. Early mobility exercises are important.

4.7.2.8 Prognosis and course

The prognosis is very good, and no recurrences are expected after uncomplicated operations.

4.7.3 Compression syndrome in the popliteal artery

This is a complex of symptoms resulting from permanent or intermittent compression of the popliteal artery by muscles and/or ligaments. As in the upper extremity, there may be venous or neural involvement in the form of a neurovascular compression syndrome (this is a rarity). The term "popliteal entrapment syndrome" is synonymous.

4.7.3.1 Anatomy

Anatomic distinctions are made between:
- Medial displacement of the popliteal artery
- Normal arterial course with compression by muscular traction
- Accessory ligaments
- Hypertrophy of the calf muscles (soleus syndrome, tendinous arch of the soleus muscle syndrome)
- Baker cysts
- Exostoses/osteochondromas of the condyles

4.7.3.2 Epidemiology

Some 1.5–5.0% of popliteal artery occlusions are due to popliteal entrapment. Athletic men in middle age are more often affected.

4.7.3.3 Clinical findings

- Unilateral peripheral circulatory disturbances/intermittent claudication in young men (usually), in the *absence* of classic risk factors
- Provocable symptoms (cessation of foot pulse on straightening of the knee with simultaneous active plantar flexion/passive dorsiflexion)
- Possible signs of peripheral embolization
- Venous/neural involvement (with paresthesias/resting pain) also possible

4.7.3.4 Diagnosis

Clinical examination

A provocation maneuver is performed during the clinical examination, with disappearance of the foot pulse on straightening of the knee with simultaneous active plantar flexion/passive dorsiflexion.

Further diagnostic imaging

- Full straightening of the knee leads to signal elimination on Doppler ultrasound/oscillography when there is compression of the popliteal artery.
- Duplex ultrasound imaging of medial displacement of the artery (medial gastrocnemius head syndrome).
- Duplex ultrasound evidence of stenosis or occlusion of the popliteal artery.
- Angiography with provocation at several levels is the gold standard.
- CT and MRI also allow imaging of topographic relationships with the surrounding structures (bones, muscles, tendinous structures; Fig. 4.7-1a, b and 4.7.2).

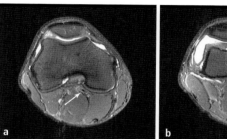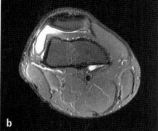

Fig. 4.7-1a, b Compression of the popliteal artery (arrow) in a provocation test (MRI).

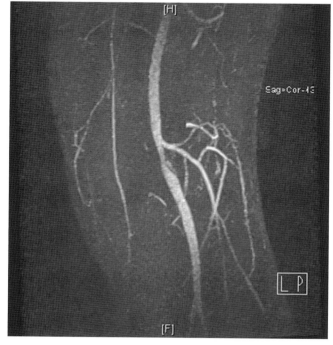

Fig. 4.7-2 Significant stenosis caused by entrapment.

Caution: the contralateral side must always be examined as well (bilateral findings are present in 30–67% of cases).

4.7.3.5   Treatment

Endovascular treatment

PTA may be considered (see section A 4.4.8), but this does not eliminate the causative compressive structure, and if a post-stenotic aneurysm is present it cannot be treated.

Vascular surgery

Vascular surgery is the treatment of choice. If the diagnosis is established early (i.e., before the development of vascular damages), transsection of the structures constricting the artery is sufficient. If the diagnosis is delayed (missed), with permanent vascular damage, then vascular reconstruction is necessary.

Surgical procedures that may be considered (see section A 4.4.8) are:
- Causal decompression (elimination of the compressive structure)
- Autologous venous bypass (P1–P3 bypass)
- Thrombectomy with an extension patch if necessary in cases of acute vascular occlusion

Risks and complications:
- Persistent motor and sensory deficits due to intraoperative injury to the neurovascular bundle
- Chronic congestion in the lower leg, due to damage to the lymphatic vessels in the popliteal fossa
- Risk of lower leg ischemia due to poor collateralization
- Risk of compartment syndrome (reperfusion damage)

Follow-up and prognosis:
- Intravenous heparinization for several days
- Oral anticoagulation for 3–6 months if appropriate
- Early mobilization exercises starting on the second or third postoperative day

4.7.3.6   Prognosis and course

There are good early and long-term results in popliteal artery compression syndrome.

References

Adson AW. Surgical treatment for symptoms produced by cervical ribs and the scalenus muscle. Surg Gynecol Obstet 1947; 85: 687–700.

Dharap AS. An anomalous muscle in the distal half of the arm. Surg Radiol Anat 1994; 16 (1): 97–99.

Gruss JD, Geissler C. Aneurysms of the subclavian artery in thoracic outlet syndrome. Zentralbl Chir 1997; 122 (9): 730–34.

Gruss JD, Hiemer W, Bartels D. Clinical aspects, diagnosis and therapy of thoracic outlet syndrome. Vasa 1987; 16 (4): 337–44.

Gruss JD, Bartels D, Tsafandakis S, Straubel H. Surgical aspects and results of treatment of the thoracic-outlet syndrome. Chirurgie 1980; 106 (6): 406–08.

Holden A, Merrilees S, Mitchell N, Hill A. Magnetic resonance imaging of popliteal artery pathologies. Eur J Radiol 2008 Jul; 67 (1): 159–68.

Lambert AW, Wilkins DC. Popliteal artery entrapment syndrome. Br J Surg 1999 Nov; 86 (11): 1365–70.

Nussbaumer P, Candrian C, Furrer M. Poplitheales Entrapment: eine seltene Ursache der Claudicatio intermittens beim jungen Patienten. Schweiz Med Forum 2002; 23: 570–72.

Ozkan U, Ouzkurt L, Tercan F, Pourbagher A. MRI and DSA findings in popliteal artery entrapment syndrome. Diagn Interv Radiol 2008 Jun; 14 (2): 106–10.

Rand T, Haumer M, Stadler A, Schoder M, Kettenbach J. PTA and stent placement distal to the superficial femoral artery. Radiologe 2006 Nov; 46 (11): 948–54.

Roos DB. New concepts of thoracic outlet syndrome that explain etiology, symptoms, diagnosis and treatment. J Vasc Surg 1979; 13: 313–21.

Roos DB. The thoracic outlet syndrome is underrated. Arch Neurol 1990; 47: 313–21.

Sanders RJ, Hammond SL, Rao NM. Diagnosis of thoracic outlet syndrome. J Vasc Surg 2007 Sep; 46 (3): 601–04.

B

Diseases of the veins

1 Venous thrombosis

1.1 Venous thrombosis in the lower extremity

Basic anatomy: Reinhard Putz
Clinical picture and conservative treatment: Knut Kröger and Frans Santosa
Doppler/duplex ultrasonography: Tom Schilling
Endovascular treatment: Ulrich Beschorner and Thomas Zeller
Surgical treatment: Michael Pillny

1.1.1 Basic anatomy

1.1.1.1 Deep venous system—lower extremity

In contrast to the superficial veins, the deep veins in the lower leg run along the corresponding arteries (Fig. 1.1-1). Together with the arteries, they lie in a firm envelope of connective tissue, which may be advantageous for ensuring the transport of blood.

In the sole of the foot, paired medial and lateral plantar veins already run along the eponymous arteries, until they join with the similarly paired posterior tibial vein. Together with the tibial artery, the posterior tibial veins rest on the deep muscles of the lower leg and—covered proximally by the soleus muscle—enter a common trunk with the veins accompanying the anterior tibial artery. The anterior tibial veins take up blood from the dorsal pedal vein, rest directly on the interosseous membrane and reach the common venous trunk through a foramen in the interosseous membrane that lies directly beneath the tibiofibular joint. The fibular veins course along the fibula. The deep veins in the lower leg contain up to around 10 paired valves.

Usually below the level of the knee joint space, the deep veins of the lower leg are generally united to form the popliteal vein, which also takes up the small saphenous vein there as well. It lies between the division of the ischial nerve into the tibial and fibular nerves and the popliteal artery, which rests on the femur in the depth. It courses proximally along with the popliteal artery in the adductor canal and winds dorsally in its course around the femoral artery, so that in the upper half of the thigh it lies medial to the artery. This is also the case in the area of the saphenous opening, where the popliteal vein may only be covered by the thin cribriform fascia of the fascia lata, depending on the thickness of the individual subcutaneous or subfascial fatty layer. At the saphenous opening, the popliteal vein takes up the veins from the confluence of the inguinal veins. The femoral vein continues through the vascular space of the retroinguinal compartment as the external iliac vein.

Numerous short perforating veins are distributed over the whole leg. They penetrate sometimes the very firm fasciae and have valves that only allow blood to flow inwards (Fig. 1.1-2). Their positions are highly variable.

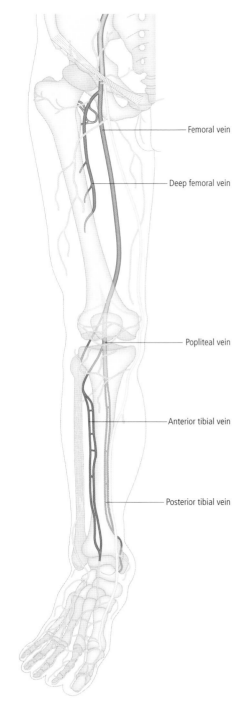

Femoral vein

Deep femoral vein

Popliteal vein

Anterior tibial vein

Posterior tibial vein

Fig. 1.1-1 Overview of the deep veins of the leg.

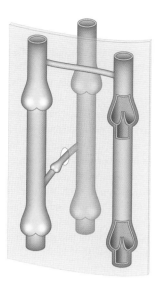

Fig. 1.1-2 Relationship between the superficial and deep veins of the lower leg.

Individual valves are also found in the large unpaired deep veins of the leg.

1.1.2 Clinical picture

Thrombosis in the deep veins is known as venous thrombosis. The size of the thrombus, its position, and its hemodynamic effect do not alter the definition; terms such as "mural thrombus in the inferior vena cava" or "partial thrombosis in the lower leg veins" only serve to describe the findings. Any thrombus in the deep venous system, no matter how small, by definition represents venous thrombosis.

1.1.2.1 Thrombosis in the lower extremity

The anatomy of the deep venous system is highly variable. The lower leg veins are usually paired accompanying veins, but ultrasound not infrequently shows as many as three or four accompanying veins. The popliteal/femoral vein is normally single but may often be doubled, at least in parts. The iliac veins and inferior vena cava can also show variations, which may remain clinically inapparent for many years. Congenital atresia of the inferior vena cava is only rarely associated with subcutaneous cavocaval anastomoses, in contrast to thrombotic occlusion. The proximal segment of the left common iliac vein crosses the proximal right common iliac artery. Congenital constrictions are found in this area (May's venous spur). Due to the mechanical interaction between the left common iliac vein and the right common iliac artery with the bony pelvic girdle, isolated pelvic vein thrombosis occurs more frequently on the left side than on the right (May-Thurner syndrome).

The prevalence of venous thrombosis in the general population is estimated at 40–180 per 100,000 annually, with an age-dependent increase. More than 50% of thromboses occur in patients with underlying malignant diseases.

Venous thrombosis is generally considered to be caused by the presence of Virchow triad—stasis, coagulation disturbance, and endothelial damage/inflammation.

1.1.2.2 Stasis

All situations involving complete or partial immobilization of the muscle pump in the calf are associated with stasis of venous blood in the legs. The main situations in which this occurs are:

- Plaster casts, bed rest, or prolonged sitting during travel by air, bus, or car where the muscular calf pump is minimized/absent.
- Fluid loss leads to unfavorable flow characteristics (i.e., viscosity) of blood with increasing hematocrit.
- Heat dilates the veins and thereby reduces the velocity of blood flow.
- Obesity and tight clothing leads to increased abdominal pressure which obstructs the outflow of venous blood.

Awareness of these higher-risk situations makes it possible to provide patients with information about physiotherapeutic methods of preventing thrombosis through active leg exercise, ensuring an adequate fluid supply, and avoiding heat and tight clothing.

1.1.2.3 Coagulation

The causes of coagulation disturbances are complex and sometimes only transient. There is an increased tendency for thrombosis to develop:

- With infection-related increases in acute-phase proteins such as fibrinogen and von Willebrand factor (factor VIII)
- At the start and end of oral anticoagulation treatment with phenprocoumon/warfarin, as these drugs also reduce the hepatic synthesis of the anticoagulant proteins C and S ahead of the reduction in the coagulant factors (II, VII, IX, and X). Overlapping administration of heparin is therefore necessary, to reduce the risk of warfarin necrosis (extensive skin necroses)
- Transient disturbances of coagulation factors in diseases involving protein loss (angiotensin III deficiency may occur in a setting of colitis or nephrotic syndrome, for example)
- Oral contraception due to the influence of hormones on the coagulation system
- Paraneoplastic coagulation disturbances due to tumor decay or tumor-associated proteins with procoagulant activity
- Congenital disturbances of individual coagulation proteins (Table 1.1-1).

1.1.2.4 Endothelium

The endothelium may be directly damaged due to local trauma, spreading inflammatory processes, and harmful chemical substances. The higher rate of thrombosis in the elderly is probably partly due to age-related endothelial changes. Blood stasis also leads to oxygen deficiency and thus disturbs the integrity of the venous endothelium, which in turn favors the development of thrombosis. Direct evidence of endothelial damage as the cause of thrombosis currently plays little if any part in the clinical assessment, but it is possible that endothelium-specific enzymes such as endothelin and adhesion molecules may become more important in the future.

Table 1.1-1 The coagulation parameters listed here only show a selection of the most frequent abnormalities. There are further descriptions for each of the individual factors that distinguish between functional disturbance, absolute deficiency, and disturbance of a coenzyme. Genetic causes for many coagulation factors can be found, and congenital and acquired syndromes can therefore be distinguished.

Coagulation disturbance	Prevalence in the normal population	Relative risk
APC resistance	5%	7
Hyperhomocysteinemia	6%	2.5
Prothrombin mutation	2%	3–4
Protein C deficiency	0.8%	3.8
Antithrombin III deficiency	0.02–0.2%	2–4
Protein S deficiency	0.7%	1–2
Antiphospholipid antibodies	2–9%	?

APC, activated protein C.

1.1.3 Diagnosis and differential diagnosis

The clinical signs of thrombosis are highly variable and range from a complete absence of symptoms—so that it is only the onset of pulmonary embolism that leads to thrombosis being diagnosed—to acute swelling in an extremity with restricted arterial perfusion (phlegmasia cerulea dolens). The major symptoms are usually:

- Local pain
- Swelling
- Livido reticularis
- Low-grade fever
- Restricted movement in the extremity

If low-grade fevers are observed, there is always a suspicion of thrombosis in hospitalized patients in intensive care units or following surgical procedures. However, in a large study including 1847 patients with suspected thrombosis, no differences between patients with or without confirmed thromboses were observed in relation to body temperature elevations.

Every deep vein thrombosis is associated with a risk of potentially massive pulmonary embolism. At the time when the thrombosis is diagnosed, more than 60% of patients already have pulmonary emboli, even if it is not clinically apparent. However, there are still no guidelines that generally recommend imaging for pulmonary embolism diagnosis (e.g., with echocardiography, scintigraphy, chest CT or MRI) in patients with thrombosis. Despite this, any patient with thrombosis should be asked about coughing, dyspnea or dyspneic episodes, or a sudden drop in performance, and if the answer is yes, then echocardiography and/or direct CT imaging should be carried out in order to exclude right ventricular strain. ECG alone does not exclude pulmonary embolism. Echocardiography also does not exclude pulmonary embolism, but makes it possible to recognize its hemodynamic significance if present.

Phlegmasia. When there is sudden occlusion of all of the deep veins in an extremity, and sometimes of the superficial veins as well, edema develops rapidly and stasis leads to disturbance of the microcirculation and ultimately of arterial perfusion. Depending on the extent of the perfusion disturbance and the speed of edema devel-

opment, a clinical distinction is made among the following manifestations:

- Phlegmasia alba dolens: pale, painfully swollen leg
- Phlegmasia rubra dolens: reddened, painfully swollen leg
- Phlegmasia cerulea dolens: cyanotic, painfully swollen leg

The diagnosis is made clinically, based on the course of the swelling and evidence of disturbed perfusion (foot pulse) and disturbed microcirculation. Phlebography is not indicated. Evidence of thrombosis should then be obtained with ultrasound, and the proximal end of the thrombus can be imaged with CT or MRI if needed. Independent of the clinical appearance, the patient is at risk of the development of hypovolemic shock and imminent loss of the extremity.

When the patient's history is being taken, inquiries should be made about risk settings that increase the likelihood of thrombosis:

- Previous deep vein thrombosis leading to a post-phlebitic syndrome.
- Immobilization or hospitalization with resultant stasis.
- Direct trauma as a marker of possible endothelial damage.
- Family history of venous thrombosis may provide a clue as to inherited thrombophilic diathesis.
- Hormone substitution/contraceptives associated with coagulation disturbances.
- Dyspnea, coughing, pleuritic chest pain, etc., indicative of possible pulmonary embolism.
- General symptoms such as weight loss, malaise, nocturnal diaphoresis raise the suspicion for paraneoplastic causes, autoimmune disease.
- In patients from the Mediterranean region, inquiries should be made about oral aphthae or genital changes consistent with Behçet disease.

There are hardly any symptoms in the area of the legs that are not capable of being attributed to thrombosis in one way or another. It is unfortunately still not established which symptoms require further imaging diagnosis and which symptoms do not, so imaging diagnosis is therefore advisable in cases of doubt.

1.1.3.1 Inspection and palpation

The clinical picture in thrombosis ranges from a completely unremarkable extremity through a swollen, warm extremity to extreme swelling, paleness, or cyanosis.

There are numerous traditionally recognized clinical signs of thrombosis, but today these no longer have any significance for demonstrating or excluding thrombosis (Table 1.1-2). When there is unclear pain, swelling, or livido, it is not acceptable for thrombosis to have been excluded by noting that some or all of the clinical signs listed were negative.

Most guidelines therefore recommend carrying out the Wells clinical pre-test probability assessment (Table 1.1-3). In everyday practice, however, this is not really helpful, as the assessment does not identify a specific group of patients who do not require further diagnostic procedures. It is also not able to identify a suspected diagnosis of thrombosis, but is only used once the suspicion has already been raised.

Table 1.1-2 Clinical signs of thrombosis that are now no longer important for diagnosing thrombosis, as they can neither confirm nor exclude a thrombosis.

Payr sign	Pain in the sole of the foot due when heavy pressure is exerted on the medial hollow of the foot
Homans sign	Pain in the calf during forced dorsiflexion of the ankle with the knee outstretched
Meyer pressure points	Pressure pain on the inner side of the edge of the tibia along the course of the anterior and posterior tibial artery
Lowenberg test	Severe pain with a pressure of 60–120 mmHg within 10–15 s with a blood pressure cuff on the lower leg
Sigg sign	The outstretched leg is slightly raised and pressure on the patella produces pain in the popliteal region
Pratt sign	Pressure pain in the popliteal region
Lisker sign	Pain on percussion of the anterior edge of the tibia and simultaneous pain-free percussion over the patella
Ducuing sign	Pain on ballottement of the relaxed calf muscles
Bisgaard sign	Pain on palpating the calcaneomalleolar region in the outstretched leg

Table 1.1-3 Assessment of the clinical probability of deep venous thrombosis (Wells et al. 2003).

Clinical characteristic	Score
Active cancer disease	1.0
Paralysis or recent immobilization of the legs	1.0
Bed rest (> 3 days); major surgery (< 12 weeks)	1.0
Pain/hardening along the deep veins	1.0
Swelling of the whole leg	1.0
Lower leg swelling > 3 cm in comparison with contralateral side	1.0
Compressible edema in the symptomatic leg	1.0
Collateral veins	1.0
Earlier documented deep vein thrombosis	1.0
Alternative diagnosis at least as probable as deep venous thrombosis	–2.0

Score ≥ 2.0: high probability of deep venous thrombosis.
Score < 2.0: low probability of deep venous thrombosis.

Table 1.1-4 Differential diagnoses.

Major symptoms	Minor symptoms	Suspected diagnosis	Diagnosis
Painful erythema	Fever, shivering fits	Erysipelas	Axillary or inguinal lymph nodes, exclusion of thrombophlebitis on ultrasound, antistreptolysin titer
Palpable hardened veins and erythema	Swelling	Thrombophlebitis	Duplex ultrasonography
Acute lancinating pain	Only on exercise	Torn muscle fiber	Ultrasound, referral for surgery
Joint-related swelling	Local pressure pain	Acute arthritis	Internal medicine and rheumatology investigation of etiology
Swelling	Stemmer sign	Lymphedema	Clinical diagnosis after exclusion of thrombosis
Swelling	Gonarthrosis, popliteal pain	Rupture of a Baker cyst	Ultrasonography
Swelling	Bilateral	Cardiac insufficiency	Echocardiography

D-Dimers. The D-dimer test is a highly sensitive, but nonspecific, laboratory parameter. D-Dimers are byproducts of coagulation and appear in increased quantities in the blood in the presence of thrombosis. Unfortunately, all inflammatory clinical pictures, cancerous conditions, and trauma or surgery also lead to increased D-dimer values. The validity of the test is therefore limited to clinically healthy patients with negative D-dimer values, and it is only in these patients that thrombosis is unlikely when there are negative D-dimer values, so that imaging can be dispensed with. In another group of patients, however, false-positive values were much more frequent and made further imaging procedures necessary. False-negative D-dimers have been reported in the first few days after casualty surgery and in patients who had already had symptoms for 2–3 weeks. In patients who are already receiving oral anticoagulation for any reason, D-dimer assessment is not suitable for excluding thrombosis.

1.1.3.2 Diagnostic imaging

Duplex ultrasonography and phlebography are complementary, rather than competing, procedures for diagnosing thrombosis and should also be used in this way.

Doppler/duplex ultrasonography

B-mode ultrasound examination technique

Compression ultrasonography using the B-mode is sufficient purely in order to exclude thrombosis. The patient should initially be supine and complete compressibility is tested starting from the iliofemoral transition cranially and caudally, with all segments of the venous system in the leg being assessed longitudinally and in narrow segments in cross-section. When there is evidence of internal structures, they should be imaged at several levels. The femoropopliteal circulatory pathway is often duplicated. Even when a vessel can be imaged with compression, attention should be given to detect any additional venous structures that are not compressible. The popliteal vein is best examined with the patient sitting and with relaxed muscles—this makes imaging easier as a result of hydrostatic filling. Imaging of the three lower leg vein groups, the gastrocnemius and soleus veins is required. When there is pain in the foot area, the plantar veins should also be checked for compressibility (for possible plantar vein thrombosis), as well as the epifascial and transfascial veins. In the area of the iliac veins and vena cava (required in cases of bilateral swelling), compression ultrasound can be carried out in B-mode, but always with supplementary Doppler ultrasound assessment in PW and color mode. The affected vessels and precise proximal and distal boundaries of the thrombus have to be imaged and described—this is important for diagnosing recurrences and evaluating later functional changes.

B-mode ultrasound assessment criteria

- Is there complete compressibility without a "residual lumen" in all segments of the epifascial, transfascial, and subfascial venous system?
- Is there an absence of internal structures?
- Is the venous lumen larger than the accompanying artery?
- Does the lumen show respiratory modulation?
- Dilation of the veins in a Valsalva test or other method of increasing the proximal pressure.
- Is the wall delicate or is there any thickening?
- Are there any ectasias? Is the lumen normal even in the epifascial veins?

PW Doppler and color duplex ultrasonography

Examination technique when exclusion of thrombosis is indicated

When an examination to exclude thrombosis is indicated, it is not obligatory to examine valvular function → an augmented signal can be used to check color filling in the vessel if necessary. Adjusted device settings: low flow optimization, including low PRF and adjusted amplification, possible change of color modes (power mode if appropriate) and color scales. In the area of the iliac vein (with an unfavorable Doppler angle), it may be necessary to use color B-flow imaging, which is less angle-dependent (with fewer artifacts than power mode).

Supplementary color duplex ultrasound assessment criteria when exclusion of thrombosis is indicated

Subfascial conducting vein system and muscular vein system:
- Is color-coded flow imaging possible in the entire vascular lumen?
- Are there any hyperperfused collaterals?
- Is there respiratory modulation of the Doppler signal?
- Is there overshoot after the Valsalva or after proximal compression?
- Is there any marginal residual perfusion in venous thrombosis?

Epifascial venous system:
- Is there color-coded flow imaging in the entire vascular lumen?
- Is the hemotachogram band-shaped, as a sign of collateral function?

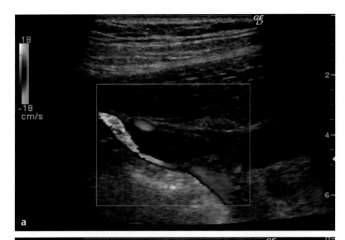

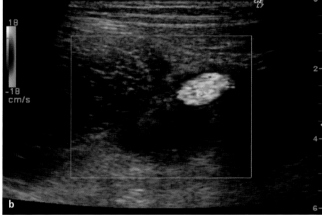

Fig. 1.1-3a, b Complete thrombotic occlusion of the external iliac vein. (a) A prolapsing thrombus plug is visible in the common iliac vein, with imaging of residual flow in the internal iliac artery. (b) An incompressible external iliac artery, with no evidence of a flow signal (with perfused external iliac artery alongside).

Transfascial venous system:
- Is there transfascial progression in thrombophlebitis or varicophlebitis?
- Is a subfascial thrombotic process ascending, suggesting "collar-stud thrombophlebitis"?

General thrombosis criteria in B-mode ultrasound:
- The vein is not free and compressible without a residual lumen.
- There is an evidence of internal structures (*caution:* reverberation echoes).
- Dilated vein.
- Hypoechogenic wall layers and thickening.
- Absence of respiratory modulation of the lumen.
- No dilation of the lumen occurs during a Valsalva maneuver.
- There is venous hypertension distal to the thrombosis, with poor compressibility or even "pseudo-incompressibility."

Thrombosis criteria on color-coded duplex ultrasound/PW Doppler ultrasound:
- A color signal is absent or there is incomplete color filling in the vein, with spontaneous and/or augmented signals (*caution:* beware of incorrect device settings, low flow-optimized settings must always be used).

- There is no respiratory modulation of the color and PW Doppler signal distal to the thrombotic occlusion.
- There are hyperperfused collaterals, with possibly band-shaped constant flow in PW mode.

Specific findings

Vena cava thrombosis

- *Caution:* duplication of the vena cava.
- Strong systolic reflux in the vena cava indicates tricuspid insufficiency. Echocardiographic diagnosis: transit thrombus, right ventricular strain and pulmonary hypertension.
- Is there any outflow obstruction of visceral and renal vascular territories? → If so, there will be dilated vessels, slow flow, zero flow, or retrograde flow, eliminated respiratory and cardiac modulation, possibly a blurred texture and progression in the size of the drained parenchyma (edematous swelling).
- Is there any evidence of a cause? Ascending iliac vein thrombosis, renal vein thrombosis, compression effects or any other local damage.
- Venous hypertension distal to the thrombosis, with poor compressibility despite a free lumen.

Iliac vein thrombosis

- Iliac vein thromboses are quite often limited at the inflow of the internal iliac vein and are therefore restricted to the external iliac vein.
- The internal iliac vein is duplicated in up to 50% of cases—evidence of this therefore does not imply a definite absence of thrombosis in a main trunk or even in all branches.

Thrombosis of the femoral vein and popliteal vein

- *Caution:* the femoral vein is duplicated in up to 30% of cases.
- Sonographic assessment may be difficult in the adductor canal; the examination should then be carried out from dorsal side if needed.

Thrombosis in the deep femoral vein

- This is often overlooked.
- It can be well imaged in longitudinal section and cross-section both with compression ultrasonography and with color duplex (Fig. 1.1-4).
- The head of the thrombus may extend beyond the femoral vein fork.

Thrombosis in conducting veins of the lower leg (Fig. 1.1-5)

- All three groups of conducting veins are fully imaged.
- A specific statement about which vein groups are affected is always required. The term "lower leg venous thrombosis" is unsatisfactory and precise details of the extent of the thrombosis are important for later diagnosis of recurrences and possibly for later diagnosis of the post-thrombotic defective state.

Thrombosis of muscular veins in the lower leg

The gastrocnemius and soleus veins have a clear anatomic correlation and can always be fully imaged. They are often affected in isolation and form the starting-point for ascending thrombosis. As

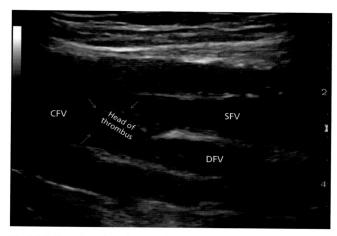

Fig. 1.1-4 Complete thrombotic occlusion of the deep femoral vein, with a thrombus plug projecting into the common femoral vein. CFV, common femoral vein; DFV, deep femoral vein; SFV, superficial femoral vein.

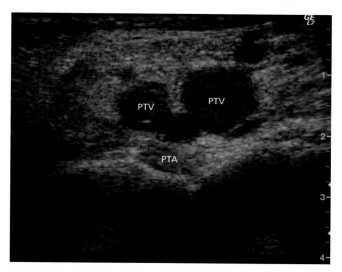

Fig. 1.1-5 Complete thrombotic occlusion of both branches of the posterior conducting vein group—incompressible, dilated conducting veins. PTA, posterior tibial artery; PTV, posterior tibial vein.

a result of the opening of the soleus veins into the fibular conducting veins and the gastrocnemius veins into the popliteal vein, there are often the corresponding coincident patterns of involvement.

Plantar vein thrombosis

When the relevant clinical findings are present (with plantar pain), there is a characteristic compression ultrasound examination with incompressible plantar veins. There is often circumscribed involvement.

Several events?

A complete examination including ipsilateral venous segments that do not currently appear to be involved, as well as the contralateral ones, should be carried out at every diagnosis of thrombosis. Occasionally, ipsilateral or contralateral signs of previous (asymptomatic or incorrectly diagnosed) thrombotic events can be found, with post-thrombotic changes. At a first diagnosis of venous thrombosis, this immediately justifies classification of the condition as recurrent thrombosis (possibly involving different treatment decisions).

Differential diagnosis

In mixed groups of patients, deep vein thrombosis (DVT) is only confirmed in approximately 20% of cases in patients presenting with suspected DVT. However, duplex ultrasound can also provide valuable assistance in verifying differential-diagnostic alternatives. Some frequent findings with leg swelling or pain include:

- Primary or secondary lymphedema
- Outflow obstruction due to compression effects (e.g., popliteal artery aneurysm, pelvic tumors; see Fig. 1.1-6)
- Bleeding (Fig. 1.1-7)
- (Ruptured) Baker cysts (Fig. 1.1-12) and other cystic space-occupying lesions (Fig. 1.1-8)
- Lipedema (Fig. 1.1-9)
- Lipedema–lymphedema (Fig. 1.1-10)
- Venous aneurysm (Fig.1.1-11)
- Heart failure (with venous pendular flow in cases of right ventricular strain and tricuspid insufficiency, Fig. 1.1-13)

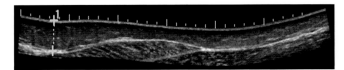

Fig. 1.1-9 Lipedema, with typically widened subcutaneous tissue and echo-complex, "cloudy" ultrasound texture (panorama image).

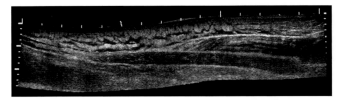

Fig. 1.1-10 Lipedema–lymphedema, with typically widened subcutaneous tissue that has a "cloudy" texture (lipedema) and almost anechogenic, septum-like areas (lymphedema).

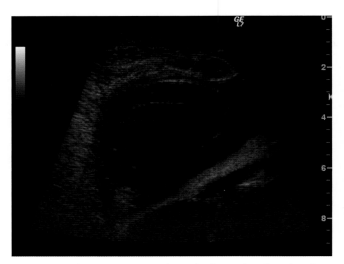

Fig. 1.1-6 A pelvic space-occupying lesion (malignant lymphoma), with compression of the external iliac vein (B flow).

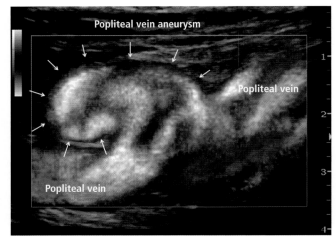

Fig. 1.1-11 Aneurysmal dilation of the popliteal vein, with local pain. The aneurysm has a typical "coffee-bean" biphasic and circular perfusion pattern (color B flow).

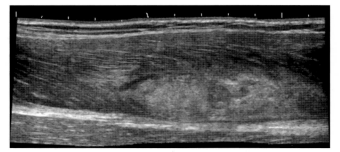

Fig. 1.1-7 Bleeding in the gastrocnemius, with a space-occupying effect and elimination of the muscle texture (panorama image).

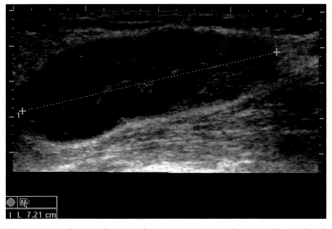

Fig. 1.1-12 A classic echo-complex space-occupying lesion in the popliteal region, with joint attachment, suggesting a Baker cyst.

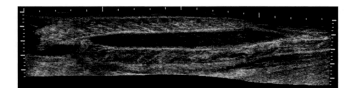

Fig. 1.1-8 A cystic space-occupying lesion between the gastrocnemius and soleus in a patient with primary chronic polyarthritis (panorama image).

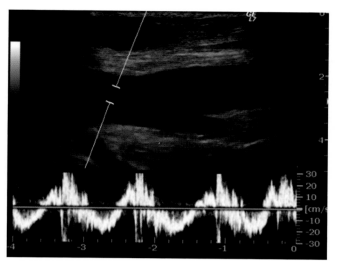

Fig. 1.1-13 A typical biphasic PW Doppler signal in the leg veins in a patient with right ventricular strain and tricuspid insufficiency.

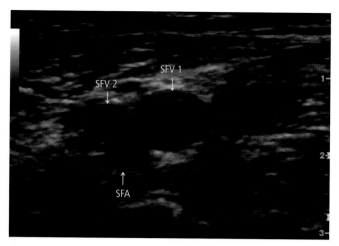

Fig. 1.1-14 Evidence of three vascular structures along the course of the femoral vessels: duplication of the femoral vein. SFV, superior femoral vein; SFA, superior femoral artery.

Pitfalls

Duplication of veins

Duplications of the femoropopliteal veins are found in up to 30% of cases. Even when there are visible and compressible veins, attention always should be given to additional incompressible structures.

Venous "pseudo-occlusion"

Proximal outflow obstruction can lead to cessation of flow and venous hypertension that can only be overcome with difficulty. This can lead to incorrect diagnosis of a thrombotic occlusion in distal venous segments. A low flow–optimized color imaging and adjusted strong compression with the transducer should therefore always be used.

Stasis effects

When an extremity is dangled for a long time, "sedimentation effects" may occur that can mimic a thrombus (Fig. 1.1-15).

Ascending phlebography

Ascending phlebography, with puncture of a dorsal foot vein, allows complete imaging of the deep venous system from the distal lower leg up to the inferior vena cava. In comparison with duplex ultrasound, it does not show the thrombus directly, but only through the filling defect created by the thrombus in the column of contrast (Fig.1-16). The following points should be noted:

- A vein at the base of the large toe should be punctured, as this allows the best inflow of contrast into the deep veins. Despite this, it is not possible in all cases to fill all three groups of veins in the lower leg evenly with contrast. If there is no filling of one group of lower leg veins, but with no further evidence of thrombosis (e.g., washing around a thrombus tip), a thrombosis should not be immediately diagnosed. Supplementary duplex ultrasound is necessary.
- The muscle veins in the gastrocnemius musculature and also the deep femoral vein cannot be directly filled with contrast from the distal direction. It is therefore possible for thromboses to be overlooked in this area.

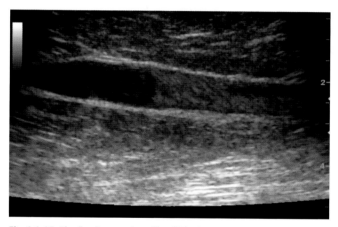

Fig. 1.1-15 The "sedimentation effect." The increased echogenicity distally should be noted (on the right in the image).

- The numerous variants of doubled or even tripled venous segments make it difficult to exclude partial thromboses in such segments with confidence.
- When thrombosis is present at several levels, there is only minor contrast filling in the pelvic veins and inferior vena cava, and the imaging procedure is often inadequate in these regions. In this case, digital subtraction angiography (DSA) can be extremely helpful. In many cases, however, it is more useful to demonstrate the level of the proximal end of the thrombus using a tomographic procedure (CT, MRI) and simultaneously exclude external compression or a tumor as the cause of the thrombosis. Phlebography findings that do not show the proximal end of the thrombus are not diagnostically adequate.

The advantage of phlebography is that it provides continuous depiction of the complete venous system in the extremity in a standardized form, with good documentation that can also be used for medicolegal purposes. Its disadvantages are its invasiveness and the exposure to radiation and contrast media that is involved.

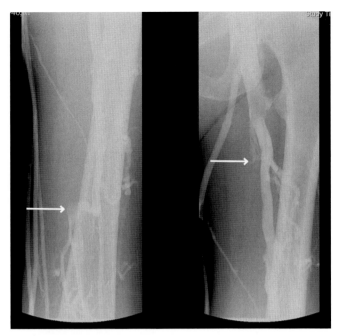

Fig. 1-16 Detail of phlebographic imaging of ascending thrombosis in the proximal superficial femoral vein. The thrombus is only visible when there is flow around it. The whole occluded segment between the arrows does not appear.

1.1.3.3 Additional diagnostic procedures

Additional diagnostic procedures in the individual patient depend on the patient's history and on the clinical findings.

- In patients with unclear general symptoms and in those with spontaneous thrombosis with no recognizable external cause, a search for a tumor should be considered. A detailed physical examination, chest x-ray, and abdominal ultrasonography are indicated for the purpose. Age-relevant screening examinations should also be completed.
- In patients with dyspnea or other unclear pulmonary symptoms such as coughing, pleuritis, etc., diagnostic workup for pulmonary embolism is useful.
- Coagulation testing to clarify a potential thrombophilic diathesis (Table 1.1-1) is indicated in all patients with recurrent thromboses and in younger patients (< 50 years of age) with spontaneous thromboses—i.e., thromboses unconnected with surgery, trauma, or tumors. With the exception of angiotensin III deficiency, for which substitution should be administered, the diagnosis of a hypercoagulable state has no relevance for acute treatment but is useful for purposes of prophylaxis against recurrence. On the other hand, transient disturbances of coagulation factors, such as those occurring with renal or gastrointestinal protein loss as a cause of thrombosis, can only be recognized if diagnostic procedures for coagulation disturbances are carried out at the time of the thrombosis. In view of the large numbers of thrombosis patients, there is no consensus regarding the need for or intensity of the diagnosis of a hypercoagulable state. However, it may provide decisive evidence in individual cases.

1.1.4 Treatment

1.1.4.1 Conservative treatment

The basic treatment consists of immediate anticoagulation and compression. Anticoagulation is administered:

- Primarily with a heparin preparation (whether fractionated or unfractionated)
- Secondarily, if there are no contraindications, with oral anticoagulation

If thrombosis is suspected, heparin should be administered immediately. This counteracts appositional growth of the thrombosis while the diagnosis is being established and the subsequent treatment procedure is being planned. Administration of a heparin preparation at a prophylactic dosage is recommended, although there have been no prospective studies on the topic.

When thrombosis is confirmed, subcutaneous or intravenous heparin administration at a therapeutic dosage should be started. For unfractionated heparin, the standard treatment is intravenous administration guided by the activated partial thromboplastin time (APTT), which should be prolonged by 1.5–2.5 times to be considered therapeutic. Low-molecular-weight heparins should be administered subcutaneously once or twice daily at dosages adjusted to body weight. It is not necessary to check treatment with low-molecular-weight heparins using anti-factor Xa. If a clinical situation with an increased bleeding risk or appositional thrombus growth makes it necessary to obtain information about the individual effect of low-molecular-weight heparins, anti-factor Xa activity can be assessed. The aim is to achieve levels of 0.4–0.8 IU/mL (3 h after administration, with twice-daily doses) or 0.6–1.3 IU/mL with once-daily administration.

Although both forms of heparin are approved for treatment of thrombosis, low-molecular-weight heparins have some advantages. Patients receiving low-molecular-weight heparin in research studies have been found to have lower recurrence rates (odds ratio 0.66–0.76), reduced mortality (OR 0.56–0.67), and fewer bleeding complications (OR 0.68–0.78).

If no further diagnostic measures (e.g., searching for tumor) or treatment measures (e.g., lysis, surgery) are required, an immediate start with oral anticoagulation treatment can be made at the same time as the heparinization. Oral anticoagulation for 3–6 months is sufficient in patients who do not have a clinically manifest pulmonary embolism and in whom the cause of the thrombosis is an obviously transient external event. If there is a second thrombotic event and continuing risk factors, anticoagulation for 1 year is useful. While there is a reasonable consensus regarding the minimum period of 3–6 months, details on the upper limit for the period of anticoagulation vary widely in the literature. In patients with idiopathic proximal thrombosis, lifelong anticoagulation treatment is recommended if the bleeding risk is justified. It is therefore not possible to give any clear recommendations for each individual case. In patients with confirmed pulmonary embolism, oral anticoagulation should only be withdrawn when there is complete normalization of right-ventricular function on ultrasound.

Rivaroxaban, a direct factor Xa inhibitor, which is available in oral form, has been approved since December 2012 for the treatment of venous thrombosis. It makes thrombosis treatment easier, as it can be used initially without prior heparin administration and it also makes a switch to oral anticoagulation with vitamin K antagonists unnecessary. The initial dosage consists of 30 mg/day for 3 weeks (2 × 15 mg/day), followed by 20 mg once a day for the rest of the treatment period. A controlled study confirmed that this form of treatment is equivalent to classic anticoagulation therapy with low-molecular-weight heparin and a vitamin K antagonist. Rivaroxaban has also been approved for prolonged secondary prophylaxis.

While the need for anticoagulation treatment has been confirmed in patients with proximal thromboses, the need for anticoagulation in those with circumscribed lower leg venous thromboses or even isolated muscular vein thromboses is a matter of controversy. Depending on the extent of the thrombosis and the patient's risk profile, anticoagulation may be dispensed with (e.g., when there is a short secondary thrombosis in otherwise active patients), but if there are additional risk factors such as immobilization or tumor, effective anticoagulation is useful. Compression therapy is indicated in all cases, independently of the intensity of the anticoagulation treatment.

Compression can be carried out with the following aids:

- Compression dressings, with multilayered dressings using short-stretch bandages: 8-cm wide bandages in the foot and ankle area, 10-cm wide bandages in the lower leg and thigh. Compression dressings can initially be placed on the swollen leg.
- Compression stockings that have a defined compression grade. These should be sized only for a slim, decongested leg and should be worn during the day by mobile patients.
- Dressing stockings. These stockings can be sterilized. They are sized to suit the swollen leg and lead to decongestion. Smaller stockings need to be prescribed as the swelling declines. After complete decongestion, a compression stocking can also be used.

Due to the swelling that is initially present with DVT, decongestion with compression dressing is necessary to begin with, extending over the proximal end of the thrombosis if possible. A short-term switch to a suitably sized dressing or compression stocking can then be carried out. Finally, a class II or III compression stocking should be worn for 6–12 months. Treatment for acute thrombosis is then completed, with conclusive thrombus organization. If there is evidence of post-thrombotic damage, lifelong continuation of the compression treatment is indicated.

In thromboses in the pelvic and thigh veins, thigh stockings are also adequate. Stockings do not provide a clear advantage, as compression of the pelvic veins is not achieved. However, they may be necessary in short, strong legs, as they stay in position better. Popliteal vein thromboses that reach to the knee joint space should also be treated with an AG stocking, as a lower leg stocking would not reach the proximal end of the thrombus. In patients with peripheral arterial occlusive disease or polyneuropathy, lower compression classes must be prescribed or compression may need to be dispensed with completely to avoid tissue damage. In individual cases, hourly decongestion treatment using controlled wrapping in awake patients, with subsequent checking for pressure points, may be helpful. Any increase in pain under a compression dressing or stocking may mean that other diseases such as peripheral arterial occlusive disease have been overlooked, or that the dressing or stocking has been incorrectly placed.

Treatment for thrombosis can be administered either on an outpatient or inpatient basis, independently of anticoagulation and compression. Inpatient treatment is indicated when there are:

- Unclear pulmonary symptoms that may already be a sign of pulmonary embolism
- Additional cardiac diseases, as these patients are able to compensate for additional minor pulmonary emboli more poorly than patients with healthy hearts
- Comprehension difficulties, as instructions are then not adequately grasped and may not be followed
- Patients who are single and cannot be treated at home, as they are not able to request assistance if clinical deterioration occurs

Outpatient treatment is possible with:
- Distal and proximal thromboses
- Older thromboses (with symptoms for more than 1 week)
- Well-informed patients who understand the treatment
- Patients who have previously been mobile

The outpatient treatment approach is also being used increasingly for proximal thromboses as well. It has been investigated in controlled studies and is reported to be just as safe and effective as inpatient care. With outpatient management, the patient's consent should always be provided in writing after information has been provided about the treatment options and the risk of fatal pulmonary embolism.

Inpatient care nowadays no longer means strict bedrest, but instead serves to allow better management of the patient, with tight check-ups. In any case, a duplex ultrasound check on the extent of the thrombus should be carried out after 2–3 days to exclude appositional growth during treatment. Thrombus growth to the level of the next afferent vein can often not be avoided, as stasis in this segment favors thrombus apposition. When there is thrombus growth beyond that, into the next-adjoining proximal venous segment, the intensity of treatment should be reconsidered and attention should be given to coagulation disturbances and paraneoplastic causes. The studies that led to acceptance of the outpatient approach in Germany were published in 1996 and only provide evidence that inpatient treatment with intravenous heparin administration and outpatient management with low-molecular-weight heparin are equivalent. They do not show that either is superior. In both treatment groups in the studies by Levine et al. (1996) and by Koopman et al. (1996), new thromboses or clinically symptomatic pulmonary embolism occurred in approximately 6% of patients (with 3 months' follow-up) and 7–8% (after 6 months' follow-up), respectively. According to an analysis by Douketis et al. (1998), the risk of fatal pulmonary embolism during treatment for acute thrombosis can be estimated at 0.4% in a patient with no signs of pulmonary embolism.

The acute symptoms, with swelling and pain, quickly resolve with correct compression. Depending on the way in which the thrombus is broken down or transformed, however, lifelong post-thrombotic damage may persist.

As the organization process can take a considerable time, it is only possible to draw conclusions about post-thrombotic damage and associated sequelae after 1 year. Post-phlebitic damage leads via swelling of the leg to trophic disturbance, with the risk of ulcer formation (see Chapter B 4 on varicose ulcers). Consistent and continuing long-term compression therapy should therefore be used to reduce the risk of ulcer formation.

As the risk of ulcer formation only applies to the lower leg, only a class II or III lower leg stocking is needed at the end of 1 year, independently of the extent of the previous thrombosis.

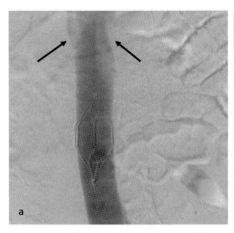
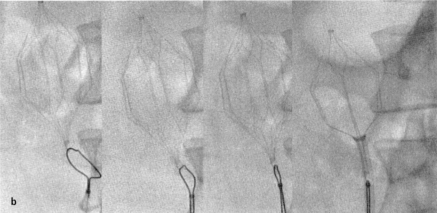

Fig. 1.1-17a, b (a) Venacavography via the left pelvic vein, with correct infrarenal positioning of the OptEase® filter. The arrows mark contrast enhancement with inflow of blood from the renal veins. (b) Removal of the OptEase® filter in the same patient as in a. The filter is captured with a snare using the hook designed for this purpose and with simultaneous advancement of the retriever sheath is withdrawn into the sheath.

Vena cava filter

Indication

Filters can be implanted in the inferior vena cava to serve as mechanical obstacles to prevent detached thrombus particles from being embolized into the lungs. Either temporary or permanent filters can be used.

Temporary filter systems (Fig. 1.1-17a, b) can be completely removed and are only used if the risk of pulmonary embolism needs to be reduced in the short term when anticoagulation is not possible such as in a perioperative period, or during fibrinolytic treatment or transportation of the patient. Permanent filter systems remain in the inferior vena cava for life and can only be removed in individual cases by means of elaborate and expensive vascular surgery. The indication for permanent filter systems is a matter of controversy, as there are no clear data on the reduction of the rate of fatal pulmonary emboli. In addition to purely temporary or permanent filters, there are also systems that take both approaches into account. These systems use a hook mechanism to recapture a permanent system and thus return the filter to the sheath for subsequent complete removal. The removal procedure can, of course, only succeed if the filter system has not become too tightly adherent to the vessel wall or it does not contain thrombus matter that might embolize when the filter system is mobilized. However, it is reported in the literature that this occurs in up to 10% of cases and that the filter systems are consequently not capable of being recovered.

Routine implantation of a vena cava filter—e.g., in high-risk patients undergoing trauma surgery in whom anticoagulation treatment is not possible—has not been shown to have any advantages with regard to the prevention of fatal pulmonary embolism.

Procedure

Depending on the length and flexibility of the system being used, the vena cava filter can be placed in the infrarenal inferior vena cava with transjugular, transbrachial, or transfemoral access under fluoroscopic guidance. If the inferior vena cava itself is thrombosed in this area, the filter system can also be positioned suprarenally. However, there is a risk of the renal veins being affected if thrombosis occurs in the filter system.

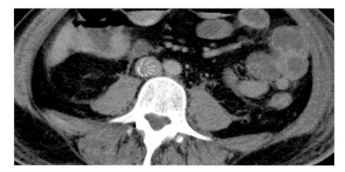

Fig. 1-18 Computed tomography of a temporary Günther Filter® implanted from the nonthrombosed side via the femoral vein. The filter is positioned infrarenally in the inferior vena cava and has not captured any thrombus, so that it can be removed without any problems.

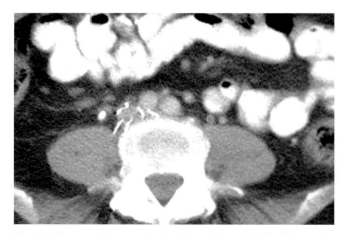

Fig. 1-19 Computed tomography of a Kimray–Greenfield Filter® that had been permanently implanted in the inferior vena cava 17 years previously. The diameter of the vena cava clearly shows post-thrombotic reduction, and individual struts have penetrated the wall of the vein.

Permanent filters are placed using self-expanding systems (Fig. 1-19). Temporary systems remain attached via the introducer system (Fig. 1-18). It is important to attach the introducer system well so that the filter system is not advanced further or withdrawn when the patient is placed in bed or repositioned.

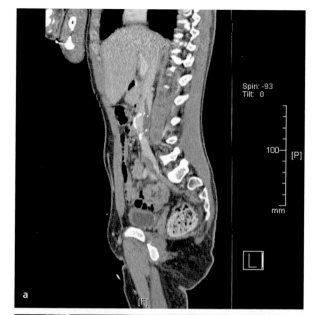

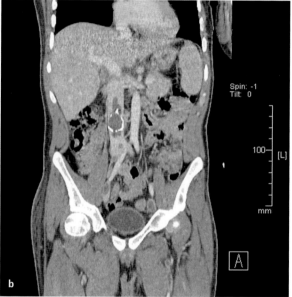

Fig. 1-20a, b Lateral (a) and ventral (b) views of an infrarenally placed OptEase Filter® with a captured embolus, in a patient with multiple trauma and left-sided thrombosis ascending into the pelvis. The filter system was not later removed.

Before the temporary filter is removed, it must be ensured that there is no embolus trapped in the filter. It is difficult to assess this with ultrasound in the relevant group of patients. Depending on the filter system, contrast imaging via the filter can be carried out. However, the safest method is angio-CT imaging (Fig. 1-20). If there are only small emboli in the filter, it can be captured using a large retriever sheath. With large quantities of thrombus, the filter has to be removed by opening the vein during vascular surgery.

Risks and complications

The value of a permanent vena cava filter in thrombosis treatment is a matter of controversy for various reasons, particularly as the filter is thrombogenic in itself and does not provide secure protection. Problems arise:

- When a vena cava filter is used in patients in whom anticoagulation cannot be administered due to an increased bleeding risk, and the filter itself thromboses
- When the vena cava filter has captured one or more washed-out thrombi and the vena cava occludes due to accumulation of thrombus material
- When filter thrombosis develops and grows through the filter, so that thrombus emerges on the proximal side of the filter and can in turn embolize without obstruction

Figures for the frequency of occlusions of the vena cava in patients with filters range from 1% for symptomatic occlusions to 25% when a systematic search is made for occlusions. The incidence of pulmonary embolism is reduced when a filter system is used, but not to zero. A study published in 2006 including 751 patients, with a mean follow-up period of 295 days, reported further symptomatic pulmonary embolism in as many as 7.5% of the patients. It is not clear whether recurrent pulmonary emboli, which have repeatedly been considered as a potential cause of cor pulmonale, can be effectively prevented with filter systems. In these cases, the focus should be on long-term oral anticoagulation treatment.

Separate complications that have been reported to occur independently of thrombotic events include venous perforation, with bleeding and damage to neighboring organs and migration of the filter system into the pulmonary circulation.

The DeWeese caval clip is an alternative to the vena cava filter. The clip is placed around the inferior vena cava using a laparotomy and completely closes the vessel. A marked post-thrombotic syndrome has to be deliberately accepted with this procedure, but it allows safe prevention of further emboli. No recent publications on this procedure are available.

Follow-up

Permanent filter systems may perforate the vessel wall or may themselves embolize as fragments and cause thrombotic occlusion after several years. The manufacturers of these systems give various recommendations regarding long-term anticoagulation, and there are therefore some patients who receive anticoagulation despite having the filter system and some who do not. The indication for additional anticoagulation, or anticoagulation treatment starting later on, depends not only on the filter system used, but also on the patient's comorbid conditions, evidence of filter thrombosis, recurrent pulmonary embolism, and pulmonary arterial hypertension, so these also need to be taken into account. Additional anticoagulation appears to reduce the mortality rate in these patients in the longer term. A retrospective analysis of 304 patients, 172 of whom did not receive long-term oral anticoagulation, showed a benefit for anticoagulation relative to event-free survival after 2 years (80.6% versus 72.3%).

Fibrinolytic therapy

Indication and optimal timing

Fibrinolysis is the only form of treatment that allows complete elimination of thrombosis while at the same time preserving the valvular system. In contrast to surgery and catheter-guided recanalization, it also reaches the large numbers of small veins in the lower legs. Despite this, the success rates achieved with lysis treatment are not convincing. The success rate for complete fibrinolysis is a maximum of 40%, associated with a treatment-associated mortality risk of around 1%. There are only few reports with long-term results, showing that successful lysis also effectively prevents post-thrombotic syndrome with ulcer formation. The indication for fibrinolytic therapy must therefore be established extremely cautiously, and the procedure should only be used in young patients with fresh thromboses. The estimated age of a thrombosis should certainly be less than 5 days, although some literature reports have described successful lysis for much older thromboses.

Procedure

There are various forms of lysis, differing in the choice of agent, dosage, and method of administration. Out of the large number of individual forms of lysis that have been promoted, only the three that were in most widespread use, at least for a time, are discussed here.

Ultrahigh-dose streptokinase (UHSK)

In this form of lysis, streptokinase is deliberately administered at a very high dosage of 9 million units (1.5 million IU/h for 6 h) so that it can penetrate the thrombus quickly and at an adequate dosage. In addition, heparinization with 1000–1500 U of unfractionated heparin per hour is administered at the same time. As is usual with streptokinase, 250,000 U is administered in a 40-mL 5% glucose solution for 20 min before the start of the actual lysis in order to neutralize potential antibodies. If necessary, the lysis procedure can be repeated on several consecutive days.

Conventional urokinase lysis

Urokinase is administered continuously, starting with a high dosage of 600,000 U over 20 min, which is then followed by prolonged treatment at 100,000 U per hour. The effect of the urokinase is clearly reflected in the fibrinogen level, which declines over time and should not be lower than 80 and 100 mg/dL. Simultaneous administration of unfractionated heparin is also used to prolong the APTT by 50%. Lysis can be continued in this form for 10–14 days.

Local lysis with recombinant tissue plasminogen activator (rt-PA)

Although rt-PA is not approved in Germany for lysis of venous thrombosis, systemic and local administration for the purpose has been investigated. Local administration via a dorsal foot vein, originally placed for phlebography, came into widespread use. A dosage of 20 or 40 mg rt-PA over 4–6 h was administered locally once per day. In addition, the patients also received intravenous heparinization aimed at prolonging the APTT by 50%.

With systemic administration, a large proportion of the fibrinolytic agent is neutralized in the blood and broken down in the liver before it can start to act at the thrombus at all. Local lysis is based on the assumption that a better effect on the thrombosis can be achieved when the fibrinolytic agent is applied at the affected extremity at lower doses. However, this is only the case if the lytic agent is delivered to the thrombus using additional measures and outflow via superficial collateral veins is prevented. To prevent the fibrinolytic from escaping from the deep veins via the perforating veins, for example, the superficial venous system has to be blocked. Depending on the extent of the thrombosis, this can be achieved by placing blood-pressure cuffs just above the ankle (80 mmHg), below the knee (60 mmHg), and above the knee (40 mmHg). Pressure in the cuffs should be maintained for the period of administration of the fibrinolytic (Fig. 1-21). One of the few studies that specifically compared the benefit of UHSK lysis and local administration of rt-PA, with a multicenter randomized design in parallel groups, has still not yet been published and is only available in the form of a doctoral dissertation. For this study, a total of 573 patients were recruited at 63 centers between April 1993 and December 1995. During the course of the study, inadequate recanalization with 20 mg rt-PA was noted and an additional third "lysis arm" with 40 mg rt-PA was introduced. Overall, rt-PA at 20 mg/6 h in 212 patients or 40 mg/6 h in 151 patients, and UHSK at 9 million IU/6 h in 210 patients were administered for up to 5 days in each case. The patient groups in the three lysis arms were homogenously distributed with regard to age, sex, body weight, level affected, general patient history and age of the thrombosis. The results are listed in Table 1.1-5, with UHSK lysis showing the best success rates, but also the highest complication rates.

Table 1.1-5 Results of a randomized comparative study with systemic administration of ultrahigh-dose streptokinase (UHSK) and local application of rt-PA at dosages of 20 mg and 40 mg (Messmer 1998).

	UHSK	20 mg rt-PA	40 mg rt-PA
Cycles	3.2	3.9	3.8
Success of lysis	74.8%	58.5%	65.6%
Severe complications	42.4%	11.3%	19.2%

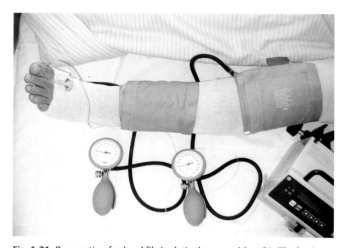

Fig. 1-21 Preparation for local fibrinolytic therapy with rt-PA. The leg is covered in a multilayered compression bandage and blood-pressure cuffs have also been placed over the Cockett and Boyd perforating veins.

A Cochrane review of the risk–benefit ratio in fibrinolytic therapy published in 2004 was based on the data from a total of 12 randomized studies, although these only included 736 patients throughout the world. The only German studies included in the review were by Schweizer et al. from 1998 and 2000. The unpublished controlled study mentioned above and the often-cited Phlefi registry were not taken into account.

The Cochrane review came to the following conclusions. Complete thrombus elimination was observed significantly more often in patients with fibrinolytic treatment than in the control group. This applied both to short-term follow-up examinations (relative risk 0.24; 95% confidence intervals 0.07–0.82; P = 0.02) and also to the later follow-up (RR 0.37; 95% CI, 0.25–0.54; P < 0.00001). A similar effect was seen for all grades of chronic venous insufficiency. After fibrinolytic therapy, there were significantly fewer cases of post-thrombotic syndrome (RR 0.66; 95% CI, 0.47–0.94; P = 0.02) and there were fewer ulcerations (RR 0.53; 95% CI, 0.12–2.43; not significant). There were also significantly more bleeding complications among patients who received fibrinolytic therapy (RR 1.73; 95% CI, 1.04–2.88; P = 0.04). The incidence of bleeding complications appears to have declined over time, as increasingly strict selection criteria were applied. Intracranial bleeding was only observed in two patients in the treatment group (RR 1.70; 95% CI, 0.21–13.70), in both cases from a study dating from 1976 and 1990 that included patients up to 75 years of age. No significant effect on mortality was found, and the data on the occurrence of pulmonary embolism and recurrent thrombosis were not conclusive. These results from the Cochrane review do not justify abandoning lysis as a treatment method for eliminating thrombus. Instead, what they actually show is the lack of adequate data. The favorable results of modern conservative thrombosis therapy are making fibrinolysis increasingly into an elective form of treatment for a very small group of patients. It may be recommended that the indication should be restricted to patients who are under the age of 50 years with thromboses no more than 5 days old.

Particularly in patients with extensive proximal thromboses and involvement of the pelvic veins and inferior vena cava, lysis therapy would be desirable. However, these are precisely the patients who also have the greatest risk of complications.

High systemic doses of the fibrinolytic agent need to be given, as large thrombus masses are present and central thrombus matter cannot be reached with local administration via a dorsal foot vein. During lysis, it is possible for proximal thrombus components that have not yet been completely dissolved to break away and embolize. To avoid this, a vena cava filter could be used, but this in turn is associated with an increased risk of bleeding due to puncture of the vein and represents another independent thrombogenic risk.

If the filter captures larger amounts of thrombus material that cannot be dissolved, the filter has to be left in place or removed surgically.

Overall, therefore, only proximal thromboses extending just into the common femoral artery can undergo lysis treatment with an acceptable level of risk (Fig. 1-22). This type of thrombosis can be reached with local lysis using 40 mg rt-PA. To eliminate thromboses in the pelvic veins or inferior vena cava, UHSK lysis would be necessary, but this is not justifiable due to the higher complication rate involved. In these cases, an interventional or surgical procedure should be considered, if treatment is possible at all.

Risks and complications

In all forms of lysis, monitoring of the circulatory parameters for blood pressure and heart rate is necessary to provide information about any deterioration in the circulatory situation due to treatment-related bleeding or pulmonary embolism. Particularly with streptokinase, allergic reactions that may even include anaphylaxis should be anticipated. Monitoring of the patient during the first 30 min, with the presence of an experienced physician and readily available epinephrine, cortisone, and intubation instruments, is therefore indicated.

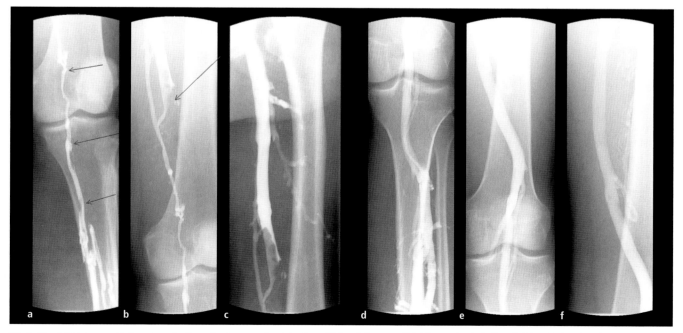

Fig. 1-22a–f Phlebographic imaging of a thrombosis ascending into the middle of the superficial femoral vein before (left) and after (right) successful fibrinolytic therapy.

Table 1.1-6 Contraindications against elective fibrinolytic treatment for thrombosis.

Complication	Cause to be considered
Bleeding	Florid gastrointestinal ulcer
	Hemorrhagic diathesis, thrombocytopenia
	Hypertension, with diastolic values > 100 mmHg
	Stroke within the previous 6 months
	Surgical procedure within the previous 4 weeks
	Arterial puncture within the last 14 days
	Aneurysms
	Tumor or metastases
	Advanced hepatic and renal disease altering the metabolization of the fibrinolytic agent
Embolism	Intracardiac thrombi (aneurysm, defect)
	Large aortic thrombi
Allergic reaction	Known intolerance, particularly for streptokinase

The findings listed in Table 1.1-6 are regarded as general contraindications for lysis. Since fibrinolytic therapy for thrombosis is always an elective procedure, rather than an emergency treatment, particular attention needs to be given to considering the contraindications.

Follow-up

Even after partly or completely successful lysis therapy, conservative treatment with anticoagulation and compression should be continued for 3–6 months. Ultrasound or phlebographic evidence of luminal patency should not lead one to overlook the fact that thrombosis is associated with endothelial damage. Healing of the endothelial damage and avoidance of recurrent thrombosis in the short term require anticoagulation treatment.

1.1.4.2   Endovascular therapy

Any form of treatment for deep vein thrombosis needs to be judged in relation to the following goals:

- Relieving pain
- Preventing progression of the thrombosis
- Preventing pulmonary thrombosis
- Preventing post-thrombotic syndrome

The treatment most often used today is purely conservative, based on systemic anticoagulation and local compression. This leads to rapid symptomatic improvement in many cases. The risk of pulmonary embolism and progression of thrombosis is also reliably reduced. However, the venous valve apparatus often remains irreversibly destroyed. In addition, there are outflow obstructions due to incomplete recanalization. The long-term prognosis with regard to the development of post-thrombotic syndrome is therefore unsatisfactory with conservative treatment. Endovascular procedures can be used to try to prevent the development of a post-thrombotic syndrome through early minimally invasive revascularization, or to achieve symptomatic improvement by eliminating outflow obstructions in both the acute and late stages.

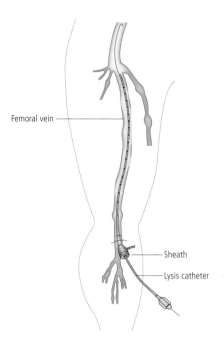

Fig. 1-23 Interventional mechanical and/or fibrinolytic therapy for a thrombosis in the superficial femoral artery. The popliteal vein is used for access, as this allows the catheter to be advanced without damaging the venous valves. (Adapted from Sharafuddin et al. 2003.)

Technique

Catheter-guided intrathrombotic thrombolysis

Systemic thrombolytic therapy harbors a high risk of severe bleeding complications. Direct application of a thrombolytic agent to the thrombus can reduce the drug dosage needed and can thus reduce the complication rate as well.

To do this, a catheter with multiple side holes (lysis catheter) is placed directly in the thrombosed segment of vein. Depending on the location of the venous occlusion, either an antegrade or retrograde access route can be chosen. The antegrade route is usually preferred, to protect the venous valve apparatus during catheter introduction. Possible puncture sites are the femoral vein in the inguinal region, for isolated pelvic vein thrombosis; and the popliteal vein, for venous thromboses at several levels (Figs. 1-23 and 1-24). For simultaneous treatment of thrombosed veins in the lower leg, antegrade puncture of one of the posterior tibial veins or retrograde puncture of the popliteal vein can also be used. If the subclavian vein is occluded, the brachial vein is a suitable access route.

To reduce the risk of local bleeding complications due to incorrect puncture, the puncture procedure is usually carried out with ultrasound guidance. A hydrophilic guidewire (e.g., 0.035-inch Terumo Glidewire®) is first introduced through a sheath with fluoroscopic guidance, and the lysis catheter is introduced directly into the thrombosed vein over the wire. The thrombolytic agent is then administered, either continuously using a syringe pump or as a bolus followed by a maintenance dose in combination with PTT-controlled local administration of unfractionated heparin.

Various thrombolytic agents at various dosages are used. A possible dosage scheme that could be used for multiple-level thromboses in normal-weight patients, for example, is rt-PA with 5–10 mg as a bolus followed by continuous infusion of 12–24 mg/24 h, or alter-

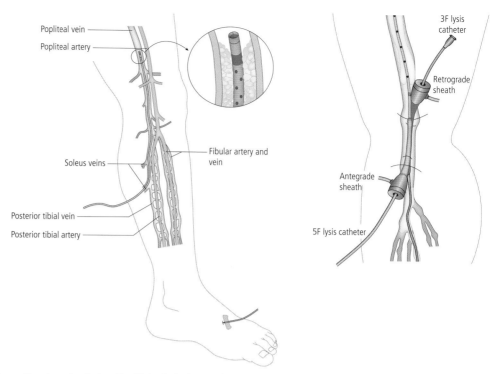

Fig. 1-24 Combined access routes for interventional mechanical and/or fibrinolytic therapy for a thrombosis in the lower leg and thigh. Left: cannulation of the posterior tibial artery via a perforating vein. Right: double cannulation of the popliteal vein, with antegrade and retrograde sheath placement. (Adapted from Sharafuddin et al. 2003.)

natively urokinase 1000–2000 IU/kg/h over 12–24 h. As a systemic increase in thrombin can also occur with local administration of fibrinolytic agents, simultaneous heparin administration is necessary in order to prevent new thrombus formation (target PTT 60–80 s). Depending on the clinical course, the success of treatment can be checked using serial duplex ultrasound examinations. Combined use with an ultrasound-emitting catheter is being tested. In this procedure, a catheter with several ultrasound-emitting probes attached to its sides (EcoSonic™, Ekos) is positioned in the thrombosed vein and the thrombolytic agent is infused via the catheter during the application of ultrasound waves. The ultrasound waves are intended to separate the fibrin bridges and thus allow better penetration of the thrombolytic agent into the thrombus, shortening the thrombolysis time. Controlled studies on the device (e.g., DUETT) are underway.

Thromboablative catheter systems

As an alternative to acute surgical thrombectomy, percutaneous thromboablative catheter systems can be used to remove particularly large thrombus masses or to achieve adequate recanalization particularly quickly. The systems that are suitable were mostly designed for arterial thromboablation and in some cases are not formally approved for use in the veins. The different anatomic conditions therefore need to be taken into account when they are used in this way. Thinner vessel walls in the veins, the presence of venous valves, and the tendency for the vessel lumen to collapse during aspiration maneuvers involve a greater risk of injury than in the arterial system. The principles involved include rheolytic aspiration (e.g., AngioJet®, Possis Medical, Inc.), mechanical aspiration (e.g., Rotarex® and Aspirex®, Straub Medical Ltd.), and laser-based or ultrasound-based thrombolysis. The Aspirex catheter (Straub Medical Ltd., Wang,

Switzerland) is available in 6F, 8F, and 10F sizes and is therefore suitable for the treatment of iliac and femoropopliteal thromboses. It is mainly used to shorten the duration of acute symptoms and thrombolysis that usually follows, or to improve the efficacy of thrombolysis.

Endovenous stents

Outflow obstructions due to incomplete recanalization or prior stenotic lesions can promote the development of post-thrombotic syndrome or recurrent thromboses. In the early and late stages of thrombotic conditions, attempts can be made to achieve complete recanalization using stent angioplasty in the venous segments affected. Due to their large diameter and relatively immobile attachment in the pelvis, the pelvic veins are well suited for this technique, but patency rates below the level of inguinal ligament are still unsatisfactory. Flexible self-expanding stents up to a diameter of 20 mm are used, since balloon-expandable stents are not suitable, due to the risk of injury to the vessel wall and later stent deformation. Access via the popliteal vein or femoral vein can be used, depending on the location of the venous segment being treated. It is usually sufficient to place a short (11-cm) 6F sheath. Sheath sizes of up to 12F may be needed for stent sizes larger than 10 mm.

In some patients with left-sided pelvic vein thrombosis, the thrombotic event is due to a spur-like stricture in the proximal iliac vein at the level of the crossing right common iliac artery (May–Thurner or Cockett syndrome). In this case, it is a good idea to advance the stent to the immediate vicinity of the iliocaval confluence or even beyond that into the distal vena cava. It is important to note here that the stenoses causing the thrombosis may be stricture-like and may sometimes only be dilatable using a cutting balloon. Direct stenting should therefore be avoided and predilation should be carried out initially, since uncorrectable incomplete stent expansion might otherwise occur.

Results

New treatment strategies for venous thrombosis can be evaluated in relation to various different goals. Purely conservative treatment based on anticoagulation and compression can in most cases adequately prevent progression of the disease and effectively prevent pulmonary embolization. In interventional treatment approaches, therefore, the focus is on successful symptomatic therapy, and in particular on the long-term results with regard to the development of post-thrombotic syndrome. Comparative analyses are made more difficult by the wide variation in symptoms, with different subjective effects on quality of life. More easily measured surrogate parameters are therefore often used, such as phlebographic patency in the venous segments treated. However, this practice can be extremely misleading, as this end point does not necessarily correlate with quality of life as a genuinely meaningful clinical result.

There have not yet been any larger randomized prospective studies to compare the efficacy of interventional forms of treatment with conservative therapy. Smaller controlled studies support the hypothesis that there is a lower rate of post-thrombotic syndromes after catheter-guided thrombolysis. However, this is counterbalanced by the potential complications, particularly bleeding. A pooled analysis of 19 smaller studies showed an average bleeding rate of 8%, with most events involving relatively harmless secondary bleeding at the puncture site. Intracranial bleeding was rare (0.2%). Fatal pulmonary emboli occurred in 0.1% of the patients. Pulmonary emboli after treatment occurred in a total of 0.9% of cases. These rates are quite comparable with the rates of thromboembolic complications that develop with purely conservative treatment. Despite this, some authors recommend the implantation of temporary vena cava filters before catheter-guided thrombolysis. Whether this leads to better results or only produces an additional source of complications has not yet been sufficiently investigated.

Only case reports have so far been published on the use of thromboablative catheter systems, as well as small series in some cases instigated by the manufacturers. The results are very promising, but the data are generally still by no means sufficient to justify routine use of these systems. Since the introduction of self-expanding stents, endovenous stent angioplasty has been an accepted treatment option for chronic venous insufficiency with occlusion or stenosis of the pelvic veins. Retrospective series including several hundred patients show patency rates of 60% to more than 90% after 1 year. Severe complications such as pulmonary embolism or severe bleeding are only rarely observed. The patients usually report marked symptomatic improvement, and venous ulcers appear to heal better (Fig. 1.1-25a–c). Hardly any longer-term results for periods of more than 5 years have been published. There is a lack of controlled studies comparing the technique with established surgical procedures such as venous patch angioplasty or Palma bypass, although these are much more invasive. The results with venous stenting below the inguinal ligament are unsatisfactory, with patency rates of less than 40% after 1 year. There are as yet insufficient data on stent angioplasties in other deep veins such as the inferior vena cava and subclavian vein.

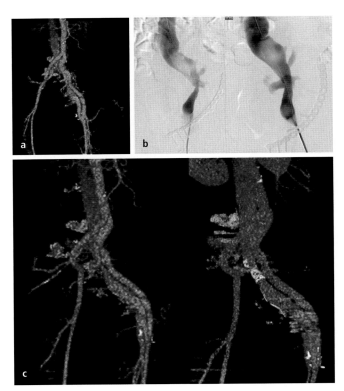

Fig. 1-25a–c **(a)** The CT shows the findings 2 years after surgical left-sided thrombectomy, with creation of an arteriovenous fistula in a patient with status post multilevel thrombosis as a sequela of a pelvic girdle fracture. Stenosis of the pelvic veins is obstructing free venous outflow and leading to arterialization of the venous system on the left side, with the development of a varicose ulcer. **(b)** Venography shows the stenosis before (left) and after (right) endovascular treatment using stent angioplasty. **(c)** The CT reconstructions make the location of the stenosis clear before (left) and after (right) stent placement following endovascular treatment.

Prospects

Interventional treatment approaches are increasingly being included in the therapeutic strategy for venous thrombosis. This is due to the increasing numbers of specialists in vascular medicine with experience in interventional vascular procedures, as well as constant improvements in the materials available. There are now sufficient data on catheter-guided thrombolysis treatment and stent angioplasty in the pelvic veins in post-thrombotic syndrome for these treatments to be offered as an alternative to conservative therapy. There is still a lack of large prospective and randomized controlled studies showing that they are definitely superior, but the results published to date are very promising. The potential complications have been identified and must be discussed with the patient. There are defined contraindications, particularly with regard to possible bleeding complications when thrombolytic agents are administered. Thromboablative catheter systems may provide an effective treatment option in special cases. However, there are insufficient data on each of the available systems for any of them to be used in routine therapy outside of research studies. It can be expected that pressure from manufacturers will lead to more research being conducted in the coming years. Multimodal approaches in which the new catheter systems are individually combined with targeted thrombolysis and venous stent angioplasty certainly hold substantial promise.

Surgical treatment options have declined in importance during the last few decades and are now mainly used only in patients with very severe clinical pictures who are at acute risk of losing the extremity (phlegmasia cerulea dolens). The less invasive interventional procedures are likely to replace vascular surgery procedures increasingly here as well. There is still a lack of comparative data.

If the superiority of interventional procedures over established conservative therapy is confirmed, it will lead to far-reaching changes in the structure of care provision. Patients with venous thrombosis will then increasingly be referred to larger, specialized vascular centers. The costs of acute care will increase. However, the incidence of high-cost long-term post-thrombotic syndromes may decline.

1.1.4.3 Surgical treatment

While anticoagulation treatment only improves the thrombophilic status and can prevent the development of ongoing thrombosis, fibrinolysis is able to eliminate the thrombus. The local causative method of treatment is venous thrombectomy, as the potentially embolic material is removed in the process and the venous valvular apparatus can be preserved in suitable cases. The results with venous thrombectomy can be substantially improved by creating an arteriovenous fistula. Late recurrences can be avoided by assessing the individual risk of thrombophilia and administering an appropriate form of risk-adjusted drug prophylaxis.

History

The development of the surgical technique of venous thrombectomy is based on the work of four surgeons: Kulenkampff, Bazy, Fründ, and Läwen. Läwen described his surgical technique in a study entitled "Further experience in surgical thrombus removal in venous thrombosis" in 1938. He carried out venous thrombectomy by opening the vessel with a direct venotomy, removing thrombi, and then re-establishing blood flow.

Kulenkampff carried out thrombectomy via a transected great saphenous vein. Fründ and Bazy, following the venous thrombectomy, also carried out ligation of the thrombectomized vein to prevent embolization of distal thrombi. The heyday of venous thrombectomy was in the 1960s, with research on and further development of the surgical technique by Brunner, May, Fogarty, Gruss, and Kunlin (*anastomose suspendue*), but it was superseded in the 1970s with the clinical introduction of heparins and in the 1980s by thrombolysis. The reasons for this included vague and not well-established indications along with a surgical technique that was inappropriate for dealing with the veins and led to poor long-term outcomes. The unsatisfactory patency rates, which led to the impression that the operation involved high risks with little success, were only improved on with the development of a more subtle technique suitable for the venous wall, routine construction of an arteriovenous fistula (or even bilateral fistulas), and modern anticoagulative drug treatment. The importance of venous thrombectomy today is best illustrated by a Medline search. In the period from 2000 to 2005, a total of 1077 articles are listed with the search term "deep venous thrombectomy" in the keywords, but only 25 with the search term "thrombectomy." Thrombectomy has thus generally lost much of its importance as a treatment method.

Indication

A questionnaire survey conducted in Germany in 1999, including 146 vascular surgery departments, showed that thrombosis in the inferior vena cava, iliofemoral circulation, embolizing thrombosis, pregnancy-associated thrombosis, and septic thrombosis were the major indications for venous thrombectomy (see Table 1.1-1). Data for a total of 6718 patients were available for the analysis; 15.9% of the patients underwent venous thrombectomy and 18.6% received fibrinolysis. The remaining 65.5% only received anticoagulation treatment. In our own department, we consider that venous thrombectomy is indicated for embolizing thromboses, regardless of their anatomic extent.

Agenesis or aplasia of the inferior vena cava is also an indication for venous thrombectomy and, if appropriate, for a prosthetic replacement, as the condition usually becomes symptomatic in the second or third decade of life and often ends at the stage of severe post-thrombotic syndrome.

Surgical technique

Complete surgical removal of a thrombus is possible only in the inferior vena cava and common and external iliac veins, as well as in the femoral vein. Thrombus can also be partly removed in the deep femoral vein.

The operation is carried out with general anesthesia, and effective anticoagulation with unfractionated heparin, which is started preoperatively, is initially continued perioperatively at a high dosage. In all patients with thrombosis proximal to the inguinal ligament, a pulmonary artery catheter (Swan–Ganz catheter) is used to monitor pulmonary artery pressure so that possible intraoperative pulmonary embolism can be detected. To reduce the risk of pulmonary embolism, positive end-expiratory pressure (PEEP) is raised to values between 12 and 18 mm H_2O and kept constantly within this range for the period of the thrombectomy. In addition, the patient is placed in an anti-Trendelenburg position until the blood flow is re-established again after the thrombectomy has been completed.

Both legs, the abdomen, and the chest are disinfected and covered with incision foil and adhesive drapes. The chest is included in the draping measures in case the procedure has to be extended to a Trendelenburg operation due to fulminant intraoperative pulmonary embolism. In procedures conducted during late pregnancy or when a simultaneous cesarean section is planned, the presence of gynecology and neonatology staff in the operating room is indispensable.

Surgical technique for isolated inferior vena cava thrombosis

When there is an isolated thrombosis in the inferior vena cava, access is via a laparotomy, with retrocolonic access to the vein. After additional administration of 5000 IU heparin, both renal veins are looped with tourniquets and thus temporarily occluded, the inferior vena cava is then occluded with soft vascular clamps below and above the ostia of the renal veins, and a longitudinal cavotomy is carried out (Fig. 1-26). This is followed by the thrombectomy maneuver in the area of the inferior vena cava and with direct visualization in both renal veins. The venotomy is closed with a continuous suture.

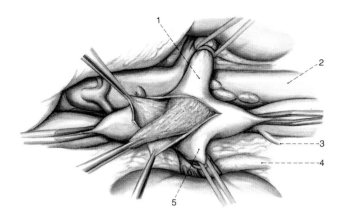

Fig. 1-26 Thrombectomy technique in the inferior vena cava, using tourniquets. 1, left renal vein; 2, aorta; 3, testicular vein/ovarian vein; 4, ureter; 5, right renal vein. (Reproduced from Kremer et al. 1989, with permission from Thieme Medical Publishers.)

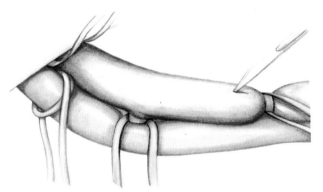

Fig. 1-27 Transfemoral access. (Reproduced from Kremer et al. 1989, with permission from Thieme Medical Publishers.)

Surgical technique for iliofemoral thrombosis

Iliofemoral thromboses, with or without a thrombus plug projecting into the lumen of the inferior vena cava, are treated using a femoral access route. Depending on whether the thrombus is unilateral or bilateral, bifemoral access may also be needed (Fig. 1-27). The vessels supplying the femoral vein are looped with tourniquets and temporarily occluded. The longitudinal venotomy is carried out in such a way as to provide an optimal overview of all of the vessels exiting from the femoral vein. Local thrombectomy is initially carried out (see Fig. 1-24), and a blockade catheter is then placed in the inferior vena cava and the thrombus is removed from the iliofemoral circulation via another thrombectomy catheter (Fig. 1-29).

A distally directed catheter thrombectomy is possible, as the valves are kept open by the thrombus and the catheter is therefore able to pass without destroying the valves. However, retrograde thrombectomy is only required if compression thrombectomy using an Esmarch bandage is not capable of eliminating thrombi located distal to the inguinal region, or does not eliminate them completely (Fig. 1-30). To assess this, the morphological completeness of the retrieved thrombus should be visually assessed (Fig. 1.28). Combined procedures with regional lysis using urokinase and subsequent thrombectomy have also been described in the literature. The indwelling venous catheter placed at the foot can also be used for phlebographic checking of the success of the treatment.

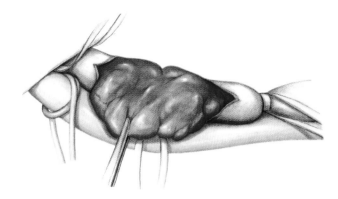

Fig. 1-28 Local thrombectomy in the area of the common femoral artery. (Reproduced from Kremer et al. 1989, with permission from Thieme Medical Publishers.)

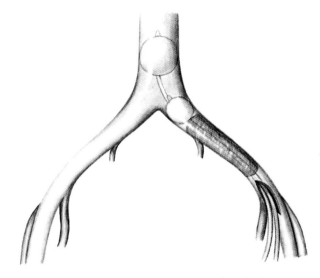

Fig. 1-29 Catheter thrombectomy using a two-unilateral catheter technique. (Reproduced from Kremer et al. 1989, with permission from Thieme Medical Publishers.)

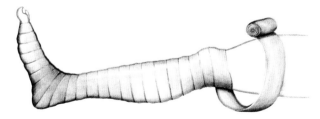

Fig. 1-30 Compression thrombectomy using an Esmarch bandage. (Reproduced from Kremer et al. 1989, with permission from Thieme Medical Publishers.)

If an outflow obstruction is still present after the thrombectomy has been completed—involving an obstruction of the ostium of the left common iliac vein, for example—an attempt can be made to eliminate it using an oval ring stripper. If this is not successful, an open thrombectomy with or without patch plasty or placement of a bypass (with the "original" Palma operation using great saphenous vein, or what is known as a "high" Palma operation with interposition of a prosthesis) can be carried out.

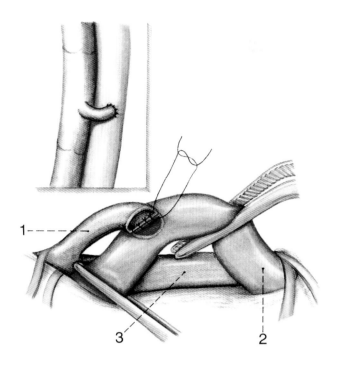

Fig. 1-31 Creation of an arteriovenous fistula. 1, side branch of the femoral vein; 2, femoral artery; 3, femoral vein. (Reproduced from Kremer et al. 1989, with permission from Thieme Medical Publishers.)

Obligatory arteriovenous fistula (AVF)

To secure the results of the operation, an arteriovenous fistula is created at the distal end point of the thrombosis in all patients. Since adequate shunt volumes are only rarely possible below the popliteal artery, the artery represents the furthest distal point for creating an arteriovenous fistula. The great saphenous vein, a side branch of the great saphenous vein, or a free venous transplant can be used for the purpose (Fig. 1-31).

The function of the fistula is to prevent recurrent thrombosis by accelerating flow in the thrombectomized segment and to increase the pressure in the venous system during inspiration.

Results

Thrombosis at several levels can serve as an example of the results with surgical treatment. Venous thrombectomy was carried out in 820 patients at the Department of Vascular Surgery at the University of Düsseldorf from 1982 to June 2005. Thrombosis at several levels, with involvement of the inferior vena cava, was found in 187 patients. Pulmonary embolism had been diagnosed in 30% of the patients before hospital admission, and unsuccessful fibrinolysis or thrombectomy had been carried out previously in 14% of them before the treatment. The perioperative mortality was 1%. Early re-occlusion, associated with occlusion of the arteriovenous fistula, was observed in 28 patients, and revision was carried out in all cases. Six months after the venous thrombectomy, and a further 3 months after surgical closure of the arteriovenous fistula, the patency rate as assessed with duplex ultrasonography or with computed tomography in a few cases was 92.9%.

Clinical and imaging follow-up (with duplex ultrasonography, light-reflex rheography, and plethysmography) was carried out in 152 pa-

tients, at a mean of 5.9 years. Thirty-three percent of the patients were free of symptoms and had no evidence of post-thrombotic syndrome. A further 38% of the patients had a mild post-thrombotic syndrome with only an occasional swelling tendency. Twenty-five percent of the patients had chronic venous insufficiency with secondary varicosis and hyperpigmentation, and 4% had varicose ulcers.

Risks and complications

The advantages of surgical thrombectomy are:
- Rapid and complete removal of thrombosis from the pelvic vein and inferior vena cava
- Complete removal of the thrombosis, reducing the further risk of pulmonary embolism
- Absence of a treatment-related bleeding risk, as in lysis therapy

The disadvantages of surgical thrombectomy are:
- Scar formation and the risk of lymphocele development
- Only incomplete thrombus removal from veins in the thigh and lower leg
- Necessity for a second operation to close the arteriovenous fistula
- The risk of additional injury to the lymphatic system, with persistent impairment of lymphatic drainage
- The risk that recurrent thrombosis in the pelvic arteries is inevitable if the thrombosis is older than supposed and can therefore not be completely removed, leading to possible later deterioration

Follow-up

Even if thrombectomy is successful, conservative treatment with anticoagulation and compression should be continued afterwards for 3 months. Despite ultrasound or phlebographic evidence of luminal patency, it must not be forgotten that thrombosis is the result of endothelial damage. Anticoagulation is needed to allow the endothelial damage to heal and to prevent short-term recurrent thrombosis. If an arteriovenous fistula has been created, it has to be closed again in the symptom-free interval. It causes circulatory stress and also represents a possible short-cut connection for paradoxical embolism.

The ideal patient who is able to benefit from this type of procedure is young and has a fresh short thrombosis in the pelvic vein. The surgical results are good in such cases, with long-term success in preventing post-thrombotic syndrome. Previous pulmonary embolism is a further indication. Patients with this type of thrombosis are rare. An isolated pelvic vein thrombosis occurs in young patients typically in the form of a pregnancy thrombosis, or when there are anomalies in the left iliac vein (pelvic vein spur) or inferior vena cava (circular atresia). This should be taken into account when planning thrombectomy.

Venous thrombectomy is thus an important pillar in the treatment of acute thrombosis and in preventing severe post-thrombotic syndrome. When the indication is established correctly and a gentle surgical technique is consistently applied, with obligatory creation of an arteriovenous fistula, the results are clearly superior to those with conservative therapy with regard to post-thrombotic syndrome, which is a serious condition. However, there are no randomized studies to provide evidence for this benefit.

References

AbuRahma AF, Perkins SE, Wulu JT, Ng HK. Iliofemoral deep vein thrombosis: conventional therapy versus lysis and percutaneous transluminal angioplasty and stenting. Ann Surg 2001; 233: 752–60.

Aguilar C, Del Villar V. Diagnostic value of D-dimer in outpatients with suspected deep venous thrombosis receiving oral anticoagulation. Blood Coagul Fibrinolysis 2007; 18: 253–7.

Arko FR, Davis CM, 3rd, Murphy EH, Smith ST, Timaran CH, Modrall JG, et al. Aggressive percutaneous mechanical thrombectomy of deep venous thrombosis: early clinical results. Arch Surg 2007; 142: 513–8.

ASTH DVT Study Group. Once-daily enoxaparin in the outpatient setting versus unfractionated heparin in hospital for the treatment of symptomatic deep vein thrombosis. J Thromb Thrombolysis 2005; 19: 173–81.

Augustinos P, Ouriel K. Invasive approaches to treatment of venous thromboembolism. Circulation 2004; 110 (9 Suppl 1): 127–34.

Belcaro G, Nicolaides AN, Cesarone MR et al. Comparison of low-molecular-weight heparin, administered primarily at home, with unfractionated heparin, administered in hospital, and subcutaneous heparin, administered at home for deep-vein thrombosis. Angiology 1999; 50: 781–7.

Beyth RJ, Cohen AM, Landefeld CS. Long-term outcomes of deep-vein thrombosis. Arch Intern Med 1995; 155: 1031–7.

Bjarnason H, Kruse JR, Asinger DA, Nazarian GK, Dietz CA Jr, Caldwell MD, et al. Iliofemoral deep venous thrombosis: safety and efficacy outcome during 5 years of catheter-directed thrombolytic therapy. J Vasc Interv Radiol 1997; 8: 405–18.

Blättler W, Heller G, Largiadèr J, Savolainen H, Gloor B, Schmidli J. Combined regional thrombolysis and surgical thrombectomy for treatment of ilio-femoral vein thrombosis. J Vasc Surg 2004; 40: 620–5.

Blum A, Roche E. Endovascular management of acute deep vein thrombosis. Am J Med 2005; 118 (Suppl 8A): 31S–36S.

Böhm K, Cor des M, Forster T, Krah K. Statistisches Bundesamt, Pressemitteilungen; Krankheitskosten 2002.

Botsios S, Erhart R, Walterbusch G. Acute gastrointestinal bleeding caused by perforation of a Greenfield caval filter into the duodenum. Dtsch Med Wochenschr 2006; 131: 2715–7.

Douketis JD, Kearon C, Bates S, Duku EK, Ginsberg JS. Risk of fatal pulmonary embolism in patients with treated venous thromboembolism. JAMA 1998; 279: 458–62.

Dovrish Z, Hadary R, Blickstein D, Shilo L, Ellis MH. Retrospective analysis of the use of inferior vena cava filters in routine hospital practice. Postgrad Med J 2006; 82: 150–3.

Enden T, Sandvik L, Klow NE, Hafsahl G, Holme PA, Holmen LO, et al. Catheter-directed venous thrombolysis in acute iliofemoral vein thrombosis—the CaVenT study: rationale and design of a multicenter, randomized, controlled, clinical trial (NCT00251771). Am Heart J 2007; 154: 808–14.

Geerts WH, Pineo GF, Heit JA, Bergqvist D, Lassen MR, Colwell CW, Ray JG. Prevention of venous thromboembolism: The Seventh ACCP Conference on Antithrombotic and Thrombolytic Therapy. Chest 126: 338S–400S.

Geffroy S, Furber A, L'Hoste P, Abraham P, Geslin P. Very long-term outcome of 68 vena cava filters percutaneously implanted. Arch Mal Coeur Vaiss 2002; 95: 38–44.

Gerhardt A, Scharf RE, Beckmann MW et al. Prothrombin and factor V mutations in women with a history of thrombosis during pregnancy and the puerperium. N Engl J Med 2000; 342: 347–80.

Gruß JD, Laubach K. Modifikation der Operationstechnik bei tiefer Becken- und Oberschenkelvenenthrombose. Thoraxchir Vask Chir 1971; 19: 509–14.

Heit JA, Melton LJ 3rd, Lohse CM, Petterson TM, Silverstein MD, Mohr DN, O'Fallon WM. Incidence of venous thromboembolism in hospitalized patients versus community residents. Mayo Clin Proc 2001; 76: 1102–10.

Husmann MJ, Heller G, Kalka C, Savolainen H, Do DD, Schmidli J, et al. Stenting of common iliac vein obstructions combined with regional thrombolysis and thrombectomy in acute deep vein thrombosis. Eur J Vasc Endovasc Surg 2007; 34: 87–91.

Interdisziplinäre S2-Leitlinien: Diagnostik und Therapie der Bein-Beckenvenenthrombose und der Lungenembolie. Vasa 2005; S 66.

Kalva SP, Wicky S, Waltman AC, Athanasoulis CA. TrapEase vena cava filter: experience in 751 patients. J Endovasc Ther 2006; 13: 365–72.

Karmy-Jones R, Jurkovich GJ, Velmahos GC et al. Practice patterns and outcomes of retrievable vena cava filters in trauma patients: an AAST multicenter study. J Trauma 2007; 62: 17–24.

Kazmers A, Groehn H, Meeker C. Do patients with acute deep vein thrombosis have fever? Am Surg 2000; 66: 598–601.

Koopman MM, Prandoni P, Piovella F et al. Treatment of venous thrombosis with intravenous unfractionated heparin administered in the hospital as compared with subcutaneous low molecular-weight heparin administered at home. The Tasman Study Group. N Engl J Med 1996; 334: 682–7.

Kremer K, Lierse W, Platzer W, Schreiber HW, Weller S. Chirurgische Operationslehre, Bd 1. Stuttgart, New York: Thieme, 1989.

Kwak HS, Han YM, Lee YS, Jin GY, Chung GH. Stents in common iliac vein obstruction with acute ipsilateral deep venous thrombosis: early and late results. J Vasc Interv Radiol 2005; 16: 815–22.

Levine M, Gent M, Hirsh J et al. A comparison of low-molecular-weight heparin administered primarily at home with unfractionated heparin administered in the hospital for proximal deep-vein thrombosis. N Engl J Med 1996; 334: 677–81.

Looby S, Given MF, Geoghegan T, McErlean A, Lee MJ. Gunther Tulip retrievable inferior vena caval filters: indications, efficacy, retrieval, and complications. Cardiovasc Intervent Radiol 2007; 30: 59–65.

Martin M. PHLEKO-/PHLEFI-Studien. Vasa 1997; 49 (Suppl): 5–39.

Matchett WJ, Jones MP, McFarland DR, Ferris EJ. Suprarenal vena caval filter placement: follow-up of four filter types in 22 patients. J Vasc Interv Radiol 1998 Jul-Aug; 9 (4): 588–93.

May R, Thurner J. [A vascular spur in the vena iliaca communis sinistra as a cause of predominantly left-sided thrombosis of the pelvic veins]. Z Kreislaufforsch 1956; 45: 912–22.

Meßmer S. Vergleich der Effektivität und Sicherheit zwischen rt-PA (lokoregionale Administration) und Streptokinase (ultra-hohe systemische Administration) bei Patienten mit akuter tiefer Beinvenenthrombose. Dissertation, Universität Freiburg, 1998.

Montero Aparicio E, Franco Vicario R, Arriola Martinez P, De la Villa FM. Inferior vena caval filter causing nephritic colic after transmural penetration of the inferior cava. Med Clin (Barc) 2007; 128: 237.

Neglen P, Hollis KC, Olivier J, Raju S. Stenting of the venous outflow in chronic venous disease: long-term stent-related outcome, clinical, and hemodynamic result. J Vasc Surg 2007; 46 (5): 979–90.

Oger E. Incidence of venous thromboembolism: a community-based study in Western France. EPI-GETBP Study Group. Groupe d'Etude de la Thrombose de Bretagne Occidentale. Thromb Haemost 2000; 83: 657–60.

Partsch H. Ambulation and compression after deep vein thrombosis: dispelling myths. Semin Vasc Surg 2005; 18: 148–52.

Partsch H. Therapy of deep vein thrombosis with low molecular weight heparin, leg compression and immediate ambulation. Vasa 2001; 30: 195–204.

Pillny M, Luther B, Müller BT, Sandmann W. Umfrage zur Therapie der tiefen Beinvenenthrombose unter den Mitgliedern der Deutschen Gesellschaft für Gefäßchirurgie. Chirurg 2002; 73: 180–4.

Quinlan DJ, McQuillan A, Eikelboom JW. Low-molecular-weight heparin compared with intravenous unfractionated heparin for treatment of pulmonary embolism: a meta-analysis of randomized, controlled trials. Ann Intern Med 2004; 140: 175–83.

Rosenthal D, Wellons ED, Levitt AB, Shuler FW, O'Conner RE, Henderson VJ. Role of prophylactic temporary inferior vena cava filters placed at the ICU bedside under intravascular ultrasound guidance in patients with multiple trauma. J Vasc Surg 2004; 40: 958–64.

Rutherford RB. Role of surgery in iliofemoral venous thrombosis. Chest 1988; 89 (Suppl 5): 434S–437S.

Schwarz T, Schmidt B, Höhlein U, Beyer J, Schröder HE, Schellong SM. Eligibility for home treatment of deep vein thrombosis: prospective study. Br Med J 2001; 322: 1212–3.

Schweizer J, Elix H, Altmann E, Hellner G, Forkmann L. Comparative results of thrombolysis treatment with rt-PA and urokinase: a pilot study. Vasa 1998; 27: 167–71.

Schweizer J, Kirch W, Koch R, Elix H, Hellner G, Forkmann L, Graf A. Short- and long-term results after thrombolytic treatment of deep venous thrombosis. J Am Coll Cardiol 2000; 36: 1336–43.

Segal JB, Streiff MB, Hofmann LV, Thornton K, Bass EB. Management of Venous Thromboembolism: A Systematic Review for a Practice Guideline. Ann Intern Med 2007; 146: 211–22.

Sharafuddin MJ, Sun S, Hoballah JJ, Youness FM, Sharp WJ, Roh BS. Endovascular management of venous thrombotic and occlusive diseases of the lower extremities. J Vasc Interv Radiol 2003; 14: 405–23.

Sillesen H, Just S, Jorgensen M, Baekgaard N. Catheter directed thrombolysis for treatment of ilio-femoral deep venous thrombosis is durable, preserves venous valve function and may prevent chronic venous insufficiency. Eur J Vasc Endovasc Surg 2005; 30: 556–62.

Siragusa S, Terulla V, Pirrelli S et al. A rapid D-dimer assay in patients presenting at the emergency room with suspected acute venous thrombosis: accuracy and relation to clinical variables. Haematologica 2001; 86: 856–61.

van Den Belt AG, Prins MH, Lensing AW, Castro AA, Clark OA, Atallah AN, et al. Fixed dose subcutaneous low molecular weight heparins versus adjusted dose unfractionated heparin for venous thromboembolism. Cochrane Database Syst Rev 2000; CD001100. 27.

van der Heijden JF, Prins MH, Buller HR. For the initial treatment of venous thromboembolism: are all low-molecular-weight heparin compounds the same? Thromb Res 2000; 100: V121–30.

Vedantham S, Millward SF, Cardella JF, Hofmann LV, Razavi MK, Grassi CJ, et al. Society of Interventional Radiology position statement: treatment of acute iliofemoral deep vein thrombosis with use of adjunctive catheter-directed intrathrombus thrombolysis. J Vasc Interv Radiol 2006; 17 (4): 613–6.

Vedantham S, Thorpe PE, Cardella JF, Grassi CJ, Patel NH, Ferral H, et al. Quality improvement guidelines for the treatment of lower extremity deep vein thrombosis with use of endovascular thrombus removal. J Vasc Interv Radiol 2006; 17 (3): 435–47; quiz 448.

Vogeley CL, Coeling H. Prevention of venous ulceration by use of compression after deep vein thrombosis. J Vasc Nurs 2000; 18: 123–7.

Vollmar J, Hutschenreiter S. The transverse crossover bypass of the pelvic veins (the „high Palma"). Vasa 1980; 1: 62–6.

Wahl WL, Ahrns KS, Zajkowski PJ et al. Normal D-dimer levels do not exclude thrombotic complications in trauma patients. Surgery 2003; 134: 529–32.

Watson LI, Armon MP. Thrombolysis for acute deep vein thrombosis. Cochrane Database Syst Rev 2004 Oct 18; (4): CD002783.

Wells PS, Anderson DR, Rodger M, et al. Evaluation of D-dimer in the diagnosis of suspected deep-vein thrombosis. N Engl J Med 2003; 349: 1227–35.

Wells PS, Forster A. Thrombolysis in deep vein thrombosis: is there still an indication? Thromb Haemost 2001; 86: 499–505.

Yale SH, Mazza JJ, Glurich I, Peters T, Mukesh BN. Recurrent venous thromboembolism in patients with and without anticoagulation after inferior vena caval filter placement. Int Angiol 2006; 25: 60–6.

1.2 Venous thrombosis in the upper extremity

Knut Kröger

Doppler/duplex ultrasonography: Tom Schilling

1.2.1 Clinical picture

In thromboses of the upper extremity, the main focus is on thrombosis of the veins in the shoulder girdle. Thrombosis ascending from distal to proximal does not typically exist in the upper extremity. Isolated thromboses of the brachial veins and radial or ulnar vein thromboses are rare.

Primary thrombosis of the shoulder girdle veins is caused by compression of the subclavian vein or axillary vein at points of physiological constriction in the shoulder girdle. In older publications, this type of thrombosis, which occurs after physical overexertion, used to be called "effort-induced thrombosis" or "Paget–von Schroetter syndrome."

Four sites of predilection from proximal to distal have been described as triggers for this type of thrombosis:

- Anterior scalene hiatus: muscular hypertrophy or incorrect insertion of the scalenus muscles may compress the subclavian artery during exertion.
- Cervical rib: in addition to the 12 thoracic ribs, there are individual cases of congenital rudimentary ribs at C7. These ribs course below the subclavian artery during development and constrict its passage through the scalenus muscles.
- Costoclavicular constriction: the subclavian vein courses between the first rib and the clavicle. Depending on movement in the shoulder joint, muscular hypertrophy or due to a statically incorrect posture, the costoclavicular space may be narrowed.
- The tendinous attachment of the pectoralis minor at the coracoid process: depending on the development of the pectoralis minor and the shape of the coracoid process, the subclavian vein—which crosses below the muscle at this point—may be compressed.

The most frequent site of constriction is the costoclavicular narrowing, although there are also a large number of pathomechanical variations. Compression of the subclavian vein in the costoclavicular area at maximum elevation and abduction may also be normal in healthy individuals. Not only elevation and abduction, which is regarded as a classic provocation maneuver, may lead to compression of the subclavian vein, but also incorrect posture with fatigue in the shoulder muscles and sinking of the shoulders with simultaneous adduction.

Among the classic causes of thrombosis included in what is known as Virchow's triad, damage to the venous wall plays an important role in primary thromboses of the shoulder girdle veins. This type of endothelial damage is an effect of recurrent compression in the area of the constriction. In contrast to the veins of the leg, immobilization due to plaster casts or confinement to bed, are less important causes of stasis. In addition, the arm and shoulder veins are shorter than the leg and pelvic veins. Venous return is easier, since the arm is at the level of the heart and the shoulder is above it. Although congenital thrombophilic parameters, such as resistance to active protein C or changes in the composition of the blood, in principle

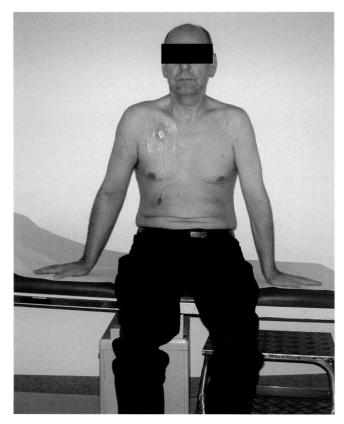

Fig. 1.2-1 The clinical picture in fresh thrombosis of the subclavian vein, with marked swelling and livid coloring in the arm.

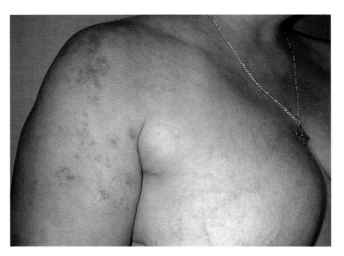

Fig. 1.2-2 The clinical picture in fresh thrombosis of the subclavian vein, with a marked collateral circulation. The small ectatic cutaneous veins in the upper arm disappear again, but the larger collateral veins in the chest area remain when there is persistent occlusion of the subclavian vein.

increase the risk of thrombosis occurring, they have greater effects on the pathogenesis of leg and pelvic vein thrombosis than thrombosis in the veins of the shoulder girdle.

The term **"secondary thrombosis of the shoulder girdle veins"** is used when the thrombosis is caused not by the classic shoulder girdle constriction syndrome or effort, but by other conditions. Iatrogenic injuries due to the use of implanted cardiac pacemakers, central venous catheters and Port-a-Cath systems in particular, play a major role here. The positioning of the central venous catheter may play a decisive role in prophylaxis against thrombosis. Precise positioning of the catheter tip in between the superior vena cava and the right atrium reduces the incidence of thrombosis. Other causes include compression of the veins by lymph nodes and tumors, clavicular fractures, surgical scars and radiation damage.

In cases of thrombosis, there is usually swelling in the arm, shoulder, or neck on the affected side and the patient reports pain. Examination of the supraclavicular and infraclavicular vascular course and the axilla is particularly painful. Livid discoloration of the arm may also occur (Fig. 1.2-1) and a venous collateral circulation may be visible prepectorally (Fig. 1.2-2). The degree of venous obstruction and speed of thrombus formation determine the clinical symptoms, which may sometimes be unobtrusive.

1.2.2   Diagnosis and differential diagnosis

In comparison with venous thrombosis in the pelvic and leg veins, there has been less intensive research on ways of diagnosing thrombosis in the shoulder girdle veins. There are therefore no clinical

pretest probabilities available and the significance of D-dimers is unclear. When there are marked clinical symptoms such as swelling, livid arm and collateral veins, the diagnosis is easily made, but the extent of the thrombosis cannot be confirmed. Imaging diagnosis is therefore needed in order to verify the thrombosis. With a sensitivity of 78–100% and a specificity of 82–100%, ultrasound is the primary option here as well.

1.2.2.1   Doppler/duplex ultrasonography

B-mode

Examination technique in B-mode

Simply to exclude thrombosis, compression ultrasonography using B-mode from the axillary vein can be carried out. The patient should primarily be examined in a supine position or sitting. B-mode compression ultrasound cannot be adequately carried out in the area of the subclavian and brachiocephalic veins and assessment with Doppler/duplex ultrasound in PW and color mode is always needed here.

B-mode ultrasound assessment criteria

For the general assessment criteria and thrombosis characteristics, see venous thrombosis of the lower extremity in section B 1.1.

PW Doppler and color duplex ultrasound

Examination technique for PW and color duplex ultrasound

A 7.5-MHz microconvex transducer can be used to assess the brachiocephalic vein and the start of the superior vena cava. If that is not available, a 3.5-MHz sector scanner with adapted programming and a 7.5-MHz linear scanner from the subclavian artery can be used distally.

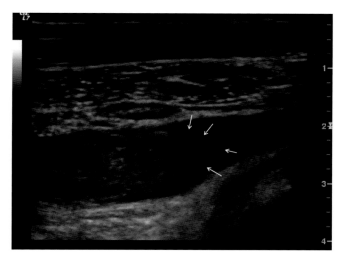

Fig. 1.2-3 Complete thrombotic occlusion of the proximal subclavian vein. The occlusion had a paraneoplastic pathogenesis in a patient with carcinoma of the pancreatic head; the distal subclavian vein is free and the "thrombus head" is visible.

Supplementary assessment criteria on color duplex ultrasound in the arm–subclavian vein system

- Checking of augmented flows and complete color filling in the distal venous segments (distal compression).
- Checking of respiratory-modulated flow and complete color filling in the subclavian and axillary veins.
- Direct imaging and indirect assessment of flow in the brachiocephalic vein, as well as indirect assessment of flow conditions in the superior vena cava (Is there triphasic flow in the inflow area?—it makes hemodynamically compromising obstruction or compression unlikely).
- The jugular veins must always be examined in thrombotic processes—ascension of the thrombus?
- In patients with status post subclavian vein thrombosis, direct sonographic assessment of the subclavian vein should be carried out, with provocation maneuvers to detect thoracic inlet syndrome. This is not useful in cases of fresh occlusion, as the effect cannot be demonstrated (Fig. 1.2-3).
- For shunt veins, see the relevant section.

1.2.2.2 Ascending phlebography

With puncture of a hand vein, ascending phlebography can display the whole deep venous system from the distal lower arm up to the superior vena cava (Fig. 1.2-4). One problem is the lack of imaging of the internal jugular vein and thrombosis of the vein which cannot always be excluded on phlebography.

Depending on the amount of contrast medium used and the extent of the thrombosis, severe dilution of the contrast may occur in the area of the superior vena cava, so that adequate differentiation of the central end of the thrombus is not always possible with certainty on phlebography. If there is suspected thrombosis in this area, CT or MRI is useful.

Short thromboses near the outlet of the subclavian vein are often well collateralized and may be overlooked by inexperienced examiners.

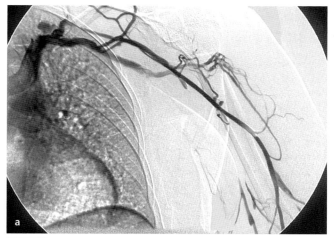

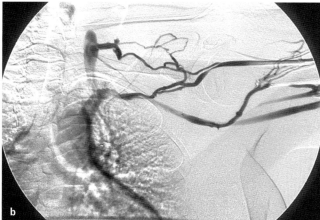

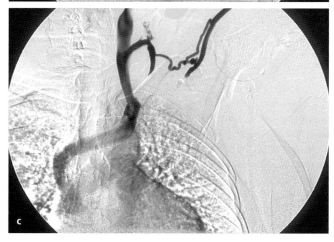

Fig. 1.2-4a–c Phlebography of the shoulder veins on the left side in a patient with recurrent swelling of the left arm and suspected costoclavicular syndrome, with a current clinical suspicion of thrombosis. (**a**) Adduction, (**b**) 90° abduction, (**c**) 150° elevation. The subclavian vein is initially patent and the internal jugular vein does not appear. With increasing abduction of the arm, the subclavian vein closes completely and the internal jugular vein appears with contrast above the collateral veins.

The most important differential diagnosis in subclavian vein thrombosis is lymphedema. When there are thromboses in the area of the jugular veins that appear as isolated painful swelling in the neck, other inflammatory processes in the area of the cervical soft tissue must always be considered.

1.2.3   Treatment

1.2.3.1   Conservative treatment

The principles of treatment are the same as in pelvic and leg vein thromboses, with immediate anticoagulation and compression (see the relevant sections). Compression should also be carried out with multilayered short-stretch compression bandages (with a 6-cm wide bandage in the hand area and an 8-cm wide bandage on the arm). Compression leads to decongestion and relieves symptoms. Since edema in the arm region resolves fairly quickly, and—in contrast to the leg—post-thrombotic damage in the subclavian vein only rarely leads to persistent functional restriction, long-term treatment with an adjusted compression sleeve is not a standard. However, it should be offered to patients with recurrent edema, depending on their individual private and occupational activities. A compression glove should then be prescribed as well in order to avoid congestion in the hand.

The duration of anticoagulation treatment should be approximately 3 months in primary thromboses. Longer periods of anticoagulation are possible, but there is no confirmed justification for this. It is also unclear whether long-term anticoagulation prevents reocclusion in patients in whom costoclavicular constriction is the cause of the thrombosis, with spontaneous recanalization. In patients with secondary thrombosis due to a central venous catheter or Port-a-Cath system, we carry out a 6-week course of treatment. In tumor patients, however, it needs to be considered whether continuing heparin administration at a prophylactic dosage after the end of the 6 weeks may be useful until chemotherapy has been completed.

Independently of anticoagulation and compression therapy, thromboses of the shoulder girdle veins can be treated either on an inpatient or outpatient basis, with the same prerequisites as for treatment of pelvic and leg vein thromboses.

Primary thrombosis

In primary thrombosis, an organic cause such as the constrictions described above should be excluded. Cervical rib can be excluded using noncontrast radiography and incorrect insertion of the scalenus muscles can be excluded by CT. Exclusion of costoclavicular constriction is difficult when the vein is thrombosed, as compression of the occluded vein cannot be imaged either on phlebography or ultrasound (Fig. 1.2-4). If there is compression of the artery with loss of the pulse when the arm is elevated, the diagnosis can be regarded as confirmed. If the arterial status is unremarkable, the diagnosis can only be made if the vein reopens. This may occur spontaneously in the course of thrombus organization or can be achieved with fibrinolytic therapy. Compression maneuvers with the patent vein then become possible.

Central venous catheter and Port-a-Cath systems

Cardiac pacemakers (Fig. 1.2-5), central venous catheters and Port-a-Cath systems (Fig. 1.2-6) are the most frequent cause of secondary thrombosis in the area of the shoulder girdle veins.

It was thought for a long time that immediate removal of the catheter or system was indicated in order to avoid promoting thrombus growth along the foreign materials and to prevent bacterial colonization of the thrombus, with a risk of septic thrombosis. However, neither of these risks appears to be particularly great, and removal

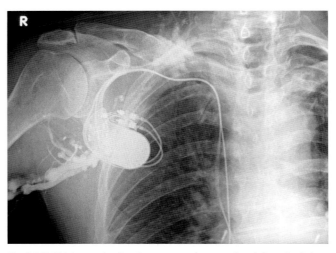

Fig. 1.2-5 Phlebography showing a pacemaker-associated thrombosis in the shoulder veins.

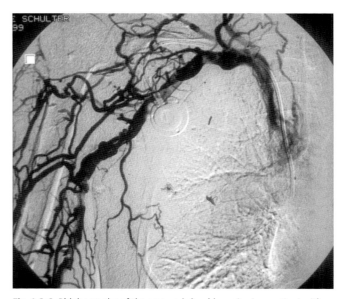

Fig. 1.2-6 Phlebography of the arm and shoulder veins in a patient with a Port-a-Cath system in place and a clinical suspicion of thrombosis. The thrombosis of the subclavian vein near the outlet is only visible in outline, but it is leading to filling of the proximal collateral veins. The contrast filling in the superior vena cava does not exclude partial thrombosis of the vena cava.

of catheter and Port-a-Cath systems therefore needs to be evaluated in the context of the overall therapy. If the patient requires the access, removal and replacement, it only represents a risk for further thrombosis. A small study in Canada has shown in 74 patients receiving chemotherapy in cases of advanced cancer that with anticoagulation treatment, it was possible to leave central venous access in place for up to 3 months after a thrombosis without the situation deteriorating (e.g., with infections, bleeding, or pulmonary embolism). Our own data from 56 patients with a Port-a-Cath system have shown that the system can still be used after thrombosis for a mean of 334 ± 409 days and that the patients were still able to undergo a mean of 9.3 ± 12.3 cycles of chemotherapy during this period.

There have been no suggestions for ways of safely removing central venous access systems without pulmonary embolism. As the thrombosis is a result of endothelial damage in the veins in these patients, most of the thrombi are adherent to the walls and there should be no reservation for removing the catheters. However, only thrombi that are hanging from the catheter material will embolize. This is consciously accepted in the case of smaller thrombi. With larger thrombi, surgical measures need to be considered, but this has not been standardized. In individual cases, it may be useful to wait and watch until a thrombus that is not adherent to the wall becomes adherent and the catheter material can then be removed with no risk of embolism.

Complications of thromboses in the shoulder girdle veins

According to the literature data, pulmonary embolism occurs in up to 20% of patients as a sequela of thrombosis in the deep arm veins. Catheter-induced thromboses are thought to be associated with a greater risk of pulmonary embolism than primary thromboses of the shoulder girdle veins. These high figures stand in contrast to clinical experience, in which pulmonary embolisms appear to occur comparatively rarely with thromboses of the shoulder girdle veins.

1.2.3.2　Interventional therapy
Thrombolytic treatment

Catheter-guided thrombolysis can completely recanalize the subclavian vein, leading to good long-term results. It is a matter of controversy whether the benefits of thrombolysis for primary thromboses of the shoulder girdle veins are real, as the classic late sequelae with post-thrombotic syndrome are also rare in spontaneous courses and do not lead to ulcer formation. There is therefore generally no consensus regarding the indication for thrombolysis in this area, nor regarding the regimen to be used. Thrombolytic treatment for isolated jugular vein thrombosis has not been reported.

Thrombolytic agents used include streptokinase, urokinase, and recombinant tissue plasminogen activator (rt-PA). More recent agents such as alteplase and reteplase have already been used successfully in individual cases. Local thrombolysis starts with intrathrombus administration of an initial loading dose and continuous low-dose intrathrombus administration is then administered for hours to days. To achieve this, a catheter is usually advanced into the thrombus via a distal arm vein under phlebographic guidance. The classic contraindication to fibrinolytic therapy, in patients with a hemorrhagic diathesis and previous surgery, needs to be taken into account.

Most experience with thrombolysis of subclavian vein thromboses has been in young, active patients who have had symptoms for less than 1 week. However, an analysis in 2007 did not confirm any specific benefits of this form of treatment in comparison with simple anticoagulation therapy. On the basis of a literature analysis, the study reports improvement in clinical symptoms in 200 of 262 patients (76%) after thrombolytic therapy and in 268 of 379 patients (70%) with anticoagulation alone (odds ratio 1.33; 95% confidence interval 0.93 to 1.91; P = 0.18).

In our own experience, the decisive problem for effective recanalization is that the thrombi are usually older than the clinical findings suggest. In addition, in patients with pectoral girdle constriction

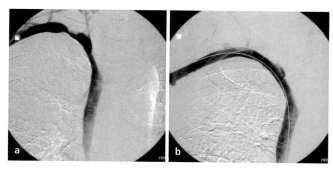

Fig. 1.2-7a, b Residual stenosis in the proximal subclavian vein on the right side after removal of a Port-a-Cath system, before and after an intervention with stent placement.

syndrome the wall of the vein has usually been damaged long before the final thrombosis, and without effective treatment for the constriction, local recurrences are inevitable. With all of the secondary catheter-associated or port-associated thromboses, thrombolysis is usually contraindicated due to the underlying disease.

Interventional techniques

Mechanical thrombectomy combined with thrombolysis has shown good results in recently published studies. These techniques shorten the duration of treatment and also the amount of thrombolytic medication required. However, it has not been confirmed that this is superior to thrombolysis alone in relation to the clinical result.

Central venous stenoses may represent a potential problem as a result of thromboses, both after spontaneous recanalization and also after thrombolytic recanalization. They reduce flow or obstruct placement of another catheter. These stenoses can be treated with angioplasty or in individual cases using stent implantation. Flexible self-expanding stents with extra-large diameters should be used for this type of intervention (Fig. 1.2-7).

In principle, implantation of a vena cava filter into the superior vena cava is also possible. However, the indication for this is not clear, since recurrent pulmonary embolisms from the upper venous circulation are comparatively rare. Hingorani and colleagues published data from a series of 72 patients in whom a Kimray–Greenfield filter was placed in the superior vena cava. A corresponding control group was lacking, but the results reported are good in that there was no clinical evidence of recurrent pulmonary embolism noted in the patients who survived their cancers for more than 4 weeks and there were no filter problems. In particular, no local thromboses and perforations of the superior vena cava with alteration of the heart or mediastinal bleeding were observed.

1.2.3.3　Surgical treatment

Purely surgical treatment for fresh thrombosis in the internal jugular vein or subclavian vein is not established, but there are considerable data on decompression therapy in patients with thromboses of the shoulder girdle veins in connection with shoulder girdle syndrome (see section A 4.7.1).

References

Ascher E, Hingorani A, Tsemekhin B, Yorkovich W, Gunduz Y. Lessons learned from a 6-year clinical experience with superior vena cava Greenfield filters. J Vasc Surg 2000; 32: 881–7.

Da Costa SS, Scalabrini Neto A, Costa R, Caldas JG, Martinelli Filho M. Incidence and risk factors of upper extremity deep vein lesions after permanent transvenous pacemaker implant: a 6-month follow-up prospective study. Pacing Clin Electrophysiol 2002; 25: 1301–6.

Gaitini D, Beck-Razi N, Haim N, Brenner B. Prevalence of upper extremity deep venous thrombosis diagnosed by color Doppler duplex sonography in cancer patients with central venous catheters. J Ultrasound Med 2006; 25: 1297–1303.

Gelabert HA, Jimenez JC, Rigberg DA. Comparison of retavase and urokinase for management of spontaneous subclavian vein thrombosis. Ann Vasc Surg 2007; 21: 149–54.

Hingorani A, Ascher E, Lorenson E, DePippo P, Salles-Cunha S, Scheinman M, Yorkovich W, Hanson J. Upper extremity deep venous thrombosis and its impact on morbidity and mortality rates in a hospital-based population. J Vasc Surg 1997; 26: 853–60.

Joffe HV, Goldhaber SZ. Upper-extremity deep vein thrombosis. Circulation 2002; 106: 1874–80.

Koksoy C, Kuzu A, Kutlay J, Erden I, Ozcan H, Ergin K. The diagnostic value of colour Doppler ultrasound in central venous catheter related thrombosis. Clin Radiol 1995; 50: 687–9.

Kovacs MJ, Kahn SR, Rodger M, Anderson DR et al. A pilot study of central venous catheter survival in cancer patients using low molecular weight heparin (dalteparin) and warfarin without catheter removal for the treatment of upper extremity deep vein thrombosis (the catheter study). J Thromb Haemost 2007; 5: 1650–3.

Kröger K, Grutter R, Rudofsky G, Fink H, Niebel W. Follow-up after Port-a-cath-induced thrombosis. J Clin Oncol 2002; 20: 2605–6.

Luciani A, Clement O, Halimi P, Goudot D, Portier F, Bassot V, Luciani JA, Avan P, Frija G, Bonfils P. Catheter-related upper extremity deep venous thrombosis in cancer patients: a prospective study based on Doppler US. Radiology 2001; 220: 655–60.

Mai C, Hunt D. Upper-extremity deep venous thrombosis: a review. Am J Med 2011; 124: 402–7.

Monreal M, Raventos A, Lerma R, Ruiz J, Lafoz E, Alastrue A, Llamazares JF. Pulmonary embolism in patients with upper extremity DVT associated to venous central lines—a prospective study. Thromb Haemost 1994 Oct; 72 (4): 548–50.

Monreal M, Munoz FJ, Rosa V, Romero C, Roman P, Di Micco P, Prandoni P. Upper extremity DVT in oncological patients: analysis of risk factors. Data from the RIETE registry. Exp Oncol 2006; 28: 245–7.

Mustafa BO, Rathbun SW, Whitsett TL, Raskob GE. Sensitivity and specificity of ultrasonography in the diagnosis of upper extremity deep vein thrombosis: a systematic review. Arch Intern Med 2002; 162: 401–4.

Rathbun SW, Stoner JA, Whitsett TL. Treatment of upper-extremity deep vein thrombosis. J Thromb Haemost 2011; 9: 1924–30.

Sajid MS, Ahmed N, Desai M, Baker D, Hamilton G. Upper limb deep vein thrombosis: A literature review to streamline the protocol for management. Acta Haematol 2007; 118: 10–8.

Usoh F, Hingorani A, Ascher E, Shiferson A, Tran V, Marks N, Jacob T. Long-term follow-up for superior vena cava filter placement. Ann Vasc Surg 2009; 23: 350–4.

2 Superficial thrombophlebitis

Basic anatomy: Reinhard Putz
Clinical picture, conservative treatment: Knut Kröger
Duplex ultrasonography: Tom Schilling
Surgical treatment: Georg Nowak, Dietrich Koch, Manuela Koch

2.1 Basic anatomy

2.1.1 Superficial venous system—lower extremity

Blood return from the dorsum of the foot is via the two veins on the sides of the foot, the lateral marginal veins. They arise from the dorsal venous network of the foot, the transverse dorsal venous arch of which often projects clearly through the skin. Blood from the sole of the foot also flows back primarily to the dorsum. This takes place through the intercapitular veins which transport the blood dorsally from the plantar venous arch through the intermetatarsal spaces.

In the area of the ankle joint, the great saphenous vein arises from the medial marginal vein in front of the medial malleolus. With many connections to superficial and deep veins, the great saphenous vein is embedded in the epifascial adipose tissue and passes upward on the medial side of the lower leg and thigh. It is accompanied by the saphenous nerve along its course in the lower leg.

Still below the knee, the great saphenous vein is joined by an anterior branch from the anterior side of the lower leg and a posterior branch that comes from the medial retromalleolar area. It is only in the area of the saphenous opening below the inguinal ligament that it passes through the fascia lata into the deeper layers and bends in a characteristic fashion into the femoral vein (Fig. 2-1).

The small saphenous vein continues as the lateral marginal vein, winds dorsally round the lateral malleolus, and also passes epifascially toward the popliteal region. After passing through the crural fascia, in varying positions, it bends into the deeper layers in the popliteal region, forming a typical narrow arch, and joins the popliteal vein. In rare cases, a larger superficial connecting branch to the great saphenous vein may continue (Fig. 2-2).

In the area of the saphenous opening, other vessels in addition to the saphenous vein join the femoral vein and together form at this point what is known as the confluence of the superficial inguinal veins, or "crosse." The superficial circumflex iliac vein comes from the iliac crest along the inguinal ligament; the external pudendal veins come from the pubic region; and the superficial epigastric vein brings venous blood from the epifascial space in the lower abdominal wall.

The numerous variants in this area that should be mentioned include in particular—in addition to duplications—a medial accessory saphenous vein and/or a lateral accessory saphenous vein that may be present. It should be expressly noted here that a very small external pudendal artery usually courses transversely from the femoral artery over the lower area of the crosse in a medial direction.

The superficial venous system is connected with the deep veins of the leg via the perforating veins, the valves of which determine the inward flow direction. Disturbances of the venous system in the legs often develop as a result of congenital factors or occupational conditions. It is characteristic of both superficial leg veins that they dilate with increasing age, with their valves causing noticeable distension and visible and palpable vascular patterns on the skin.

2.2 Clinical picture

Superficial thrombophlebitis is thrombosis in the subcutaneous epifascial veins as opposed to deep vein thrombosis.

There are no generally valid data on the frequency of superficial thrombophlebitis, since in contrast to deep vein thrombosis it is regarded as a benign condition with a low risk of pulmonary embolism. Superficial thrombophlebitis in the brachial veins after venous indwelling catheter placement or blood sampling is the most frequently seen form, followed by thrombophlebitis in older people with a history of varicosis (varicophlebitis).

The cause of superficial thrombophlebitis is generally regarded as the Virchow triad, with stasis and disturbances of coagulation and of the endothelium. In addition, as in deep vein thrombosis, an underlying malignancy always needs to be considered when superficial thrombophlebitis is found without an external cause.

2.2.1 Varicophlebitis

As the word suggests, varicophlebitis occurs when thrombophlebitis develops in a vein that already has varicose changes. On the one hand, thrombophlebitis of this type may be quite extensive, depending on the extent of the varicosis. On the other hand, however, it often remains strictly limited to a side branch of the great saphenous vein. This form of phlebitis represents some 90% of all cases of phlebitis in the leg. As varicosis increases with age, the frequency of varicophlebitis also increases.

Etiologically, the focus is on stasis as the cause. Patients with varicosities are advised to avoid heat (e.g., in thermal baths or saunas), as warmth promotes stasis as a result of venous dilation. However, there are no clear research data to support this claim. Local trauma in an area of varicosis might also possibly lead to superficial thrombophlebitis via endothelial injury.

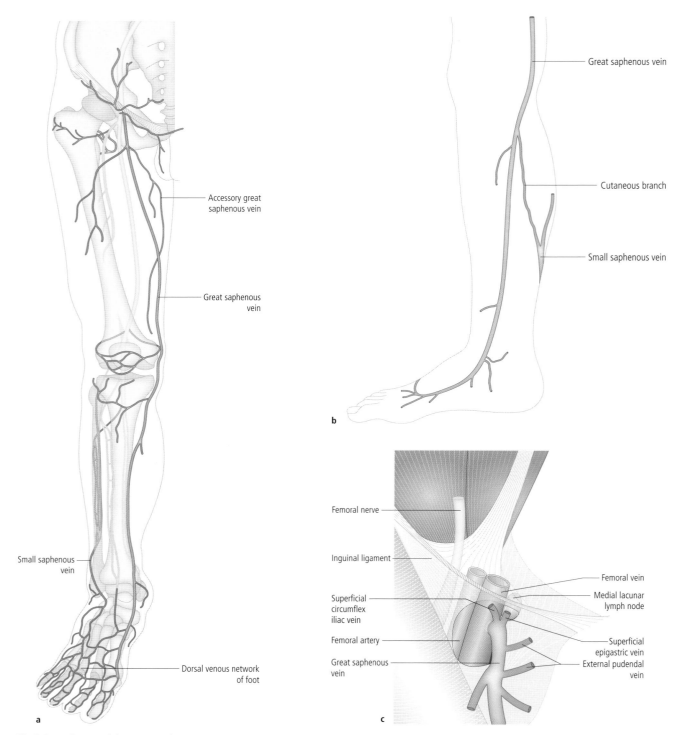

Fig. 2-1a–c Course of the great saphenous vein.

The major symptoms are local pain, palpable subcutaneous resistance, reddening, and hyperthermia. When there are marked findings, accompanying edema in the extremity, low-grade fevers, and restricted movement of the extremity may be seen.

As the distinction between the clinical pictures of superficial thrombophlebitis and deep vein thrombosis suggests, it is questionable from the anatomic point of view to regard the deep and superficial venous systems as separate. The two venous systems form an ana-

tomic and functional unit, and thrombotic changes can spread from one system to the other in the transitional areas (the perforating veins and the ostia of the great and small saphenous veins). This imprecision in terminology leads to terms such as "collar-stud phlebitis," when thrombophlebitis in the great saphenous vein extends beyond the saphenofemoral junction into the common femoral vein. In this case, it is deep vein thrombosis.

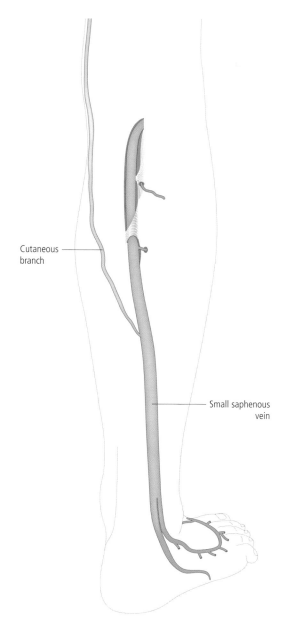

Fig. 2-2 Course of the small saphenous vein.

Cutaneous branch

Small saphenous vein

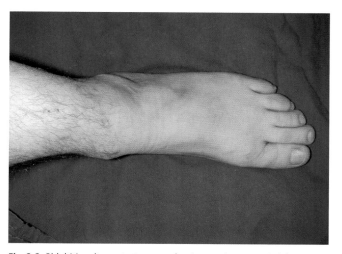

Fig. 2-3 Phlebitis saltans starts as a rather inconspicuous, painful erythema.

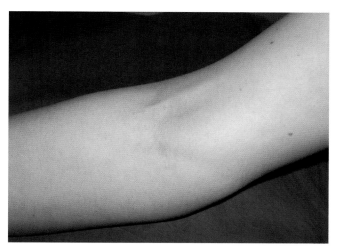

Fig. 2-4 Mondor phlebitis on the inside of the left elbow.

2.2.2   Thrombophlebitis saltans et migrans

Superficial thrombophlebitis in changing locations (saltans et migrans) occurs in previously unaltered veins. It is therefore usually small in extent and does not involve the large subcutaneous conducting veins (Fig. 2-3). The course also varies. Several small thrombophlebitides may arise simultaneously or in sequence. The course may be episodic, and the upper extremity may also be involved. Sudden appearance in various different locations is known as "saltatory," and a slowly spreading form is called "migrating." Etiologically, the focus is on inflammatory phenomena in the wall of the vein that form part of the symptomatic complex of other underlying diseases. When superficial thrombophlebitis shows this type of course, it is therefore always necessary to inquire into possible underlying disease and carry out more extensive diagnostic testing. Simultaneous involvement of visceral and intracranial veins has also been reported. Typical underlying etiologies include malignancies, autoimmune diseases (e.g.,

lupus erythematosus, Wegener disease, Behçet disease, and thromboangiitis obliterans). In contrast to deep vein thrombosis, middle-aged men are the patients most frequently affected by this type of phlebitis.

2.2.3   Mondor disease

This is an atypical form of thrombophlebitis that preferentially occurs in the arm. It is always associated with the thoracoepigastric veins, although this form has only rarely been described in the literature during the last 20 years. The course is marked by a typical hardening and contraction of the veins, with funicular scarring, which may persist in the longer term (Fig. 2-4). Although there have been case reports of this condition in connection with underlying malignancies such as breast carcinoma, the cause is still not known. Mondor phlebitis has also been reported to occur with trauma or inflammatory liver diseases (Denzel and Lang 2001), for example. The cause is often idiopathic.

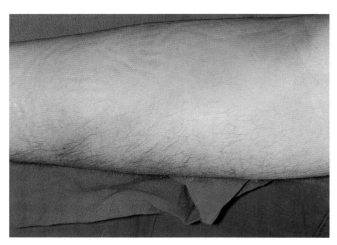

Fig. 2-5 Marked phlebitis in the arm after a venous indwelling catheter. Here again, compression is the treatment of choice.

2.2.4   Catheter-associated thrombophlebitis

All indwelling venous cannulas or catheters can induce thrombophlebitis. The major causes are direct irritation of the venous wall, which may be mechanical or toxic (with hyperosmolar solutions) (Fig. 2-5). Rarer causes include allergic reactions to the catheter material, coagulation disturbances, and introduction of pathogens.

2.3   Diagnosis and differential diagnosis

The major symptoms will typically have developed within the space of a few hours and should be definitively attributable to the course of a subcutaneous vein. In addition, the patient should be asked about:

- Pre-existing varicosis: varicophlebitis
- Immobilization or direct trauma as a possible cause
- Previous thrombophlebitis in the arms or legs that might suggest an episodic course, as evidence of autoimmune diseases or thromboangiitis obliterans
- Cases of superficial thrombophlebitis or deep vein thrombosis in the family, suggesting a thrombophilic diathesis
- Dyspnea, suggesting pulmonary embolism
- General symptoms such as weight loss, sudden drop in performance, or nocturnal sweating, suggesting a paraneoplastic cause
- Oral aphthae or genital changes in patients from the Mediterranean region, as a manifestation of Behçet disease

2.3.1   Inspection and palpation

- Subcutaneous resistance that is painful on pressure and displaceable
- Erythematous and warm skin
- Varicosities or trophic disturbances, as signs of chronic venous insufficiency: varicophlebitis
- Multiple small superficial thrombophlebitis sites up to a few centimeters in size and of varying age, with otherwise normal skin coloring: thrombophlebitis saltans
- Thrombophlebitis gradually spreading from distal to proximal in a vein showing no varicose dilation: thrombophlebitis migrans
- Palpable pulse: important for later compression treatment

In Mondor thrombophlebitis, the signs of inflammation may be very slight and the development of a painful, indurated and wire-like cicatricial strand with retracted skin may predominate.

Involvement of the deep veins via perforating veins (Fig. 2-6) and via the junction of the great and small saphenous veins in the leg, or of the cephalic and basilic veins in the arm, must be excluded. If the great or small saphenous veins are directly affected, involvement of the deep veins is present in up to 15% of cases. If only the side branches are involved, there is still deep vein involvement in 5%. If there is any evidence of deep vein involvement, then phlebothrombosis is present and needs to be treated as such.

Not every cutaneous or subcutaneous area of reddening and induration is synonymous with phlebitis. Possible differential diagnoses are listed in Table 2-1.

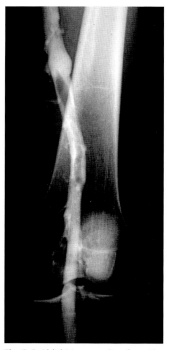

Fig. 2-6 Phlebitis ascending from the small saphenous vein into the deep venous system.

Table 2-1 Differential diagnosis of phlebitis.

Major symptoms	Minor symptoms	Suspected diagnosis	Diagnosis
Painful erythema	Fever, shivering fits	Erysipelas	Axillary or inguinal lymph nodes, exclusion of thrombophlebitis on ultrasound, antistreptolysin titer
Painful subcutaneous node	Itching	Insect sting	Dermatological consultation
Extensive local painful erythema	Slightly raised, indurated	Erythema nodosum	Internal medicine etiological investigation

2.3.2   Doppler and duplex ultrasonography

Although thrombophlebitis is mainly diagnosed clinically, color duplex ultrasonography with a 5-MHz or 7-MHz transducer should be carried out when there are marked findings. This is the only way of safely assessing the extent of the thrombophlebitis. A prospective registry in France showed in 844 patients with symptomatic superficial thrombophlebitis that as many as 210 (24.9%) already also had thrombosis in the deep leg veins or symptomatic pulmonary embolism.

2.3.2.1   Examination technique

High-frequency linear scanners should be used, initially with slight application pressure to avoid compressing the vessels (precise low-flow-optimized device setting). The following details should be investigated:

- Is there any intraluminal thrombus?
- Where are the proximal and distal boundaries of the thrombus (may go well beyond the area noted externally in the clinical examination)? Is the thrombus adherent to the wall?
- Are there any signs of transfascial progression via perforating veins, with involvement of subfascial conducting veins and muscular veins?
- Are there any signs of transfascial progression via the junction regions, with thrombus plugs or subfascial spread?
- Are there any signs of periphlebitis (hypoechoic perivascular structures)?
- Are there any signs of earlier changes in the epifascial venous system?

2.3.2.2   Differential diagnosis

- Thrombophlebitis: thrombotically occluded—previously normal-lumen vein (Fig. 2-7)
- Varicophlebitis: signs of previous ectasia/varicosities in the affected segment (Fig. 2-8)
- Thrombophlebitis *en fil de fer* (Mondor disease): cord-like (peri-)phlebitis, particularly in the area of the chest wall, but also in other locations resulting in a very narrow thrombosed lumen
- "Collar-stud thrombophlebitis": transfascial outgrowth of a phlebothrombosis via perforating veins into the epifascial venous system

2.3.3   Further diagnostic procedures

Further diagnostic procedures depend on the individual patient and the history or clinical findings:

- In older people with varicophlebitis and weight loss, a search for a tumor is indicated.
- In younger people with other forms of superficial thrombophlebitis, attention should be directed to clarifying autoimmune diseases. In younger men, a search should always be made for thromboangiitis obliterans, and the arterial system in the lower legs and forearms must be examined.
- In Mondor thrombophlebitis, breast carcinoma should be excluded.

Biopsy sampling in thrombophlebitis saltans often does not provide any further diagnostic information.

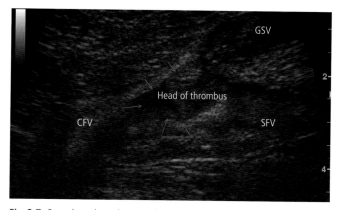

Fig. 2-7 Complete thrombotic occlusion of the great saphenous vein, with progression via the crosse and thrombus plugs in the common femoral vein (B-flow). CFV, common femoral vein; GSV, great saphenous vein; SFV, superficial femoral vein.

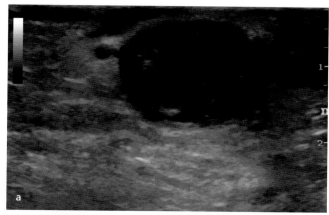

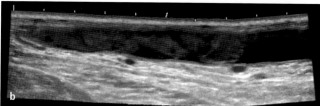

Fig. 2-8a, b Previous marked varicosis in a patient with Klippel–Trénaunay syndrome—evidence of very hypoechoic (fresh?) thrombi and varicophlebitis. (**a**) Transverse, (**b**) longitudinal.

2.4   Treatment

2.4.1   Conservative treatment

Conservative treatment is based on compression and anticoagulation therapy. Compression is achieved with:

- Dressing with a short-stretch compression bandage
- Support stocking
- Compression stocking

As there is often edema associated with the early presentation, initial placement of a compression bandage extending past the proximal end of the thrombophlebitis is indicated in order to promote decongestion. After a short interval, a switch can then be made to an appropriate support or compression stocking, which should certainly be worn for 4–6 weeks after clinical healing has been achieved. A zinc gelatinous bandage can also be placed instead of a compression bandage, but it does not offer any particular advantages. For local treatment of an accompanying sterile inflammatory reaction, an anti-inflammatory ointment can be applied underneath the compression dressing. There is no evidence that this form of treatment has any advantages, but some patients report reduced pain. In phlebitis in the arm, which is often due to indwelling venous cannulas, the widely used ethacridine (Rivanol) and alcohol dressings are not indicated; they only achieve superficial disinfection and usually dry out rapidly. A compression dressing is also helpful in this type of phlebitis. Fears of spreading infection are not justified and there are no data providing any evidence for it. If pus is clearly draining from the puncture site, then the puncture site should be explored and if necessary incised; additional short-term antibiotic treatment is then useful and the compression dressing should be exchanged daily so that the course of the infection can be assessed.

Additional special considerations:

- In varicophlebitis, the question of the basic treatment for varicosis needs to be clarified once healing has been achieved.
- In thrombophlebitis saltans or migrans, compression treatment is only indicated with some qualifications, as the small veins with inflammatory changes cannot be compressed. Particularly when phlebitis occurs in the region of the foot, compression dressings tend to cause pain (Fig. 2-3). For phlebitis in the calf, compression should be attempted. A search should be made for autoimmune diseases and vasculitis as causes of this type of phlebitis.
- In Mondor thrombophlebitis, adequate compression is not possible simply because of the location.
- When there are general symptoms such as weight loss, a search for a tumor is also indicated. Otherwise, the association with tumor should include at least clinical observation of the patient to monitor for signs of possible tumor—by the family physician, for example.
- Whenever there is an increase in pain under the compression dressing or stocking, other diseases, such as peripheral arterial occlusive disease, that may have been overlooked need to be considered, or the dressing or stocking may have been placed incorrectly.

Although superficial thrombophlebitis results in pulmonary embolism less frequently in comparison with phlebothrombosis, it is a possibility that needs to be considered. Diagnostic assessment for pulmonary embolism is indicated particularly in patients with pulmonary symptoms in whom thrombophlebitis appears as a secondary and incidental finding.

Anticoagulation. Additional administration of heparin is not necessary in cases of circumscribed superficial thrombophlebitis, as the mortality due to pulmonary embolism in connection with thrombophlebitis is low. In the randomized and double-blinded CALISTO study, 3002 patients with thrombophlebitis in the superficial venous system received either 2.5 mg fondaparinux or a placebo for 45 days. As Table 2-2 shows, there were no differences in the mortality rates on days 47 or 77 (0.1% in both groups). Although more cases of venous thromboembolism occurred in the placebo group overall (0.2% vs. 1.3%; 95% CI, 50 to 95; $P < 0.001$), the number of pulmonary embolisms without fondaparinux was very low at 0.3% and none of the pulmonary embolisms was fatal. However, the following exceptions to this rule apply and may make subcutaneous heparin administration for a few days useful or even necessary. The period of heparin administration depends on the clinical course.

- When there is evidence of deep venous involvement, a thrombosis is present and needs to be treated as such. After initial heparinization, anticoagulation follows for 3 months.
- When there is duplex ultrasound evidence that the extent of the thrombophlebitis is increasing despite a compression dressing, heparin should be administered (at a prophylactic dosage) to stop any further expansion.
- Heparin should also be administered when there is thrombophlebitis of the proximal great or small saphenous vein that extends to the ostia of the veins. In these cases, an attempt should be made, if possible, to prevent spread into the deep venous system (short-term double prophylactic dosage or even therapeutic dosage of a low-molecular-weight heparin).
- The same applies to involvement of a perforating vein. Here again, spread into the deep venous system leading to thrombosis must be prevented.

Table 2-2 Results of the CALISTO study on anticoagulation in patients with phlebitis.

End point	Fondaparinux (n = 1502) No. of events (%)	Placebo (n = 1500) No. of events (%)	Absolute risk reduction Proportion in % (95% CI)	P value
Day 47				
Death[‡]	2 (0.1)	1 (0.1)	0.1 (–0.2 to 0.3)	1.00
Pulmonary embolism	0	5 (0.3)	–0.3 (–0.6 to 0.0)	0.03
Deep leg vein thrombosis	3 (0.2)	18 (1.2)	–1.0 (–1.6 to –0.4)	< 0.001
Day 77				
Death[‡]	2 (0.1)	1 (0.1)	0.1 (–0.2 to 0.3)	1.00
Pulmonary embolism	0	6 (0.4)	–0.4 (–0.7 to –0.1)	0.02
Deep leg vein thrombosis	4 (0.3)	19 (1.3)	–1.0 (–1.6 to –0.4)	0.001

‡ There were two cases of death in the fondaparinux group due to tumor disease, and one in the placebo group due to acute cardiac failure.

In thrombophlebitis saltans, a trial of acetylsalicylic acid (dosage 1 g/d) is indicated to slow or prevent a recurrent episodic course. There have been no recent controlled studies on this procedure. The typical course of superficial thrombophlebitis is benign. Many veins remain permanently closed and are later no longer visible on ultrasound. This cicatricial process is similar to that resulting from sclerotherapy.

In varicophlebitis that is not adequately compressed, the thrombus sometimes becomes organized in the vein, retracting and calcifying. These residues are permanently visible on ultrasound and on non-contrast radiography. Thrombophlebitis that goes unnoticed can thus lead to deteriorating varicosities over many years.

In thrombophlebitis migrans or saltans, the veins remain closed after healing. Mondor-type thrombophlebitis is usually a unique and self-limiting phenomenon, whereas thrombophlebitis migrans can have an episodic course.

2.4.2   Endovascular therapy

Interventional therapy is not carried out for superficial thrombophlebitis, as it tends to have a benign course.

2.4.3   Surgical treatment

Treatment for acute superficial thrombophlebitis is generally conservative therapy. The aims in surgical interventions are:

- To prevent further progression into the deep venous system, with the potential complication of deep venous thrombosis, and to avoid the risk of pulmonary embolism
- To shorten the painful course of the condition

In clinical practice, the majority of patients present with a delay of several days to weeks. Even using a combination of the patient's history, which is not always informative, and the ultrasound findings, an experienced examiner can still only roughly estimate the age of the changes seen.

2.4.3.1   Diagnosis and preparations

In addition to the usual preparations for surgery, imaging is crucially important. For quality control, it is preferable for the surgeon to do the duplex ultrasound examination personally.

The operation is carried out with heparin prophylaxis, with the patient in the reversed Trendelenburg position and with positive end-expiratory pressure (PEEP) ventilation, as a postponed surgical emergency procedure within 24 h of diagnosis.

2.4.3.2   Indication

Superficial thrombophlebitis treatment is mainly conservative, as discussed above. Decongestion using surgical measures is only required in individual cases, including imminent sepsis—e.g., after infection from an indwelling catheter.

Varicophlebitis

It is important to take the various locations (crural, femoral) and types of spread (epifascial, transfascial) into account here initially. The following stages of progression are distinguished (based on Steckmeier):

- Type I: variceal thrombosis in the saphenous veins without involvement of the ostia
- Type II: thrombus extending to the level of the ostium
- Type III: thrombus extending beyond the ostium into the deep vein
- Type IV: migration of the thrombus via a perforating vein into the deep veins

If a long section of the trunk of the great or small saphenous vein is involved and the thrombus extends near the ostium of each vein into the deep system, surgery can be useful to shorten the painful course and prevent progression. Imminent or manifest spread of the thrombus into the deep venous system, with a thrombus near the ostium or already extending transfascially, with the risk of embolism, indicates surgery. Both at the level of the popliteal ostium and at the saphenofemoral junction, a thrombus crossing the boundary is located in a vascular segment associated with movement, and there is a risk of the thrombus shearing off and causing pulmonary embolism. By contrast, a thrombus floating freely in the superficial femoral artery does not represent a conclusive indication for surgery. The authors recommend a conservative approach for types I and IV, with treatment of the epifascial system after the phlebitis has healed. For stages II and III, emergency surgery is recommended. Some authors make their approach dependent on the distance of the thrombus tip from the ostium (within 5 cm or 10 cm of the level of each ostium into the deep system). The decisive aspect for treatment is monitoring the course of expansion, as progressive findings may be observed even after the start of conservative treatment with a compression dressing and heparinization.

2.4.3.3   Surgical methods

Local surgical measures

When there are clearly fresh, circumscribed findings and a short patient history, a stab incision with cryoanalgesia can be carried out. Fresh coagulum can be expressed, and pain is markedly reduced. This approach is mainly used in cases of variceal thrombosis. Staged varix removal should follow resolution of acute symptoms. Otherwise, recanalization of the affected saphenous vein can be expected, with recurrent phlebitis.

High saphenous ligation

When ligation near the ostium is carried out during surgery, projection of the thrombus into the deep system must be definitively excluded; otherwise, the ligation might cause thrombus fragments to break off. Particularly with this procedure, it is therefore desirable for the surgeon to personally carry out a duplex examination shortly before the operation.

With high saphenous ligation, only the saphenofemoral ostium is closed by ligation initially. The vein remains in place and is only treated in a staged way after the acute episode has healed. However, there is a risk of recurrent phlebitis if the remaining vein recanalizes. In this procedure, it should be borne in mind that the subsequent operation at the junction must be regarded as repeat surgery for recurrence. Near the junction, there is therefore not only postphlebitic but also postoperative scarring, which makes the procedure more difficult and unnecessarily increases the surgical risk. If postoperative oral anticoagulation treatment is indicated, the subsequent procedure will also have to be delayed by up to 3 months.

Narath operation

This method involves complete treatment of the findings in a single session: thrombectomy at the saphenofemoral junction via a longitudinal incision near the junction in the great saphenous vein or small saphenous vein. Ideally, it is possible to remove the thrombus completely with the forceps via this longitudinal incision. In case of doubt, a careful Fogarty maneuver can be added.

The procedure is completed with crossectomy and extirpation of the vein via single skin incisions along the course as far as the proximal lower leg.

2.4.3.4   Follow-up treatment

The postoperative treatment recommendations again vary widely, ranging from administration of low-molecular-weight heparin for a few weeks to oral anticoagulation treatment for 3–6 months. In cases of fresh, circumscribed varicophlebitis without involvement of the deep veins, a period of 14 days' treatment with low-molecular-weight heparin or fondaparinux at therapeutic dosages is sufficient. If additional typical thrombophilia risk factors are present, oral anticoagulation for 3 months is justified.

References

Belcaro G, Nicolaides AN, Errichi BM, Cesarone MR, De Sanctis MT, Incandela L, Venniker R. Superficial thrombophlebitis of the legs: a randomized, controlled, follow-up study. Angiology 1999; 505: 23–9.

Blum F, Gilkeson G, Greenberg C, Murray J. Superficial migratory thrombophlebitis and the lupus anticoagulant. Int J Dermatol 1990; 29: 190–2.

Bollinger A, Gemperli M. Treatment of thrombophlebitis saltans using acetyl-salicylic acid in microcapsules. Vasa 1972; 1: 143–4.

Cesarone MR, Belcaro G, Agus G et al. Management of superficial vein thrombosis and thrombophlebitis: status and expert opinion document. Angiology 2007; 58 (Suppl 1): 7S–14S.

Chanet V, Amarger S, Pons B, Dechelotte P, Ruivard M, Philippe P. Nodular thrombophlebitis and granulomatous systemic disease. Rev Med Interne 2007 Mar; 28 (6): 416–9.

Chengelis DL, Bendick PJ, Glover JL, Brown OW, Ranval TJ. Progression of superficial venous thrombosis to deep vein thrombosis. J Vasc Surg 1996; 24: 745–9.

Cox EM, Siegel DM. Mondor disease: an unusual consideration in a young woman with a breast mass. J Adolesc Health 1997; 21: 183–5.

Denzel C, Lang W. Diagnosis and therapy of progressive thrombophlebitis of epifascial leg veins. Zentrbl Chir 2001 May; 126 (5): 374–8. German.

Decousus H, Prandoni P, Mismetti P, Bauersachs RM, Boda Z, Brenner B, Laporte S, Matyas L, Middeldorp S, Sokurenko G, Leizorovicz A; CALISTO Study Group. Fondaparinux for the treatment of superficial-vein thrombosis in the legs. N Engl J Med 2010; 363: 1222–32.

Decousus H, QuPERLI, Presles E, Becker F, Barrellier MT, Chanut M, Gillet JL, Guenneguez H, Leandri C, Mismetti P, Pichot O, Leizorovicz A; POST (Prospective Observational Superficial Thrombophlebitis) Study Group. Superficial venous thrombosis and venous thromboembolism: a large, prospective epidemiologic study. Ann Intern Med 2010; 152: 218–24.

Di Nisio M, Wichers I, Middeldorp S. Treatment for superficial thrombophlebitis of the leg. Cochrane Database Syst Rev 2007m Apr 18; (2): CD004982.

Hach W. Venenchirurgie. Stuttgart: Schattauer Verlag, 2006.

Holle-Robatsch S, Fink AM, Schubert C, Steiner A, Partsch H. Mondor phlebitis associated with hepatitis C. Vasa 2001; 30: 297–8.

Kalodiki E, Nicolaides AN. Superficial thrombophlebitis and low-molecular-weight heparins. Angiology 2002; 53: 659–63.

Kock HJ, Krause U, Albrecht KH, van der Laan E, Rudofsky G, Eigler FW. Crossectomy in ascending superficial thrombophlebitis of the leg veins. Zentrbl Chir. 1997; 122 (9): 795–800.

Lazarides MK, Georgiadis GS, Papas TT, Nikolopoulos ES. Diagnostic criteria and treatment of Buerger's disease: a review. Int J Low Extrem Wounds 2006; 5: 89–95.

Marchiori A, Mosena L, Prandoni P. Superficial vein thrombosis: risk factors, diagnosis, and treatment. Semin Thromb Hemost 2006; 32: 737–43.

Mayor M, Buron I, de Mora JC, Lazaro TE, Hernandez-Cano N, Rubio FA, Casado M. Mondor's disease. Int J Dermatol 2000; 39: 922–5.

Murgia AP, Cisno C, Pansini GC, Manfredini R, Liboni A, Zamboni P. Surgical management of ascending saphenous thrombophlebitis. Int Ang 1999 Dec; 18 (4): 343–7.

Naschitz JE, Kovaleva J, Shaviv N, Rennert G, Yeshurun D. Vascular disorders preceding diagnosis of cancer: distinguishing the causal relationship based on Bradford-Hill guidelines. Angiology 2003; 54: 11–7.

Noppeney T, Noppeney J, Winkler M, Kurth I. Acute superficial thrombophlebitis—therapeutic strategies. Zentralbl Chir 2006; 13: 51–6.

Rohrbach N, Mouton WG, Naef M, Otten KT, Zehnder T. Wagner HE. Morbidity in superficial thrombophlebitis and its potential surgical prevention. Swiss Surg 2003; 9 (1): 15–7.

Talhari C, Mang R, Megahed M, Ruzicka T, Stege H. Mondor disease associated with physical strain: report of 2 cases. Arch Dermatol 2005; 141: 800–1.

Verrel F, Steckmeier B, Parzhuber A, Rauh G, Tato F. Ascending varicose vein phlebitis—classification and therapy. Langenbecks Arch Chir Suppl Kongressbd. 1998; 115: 1237–9.

Verrel F, Spengel FA, Steckmeier B. Stage-adapted therapy concept in ascending thrombophlebitis. Zentrbl Chir 2001 Jul; 126 (7): 531–6.

3 Varicosis

Clinical picture: Helene Arns
Doppler and duplex ultrasonography: Tom Schilling
Conservative treatment: Helene Arns
Endovascular treatment: Michael Offermann
Surgical treatment: Georg Nowak, Dietrich Koch, Manuela Koch

3.1 Clinical picture

Varicose veins and varices arise as a result of weakness in the wall of a vein in the superficial venous system, which progresses due to adverse influencing factors—e.g., the patient has an occupation that involves constant standing, pregnancy or obesity—and leads to venous dilation and subsequent insufficiency of the venous valves.

The lower extremities primarily are affected. Venous varicosity is a frequent condition. According to the results of the Bonn Vein Study in 2003, it occurs in one in six men and one in five women. The view that varicosis is a disease mainly affecting women is therefore incorrect. Nor is it a disease only seen in older people, although its frequency and extent increase considerably with age.

A distinction is made between *primary* and *secondary* varicosities. There is no clear single cause for the primary pathogenesis of varicosity, and it is thought that there may be a genetic predisposition to weakness in the venous wall ("phlebasthenia"). In rare cases, primary varicosity is due to congenital vascular malformations. Secondary varicosity can arise as a sequela of deep vein thrombosis, for example.

Conditions that require medical treatment include varicosity of the great or small saphenous veins, and also varicosis of the side branches, depending on their extent—e.g., the medial and lateral accessory saphenous vein—and varicosity of the perforating veins.

Reticular varicosity and spider veins are a cosmetic problem and are therefore treated for that reason when patients request it. There are only a few cases here in which the findings, such as spider veins extending over a large area, may create problems such as bleeding after trauma or itching.

Medically relevant findings can be clearly diagnosed with imaging procedures. Decision-making regarding the need for varicose vein treatment and the indication for conservative or surgical therapy is a matter for specialists qualified in phlebology and depends, among other things, on the patient's symptoms and the precise pattern of findings. More recently the aim has been to treat varicosity at an early stage in order to prevent complications and the sequela of chronic venous insufficiency.

3.2 Clinical findings

Many people have varicose veins but are free of symptoms, are not concerned about any aesthetic disturbance, and consequently do not see any need to visit a physician. However, if symptoms do lead the patient to consult a family physician or specialist, they may vary in their specificity. Less specific forms include leg cramping, a feeling of heaviness or pain in the legs, leg fatigue depending on the patient's everyday exposure to stress, and a tendency for swelling to develop, particularly in the lower legs and ankles. Specific symptoms reported include a feeling of warmth and itchiness in the area of a visible varicose vein, nonhealing eczema (which may have been treated for several years previously as a case of circumscribed psoriasis), venous inflammation, and "ulcerated leg." Due to their "weaker" type of connective tissue and greater attention to health problems and unacceptable cosmetic outcomes, women tend to present for medical treatment more often than men.

From the medical point of view, the clinical signs of varicosity consist of visible and palpable varices in the saphenous veins and side branches, "blow-out" phenomena in the area of the perforating veins, coronal venectasia, dermatosclerosis, and stasis dermatitis particularly in the distal segments in the legs, varicophlebitis, and varicose ulcer. The frequency of varicose ulcer has markedly declined in comparison with surveys conducted 20 years ago. Despite this, "maximum" findings with primary or secondary varicosis that has already been present for years or decades are still quite a common and challenging clinical picture.

The clinical, etiologic, anatomic, and pathophysiologic (CEAP) classification of varicosis is now used to document clinical findings in varicosis in a scientifically comparable way (Table 3-1).

Table 3-1 The clinical, etiologic, anatomic, and pathophysiologic (CEAP) classification of varicose veins.

C0	No visible signs of venous disease
C1	Spider veins and reticular varices
C2	Varicosity with no signs of chronic venous insufficiency
C3	Varicosity with edema but without skin changes
C4	Varicosity with skin changes (pigmentation, eczema, dermato-liposclerosis, atrophie blanche)
C5	Varicosity with scarring in varicose ulcer
C6	Varicosity with florid varicose ulcer

3.3   Diagnosis

The diagnosis is based on the patient's history and clinical findings. Important patient history details may include previous vascular disease, information about a familial disposition, concomitant diseases such as diabetes mellitus, previous treatments, and evaluation of the treatment results. The clinical examination must include palpation of the pulse in the feet and in the area of the posterior tibial artery and dorsalis pedis artery, and also the popliteal and femoral arteries when appropriate, to ensure that existing arterial occlusive disease is not overlooked.

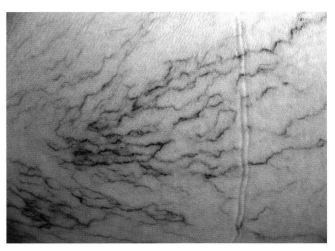

Fig. 3-1 Spider veins.

3.3.1   Functional diagnosis

Diagnostic procedures, such as light reflection rheography (LRR) and photoplethysmography (PPG), are easily conducted examinations for assessing venous reflux. During a standardized sequence of maneuvers, the venous filling time in the dermal venous plexus is measured as a diagnostic parameter and recorded on a graph. If the filling time is too short by definition, there is a suspicion of varicosities. This method is prone to error; pharmacies sometimes offer it as a service, but the information obtained can at best only provide general guidance.

Venous occlusion plethysmography (VOP) makes it possible to assess the capacity and outflow of the veins. In this examination method, the patient has to be able to be supine for several minutes and must be able to tolerate the pneumatic cuff. Reduced venous capacity and outflow may suggest an acute or older occlusion in the venous system.

Invasive phlebodynamometry (PD) to measure peripheral venous pressure and provide quantitative information about the restriction of venous function is only recommended in special situations.

3.3.2   Doppler and duplex ultrasonography

No matter how clear the clinical findings of varicosities may be, imaging diagnosis and documentation of the findings are necessary to obtain a complete and reproducible examination result. Color duplex ultrasonography is now the standard and it allows multiple confirmation of a diagnosis with morphological imaging on B-mode ultrasound, depiction of the frequency range as a Doppler signal, and color coding of venous flow information. Morphological

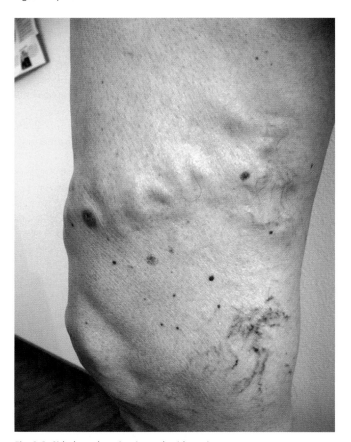

Fig. 3-2 Side-branch varicosity and spider veins.

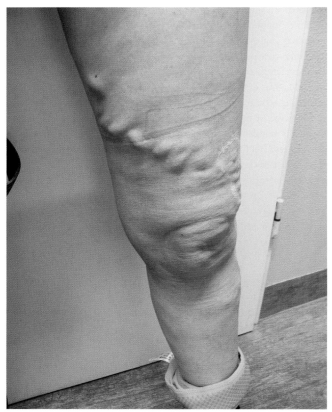

Fig. 3-3 Saphenous and side-branch varicosity.

Table 3-2 Staging of saphenous varicosity (adapted from Hach).

Great saphenous vein	Stage	Small saphenous vein
Insufficiency of ostial valves	I	Insufficiency of ostial valves
Insufficiency of venous valves with retrograde blood flow to above the knee	II	Insufficiency of venous valves with retrograde blood flow to the mid-calf
Insufficiency of venous valves with retrograde blood flow to below the knee	III	Insufficiency of venous valves with retrograde blood flow to the ankle region
Insufficiency of venous valves with retrograde blood flow to the ankle region	IV	

and functional criteria can thus be analyzed and documented in a *single* noninvasive examination procedure. Examining the patient in a standing position is recommended. The Valsalva test can be used to cause retrograde blood flow in the saphenous veins. However, many patients are not able to effectively carry out Valsalva, in which case the examiner then has to create retrograde blood flow by applying pressure to the leg, so that any possible reflux can then be assessed on ultrasound. A systematic procedure is recommended in every duplex ultrasound examination: for example, initial bilateral assessment of the great saphenous vein at the saphenofemoral junction (also known as the "crosse" or confluence), then bilateral assessment of the small saphenous vein at the saphenopopliteal junction. The distal insufficiency point, i.e., the distal-most point of the insufficient venous segment, must be identified (Table 3-2). This is used as a reference point for planning of appropriate treatment, in this case, surgical treatment in particular for saphenous varicosities. Other hemodynamically important segments of saphenous varicosities, side branch or perforating vein varicosities are then checked depending on the initial findings.

The deep venous system always has to be included in the assessment to ensure that any post-phlebitic syndrome is not missed. Residual/recanalized partial occlusions of previously completely thrombosed deep veins, or residual venous valve damage after satisfactory recanalization of a thrombosis, must be documented and taken into account during treatment planning. Depending on the results of the clinical and Doppler preliminary venous examination, the arterial system in the legs may also require duplex ultrasound examination.

3.3.2.1 Examination technique

The basis for this is B-mode and color duplex examination, as described in the chapter on phlebothrombosis (Chapter B 1), plus:

- Measurement of the lumen of the epifascial veins (varicosities defined as epifascial vein ectasia)
- Checking of normal valvular function in the epifascial, transfascial, and subfascial venous system, with proximal compression maneuvers (manual or Valsalva), or distal compression/decompression.

Reflux examinations are always carried out with the patient standing (seated only if unable to stand) since in the supine position there is inadequate sensitivity due to the lack of hydrostatic loading. Adjusted device setting with low-flow optimization, including a

low PRF should be performed. Adjusted enhancement, or a switch to color modes (power mode if appropriate) and color scales are done as necessary. The transfascial perforating veins are best imaged starting from the subfascial veins, with proximal/distal compression/decompression maneuvers. When the muscles are tensed, perforating veins may show insufficiency that cannot be demonstrated in the relaxation phase, such that a supplementary examination of the perforating veins may therefore be needed with the patient standing on tiptoes.

3.3.2.2 Differential diagnosis

Secondary varicosities in:

- Post-thrombotic syndrome
- Proximal outflow obstruction(s) with compression effects
- Hyperperfusion, for example in patients with arteriovenous fistulas.

3.3.2.3 Specific findings

Epifascial (intrafascial) venous system

- Is the lumen normal? If there is reflux with a normal lumen, then varicosities (defined as luminal dilation) is not really present, but rather only a form of valvular insufficiency, which should be described as that.
- Identification of the proximal insufficiency point:
  - Are there any valvular insufficiencies and thus reflux in the junction regions of the great and small saphenous veins during a Valsalva maneuver and/or abdominal compression? If yes, the condition meets the definition of complete saphenous varicosity.
  - Is there reflux in or from the veins in the confluence?
  - If the junction regions are sufficient: is there reflux along the course of the saphenous veins with the provocation measures mentioned above or during compression/decompression maneuvers? If yes, then it needs to be determined whether it is coming from perforating veins (incomplete saphenous varicosities of the perforating type), or from side branches (incomplete saphenous varicosities of the side branch type), or from a Giacomini anastomosis (incomplete saphenous varicosities of the dorsal type).
  - If there is isolated side branch varicosity in the lateral accessory saphenous vein, the junction type has to be differentiated, as there are treatment implications: supravalvular inguinal (via the junction valve of the greater saphenous vein—i.e., that valve is sufficient); infravalvular inguinal (under the junction valve—i.e., that valve is correspondingly insufficient); or femoral (entering the greater saphenous vein along its course).
- Identification of the distal insufficiency point (extent of reflux):
  - HACH classification when there is complete saphenous varicosity (greater saphenous vein: HACH I–IV, small saphenous vein: HACH I–III).
  - In cases of incomplete saphenous varicosity, the recirculation route should be described and defined.
- Are there side branch insufficiencies or junctional variants of the side branches, particularly in the greater saphenous vein?

Transfascial venous system

Are the vessels paired, are they fusiform (so far as can be assessed)? Is the course from distal and epifascial to proximal and subfascial, with an acute junction angle (≤ 60°)?

■ Is the flow only from epifascial to subfascial? Is the reflux > 0.5 s?

■ Are there any afferent perforating veins with incomplete saphenous varicosity?

■ Are there any secondary transfascial insufficiencies in primary varicosity or post-thrombotic syndrome?

■ Are there afferent perforating veins in the periulcerous region in cases of varicose ulcer?

Subfascial venous system

■ Are there any signs of secondary subfascial decompensation in primary varicosis?
  – Normal wall structures and valvular morphology
  – Possible ectasia
  – Reflux with provocation maneuvers

■ Are there any signs of a post-thrombotic subfascial defective state, possibly resulting in secondary varicosity?
  – Wall thickening and possible residual thromboses
  – Irregular lumen with ectasia and lumen narrowing
  – Segmental flow velocity differences
  – Reflux on provocation maneuvers

3.3.3 Further invasive diagnostic procedures

Phlebography and pressure phlebography have been rendered virtually obsolete by color duplex sonography. In rare cases of primary, recurrent, or secondary varicosity, in post-thrombotic syndrome, contrast imaging may provide additional information about the findings for a physician conducting conservative or surgical treatment. In our own clinical experience, phlebography in the region of the lower leg is often only of limited use and can only provide valid imaging information when carried out by a radiographic specialist. The contrast is often not transported as far as the distal segments in the legs. Deep and superficial lower leg veins are interpreted as being occluded, or their reflux behavior cannot be assessed. However, an experienced ultrasonographer with suitable equipment can demonstrate and functionally test every vessel right up to the distal leg segments.

Computed tomography and magnetic resonance imaging are rarely used, and only for specialized examinations. Pelvic vein thrombosis, for example, might be an indication for CT or MRI.

3.4 Treatment

3.4.1 Conservative treatment

Not many patients, and not all physicians, are aware of the need to treat venous varicosity. Patients often believe the varicosity that is not causing any symptoms does not need to be treated. Unfortunately, this view is still held by many physicians as well even today, and physicians still tend to give the overall clinical picture too little attention. Even in the case of complications, referral to a specialist is often significantly delayed. Although awareness of the necessity to treat varicose veins has improved and efforts are made to achieve early treatment, severe disease courses are still quite common. Asymptomatic varicosities should be treated in order to prevent progression of the disease with associated complications. The aim when treating symptomatic varicosities is to relieve symptoms by improving the hemodynamics and to improve the clinical picture or cure the condition. In varicose veins, and varicophlebitis in particular, there is a high risk of deep vein thrombosis, which can trigger pulmonary embolism with potentially fatal consequences. A post-thrombotic syndrome that gradually develops over several years can have sequelae that are difficult to treat, such as varicose ulcers.

In principle, the aim should be to provide definitive surgical or laser-surgical treatment for varicosis. With specific patterns of findings or factors involving the patient's state of health or views about treatment, conservative or temporary conservative treatment may be preferred.

3.4.1.1 Exercise therapy

The simplest supportive treatments for patients with varicosis include raising the legs, doing walking exercises for the veins, and specialized venous physiotherapy. Stimulating the muscle–joint venous pump leads to emptying of the distally overloaded venous segments and improves venous backflow.

3.4.1.2 Local and systemic venous therapeutic agents

Over-the-counter local therapeutic agents such as horse-chestnut gel have a temporary cooling effect on the skin and are therefore found to be pleasant in the often hyperthermic skin areas affected by varicosis. It may also be possible to achieve this effect with cold packs.

In comparison with a placebo, a slight volume reduction in the edematous leg has been demonstrated with the numerous over-the-counter systemic venous therapeutic agents, such as flavonoids (e.g., red vine leaves) and triterpene saponins (e.g., horse chestnut). This slight reduction in edema may be useful *in addition* to other treatment measures and is often reported to relieve symptoms in varicosis with congestive symptoms, particularly in older patients. Many patients unfortunately regard taking "vein tablets" as a way of avoiding a visit to the physician in good conscience and patiently continue self-treatment. The high cost of over-the-counter venous drugs generally bears no relation to their actual benefit.

3.4.1.3 Compression stocking

Wearing a compression stocking is an effective form of treatment for varicosities. The compression stocking has to be individually fitted and worn daily.

The stocking can be removed at night, and venous backflow is then adequately improved by raising the legs. When the patient is sitting, standing, or walking during the day, the compression pressure exerted by the stocking reduces the diameter of the veins and accelerates venous and lymphatic backflow, as well as improving venous valvular function. Ideally, this restores the physiological backflow of blood and thus makes it possible to initially avoid surgical treatment for the varicosis. A few absolute contraindications need to be observed: advanced peripheral arterial occlusive disease, decompensated cardiac insufficiency, septic phlebitis, and phlegmasia cerulea dolens.

Compression stockings are available with various compression classes (classes 1–4), various lengths (e.g., knee-high, thigh-high, and pantyhose), two possible weave types (flat-knit and round-knit), and various materials (e.g., polyamide, elastane, and cotton). After measurement of the patient's defined leg length by the suppliers, either a standard compression stocking can be immediately provided or an individualized, custom-made stocking can be ordered. Depending on the findings of varicosity and the patient's personal situation, compression stockings can be prescribed by the physician, with a precise specification. Compression stockings are effective, but require consistent and active involvement by the patient. To achieve this, a detailed explanation of the way in which the stocking functions has to be given and the way to use it needs to be demonstrated by the supplier and later checked and discussed in the physician's office. Physicians should already have used a compression stocking themselves so that they can understand and assess any difficulties the patient may be having. One study showed that problems with compliance resulted from the stockings being "awkward to put on" and "uncomfortable to wear." Objections on aesthetic grounds only played a minor role. Putting compression stockings on and taking them off requires effort and mobility, even when prescribable aids made of fabric or steel are used. Instead of the compression class 2 that is indicated as a standard (approximately 23–32 mmHg pressure in the captured area), it is justified to switch to compression class 1 in older patients. By contrast, advanced findings with chronic venous insufficiency may make a stocking with compression class 3 necessary; this is more easily achieved by adding stockings, with one class 2 stocking and a class 1 stocking worn on top of it. If this is not possible—in a patient with chronic polyarthritis, for example—then assistance provided by an outpatient nursing service should be discussed.

Particularly in summer, when symptoms of venous insufficiency increase due to the heat, patients' willingness to cooperate declines and compression stockings tend to be left off. This can lead to complications or progression of the disease. Continuing communication with the patient is important—e.g., during the regular check-ups that are needed particularly for conservative treatment and when a new prescription for compression stockings is needed.

3.4.1.4 Compression dressing

Older patients are often able to treat their painful chronic venous insufficiency consistently by putting on compression dressings themselves and are often able to develop an effective dressing technique with them. When applied in the correct way, compression dressings are an alternative to compression stockings. The type of compression bandage used at home is often not fully suitable and is often not prescribed by physicians for a specific condition. Elastic long-stretch compresses are often used, which apply excessive tension to the tissue and may hamper treatment. Reusable elastic short-stretch compresses can be recommended. Ideally, the compression dressing should be applied by a competent nurse-practitioner or nursing service. With several bandaging techniques, there are a few principles that need to be observed, such as including the heel and reducing the pressure from distal to proximal. Some outpatient nursing services also use unsuitable dressing material, or due to pressure of time or inadequate training place ineffective or damaging dressings. This needs to be checked and the compression dressing may then need to be abandoned in favor of a compression stocking, which is more effective.

It has been shown that consistent application of compression measures can effectively relieve symptoms and can largely prevent the complications of varicose disease or allay them.

3.4.1.5 Sclerotherapy

Sclerotherapy holds an intermediate place between conservative and surgical treatment for varicosities. The procedure uses fluid or foamed sclerosing agents at various dosages. For small-caliber varicoses, the preferred field for sclerotherapy, the spider-veins can be easily eliminated with fluid sclerosants, but a sclerosant foam is better for reticular varices. For large-caliber findings such as side branch varices, perforating vein varices, or (less frequently) saphenous and recurrent varicosities, with recurrence at the saphenofemoral junction, there has been a revival in the use of foam sclerosis in recent years. In large vessels, foam sclerosis with duplex ultrasound guidance is carried out. The advantage of foam sclerosis in comparison with sclerosis using a fluid agent, usually polidocanol, is that it is easier to distribute the foam bubbles more evenly in the vessel. The foam is produced using various techniques with a specific mixing ratio of sclerosant to air (e.g., 1:4). Using a needle to inject the substance, which is toxic to tissue, produces local endothelial damage and leads to obliteration and fibrosis of the varix. The resulting thrombus is broken down over a period of weeks or a few months, depending on the size of the varix. Over the longer term, the varicose vein becomes transformed into a strand of connective tissue. Recent studies have shown that when saphenous varicosis is sclerosed using foam, the recurrence rate appears to be lower than when a fluid sclerosant is used. However, complications such as phlebitis appear to occur more frequently. Further studies are required.

The procedure is inexpensive and causes little stress to the patient. The patient must be informed beforehand about the procedure and potential complications, which are only very rarely severe, and written consent must be obtained. Potential complications include allergic reactions, migraine-like symptoms, scintillating scotoma, skin necrosis, excessive sclerotic reactions (thrombophlebitis), permanent pigment disturbance, matting, neural damage, venous thromboembolism, and damage caused by intra-arterial injection. Contraindications to sclerosis include allergy against the sclerosant, bedridden status, and acute superficial or deep leg vein thrombosis. A maximum foam volume of 10 mL per session can be recommended, which is only reached when larger varices are being sclerosed. Anesthesia is not required, and the treatment is usually carried out with the patient in a recumbent position. Treatment for large varices can be safely guided using duplex ultrasonography—from the correct location for the needle insertion site and continuing to distribution of the foam in the vessel. When there is a normal course of healing, the patient does not experience any pain-related movement restrictions. Depending on the extent of the treatment, the patient needs to wear compression dressings and compression stockings, usually for a few days to weeks. Immediately after treatment, the patient should walk up and down in the office for 15–30 min to distribute the sclerosant further in the vascular system by stimulating the muscle–joint pump, and so that medical care is available in case of allergic reactions. Intensive exercise, hot baths, visits to the sauna, and sun exposure should be avoided in the first few weeks after sclerotherapy to prevent excessive reactions such as phlebitis.

Experience and practice are necessary to "hit" small-caliber and large-caliber varices well and adequately and to achieve successful sclerosis without complications and with the correct choice of dosage and agent. Treatment should therefore be carried out in several sessions if appropriate. During healing of the thrombus or "iatrogenic phlebitis," any larger intravascular coagulant can be expressed in order to accelerate healing and avoid permanent hyperpigmentation. It should be emphasized again that a duplex ultrasound examination of the veins must be carried out before every sclerosis treatment. Even spider-veins that have an insignificant appearance may be due to underlying saphenous varicosis, which then has to be given priority treatment. In the usual approach, the saphenous varicosity is first treated surgically or with laser surgery, and the remaining side branch varicosities, reticular varices, and spider veins are then sclerosed afterwards.

The very high aesthetic expectations that patients nowadays have may lead to conflicts in therapeutic decision-making. For example, although from the medical point of view foam sclerosis might be sufficient in a patient with only moderate varicosity of the lateral accessory vein, the possibility of permanent unattractive hyperpigmentation on the thigh might lead one to consider a ligation and mini-phlebectomy as a suitable form of treatment instead. An individualized and detailed discussion with the patient and conclusive written consent for the desired procedure are important.

3.4.2 Endovascular therapy/endoluminal treatment

Surgical efforts to achieve reliable treatment of varicose veins have a long history, and there is an equally long list of published procedures that have been developed for the purpose. Starting around 1890, for example, Trendelenburg carried out ligation of the saphenofemoral junction without stripping the great saphenous vein. Ligation and stripping of the great saphenous vein later emerged as the most promising procedure, but even this method did not lead to complete freedom from recurrences.

Increasingly aggressive ligation with stripping also did not lead to the desired results. Even in 2000, a recurrence rate of 30% in patients treated over a 35-year period was reported (Fischer et al. 2000). In 2002, Mumme et al. reported on quality problems in primary procedures, with 66.9% of procedures for recurrences being required due to incomplete primary interventions (Mumme et al. 2002).

In the early 2000's, endoluminal methods such as VNUS Closure™ (radiofrequency ablation, RFA), in which a high-frequency catheter is used to release heat in the insufficient vein, leading to thermal damage to the vessel wall and secondarily to contraction of the vessel wall and adhesion of the vessel; and endoluminal laser treatment of varicose veins were the first examples of a new generation of nonsurgical techniques for the treatment of varicosis.

These procedures call into question several fundamental pillars of traditional venous surgery that were previously thought to be incontrovertible:

- With the exception of an insufficient saphenous vein, none of the branches entering in the area of the saphenofemoral junction is treated or occluded.
- The treatment induces artificial thrombosis in the vein being treated in the vicinity of the saphenofemoral junction.

After more than 10 years, various randomized studies have now provided good evidence of the advantages of endoluminal procedures in comparison with stripping. The most significant differences for patients are:

- A shorter period of convalescence until complete health is restored
- Reduced postoperative symptoms
- Improved quality of life

3.4.2.1 Technique

Endoluminal obliteration procedures are all based on the same principle. With continuous ultrasound guidance, a catheter (VNUS®) or glass fiber (laser) is introduced into the insufficient vessel from the distal location and placed in the superficial venous system near the relevant deep junction, or at the ostium of the insufficient perforating vein. While the catheter or glass fiber is being withdrawn, heat is released into the vein. However, the actual mechanism of effect varies.

RF VNUS Closure™

In the VNUS Closure™ procedure, there should be no blood left in the vessel if possible, and wrapping with Esmarch bandages (VNUS Closure™) or an extreme Trendelenburg position is therefore required. The generator in the RFA procedure produces microwaves that are released by electrodes at the tip of the catheter into the venous wall, where they set water molecules in a state of increasing oscillation; the catheter tip should therefore be placed as close as possible to the venous wall. The actual temperature is measured at the site of action, compared with the target value selected by the operator, and the energy is controlled using a control circuit in such a way that the temperature is held constant for a specific time. The energy produced by the generator is thus released in the form of heat on the wall of the vein, where it creates an immediate contraction effect due to thermal damage to collagen and denaturing of the endothelium, followed by inflammatory and degenerative processes that lead to occlusion of the vein and scar formation.

The hardware used for the catheter procedure (RFA/VNUS Closure™) remained unchanged for many years and is basically only available from a single manufacturer (VNUS™ Medical Technologies, Inc.) (Fig. 3-4).

The catheter technique has been undergoing further development for several years now, with the introduction of the ClosureFast® catheter. Disadvantages of the traditional Closure® procedure inherent to the method included the much longer time required for the closure procedure, along with the bloodlessness required in the vessel. With the development of the new catheter, these two disadvantages have been resolved.

Instead of delicate electrodes, the ClosureFast™ catheter has a heating element 7 cm long at its tip, with which sequential treatment (i.e., no longer continuous) is applied in 7-cm steps with minor overlapping (95–120°C, 20-s treatment interval). This requires:

- The generator, which produces the defined energy released at the catheter tip in the form of microwaves
- The catheter (Closure™ 4F and 8F, ClosureFast™ 7F) (Fig. 3-5)
- An introducer set

All three components are normally supplied by the manufacturer, usually in complete sets with various lengths and diameters. A (color) ultrasound device with a high-resolution transducer (preferably 7.5 MHz or more) is also needed.

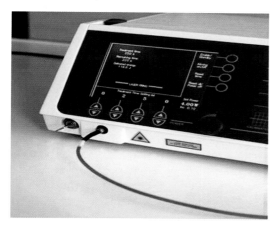

Fig. 3-4 Diode laser.

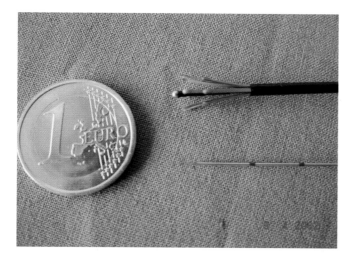

Fig. 3-5 Size comparison: an 8F VNUS Closure™ catheter and a 600-μm laser fiber tip in a metal sheath.

Laser (EVL, ELVES, ELT)

In contrast to the ClosureFast® procedure, it is absolutely necessary for blood to be present in the vessel (at least with lasers that work with a wavelength adapted to hemoglobin). When lasers are used, hemoglobin acts as a chromophore, absorbing the monochrome (usually) infrared light produced by the connected laser and thereby producing massive heat. The actual temperature is not precisely known, but may be up to 1000°C in the plasma, although it already declines exponentially even after only a few millimeters. The components of the blood evaporate in the form of billions of tiny bubbles that damage the endothelium in such a way that an artificial thrombotic occlusion is produced.

While the VNUS Closure™ procedure remained unchanged for many years, lively competition developed among the laser manufacturers and led not only to a large number of companies entering the market, but also to divergent philosophies regarding the optimal wavelength and energy for the energy source. In the early phase, lasers with a wavelength of 940 nm were mainly used, but devices with a wide range of wavelengths from 810 m to approximately 1200 nm became available later as well. Pulsed applications are in competition with applications involving continuous energy release, and energies of between 8 W and 35 W are in use. The following components are required:

- A laser (usually diode) that uses various energies to produce monochrome light (e.g., 810, 940, 980, 1064 nm with Nd:Y, 1064 nm with Nd:YAG) at the laser-fiber tip in the vessel
- Suitable laser fiber
- Suitable introducer set

The first three components are usually supplied by the manufacturer, with the laser fiber and set being available with various lengths and diameters. It should be noted that individual diode laser manufacturers (probably for competition reasons) ensure, by modifying the adapter used to connect the laser fiber to the diode laser, that only fibers manufactured by their own company can be used with the device concerned. Other items needed are:

- An ultrasound device, preferably color duplex, with accessories allowing constant sterile monitoring of the position of the catheter or glass fiber during the procedure
- Protective glasses for everyone in the operating room (Fig. 3-6), including the patient

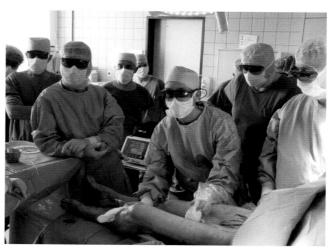

Fig. 3-6 Protective glasses must always be worn during a laser operation.

Note: When class 3B and 4 lasers are used (in accordance with European standard EN 60825-1) or 3b and 4 (in accordance with German standard DIN VDI 0837), a laser protection officer must be appointed in writing by the company. The company can also carry out this duty itself. The basis for the appointment is paragraph 6 of professional association regulation B 2. Laser protection officers must have adequate specialist knowledge. The laser protection officer must regularly check that the emergency shut-off switch is working and must clearly mark laser protection areas. Scientific studies have shown that the eyelid closure reflex (which usually occurs within 0.25 s; longer irradiation damages the eye) was adequate in fewer than 20% of individuals tested. It cannot usually be assumed, therefore, that the eyelid closure reflex will be able to protect the eyes.

It is therefore necessary to put up signs indicating laser operations, as well as standardized illuminated signs in front of the operating room that must be switched on when the laser is being used. Highly reflective surfaces in the operating room and instruments with highly reflective surfaces are also unsuitable.

Endovenous bipolar radiofrequency-induced thermotherapy (RFITT)

Another procedure for endoluminal thermoablation of varicose veins has been available from the Olympus/Celon companies since about 2007 and is known as endovenous bipolar radiofrequency-induced thermotherapy (RFITT). In RFITT (also called the Celon® method), the wall of the vein is heated using high-frequency alternating current (creating a microwave effect similar to that of VNUS®), thereby causing tissue shrinkage. The difference between this and the other procedures lies in the reduced thermal burden on the tissue structures (ca. 85–95°C; VNUS®, ClosureFast® 100–120°Cl; laser 700–900°C).

In combination with continuous impedance measurement, the application time in the venous wall can be technically optimized. The operator receives information about the optimal area of application via an acoustic signal. Tumescent anesthesia, as in the other procedures, is not necessary.

At the time of writing (early 2012), widespread experience in hundreds of patients confirmed the anticipated success of the method, particularly with regard to heat-related side effects, but a randomized study comparing the procedures was not yet available.

Steam catheter

The Gutmann company, the distributor in Germany, has been offering a new catheter development involving steam vein sclerosis (SVS) since around 2009.

The technique is also based on the principle of achieving vascular occlusion by causing thermal damage to the tissue. In the SVS procedure, however, the heat required is delivered to the vessel in impulses via pressurized steam. A compressor forces small amounts of sterile water out of an attached reservoir toward the catheter tip. On the way there, the droplets are heated to 120°C so that small, almost spherical clouds can be sprayed at the catheter tip from two diametrically arranged microholes to directly heat the vein wall (as in scalding).

The theoretical advantages of this are obvious, since only water is left over after the "burning." In fact the hot steam immediately condenses on the much cooler venous wall and is transported away in the form of water drops. Toxic or allergic side effects are therefore excluded.

In addition, the method also has the advantage that it is not in principle limited by the diameter of the vessel (e.g., approximately 12 mm with ClosureFast). The nearly spherical steam cloud can even reliably close severely dilated vessels with diameters of 25 mm. Also worth mentioning is the option of using the method in large side branches; the extremely thin catheter can be introduced into the varix via a Braun cannula, for example, and can occlude the side branch with one or two shots of steam.

However, extreme care is also required with this apparently "ecological" technique. The pressurized steam transports a substantial amount of energy. The catheter tip must never be placed too close to the deep vein. In addition, no "hot water" can be allowed to travel in a retrograde direction from the puncture site. This has happened in two patients, who suffered very circumscribed scalding of the skin (although it was completely reversible).

In addition, the discrepancy in weight between the feather-light catheter and the nearly 500 g heavy connecting cable, which takes some getting used to, also gives rise to some potential difficulty. The slightest change in the position of the heavy cable can lead to substantial unintentional dislocation of the catheter tip and makes cautious handling necessary.

Unfortunately, the manufacturer has so far failed to have the method evaluated in a research study in comparison with any of the established procedures. The company has also shown few signs of allowing any of the urgently needed improvements suggested by users

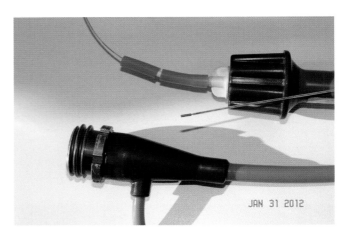

Fig. 3-7 SVS steam catheter—tricky: a microcatheter with a maxi-sized connecting cable.

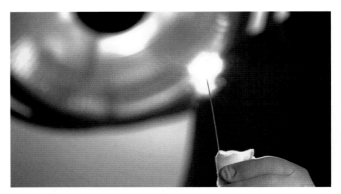

Fig. 3-8 SVS steam catheter: a cloud of tensed steam at 120°C.

to be incorporated into serial production. In addition to the author, several other users have also reported that the metal catheter tip was already buckled when it was taken out of the packaging, and in one case even became detached from the catheter (in the tissue).

Despite this, the author's experience with approximately 100 applications has been generally positive. The rates of satisfaction and occlusion are similar to those with the other methods, so that it would be regrettable if the steam catheter were to fail due to a lack of product optimization.

ClariVein

The latest new development on the fiercely competitive market for endoluminal venous surgical procedures is the ClariVein catheter (for scleromechanical varix obliteration). The technique basically combines two familiar treatment approaches: an endoluminal catheter technique in combination with a sclerotherapy procedure, with a sclerosant (Aethoxysclerol) being applied via a narrow-lumen catheter at the site of effect.

To increase the safety of the chemotoxic occlusion process, the procedure's originators at Yale University (New Haven, CT) developed a special feature: the catheter contains a minimally thin steel wire, the slightly angled tip of which can be extended at the site of action and rotated using a flange-mounted electrical drive on the handpiece. This roughens the intima in order to prepare the way for safe occlusion using Aethoxysclerol, which is introduced in a dosed fashion via a syringe that is also mounted on the handpiece. At the same time, the rotating wire atomizes the sclerosant like a whisk in order to distribute it evenly.

Although the technique appears to be similar to the endoluminal procedures mentioned above, there are considerable differences. This is truly a procedure that allows "lunchtime surgery." Whereas the goal for most surgeons is to relieve the patient in a single session not only of the cause of varicosis (eliminating the reflux segment) but also to carry out additional, usually microsurgical, procedures to remove visible varices, with ClariVein it is actually only the reflux that is treated. It is assumed that the associated varices will resolve entirely or partly in the majority of the patients, so that there is either no need for follow-up treatment or it can be carried out with sclerotherapy after a few months. This means that those patients in

whom normalization of intravenous epifascial pressures does actually lead to normal findings will be able to benefit maximally from ClariVein. (Other patients will require subsequent measures in one form or another.) The procedure only requires local anesthesia in the area of the puncture site—at least 2 mL mepivacaine (Scandicain) 2%—and is otherwise pain-free. The rotating wire is only perceived by the patient as a vibration in the tissue.

In addition, patients can put on a class 2 thigh compression stocking immediately after the operation and can leave the building and return to normal everyday life 30 minutes after the procedure—which patients who have received this treatment find remarkable.

The method is a new one, and findings confirmed by independent research are not yet available. Despite this, initial observations by the author over a 6-month period in 25 patients, as well as approximately 1000 cases treated in the Netherlands, show excellent results, raising hopes for the future.

The technique still requires a few detailed improvements (e.g., optimized attachment of the syringe to the handpiece, adequate disposal facilities for the batteries, and a market-rate price (currently approx. € 400 as a single-use article), but the manufacturer appears to be cooperative and there are therefore grounds for hope.

By contrast, there is little hope of health-care funding bodies accepting the costs, and in a period of declining resources even private insurance companies have declined payment. This could lead to a method that has considerable advantages being unnecessarily limited, which would be particularly regrettable in view of the economic damage resulting from working hours unnecessarily lost through varicosities.

3.4.2.2 Indication for the procedure

The indications for an endoluminal procedure are the same as those for conventional surgical procedures. If a surgical operation is not indicated, an endoluminal procedure is usually also not indicated.

3.4.2.3 Preliminary examinations

The preliminary examinations are also identical with those used for an open surgical procedure. However, the endoluminal surgeon should if possible carry out detailed duplex ultrasonography personally in order to assess whether the ultrasound anatomy makes an endoluminal procedure possible at all.

Unfavorable conditions for catheter and laser procedures are:
- Very short occlusion lengths
- Extremely tortuous vessels
- Funnels after previous operations
- Doubled and inaccessible vessels (Rabe et al. 2003)

3.4.2.4 Patient information

The patient information discussion is usually more extensive than is necessary for ligation with stripping. Although the endoluminal procedure can now be described without reservations as an established alternative to resection, the choice of procedure should be left to the patient—not least because of the considerable flaws in reimbursement for catheter and laser operations resulting from current

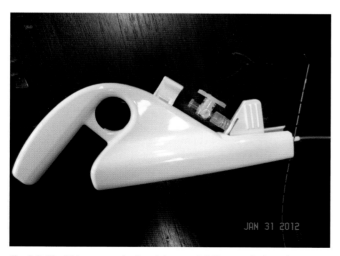

JAN 31 2012

Fig. 3-9 ClariVein: a complex handpiece and delicate technique, but gentle and effective.

health-care policies. For example, endoluminal procedures with very few exceptions are not currently reimbursed by public health-insurance companies. In addition to a standardized information sheet for ligation with stripping, it can therefore be recommended that a separate information sheet for the endoluminal procedure should be provided, as well as information about the cost and reimbursement situation.

To provide information about potential specific side effects and risks of the endoluminal part of the procedure, it is indispensable to mention:

- Heat injury to the skin (in particular) due to the heat applied
- Areas of hematoma due to perforation of the vessel resulting from the heat
- Heat-related neural irritation, particularly with procedures in the area of the great saphenous vein
- Possible incomplete occlusion or reopening of the vessel after the procedure, which may lead to renewed reflux

More general, purely statistical risks include:

- Inflammation, wound healing disturbances
- Bleeding complications (depending on anticoagulation or antiplatelet treatment)
- Thrombosis and pulmonary embolism due to the patient's individual risk profile (e.g., a known congenital coagulation defect)

The discussion should also touch on:

- Information about prophylaxis against deep vein thrombosis (physical and drug measures)
- Explanations of why drug prophylaxis against thrombosis is not necessary (including written documentation)
- Heparin-specific information (e.g., heparin-induced thrombocytopenia)
- Cosmetic considerations (postoperative development of spider veins varices, matting, pigmentation)

The question of what to do if the laser procedure cannot be completed intraoperatively should also be discussed. In this case, the patient's preference needs to have been defined and documented before the procedure—e.g., abandoning the procedure and switching to a different one. Alternative procedures therefore also have to be discussed beforehand as well.

3.4.2.5 Perioperative prophylaxis against thromboembolism

The extent and magnitude of perioperative prophylaxis against deep vein thrombosis should basically follow the recommendations of the interdisciplinary guideline on perioperative prophylaxis against thrombosis.

Low-molecular-weight heparin or a similar preparation at a prophylactic dosage for approximately 7 days should therefore be sufficient for the requirements if indicated.

There is no current evidence that it is absolutely necessary to administer perioperative prophylaxis against thrombosis independently of the individual risk—i.e., purely because of the endoluminal procedure as such.

3.4.2.6 Anesthetic procedure

There are also no relevant differences from the traditional surgical technique with regard to the anesthetic procedure. In the author's view, it is best to follow the patient's own preference. Conversely, this means that the surgical unit must be capable of offering all of the customary anesthetic procedures, so that medical recommendations are not based on a logistic or financial rationale.

Local anesthesia

Classic local anesthesia for a strictly circumscribed area of anesthesia is not really possible.

Tumescent anesthesia

Tumescent anesthesia is regarded as the procedure of choice by many authors. The combined effect of anesthesia, compression of the vessel, and perivascular cooling or isolation is regarded as ideal. This form of anesthesia can certainly be recommended in patients who have no difficulties about being conscious during the operation.

Tumescent anesthesia is unquestionably an elegant approach if it has also been agreed between the patient and surgeon preoperatively that only the proximal reflux segment should be closed, and that one should then wait to see whether the dependent side branches regress sufficiently for there to be a chance of dispensing with a second procedure, or of sclerosing the remaining branches. However, if the patient is rather anxious and does not wish to be aware of anything during the procedure, that represents an argument against tumescent anesthesia. Tumescent anesthesia can also not be recommended if one is trying to use a single session both to close the proximal reflux segment and also to eliminate possibly substantial side branch varicosity with a supplementary procedure at the same time.

Regional and conduction anesthesia

The endoluminal procedure can of course also be carried out with conduction anesthesia or spinal anesthesia. However, this eliminates the various advantages associated with immediate mobilization of the patient after the operation (i.e., prophylaxis against thrombosis, rapid discharge, improved quality of life).

Prophylaxis against thrombosis and spinal anesthesia

The guideline on regional anesthesia near the spine during thrombosis prophylaxis/antithrombotic therapy was revised quite some time ago. According to the guideline, not only placement of an epidural catheter but also its removal are capable of inducing bleeding. When a therapeutic dosage of heparin is being administered, this type of anesthesia is still contraindicated. Otherwise, a delay after the last dose of the antithrombotic agent is recommended. Using fondaparinux (Arixtra®) instead of a low-molecular-weight heparin might improve the situation. In accordance with approval requirements, fondaparinux is basically administered 6–8 h postoperatively, with no reduction in the quality of DVT prophylaxis.

General anesthesia

In patients who have reservations about the above procedures and who would prefer to be unconscious during the operation, general anesthesia is the method of choice. General anesthesia can be expressly recommended if closure of the reflux segment as well as any dependent varicosis are to be carried out in a single session by combining two or more procedures (with endoluminal laser proximally, distal dissection of a perforating vein, and microphlebotomy of side branches).

3.4.2.7 Operation

In the author's view, the aim in any procedure for an insufficient and varicose vein should always be to simultaneously eliminate the reflux segment, while also removing all other relevant variceal findings in the form of side branches or insufficient perforating veins. A combination of several procedures in the same session is therefore usually carried out.

However, it should also be mentioned that many centers act on the philosophy that one should use the minimal procedures possible. Attempts are therefore made to achieve regression of dependent varices by closing the proximal reflux segment, and this is successful in some cases. However, if it does not succeed, another procedure—or even a series of further procedures—will be necessary.

Setup

For quality management purposes and to provide a reproducible process quality, the setup for the procedure is always the same, no matter which leg or which vein is involved.

If right-handed, the surgeon stands at the patient's right and opposite to the ultrasound device. The sheath and catheter/laser fiber are introduced continuously, with the transducer held in the left hand. Before this, one should have an approximate idea of how far the puncture site is from the junction region so that, as a double safety measure, it can be ensured that the catheter/glass fiber tip is not inadvertently advanced too deep (into the common femoral artery or popliteal artery), as this could have fatal consequences.

Operating time

The learning curve here is fairly flat. It is probably only after 100–200 procedures that one has experienced all of the possible complications and pitfalls. During the initial period, the procedure can be extremely difficult and prolonged in the following situations:

- Corpulent patients
- Veins located deeply
- Even only slight tortuosity
- Very small shifts in the course of the vein

With increasing routine and confidence, the user is gradually able to reduce the length of the purely luminal part of the procedure to approximately 15 min, depending on the length of the vascular segment to be obliterated and the type of anesthesia being used. The more conventional part, with microphlebotomy, foam sclerotherapy, or dissection of perforating veins is additional to this, so that a block of 45–60 min can be generally assumed.

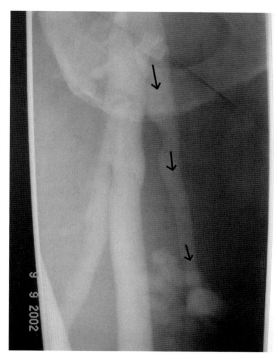

Fig. 3-10 Short vessel stump: an unfavorable indication, particularly at the start of the learning curve.

Procedure

After cleaning of the extremity, it is draped in the same way as during stripping, so that the inguinal region/popliteal region can be reached without problems (with the transducer). Mapping of the vein being treated should then always be repeated. It is particularly important for the quality of the procedure and the results to recognize or not to overlook any limiting factors:

- Doubled insufficient vessels
- Large insufficient perforating veins
- Tortuosity of the vessel
- Ectatic vascular segments
- Large side branches with strong inflow

Overlooking any unfavorable anatomy or initial situations can nullify what was thought at first to be a good procedural result (Fig. 3-10). When several insufficient vessels are present, for example, it must therefore always be ensured that they will all be accessible with the catheter or laser fiber. If only one is obliterated, then "recurrent" varices will predictably develop.

Access routes

Following mapping, access to the insufficient vein is obtained in the distal leg. After the sheath or set has been introduced, the catheter or laser fiber is then advanced proximally with ultrasound guidance.

Seldinger technique

Once one has learned how to puncture *one* vessel with ultrasound guidance, one is able to do the same with *any* vessel. The principle when obtaining access to a peripheral vein is identical to that in the subclavian or femoral artery:

- Oblique puncture with ultrasound guidance
- Introduction of a guidewire
- Advancing a size-adapted sheath over the wire
- Removal of the wire
- Introduction and placement of the catheter or laser fiber

Direct access/phlebotomy

Alternatively, direct access to the vessel under vision is possible with a microsurgical phlebotomy. The vessel, at an ideal site located using duplex ultrasonography, is raised above the skin level via a 2-mm micro-access with the appropriate instruments, and the sheath is then introduced into the vein under direct vision.

The advantage of this method clearly lies in the ability to ligate the affected vein distally, so that blood flow from the distal direction, with all the disruptive side effects from the heat-treated vessel, is minimized or stopped. Here again, the learning curve is fairly flat. It takes time to learn how to expose a deep-lying vein quickly even in voluminous legs.

On the other hand, the author's own experience in some 1700 operations shows that this access route is always possible, in contrast to the Seldinger technique.

3.4.2.8   Great saphenous vein/small saphenous vein

The tip of the laser fiber/catheter should be positioned approximately 1.5–2.0 cm from the junctional region (Fig. 3-11). Ideally, junctional branches that drain distally or pudendally should be left untouched. Unobstructed outflow from these vessels is an important side effect that prevents any thrombus present from spreading beyond the level of the end of the great saphenous vein into the junction and thus the deep veins. The catheter/laser fiber is withdrawn during heat application in accordance with the manufacturer's recommendations:

- VNUS Closure™: 15 s after reaching a stable temperature of approximately 85°C, the catheter is withdrawn at a speed of approximately 2–3 cm/min. The actual temperature should not deviate by more than 3°C below the target value.
- ClosureFast™: 20 s after a stable temperature of 120°C is reached, the catheter is left for 20 s each in one position and then pulled approximately 6.5 cm further, corresponding to a marking on the catheter, so that the next 7-cm segment can be treated with an overlap of about 0.5 cm.
- ELV: the basic question when a laser is used for endoluminal occlusion of an insufficient vessel is how much energy should be applied.

It is not difficult to follow the fairly straightforward facts involved in the effect: the greater the energy applied, the greater the potential side effects, and the less energy, the fewer the side effects—although the risk of incomplete occlusion and rapid recanalization will then be greater. Complicating matters is the fact that it is not just the amount of energy applied in total by the end of an operation that plays a role, but also the amount applied per square centimeter during the procedure. A withdrawal speed that is too rapid may lead to too low a dosage in some segments, but this may be concealed by increased amounts released in other segments due to slower withdrawal there.

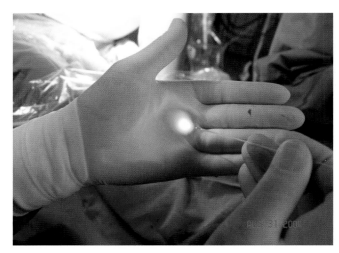

Fig. 3-11 Testing the laser fiber before the operation. An intact fiber must always produce a circular dot of light from the pilot laser.

In the search for an optimal procedure, some authors have advocated using a constant energy density of approximately 80 J/cm, with good postoperative and short-term results. Proebstle et al. (2006) proposed that the energy dosage should be adjusted to the size of the vessel diameter. The standardized protocol used by the present author involves the release of 100 J/cm in the first 10 cm of a vessel, followed by 50 J/cm each per further centimeter of length. This type of energy application is based on the following considerations:

- The first few centimeters proximally have to be securely occluded in order to resist reflux permanently.
- The vascular diameter declines from proximal to distal.

In this way, the total energy amounts administered in one leg after a typical great saphenous vein occlusion over a length of 30 cm will be approximately 2000–2500 J.

3.4.2.9   Insufficient perforating veins

It is important to treat insufficient perforating veins in order to heal ulcers in their surroundings, but the acceptability of subfascial endoscopic perforate surgery (SEPS) is declining. Endoluminal catheter or laser occlusion is therefore becoming an attractive alternative. In London, Whiteley et al. (2003) reported on treatment with a VNUS Closure™ catheter in 770 insufficient perforating veins in 506 legs, with an occlusion rate of 76% after 2 years. However, this approach represents a fairly advanced form of endoluminal therapy. Treatment of insufficient perforating veins is thus not a procedure for beginners. The ultrasound skills the operator requires are even greater than those needed for treatment of the great or small saphenous veins. A very good capacity for three-dimensional thinking is required. The distance from the deep vein should be at least 5 mm, although there have been reports of a 3-mm margin being used without deep vein thromboses occurring (Noppeney and Nüllen 2005). The procedure has limitations if the course of the perforating veins is not very straight.

3.4.2.10 Pitfalls

Incorrect puncture/poor positioning

Incorrect puncture of the vessel is not initially a problem specific to the endoluminal procedure. However, there may be considerable damage if incorrect positioning of the catheter/laser fiber is not noticed. Particularly in corpulent patients, the differences in ultrasound impedance between the vessel wall and the catheter/fiber, for example, are often very slight. They are therefore difficult to distinguish and resemble those in the various layers of adipose tissue. After a tumescent anesthetic has been injected, precise identification of a laser-fiber tip, for example, often becomes almost impossible. This means that it is extremely important to ensure continuous localization of the instrument inside the lumen, and the high degree of ultrasound skill required of the surgeon is therefore understandable.

Penetration depth

Most of the laser-fiber sets available from manufacturers include introducer elements (sheaths) that have length markings with a centimeter scale, although more inexpensive versions may not include this. Particularly with the latter type, additional marking of the penetration depth of the sheath—e.g., using a sterile plaster strip—may be helpful, as it mechanically prevents the sheath from being advanced to a deeper level than previously measured.

Energy dosage

Particularly with the laser, it is important to note and check the correct adjustment of the device. Even when the method is correctly carried out, the incidence of extensive hematomas due to the vascular wall being perforated by a laser-fiber tip that is in contact with it cannot be reduced below a statistical minimum. In the vicinity of the saphenofemoral junction, inadvertent application of excessively high energy involves potentially severe collateral damage in the deep veins.

In slim individuals, excess energy in the area of the great saphenous vein, which rests on the adductor muscles, can cause severe soft-tissue pain.

Every user's protocol list should therefore include a check-off item to ensure that the energy adjustment is verified before the laser is activated.

Decoupling/fiber break

In most laser-fiber systems, the laser fiber and the guide tube are connected with a Luer-Lok seal. Nevertheless, attention is needed to ensure that the two systems do not become uncoupled intraoperatively. This would mean that applying traction to the laser fiber would leave the tip of the fiber in the sheath, and the energy released would evaporate without effect and potentially perforate the sheath. The procedure would inevitably fail (Fig. 3-12).

If a fiber break between the laser and the patient is not noticed, there is a high risk of retinal injury due to nondirectional incident laser light (Fig. 3-11). Experience shows that laser-protection glasses are not worn in some operating rooms. As long as the fiber tip is inside the vein, nothing can actually happen. However, if the fiber outside the vein, between the diode laser and the patient, becomes kinked

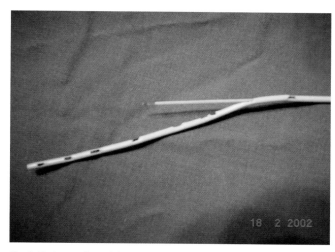

Fig. **3-12** Decoupling of the laser fiber and sheath.

and breaks without it being noticed, the scattered radiation that escapes will pose a threat to the eyes. At an energy level of 12 W, a diode laser produces 105 times as much energy as is needed to cause permanent damage to the retina.

Double veins/side branches

Venous reflux in a doubled vein that is not treated inevitably leads to failure. Venous inflow from very strong side branches that lie below the puncture site after access is obtained with the Seldinger technique, and which are not selectively ligated, can lead to inadequate surgical results.

During intraoperative vein mapping, all of the side branches have to be noted and selectively dealt with. The same applies to insufficient perforating veins along the course of the occlusion segment.

3.4.2.11 Recurrence

There is no standard definition of a recurrence following variceal surgery. After an endoluminal procedure, the term "recurrence" actually describes renewed reflux into a vessel that has not been occluded, or only partially, or which has completely or partially recanalized.

If the operated vessel is not completely closed or partly recanalizes, although it does not show any pathological reflux, then no further treatment is initially needed, and only monitoring of the course is required. However, if there is a need for a secondary corrective procedure due to renewed reflux (a "servicing operation"), then the present author believes the greatest advantages of the endoluminal procedure in comparison with ligation and stripping come into play:

- The secondary procedure has the same level of risk as a primary procedure.
- All treatment options are still available, with no change.

Among the author's patients, a secondary intervention is needed in approximately 4–5% of patients who have undergone the procedure. Complete recanalization or complete nonocclusion are the exceptions. A combination of proximal duplex-guided foam block sclerosis and distal microphlebectomy has proved to be a very elegant approach in such cases. As the insufficient vessel usually becomes contorted during the first operation as a result of the heat, and shows septa or stenoses, a second endoluminal treatment is no longer possible. A regular ligation would also theoretically be possible at the same level of risk as in a primary procedure, but this can practically be avoided. However, if a crossectomy is unavoidable in exceptional cases, the operator can expect that the energy released in the vicinity of the vessel during the first endoluminal procedure will have led to adhesions similar to those in phlebitis, so that blunt dissection will have its limits.

3.4.2.12   Follow-up

Patients who have undergone catheter or laser operations do not require any special form of follow-up. Treatment is based on compression therapy, with a compression dressing placed in the operating room and a class 2 compression stocking being worn for a few weeks. The need for postoperative prophylaxis against thrombosis depends on the individual patient's risk staging (see above). A standardized and consistently followed protocol is needed to allow reliable prediction of the quality of the processes and results of the procedures. The protocol used by the present author, for example, includes clinical check-ups and ultrasound checks on days 3, 14, and 42, and thereafter every 6 months for 3 years.

3.4.2.13   Conclusions and prospects

A conclusive evaluation was not possible when the first edition of this book was published. In the meantime, however, considerably larger data sets are becoming available from constantly growing numbers of treatments. In the USA in 2010, for example, approximately 80% of all varix operations were being carried out endoluminally. In the Netherlands, where the health-care system envisages reimbursement for the diagnosis (varicosis) independently of the method of treatment used, approximately 1000 patients in Eindhoven were treated with good results within a 12-month period using the ClariVein technique, which still lacks validated research. The fact is that all of the methods are associated with almost identical outcome results. The efficacy, side effects and patient satisfaction rates are comparable and only vary relatively slightly.

For various reasons—and partly because the term "laser" is much more acceptable and attractive for therapists and patients—laser treatment enjoyed a dazzling and triumphant progress in comparison with the radiofrequency catheter at the turn of this century. In the meantime, however, with the ClosureFast® catheter, Covidien has been able to recover ground that was lost.

It is hoped that reason will ultimately triumph and that the Federal Joint Committee (*Gemeinsamer Bundesausschuss,* GBA) in Germany and funding bodies will be motivated by the positive long-term results with all of the endoluminal procedures to include these procedures in their catalogues and provide adequate reimbursement for them in the outpatient environment, so that less well-off, non-private patients will also be able to benefit from the advantages of these methods.

3.4.3   Surgical treatment

The quality of variceal surgery is capable of improvement—and the first step here is for surgeons to ask themselves whether they personally are able to give this hemodynamically significant alteration the attention and care it deserves. Varicectomy needs to be raised from the side role to which it has been relegated, to the status of a serious operation. The procedure, dubbed as a "typical beginner's operation," must certainly not be transferred to young assistants for them to use it to practice their surgical skills at their own responsibility. After all, there have been occasional case reports on extirpation of the superficial femoral artery during varicectomy.

Varicectomy is mainly an operation on insufficiency points. However, if the surgeon does not also act as a well-informed examiner preoperatively, the probability of inadequate surgical treatment increases. It is the surgeon's responsibility to carry out preoperative color duplex ultrasonography, in order to be able to carry out the procedure in a stage-appropriate way from the anatomical and functional viewpoints.

3.4.3.1   Indication

When there is confirmed insufficiency of the junction or saphenous veins, the following classic symptoms are reported:

- Feeling of heaviness
- Congestion symptoms
- Tendency to swell
- Itching
- Tendency to develop cramp
- Aesthetic impairment

In most cases, these symptoms alone justify the indication for staged surgery. This applies both to young patients and also to the elderly who are unsatisfied with compression treatment alone.

Absolute indications are:

- Trophic disturbances in the skin
- Varicophlebitis
- History of variceal bleeding
- Varicose ulcer on the leg

Absolute contraindications:

- Fresh deep thrombosis
- Higher-grade arterial occlusive disease

Relative contraindications:

- Post-thrombotic disease pictures
- General condition
- Extent of obesity and potential problems involved

Preoperative healing of a varicose ulcer is not required. Perioperative administration of antibiotics is useful. When the indication for this elective procedure is being assessed, consideration should also be given to whether it should be carried out on an outpatient or inpatient basis. Factors that play a role here are:

- Comorbid conditions
- Risk factors
- Quality of communication with the patient and adequate compliance

- Patient's social environment
- Potential anesthesia problems
- Patient's preferences and sense of safety

3.4.3.2 Preliminary examinations

The standard preoperative examination requires an imaging procedure. Color duplex ultrasonography is currently adequate in the hands of an experienced examiner in most cases. This method is usually capable of identifying the areas of insufficiency and special anatomic characteristics. If the imaging does not offer the level of safety required—e.g., due to post-thrombotic changes—then phlebography is indicated in addition.

Light reflection rheography or phlebodynamometry can provide information about hemodynamic effects. In addition, a partial blood count and coagulation status, as well as a chest x-ray (as specified by the anesthetist) are required.

3.4.3.3 Patient information

Sufficient time should be assigned to the information discussion, as a confidence-building measure. Up-to-date information sheets are always helpful, but they should be supplemented with information about specific individual considerations, including a sketch if necessary. The discussion should provide information about:

- Inflammation and wound healing disturbances
- Bleeding complications (depending on whether anticoagulation or antiplatelet treatment has been given)
- Thrombosis and pulmonary embolism, as well as the patient's individual risk profile (is there a known congenital coagulation defect?)
- Information about prophylaxis against risk factors (physical and medical methods)
- Explanation and documentation of why drug treatment for prophylaxis against thrombosis is not necessary
- Otherwise: information about heparin (including heparin-induced thrombocytopenia)
- Recurrent varicosis
- Nerve lesions (saphenous nerve, sural nerve) and their clinical effects
- Cosmetic considerations (postoperative development of spider veins, matting, pigmentations)
- Cicatricial keloid, pigmentations

3.4.3.4 Perioperative prophylaxis against thromboembolism

A standardized approach is not advisable. The range of perioperative complications extends from heparin-induced thrombocytopenia (HIT), on the one hand, to fulminant pulmonary embolism on the other. The main agents used are low-molecular-weight heparins, as well as synthetic preparations (fondaparinux) more recently.

The guidelines published by the various societies emphasize individualized risk stratification. Each patient requires individual attention relative to specific individual risk factors and the surgical procedure. The *expositional* risk has to be distinguished from the *dispositional* risk here. Expositional risk results from the extent and duration of the planned procedure and the surgical trauma. Dispositional risk describes the patient's individual starting point (including age, body mass index, hormone treatment, internal medicine risks, immobility, congenital coagulation defects). During the information discussion, the general nature and risks of drug treatment for prophylaxis against thrombosis are mentioned and noted in writing. Low-molecular-weight heparins, the HIT risk with which is much lower than that of unfractionated heparin, are typically used today. When there is manifest renal insufficiency, attention should be given to the risk of accumulation.

Depending on the drug being used, prophylaxis can also be started postoperatively (with fondaparinux). The incidence of postoperative thromboses is no higher with this agent in comparison with preoperative administration of low-molecular-weight heparins, but the incidence of surgery-related hematomas is thought to be lower. Prolonged drug prophylaxis must be continued until an unobstructed gait is achieved. Other usual postoperative measures such as compression therapy and early mobilization are, of course, also carried out.

3.4.3.5 Anesthetic procedure

The anesthetic procedure should be selected in accordance with the extent of the planned operation and the perioperative situation. In addition, the patient's preferences and ability to cope with events in the operating room also need to be taken into account.

Local anesthesia

Local anesthesia appears appropriate for limited treatment of a side branch or perforating vein. In slim patients, it may also be possible to carry out a ligation with local anesthesia.

Tumescent anesthesia

Tumescent anesthesia is a widely used method for liposuction in plastic surgery. For vein surgery, it appears to be a comfortable form of anesthesia with a low complication rate and a high level of patient satisfaction. The longer preparation time appears to be a disadvantage. In addition, absorption of the fluid occurs in the operating field and potential bleeding sources may be more difficult to identify. However, the infiltrated fluid makes extraction easier.

Regional anesthesia

In the form of spinal anesthesia, this is the method many patients prefer as an alternative to general anesthesia. Administering concomitant sedation increases patient comfort. Disadvantages include the prolonged period of immobility and postoperative monitoring needed, as well as potentially delayed urinary disturbances (after the patient has returned home). If the operation is carried out on an outpatient basis, spontaneous urination must be achieved prior to discharge.

Thrombosis prophylaxis and spinal anesthesia

An adequate time delay for perioperative thrombosis prophylaxis needs to be observed when spinal anesthesia is used. Unfractionated heparin should be administered on the evening before the operation.

General anesthesia

Intubation anesthesia and anesthesia with a laryngeal mask may be mentioned here. Patients' fears about "not waking up any more" are sometimes greater than their fear of the operation itself.

3.4.3.6 Operation

The aim of surgical treatment is to improve venous hemodynamics by:
- Eliminating the insufficiency points
- Removing the diseased venous segments in a stage-appropriate procedure

If complete saphenous varicosity is present, complete ligation of the great and small saphenous veins near the ostium is indicated. If there is incomplete saphenous varicosity, interruption of the proximal insufficiency point—e.g., the perforating vein of the adductor canal (Dodd perforator)—is required.

3.4.3.7 Great saphenous vein

The individual steps are as follows:
- Transverse inguinal incision lateral to the adductor insertion
- Identification and mainly blunt dissection close to the great saphenous vein, while protecting the lymphatic vessels
- Identification of the saphenofemoral junction
- Ligation
- Transection of the great saphenous vein
- Precise ligation of the junction with nonresorbable sutures
- Introduction of the stripping probe
- Side branch extraction (with the hook method, Fig. 3-13)
- Distal diversion and stripping of the great saphenous vein while preserving competent parts.

The guidelines recommend interrupting any branches that enter the main vein separately at the level of the junction. The invagination technique is preferable, as it causes less trauma. The advantage of selective treatment for insufficient crural perforating veins has not been definitively confirmed.

If the Babcock method is used, it is helpful to have probe heads with threaded tips onto which a second wire probe can be attached. This allows the head to be withdrawn through the inguinal region again. If avulsion of the vein occurs, a second attempt can then be made with this probe (Fig. 3-14a–d).

The risk of the great saphenous vein avulsing can be reduced if the side branches are transected and removed before the stripping procedure. It is not usually necessary to place a Redon drain; if a drain is placed, it can be introduced from the inguinal direction as far as the great saphenous vein channel.

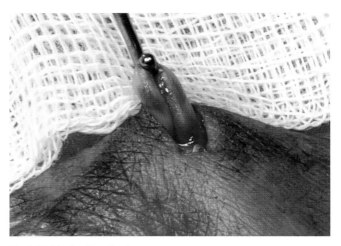

Fig. 3-13 The hook method.

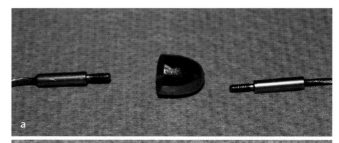
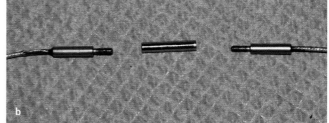
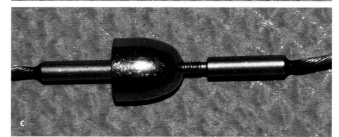
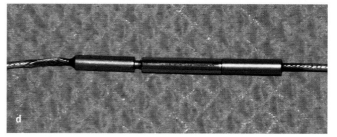

Fig. 3-14a–d Connecting two probes using a probe head with a thread or adapter.

3.4.3.8 Small saphenous vein

Preoperative marking of the ostium of the small saphenous vein into the popliteal vein with ultrasound guidance is obligatory. Otherwise, if a variant location is encountered, the procedure becomes unnecessarily difficult and in some cases an early "recurrence" follows. The marking should be placed at a site at which the small saphenous vein courses as closely as possible to the fascia. This makes it easier for an as-yet inexperienced surgeon to locate the small saphenous vein, which can then be followed deeper.

The transverse incision a few centimeters long near the knee joint opens the way to the fascia. The vein can often be identified before the fascia is opened. Incision of the fascia is carried out longitudinally on the leg—i.e., at right angles to the course of the fibers. This makes it possible if necessary to extend the incision centrally or peripherally. The femoropopliteal vein is ligated and transected. Blunt dissection exposes the small saphenous vein near the ostium. In the same way as with the great saphenous vein, the small saphenous vein is looped and followed deeper to the popliteal vein. Due to narrow anatomic conditions, it may be challenging to demonstrate the saphenopopliteal junction. It is preferable to demonstrate the junction with the popliteal vein, but it should not be achieved forcibly.

If a Giacomini vein is present, it is also probed as far as its junction with the great saphenous vein and then interrupted there. This junction is also closed flatly with nonresorbable suture material. Extirpation is carried out in the same way as in the great saphenous vein. If the small saphenous vein cannot be probed in the retrograde direction—e.g., following phlebitis—it can be identified in the distal lower leg behind the lateral malleolus and probed in the antegrade direction.

Inadvertent slippage into a deep vein—e.g., via a perforating vein—must be avoided at all costs in this process. Due to the spatial constriction, the invagination technique is preferable. The incidence of injury to the sural nerve can be reduced by carrying out a gentle maneuver. Finally, after the other usual concluding procedures, the fascia must be closed carefully. Otherwise, there may be undesirable bulging in the popliteal region, which is unwelcome both to the surgeon and to the patient.

3.4.3.9 Perforating veins (Dodd and Cockett)

Two frequently diagnosed perforating veins may be mentioned here as examples: the Dodd vein in the thigh and the Cockett veins in the lower leg. In incomplete saphenous varicosity, an insufficient Dodd vein as a proximal insufficiency point can grow to reach a substantial caliber, and if it is not recognized can lead to considerable bleeding during extirpation of the great saphenous vein. Preoperative examination of the whole femoral course of the great saphenous vein is therefore advisable. The Dodd perforating vein is also often the starting point for insufficiency in a residual vein after a previous varicectomy. It should also be marked with ultrasound guidance and selectively treated via a separate incision on the medial thigh. As atraumatic a surgical technique as possible should be ensured, particularly in adipose thighs. Following the vein deeper should, if possible, demonstrate the segment near the fascia, where transection with ligatures is carried out.

Crural Crockett veins can often be recognized by their blowout when the patient is standing. When the patient is recumbent, a fascial gap can be palpated at this site. A longitudinal incision is made, followed by demonstration near the fascia and transection as described above.

If skin conditions obstruct direct surgical access and prolonged treatment for wound healing disturbances can otherwise be expected, endoscopic subfascial dissection of perforating veins (ESDP) can be used. This makes it possible to proceed at a distance from the damaged areas with monitor assistance or under direct vision.

3.4.3.10 Alternative surgical methods

Examples that may be mentioned are:
- Outpatient conservative and hemodynamic treatment for venous insufficiency *(cure conservatrice et hémodynamique de l'insuffisance veineuse en ambulatoire, CHIVA)*
- External valvuloplasty/bandaging

CHIVA

The aim in the CHIVA surgical method is to reduce the blood volume in the recirculation cycle. In contrast to the classical theory, four venous networks are distinguished (R1–R4), which are connected with each other by shunts. Preoperative preparation involves a finely detailed duplex ultrasound examination. A refluxing junction is ligated, but there is no ligation in the classic form, so that circulation via the side branches is preserved. Reflux in the saphenous vein is reduced by the amount coming from the common femoral vein. The distal insufficiency points are also preserved to allow recirculation into the deep venous system. The aim of the alternative methods is to preserve the veins and achieve a normalization of the venous diameter.

External valvuloplasty/bandaging

External valvuloplasty or bandaging involves external constriction in the area of the ostium of the great saphenous vein. This is intended to restore the closing capacity of the central venous valve and preserve the vein as a replacement vessel for any bypass operations that may be required later. According to the guidelines published by the German Phlebology Society, a conclusive assessment of this method and its results is not yet possible due to insufficient data.

3.4.3.11 Surgical treatment for recurrence

A recurrence is a renewed development of reflux in an area in which surgery has been carried out previously. Reported rates of "recurrence" are in the range of 6–60%. The proportion of actual recurrences is in the range of 8–14%. According to the German Society for Vascular Surgery's quality assurance project for variceal surgery, the rate of recurrent procedures is approximately 15%. The term "recurrence" should only be used if a correctly conducted ligation has been carried out. In cases in which the crossectomy has not been fully completed, it is more appropriate to speak of a pseudorecurrence.

Surgery to treat recurrences must be regarded as a demanding vascular surgery procedure. The duration of the operation may be markedly prolonged. The patient should be informed about the increased complication rate (with nerve lesions and injury to the large vessels).

Causes

Recurrences are caused by:

- Incomplete previous surgery
- Progressive disease
- Neoangiogenesis

Neoangiogenesis in particular, which develops from endothelium at the vessel stump, is attracting increasing attention as a cause of recurrences. The vascular endothelial growth factor (VEGF) receptor appears to play an important role in the etiology and pathogenesis of neovascularization after crossectomy. If the stump is left very short, the endothelium presents with an open funnel shape for the sprouting of new vessels. By contrast, if the stump is left long, the epithelial layers are able to adhere to each other and the exposed endothelial surface area is reduced.

Research is currently being conducted to examine whether the radical ligation that is currently regarded as the standard procedure actually prevents recurrences or may even have a causative influence on neoangiogenesis. Until reliable data become available, the following measures are recognized methods of preventing recurrences even during the first operation:

- Complete ligation
- Transection of side branches up to the first branching
- Additional ligation of side branches that have direct ostia within 2 cm into the common femoral vein
- Flat transfixion ligature with nonresorbable suture material
- Leaving a long stump and suturing of the stump end

Indication

- Typical symptomatic picture
- Constant reflux into a larger side branch transfascially
- Incomplete previous operation with side branches left
- Stump diameter > 5 mm

Inguinal reflux that is only via an inguinal variceal bed does not require surgical treatment.

Diagnosis

Color duplex ultrasonography is indispensable and provides adequate functional, anatomic, and hemodynamic information in most cases. Preoperative ultrasound-guided marking is also imperative in case of a popliteal recurrence. This often lies outside the area of the first operation, so that adhesion-free access is possible. Phlebography can also be carried out in case of doubt.

Operation

Inguinal

The transverse inguinal incision is made slightly lateral to the first incision, over the palpable superficial femoral artery. The fascia is demonstrated lateral to the lymphatic vessels and is opened longitudinally. The fascia can be lifted ventrally using sharp wound retractors, so that the site is stretched and the saphenous stump can be demonstrated for a few centimeters cranially and caudally. The common femoral vein is only dissected sufficiently to allow vessel clamps to be applied in case of bleeding.

The saphenous stump is carefully circled with an Overholt clamp and double nonresorbable ligatures are applied a few millimeters apart. The stump is only transected if adequate mobilization of the stump ends can be achieved and slippage of the ligatures can be avoided. In a favorable situation, residual side branches can be treated using the same access. However, this leads to more complications. Wound closure starts with closure of the fascia.

Popliteal

A repeat operation in the popliteal fossa is a surgically demanding procedure. Scarring and the close anatomic vicinity of large vessels and nerves mean that there are a large number of potential complications. Preoperative diagnosis by the surgeon is therefore very important. Inflow from a site outside of the cicatricial area is often found to be the cause of the recurrence. This can then be easily treated with scar-free access.

Dissection through the old scar may be prolonged and unclear, as the venous convolutions that are often present are thin-walled and bleeding can obstruct progress. The goal here is of course again to control reflux inflow directly at the popliteal vein using a nonresorbable transfixion ligature. However, this goal should not be forcibly pursued, as injury to the popliteal vein leads to an unclear situation that requires both an experienced surgeon and suitable surroundings. If there was no fascial closure or secondary dehiscence occurred after the first operation, the resulting adhesions may be substantial. If fascial closure is not possible after the repeat operation, a Mersilene mesh can be implanted as a substitute.

References

Baier P-M. Zur Chirurgie der poplitealen Rezidivvarikosen. Gefäßchirurgie 2006; 11: 195–202.

Fischer R, Chandler JG, De Maeseneer MG, et al. The unresolved problem of recurrent saphenofemoral reflux. J Am Coll Surg 2002; 195: 80–94.

Fischer, R, Linde, N, Duff, C. Der klinische Verlauf nach der Strippingoperation – Ergebnisse einer Nachkontrolle nach 34 Jahren. Vasomed 2000; 12: 152–60.

Fischer R, Kluess HG, Frings N, Duff C. Der aktuelle Stand der Magnakrossenrezidiv-Forschung. Phlebologie 2003; 3: 54–9.

Frings N, Glowacki P, Nelle A, Tran VTP. Prospektive Studie zur Verhinderung der Neoangiogenese nach Magna-Crossektomie. Zentralbl Chir 2001; 126: 528–30.

Frings N, Tran van Thann P, Glowacki P, Subasinghe Ch. Komplikationen in der Varizenchirurgie und Strategien zu ihrer Vermeidung. Phlebologie 2002; 1: 26–37.

Frings N, Nelle A, Tran van Thann P, Glowacki P. Unvermeidbares Rezidiv und Neoreflux nach korrekter Vena-saphena-magna-Krossektomie: Neovaskularisation? Phlebologie 2003; 4: 96–100.

Gerard JL, Desgranges P, Becquemin JP, et al. Feasibility of ambulatory endovenous laser for the treatment of greater saphenous varicose veins: one-month outcome in a series of outpatients. J Mal Vasc 2002; 27: 222–5.

Gloviczki P, Bergan JJ, Rhodes JM, et al. Mid-term results of endoscopic perforator vein interruption for chronic venous insufficiency: lessons learned from the North American subfascial endoscopic perforator surgery registry. The North American Study Group. J Vasc Surg 1999; 29: 489–502.

Goldman MP, Mauricio M, Rao J. Intravascular 1320 nm laser closure of the great saphenous vein: a 6 to 12 months follow-up study. Dermatol Surg 2004; 30: 1380–5.

Hach W. Stammvarikose der V. saphena magna. Aus: Die primäre Varikose. In: Venenchirurgie. Abdruck. Phlebologie 2006; 148–56.

Hach W. Venenchirurgie. Stuttgart: Schattauer Verlag, 2006.

Hach W, Hach-Wunderle V, Nestle W. Die Insuffizienz der Cockett-Vv.-perforantes und die operative Behandlung. Gefäßchirurgie 2000; 5: 130–7.

Hach W, Hach-Wunderle V. Das Stripping und die Konkurrenzverfahren zur chirurgischen Behandlung der Stammvarikose. Gefäßchirurgie 2000; 5: 56–61.

Hach W, Hach-Wunderle V. Die Aufklärung zur Thromboseprophylaxe mit Heparin in der Venenchirurgie. Gefäßchirurgie 2001; 6: 219–26.

Hach W. Was ist CHIVA? Gefäßchirurgie 2002; 7: 244–50.

Heidrich M, Balzer K. Die konventionelle operative Therapie der Stammvenen. Gefäßchirurgie 2006; 11: 45–60.

Hermanns H-J. Adipositas und Varizenchirurgie. Gefäßchirurgie 2007; 12: 24–52.

Hinchliffe RJ, Ubhi J, Beech A, et al. A prospective randomised controlled trial of VNUS Closure versus surgery for the treatment of recurrent long saphenous varicose veins. Eur J Vasc Endovasc Surg 2006; 31: 212–8.

Interdisziplinäre Leitlinie der Deutschen Gesellschaft für Chirurgie, Dt. Ges. f. Unfallchirurgie, Dt. Ges. f. Orthopädie und orthopädische Chirurgie, Dt. Ges. f. Viszeralchirurgie, Dt. Ges. f. Thorax-, Herz- und Gefäßchirurgie, Dt. Ges. f. Gefäßchirurgie, Dt. Ges. f. Kinderchirurgie, Ver. d. Dt. Plastischen Chirurgen, Dt. Ges. f. Gynäkologie und Geburtshilfe, Dt. Ges. f. Urologie, Dt. Ges. f. Neurochirurgie, Dt. Ges. f. Anästhesiologie und Intensivmedizin, Ges. f. Thrombose- und Hämostaseforschung, Dt. Ges. f. Angiologie, Dt. Ges. f. Phlebologie, Dt. Ges. f. Hämatologie und Onkologie, Dt. Dermatologische Ges., BV d. Dt. Chirurgen, BV Dt. Anästhesisten, GFB, Phlebologie 2003; 32: 164ff; FRAUENARZT 2003; 44: 1013ff.

Jones L, et al. Neovascularisation is the principal cause of varicose vein recurrence: results of a randomized trial of stripping the long saphenous vein. Eur J Vasc Endovasc Surg 1996; 12: 442–5.

Kabnick LS. Outcome of different endovenous laser wavelengths for great saphenous vein ablation. J Vasc Surg 2006; 43: 88–93.

Kluess H, Noppeney T, Gerlach H, Braunbeck W, Ehresmann U et al. Leitlinie zur Diagnostik und Therapie des Krampfaderleidens. Phlebologie 2004; 33: 211–1.

Lurie F, Creton D, Eklof B, et al. Prospective randomized study of endovenous radiofrequency obliteration (Closure) versus ligation and stripping in a selected patient population (EVOLVES study). J Vasc Surg 2003; 38: 207–14.

Lurie F, Creton D, Eklof B, et al. Prospective randomized study of endovenous radiofrequency obliteration (Closure) versus ligation and vein stripping (EVOLVeS): two-year followup. Eur J Vasc Endovasc Surg 2005; 29: 67–73.

Merchant RF, DePalma RG, Kabnick LS. Endovascular obliteration of saphenous reflux: A multicenter study. J Vasc Surg 2002; 35: 1190–6.

Miszcak ZT, Baier P-M. Varizenoperation beim älteren Menschen. Vasomed 2008; 1: 3–17.

Mumme A, Olbrich S, Barbera L, Stücker M. Saphenofemorales Leistenrezidiv nach Stripping der Vena saphena magna: technischer Fehler oder Neovaskularisation? Phlebologie 2002; 31: 38–41.

Mundy L, Merlin TL, Fitridge RA, et al. Systematic review of endovenous laser treatment for varicose veins. Br J Surg 2005; 92: 1189–94.

Myers KA, Ziegenbein RW, Zeng GH, et al. Duplex ultrasonography scanning for chronic venous disease: patterns of venous reflux. J Vasc Surg 1995; 21: 605–12.

Navarro L, Min R, Boné C. Endovenous laser: a new minimally invasive method of treatment of varicose veins—preliminary observations using an 810 nm diode laser. Dermatol Surg 2001; 27: 117–22.

Noppeney T, Nüllen H. Die Rezidiv-Varikose – was ist das? Gefäßchirurgie 2005; 10: 424–7.

Noppeney T, Eckstein HH, Niedermeier H, Umscheid T, Weber H. Ergebnisse des Qualitätssicherungsprojektes Varizenchirurgie der Deutschen Gesellschaft für Gefäßchirurgie 2005; 10: 121–8.

Offermann M, VNSU vs ELVES. Vortrag, geh. anlässl. des Nordwestdeutschen Gefäßchirurgen-Kongress. Hamburg, 2003.

Pichot O, et al. Role of duplex imaging in endovenous obliteration for primary venous insufficiency. J Endovasc Ther 2000; 7: 451–9.

Pierik EG, van Urk H, Wittens CH. Efficacy of subfascial endoscopy in eradicating perforating veins of the lower leg and its relation with venous ulcer healing. J Vasc Surg 1997; 26: 255–9.

Proebstle TM, Lehr HA, Kargl A, et al. Endovenous treatment of the greater saphenous vein with a 940-nm diode laser: thrombotic occlusion after endoluminal thermal damage by laser-generated steam bubbles. J Vasc Surg 2002; 35: 729–36.

Proebstle TM, Krummenauer F, Gul D, et al. Nonocclusion and early reopening of the great saphenous vein after endovenous laser treatment is fluence dependent. Dermatol Surg 2004; 30: 174–8.

Proebstle TM, Moehler T, Herdemann S. Reduced recanalization rates of the great saphenous vein after endovenous laser treatment with increased energy dosing: definition of a threshold for the endovenous fluence equivalent. J Vasc Surg 2006; 44: 834–9.

Rabe E, Pannier-Fischer F, Bromen K et al. Bonner Venenstudie der Deutschen Gesellschaft für Phlebologie. Phlebologie 2003; 32: 1–14.

Rabe E, Pannier F, Gerlach H, Breu FX, Guggenbichler S, Wollmann JC. Leitlinie Sklerosierungsbehandlung der Varikose. Phlebologie 2008; 37: 27–34.

Rautio T, Ohinmaa A, Perälä J, et al. Endovenous obliteration versus conventional stripping operation in the treatment of primary varicose veins: a randomized controlled trial with comparison of costs. J Vasc Surg 2002; 35: 958–65.

Reidenbach H-D, Dollinger K, Hofmann J. Überprüfung der Laserklassifizierung unter Berücksichtigung des Lidschlussreflexes. Schriftenreihe der Bundesanstalt für Arbeitsschutz und Arbeitsmedizin; Fb 985. Bremerhaven: Wirtschaftsverlag NW, 2003.

Rewerk S, Noppeney T, Nüllen H, Winkler M. Neoangiogenese als Rezidivursache nach Krossektomie der primären Stammvarikose. Gefäßchirurgie 2008; 13: 130–4.

Rewerk St, Meyer AJ, Duczek C, Winkler M, Noppeney T, Nüllen H, Gruber A, Willeke F. Pathogenese der Neovaskularisation (Venoneuronale Regeneration) nach der Krossektomie. Welche Rolle spielt die NGF-VEGF-VEGFR-Kaskade? Meeting Abstract. 124. Kongress der Deutschen Gesellschaft für Chirurgie, München: 4.5.2007.

Rutherford EE, Kianifard B, Cook SJ, et al. Incompetent perforating veins are associated with recurrent varicose veins. Eur J Vasc Endovasc Surg 2001; 21: 458–60.

Schweiger H, Schnell O, Sturm J. Das Schicksal der Restsaphena nach stadiengerechter Varizenoperation. Gefäßchirurgie 2002; 7: 13–6.

Stötter L, Schaaf I, Bockelbrink A. Comparative outcomes of radiofrequency endoluminal ablation, invagination stripping, and cryostripping in the treatment of great saphenous vein insufficiency. Phlebology 2006; 21: 60–5.

Stücker M, Reich S. Evidenzbasierte Daten zur Wirksamkeit der Pharmakotherapie bei chronisch-venöser Insuffizienz. Vasomed 2007; 19 (1): 32.

Timperman PE, Sichlau M, Ryu RK. Greater energy delivery improves treatment success of endovenous laser treatment of incompetent saphenous veins. J Vasc Interv Radiol 2004; 15: 1061–3.

Timperman PE. Prospective evaluation of higher energy great saphenous vein endovenous treatment. J Vasc Interv Radiol 2005; 16: 791–4.

Verrel F, Steckmeier B, Parzhuber A, Spengel FA, Rauh G, Reininger CB. Ascending varicophlebitis: classification and treatment. Gefäßchirurgie 1999; 13–9.

Weiss RA. RF-mediated endovenous occlusion. In: Weiss RA, Feied CF, Weiss MA, (eds.) Vein diagnosis and treatment: a comprehensive approach. New York, NY: McGraw-Hill Medical Publishing, 2001; 211–21.

Weiss RA, et al. Controlled radiofrequency endovenous occlusion using a unique radiofrequency catheter under Duplex guidance to eliminate saphenous varicose vein reflux: A 2-year follow-up. Dermatologic Surgery Jan 2002; 28: 1: 38–42.

Wienert V, Gerlach H, Gallenkemper G et al. Leitlinie Medizinischer Kompressionsstrumpf (MKS). Phlebologie 2006; 35: 315–20.

Wienert V, Waldermann F, Zabel M, Rabe E, Jünger M. Leitlinie Phlebologischer Kompressionsverband. Phlebologie 2004; 33: 131–4.

Whiteley MS HJ, Price BA, Scott MJ, et al. Radiofrequency ablation of refluxing great saphenous systems, Giacomini veins, and incompetent perforating veins using VNUS closure and TRLOP technique. Phlebology 2003; 18: 52.

4 Venous ulcer

Clinical picture: Helene Arns
Duplex ultrasonography: Tom Schilling
Conservative treatment: Helene Arns
Surgical treatment: Hans Joachim Hermanns

4.1 Clinical picture

The term "ulcerated leg" basically refers to venous (varicose) ulcer, arterial ulcer, and mixed arterial and venous ulcer. More rarely, the pathogenesis of an ulcer involves marked lymphedema, vasculitis, and pyoderma gangraenosum. Stage C6 in the CEAP classification is diagnosed much less often in the physician's office today than it was 30 years ago, as patients are now better informed and physicians decide at an earlier stage that there is an indication for treatment of venous insufficiency and diagnosis or treatment of deep vein thrombosis. According to the results of the Bonn Vein Study in 2004, there are approximately 100,000 cases of florid ulcer due to venous diseases. An estimated 25,000 of these ulcers must be classed as treatment-resistant according to the definition given in the guideline on venous ulcer (Fig. 4-1a, b). Even today, they still represent a considerable therapeutic challenge. The patient's history and the ordeal of the condition usually extend over years and even decades without permanent ulcer healing, and substantially reduce the quality of life of those affected. In economic terms, treatment for venous ulcer creates very considerable costs.

Venous ulcer is a loss of substance in the area of the distal lower leg that arises due to damage to the venous valves that has persisted for years or decades and involves progressive findings, with several injuries to the venous valves in the area of the subfascial, transfascial, and/or epifascial veins. This venous valve defect usually results from untreated saphenous vein insufficiency (primary varicosis) or a previous deep vein thrombosis in the leg (post-thrombotic syndrome with secondary insufficiency). As a sequela of venous valve insufficiency and inadequate recanalization of thrombosed venous segments, return flow of the blood from the lower leg to the heart is restricted. The venous reflux of blood and/or outflow blockage by a residual obstruction in a deep vein leads to "ambulatory hypertension" and venous hypervolemia in the subsequent venous segment. In the later course of the disease, the next distal venous valve also becomes insufficient, and so on. The volume and pressure load on the tissue leads, via disturbed microcirculation, to pathological tissue changes that can lead—through the stages of spider veins, saphenous and side branch varicosities, and edema and dermatoliposclerosis—to florid venous ulcer. In pathophysiological terms, this is a chronic inflammatory process affecting not only the ulcer wound, but also the tissue surrounding the ulcer to various extents.

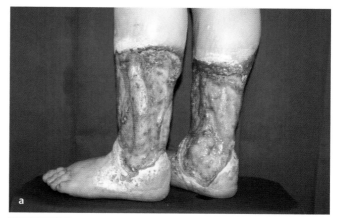

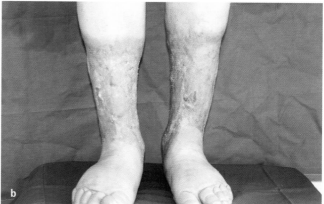

Fig. 4-1a,b (a) Bilateral post-thrombotic venous ulcer that had persisted for 45 years. (b) Results after shave therapy.

4.2 Clinical findings

For these mostly older patients, it is often a minor bruise or insect sting that "suddenly" gives rise to the ulcer. The "wound," which may be moist and is often very painful, causes the patient to visit the physician. The skin region, which has previously had sclerotic atrophic changes, has often been observed without treatment for many years. A few patients present to specialists with large ulcer findings and a history of previous treatment lasting months or years. The treatment may have been carried out only at home, or with medical care over a longer period. Healing of the ulcer may have occurred at some point in the intervening period, but a recurrent and treatment-resistant ulcer is now found. Due to the increasing size and odor, and the severe restriction of the patient's quality of life, phlebological and vascular surgery treatment is initiated.

Recognizable clinical signs of advanced chronic venous insufficiency (see the CEAP classification) include:

- Spider veins over an extensive area on the borders of the feet, which are described as "paraplantar varicose corona."
- Large reddish-brown hyperpigmentations and dermatoliposcleroses around the ulcer, or extending to cover the whole distal lower leg to mid-calf, which may form a cuff shape around the whole circumference.
- Accompanying "congestion dermatitis" near the ulcer. The skin surface is parchment-thin in areas and sensitive to the smallest injuries.
- Net-shaped hypopigmented areas that have developed over a long period in the area of the dermatosclerosis, known as *atrophie blanche*.
- Marked saphenous and side branch varicosities in the whole leg. Veins showing varicose changes are often visible right down to the base of the ulcer.

Venous ulcer usually occurs in the distal lower leg—e.g., in the area of the distal insufficiency point of a primary or secondary varicosity. When there is advanced insufficiency of the great saphenous vein, it forms (corresponding to the vein's anatomy) in the area of the medial malleolus; when there is marked insufficiency of the small saphenous vein, it forms on the lateral malleolus at the foot. In the presence of side branch varicosity or perforating vein insufficiency, or with a pathogenesis of deep vein thrombosis, the findings may have various locations. The site, extent, and depth are decisive for the pain symptoms caused by the ulcer. Physiological rolling of the foot may be limited due to pain, and may even involve an arthrogenic congestion syndrome. The patient avoids walking movements, which in turn obstructs the activation of the muscle–joint pump, making healing of the ulcer more difficult and potentially leading to further deterioration in the condition. Lymph also collects, exerting further pressure on the ulcer and the surrounding tissue.

4.3 Diagnosis

4.3.1 Clinical diagnosis

It is important to take a detailed patient history on the origin of the ulcer, its frequency of recurrence, previous diseases such as deep vein thromboses, phlebitis, and prior or existing saphenous varicosis. Inquiries should be made about any familial predisposition to chronic venous insufficiency, coagulation disturbances, and accompanying diseases such as diabetes mellitus, peripheral arterial occlusive disease (PAOD), and cardiac or renal insufficiency. Information about previous ulcer treatment, including application of ointments subjectively felt to offer "guaranteed success," that may have led to healing of the ulcer years before, should be taken seriously and discussed with the patient in order to encourage good collaboration. Information about previous treatments and details may allow intolerance of external treatment agents to be taken into account if they

are noted in an allergy ID booklet. Tetanus protection should be in place or may need to be updated.

The patient should be asked about mobility and it should be assessed, as this is important for understanding the cause of the ulcer and the approach to later treatment. Joint disease, marked obesity, and ulcer pain are important influencing factors here. In patients who are employed, inquiries should be made about work done in a standing position, and maintenance of fitness to work should be taken into account during later treatment planning to ensure that patients are able to keep their jobs.

Precise description and documentation of the ulcer are necessary before the first treatment. The assessment should include its size measured in centimeters, its depth, a description of any bacterial colonization, and necrotic parts of the ulcer. Findings in the surrounding skin and signs of visible varicosis must also be documented. A palpable arterial foot pulse, if this is possible relative to the location of the ulcer, suggests that PAOD can be largely excluded.

Particularly in an outpatient practice, a smear should be taken to exclude resistant bacteria (e.g., methicillin-resistant *Staphylococcus aureus*, MRSA) if antibiotic treatment is necessary, although this is rarely the case. Particularly in venous ulcers that have been present for a long time, the possibility of a malignant pathogenesis must be considered, and taking a biopsy for histopathological examination may be needed. When the ulcer findings extend very deeply, an x-ray may be needed to exclude bone involvement.

Measuring the circumference of the legs, always in comparison with the contralateral side, provides important information for the later effectiveness of treatment. Photographic documentation (including a measurement scale for reference) should be carried out to allow the course to be checked by the physician and the patient and for any correspondence with insurance companies if needed.

4.3.2 Diagnostic imaging

Diagnostic imaging is carried out in the same way as for venous insufficiency. Functional examination procedures that may provide guidance include light reflex rheography to assess venous reflux and vein occlusion plethysmography to assess venous capacity and venous outflow. Flow information about the venous valves can be obtained using Doppler ultrasonography, which also allows assessment of arterial perfusion in the legs. If there is a suspicion of PAOD in the arterial findings, it should be given special attention during subsequent color duplex ultrasonography, which is the major examination method for diagnosing venous ulcers.

4.3.2.1 Duplex ultrasonography

Examination technique

The examination technique corresponds to that used when examining the arteries and veins in the leg (see the discussion there). After arterial perfusion abnormalities have been excluded, a detailed diagnostic approach is used to explore the possible causes of venous hypertension. In particular, attention needs to be given to afferent perforator veins, which may be able to maintain local venous hypertension and thus ulceration even after the trunk and branch varices have been cleared.

Differential diagnosis

Although > 70% of chronic wounds and ulcers in the area of the legs are of venous origin, many other causes are also found. The following are relevant for duplex ultrasound differential diagnosis and must be clarified (see the corresponding sections for details of the examination):

- Arterial insufficiency
- Chronic venous insufficiency:
  - Post-thrombotic syndrome
  - Primary varicosities:
    - Secondary subfascial decompensation in primary varicosities)
    - Perforating vein insufficiency (Fig. 4-2)
  - Secondary varicosities:
    - Post-thrombotic syndrome with secondary varicosities
    - Proximal outflow obstruction
    - Congenital arteriovenous malformations/angiodysplasias (atresia, valvular defects, multiple arteriovenous shunts)
    - Acquired arteriovenous fistulas
- Lymphedema
- Secondary causes (including liver diseases, cardiac diseases, intra-abdominal tumors, insufficient joint–muscle pump (edema without venous hypertension)

Rarely, phlebography or ascending phlebography with a Valsalva maneuver may be necessary to obtain additional information about the findings in patients with atypical courses of varicosities and recurrent varicosities, secondary varicosities in post-thrombotic syndrome, or in patients in whom ultrasound assessment is difficult. However, phlebography combined with contrast injection is no longer required as an imaging procedure to determine the pathogenesis of venous ulcers. In practiced hands, color duplex ultrasonography is equally valid and in the area of the lower leg is often actually better. Duplex ultrasonography does not involve any radiation exposure and can be repeated at any time without causing pain.

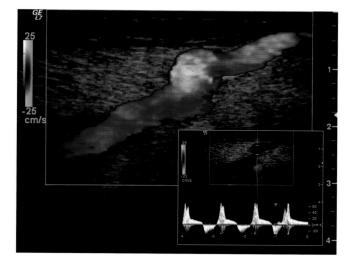

Fig. 4.2 Chronic varicose ulcer, with evidence of an insufficient perforating vein and incessant reflux as the cause of locally persistent venous hypertension despite clearing of varicosities in the main trunk and side branches.

4.4 Treatment

4.4.1 Conservative treatment

Once diagnosis is completed, treatment is planned in accordance with the findings, taking into account the patient's individual diseases and life situation. Fast and permanent healing of the venous ulcer should always be attempted, and this can often be achieved by treatment of the inciting cause, using surgical or laser therapy for insufficiency. Conservative treatment for venous ulcer may be indicated when there is a marked post-thrombotic syndrome, in older patients with a high level of surgical risk, and if the patient declines surgery. Conservative therapy is often also carried out temporarily to reduce the size of large ulcer findings and allow later surgery for the underlying condition with a reduced risk of infection.

4.4.1.1 Compression treatment

Successful treatment for varicose ulcer depends on collaboration and compliance on the part of the patient. The patient should therefore receive information about the general context of the disease picture, expressed in an easily understood way, and it should be clear that it may take a long time to cure a condition that has developed over months or years. In most cases, treatment can be carried out in an outpatient setting.

The basis of conservative treatment for varicose ulcer is medical compression therapy, which is only contraindicated in a few exceptional cases: patients with advanced peripheral occlusive disease (malleolar artery occlusive pressure less than 60–80 mmHg), decompensated cardiac insufficiency, septic phlebitis, and phlegmasia cerulea dolens. In its traditional form, compression therapy involves a specially wrapped compression dressing that is used for specific types of bandaging. Reusable short-stretch elastic bandages, which provide the necessary "working pressure" and low "resting pressure" on the leg, are very suitable. The compression dressing reduces the diameter of the vein, bringing the insufficient venous valves closer together. Venous backflow, lymph drainage, and pathological disturbances of microcirculation are improved by the compression pressure, which declines from distal to proximal. Elastic long-stretch bandages or zinc gelatinous bandages, which are hardly elastic at all, are not really suitable for these requirements.

A specialized "ulcer compression stocking" for the lower leg, consisting of a skin-compatible light understocking to which wound coverings and a specially knit class 2 compression stocking are attached, is a modern compression procedure. Objective studies have shown that these special ulcer stockings have compression and treatment effects that are at least as good as a compression dressing. In practice, use of the compression stocking is particularly appropriate if the ulcer is not larger than a specific size or if it has been reduced to a certain size by initial compression therapy with dressings.

The advantage here is that patients can apply the stocking independently if they are sufficiently mobile and strong. Alternatively, the stocking can be applied by a nursing service, allowing effective home care for the condition. Apart from interim check-ups, the patient is independent and can continue to work without interruption. The use of the stocking must be demonstrated to patients and practiced with them. Both the sensation when wearing a compression dressing and the compression stocking should be discussed. Compression can be perceived as a relief, but pressure pain is often also felt initially in the direct vicinity of the ulcer.

4.4.1.2   Analgesia

Any pain caused by the ulcer should be adequately treated with analgesia and anti-inflammatory therapy. Nonsteroidal anti-inflammatory drugs (NSAIDs) are suitable, and can be used for a longer period provided contraindications are taken into account. Stronger pain therapy is only required in rare cases and should be prescribed in accordance with the World Health Organization grading scheme. Decongestion treatment with compression therapy is carried out with the leg resting and raised, and can be particularly promoted as well by activating the muscle–joint pump—i.e., by having the patient do normal walking. Adequate pain therapy is important here. The behavior often seen in older patients is that pain is tolerated in order to avoid taking medication and leads to reduced mobility, which has unfavorable effects on the treatment. Footdrop and an arthrogenic congestion syndrome may be long-term sequelae.

4.4.1.3   Local treatment

The importance of local treatment for venous ulcer is generally overestimated. Nevertheless, new types of wound coverage keep being developed by pharmaceutical companies for the wound environment in venous ulcers, the aim being to achieve more rapid healing. The venous ulcer and the surrounding skin often show severe inflammatory changes both due to the patient's own treatments and previous medical treatment, and contact allergic reactions are seen when some external agents are used.

An extensive study on local treatment for venous ulcer showed that keeping the wound moist with physiological saline alone promotes healing and reduces pain, leading to a clearly beneficial treatment effect. The study found no clear benefit for many of the expensive and even extremely expensive wound coverings that are commercially available, such as fat gauze, foams, hydrocolloids, or alginates. Particularly due to the cost, they are only of limited usefulness for outpatient treatment. Despite this, our own experience shows that when the patient's individual condition is taken into account—in contrast to a large and inhomogeneous group of patients receiving varyingly good compression treatment—a specifically selected wound covering can be more effective than saline treatment alone. Examples that might be mentioned here are silver-containing wound dressings in ulcers with bacterial colonization and foam dressings in conditions with severe discharge. A moist wound environment is important for wound healing in all cases. To ensure patient compliance, good tolerability and reduced pain are required. As a matter of principle, the wound dressing should cover only the ulcer and not the surrounding skin. Hydrocolloid dressings in particular, which extend beyond the edges of the ulcer, cause unfavorable maceration of the surrounding skin and thus often actually lead to an enlargement of the condition. Depending on the findings, the surrounding skin should be treated at low dosage with external agents, such as zinc paste or (briefly) corticoids. Generally, the increased sensitivity of the tissue to externally applied substances, present in advanced chronic venous insufficiency, needs to be taken into account. In particular, experimenting with constantly changing wound dressings, potentially combined with treatment by different physicians, should be avoided.

The planned duration of dressing placement may lead to different types of wound treatment. A compression dressing for local ulcer treatment with NaCl has to be changed almost daily to ensure that the ulcer base does not dry out too much and cause pain. Dressings with wound coverings that include active agents, such as foams, alginates, etc., can and should be left in place for several days to create an optimal wound environment. The patients only have to return twice weekly for a dressing change. This requires a suitable compression bandage material and a professional wrapping technique, of course. An elastic short-stretch bandage can guarantee effective compression in a mobile leg for 1–2 days, and an adhesive bandage may allow effective compression for several days.

4.4.1.4   Wound debridement

When dressings are exchanged, cleaning or rinsing of the ulcer may be indicated. A sterile saline solution or drinking water are equally suitable for this, as several controlled studies have shown. Any necrotic tissue at the base and edges of the ulcer obstructs wound healing. Crusting often simulates apparent healing of a venous ulcer. So far as is possible in relation to the size of the lesion and the pain symptoms, necrotic tissue can be carefully removed with sterile forceps or a sharp spoon. The value of removing crusts should be explained to patients, as "ruining" an apparently successful healing process is liable to meet with incomprehension.

Gels that have a local anesthetic effect only offer a slight reduction in pain during wound healing. The options for conservative treatment here are generally limited. If more extensive wound debridement is required, a surgical intervention should be considered.

4.4.1.5   Lymph drainage

If decongestion of the leg using compressing dressings or stockings does not lead to satisfactory and successful treatment, or if there is no visible progress in ulcer healing in an area of marked dermatoliposclerosis, concomitant lymph drainage may be useful as an additional treatment measure. Manual lymph drainage is preferable here rather than machine lymph drainage (machine-aided intermittent compression). Manual treatment by a specially trained lymph therapist, particularly with targeted treatment of the ulcer margin and with variable pressure, accelerates decongestion and thus ulcer healing as well. However, effective decongestion and faster improvement in the condition can also be achieved with machine-aided compression treatment as well. In this procedure, the patient pulls a multiple-chamber lymph drainage device—e.g., in the shape of a boot—over the affected leg. The lymph boot causes motor-controlled pressure waves to move evenly from the distal to the proximal extremity, promoting removal of the lymph burden. Compression dressings or stockings must always be placed after both types of physiotherapy procedure in order to maintain and enhance the treatment effect.

4.4.1.6 Physiotherapy

Physical exercise therapy may be useful if a patient does not have the mobility to activate the muscle–joint pump, if pain-related avoidance of the necessary movement has led to functional stiffness in the ankle joint, or if there are pareses in the area of the lower leg.

4.4.1.7 Sclerotherapy

Sclerotherapy with fluid or foamed sclerosing agents may be useful for nonsurgical elimination of varicose venous segments in the area of the ulcer. When sclerosis is successful, the varix thromboses a few days after the treatment and is broken down into a connective tissue-like strand over a period of days to weeks. Venous hypervolemia in the ulcer area is reduced, venous return is improved to some extent, and healing of the lesion is thereby promoted. The procedure itself is not painful, but varicophlebitis needs to be taken into account as a potential complication that may have a temporary negative effect on pain symptoms and on the ulcer. The patient should receive information about the procedure and potential complications and should provide written consent. For insufficient veins with the size of a side branch or saphenous varicosity, treatment with foamed sclerosants is preferable to a liquid drug agent. The foamed agent spreads more easily and evenly on the vascular walls in the varix, triggering vascular spasm and subsequent thrombosis more effectively. A liquid sclerosant is suitable enough for eliminating small varices. Compression therapy continues as before after sclerotherapy.

4.4.1.8 Course

If the venous ulcer has healed after several weeks' treatment and etiologic treatment for the disease is not planned or not possible, lifelong compression therapy has to be continued to prevent recurrent ulcer. A class 2 compression stocking is a practical and sufficiently effective method here, and must be worn up to the knee or up to the thigh, depending on the general state of chronic venous insufficiency in the leg. A marked reduction in the rate of ulcer recurrence has been demonstrated when compression stockings are worn, particularly with specially manufactured ulcer stockings. A local increase in compression in the area of the healed ulcer—e.g., in the retromalleolar space—can be achieved by placing an inlay or sewing a pad into the compression stocking.

Wearing a compression stocking is particularly important in summer, even though it may be uncomfortable for the patient, as deterioration in concomitant lymphatic and venous edema may develop, with a risk of recurrent ulcer. If it is not possible for the patient to put on a class 2 compression stocking or two class 1 stockings on top of each other without assistance, then help needs to be provided by relatives or by a nursing service. Here again, it is important to ensure effective communication with the patient, with a persuasive appeal for help in stabilizing the condition and thereby maintaining the patient's own quality of life.

A healed venous ulcer (C5 in the CEAP classification) should be checked by a specialist at regular intervals—e.g., every 6 or 12 months. This helps prevent recurrent ulcers and allows early treatment if they develop.

With venous ulcers that are resistant to conservative treatment, surgical methods of ulcer treatment have to be considered.

4.4.2 Surgical treatment

The indication for a surgical procedure should only be assessed if, after all conservative measures have been exhausted, no healing tendency is noted after 3 months or an ulcer has not healed after 12 months.

Surgical treatment for venous ulcers is based on three approaches:

■ Eliminating reflux in insufficient venous segments using vein surgery or endovenous occlusion procedures
■ Fascial surgery (paratibial fasciotomy, fasciectomy)
■ Ulcer surgery

4.4.2.1 General preoperative diagnosis

The basic diagnostic procedures for assessing surgical measures involve all the principles of noninvasive vascular diagnosis. Assessment of vascular status should cover both the venous and arterial circulation. An imaging procedure is required at this point at the latest. This provides prognostically and therapeutically important assignment of the ulcers to:

■ Primary and secondary varicosis
■ Deep conducting vein insufficiency
■ Post-thrombotic syndrome
■ Other forms, in combination with arterial diseases

Duplex ultrasonography has now replaced invasive methods, such as ascending phlebography with a Valsalva maneuver, and is the standard method. In special cases, such as ulcers in a patient with complex venous malformations or in extensive post-thrombotic syndromes, it may be helpful to use both procedures. If there are insufficient epifascial or transfascial reflux segments in post-thrombotic venous ulcer for which surgical elimination would be hemodynamically useful, functional and morphologic examination methods can be combined. Ultrasound-guided, targeted compression of insufficient venous segments and simultaneous phlebodynamometry allow precise prognostic assessment of the improvement in venous hemodynamics after reflux treatment (Fig. 4-3). If the venous pressure is unchanged after this maneuver or even declines, then effective surgical treatment at low risk is possible for secondary varicosity in a patient with post-thrombotic syndrome.

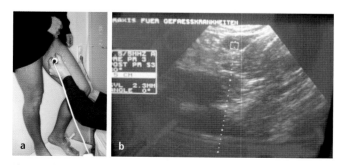

Fig. 4-3a, b Ultrasound-guided venous pressure measurement in post-thrombotic syndrome.

4.4.2.2 Specialized preoperative diagnosis

MRI of the lower leg

Diagnostic information about morphological and functional changes in the subfascial space is important for specific issues and surgical approaches involving the deep fascia of the leg (paratibial fasciotomy, fasciectomy). Preoperative MRI diagnosis of both legs (to compare sides), or alternatively CT diagnosis, is important to provide evidence of a chronic venous compartment syndrome. CT and MRI are equivalent for demonstrating thickening of the cutis and increased density in the subcutis. Fluid (e.g., edema) is better imaged with MRI, which also allows clear differentiation between sclerosis and fluids. Muscular changes such as fatty degeneration and involution of the musculature are also better seen with MRI (Fig. 4-4a, b).

Compartment pressure measurement

Pressure measurements in muscular compartments are carried out both in acute diseases caused by severe trauma (acute compartment syndrome) and in chronic pressure increases, particularly in muscle compartments in the lower leg. According to Hach's pathogenetic

concepts, chronic venous compartment syndrome in patients with severe chronic venous disease is the cause of persistent and recurrent venous ulcers in the legs. The treatment consists of measures to decompress the fascia (fasciotomy and fasciectomy). The dorsal compartments in the lower leg are particularly affected by pressure increases. Measurements in the deep dorsal compartment, which can be reached using a Gerngroß paratibial transmembrane access route (interosseous membrane), provide the best prognostic value. Various direct and indirect measurement procedures are available. Mechanoelectric methods are nowadays preferred. Compartment pressure measurements are only carried out in specialized wound centers since an invasive puncture procedure with potential complications is involved and the relevant technical equipment is required.

Histology

If suspicious and treatment-resistant local findings are present, biopsy samples should be taken from various ulcer areas. In rare cases, it is possible for squamous cell carcinoma to develop against the background of venous ulcer in the leg (Fig. 4-5a, b).

Identifying pathogens and resistance assessment

Assessment of the bacterial spectrum and antibiotic sensitivity testing are recommended as part of the preoperative planning. Ulcers in which there is an indication for surgery have often left the stage

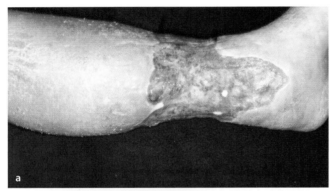

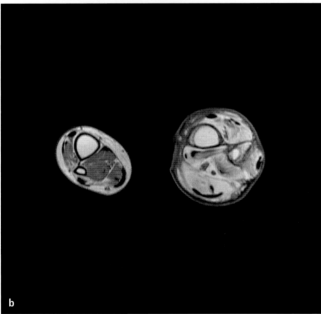

Fig. 4-4a, b (a) Treatment-resistant post-thrombotic venous ulcer (gaiter ulcer). (b) MRI of the lower leg in gaiter ulcer. Left: the ulcer region, with dermatosclerosis, subfascial edema, and lipomatous involution of the musculature. Right: normal findings.

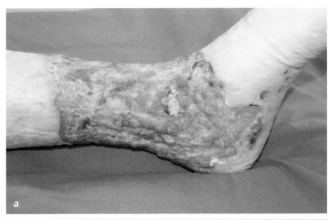

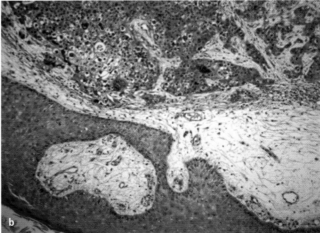

Fig. 4-5a, b (a) Squamous cell carcinoma against a background of many years of venous ulcer. (b) Histological findings: squamous cell carcinoma in a primary venous ulcer.

of contamination and colonization and show clear signs of infection, accompanied by a marked increase in pain that makes the decision in favor of surgery compelling. Information about any MRSA colonization in particular is also absolutely necessary for purpose of hygiene planning.

4.4.2.3 Endovenous occlusion procedures and venous surgery

In cases of venous ulcer caused by primary insufficiency, the elimination of the insufficient epifascial or transfascial venous segments usually leads to permanent ulcer healing without any other measures being needed. However, if the ulcerations are more extensive and spontaneous healing is doubtful, local ulcer surgery methods can be combined with the surgical treatment. Shave treatment with simultaneous mesh graft plasty during the same procedure can be recommended.

In addition to classic venous surgery, modern endovenous procedures (laser therapy, radiofrequency therapy, and foam sclerosis) now offer good alternative treatment options. Which procedure is to be used should always be decided in the individual case using the specific pattern of findings.

Variceal surgery provides satisfactory long-term results in relation to ulcer healing and recurrence rates. Data for the endovenous procedures are currently lacking due to the short follow-up periods so far available. However, equivalent ulcer healing rates can be expected. Particularly with special patterns of findings, such as a combination of venous ulcer with extreme obesity, the less-invasive procedures can be used to reduce surgical and postoperative risks.

4.4.2.4 Perforating vein surgery

Surgical treatment for insufficient perforating veins has always played an important role in the hemodynamic view of ulcer development. As a result of the short connections between the deep and superficial veins, existing insufficiency can cause a substantial shift in blood volume into the epifascial system. This leads to edema development and trophic disturbances, and even ulcerations. Open surgical procedures (e.g., the Linton operation) to eliminate these perforating veins, with a longitudinal paratibial incision and selective ligation of all of the perforating veins, have been abandoned due to the resulting severe trauma, frequently disturbed wound healing, and lymphatic complications.

Today, insufficient perforating veins with minor trophic disturbances are dissected or ligated directly epifascially. If there is advanced dermatolipofasciosclerosis in the ulcer area that makes direct access difficult, subfascial methods are available. In addition to uncontrolled subfascial dissection with a finger, spatula, or scissors, there is the technique of endoscopic subfascial dissection of perforating veins (ESDP), introduced by Hauer in 1985. This procedure made it possible to locate a paratibial access site in healthy areas of skin at a distance from the actual ulcer and trophic periulcerous changes. The perforating veins are then transected or ligated with clips under endoscopic visual control. Various technical variants have been developed. Starting with direct visualization (Hauer and Fischer), video-assisted instrument sets were rapidly developed (Sattler, Gasser et al.). Developments with the procedure reached their climax in 1993, when the Research Group for Endoscopy and Fasciotomy in Venous Surgery was founded by Fischer and Hach.

Evidence-based studies and clinical results in recent years have led to a critical view of the method. In addition to postoperative disturbances that sometimes persist (such as sensory deficits, a tendency to develop edema, pain, and subfascial infection), recurrence rates of 40–75% have been reported after ESDP. The indication should now be established very strictly and should only be considered for insufficient perforating veins in clinical stages C4–C6.

On the basis of figures available from the German Society for Vascular Surgery's varix quality assurance survey for the last 5 years, only 0.8% of insufficient perforating veins that are diagnosed are now treated endoscopically.

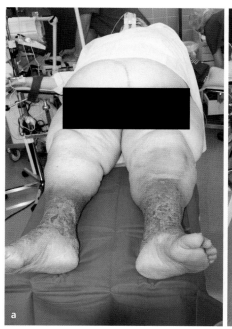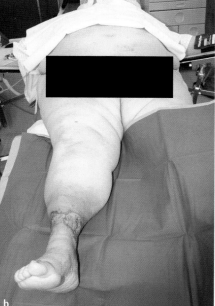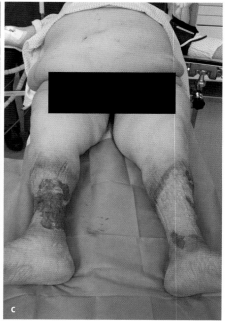

Fig. 4-6a–c Venous ulcer in extreme obesity.

4.4.2.5 Hach paratibial fasciotomy

Paratibial fasciotomy was developed by Hach and has become an established part of the repertory of surgical procedures. It led to the pathogenetic concept that chronic venous compartment syndrome (CVCS) is the cause of recurrent or treatment-resistant venous ulcerations. Dividing the deep fascia of the leg and opening the subfascial compartments is intended to produce decompression, leading to faster healing.

Technique

The skin, subcutis and deep fascia are opened with a paratibial incision 3–5 cm long. The fascia is then split with scissors or with the Hach fasciotome (Martin Ltd.) as far as the medial malleolus. When perforating veins are dissected during the fasciotomy, torrential bleeding can occur and needs to be controlled in order to avoid subfascial hematomas. Splitting of the fascia in the proximal direction usually follows. The fasciotomy can also be carried out endoscopically and combined with perforating vein treatment. Placement of a wound drain (in case of secondary bleeding) and perioperative antibiotic prophylaxis (against subfascial infection) can be recommended.

Clinical results

There have as yet been no study results or publications on the value of isolated fasciotomy in the treatment of venous ulcer or permanent subfascial decompression. However, Hach and colleagues have demonstrated the positive effects of their method in the incomplete and unpublished PAFAS study. Langer et al. (1995) carried out compartment pressure measurements 6 months before and after patients underwent fasciotomy. The raised preoperative pressure values declined after the fasciotomy, but were higher than the preoperative baselines values again 6 months later. However, the ulcers cleared up normally. The importance of the fasciotomy and temporary reduction of compartment pressure here has not yet been adequately clarified. The method is still basically empirical.

Prospects

According to the German Society for Vascular Surgery's varix quality assurance survey, there is a declining trend among users for this surgical procedure as well. Approximately 1.2% of all venous procedures now involve paratibial fasciotomy. Relative to the indication range of C4–C6, 10% of patients undergo paratibial fasciotomy. The proportion was still 12.8% in 2001, but fell to 7.1% in 2004. The indication for paratibial fasciotomy should now be established strictly, and morphological and functional subfascial changes should be confirmed before the procedure, using MRI and compartment pressure measurement.

4.4.2.6 Shave therapy

As a tangential and exclusively suprafascial method of necrectomy and fibronectomy, shave therapy is one of the local methods of ulcer treatment. Due to the good to very good long-term results and minor trauma in comparison with other local surgical procedures, it is now the method of choice in surgical therapy for treatment-resistant venous varicose ulcers. Hynes was already carrying out shave treatments in 1956 for plastic surgery procedures (e.g., chronic radiation dermatitis). In 1987, Quaba et al. reported on successful therapy for treatment-resistant venous ulcers using "layered shaving." However, the procedure became scientifically established through the work of Schmeller and colleagues in 1994–1999.

Technique

Using hand dermatomes (Schmeller, Quaba) or machine dermatomes, all suprafascial necroses and fibrotic components in the ulcer area are removed layer by layer until rich capillary bleeding develops at the base of the wound. This creates a fresh wound. To prevent step formation, the wound surface should be as flat as possible. It is now recommended to use battery-powered or wave-powered dermatomes. These allow more precise removal of necroses and easier handling. Layer thicknesses of 0.3–0.4 mm can be recommended. These mean that one does not reach deeper tissue layers too quickly, which can be associated with a risk of injury to structures (such as the joint capsule apparatus or Achilles tendon).

The donor skin is taken from the diseased leg if possible. Here again, layer thicknesses of 0.3–0.4 mm are beneficial. Hemostasis in the donor-site area and in the former ulcer area is carried out with epinephrine-saturated compresses. If sufficient skin is available, the mesh ratio should be 1:1.5. Thicker mesh skin graft leads to poorer healing-in, and a larger mesh ratio (1:3) tends to lead to poorer stress tolerance in everyday life. The donor skin can be attached with stay sutures, tissue glue, or self-adhesive wound dressings.

Clinical results

Long-term results showing complete healing rates of 70–80%, with follow-up periods of up to 84 months (mean) after shave therapy and simultaneous mesh graft plasty have not yet been achieved with any other procedure (Table 4-1). Creating a fresh wound leads to problem-free healing even of treatment-resistant ulcers with an ulcer history of more than 40 years. The mean duration of the ulcer disease in these patients was approximately 16 years before the surgical treatment. Comparable procedures, such as wound conditioning by cultivating granulation tissue and subsequent mesh graft plasty, led to much poorer results and healing rates (30–50%). Granulation tissue as a secondary tissue represents an unfavorable transplant bed. Fasciectomy also only shows long-term healing rates of approximately 50% (Table 4-2).

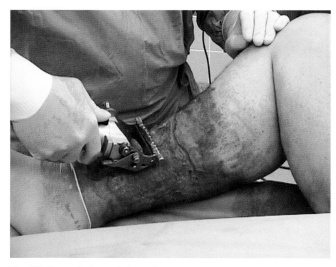

Fig. 4-7 The technique of shave therapy.

Table 4-1 Author's own long-term results with shave therapy (in Krefeld, Germany).

	Dec. 2000	Jun. 2001	Feb. 2002	Mar. 2003	Mar. 2004	Mar. 2005	Mar. 2006	Mar. 2007
Patients	60	74	88	111	151	193	244	278
Legs	71	88	105	140	189	249	320	363
Shave treatments	14	120	149	207	270	335	382	451
Ulcer duration (years)	15.1	15.3	16.1	16.3	16.0	16.3	16.6	16.4
Healed	77.5%	81.0%	88.0%	82.0%	80.0%	79.2%	77.5%	79.6%
Residual ulcer	14.0%	9.0%	6.5%	10.0%	12.6%	8.4%	9.7%	8.2%
Recurrence	8.5%	10.0%	5.5%	8.0%	7.4%	12.4%	12.8%	12.2%
Follow-up (months)	9.5	13.5	18.5	26.6	34.0	43.3	51.5	57.4

Table 4-2 Comparative results with surgical ulcer treatment.

	Schmeller	Hermanns	Popescu	Schwahn-Schreiber
Surgical procedures	Shave	Shave	Shave	Fasciectomy
Patients	12	244	28	10
Legs	17	320	30	14
Follow-up period (months)	84	51.5	24	84
Healing	70.6%	77.5%	72.0%	50.0%
Year	2006	2006	2003	2006

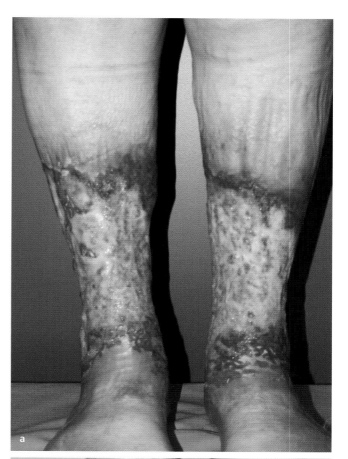

Recurrences

If recurrences develop after shave therapy, other treatment options are available for these patients. Initially, a repeated and extended necrectomy is justified after a balanced assessment of the lesion, and this can also be done in combination with a simultaneous vacuum-assisted closure (VAC) procedure. VAC treatment up to the first dressing change can further promote healing-in of the transplant. Many recurrences then heal permanently without any further measures being needed. If repeat recurrences develop or transfascial necroses have already developed, excision of the lesion, including the fascial structures as a partial or crural fasciectomy, should be carried out. In this method, the transplant bed consists of subfascial structures (musculature, tendons, and bone).

Complications

Postoperative disturbances after shave therapy in a total of 500 procedures consisted of: two septic fever episodes, four cases of erysipelas, one lymph fistula, and one case of pneumonia. In a patient with many years of drug dependency, fulminant necrotic fasciitis developed in the third postoperative week, which led to death in a setting of recurrent deep vein thrombosis resulting in a pulmonary embolism. However, this complication cannot be regarded as procedure-specific.

Twenty-one percent of the patients were aged 80–99 years at the time of the operation. All of these patients were able to cope with the surgical measures without difficulties, and they had healing results that were just as good as those in the younger patients.

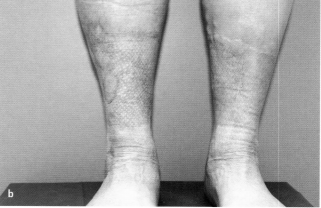

Fig. 4-8a, b Long-term postoperative results 8 years after shave therapy.

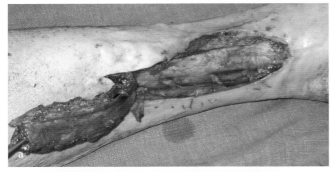

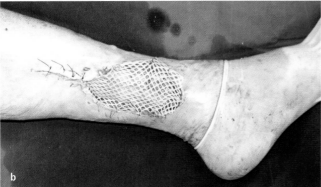

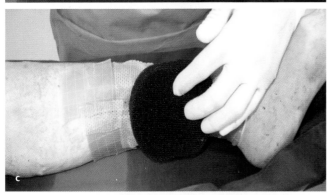

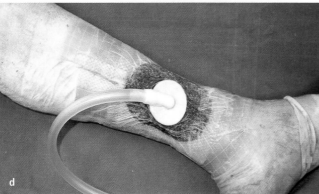

Fig. 4-9a–d Recurrent ulcer: fasciectomy, simultaneous mesh graft plasty, and vacuum-assisted closure treatment.

Postoperative and post-hospital treatment

Limited bed rest (with visiting the toilet and washing permitted) is required to begin within the postoperative period up to the first dressing change (on day 4 or 5). This is followed on days 7–10 by complex physical decongestion treatment in all of the patients, consisting of manual lymph drainage and machine-aided intermittent

compression treatment. This leads to stabilization of the surgical results by providing protection against edema, and it also protects the transplant, which has only a few lymphatic capillaries, against recurrent lesions. Physiotherapy, particularly to mobilize stiff ankle joints in patients with arthrogenic congestion syndrome, should be an integral part of the treatment plan.

Prospects

It is essential for good long-term results to have a standardized post-hospital plan. Compression therapy, usually with class 2 compression stockings, should be continued permanently for the rest of the patient's life. Prophylaxis against edema in the affected extremities can be used to protect the transplant, with daily machine-aided intermittent compression treatment. Patients should have their own devices prescribed for them. Providing patient training in ways of coping with the chronic disease (skin care, dressing technique, use of the compression stocking) and involving outpatient nursing services lead to a high level of patient motivation and are decisive for the long-term prognosis.

4.4.2.7   Hach fasciectomy

Fasciectomy was also developed by Hach and colleagues. Excising the ulcer region, including periulcerous dermatoliposclerosis and involved fascial segments (en bloc resection), results in opening of the subfascial space. According to the theory, removal of the diseased area should lead to decompression of the subfascial structures and their subsequent regeneration. If the changes are regionally limited, what is known as a partial fasciectomy is carried out, whereas if there are extensive changes (gaiter ulcer), the procedure is called circular or crural fasciectomy.

Technique

Due to the strong bleeding tendency and to provide a better overview, the procedure is mainly carried out in a state of relative ischemia achieved by placing a Lövquist cuff. Areas of trophic disturbance (dermatolipofasciosclerosis) are removed, including the deep fascia, and a transplant bed is created for the prepared mesh skin, without damaging tendon sheaths, periosteum, or muscle fascia. Once the ischemia has been reduced, extensive hemostasis is carried out, sometimes requiring purse-string ligation and epinephrine-saturated compresses. The split skin is then applied and fixed. The subsequent postoperative procedure is the same as that for shave therapy.

Clinical results

In comparison with shave therapy, the method causes greater trauma and the operating time is longer as more dissection effort is required. As a result of the potential for intraoperative injury to subfascial structures such as tendon sheaths and periosteum, partial rejection of the transplant occurs more frequently. Repeat procedures with second transplantations or secondary healing of residual lesions lead to prolonged hospitalization periods and longer healing courses. Step formation in the transplant area, which sometimes normalizes later, is a cosmetic disturbance. Overall, the published long-term results, with healing rates of 50% after 84 months, are clearly inferior to those with shave therapy.

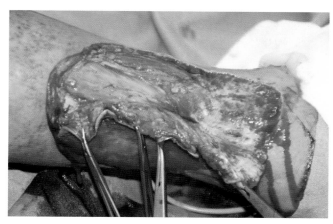

Fig. 4-10 Partial fasciectomy.

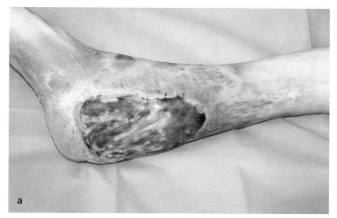

a

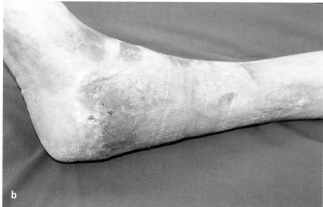

b

Fig. 4-11a, b (a) Recurrent ulcer after free muscle flap transplantation. (b) Results after a shave operation for ulcer in the muscle transplant.

Prospects

The range of indications for crural fasciectomy has changed in recent years due to the good results obtained after shave therapy. Primary crural fascial resections in ulcerations with exclusively epifascial locations have now become rare. If transfascial necroses with exposed tendon parts are present primarily, they can be successfully treated using resection of the lower leg fascia, including the necrotic tissue and tendon parts. Multiple recurrences after shave therapy and marked metaplastic ossifications, which represent a technical obstacle to tangential necrectomy due to extreme calcification, are now regarded as indications for fasciectomy.

4.4.2.8 Other procedures

Homans operation

The en bloc excision of a local ulcer in the lower leg, including the affected fascia, first carried out by Homans in 1916, corresponds to today's partial fasciectomy.

Free muscle transposition plasty

Free muscle flap plasties for covering chronic defects in the lower leg caused by venous diseases are only rarely carried out. Transplantation based on a defect disturbed by fibrosis and sclerosis is unpromising. Since the introduction of VAC treatment in combination with split-skin transplantation, this elaborate plastic surgery procedure is hardly indicated any more. It should also be noted that large parts of the muscle flap are hypesthetic or anesthetic, and new ulcerations may develop as a result of pressure lesions (in the shoe area).

Hach lateral muscle transposition plasty

This is a surgical method for ulcers in the lateral distal lower leg (in the lateral malleolus region). After resection of the necroses, the exposed distal fibula is covered with the surrounding musculature after it has been mobilized. The musculature thus serves as the transplant bed. Alternatively, shave therapy can be carried out for ulcerations in this location, with simultaneous mesh graft plasty and VAC therapy.

4.4.2.9 Follow-up treatment

Treatment-resistant venous ulcer is rarely a result of primary varicosity. Instead, there are permanent problems, with the presence of irreparable damage in the deep venous system involving a postthrombotic syndrome, or a conducting vein insufficiency with a different pathogenesis. Long-term treatment success after surgical therapy can therefore only be achieved with consistent follow-up treatment. With every method of surgery, measures to provide protection against edema, such as long-term compression therapy, usually with compression stockings, continued decongestion therapy, and lifestyle changes (e.g., weight loss) are important factors in achieving lasting success.

References

Eckstein HH, Niedermeier HP, Noppeney T et al. Kommission für Qualitätssicherung Deutsche Gesellschaft für Gefäßchirurgie. Auswertungen Qualitätsmanagement „Varizen".

Fischer R, Schwahn-Schreiber Ch, Sattler G, Duff C. Die Indikation zur subfaszialen endoskopischen Perforantensanierung hat sich geändert. Phlebologie 2004; 33: 145–8.

Gaber Y, Gehl HB, Schmeller W. Magnetresonanz- und Computertomographie vor und nach Shave-Therapie venöser Ulzera. Phlebologie 1999; 28: 87–92.

Gallenkemper G, Ehresmann U, Hermanns HJ, Herouy Y, Kahle B, Jünger M, Rabe E, Scharfetter-Kochanek K, Schwahn-Schreiber C, Stücker M, Vanscheidt W, Waldermann F, Wilm S. Leitlinie zur Diagnostik und Therapie des Ulcus cruris venosum. Phlebologie 2004; 33: 166–85, Phlebologie 2008; 37: 308–29.

Hach W, Gerngroß H, Präwe F, Sterk J, Willy Ch, Hach-Wunderle V. Kompartmentsyndrom in der Phlebologie. Phlebologie 2000; 29: 1–11.

Hach W, Hach-Wunderle V. Neue Aspekte zum chronisch venösen Kompartmentsyndrom. Gefäßchirurgie 2001; 6: 164–9.

Hach W. Das arthrogene Stauungssyndrom. Gefäßchirurgie 2003; 8: 227–33.

Hach W. Wie es zur paratibialen Fasziotomie kam. Phlebologie 2004; 33: 110–4.

Hach W, Gruß JD, Hach-Wunderle V, Jünger M. Venenchirurgie. Leitfaden für Gefäßchirurgen, Angiologen, Dermatologen und Phlebologen. 2. Auflage. Stuttgart: Schattauer, 2007.

Hermanns HJ, Hermann V, Waldhausen P, Gallenkemper G. Lebensqualität vor und nach Shave-Therapie bei therapieresistenten Ulcera cruris. Vasomed 2000; 12 (4): 162.

Hermanns HJ, Gallenkemper G, Waldhausen P, Hermann V. Rezidivulcera nach Shave-Therapie – die Negativbilanz. Vasomed 2001; 13 (4): 154.

Hermanns HJ, Gallenkemper G, Kanya S. Langzeitergebnisse nach Shave-Therapie des therapieresisten Ulcus cruris. Vasomed 2003; 15 (4): 160–1.

Hermanns HJ, Gallenkämper G, Kanya S, et al. Die Shave-Therapie im Konzept der operativen Behandlung des therapieresistenten Ulcus cruris venosum. Phlebologie 2005; 34: 209–15.

Hermanns HJ. Die endoskopisch subfasziale Dissektion von Perforansvenen (Kommentar). Phlebologie 2006; 35: 92–3.

Hynes W. „Shaving" in plastic surgery with special reference to the treatment of chronic radiodermatitis. British Journal of Plastic Surgery 1959; 12: 43–54.

Kahle B. Ergebnisse der Schaumsklerosierung bei Ulcus cruris venosum. Vasomed 17. Jahrgang 1/2005: 21.

Kluess HG, Noppeney T, Gerlach H, Braunbeck W, Ehresmann U, Fischer R, Hermanns HJ, Langer Ch, Nüllen H, Salzmann G, Schimmelpfennig L. Leitlinie zur Diagnostik und Therapie des Krampfaderleidens. Phlebologie 2004; 33: 211–21.

Langer CH, Fuhrmann J, Grimm H, Vorpohl U. Orthostatische Kompartmentdruckmessung nach endoskopischer Fasziotomie. Phlebologie 1995; 24: 163–7.

Perrin M. Place de la chirurgie dans le traitement de l'ulcère veineux de jambe. Encyclopédie Médico-Chirurgicale 2004: 43–169-H.

Popescu M, Haug M. Eine einfache und effektive Behandlung des persistierenden venösen Ulcus cruris. Vasomed 2003; 15: 62–5.

Quaba AA, McDowall RAW, Hackett EJ. Layered shaving of venous leg ulcers. British Journal of Plastic Surgery 1987; 40: 68–72.

Rabe E, Pannier-Fischer F, Bromen K, Schuldt K, Stang A, Poncar Ch, Wittenhorst M, Bock E, Weber S, Jöckel KH. Bonner Venenstudie der Deutschen Gesellschaft für Phlebologie. Phlebologie 2003; 32: 1–14.

Ramelet AA, Schmeller W, et al. Management of leg ulcers. Curr Probl Dermatol, Basel: Karger, 1999, Vol 27: 182–9.

Schmeller W, Schwahn-Schreiber C, Hiss U, Gaber Y, Kirschner P. Vergleich zwischen Shave-Therapie und cruraler Fasziektomie bei der Behandlung „therapieresistenter" venöser Ulzera. Phlebologie 1999; 28: 35–60.

Schmeller W, Gaber Y. Behandlung therapieresitenter venöser Ulzera mittels Shave-Therapie. Deutsches Ärzteblatt 2000; Heft 38: Seite B 2107–10.

Schmeller W, Gaber Y. Persistierendes Ulcus cruris und chronisches venöses Kompartmensyndrom – Gibt es wirklich einen kausalen Zusammenhang? Phlebologie 2001; 30: 75–80.

Schmeller W, Schwahn-Schreiber Ch, Gaber Y. Langzeitergebnisse nach Shave-Therapie bzw. Fasziektomie bei persistierenden venösen Ulzera. Phlebologie 2006; 35: 89–91.

Van Rji AM, Hill G, Gray C et al. A prospective study of the fate of venous leg perforators after varicose vein surgery. J Vasc Surg 2005; 42: 1156–62.

Wienert V, Gerlach H, Gallenkemper G et al. Leitlinie Medizinischer Kompressionsstrumpf (MKS). Phlebologie 2006; 35: 315–20.

Wienert V, Waldermann F, Zabel M, Rabe E, Jünger M. Leitlinie Phlebologischer Kompressionsverband. Phlebologie 2004; 33: 131–4.

Wienert V, Partsch H, Gallenkemper H et al. Leitlinie: Intermittierende pneumatische Kompression (IPK oder AIK). Phlebologie 2005; 34: 176–80.

5   Portal vein thrombosis, splenic vein thrombosis

Clinical picture: Thomas Frieling
Clinical findings: Thomas Frieling
Diagnosis and differential diagnosis: Thomas Frieling
Treatment: Thomas Frieling
Interventional treatment: Philip Hilgard and Claus Nolte-Ernsting

5.1   Clinical picture

The incidence of portal vein thrombosis in the general population is approximately 0.05%. It occurs in association with liver cirrhosis in up to 16% of cases, after liver transplantation in up to 14%, with Budd–Chiari syndrome in up to 22%, and with liver cirrhosis and malignancies in up to 34%. The cause of portal vein thrombosis remains unclear in approximately 50% of cases (idiopathic portal vein thrombosis). The remainder of the cases are attributed to various types of cancer (including hepatocellular carcinoma, pancreatic carcinoma, gastric carcinoma, colonic carcinoma, peritoneal carcinosis, and myeloproliferative diseases), inflammatory conditions (including pancreatitis), thrombocytosis, polycythemia, coagulation disturbances (e.g., protein S deficiency, protein C deficiency, angiotensin III deficiency, activated protein C resistance), pregnancy, and contraceptives.

Splenic vein thromboses are rare events. Precise figures on the incidence are not available. Splenic vein thrombosis is caused by pancreatitis or a pancreatic tumor in approximately 70% of cases (Fig. 5-1). Other causes include trauma, surgical complications, pancreatic pseudocysts, malignancies (including renal carcinomas and lymphomas), thrombocytosis, polycythemia, coagulation disturbances (protein S deficiency, protein C deficiency, activated protein C resistance), pregnancy, oral contraceptives, appendicitis, sepsis, radiotherapy, variceal sclerotherapy, and thrombosis of the leg and pelvic veins.

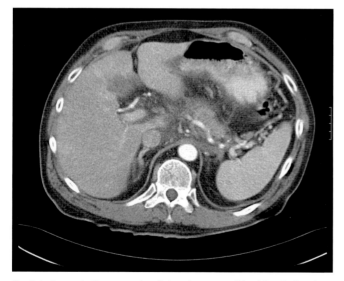

Fig. 5-1 Computed tomography of chronic pancreatitis with splenic vein thrombosis. (Picture courtesy of Prof. V. Fiedler, Institute of Radiographic Diagnosis, Helios Hospital, Krefeld, Germany.)

5.2   Clinical findings

Acute portal vein thrombosis is only rarely associated with the symptoms of acute abdomen, and usually remains asymptomatic. The clinical findings and prognosis in chronic portal vein thrombosis are determined by the underlying disease and extent of portal hypertension involved—i.e., esophageal variceal bleeding, congestive gastropathy, splenomegaly, hypersplenism (20% with thrombocytopenia, 15% with leukopenia, 10% with hemolytic anemia). Ascites, hepatorenal or hepatopulmonary syndrome, and encephalopathy do not usually occur when there is no impairment of hepatic function in portal vein thrombosis.

Splenic vein thrombosis is also often asymptomatic. Abdominal pain is mainly caused by the splenomegaly observed in approximately 50% of cases. Esophageal fundic varices may develop after 2–3 weeks.

5.3   Diagnosis and differential diagnosis

Exploratory examinations are carried out with ultrasonography and duplex ultrasonography. Abdominal ultrasound reveals a dilated and thrombosed portal vein or splenic vein, with hyperechoic material in the lumen. In addition, there is often dilation of the hepatic arteries, splenomegaly, dilated visceral collateral veins, and cavernous transformation.

The method of choice is color duplex ultrasonography. Typical signs of portal vein thrombosis or splenic vein thrombosis include evidence of hyperechoic material in the portal vein lumen, absent flow, flow past a thrombus, or inverse flow. Color duplex ultrasonography now has a sensitivity of nearly 100% for portal vein thrombosis. In splenic vein thrombosis, angiography (splenoportography) can establish the diagnosis in approximately 100% of cases. The characteristic finding is contrast filling of the splenic vein in late-phase arteriography, whereas the portal vein is patent.

Computed tomography (CT) is indicated in patients with symptoms of ileus and pancreatitis (Fig. 5-1). The CT scan shows an intravascular filling defect after contrast administration, increased density in the area of the venous wall, collateral circulation, and cavernous transformation. The sensitivity of CT, at 75%, is slightly lower than that of magnetic resonance imaging (MRI) but higher than that of ultrasonography.

Endoscopy reveals the signs of portal hypertension, with esophageal and fundic varices and congestive gastropathy. On indirect arterial portography using the digital subtraction angiography (DSA) technique, portosystemic and portoportal collaterals are seen, with angiographically normal imaging of the hepatic veins.

The differential diagnosis should include the causes of portal hypertension listed in the following chapter. These also include tumor involvement of the portal vein. Hepatic cysts, which may simulate cavernous transformation, should also be considered.

5.4 Treatment

Basic treatment for portal vein thrombosis and splenic vein thrombosis consists of effective anticoagulation with heparin and medication to reduce portal vein pressure using nitrates or β-blockers. Recanalization with cavernous transformation of the portal vein often occurs over the course of time, with substantial normalization of flow conditions. On endoscopy, esophageal and fundic varices can be treated with rubber-band ligation or sclerotherapy using ethoxysclerol or Histoacryl®. In cases of acute bleeding, portal vein pressure can be reduced briefly with somatostatin, octreotide, or terlipressin. Endoscopic hemostasis is successful in 90–95% of cases. Placement of a transjugular intrahepatic portosystemic shunt (TIPSS; see Chapter B 6) can also be done on an emergency basis in patients with acute portal vein thrombosis. The mortality rate in emergency situations is nearly 50%.

If all internal-medicine options have been exhausted, symptomatic portal vein thrombosis can be treated with portosystemic shunt surgery (distal splenorenal shunt, mesocaval shunt). The surgical mortality rate with shunt operations is up to 13%; the long-term survival rate after 4 years is approximately 60% and is mainly determined by the underlying disease.

Splenectomy is the treatment of choice in acute splenic vein thrombosis. However, it is contraindicated if portal vein thrombosis is also present. The prognosis depends on the underlying disease, and the course of the condition depends on the development of portal hypertension. Approximately 50% of patients with splenic vein thrombosis develop gastroesophageal varices. Early splenectomy prevents this complication from developing.

5.4.1 Interventional therapy for portal vein thrombosis

5.4.1.1 Introduction

Although portal vein thrombosis (PVT) in the absence of underlying malignant disease (particularly hepatocellular carcinoma) is relatively rare, it may substantially complicate the course of liver cirrhosis due to the resulting severe portal hypertension. Typical complications of portal hypertension with or without portal vein thrombosis include:

- Treatment-refractory ascites
- Esophageal and gastric fundus varices with bleeding
- Hepatorenal syndrome

Interventional treatment for portal vein thrombosis, as a minimally invasive alternative to surgical shunt placement, is a relatively new therapeutic approach that currently *does not* have a secure evidence base in the form of controlled studies. The following recommendations are thus based on small, uncontrolled studies or case series, as well as the authors' personal experience.

When an interventional treatment procedure is being selected, the acuteness of the condition needs to be taken into account—i.e., the age of the thrombosis, its etiology and pathogenesis, as well as underlying hepatic function. Before any interventional treatment is carried out, the cases of patients with PVT should be discussed on an interdisciplinary basis with gastroenterologists with hepatology experience, radiologists, and surgeons in order to clarify the options for one of the established surgical treatments for PVT—e.g., a Warren splenorenal shunt. Surgery is the treatment of choice, particularly in chronic PVT in the absence of liver cirrhosis (Parikh et al. 2010; Ponziani et al. 2010) and need not be discussed here.

With regard to interventional therapy for PVT, several procedures are now available that can be used in a variety of situations, and even sequentially in individual cases (De Santis et al. 2010; Ferro et al. 2007; Hollingshead et al. 2005; Safieddine et al. 2007; Senzolo et al. 2007; Wang et al. 2010):

- Short-term or long-term systemic venous fibrinolytic therapy
- "Local" long-term visceral fibrinolytic therapy via the superior mesenteric artery and/or splenic artery
- Recanalization of the portal vein with local lysis and/or stent implantation via a transjugular intrahepatic portosystemic stent shunt (TIPSS)

5.4.1.2 Systemic (venous) and local visceral lytic therapy via the superior mesenteric artery

Indications

- Fresh portal vein thrombosis no more than 2 weeks old (Fig. 5-2)
- Portal vein thrombosis, no more than 2 weeks old, as a sequela of Child stage A liver cirrhosis with no evidence of hepatocellular carcinoma

Contraindications

- Malignant portal vein thrombosis
- Portal vein thrombosis over 2 weeks old
- Chronic portal vein thrombosis with cavernous transformation (small-lumen venous collaterals in the hilum of the liver alongside the thrombosed portal vein)
- General contraindications against fibrinolytic therapy (even in intra-arterial fibrinolytic therapy, the major part of the thrombolytic agent administered is systemically active, so that the same contraindications apply; Table 5-1)

Technique and administration of intravenous systemic fibrinolytic therapy

Systemic administration of the thrombolytic agent is carried out via a peripheral or central venous indwelling catheter. The fibrinolytic therapy should always be carried out in a monitored intensive-care setting.

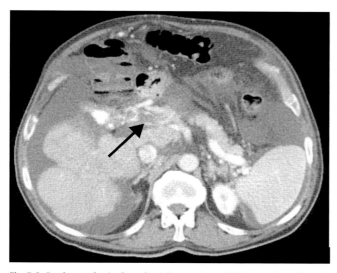

Fig. 5-2 Fresh portal vein thrombosis in a patient with liver cirrhosis (arrow).

Table 5.1 Contraindications against drug-based fibrinolytic therapy.

Absolute contraindications	Relative contraindications
Craniocerebral trauma < 3 months with significant neurologic deficit	Coma or stupor
History of intracranial hemorrhage	Active gastric ulcer
Known cerebral tumor or intracranial vascular malformation	Aortic aneurysm, aortic dissection
Intra-abdominal or intrathoracic hemorrhage < 6 months	Limited hepatic function, warfarin therapy
Ischemic stroke < 3 months	Colitis of any cause
Surgical procedure < 10 days	Metastatic carcinoma or lymphoma
Arterial hypertension not controlled with drug treatment, with systolic blood pressure > 185 mmHg or diastolic pressure > 110 mmHg	Surgical procedure or organ biopsy < 30 days
Severe hemorrhagic diathesis or coagulopathy	Arterial puncture in a noncompressible position < 7 days
	Gastrointestinal bleeding < 30 days
	Pregnancy or delivery < 30 days
	Known allergy to urokinase

- Short-term thrombolysis with **tissue plasminogen activator**: administration of alteplase 0.9 mg/kg body weight (maximum dosage 90 mg) (r-TPA = Actilyse®)
  - 10% of this as an intravenous bolus and
  - 90% immediately thereafter as an infusion over 1 h
  - No antithrombotic agents (heparins) for 24 h after thrombolysis
- Long-term thrombolysis with **urokinase**: continuous infusion of urokinase 15,000–50,000 IU per hour for 5–7 days, with compulsory intensive-care monitoring (max. dosage 90 mg):

- Control of dosage via fibrinogen (no less than 50 mg/dL, ideally 50–100 mg/dL)
- Concomitant partial thromboplastin time (PTT)-guided anticoagulation treatment (continued for approx. 60 to max. 80 s) with unfractionated intravenous heparin (to allow for rapid reversal if necessary)

While short-term thrombolysis with tissue plasminogen activator is only capable of inducing recanalization in very fresh thromboses (with start of symptoms up to a maximum of 48 h previously), long-term urokinase fibrinolysis may be successful in individual cases even with thromboses as old as 2 weeks. In the frequently observed cases with a subacute course and consequently unclear time of onset of thrombosis, but with imaging evidence of "fresh" thrombus (no cavernous transformation, thrombus not organized), urokinase fibrinolysis is therefore preferable.

Technique and administration of "local" visceral fibrinolytic therapy via the superior mesenteric vein and/or splenic vein

- Catheter access of the superior mesenteric artery and placement of a microcatheter in the main trunk. Alternatively, in cases of isolated splenic vein thrombosis, access of the splenic artery is also possible via the celiac trunk. Percutaneous arterial access is usually obtained via the common femoral artery. Figure 5-3 demonstrates catheters in the hepatic and splenic arteries (local treatment had not been possible in the case shown).
- In patients with chronic portal vein thrombosis against a background of liver cirrhosis, a spontaneous splenorenal shunt is often present and a targeted search for it should be made using imaging techniques (Fig. 5-3). As an alternative, direct angiographic access of the splenic vein or hepatic portal vein may be attempted via a splenorenal shunt (access via femoral vein → renal vein → shunt vein → splenic vein).
- After catheter placement in the desired position, long-term fibrinolysis is carried out with urokinase (see above for dosage) and intensive-care monitoring.
- The fibrinolysis treatment must be interrupted immediately if there are any clinical signs of hemorrhage or an unexplained fall in the hemoglobin level is noted.

5.4.1.3 Interventional therapy (local fibrinolysis, thrombectomy, balloon angioplasty and/or stenting) via a transjugular intrahepatic portosystemic shunt (TIPSS)

Indications

- Portal vein thrombosis that is idiopathic or has developed in the context of liver cirrhosis, with no relevant cavernous transformation and with a main portal vein trunk that can be well demonstrated on ultrasound, including the portal vein bifurcation
- Unsuccessful venous or local visceral fibrinolytic therapy for acute portal vein thrombosis (< 2 weeks)
- Chronic portal vein thrombosis with cavernous transformation (only in exceptional cases)

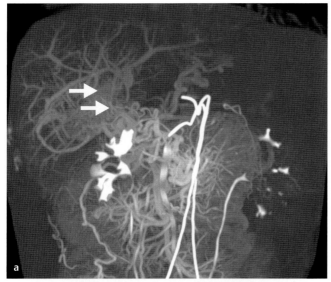

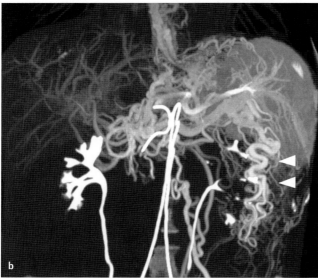

Fig. 5-3a, b Older portal vein and mesenteric vein thrombosis with marked cavernous transformation (arrow) and spontaneous splenorenal shunt (arrowheads) in a patient with no liver cirrhosis. Magnetic resonance angiography to clarify the vascular anatomy, with direct administration of contrast into the hepatic artery (**a**) and splenic artery (**b**).

Contraindication

- Malignant portal vein thrombosis

Technique and administration of interventional therapy for PVT via TIPSS

- Transcatheter access of the portal vein via jugular vein
  - Access of the right internal jugular vein and placement of a 9F sheath using the Seldinger technique
  - Retrograde placement of a steerable (i.e. angled) catheter with a hydrophilic wire into the right hepatic vein
  - Introduction of a rigid guidewire into the right hepatic vein via previously placed catheter
  - Introduction into the right hepatic vein over the rigid guidewire of a puncture needle approx. 55 cm long with a pre-bent tip (modified Ross needle)

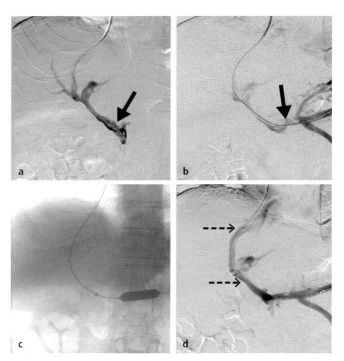

Fig. 5.4a–d Transjugular portography, TIPSS placement and balloon angioplasty in a patient with partial thrombosis of the portal and splenic veins. (**a**, **b**) Diagnostic transjugular portography, showing the thrombus and consequently reduced diameter of the main trunk of the portal vein (arrow). (**c**) Balloon angioplasty of the thrombotic parts of the vessel. (**d**) Portography after placement of the TIPSS (dashed arrows).

- Removal of the guidewire, and subsequent puncture of the right main branch of the portal vein, ideally approx. 0.5–1.5 cm distal to the portal vein bifurcation using real-time ultrasound and fluoroscopic guidance; care must be taken to ensure that there is adequate parenchymal coverage of the puncture entry site (otherwise there is a danger of intra-abdominal hemorrhage). During the puncture procedure into the thrombotic branch of the portal vein, ultrasonography must allow continuous identification of the position of the tip of the puncture needle relative to the intended puncture site in the portal vein.
- *Caution:* Puncture of the portal vein from the transjugular direction and advancement of the guidewire may be very difficult, due to the absence of blood backflow resulting from the thrombosis. If necessary, an attempt may also be made to carry out a percutaneous ultrasound-guided puncture of the right branch of the portal vein, with subsequent wire placement.
- After successful puncture and access of the main trunk of the portal vein with a flexible hydrophilic wire and removal of the puncture cannula, a 5F angiography catheter can be advanced into the perfused section of the portal vein trunk (or into the splenic vein if appropriate), and direct portography can be carried out, with direct portal vein pressure measurement if needed.
- Transjugular introduction of a rigid guidewire into the portal vein, over which all subsequent intervention steps can be carried out.

- Local intraportal catheter thrombectomy or catheter fibrinolysis via the transjugular access route, if necessary, after definitive portal vein puncture (usually before placement of the intrahepatic stent, to minimize the risk of pulmonary embolism); see Fig. 5-4. The following measures may be considered here:

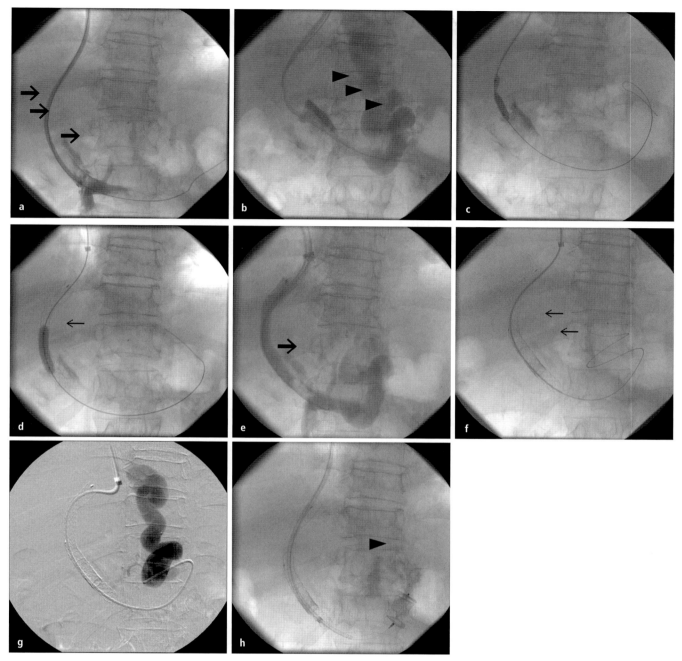

Fig. 5-5a–h Transjugular portography, TIPSS placement, and closure of a large gastric varix in a patient with liver cirrhosis, nonmalignant portal vein thrombosis. Subsequently, massive portal hypertension was noted clinically, with grade 3 esophageal varices and treatment-refractory ascites. (**a**) Diagnostic transjugular portography, showing the thrombus (arrows) and occluded portal vein downstream from it. (**b**) A large gastric varix (arrowheads), arising from the splenic vein. (**c**) Dilation of the TIPSS tract using a balloon (8 mm) and (**d**) dilation of the newly placed TIPSS (arrow). (**e**) Portography after TIPSS placement, with persistent thrombus in the distal segment of the portal vein (arrow). (**f**) Extension of the TIPSS into the distal portal vein using a stent-in-stent technique (arrows) and probing/demonstration (**g**) of the gastric varix. (**h**) Status post occlusion of the gastric varix using an 18-mm Amplatz occluder (arrowhead).

– If the thrombosis is very fresh, an attempt at aspiration thrombectomy may be made with a wide-lumen aspiration catheter (e.g., 8F).

– Attempt at catheter thrombectomy (e.g. rheolytic).

– In case of fresh thromboses, local short-term fibrinolytic therapy (e.g., pulse spray) with tissue plasminogen activator (see above for dosage), or rarely, long-term fibrinolysis with urokinase may be possible.

– In older and organized thromboses, balloon dilation is carried out in the partly or completely obliterated portal vein (diameter

8–10 mm, see Fig. 5-4) to fragment the thrombus and prepare for subsequent scaffolding with a TIPSS stent (see Fig. 5-5).

■ Placement of the TIPSS in the parenchymal tract using a self-expanding stent prosthesis covered with polytetrafluoroethylene (PTFE)

– After the interventions described above, the parenchymal tract is dilated to 8 mm.

– Using a transjugularly introduced measuring catheter, the length of the TIPSS tract and the stent length to be implanted are measured. Depending on the extent of the portal vein thrombosis, a stent length extending possibly into the venous confluence (or perhaps even beyond it) needs to be planned. As the available stent length is limited by the manufacturers, two or several overlapping stents sometimes have to be implanted in order to recanalize the entire thrombotic segment of the portal vein (Fig. 5-5). *Caution:* to prevent hepatic vein stenoses (i.e. the TIPSS outflow tract), the stent must also not be too close to the hepatic veins.

- Transjugular exchange of a long 10F TIPSS sheath into the main portal vein trunk.
- Introduction of the TIPSS-specific devices and, after the position has been checked, fluoroscopy-targeted release of the covered stent. The nominal stent diameter should be 10 mm.
- After complete implantation of the covered stent(s), the lumen can be further enlarged using a balloon catheter (a balloon diameter of 8 mm is usually sufficient, but if ascites, for example, persists afterward, the covered stent can be dilated up to the full 10 mm to its nominal diameter in a subsequent session).
- Final portography (with/without portal vein pressure measurement) is then performed.
- Removal of the instruments and placement of an internal jugular central venous catheter as needed.

After TIPSS placement, the patient requires intensive-care monitoring for 24 h to allow early detection of any risk of intra-abdominal hemorrhage. The TIPSS causes an immediate and marked increase of blood flow in the portal vein, and therefore the possibility that, with appropriate anticoagulation (acetylsalicylic acid [ASA] and heparin [initially at a therapeutic dosage]), that the previously thrombosed portal vein may remain permanently patent in most cases after the local intervention (e.g. lysis, balloon angioplasty, and stenting of the portal vein). Particularly in patients with liver cirrhosis with an option for future liver transplantation, placement of a TIPSS and/or portal vein stent should be carried out in close consultation with a hepatologist or surgeon with transplantation experience, since stent implantation extending well into the main trunk of the portal vein (e.g. extending beyond the venous confluence) can sometimes impair the technical feasibility of liver transplantation. Follow-up ultrasound examinations of the TIPSS are carried out weekly for the first 4 weeks, every 6 weeks for the first 6 months, and thereafter every 3–6 months. If there are clinical (upper gastrointestinal bleeding, recurrent increasing ascites, etc.) and/or ultrasound signs of TIPSS occlusion, a repeat intervention must be carried out at the earliest opportunity, with an attempt to recanalize the TIPSS. Hepatic encephalopathy is a possible complication (particularly in patients with liver cirrhosis), but it can typically be controlled both in the acute phase and long-term using medication in accordance with hepatology recommendations (e.g. lactulose, paromomycin, or rifaximin and ornithine aspartate). When hepatic encephalopathy is refractory to drug treatment, placement of a reduction stent in the TIPS stent prosthesis may be considered.

References

De Santis A, Moscatelli R, Catalano C, Iannetti A, Gigliotti F, Cristofari F, Trapani S, et al. Systemic thrombolysis of portal vein thrombosis in cirrhotic patients: a pilot study. Dig Liver Dis 2010; 42: 451–5.

Ferro C, Rossi UG, Bovio G, Dahamane M, Centanaro M. Transjugular intrahepatic portosystemic shunt, mechanical aspiration thrombectomy, and direct thrombolysis in the treatment of acute portal and superior mesenteric vein thrombosis. Cardiovasc Intervent Radiol 2007; 30: 1070–4.

Hollingshead M, Burke CT, Mauro MA, Weeks SM, Dixon RG, Jaques PF. Transcatheter thrombolytic therapy for acute mesenteric and portal vein thrombosis. J Vasc Interv Radiol 2005; 16: 651–61.

Parikh S, Shah R, Kapoor P. Portal vein thrombosis. Am J Med 2010; 123: 111–9.

Ponziani FR, Zocco MA, Campanale C, Rinninella E, Tortora A, Di Maurizio L, Bombardieri G, et al. Portal vein thrombosis: insight into physiopathology, diagnosis, and treatment. World J Gastroenterol 2010; 16: 143–55.

Safieddine N, Mamazza J, Common A, Prabhudesai V. Splenic and superior mesenteric artery thrombolytic infusion therapy for acute portal and mesenteric vein thrombosis. Can J Surg 2007; 50: 68–9.

Senzolo M, Patch D, Cholongitas E, Burroughs AK. Transjugular intrahepatic portosystemic shunt for portal vein thrombosis with and without underlying cirrhosis. Cardiovasc Intervent Radiol 2007; 30: 545; author reply 546.

Wang MQ, Guo LP, Lin HY, Liu FY, Duan F, Wang ZJ. Transradial approach for transcatheter selective superior mesenteric artery urokinase infusion therapy in patients with acute extensive portal and superior mesenteric vein thrombosis. Cardiovasc Intervent Radiol 2010; 33: 80–9.

6 Portal hypertension

Thomas Frieling

6.1 Clinical picture

Portal hypertension is a syndrome characterized by a chronic increase in portal vein pressure. According to earlier studies, at least 60% of patients with liver cirrhosis develop portal hypertension with esophageal varices or ascites during the course of the disease. The various causes of portal hypertension are listed in Table 6-1. If the pressure gradient between the portal vein and hepatic veins is more than 10 mmHg, a collateral circulation develops, with the formation of esophageal varices and fundic varices near the gastric cardia (afferent flow via the gastric veins or short gastric veins to the esophageal veins, efferent flow via the azygos vein to the superior vena cava). Hemorrhoids also develop (with afferent flow via the inferior mesenteric vein and rectal vein and efferent flow via the anal veins and iliac vein to the inferior vena cava), as do paraumbilical veins with the development of caput medusae (with afferent flow via the left portal vein branch to the epigastric veins, which form connections with the superior and inferior caval veins), collaterals between the surface of the liver or spleen and the diaphragm, in the retroperitoneal space, between the omentum and the anterior abdominal wall, and the formation of a spontaneous splenorenal shunt (with portal vein blood flowing directly from the splenic vein or from diaphragmatic, pancreatic, or gastric veins to the left renal vein). Collaterals to the omentum and the anterior abdominal wall may be injured during laparoscopy, and this can lead to severe secondary bleeding.

6.2 Clinical findings

The clinical findings in patients with portal hypertension depend on the underlying disease and the complications of hypertension (Table 6-2). For example, bleeding from esophageal or fundic varices occurs in 30–40% of cases (Fig. 6-1). There is an increased risk of bleeding in patients with previous variceal bleeding, with large varices (> 5 mm), red spots (dilated superficial venous plexus on the varices), combined esophageal and fundic varices, and in those with limited liver function (Child class C). Congestive gastropathy is also often seen, as is splenomegaly with hypersplenism (20% thrombocytopenia, 15% leukopenia, 10% hemolytic anemia). If liver function disturbances are also present, ascites or hepatorenal syndrome may develop, often triggered by bleeding, spontaneous bacterial peritonitis, nephrotoxic drugs, or uncontrolled diuretic treatment. Type I hepatorenal syndrome develops rapidly and progressively within 1–2 weeks, and the mean survival time without treatment is

Table 6-1 Causes of portal hypertension.

Prehepatic portal hypertension (portal vein or splenic vein thrombosis)	■ Tumor diseases (e.g., hepatocellular carcinoma, pancreatic carcinoma, gastric carcinoma, colon carcinoma, peritoneal carcinosis, myeloproliferative diseases) ■ Inflammation (e.g., pancreatitis) ■ Thrombocytosis, polycythemia, coagulation disturbances (protein S, protein C, angiotensin III deficiency) ■ Pregnancy, oral contraceptives
Intrahepatic portal hypertension	■ Presinusoidal: schistosomiasis, congenital hepatic fibrosis, primary biliary cirrhosis, sarcoidosis, chronic intoxication with vinyl chloride, arsenic, or copper ■ Sinusoidal: alcoholic liver cirrhosis, virus-induced liver cirrhosis ■ Postsinusoidal: thrombosis of the intrahepatic veins (Budd–Chiari syndrome), hepatic vein occlusive disease (obliterative hepatic endophlebitis), membrane stenotic occlusions in the hepatic veins or inferior vena cava, often oral contraceptives, polycythemia, coagulation disturbances, and tumor compression of the hepatic veins
Posthepatic portal hypertension	■ Right cardiac insufficiency ■ Obstruction of the inferior vena cava proximal to the hepatic vein ostia ■ Constrictive pericarditis

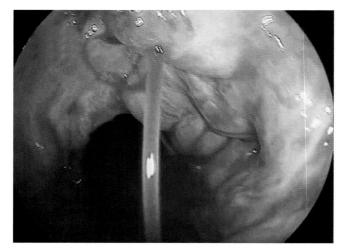

Fig. 6-1 Portal hypertension and esophageal variceal bleeding.

Table 6-2 Sequelae of portal hypertension.

Esophageal varices, fundic varices, gastric varices
Ascites
Congestive gastropathy
Hypersplenism, hypersplenic syndrome
Hepatorenal syndrome types I and II
Hepatopulmonary syndrome

Table 6-3 Characteristics of hepatorenal syndrome.

Major criteria

- Advanced liver disease with portal hypertension
- Low glomerular filtration rate with creatinine > 1.5 mg/dL or creatinine clearance < 40 mL/min
- No other triggering factors (shock, infection, nephrotoxic drugs, gastrointestinal/renal fluid losses)
- No sustained renal function improvement after withdrawal of diuretics and fluid administration (1.5 L NaCl 0.9%)
- No proteinuria (< 500 mg/dL), no primary renal disease

Additional criteria

- Urinary output < 500 mL/24 h
- Low urinary sodium (< 10 mmol/L)
- Urinary osmolality > plasma osmolality
- Erythrocyturia < 50 per high-powered field
- Hyponatremia < 130 mmol/L

Table 6-4 Measurement parameters for color duplex ultrasonography.

Parameter	Normal values
Peak systolic velocity (PSV)	20–30 cm/s
Time-averaged maximum velocity (TAV_{max})	9–105 cm/s
Time-averaged mean velocity (TAV_{mean})	13–22 cm/s
Blood flow volume (BF)	694–1066 mL/min
Diameter	10.9 ± 1.6 mm
V_{max}	20.4 ± 4.7 cm/s
V_{min}	14.0 ± 3.6 cm/s
V_{max}–V_{min}	6.5 ± 3.2 cm/s

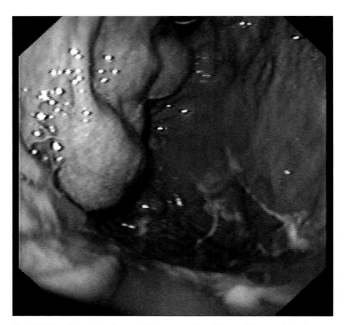

Fig. 6-2 Fundic varices in portal hypertension. View of the cardia in inversion.

less than 2 weeks. By contrast, type II has a moderate and insidious course, with a more favorable prognosis. Table 6-3 lists the characteristics of hepatorenal syndrome.

In addition to hepatorenal syndrome, hepatopulmonary syndrome may also develop in 5–15% of cases. The characteristic features are inadequate vasodilation in the pulmonary (pre-)capillaries and hyperdynamic circulation, functional right–left shunts that improve with oxygen ventilation, failure of the Euler–Liljestrand reflex, and arterial hypoxemia < 70 mmHg, which deteriorates with exercise and when the patient is standing. The clinical findings include dyspnea, peripheral cyanosis, and clubbing in the fingers. In type I hepatopulmonary syndrome, diffuse arterial anastomoses are seen over the whole lung, while circumscribed findings are seen in type II.

6.3 Diagnosis and differential diagnosis

In addition to the clinical examination, which shows typical signs of liver cirrhosis (ascites and splenomegaly), abdominal ultrasonography (for liver cirrhosis, splenomegaly, ascites, dilated portal vein, dilated visceral collateral veins) is the method of choice and also allows identification of Budd–Chiari syndrome (with thromboses and membrane occlusion in the hepatic vein and inferior vena cava). The optimal assessment point for color duplex ultrasonography is located intercostally, before the division into the two intrahepatic branches at the confluence. The insonation angle should be less than 60°. The parameters measured are peak systolic velocity (PSV), end-diastolic velocity (EDV), time-averaged maximum velocity (TAV_{max}), time-averaged mean velocity (TAV_{mean}), resistance index (RI), pulsatility index (PI), blood flow volume (BF), diameter, V_{max}, V_{min}, and V_{max}–V_{min}. Table 6-4 shows the normal values for several parameters.

In patients with portal vein hypertension, flow in the portal vein may be slower or reversed (hepatofugal flow). In Budd–Chiari syndrome, flow signals are absent in the area of the hepatic veins or inferior vena cava. Dilation of the hepatic veins or inferior vena cava without caliber changes during respiration or a Valsalva maneuver is an indirect sign of venous obstruction.

Endoscopy shows esophageal or fundic varices and congestive gastropathy (Fig. 6-2). Computed tomography, magnetic resonance imaging, indirect arterial portography using the DSA technique, and venography of the hepatic veins and inferior vena cava is usu-

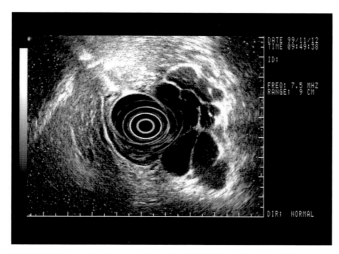

Fig. 6-3 Endoscopic ultrasound imaging of fundic varices. Anechoic vascular structures are seen in the wall of the cardia and gastric fundus.

Table 6-5 Differential diagnosis of portal hypertension.

Changes	Differential diagnoses
Esophageal and fundic varices	▪ "Downhill" varices in the proximal third of the esophagus with right cardiac insufficiency or mediastinal processes with flow impairment in the inferior vena cava ▪ Mediastinal tumors with esophageal involvement, esophageal carcinoma ▪ Abdominal processes with cardial and fundic involvement, cardial gastric carcinoma ▪ Splenic vein thrombosis ▪ Arteriovenous splenic fistula
Ascites	▪ Right cardiac insufficiency, constrictive pericarditis ▪ Peritoneal carcinosis ▪ Marked hypoalbuminemia ▪ Tuberculosis ▪ Pancreatic ascites ▪ Secondary bacterial peritonitis ▪ Nephrotic syndrome, nephrotic ascites ▪ Primary or secondary intestinal lymphangiectasia
Splenomegaly, hypersplenic syndrome	▪ Hematological diseases (e.g., myeloproliferative diseases, malignant lymphomas, hemolytic anemia) ▪ Rheumatological diseases (e.g., juvenile rheumatoid arthritis, Felty syndrome) ▪ Amyloidosis

ally reserved for special investigations (including hepatic tumors, Budd–Chiari syndrome, and occlusion of the inferior vena cava). Esophageal and fundic varices can also be visualized with endoscopic ultrasonography (Fig. 6-3). Differential diagnostic conditions that may simulate portal hypertension clinically are listed in Table 6-5—esophageal fundic varices, ascites, splenomegaly, and hypersplenism.

6.4   Treatment

Conservative treatment for portal hypertension involves drug treatment to reduce portal vein pressure, with nitrates and β-blockers. The aim is to achieve a portal vein pressure < 10 mmHg. The clinical sign of adequate adjustment with β-blockers is a reduction in the baseline heart rate at rest by 20%. Intravenous administration of somatostatin analogues (octreotide) and Glycylpressin (terlipressin) can be used for drug treatment of acute variceal bleeding and for rapid reduction of portal vein pressure.

Esophageal varices are treated endoscopically using rubber-band ligation (Fig. 6-4), or less often with sclerotherapy using ethoxysclerol. Fundic varices can be treated by injecting Histoacryl, which polymerizes in the varices. In comparison with the transjugular intrahepatic portosystemic shunt (TIPSS), portosystemic shunt operations (with a distal splenorenal shunt, portocaval or mesocaval shunt) have declined in importance due to their high complication rates.

In TIPSS placement, after transjugular access via a hepatic vein, the right portal vein branch is usually punctured with ultrasound and fluoroscopic guidance (Fig. 6-5). After this, the puncture channel

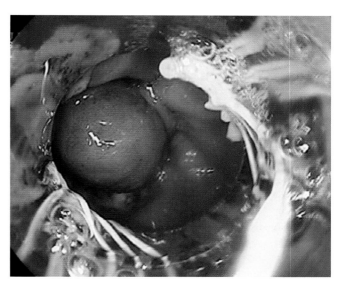

Fig. 6-4 Rubber-band ligation of esophageal varices in a patient with portal hypertension. The image shows an endoscopic view of a ligated esophageal varix (blue rubber band).

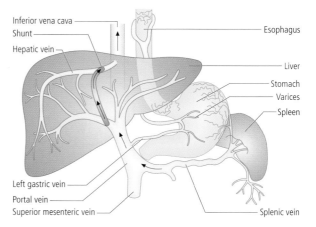

Fig. 6-5 Diagram of the transjugular intrahepatic portosystemic shunt (TIPSS) procedure.

Table 6-6 Indications and contraindications for transjugular intrahepatic portosystemic shunt (TIPSS) placement.

Indications for TIPSS placement	■ Endoscopically untreatable esophageal and fundic varix recurrent bleeding ■ Treatment-refractory ascites ■ Hydrothorax ■ Hepatorenal syndrome ■ Budd–Chiari syndrome ■ Fresh portal vein thrombosis
Contraindications against TIPSS placement	■ Thrombotic occlusion of the internal jugular vein or vena cava ■ Cavernous transformation of the portal vein ■ Polycystic liver ■ Advanced liver failure ■ Encephalopathy ■ Hepatic metastases ■ Consumption coagulopathy ■ Severe cardiac insufficiency (caution: shunt volumes) ■ Hepatocellular carcinoma (relative contraindication)

is dilated to 8–12 mm and the connection thereby created is maintained using a metal stent. Probing the portal vein also allows Histoacryl sclerotherapy for esophageal varices. Functionally, the TIPSS represents a portocaval side-to-side shunt, with the advantages that it can be carried out without surgery and that the diameter can be selected variably.

The main indications and contraindications for TIPSS are presented in Table 6-6. TIPSS is more effective in preventing recurrent bleeding than endoscopic treatment (recurrent bleeding rate with TIPSS 19% vs. endoscopy 47%). By contrast, the rate of encephalopathy is higher after TIPSS (34% vs. 19%). The procedure-related mortality rate is 2%, and the complication rate is 10%. The most frequent and dangerous complication is the development of encephalopathy

(15–30%). The prognosis in patients with advanced liver disease (Child C) and esophageal variceal bleeding is poor, with a 30-day mortality rate of up to 60%. Ascites, intubation, a low Quick value, an elevated creatinine level and leukothrombopenia are independent risk factors. Shunt stenoses that develop during the first year after TIPSS placement can be dilated. Early occlusion due to shunt thromboses (10%) should be prevented by administering heparin initially and aspirin later.

TIPSS placement can also be carried out as an emergency procedure. Primary hemostasis is successful in 90% of cases. However, the mortality in emergency situations is nearly 50%.

References

Brothers TE, Stanley JC, Zelenock GB. Splenic arteriovenous fistula. Int Surg 1995; 80: 189–94.

Ignee A, Gebel M, Caspary WF, Dietrich Ch F. Duplexsonographie der Lebergefäße – eine Übersicht. Z Gastroenterol 2002; 40: 21–32.

Jäger KA, Landmann L (eds). Praxis der angiologischen Diagnostik: Stufendiagnostik und rationelles Vorgehen bei arterieller und venöser Durchblutungsstörung. Berlin, Heidelberg, New York: Springer, 1994.

Jensen DM. Endoscopic screening for varices in cirrhosis: findings, implications, and outcomes. Gastroenterology 2002; 122: 1620–30.

Lankisch PG. The spleen in inflammatory pancreatic disease. Gastroenterology 1990; 98: 509–16.

Levine JS, Klör H-U, G Oehler (eds.). Gastroenterologische Differentialdiagnostik. Stuttgart, New York: Schattauer, 1995.

Ludwig M (ed.). Angiologie in Klinik und Praxis. Stuttgart: Thieme, 1998.

Maier K-P (ed.). Hepatitis – Hepatitisfolgen. Stuttgart: Thieme, 2000.

Rieger H, Schoop W (eds). Klinische Angiologie. Berlin, Heidelberg, New York: Springer, 1998.

Rupp KD, Hohlbach G. Der Mesenterialinfarkt als seltene Differentialdiagnose des akuten Abdomens. Chir Gastroenterologie mit interdisziplinären Gesprächen 1991: 19–23.

Siegenthaler W (ed.). Klinische Pathophysiologie. Stuttgart: Thieme, 2001.

7   Diseases of the superior vena cava and its major afferent vessels

Dierk Vorwerk
Duplex ultrasonography: Tom Schilling

Depending on the etiology, obstruction may affect the superior vena cava, the brachiocephalic vein, subclavian vein and axillary vein, either separately or together. The clinical relevance depends on the extent of the condition.

7.1   Etiology

Congenital. Aplasia of the superior vena cava is a congenital condition. There are numerous variants, such as persistent left superior vena cava. Venous strictures are also congenital (congenital web; see section D 3.1).

Inflammatory diseases are caused by:
■ Stenoses due to radiotherapy
■ Fibrosing mediastinitis
■ Tuberculosis
■ Histoplasmosis
■ Mediastinal spread of necrotic pancreatitis
■ Thrombosis in acute mediastinitis

Traumatic conditions include thrombosis and cicatricial stenosis due to atrial catheters, central venous catheters, pacemaker cable, and Paget–von Schroetter syndrome (stress thrombosis of the subclavian vein).

Tumor-related. Compression by mediastinal space-occupying lesions and metastases, with or without thrombosis, is a tumor-related condition. There are also endoluminal tumors and secondary tumor thromboses from the inferior vena cava (hypernephroma).

7.2   Clinical findings

The clinical findings depend on the speed of etiological development, the capacity for compensation, and other causes such as the presence of an arteriovenous shunt. Simple constrictions in the superior vena cava and its major efferent vessels are often asymptomatic, but represent anatomic sites of predilection for thrombotic deposits and may decompensate when increased flow occurs—e.g., after the creation of an arteriovenous fistula for dialysis purposes.

When there is only unilateral obstruction of the main afferent vessels, swelling of the corresponding extremity, with venous marking, is the principal finding. If there is an arteriovenous shunt in the same extremity, massive swelling of the arm may occur, with inability to close the hand, pain, and in the worst case superimposed thrombosis as a venous compartment syndrome as well.

When there is obstruction of the superior vena cava, the symptoms may be variable, ranging from a mild increase in venous marking when there is good compensation via chest wall collaterals and the azygos system to severe upper inflow congestion. The upper inflow congestion that occurs particularly in cancer patients is characterized by swelling of the face and upper extremities, possible chemosis and eyelid edema, cyanosis, dyspnea, and headache. In severe cases, this can develop into an acute emergency situation.

7.3   Diagnosis

7.3.1   Duplex ultrasonography

7.3.1.1   Examination technique

The proximal subclavian vein, brachiocephalic (innominate) vein and proximal superior vena cava can be imaged from supraclavicular and jugular sites, preferably with a 7.5-MHz microconvex probe. If the latter is not available, an adapted programmed low-frequency convex probe can be used, and distally a (5)–7.5–(10)-MHz linear probe. If a thoracic inlet syndrome is suspected, the relevant provocation tests can be carried out with duplex ultrasound interrogation of the subclavian vein.

In addition to demonstration of flow on color duplex ultrasound, analysis of the pulsed-wave (PW) Doppler signal is essential. Mediastinal veins in the vicinity of the heart show a classic triphasic flow profile (maximum flow with atrioventricular valve closure, brief return flow during atrial filling, maximum flow during tricuspid opening). Respiratory variation is superimposed, and if there is no evidence of strong variation then a suspicion of flow obstruction downstream from the probe point is raised. Indirect evidence of compromised flow in the vena cava can therefore be obtained when the afferent veins are examined.

7.3.1.2   Differential diagnosis

Thrombosis or compression effect in the superior vena cava:

■ Thrombosis: thrombi can often be demonstrated in the afferent veins as well.

■ Compression effects: only indirect signs of flow obstruction via restricted cardiac and respiratory signal variation, with no direct evidence of thrombus (Fig. 7-1).

7.3.1.3   Specific findings

■ Subclavian vein thrombosis: see phlebothrombosis in the upper extremity.

■ Jugular vein thrombosis: frequently involved when there is proximal thrombotic outflow obstruction, or may be induced by iatrogenic puncture and/or introduction of foreign bodies. In isolated thromboses of the jugular vein, there is often simultaneous involvement of the upper venous angle.

■ Brachiocephalic vein thrombosis: often associated with arm vein thromboses, or in isolation with suspicion of iatrogenic foreign bodies (pacemaker lead, infusion port, central venous catheter) or paraneoplastic etiologies. In these cases, there is classic disturbed respiratory and cardiac variation of the veins distal to the lesion.

■ Superior vena cava thrombosis: it is often not possible to image this directly, and in such cases only indirect signs of flow obstruction are found, with restricted cardiac and respiratory variation. If the brachiocephalic veins are also thrombosed, then coincident superior vena cava thrombosis can be neither confirmed nor excluded using duplex ultrasonography, since direct and indirect imaging signs are unreliable.

7.3.2   Phlebography

Phlebography is the gold standard and is best done using the digital subtraction angiography (DSA) technique with bilateral venous puncture with an indwelling venous cannula (18 G) and simultaneous bilateral injection.

7.3.3   Computed tomography

Computed tomography of the chest is used to identify the anatomic cause (e.g., tumor) and for precise assessment of the extent of the thrombosis. Contrast (70–100 mL) should not be injected on the affected side, if possible. Imaging using a multislice technique with coronary reconstruction and machine injection is now the method of choice.

In subclavian thrombosis, *ultrasound diagnosis* using color duplex methods is possible, but the central extent can often not be precisely assessed. *Magnetic resonance imaging* procedures are becoming increasingly important as an alternative to CT and phlebography.

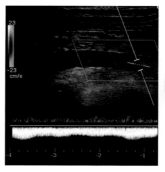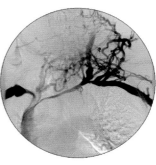

Fig. 7-1 Differential diagnosis in the proximal arm/mediastinal venous thromboses. Clinical signs of swelling in the arm and a cordal PW Doppler signal with absent cardiac and respiratory variation when a completely perfused left subclavian vein is demonstrated allow a diagnosis of proximal outflow obstruction. If the hemodynamics of the contralateral arm are unremarkable, involvement of the vena cava can be excluded. The remaining differential diagnosis is either thrombosis or compression/infiltration with a known thymus carcinoma. Phlebography confirms a tumor compression effect.

7.4   Treatment

Treatment approaches depend on the clinical picture and its severity and cause. No treatment is required for compensated lesions.

7.4.1   Paget–von Schroetter syndrome

The treatment includes full heparinization, raising of the extremity, and a search for the anatomic cause (e.g., cervical rib). Alternatively, thrombolysis followed by anticoagulation can be carried out. Thrombolysis should only be used in acute situations with a very short history, as the effectiveness of the treatment is severely limited when thromboses are several days old. The patient should be experiencing a high level of pain for an invasive procedure to be justified, since in principle a benign course can be expected. The contraindications against lysis treatment must be strictly observed. Once a suitable nonthrombosed elbow vein has been identified, it is punctured in sterile conditions (best done with ultrasound guidance in an edematous arm), and a 5–6F sheath is introduced. A catheter with a side hole and a hydrophilic guidewire are passed through the occlusion, and the catheter is slowly withdrawn through the occlusion, with the thrombus being "vaccinated" with 5–10 mg recombinant tissue plasminogen activator (rTPA). The catheter is then positioned in the occlusion, and continuous lysis at 1 mg rTPA/h is administered for a maximum of 24 h. Alternatively, a multiple-hole catheter that has outlet holes along a length equivalent to the lysis segment can be used. It is important here that the active length of the catheter should not exceed the length of the thrombosis, as lysate would then be lost in the free venous segment. It is also important to attach the sheath to the skin using a suture, place sterile draping, and provide adequate heparinization for the patient during the lysis procedure.

The effectiveness of other endoluminal treatment approaches such as mechanical thrombectomy, balloon dilation, and stent implantation has not yet been studied in detail.

7.4.2 Central venous stenoses and occlusions with dialysis shunts

7.4.2.1 Endovascular therapy

With stenoses, balloon dilation alone using a large balloon diameter (12–15 mm) can be attempted. If there is still a hemodynamically relevant stricture, stent implantation should be carried out. Large-lumen self-expanding stents (diameter 12–16 mm) should be used. In chronic occlusions, thrombolysis is not usually necessary. With fresh thromboses, reducing the size of the thrombus using intravenous thrombolysis can be attempted, but stent implantation can also fix the thrombus in place locally, so that lysis is not required. Following endoluminal procedures, recurrent stenoses often develop (as long as the shunt connection exists), which can be treated endoluminally. In principle, these recanalization techniques can also be used to reopen the vessel to provide access routes for indwelling venous catheters.

Access routes

Despite the large sheath diameter needed, at 9–12F, it is possible to place it in the stricture from the arm via the shunt. A femoral access site can be used as an alternative route. This is necessary when it is not possible to probe a lesion via the brachial or jugular routes. In patients with narrow arm veins or very rigid lesions that obstruct easy passage of the stent, a pull-through technique can also be used in which the wire from a transbrachial access site is captured from the femoral direction in the inferior vena cava and led out. Traction can then be applied at both ends of the wire to make passage easier. Long wires are needed in this procedure.

Technique

There are only minor differences in the stent implantation technique used when malignant or benign obstructions are present. The procedure is therefore described here for both clinical pictures. Initially, puncture of a suitable elbow vein on the shunt site is carried out with an 18-G indwelling catheter, and the vein is probed using a hydrophilic guidewire. After placement of a 6F sheath, the stenosis or occlusion is probed using a multipurpose catheter (e.g., Headhunter, 4F or 5F). In complete occlusions, a slightly stiffer straight guidewire may be helpful. After the occlusion or stenosis has been passed, the catheter can be advanced via the right atrium into the inferior vena cava; the guidewire is then exchanged for a long (ca. 200–300 cm) and more rigid guidewire (e.g., Amplatzer®). If primary balloon dilation is to be carried out, large-lumen balloons with a diameter of 14–18 mm should be used. Before stent implantation, a suitable sheath (6–11F, depending on the type and diameter of the stent) has to be implanted. This is also easily done via the elbow vein with adequate local anesthesia; the sheath should be advanced into the brachial vein slowly.

The stent is then implanted. Preparing a reference angiography series in the same position beforehand can be recommended so that the lesion can be located exactly, allowing precise positioning. Angiography can therefore be done either via a catheter introduced in parallel or via a guide catheter (e.g., 6F) introduced coaxially with a Y connector.

The stents used should be self-expanding, with a diameter slightly larger (1–2 mm) than that of the target vein. In the superior vena cava, this may mean a stent diameter of 22 mm. When a Wallstent is used, the shortening of the stent after deployment needs to be taken into account when selecting the length and when placing it. With benign lesions, the stent should be precisely sized, so that if possible it does not project over the ostial segments of important branches such as the internal jugular vein. With malignant lesions, a more generous approach can be taken due to the patient's limited life expectancy.

7.4.2.2 Surgical treatment

Surgical bypass techniques may be considered as an alternative to endoluminal procedures. However, these are elaborate, always individualized, and difficult, although the results are durable.

7.4.3 Malignant obstructions with superior inflow congestion

The treatment of choice is stent implantation in the superior vena cava. This provides better results than radiotherapy with regard to the speed with which clinical symptoms resolve, as well as durability (Figs. 7-2–7-6). Only one venous axis (the brachiocephalic vein on the right or the superior vena cava on the left) has to be reopened. If there is no bilateral jugular vein thrombosis, this is in most cases sufficient to ensure recirculation, and the symptoms resolve within a few hours.

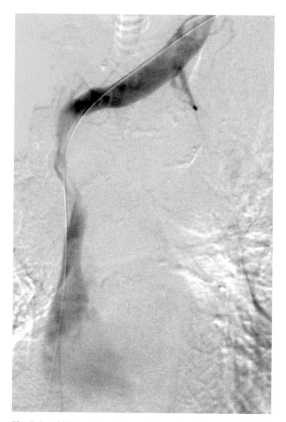

Fig. 7-2 A high-grade malignant stenosis of the superior vena cava due to tumor compression.

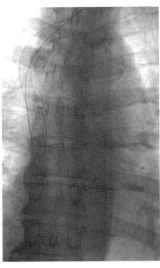

Fig. 7-3 After primary stent implantation, the stent is still tapered in the stenosis.

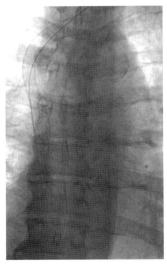

Fig. 7-4 Following balloon dilation, the stent expands to the desired diameter.

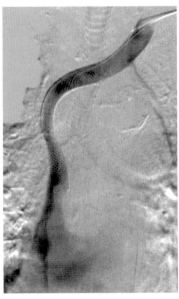

Fig. 7-5 Angiography shows good central outflow.

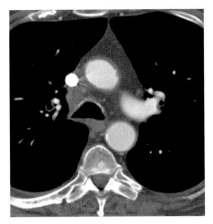

Fig. 7-6 Computed tomography shows normal expansion of the stent in the superior vena cava.

When there is only stenosis, primary stent implantation followed by balloon dilation is sufficient. When thromboses are also present, some authors recommend prior thrombolysis, but during primary stenting this can be dispensed with, as there is only a slight risk of embolization.

The ends of the stent should span the obstruction generously and should not end within the obstructed vascular segment. The central end of the stent should not extend into the right atrium, as there would otherwise be a risk of atrial perforation with pericardial tamponade. The stent can be implanted from the brachial or femoral direction. The diameter selected for the stent should be as large as possible to allow firm positioning.

Alternatively, radiotherapy may be considered in order to reduce the tumor size. However, the effect of this is delayed. A combination of endoluminal resection and radiotherapy is also possible. Surgical procedures have no place in this type of palliative approach.

Patients with malignant superior inflow congestion should undergo heparinization at therapeutic dosages with subcutaneous heparin analogues, in order to prevent recurrent thrombosis. This is not necessary in dialysis patients, due to the good flow resulting from the shunt connection.

References

Haage P, Vorwerk D, Piroth W, Schuermann K, Guenther RW. Treatment of hemodialysis-related central venous stenosis or occlusion: results of primary Wallstent placement and follow-up in 50 patients. Radiology 1999 Jul; 212 (1): 175–80.

Landry GJ, Liem TK. Endovascular management of Paget-Schroetter syndrome. Vascular 2007 Sep–Oct; 15 (5): 290–96.

Rajan DK, Saluja JS. Use of nitinol stents following recanalization of central venous occlusions in hemodialysis patients. Cardiovasc Intervent Radiol 2007 Jul–Aug; 30 (4): 662–67.

Smayra T, Otal P, Chabbert V, Chemla P, Romero M, Joffre F, Rousseau H. Long-term results of endovascular stent placement in the superior caval venous system. Cardiovasc Intervent Radiol 2001 Nov–Dec; 24 (6): 388–94. Epub 2001, Oct 17.

Wilson E, Lyn E, Lynn A, Khan S. Radiological stenting provides effective palliation in malignant central venous obstruction. Clin Oncol (R Coll Radiol) 2002 Jun; 14 (3): 228–32.

C

Inflammatory vascular diseases

1 Diagnosis and classification of vasculitides

Bernhard Hellmich

1.1 Clinical picture and definition

Vasculitis is an inflammation of the blood vessels, which may be an independent clinical picture (primary vasculitis) or may arise as a sequela of another disease (secondary vasculitis). Vasculitides may be limited to a single organ system (e.g., cutaneous vasculitis), but usually appear in several organs (primary systemic vasculitis). This chapter presents the general foundations of diagnosis and treatment for vasculitides, while the individual clinical pictures will be discussed beginning with Chapter C 2.

1.2 Diagnosis

A combination of the history details given by the patient, the clinical findings, serology, imaging diagnosis, and histological findings leads to the diagnosis of vasculitis (Hellmich et al. 2004). Initially, a detailed history should be taken and a thorough physical examination is required. It is only after vasculitis has been diagnosed that precise assignment to a disease entity (classification) can be carried out using classification criteria (Jennette et al. 1994). There are as yet no generally accepted diagnostic criteria, but these are currently being developed in a multinational research project (DVCAS).

1.2.1 History

A picture of chronic inflammation that does not respond to antibiotics is typical. Organ-specific diagnosis is important, with a determined search for major symptoms—e.g., infarction (heart, mesenteric vessels, brain), red eye (episcleritis), painful exanthema (cutaneous vasculitis), blood-tinged rhinorrhea (Wegener disease), pareses or sensory disturbances (neuropathy), abdominal angina (mesenteric ischemia), hemoptysis (alveolar capillaritis), headache (central nervous system), rheumatic symptoms, etc. In addition, predisposing factors in the patient's history (tumor, infections, medication) should be investigated.

1.2.2 Clinical findings

During the clinical examination, a targeted search should be made for typical manifestations such as painful purpura, particularly in the distal region (lower legs, ankles), signs of ischemia, conjunctivitis, exophthalmos, difficulty in walking/sensory disturbance (polyneuropathy), and edema (glomerulonephritis). Functional tests (walking test, sensory examination, hearing test, eye test) and examinations by other consultants (e.g., ear, nose and throat specialist, ophthalmologist, and neurologist) provide further information about potential organ manifestations (Hellmich et al. 2005).

1.2.3 Serology

A distinction is made between diagnosis-associated parameters such as antineutrophilic cytoplasmic antibody (ANCA) and cryoglobulins, on the one hand, and activity parameters (C-reactive protein, complements) and organ-specific parameters (creatinine, urinary sediment) on the other. There are no laboratory parameters (not even ANCA) that are able to confirm a diagnosis of vasculitis.

1.2.3.1 Diagnosis-associated parameters

On indirect immunofluorescence testing, antineutrophilic cytoplasmic antibodies (ANCA) show cytoplasmic (c-ANCA) or perinuclear (p-ANCA) fluorescence. Detailed specification using enzyme-linked immunosorbent assay (ELISA) then reveals the target antigens, although only antiproteinase 3 antibodies (c-ANCA) and antimyeloperoxidase antibodies (p-ANCA) are specific for diagnosing vasculitis. In Wegener disease (c-ANCA/PR3-ANCA), microscopic polyangiitis (p-ANCA/anti-MPO-ANCA, or more rarely c-ANCA) and Churg–Strauss syndrome (p-ANCA/anti-MPO-ANCA), ANCA is found at varying frequencies depending on the activity stage and disease stage. Combined assessment with immunofluorescence and ELISA provides the highest levels of sensitivity and specificity, and according to the consensus guidelines this is now the standard for ANCA diagnosis (Savige et al. 2003). New procedures such as capture-and-anchor ELISA may provide greater specificity than previous ELISA techniques (Csernok et al. 2004).

Other disease-associated parameters include the cryoglobulins (in hepatitis C-associated and essential cryoglobulinemic vasculitis), pathogen serology (hepatitis B surface antigen, hepatitis C virus RNA/antibodies, human immunodeficiency virus serology), and the differential blood count (with eosinophilia in Churg–Strauss syndrome).

1.2.3.2 Surrogate parameters for organ involvement

Assessment for potential organ involvement should include a urinary examination for dysmorphic erythrocytes and albuminuria (each of which suggests glomerulonephritis), renal function testing, transaminases (hepatic involvement, hepatitis) and creatine kinase (CK; vasculitis in the skeletal muscle, myositis, myocardial infarction in coronary arteritis).

1.2.3.3 Activity-associated parameters

In florid vasculitis, the erythrocyte sedimentation rate (ESR) and CRP are almost always raised. However, both parameters are nonspecific and may also be raised in infections. In case of doubt, procalcitonin assessment may be helpful, as it is only raised in bacterial infections. Complement levels (C3, C4, CH50) are lowered in immune complex vasculitides. ANCA titers vary with disease activity. An increase in ANCA by more than three titer steps is predictive of an increased risk of recurrence, but does not in itself justify more intensive treatment.

1.2.4 Imaging diagnosis

Angiography or *magnetic resonance angiography* is indicated in cases of vasculitis in medium-sized or large vessels when there are clinical signs of ischemia (e.g., necrosis, weak pulse). Magnetic resonance angiography (MRA) is less invasive, but the resolution is often too low with the smaller vessels. Typical findings include aneurysms and segmental stenoses (which are not specific for the type of vasculitis).

Magnetic resonance imaging (MRI) of the brain and skull is useful if there is a suspicion of central nervous system involvement (with focal lesions) and to identify granulomas or sinusitis.

High-resolution computed tomography (HRCT) of the lungs is a highly sensitive method of demonstrating infiltrates and granulomas (and is indicated when there is a suspicion of pulmonary involvement).

Bronchoscopy with bronchoalveolar lavage (BAL) should be carried out to clarify unclear findings on pulmonary HRCT and to differentiate between infection (bacteriology with special stains—e.g., for *Pneumocystis carinii*) and disease activity of the vasculitis. Typical BAL findings in vasculitis include sterile neutrophilic alveolitis, erythrocytes, and/or iron-transporting macrophages (alveolar hemorrhagic capillaritis) or eosinophilic alveolitis (Churg–Strauss syndrome) (Schnabel et al. 1999).

1.2.5 Histology

Biopsy evidence of vasculitis confirms the diagnosis and is the gold standard procedure. Vasculitis is defined histologically as infiltration of inflammatory cells into the vessel wall with fibrinoid necrosis. The biopsy should always be taken from pathologically altered tissue—e.g., skin, kidney, nasal mucosa, or lung. Imaging procedures should be used to select the biopsy site (e.g., muscle MRI, cranial MRI, angiography, HRCT). If biopsy is not possible or the results are negative, surrogate parameters for typical organ changes may be diagnostic when there is a typical clinical picture (e.g., glomerular erythrocyturia and proteinuria), as well as serological parameters (e.g., ANCA).

1.3 Subdivision and classification of vasculitides

1.3.1 Subdivision of vasculitides

It is only once a diagnosis of vasculitis has been established (see above) that assignment (classification) to a specific clinical picture can be carried out. An initial distinction is made between whether the vasculitis has developed as an independent clinical picture (primary vasculitis) or as a sequela of another disease (secondary vasculitis). Secondary vasculitides are further differentiated according to the triggering factor (e.g., infection, medication) or associated disease (e.g., tumor), and classification criteria have been formulated to distinguish between the primary vasculitides.

1.3.2 Classification criteria for primary systemic vasculitides

Criteria for classifying primary vasculitides were published by the American College of Rheumatology (ACR) in 1990. Individual clinical pictures were later defined in more detail at a consensus conference held in Chapel Hill, North Carolina, in 1992. The primary vasculitides were classified according to the size of the vessels affected (vasculitides in small, medium-sized and larger vessels), as the diseases included in these subgroups have common clinical characteristics (Table 1-1). The Chapel Hill Consensus Conference distinguished microscopic polyangiitis as a separate clinical picture from polyarteritis nodosa (Jennette et al. 1994). ANCA-associated vasculitides, characterized by evidence of antineutrophilic cytoplasmic antibodies (ANCA) and showing many similarities in their clinical manifestations, were differentiated within the group of small-vessel vasculitides.

Two recent studies have shown that both the ACR criteria and the Chapel Hill definitions are unsuitable for primary diagnosis of the primary vasculitides. When these criteria were used for diagnosis, a substantial number of patients received false-positive diagnoses, on the one hand, while on the other several patients with vasculitis were not identified. The criteria can therefore only be used if the diagnosis of vasculitis is already established.

Table 1-1 Definition of primary vasculitides (Chapel Hill Consensus Conference, 1992).

Vasculitis in large vessels	Vasculitis in medium-sized vessels	Vasculitis in small vessels
Giant cell arteritis	Polyarteritis nodosa	Wegener disease*
Takayasu arteritis	Kawasaki syndrome	Microscopic polyangiitis* Churg–Strauss syndrome* Cryoglobulinemic vasculitis Henoch–Schönlein purpura Cutaneous leukocytoclastic angiitis

* Antineutrophilic cytoplasmic antibody (ANCA)-associated vasculitides.

1.4   Treatment

1.4.1   Foundations of treatment

Treatment schemes that have been tested in controlled, double-blind studies are only available for a few of the vasculitides. Various factors therefore need to be taken into account when deciding on a specific therapeutic approach.

1.4.2   Type of disease

1.4.2.1   Primary vasculitides

In vasculitides affecting large vessels, as well as cutaneous vasculitides, glucocorticoids as a monotherapy are often initially sufficient. Particularly in small-vessel vasculitides with multiple-organ involvement, glucocorticoids alone are not adequate for inducing remission, and it is therefore often necessary to administer cyclophosphamides.

1.4.2.2   Secondary vasculitis

In the secondary vasculitides, options for causal treatment of the underlying disease should initially be tested—e.g., antiviral therapy in HCV-associated or HIV-associated vasculitis. If the vasculitis has been caused by drug treatment, the causative agents should be withdrawn.

1.4.3   Extent of vasculitis

1.4.3.1   Limited course

If the vasculitis is limited to one or only a few organ systems, less aggressive treatment is often sufficient. An example of this would be exclusive involvement of the otorhinolaryngeal tract in Wegener disease (known as the initial phase); less aggressive treatment with sulfamethoxazole/trimethoprim is possible here.

1.4.3.2   Generalized course

The individual prognosis usually deteriorates along with the number of organs affected. With multiple-organ involvement, cyclophosphamide therapy is usually required initially.

1.4.4   Organ involvement

Some manifestations of the disease with an unfavorable prognosis require immediate powerful immunosuppressive treatment, usually with cyclophosphamide, even if no inflammatory activity of the vasculitis is evident in the area of other organs. Prognostically unfavorable signs are rapid and progressive glomerulonephritis, alveolar hemorrhage, and extensive signs in the heart or central nervous system. Impending failure in an individual organ (e.g., peripheral necrosis) also represents an indication for more intensive treatment, even when other manifestations of the disease are absent. Less prognostically relevant signs, such as cutaneous involvement, are often amenable to less intensive forms of treatment.

1.4.5   Vasculitis activity

The goal of treatment may be either to reduce disease activity (remission induction) or to avoid a recurrence once a remission has been achieved (remission maintenance).

1.4.5.1   Induction therapy

The standard for induction therapy in systemic vasculitis with active generalized disease is treatment with what is known as the "modified Fauci scheme" (cyclophosphamide + prednisolone), particularly when there is multiple-organ involvement or a risk of organ failure. In vasculitides of larger vessels (giant cell arteritis, Takayasu arteritis), glucocorticoid therapy is usually sufficient. In limited courses of Wegener disease, methotrexate (MTX) is equivalent to cyclophosphamide (CYC). In ANCA-associated vasculitides, rituximab is as effective as CYC, but in comparison with time-limited CYC therapy it does not appear to be associated with fewer side effects as was hoped.

Induction therapy with CYC is primarily administered as an intravenous pulse therapy, due to its lower toxicity, and is limited to 3–6 months, as the risk of drug-induced early or late complications (e.g., cytopenia, hemorrhagic cystitis, bladder carcinoma) increases along with the period of treatment. Remission-inducing treatment is stopped as soon as the activity of the principal organ manifestation has markedly declined (partial remission) or if there are no further signs of inflammatory activity with the vasculitis (full remission).

1.4.5.2   Maintenance therapy

A switch is made to less aggressive therapy to prevent recurrences after stable partial remission or full remission has been achieved. For most types of vasculitis, there have been hardly any controlled studies comparing individual drugs, and only general recommendations can therefore be given at present. For MTX, azathioprine, and leflunomide, data are available from randomized studies on the ANCA-associated vasculitides, and these agents can therefore be regarded as the major drugs. According to recent research results, mycophenolate mofetil is less effective than azathioprine in ANCA-associated vasculitides.

1.4.5.3   Procedure for unsatisfactory response to standard treatment

Possible options in refractory courses are:
- Plasmapheresis: particularly in patients with renal insufficiency and immune complex-mediated vasculitides (e.g., cryoglobulinemic vasculitis)
- Tumor necrosis factor (TNF) inhibitors (e.g., infliximab): can be used in addition to the standard treatment in ANCA-associated vasculitis; benefit in other forms of vasculitis doubtful
- Intravenous immunoglobulins (400 mg/kg body weight/d for 5 days, repeated after 4 weeks if appropriate): documented efficacy in Kawasaki syndrome and ANCA-associated vasculitides
- Rituximab (monoclonal anti-CD20 antibody), anti-CD52, anti-CD4: in ANCA-associated vasculitides

- 15-deoxyspergualin (gusperimus, NKT-01) in Wegener disease
- Cyclophosphamide: intensified Fauci scheme (leukocyte-adjusted administration of cyclophosphamide, high toxicity, now usually avoidable)

1.4.6 Drugs and treatment protocols

1.4.6.1 Glucocorticoids

Value of treatment in vasculitis

Glucocorticoids are the drugs of choice for acute treatment. They provide the fastest onset of action of all immunosuppressive agents. Long-term use is limited due to side effects and is therefore only possible at low dosages.

For single-agent treatment, glucocorticoids are the agent of choice in initial therapy for temporal arteritis, Takayasu arteritis, and mild courses of Churg–Strauss syndrome. In most forms of systemic vasculitis, glucocorticoids are not suitable as the sole form of primary therapy for inducing remission. Glucocorticoids are an important component of combination treatment, along with other immunosuppressive agents such as cyclophosphamide.

Drugs and dosages

The most frequently used agents are prednisolone and methylprednisolone. Equivalent doses: 5 mg prednisolone corresponds to 4 mg methylprednisolone. Due to the circadian rhythm of cortisol secretion, the whole dose should be administered in the morning, or with a smaller dose in the evening when there is a high level of disease activity.

The usual *forms of administration* are listed below.

Pulse (bolus) therapy

- 250–1000 mg/d i.v. as a short-term infusion for 3 days to a maximum of 5 days
- *Indication:* potentially life-threatening signs (e.g., alveolar hemorrhagia, cardiac dysrhythmia with hemodynamic effects) or imminent threat to a vital organ (e.g., renal failure in rapidly progressive glomerulonephritis, loss of sight in temporal arteritis, etc.)

High-dose therapy

- 1.0–1.5 mg/kg body weight prednisolone
- *Indication:* for inducing remission
- In systemic vasculitis, usually combined with an immunosuppressant

The high glucocorticoid dosage is the major factor responsible for the high rate of infection during remission induction with the Fauci scheme (in combination with cyclophosphamide). A reduction in the Cushing threshold dosage (7.5 mg prednisolone equivalent) should therefore be attempted within the first 3 months (modified Fauci scheme). The dose reduction depends on the disease activity—e.g., initially by 10 mg every 3 days; below 50 mg/d, by 5–10 mg/week; below 20 mg, by 2.5–5.0 mg/week, down to 7.5 mg/d.

Low-dose therapy

- Below the Cushing threshold dosage (7.5 mg/d)
- *Indication:* in combination with immunosuppressants (azathioprine, MTX, etc.) for remission maintenance
- Aim: tapering during the further course, but this is often not possible
- Consequently: reduction by 1 mg/month to the lowest effective dosage

Side effects

Glucocorticoids lead to increased susceptibility to infections, particularly when combined with immunosuppressants. Glucocorticoids may suppress signs of infection such as fever, and severe infections may therefore not be initially recognized clinically.

Due to the risk of glucocorticoid-induced osteoporosis, prophylactic treatment with a combination of vitamin D (1000 IU/d) and calcium (1000 mg/d) should always be administered. In long-term treatment, bisphosphonates (e.g., alendronate, risedronate) should also be added, depending on bone mineral density (see the osteology guidelines). Other typical side effects are listed in Table 1-2.

Side effects of glucocorticoids depend on the dosage and duration of treatment. In long-term administration of dosages higher than 7.5 mg/d, there is a markedly increased risk of side effects, but the risk of osteoporosis is already increased at dosages over 2.5 mg/d. Reducing the glucocorticoid dosage in accordance with disease activity is the best way of preventing side effects.

Table 1-2 Adverse effects of systemic glucocorticoids.

Infections
Glucocorticoid-induced osteoporosis
Iatrogenic Cushing syndrome
Steroid-induced diabetes mellitus
Fluid retention
Skin atrophy, steroid acne, wound healing disturbances
Cataract, glaucoma
Psychological changes (known as "steroid psychosis")
Muscle weakness, steroid myopathy

1.4.6.2 Cyclophosphamide

Value of treatment in vasculitis

Cyclophosphamide (CYC) is the drug of choice for inducing remission in patients with systemic vasculitis. CYC is the agent with the best-documented efficacy and it can be lifesaving in severe courses with impending organ failure. Due to the severity and frequency of the side effects, it can only be administered for limited periods.

Treatment schemes and dosages

Oral long-term cyclophosphamide therapy—modified Fauci scheme (NIH standard)

Oral cyclophosphamide therapy (2 mg/kg body weight/d p.o. + prednisolone 1 mg/kg body weight; for dose reduction, see above) is the standard for inducing remission in generalized Wegener disease and other ANCA-associated forms of vasculitis (Hoffman et al. 1992). Efficacy has also been documented for polyarteritis nodosa. The onset of effect can be expected after 2–4 weeks. The treatment period is 3–6 months, and when remission begins a switch can be made to less toxic substances (azathioprine, MTX). Oral mesna can be administered as an accompanying drug (2 mg/kg body weight), distributed over three daily doses, for prophylaxis against cystitis (Reinhold-Keller et al. 2000).

Intensified oral cyclophosphamide treatment—intensified Fauci scheme

Intensified CYC treatment (cyclophosphamide 3–4 mg/kg body weight/d p.o.; prednisolone 1 g for 3 days i.v., then 1 mg/kg body weight; for dose reduction, see above) is indicated when vasculitis progresses during administration of the standard dosage. A decline in leukocytes can be expected after 6–8 days, and dose adjustment is then required. Due to bone-marrow depression, intensified treatment can only be administered for a limited period (4–8 weeks), and it is now being used increasingly rarely, as alternative treatments such as infliximab or rituximab are available for refractory cases.

Cyclophosphamide treatment (CYCLOPS scheme)

Data from the CYCLOPS study have shown that cyclophosphamide bolus therapy for multiple-organ involvement leads to remission rates similar to those seen with long-term oral therapy (de Groot et al. 2001). In addition, the rate of severe side effects (Table 1-3) with bolus treatment is lower, as a lower cumulative CYC dosage is required.
- **Administration:**
  - Cyclophosphamide 15 mg/kg body weight in weeks 0, 2, and 4, and then every 3 weeks i.v. as a short-term infusion
  - Prednisolone 100 mg i.v.
  - Parenteral fluid administration: 1–2 L NaCl 0.9% i.v. for 4–6 h
  - Mesna (Uromitexan®) in three daily doses at 0, 4, and 8 h for prophylaxis against cystitis
- Treatment period: six cycles, followed be reassessment of disease activity

Table 1-3 Adverse effects of cyclophosphamide.

Frequent	Rarer
■ Infections: often severe, occasionally fatal; high steroid dosage usually a major contributing factor; often associated with leukopenia ■ Infertility: teratogenic—contraception required during treatment	■ Hemorrhagic cystitis: associated with an increased risk of urothelial carcinoma; prophylaxis with mesna is recommended (see text) ■ Urothelial carcinoma ■ Myelodysplastic syndrome ■ Hair loss, thrombocytopenia, nausea, very rarely pulmonary fibrosis

Treatment monitoring

- Blood count:
  - In long-term therapy, daily to begin with; if the leukocyte count is stable after 10–12 days' treatment, three times per week. Treatment is interrupted if there is granulocytopenia < 2000/μL.
  - With bolus treatment, on days 8, 10, and 12 after bolus administration (leukocyte nadir).
  - If there is persistent agranulocytosis, recombinant human granulocyte colony-stimulating factor (rhG-CSF) is administered until neutrophilia over 1000/μL is reached.
- Urinary status and sediment: if nonglomerular erythrocyturia is noted (with suspected cystitis), treatment should be interrupted and a cystoscopic examination should be carried out.

1.4.6.3   Methotrexate

Value in vasculitis treatment

Methotrexate (MTX) is less effective for immunosuppression than cyclophosphamide and has much lower long-term toxicity (Table 1-4). MTX in combination with glucocorticoids is the treatment of choice for inducing remission in patients with ANCA-associated vasculitis at a localized or early systemic disease stage (with no renal involvement and no involvement of other organs) (de Groot et al. 2005). MTX can also be used for remission maintenance in Wegener disease, although renal recurrences appear to be relatively frequent in comparison with azathioprine. In giant cell arteritis, MTX can be administered to reduce the glucocorticoid dosage.

Table 1-4 Adverse effects of methotrexate.

Interstitial alveolitis: in up to 5% of patients; potentially life-threatening; may occur either early or late; diagnosis: HRCT, BAL (lymphocytic alveolitis); interruption of treatment required; treatment with high-dose prednisolone
Infections: more rarely than with cyclophosphamide; frequent Pneumocystis carinii pneumonia, fungal infections
Pancytopenia, agranulocytosis: often due to dosage errors (e.g., with daily MTX administration)
Raised transaminases
Miscarriage, deformities: contraception required up to 3 months after the end of treatment
Nausea, vomiting
Stomatitis, hair loss
BAL, bronchoalveolar lavage; HRCT, high-resolution computed tomography; MTX, methotrexate.

Dosage and method of administration

As the resorption rate is highly variable between individuals, MTX (0.3 mg/kg once per week) is preferably administered parenterally (i.v. or s.c.). Administration of folic acid (5–10 mg) 24 h later p.o. reduces the side effects (e.g., raised transaminases). MTX is eliminated renally and is therefore contraindicated in patients with renal insufficiency.

Treatment monitoring

- History and examination: fever, coughing (*caution:* pneumonitis), dyspnea, stomatitis.
- Laboratory tests: differential blood count, transaminases, γ-glutamyltransferase, creatinine.
- Weekly for the first month, every 14 days up to the third month, and thereafter once monthly.
- Treatment is interrupted in case of pneumonitis, neutropenia, thrombopenia, aplastic anemia, an increase in transaminases by a factor of three, and raised creatinine.
- In case of agranulocytosis, 12 mg calcium folinate (e.g., leucovorin) every 3 h i.v.
- The effect is enhanced and toxicity is potentiated with simultaneous administration of MTX and sulfamethoxazole/trimethoprim. This combination should be avoided if possible.

1.4.6.4   Azathioprine

Value in vasculitis treatment

In contrast to MTX, hardly any data are available on the use of azathioprine (AZA) in remission-inducing treatment. It is therefore mainly used for remission maintenance therapy. In ANCA-associated vasculitis, AZA after remission-inducing therapy with cyclophosphamide (Fauci scheme) for 3 months is as effective in maintaining remission as continuing cyclophosphamide therapy for a further 12 months, probably with lower long-term toxicity (Jayne et al. 2003). In two randomized studies, AZA was found to be as effective as MTX, and was superior to MMF, with regard to reducing the risk of recurrence.

Dosage and method of administration

AZA can also be administered in patients with renal insufficiency. The dosage for remission-maintenance treatment is 2–3 mg/kg body weight p.o.; when the creatinine clearance is < 20 mL/min, the maximum dosage is 1.5 mg/kg body weight/d. In treatment-refractory cases, azathioprine can be administered at high doses as a pulse therapy (1.2 g i.v. for 24 h every 4 weeks, 150 mg p.o. in weeks 2 and 3), but only case reports are available on this. The risk of side effects (Table 1-5) is higher when the enzyme thiopurine methyltransferase (TPMT) shows reduced activity, and enzyme activity assessment may therefore be helpful before the start of treatment.

Table 1-5 Adverse effects of azathioprine.

Gastrointestinal: nausea, vomiting, diarrhea, raised transaminases
Blood count: leukopenia, thrombopenia, anemia
Infections
Drug-induced fever
Rarely: hair loss, alveolitis, exanthema
Miscarriage, deformities: contraception required up to 6 months after the end of treatment

Treatment monitoring

- History and examination: fever, stomatitis, diarrhea, nausea.
- Laboratory tests: differential blood count, transaminases, γ-glutamyltransferase, creatinine, urinary status.
- Weekly for the first month, every 14 days up to the third month, and thereafter once monthly.
- Treatment is interrupted in case of pneumonitis, neutropenia, thrombopenia, aplastic anemia, an increase in transaminases by a factor of three, and raised creatinine.

1.4.6.5   Other agents and treatment procedures

The following drugs are not usually the agents of first choice, as larger controlled studies are not yet available. They are reserved for alternative treatment for special indications:

- Cyclosporine (3–5 mg/kg body weight/d): e.g., for remission maintenance after kidney transplantation
- Leflunomide (20–40 mg/d p.o.): remission maintenance in Wegener disease
- Mycophenolate mofetil: remission maintenance in Wegener disease and microscopic polyangiitis
- Trimethoprim/sulfamethoxazole:
  - Initial phase in Wegener disease: dosage 2 × 960 mg/d p.o.
  - For prophylaxis against *Pneumocystis carinii* in the Fauci scheme with high glucocorticoid dosages: dosage 960 mg three times per week p.o.
- Intravenous immunoglobulins (2 g/kg body weight for 3–5 days) in refractory courses
- Rituximab (750 mg/m^2 body surface in weeks 1, 2, 3, and 4) in refractory ANCA-associated vasculitis
- Infliximab (5 mg/kg i.v. in weeks 0, 1, 2, 4, 8)
- Plasmapheresis (see above)

2 Giant cell arteritis

Bernhard Hellmich
Duplex ultrasound technique: Tom Schilling

2.1 Clinical picture

Giant cell arteritis (synonyms: temporal arteritis, Horton disease) is a vasculitis of the aorta and its branches, the histological correlate for which is granulomatous vasculitis with evidence of giant cells. Giant cell arteritis often becomes manifest at the temporal artery and usually occurs in patients over the age of 50. Involvement of the aorta and neighboring vessels is now being diagnosed more frequently as a result of improved modern imaging techniques.

2.1.1 Epidemiology

Giant cell arteritis is the most frequent form of primary vasculitis in northern Europe and the United States. In northern Germany, the prevalence is 80 per one million population. The disease usually first develops in patients over the age of 50 years. Giant cell arteritis occurs much more frequently in elderly patients (with an incidence of 49 per 100,000 population in those over 80 years of age). Women are affected three times more often than men. In Scandinavia, giant cell arteritis occurs twice as frequently as in southern Europe.

2.1.2 Etiology and pathogenesis

The cause of the disease is not known. As in other autoimmune diseases, there is a genetic predisposition; an association with HLA-DRB1-04 has been reported. In addition, oligoclonal expression of lymphocytes in the vascular wall is seen, suggesting an antigen-driven process. The CD4$^+$ T cells in the adventitia mainly produce interferon-α, so that there is a Th1 cytokine profile. Damage to the media appears to be induced by macrophages. Intimal proliferation is also induced by macrophages and by the giant cells. The role of viruses and bacteria in inducing the immune reaction is still unclear. In biopsies from the temporal artery, evidence of parvovirus B19 DNA in 54% of cases has been reported. Evidence of *Chlamydia pneumoniae* DNA in temporal biopsies has also been reported.

2.1.3 Histopathology

Histopathological findings include the following, depending on the disease stage:
- Granulomatous arteritis (mononuclear infiltrate in the media, multinuclear giant cells in the external elastic membrane)
- Nongranulomatous arteritis (mononuclear infiltrate in the intima, intimal proliferation)
- Cicatricial stage (fibrosis in the media and intima)

2.2 Clinical findings

The severity of the symptoms varies. Up to 40% of the patients do not have the typical pattern of symptoms. Typical major findings in giant cell arteritis are:
- Unilateral or bilateral diffuse headache (frequency 70%)
- Visual disturbances (frequency 30%): scotoma, amaurosis fugax, loss of sight, possible blindness
- Temporal artery indurated and painful on pressure (frequency 45%)
- Pain when chewing—masticatory claudication (frequency 40%)
- Tongue pain, dysphagia
- General symptoms (B symptoms), often at the start of the disease
- Proximal myalgia in 40–60% of patients (polymyalgia rheumatica)
- Symptoms of peripheral ischemia in stenoses of aortic arch vessels
- Scalp or tongue necrosis
- Rarely arthralgia or arthritis

2.3 Diagnosis

2.3.1 Clinical examination

The typical major finding is a temporal artery that is painful on pressure and painfully indurated (either unilaterally or bilaterally). When there is vasculitis of the vessels near the aorta, there are also stenotic murmurs over the large vessels, or a difference in blood pressure from the contralateral side. Visual disturbances or blindness occur when the branches supplying the eyes are affected. Necrosis of the scalp is rare.

2.3.2 Diagnostic testing

2.3.2.1 Laboratory diagnosis

A severely elevated erythrocyte sedimentation rate and raised C-reactive protein are usually present. No specific serological parameters or antibodies are known.

2.3.2.2 Color duplex ultrasonography

Due to the segmental involvement, longitudinal and transverse examinations of both temporal artery trunks and the frontal and parietal branches are necessary. This requires a high-resolution linear scanner (ideally 10 MHz or more). The typical finding in giant cell arteritis is a hypoechoic halo (Fig. 2-1) surrounding the vessel lumen (Schmidt et al. 1997). In a prospective study of patients with a clinical diagnosis of giant cell arteritis, this finding was 100% specific for the presence of histologically documented intramural inflammation. Vascular stenoses and occlusions are also seen (but are less specific).

The accuracy of color duplex ultrasound is highly examiner-dependent. Unless the ultrasound findings are extremely clear, biopsy is still the gold standard for diagnosis. Ultrasonography is mainly used to screen for atypical symptoms and to select the biopsy site.

Technique of duplex sonography

All of the branches of the superficial temporal artery are insonated using a high-frequency transducer, longitudinally and in cross-section, with only slight probe pressure. The typical examination technique for each region can otherwise be used, even when the superficial temporal artery is involved, often with simultaneous involvement of the aorta and aortic branches near the trunk. If involvement of the ocular vessels is suspected, direct insonation of the ophthalmic artery, central retinal artery, and choroid vessels can be carried out with a high-frequency probe (≥ 7.5 MHz) with the patient's eye closed (Fig. 2-2). During ultrasonography of the eye, it is important to apply minimal pressure and use the optic nerve as a landmark, adjusting the device with a low mechanical index of < 0.3 if possible. The examination time should be as short as possible, and pulsatility (reduced?) and acceleration time (prolonged?) can be used as classic signs of post-stenotic/occlusive flow.

A common pathognomonic sign in large-vessel vasculitis with the histological pattern of giant cell arteritis is a relatively homogeneous, hypoechoic widening of the intima–media thickness (Fig. 2-3), but with clear segmental involvement ("macaroni sign," or in cross-section at the superficial temporal artery "halo" phenomenon). Any stenoses should be graded in accordance with the usual location-related stenotic criteria (peak velocity ratio).

Differential diagnosis

When there is a widened boundary-zone reflex:
- Metabolic disturbances
- Hypertension
- Diabetes mellitus
- Nicotine abuse
- Inflammatory edema in the vascular wall with a different cause

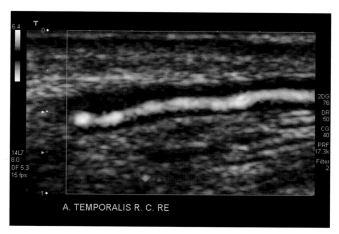

Fig. 2-1 Typical findings in giant cell arteritis, showing a hypoechoic halo surrounding the vascular lumen.

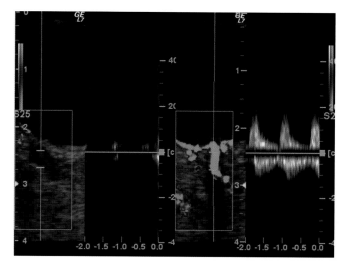

Fig. 2-2 Left: rudimentary residual perfusion of the central retinal artery in a patient with giant cell arteritis with involvement of the ophthalmic artery. Right: normal hemodynamic and color-duplex ultrasound findings in the central retinal artery and choroid vessels (imaging with pulsatile flow detection, PFD).

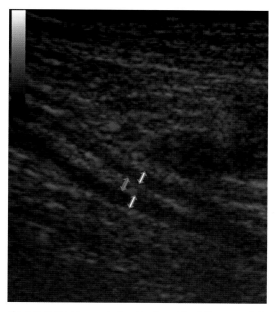

Fig. 2-3 Typical hypoechoic widening of the intima–media in the subclavian artery, with narrowing of the lumen, in a patient with large-vessel vasculitis.

2.3.2.3   Positron emission tomography

[15]Fluorodeoxyglucose positron emission tomography (FDG-PET) allows imaging of florid arteritis in the aorta and nearby vessels in patients with giant cell arteritis (Fig. 2-4) (Blockmans et al. 2000). Due to its high cost, FDG-PET is not a standard procedure, and instead it should be used in a targeted way if there are signs of aortitis—e.g., with evidence of an aortic aneurysm, very high serological inflammatory parameters, or a delayed response to glucocorticoid therapy. The prognostic relevance of aortitis imaged using PET is as yet unclear, and studies are currently being conducted to evaluate this. It is particularly unclear whether patients with positive PET findings require further intensive therapy despite clinical and serological remission. The resolution available with FDG-PET is usually too low for imaging of isolated temporal arteritis. PET-CT allows more precise anatomic correlation.

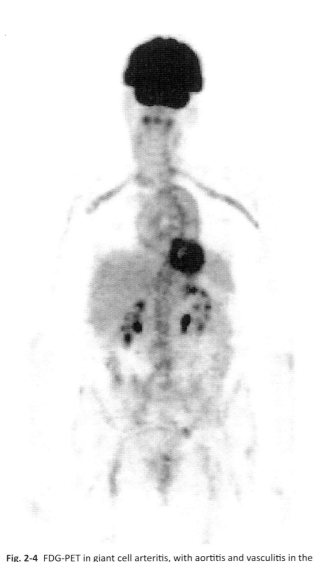

2.3.2.4   Magnetic resonance angiography/angio-CT

Magnetic resonance angiography (MRA) is used to demonstrate changes (especially stenoses) in extracranial vessels, particularly the aortic arch. Its specificity with regard to inflammatory activity (edema in the vessel wall) is much lower than that of PET. The two techniques are therefore complementary: FDG-PET provides information about florid inflammatory processes, while MRA shows their anatomic effects (e.g., aneurysm, stenosis).

2.3.2.5   Angiography/digital subtraction angiography (DSA)

DSA is mainly indicated when an intervention is planned (e.g., percutaneous transluminal angioplasty, PTA). Ultrasonography, MRA, and PET are less invasive or more specific procedures for diagnosing stenoses and disease activity.

2.3.2.6   Temporal artery biopsy

Temporal artery biopsy is the gold standard for confirming a diagnosis of giant cell arteritis, and it is also helpful in distinguishing the condition from other forms of systemic vasculitis involving the temporal artery. In addition to the findings mentioned above (section 2.3.1), there is often small-vessel vasculitis in the vasa vasorum and no fibrinoid necrosis, in contrast to polyarteritis nodosa. Selecting the biopsy site using duplex ultrasonography improves the diagnostic yield. With a typical clinical picture *and* clear ultrasound findings, a biopsy is now typically unnecessary.

2.3.3   Differential diagnosis

Temporal artery vasculitis is not specific for giant cell arteritis (Table 2-1 lists classification criteria) and may also occur with other forms of systemic vasculitides (Table 2-2).

Table 2-1 Classification criteria for giant cell arteritis (ACR 1990).

■ Age at disease onset ≥ 50 years
■ First onset or new type of headache
■ Pressure pain, swelling or reduced pulse in the temporal artery
■ Increased ESR: ≥ 50 mm in the first hour
■ Biopsy: vasculitis with mononuclear cell infiltration or granulomatous inflammation, usually with multinuclear giant cells

Three of the five criteria have to be met for classification (sensitivity 93.5%, specificity 91.2%)
ESR, erythrocyte sedimentation rate.

Fig. 2-4 FDG-PET in giant cell arteritis, with aortitis and vasculitis in the subclavian artery bilaterally.

Table 2-2 Differential diagnosis of temporal arteritis.

Major symptoms	Minor symptoms	Suspected diagnosis	Diagnosis
Blood-pressure difference in the arms > 10 mmHg Aortic stenosis Age < 40 years	Discontinuous segmental involvement Renal artery stenosis	Takayasu arteritis	MRA or DSA
Pressure pain in the temporal artery Age > 50 years	Shoulder stiffness Histology: vasculitis in vasa vasorum	Giant cell arteritis	Temporal artery biopsy
Angiography: aneurysms in medium-sized vessels	Mesenteric vessels often involved Peripheral neuropathy Histology: fibrinoid necrosis	Polyarteritis nodosa	Angiography
Crusted rhinitis	Pulmonary masses	Wegener disease	c-ANCA
Purpura, neuropathy	Hepatitis C	Cryoglobulinemia	Cryoglobulins

c-ANCA, cytoplasmic antineutrophil cytoplasmic antibodies; DSA, digital subtraction angiography; MRA, magnetic resonance angiography.

2.4 Treatment

2.4.1 Drug treatment

2.4.1.1 Glucocorticoids

Glucocorticoids are the standard treatment in the acute stage of giant cell arteritis, as they act rapidly and safely. Prednisolone is administered at a dosage of 1 mg/kg initially, or 250 mg prednisolone i.v. for 3 days if there is imminent loss of sight or neurological complications. A dose reduction of 10 mg every 2 weeks is initially carried out; from 30 mg, 5 mg/week down to 7.5 mg/d; then by 1 mg/month to the lowest effective dosage. When there are visual disturbances, glucocorticoid therapy has to be started without delay. If the treatment is not started within 24 h, amaurosis usually becomes irreversible. The high dosages required, high recurrence rates of more than 60% during long-term therapy, the long duration of treatment averaging 2 years, and the side effects of long-term administration are all arguments in favor of additional steroid-sparing treatment.

2.4.1.2 Methotrexate (MTX)

A meta-analysis of three randomized studies on the use of MTX in patients with giant cell arteritis showed a significant reduction in the recurrence rate and a reduction in glucocorticoid requirements (Mahr et al. 2007). As the absolute effects were comparatively slight, this is indicated particularly when there is a high level of inflammatory activity and/or when there are other risk factors for glucocorticoid-induced side effects (e.g., osteoporosis and diabetes mellitus). In the same way as in treatment for other forms of vasculitis, higher dosages (0.3 mg/kg MTX once per week + prednisolone) may be more effective than the 10 mg/week that has been studied in the treatment of giant cell arteritis.

2.4.1.3 Cyclophosphamide

This is indicated with fulminant courses (e.g., with a large aortic aneurysm) and when there is no response to MTX and prednisolone.

2.4.1.4 Acetylsalicylic acid (ASA)

Two large retrospective studies with ASA 100 mg/d have reported a reduced incidence of cardiovascular events in patients with giant cell arteritis (Nesher et al. 2004). In combination with prednisolone, there is an increased risk of gastrointestinal ulcers, and prophylaxis (with proton-pump inhibitors) is therefore recommended.

2.4.2 Endovascular treatment

Endovascular treatment procedures should be considered particularly at the noninflammatory stage if no further effect of immunosuppressive treatment can be expected (Both et al. 2006). Various interventional and vascular reconstruction procedures can be used (see under Takayasu arteritis).

2.5 Prognosis and course

Life expectancy is not substantially reduced. Disease-specific factors such as the duration of the disease and age at first manifestation or clinical manifestation do not affect the mortality.

3 Takayasu arteritis

Bernhard Hellmich

3.1 Clinical picture

Takayasu arteritis is a granulomatous vasculitis affecting the aorta and its branches, with a predilection for the aortic arch and its branches (Table 3-1). The age at first manifestation is usually under 40.

Table 3-1 Classification criteria for Takayasu arteritis (ACR 1990).

- Age at disease onset < 40 years
- Symptoms of claudication in the extremities
- Weakened pulse in one or both brachial arteries
- Blood-pressure difference (systolic) between the arms > 10 mmHg
- Flow murmur over the aorta or subclavian vein
- Pathological angiography findings

Three of the six criteria have to be met for classification (sensitivity 90%, specificity 98%)

3.1.1 Epidemiology

Takayasu arteritis occurs throughout the world, but the prevalence/incidence is highest in eastern Asia. The prevalence in northern Germany is 4.4 per million. The first manifestation is usually in the second or third decade of life, and 80–90% of those affected are women.

3.1.2 Etiology

There is no standard explanation of the pathogenesis. The following possibilities have been considered:
- Genetic predisposition:
  - Association with HLA-Bw52 in the eastern Asian population; in Western populations, there are inconsistent immunogenetic findings and there is no association with HLA-Bw52
  - Association with complement allotypes C4A2 and C4BQO

- Cellular immune reactions: activation of $CD4^+$ T cells, altered T-cell receptor repertoire, evidence of $\gamma\delta$ T cells
- Endocrine immune reaction: activation of endothelial cells, production of anti-endothelial cell antibodies

3.1.3 Histopathology

Takayasu arteritis is a granulomatous polyarteritis:
- Active vasculitis: granulomas with multinuclear giant cells and lymphocytic infiltrates
- Inactive disease: fibrosis in the vessel wall, occasional mural thrombi

3.2 Clinical findings

The major symptoms of Takayasu arteritis are:
- Movement-dependent shoulder–arm pain
- Intermittent claudication in the arms and legs
- Bilateral difference in blood pressure in up to 65% of patients
- Arterial hypertension in 40–70% of cases (associated with stenosis of the renal artery)
- Generalized symptoms, often at the start of the disease
- Visual disturbances (in 30% of patients), amaurosis fugax, with involvement of the carotid artery
- Cardiac symptoms (exertional dyspnea, angina pectoris, palpitations)
- Arthralgia and myalgia in up to 55% of the patients

Table 3-2 Differential diagnosis of temporal arteritis.

Major symptoms	Minor symptoms	Suspected diagnosis	Diagnosis
Blood-pressure difference in the arms > 10 mmHg Aortic stenosis Age < 40 years	Discontinuous segmental involvement Renal artery stenosis	Takayasu arteritis	MRA or DSA
Pressure pain in the temporal artery Age > 50 years	Shoulder stiffness Histology: vasculitis in vasa vasorum	Giant cell arteritis	Temporal artery biopsy
History of syphilis	Continuous involvement Usually only thoracic aorta involved	Syphilitic aortitis	TPHA test MRA or DSA

DSA, digital subtraction angiography; MRA, magnetic resonance angiography; TPHA, Treponema pallidum hemagglutination.

3.3 Diagnosis

3.3.1 Clinical examination

Typical major findings in Takayasu arteritis are stenotic murmurs over the large vessels, particularly at the aortic arch branches, bilateral differences in blood pressure (comparative measurements should always be carried out on both sides in the arms and legs), weakened pulse, diastolic murmur over the aortic valve (aortic insufficiency due to valvular ring dilation in up to 20% of patients), and cutaneous manifestations (pyoderma gangrenosum or erythema nodosum in 15% of patients). Possible differential diagnoses are listed in Table 3-2.

3.3.2 Laboratory and imaging diagnosis

3.3.2.1 Laboratory diagnosis

There are no specific serological parameters (*Treponema pallidum* hemagglutination test if syphilitic aortitis is possible). There is little correlation between disease activity and acute-phase parameters.

3.3.2.2 Angiography/Digital subtraction angiography (DSA)

Angiography used to be regarded as the gold standard for diagnosis and assessment of the course, but it provides no information about inflammatory activity, and monitoring of the course is therefore necessary. Typical findings are:
- Long stenoses in the aorta, proximal stenosis at the brachiocephalic vessels
- Involvement of the pulmonary artery in up to 70% of cases
- Rarely, aneurysmal dilation (15%)
- Discontinuous segmental involvement

3.3.2.3 Magnetic resonance angiography

Magnetic resonance angiography (MRA) can also demonstrate the quality of the arterial wall and thus not only the extent of the disease but also disease activity. As MRA is also less invasive and iodine-containing contrast is not required, it is preferable to conventional angiography if available. The renal arteries and pulmonary vessels should also be imaged. Typical findings include:
- In active disease: increased contrast uptake, high signal intensity on T2-weighted sequences
- Thickening of the walls
- Neovascularization in thickened vascular wall segments
- Mural thrombi in up to 60% of patients

3.3.2.4 Ultrasonography/echocardiography

Duplex ultrasonography usually only provides inadequate imaging of the thoracic aorta, which is most often involved. Ultrasound is therefore not capable of replacing angiography or MRA, although it is suitable for noninvasive checking of the course in some conditions. *Echocardiography* can identify regurgitation in the area of the aortic valve and aortic ring dilation.

3.3.2.5 PET/PET-CT

The majority of patients with TA show increased uptake in the aorta and neighboring vessels on PET or PET-CT. However, recent research suggests that the correlation between the PET findings, serology, and the clinical assessment of disease activity is often poor (Arnaud et al. 2009).

3.4 Treatment

There have been no controlled studies on the treatment of Takayasu arteritis. Treatment recommendations are mainly based on retrospective investigations.

3.4.1 Drug therapy

3.4.1.1 Glucocorticoids

Glucocorticoids are the agents of choice. However, complete remission is only achieved in 50% of cases with glucocorticoid monotherapy. Dosage recommendations:
- Initial therapy: prednisolone 1 mg/kg, with dose reduction depending on the response
- Maintenance therapy: low-dose treatment (e.g., 5 mg/d) reduces the frequency of recurrences

3.4.1.2 Methotrexate (MTX)

In a study including 16 patients, methotrexate in combination with glucocorticoids led to remission in 81% of cases. The dosage is 0.3 mg/kg once per week + low-dose prednisolone (depending on the clinical findings).

3.4.1.3 Cyclophosphamide (CYC)

Cyclophosphamide administration is indicated in fulminant courses and when there is no response to MTX and prednisolone.

3.4.1.4 Supportive medication

Due to the high incidence of mural thrombi, it is useful to administer platelet inhibitors (e.g., acetylsalicylic acid). β-Blockers may slow or stop the progression of left ventricular hypertrophy and are particularly effective in cases of aortic insufficiency.

3.4.2 Endovascular treatment

Particularly in the noninflammatory stage, endovascular treatment procedures should be considered if no further effect of immunosuppressive treatment can be expected.

3.4.2.1   Percutaneous catheter angioplasty

The initial success rate is 55–90%, but recurrent stenoses are seen in up to 50% of cases after 5 years. Indication: segmental renal artery stenoses, stenoses in branches of the aorta with a clinical correlate.

3.4.2.2   Stent implantation

The primary results are better than with percutaneous transluminal angioplasty alone. In a smaller study including six patients, no recurrent stenoses were seen on angiography after 6 months. Indication: renal artery stenosis, symptomatic stenosis, aortic aneurysm.

3.4.2.3   Vascular surgery

Thromboendarterectomy is associated with a high rate of recurrence in Takayasu arteritis and is therefore not a standard procedure. There is an indication for bypass placement/vascular reconstruction if substantial ischemic symptoms occur in the chronic, noninflammatory stage. Much poorer results are seen in cases of active vasculitis.

3.5   Prognosis and course

The 5-year survival rate is approximately 80–90%. The prognosis is poorer in patients with aortic valve insufficiency, aneurysms, and arterial hypertension.

4   Polyarteritis nodosa

Bernhard Hellmich

4.1   Clinical picture

Polyarteritis nodosa (PAN) is defined as a necrotizing vasculitis in medium-sized vessels (medium-sized and small arteries) (Table 4-1). By definition, polyarteritis nodosa therefore does not include glomerulonephritis or vasculitis of small vessels (capillaries, arterioles).

Table 4-1 Classification criteria for polyarteritis nodosa (ACR 1990).

■ Weight loss > 4 kg
■ Livedo reticularis
■ Pain or pain on pressure in the testicles
■ Diffuse myalgia
■ Mononeuropathy or polyneuropathy
■ Diastolic blood pressure > 90 mmHg
■ Urea > 40 mg/dL, creatinine > 1.5 mg/dL
■ Hepatitis B infection (HBsAg or antibodies positive)
■ Angiography: occlusions or aneurysms in visceral arteries
■ Histology: granulocytes in the vessel walls in small or medium-sized arteries

Three of the 10 criteria have to be met for classification (sensitivity 82%, specificity 87%)

4.1.1   Epidemiology

The annual incidence is approximately 5–9 per million population. PAN is probably in fact even rarer than this, as many patients with microscopic polyangiitis were earlier classified as having polyarteritis nodosa. The first manifestation appears most often over the age of 40, and men are affected three times more often than women.

4.1.2   Etiology and pathogenesis

The etiology is unknown in most cases. In a subgroup of patients, hepatitis B virus infection is a triggering factor; hepatitis B surface antigen is positive in up to 30% of patients.

Pathogenesis. PAN is an immune complex vasculitis:
■ Circulating immune complexes activate complement and granulocytes.
■ Endothelial damage is caused by the activated neutrophilic granulocytes.
■ Immune complex deposits collect on the vascular wall.

4.2   Clinical findings

The clinical symptoms are variable and depend on the disease stage and the organs affected (Table 4-2).

Table 4-2 Clinical findings in polyarteritis nodosa.

Organ manifestation	Major symptoms	Frequency
General symptoms	Fever, weight loss, nocturnal sweating	70%
Mononeuritis multiplex, polyneuropathy	Peroneal nerve weakness, hyposensitivity	50–70%
Gastrointestinal tract: mesenteric arteries	Bloody diarrhea, abdominal angina, mesenteric infarction, hepatic and splenic infarction	25–40%
Joints	Arthralgia, arthritis, myalgia	20–50%
Kidneys: renal vasculopathy	Arterial hypertension, renal artery stenosis	≈ 70%
Heart	Angina pectoris, myocardial infarction, dyspnea	≈ 50%
Skin	Palpable purpura, skin necroses, gangrene, nodules, livedo reticularis	40%
Central nervous system	Epilepsy, psychosis	< 10%

4.3   Diagnosis

4.3.1   Clinical examination

The clinical symptoms are variable and depend on the organs affected (Table 4-2).

4.3.2   Laboratory diagnosis

The erythrocyte sedimentation rate (ESR) and C-reactive protein (CRP) levels are nonspecifically increased. There are no specific antibodies. Antineutrophilic cytoplasmic antibody (ANCA) is positive in approximately 10% of cases (usually p-ANCA). Pathogen diagnosis should be carried out to exclude other secondary immune complex vasculitides: HB_sAg (positive in up to 30% of cases), hepatitis C virus (HCV), and human immunodeficiency virus (HIV) serology.

4.3.3   Biopsy/histology

A biopsy should always be attempted in order to provide histological confirmation of the diagnosis. The typical finding in PAN is necrotizing vasculitis in medium-sized vessels with evidence of immune complex deposition. Biopsies are best taken from skin and muscle in macroscopically involved areas. Magnetic resonance imaging (MRI) of the musculature may make it easier to select the biopsy site (alternatively, a sural nerve biopsy can be taken in patients with severe polyneuropathy and pathological nerve conduction velocity findings).

4.3.4   Imaging diagnosis

4.3.4.1   Angiography/DSA

If indicated (with symptoms of ischemia), and depending on the patient's history and clinical findings, angiography of the legs and pelvic region, coronary angiography, or mesenteric arteriography may be useful.

Typical findings in PAN are microaneurysms and tapering or segmental stenoses with no signs of atherosclerosis. These angiographic findings are typical of vasculitis, but not specific for polyarteritis nodosa.

4.3.4.2   Ultrasonography/duplex ultrasonography

Duplex ultrasonography is indicated to identify renal artery stenosis in all patients with arterial hypertension and/or renal insufficiency, as well as for identifying splenic and hepatic infarction.

Table 4-3 Differential diagnosis of polyarteritis nodosa.

Major symptoms	Minor symptoms	Suspected diagnosis	Diagnosis
Mononeuritis, abdominal angina	Arterial hypertension	Polyarteritis nodosa	Biopsy: immune complex vasculitis in medium-sized vessels, HB$_s$Ag positive
Pulmonary nodules, blood-tinged rhinorrhea	Episcleritis, palpable purpura	Wegener disease	Biopsy: granulomas, c-ANCA/anti-PR3 positive
Pulmonary-renal syndrome	Gastrointestinal symptoms	Microscopic polyangiitis	Biopsy: no granulomas, p-ANCA
Bronchial asthma, nasal polyposis	Polyneuropathy	Churg–Strauss syndrome	Eosinophils: > 10%
Erosive polyarthritis	Purpura, neuropathy	Rheumatoid vasculitis	X-ray of joints, rheumatoid factors positive, complement ↓
Polyneuropathy, hepatitis	Purpura	Cryoglobulinemic vasculitis	HCV positive, cryoglobulins

Anti-PR3, antiproteinase 3; c-ANCA, cytoplasmic antineutrophilic cytoplasmic antibody; HB$_s$Ag, hepatitis B surface antigen; p-ANCA, perinuclear antineutrophilic cytoplasmic antibody; HCV, hepatitis C virus.

4.3.5   Differential diagnosis

The most important differential diagnoses (Table 4-3) are vasculitides of small vessels, which may also affect medium-sized vessels. Histological findings or surrogate parameters for small-vessel vasculitis (e.g., glomerulonephritis, pulmonary capillaritis) exclude polyarteritis nodosa. Secondary vasculitides also have to be distinguished from polyarteritis nodosa.

4.4   Treatment

4.4.1   Inducing remission

Long-term cyclophosphamide treatment (Fauci scheme, NIH standard) for 3–6 months is the standard, particularly when there are organ-threatening signs (e.g., focal neuropathy with paresis) (Guillevin et al. 2003). This is accompanied by prednisolone administration (initially 1 mg/kg body weight/d; in cases of imminent organ failure, 250 mg–1 g/d i.v.; dose reduction depending on disease activity). If there is no imminent threat of organ failure, methotrexate can be used as an alternative.

4.4.2   Remission maintenance

There is no general standard as in remission-induction treatment. Recurrences are seen less often than in small-vessel vasculitides. If partial or full remission is achieved after cyclophosphamide treatment, azathioprine may be administered (2–3 mg/kg/d; also possible in cases of renal insufficiency), or alternatively methotrexate (0.3 mg/kg/d i.v.; only with normal renal function).

4.4.3   Hepatitis B virus-associated polyarteritis nodosa

In hepatitis B-associated PAN, the aim should be to treat the cause by eliminating the pathogen. According to a protocol used by the French vasculitis research group, primary treatment of the vasculitis using high-dose prednisolone for 2 weeks (week 1, 1 mg/kg, followed by reduction), with subsequent treatment for hepatitis B with lamivudine (100 mg/d) in combination with plasmapheresis leads to high remission rates (Guillevin et al. 2004).

4.5   Prognosis and course

The 5-year survival rate is 80% with immunosuppressive therapy. The recurrence rate is lower than with other forms of vasculitis, at 20% (Guillevin et al. 1996). In HBV-associated polyarteritis, seroconversion is successful in over 50% of cases, and recurrences are then only seen in 10% of the patients.

5 Kawasaki syndrome

Bernhard Hellmich

5.1 Clinical picture

Kawasaki syndrome (synonym: mucocutaneous lymph node syndrome) is a highly febrile disease of childhood characterized by a typical combination of cutaneous and mucosal signs and lymph node swelling. As cutaneous vasculitis and vasculitis of the coronary arteries are found in nearly all of the patients, the disease is now assigned to the systemic vasculitides.

5.1.1 Epidemiology

The annual incidence in Japan is 80 per 100,000 population, and in the United States 10 per 100,000 population. It first becomes manifest usually before the fifth year of life, with a peak at the age of 18 months. Boys are more often affected than girls (1.5:1).

5.1.2 Etiology and pathogenesis

The etiology is not known; bacterial superantigens may play a role. Histology shows infiltration of smaller and medium-sized arteries in coronary vasculitis.

5.2 Clinical findings

A distinction is made between pathognomonic cutaneous symptoms and optional minor symptoms (Table 5-1). According to the 1990 American Heart Association (AHA) criteria, fever and at least four additional cutaneous symptoms are required for diagnosis.

5.3 Diagnosis

The diagnosis is made clinically using the AHA criteria.

5.3.1 Laboratory diagnosis

The erythrocyte sedimentation rate (ESR) and C-reactive protein (CRP) levels are nonspecifically increased. There are no pathognomonic antibodies.

5.3.2 Electrocardiography

Cardiac dysrhythmia is frequently seen when there is myocardial involvement, with S–T interval changes, pericardial and coronary involvement.

5.3.3 Echocardiography

Echocardiography provides evidence of proximal coronary aneurysms (coronary angiography may provide supplementary information) and is used to document myocardial contraction disturbances.

5.3.4 Differential diagnosis

The most important differential diagnosis in Kawasaki syndrome is Schönlein–Henoch purpura (see Chapter 11). When the principal manifestation is vasculitic, the differential diagnoses are the same as in polyarteritis nodosa (Table 4-3). Other differential diagnoses are listed in Table 5-2.

Table 5-1 Major and minor symptoms of Kawasaki syndrome.

Major symptoms	Minor symptoms
■ Fever 39–41°C of unclear cause for at least 5 days	■ Cardiac manifestation: initially panmyocarditis, later coronary vasculitis with development of aneurysms; clinically, angina pectoris, myocardial infarction, cardiac insufficiency
■ Bilateral conjunctival infection	■ Renal involvement: proteinuria and erythrocyturia
■ Reddening and swelling of the lips, reddening of oral mucosa and tongue	■ Oligoarthritis or polyarthritis
■ Edematous swelling with erythema on the palms of the hand and soles of the feet, with scaling on tips of fingers and toes in second week of disease	■ Central nervous system involvement: cephalalgia, meningism
■ Exanthema, mainly on trunk	■ Abdominal symptoms, vomiting
■ Mainly cervical lymph node swelling, size > 1.5 cm	

Table 5-2 Differential diagnosis of Kawasaki syndrome.

Major symptoms	Minor symptoms	Suspected diagnosis	Diagnosis
Fever for 5 days	Lymph node swelling Exanthema + enanthema	Kawasaki syndrome	Clinical findings: AHA criteria
Palpable purpura Glomerulonephritis	Diffuse abdominal pain	Schönlein–Henoch purpura	Complement ↓ IgA in serum ↑
Generalized exanthema	Bacterial infection Medication history	Lyell syndrome	Clinical findings History

AHA, American Heart Association.

5.4   Treatment

5.4.1   Intravenous immunoglobulin (IVIG)

IVIG is the treatment of choice. Immediate administration is indicated in the acute phase (2 g/kg body weight as a single dose), and this reduces the development of coronary aneurysms by more than 80%.

5.4.2   Acetylsalicylic acid (ASA)

ASA 80–100 mg/kg body weight p.o. should be administered in the acute phase until the patient is free of fever. In coronary artery aneurysms, low-dose ASA (5–10 mg/kg body weight/d) for platelet inhibition is useful.

5.4.3   Therapy for treatment-refractory courses

- Second dose of IVIG
- Pentoxifylline in addition, if appropriate (20 mg/kg daily)
- Prednisolone 2 mg/kg/d, reduced after 2 weeks if a response is seen, depending on clinical symptoms

5.5   Prognosis and course

The prognosis depends on the presence of coronary involvement. Complications include coronary thromboses and malignant cardiac arrhythmia. The mortality since the introduction of IVIG has been 0.3% (previously > 3%). Recurrences are possible, but are very rare in comparison with other systemic forms of vasculitis.

6 Wegener granulomatosis

Bernhard Hellmich

6.1 Clinical picture

Wegener disease (synonym: Wegener granulomatosis) is defined as a granulomatous inflammation of the respiratory tract, with necrotizing vasculitis mainly affecting smaller vessels (Table 6-1). Wegener granulomatosis is the most frequent of the ANCA-associated forms of vasculitis (Reinhold-Keller et al. 2005).

Table 6-1 Classification criteria for Wegener granulomatosis (ACR 1990).

■ Inflammation in the nose/mouth with blood-tinged or purulent nasal secretion and/or oral ulcers
■ Nodules, fixed infiltrates or cavities on chest x-ray
■ Microhematuria (> 5 erythrocytes/high-powered field) or evidence of erythrocyte casts
■ Biopsy evidence of granulomatous inflammation (intravascular, perivascular, or extravascular)

Two of the four criteria have to be met for classification (sensitivity 92%, specificity 88%).

6.1.1 Epidemiology

The annual incidence in Germany is approximately 10 per 1 million population, with a prevalence of up to 50 per 1 million population (Reinhold-Keller et al. 2005). The disease can become manifest at any age, most frequently over the age of 40.

6.1.2 Etiology and pathogenesis

The etiology is not known. The condition may be induced by bacterial superantigens *(Staphylococcus aureus)* in the respiratory tract mucosa. It starts with a granulomatous inflammation of the respiratory tract (initial phase), which after a variable period of time usually progresses to generalized vasculitis (the generalization phase). In patients with Wegener granulomatosis, antigen-presenting dendritic cells activate the PAR-2 receptor via the ANCA target antigen PR-3, triggering interferon-γ secretion and thereby promoting the development of granulomatous inflammation (Csernok et al. 2006). During the generalization phase, T-cell activation then probably leads to maturation and activation of plasma cells and thus to the development of ANCA. ANCAs and cytokines then cause activation of neutrophilic granulocytes, which lead to endothelial damage (Gross 1999).

6.1.3 Histopathology

The histological findings depend on the disease stage:

■ Initial phase: granuloma formation in the respiratory tract, immunohistochemically T cells with Th1 cytokine patterns

■ Generalization phase: vasculitis in small and sometimes also medium-sized vessels, with a Th1 cytokine pattern

6.2 Clinical findings

The clinical symptoms are variable and depend on the disease stage and organs affected (Table 6-2). While the localized phase of the disease, with mainly ear, nose, and throat findings, is often not recognized for a long period, pulmonary and renal involvement usually leads to diagnosis (Reinhold-Keller 2000). Systemic vasculitis may become evident in numerous organs—e.g., in the form of ischemic colitis (Fig. 6-1).

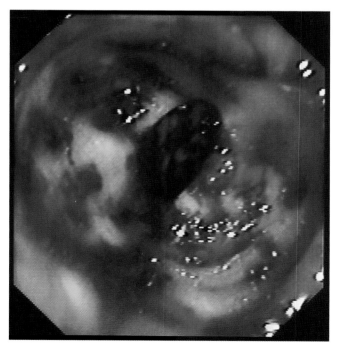

Fig. 6-1 Ischemic colitis.

Table 6-2 Clinical findings in Wegener disease.

Organ manifestation	Major symptoms	Frequency
Lungs	Dyspnea, rarely hemoptysis	85%
Ear, nose, and throat	Blood-tinged rhinorrhea, endonasal crust formation, sinusitis, hearing loss, subglottic stenosis	95%
Glomerulonephritis	Edema, microhematuria	80%
Joints	Arthralgia, arthritis, myalgia	70%
Eyes	Episcleritis, conjunctivitis, retrobulbar granuloma	Up to 60%
General symptoms	Fever, weight loss, nocturnal sweating	> 50%
Cutaneous vasculitis	Palpable purpura, cutaneous necroses, nodules	Up to 50%
Polyneuropathy	Peroneal nerve weakness, hyposensitivity	20%
Central nervous system	Epilepsy, psychosis	< 10%
Gastrointestinal tract	Bloody diarrhea, tenesmus	< 10%

6.3   Diagnosis

6.3.1   Clinical examination

The clinical symptoms depend on the organ involvement (Table 6-2). During the initial phase, the clinical symptoms involve the ear, nose, and throat and/or pulmonary changes, while in the generalization phase the picture is one of systemic small-vessel vasculitis. Saddle nose is a typical symptom in patients with a prolonged course.

6.3.2   Diagnostic testing

6.3.2.1   Laboratory diagnosis

Antineutrophilic cytoplasmic antibodies (ANCAs)

ANCAs showing cytoplasmic fluorescence on fluorescent microscopy (c-ANCAs) and reactivity with proteinase 3 (PR3) on enzyme-linked immunosorbent assay (ELISA) are characteristic of Wegener disease (Csernok et al. 1990). The highest levels of sensitivity and specificity are achieved with a combination of fluorescence microscopy (c-ANCA) and ELISA (anti-PR3 antibodies). ANCAs are a sensitive marker for disease activity. c-ANCA/anti-PR3 antibodies are positive during the generalization phase in 95% of patients, but only in 50% during the initial phase. False-positive ANCA findings rarely occur (e.g., in infectious diseases). The ANCA test is therefore not capable of replacing histological confirmation of the diagnosis.

Urinary diagnosis, renal function

- Urinary status and sediment: dysmorphic erythrocyturia suggests a glomerular origin of the erythrocyturia, and a targeted microscopic examination is therefore needed.
- Proteins in 24-hour urine: there is increased elimination in glomerulonephritis, but also in nephrotic syndrome without inflammatory activity.
- Urinary protein differential analysis (electrophoresis): distinguishes between glomerular proteinuria (only albumin elimination), tubular proteinuria, and prerenal proteinuria.
- Creatinine, urea, creatinine clearance: monitoring of renal function.
- In nondysmorphic erythrocyturia during cyclophosphamide treatment, hemorrhagic cystitis should be considered.

Acute-phase parameters

The erythrocyte sedimentation rate (ESR) and C-reactive protein (CRP) are raised in active disease, but in infections as well. If a concomitant infection is possible, a procalcitonin assessment should be carried out (only raised when there is infection).

6.3.3   Biopsy/histology

A biopsy should always be attempted in order to allow histological confirmation of the diagnosis. Typical findings are granulomas and/or necrotizing vasculitis without immune complex deposition (pauci-immune vasculitis). A biopsy can be taken from macroscopically involved nasal mucosa. Alternatively, a renal biopsy is possible if there are abnormal urinary findings (this is sensitive, but associated with more complications) or a pulmonary biopsy (less sensitive). If histological confirmation is lacking, surrogate markers for major organ involvement (e.g., dysmorphic erythrocyturia, glomerular proteinuria) in combination with positive ANCA findings make the diagnosis probable.

6.3.4   Imaging diagnosis

6.3.4.1   Chest x-ray and high-resolution computed tomography (HRCT) of the chest

Nodules, infiltrates, and cavities are typical findings in Wegener granulomatosis (Fig. 6-2). Pathological findings require further clarification with bronchoscopy and bronchoalveolar lavage (BAL).

6.3.4.2   MRI of the skull

Magnetic resonance imaging (MRI) is used to identify inflammatory activity in the otorhinolaryngeal region (e.g., sinusitis, granuloma), to diagnose central nervous system involvement (with microinfarctions), and to clarify exophthalmos (retrobulbar granuloma).

6.3.5   Differential diagnosis

A diagnosis of Wegener granulomatosis is only possible with a combined assessment of the patient's history, the clinical, laboratory (ANCA), and diagnostic findings, and the histological findings (Tables 6-2 and 6-3).

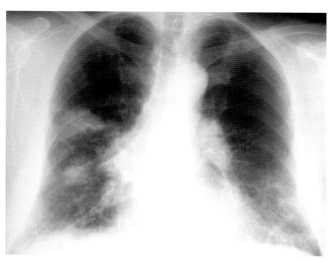

Fig. 6-2 Nodules, infiltrates, and cavities are typical findings in Wegener granulomatosis.

6.4 Treatment

Treatment depends on the stage, activity, and extent of the disease (Table 6-4).

6.4.1 Initial phase (localized Wegener granulomatosis)

Trimethoprim/sulfamethoxazole (2 × 960 mg/d) is only indicated when there is isolated otorhinolaryngeal involvement and if there are no signs of vasculitis or general symptoms. It leads to sustained remission in two-thirds of the patients. Methotrexate (MTX; 0.3 mg/ kg/week) is the treatment of choice when there is greater disease activity and/or pulmonary involvement.

6.4.2 Early systemic phase

The results of the NORAM study showed that in early systemic Wegener granulomatosis (Table 6-4), MTX (0.3 mg/kg/week) leads to similar remission rates in comparison with cyclophosphamide (CYC), but it is associated with fewer side effects (de Groot et al. 2005).

6.4.3 Generalization phase

6.4.3.1 Inducing remission

The accepted standard for many years was cyclophosphamide therapy (Fauci scheme, NIH standard) for 3–6 months, particularly with locally destructive and organ-threatening manifestations (Jayne et al. 2003). However, in comparison with long-term oral therapy, cyclophosphamide bolus treatment (with the CYCLOPS scheme) leads to a similar remission rate, while being less toxic (de Groot et al. 2001). Prednisolone is always administered as an accompanying medication (initially 1 mg/kg body weight/day, with imminent organ failure 250 mg–1 g/d i.v., dose reduction depending on disease activity). Rituximab is as effective as CYC for induction therapy, but does not provide any safety benefit in the short term. Rituximab is therefore an alternative for first-line therapy if there are contraindications to CYC administration. There are as yet no validated long-term data on treatment with rituximab in patients with antineutrophil cytoplasmic antibody (ANCA)-associated vasculitis (AAV).

When there is severe renal involvement, accompanying plasmapheresis (seven times in 14 days) reduces the rate of renal failure requiring permanent dialysis (Jayne et al. 2007).

Table 6-3 Differential diagnosis of Wegener disease.

Major symptoms	Minor symptoms	Suspected diagnosis	Diagnosis
Pulmonary nodules Blood-tinged rhinorrhea	Episcleritis, palpable purpura	Wegener disease	Biopsy: granuloma, c-ANCA/anti-PR3
Pulmonary-renal syndrome	Gastrointestinal symptoms	Microscopic polyangiitis	Biopsy: no granuloma, p-ANCA
Bronchial asthma Nasal polyposis	Polyneuropathy	Churg–Strauss syndrome	Eosinophilia: > 10%
Granulomatous lymphadenopathy	Interstitial pulmonary changes	Sarcoidosis	ANCA negative
Polyneuropathy, hepatitis	Purpura	Cryoglobulinemic vasculitis	HCV positive, cryoglobulins

ANCA, antineutrophilic cytoplasmic antibody; anti-PR3, antiproteinase 3; c-ANCA, cytoplasmic antineutrophilic cytoplasmic antibody; p-ANCA, perinuclear antineutrophilic cytoplasmic antibody; HCV, hepatitis C virus.

Table 6-4 Disease stages in antineutrophilic cytoplasmic antibody (ANCA)-associated vasculitides.

Stage	Systemic vasculitis outside the otorhinolaryngeal tract and lungs	Organ-threatening or life-threatening	Other definitions	Serum titer (µmol/L)
Localized	–	–	No B symptoms, ANCA usually negative	< 120
Early systemic	+	–	B symptoms present, ANCA + or –	< 120
Generalized	+	+	ANCA +	< 500
Severe	+	+, organ failure	ANCA +	> 500

6.4.3.2   Refractory situation

The standard treatment does not lead to remission in approximately 10% of the patients. Small open studies have shown that additional administration of infliximab (5 mg/kg) or rituximab (375 mg/m²) is beneficial in these refractory cases (Hellmich et al. 2006). When there is a fulminating course and cyclophosphamide treatment using the NIH standard has failed, an intensified Fauci scheme can also be administered temporarily (3–4 mg/kg/d p.o.).

6.4.3.3   Remission maintenance

If partial or full remission is achieved after cyclophosphamide therapy, continued immunosuppressive treatment reduces the risk of recurrences. Without remission maintenance therapy, the recurrence rate is over 70%. The CYCAZAREM study led to the establishment of azathioprine (dose 2–3 mg/kg/d) as the standard form of remission maintenance therapy (Jayne et al. 2003). Alternatively, there is now also evidence from randomized studies that methotrexate and leflunomide are effective (Metzler et al. 2007). Administration of mycophenolate mofetil leads to a higher recurrence rate in comparison with azathioprine.

6.4.4   Supportive therapy

Low-dose trimethoprim/sulfamethoxazole (960 mg two to three times per week) should be administered for prophylaxis against *Pneumocystis carinii* infection (however, caution is needed with methotrexate, as there is cumulative toxicity). Subglottic stenoses can be dilated endoscopically. Steroid-containing eyedrops are useful in episcleritis.

6.5   Prognosis and course

The prognosis depends on organ involvement; renal and pulmonary involvement is unfavorable. The survival rate is approximately 80% (median 6–8 years) when the Fauci scheme is used. Recurrences are observed in up to 70% of the patients within 5 years. Treatment-associated complications (opportunistic infections, increased risk of urinary bladder carcinoma with cyclophosphamide) are prognostically unfavorable.

7 Microscopic polyangiitis

Bernhard Hellmich

7.1 Clinical picture

Microscopic polyangiitis is defined as a necrotizing vasculitis, which in contrast to polyarteritis nodosa mainly affects small vessels (Table 7-1). Like Wegener disease and Churg–Strauss syndrome, microscopic polyangiitis is one of the antineutrophilic cytoplasmic antibody (ANCA)-associated forms of vasculitis and is also characterized by an absence of immune complex deposits. In contrast to Wegener disease, however, there is no clinical or histological evidence of granulomatous changes. Glomerulonephritis is almost always present.

Table 7-1 Definition of microscopic polyangiitis (Chapel Hill Consensus Conference 1992).

- Necrotizing vasculitis with little or no immune complex deposition
- Small vessels always involved (capillaries, venules, arterioles)
- Involvement of smaller and medium-sized arteries is possible
- Necrotizing glomerulonephritis is very frequent
- Pulmonary capillaritis is frequent

7.1.1 Epidemiology

The incidence of microscopic polyangiitis (MPA) is approximately two to four per 1 million population, and it is therefore half as frequent as Wegener disease. It may become manifest at any age, most frequently in those aged over 50.

7.1.2 Etiology and pathogenesis

The etiology of the disease is not known. As in Wegener disease, it is assumed that ANCA plays a major role in the pathogenesis (see section C 6.1.2).

7.2 Clinical findings

The major symptom of MPA is glomerulonephritis, which occurs in nearly all patients. Pulmonary-renal syndrome, with rapidly progressive glomerulonephritis and alveolar hemorrhage, occurs more often with microscopic polyangiitis than in other ANCA-associated forms of vasculitis and requires immediate therapeutic intervention. Involvement of the gastrointestinal tract is more frequent than in other types of ANCA-associated vasculitides.

7.3 Diagnosis

7.3.1 Clinical examination

The clinical symptoms depend on the organ involvement (Table 7-2).

Table 7-2 Clinical findings in microscopic polyangiitis.

Organ manifestation	Major symptoms	Frequency
Glomerulonephritis	Edema, microhematuria	> 90%
Lungs	Dyspnea, coughing	50–70%
Alveolar hemorrhage	Hemoptysis	10–50%
Gastrointestinal tract	Bloody diarrhea, tenesmus, pancreatitis	30%
Eyes	Episcleritis, conjunctivitis	20%
General symptoms	Fever, weight loss, nocturnal sweating	> 50%
Cutaneous vasculitis	Palpable purpura, cutaneous necroses, nodules	Up to 50%
Polyneuropathy	Peroneal nerve weakness, hyposensitivity	60–70%
Joints	Arthralgia, arthritis, myalgia	10%
Ear, nose and throat	Sinusitis	13%

7.3.2 Diagnostic testing

7.3.2.1 Laboratory diagnosis

Antineutrophilic cytoplasmic antibodies (ANCAs)

ANCAs are positive in 80% of patients with active disease. In contrast to Wegener disease, p-ANCAs (in 60% of patients) are found more frequently than c-ANCAs (in 20% of patients). The target antigen of p-ANCAs in microscopic polyangiitis is myeloperoxidase (MPO).

Urinary diagnosis, renal function

Due to the frequent renal involvement, detailed diagnostic procedures should be carried out. The approach is the same as the procedure used for Wegener granulomatosis (urinary sediment, dysmorphic erythrocytes, creatinine, etc.).

7.3.3 Biopsy/histology

Biopsy should always be attempted in order to confirm the diagnosis. Typical findings: nongranulomatous necrotizing vasculitis in small vessels without immune complex deposition (pauci-immune vasculitis). A renal biopsy should usually be taken if there are abnormal urinary findings, as this is also relevant for the prognosis (scarring versus active glomerulonephritis). If histological confirmation is not possible, surrogate markers for major organ involvement (e.g., dysmorphic erythrocyturia, glomerular proteinuria) in combination with positive ANCA findings can make the diagnosis probable.

7.3.4 Imaging diagnosis

7.3.4.1 Chest x-ray and high-resolution computed tomography (HRCT) of the chest

Typical findings include alternating infiltrates (in contrast to Wegener disease, there are no granulomas or cavities). Pathological findings should be clarified using bronchoscopy and bronchoalveolar lavage. In contrast to other forms of vasculitis, MPA can lead to the development of pulmonary fibrosis.

7.3.4.2 Bronchoalveolar lavage (BAL)

BAL is indicated when there is evidence of infiltrates on HRCT (alveolar hemorrhage vs. alveolitis vs. pathogen-related pneumonia vs. drug-induced pneumonitis) and to clarify hemoptysis (alveolar hemorrhage or bleeding from the otorhinolaryngeal tract?). Iron-loaded macrophages on BAL samples suggest previous alveolar hemorrhage.

7.3.4.3 MRI of the skull

Magnetic resonance imaging (MRI) is helpful for identifying inflammatory activity in the otorhinolaryngeal region and for diagnosing central nervous system involvement (with microinfarctions).

7.3.5 Differential diagnosis

The major differential diagnoses are the same as in Wegener disease (Table 6-3). It is often difficult to distinguish the condition from Wegener disease, as both conditions are ANCA-associated, affect the small vessels, and often show involvement of the lungs and kidneys. If there is an absence of granulomatous changes (clinically and/or histologically), the conditions should be classified as microscopic polyangiitis.

7.4 Treatment

Treatment depends on the stage, activity, and extent of the disease and corresponds to the recommendations for treatment of Wegener granulomatosis (see section C 6.4), with one exception: there is no indication for the use of trimethoprim/co-trimoxazole in MPA.

7.5 Prognosis and course

The prognosis depends on organ involvement; renal and pulmonary involvement are unfavorable. The 5-year survival rate is 75%. With alveolar hemorrhage, however, the mortality rate increases by a factor of eight. Recurrences are observed in up to 5% of the patients within 5 years, and regular clinical and laboratory check-ups are therefore useful.

8 Churg–Strauss syndrome

Bernhard Hellmich

8.1 Clinical picture

Churg–Strauss syndrome (CSS) is defined as a necrotizing vasculitis in small and medium-sized vessels, of unknown etiology, the histological correlate of which is an eosinophilic inflammation preferentially affecting the respiratory tract. The disease is usually associated with bronchial asthma and blood eosinophilia. Churg–Strauss syndrome is one of the antineutrophilic cytoplasmic antibody (ANCA)-associated forms of vasculitis (Table 8-1).

Table 8-1 Classification criteria for Churg–Strauss syndrome (ACR 1990).

- Bronchial asthma
- Blood eosinophilia (> 10%)
- Mononeuropathy/polyneuropathy
- Wandering or transient pulmonary infiltrates
- History of or manifest chronic sinus conditions
- Histology: extravascular tissue eosinophilia around arterioles and venules

Four of the six criteria have to be met for classification (sensitivity 85%, specificity 100%).

8.1.1 Epidemiology

The annual incidence is 1–2.4 per million population, and CSS is thus much rarer than Wegener disease and microscopic polyangiitis. The prevalence is approximately 1.3 per 100,000 population (in Norway). The condition can become manifest at any age.

8.1.2 Etiology and pathogenesis

The etiology of CSS is not known. The results of a large crossover study have shown an association with asthma drugs, particularly leukotriene receptor antagonists (e.g., montelukast). However, this may only reflect the deterioration of asthma before the outbreak of CSS. Immunological processes appear to play an important role in the pathogenesis as a contributing cause (Hellmich et al. 2003). In the active stage of disease, evidence of p-ANCA/MPO-ANCA is found in 50% of the patients. In addition, overexpression of Th2 cytokines such as interleukin-5 appears to be important. Histopathologically, necrotizing pauci-immune vasculitis, extravascular eosinophilic infiltrates, and granulomas are found.

8.2 Clinical findings

The extent of the symptoms varies and depends on the organs affected (Table 8-2).

Table 8-2 Symptoms of Churg–Strauss syndrome.

Organ manifestation	Major symptoms	Frequency
Lungs	Bronchial asthma	100%
Ear, nose, and throat	Sinusitis	> 50%
Polyneuropathy	Peroneal nerve weakness, hyposensitivity	70–80%
Cutaneous vasculitis	Palpable purpura, cutaneous necroses, nodules	65%
Heart: myocarditis, pericarditis	Cardiac dysrhythmia, angina pectoris	10–15%
Joints	Arthralgia, arthritis, myalgia	60%
Glomerulonephritis	Edema, microhematuria	10–25%
General symptoms	Fever, weight loss, nocturnal sweating	70%

8.3 Diagnosis

8.3.1 Clinical examination

The clinical symptoms depend on the organ involved (Table 8-2). In the prodromal phase, there is often only bronchial asthma, allergic rhinitis, and nasal polyposis (Hellmich et al. 2006).

8.3.2 Diagnostic testing

8.3.2.1 Laboratory diagnosis

- Differential blood count: usually massive eosinophilia
- c-ANCA (target antigen PR3) or p-ANCA (target antigen MPO): positive in approximately 50% of patients
- Erythrocyte sedimentation rate (ESR), C-reactive protein (CRP): nonspecifically raised
- Immunoglobulin E (IgE), eosinophil cationic protein (ECP) raised

Table 8-3 Differential diagnosis of Churg–Strauss syndrome.

Major symptoms	Minor symptoms	Suspected diagnosis	Diagnosis
Bronchial asthma Nasal polyposis	Polyneuropathy Pulmonary infiltrates	Churg–Strauss syndrome	Biopsy: vasculitis
Blood eosinophilia		Hypereosinophilic syndrome	Biopsy: no vasculitis
Pulmonary nodules Sinusitis	c-ANCA/anti-PR3 antibodies positive	Wegener disease	Eosinophilia: < 10%
Abdominal symptoms	Transient eosinophilic pulmonary infiltrate	Helminthic infection (e.g., ascariasis)	Fecal examination for helminth eggs
B symptoms	Splenomegaly	Acute myeloid leukemia	Excess blast cells in blood and contrast medium

Anti-PR3, antiproteinase 3; c-ANCA, cytoplasmic antineutrophilic cytoplasmic antibody.

- Urinary status and sediment: dysmorphic hematuria and proteinuria in glomerulonephritis
- Creatinine, urea: raised in glomerulonephritis
- Fecal examination for helminth eggs, to exclude eosinophilia due to helminthic infection

8.3.2.2   Electrocardiography (ECG)

ECG often shows cardiac dysrhythmia when there is myocardial involvement and S–T interval changes when there is pericardial involvement. Myocardial involvement can also be demonstrated using cardiac magnetic resonance imaging.

8.3.2.3   Chest x-ray and high-resolution computed tomography (HRCT) of the chest

Migratory infiltrates often correlate with eosinophilic alveolitis, and nodules that do not fade correlate with granulomas. Bronchoalveolar lavage can be performed for differential diagnosis of pulmonary changes (eosinophilic alveolitis with pulmonary activity).

8.3.2.4   Biopsy

Biopsy should always be attempted to allow histological confirmation of the diagnosis. Possible biopsy sites include the skin in purpura, the sural nerve in polyneuropathy, the gastrointestinal tract, or the lungs (invasive).

8.3.3   Differential diagnosis

Other diseases that may be associated with eosinophilia have to be excluded (Table 8-3).

8.4   Treatment

8.4.1   Glucocorticoids

Monotherapy with glucocorticoids is the standard treatment. For initial therapy, prednisolone is administered at 1 mg/kg. Dose reduction is carried out depending on the clinical response. Low doses (< 5 mg) are often required for long-term treatment of bronchial asthma (Hellmich and Gross 2004). As recurrences are quite frequent, glucocorticoid-sparing therapy should be initiated early in the treatment plan.

8.4.2   Immunosuppressants

As in other ANCA-associated types of vasculitis, combination therapy with powerful immunosuppressive agents should be administered primarily when there are prognostically unfavorable disease manifestations (renal involvement, cardiomyopathy, involvement of the gastrointestinal tract or central nervous system). For inducing remission, administration of cyclophosphamide as a bolus dose or as long-term therapy plus prednisolone has been established in research studies (Guillevin et al. 1999). Methotrexate (MTX) is an alternative if there are no organ-threatening signs (Metzler et al. 2004).

8.4.3   Interferon-α

In fulminant courses and when there is no response to cyclophosphamide/prednisone, remission can often be induced with interferon-α (dosage 10,000–30,000 IU s.c. three to five times per week) (Tatsis et al. 1998). However, long-term administration is limited by side effects.

8.5   Prognosis and course

The prognosis depends on the organ involvement (mean survival after 6.5 years 72%) and is generally better than in Wegener disease.

9 Cryoglobulinemic vasculitis

Bernhard Hellmich

9.1 Clinical picture

Cryoglobulinemic vasculitis is an immune complex vasculitis mainly affecting small vessels.

9.1.1 Etiology and pathogenesis

In essential-mixed cryoglobulinemia (ECV), chronic hepatitis (usually hepatitis C) is now often found thanks to optimized detection methods, and ECV is therefore now included among the secondary vasculitides (Lamprecht et al. 1999, 2001). Blood proteins that are unstable on cooling can increase the viscosity of the blood on cooling to 30°C and can form immune complexes with monoclonal IgM rheumatoid factor and polyclonal IgG plus complement (mixed cryoglobulinemia), leading to endothelial damage. Three types of cryoglobulinemia are now distinguished on the basis of different precipitation properties:

- *Type I cryoglobulins* consist of monoclonal proteins alone and appear in the various types of monoclonal gammopathies (e.g., plasmacytoma).
- *Type II cryoglobulins* consist of several classes of immunoglobulin (mixed cryoglobulins), with monoclonal components being present alongside polyclonal elements.
- *Type III cryoglobulins* have a purely polyclonal structure.

In type II and III cryoglobulins, one of these immunoglobulin classes always has rheumatoid factor characteristics (IgM, anti-IgG). During viral infection (hepatitis B, C), bacterial infection, and parasitic infection, as well as in collagenoses (e.g., systemic lupus erythematosus, Sjögren syndrome), type II cryoglobulinemia develops, as well as type III cryoglobulinemia in some cases.

9.2 Clinical findings

The clinical findings always show palpable purpura—e.g., in the area of the lower extremity, as well as on the extensor sides of the upper extremities and on the buttocks. Joint symptoms are highly variable. Polyarthritis may be present. Polyneuropathy and glomerulonephritis often develop.

9.3 Diagnosis

The diagnostic procedure is the same as that for other types of small-vessel vasculitis. Serologically, positive rheumatoid factor and complement reduction (C4, C3, CH50) are seen in addition to positive evidence of cryoglobulinemia. Hepatitis C has to be excluded. The further diagnostic procedures depend on the clinically guiding symptoms.

9.4 Treatment

In ECV as well, treatment is basically carried out relative to the underlying disease. In milder courses—i.e., when there is no severe organ involvement—a trial of therapy with interferon-α (3 million IU/week) and ribavirin can be made if there is underlying hepatitis C. In severe courses (e.g., with renal function disturbance), plasmapheresis is often necessary. Immune suppression and plasmapheresis are also carried out in the acute stage. Successful treatment of type II cryoglobulinemia due to hepatitis B or C infection is possible with interferon-α2a. The other types require combination therapy with glucocorticoids and cytotoxic agents (cyclophosphamide). A new treatment approach involves administration of rituximab (Lamprecht et al. 2003).

9.5 Prognosis and course

The prognosis in ECV crucially depends on renal involvement (severity of glomerulonephritis) and the underlying disease (e.g., plasmacytoma).

10 Cutaneous leukocytoclastic vasculitis

Bernhard Hellmich

10.1 Clinical picture

Cutaneous leukocytoclastic vasculitis is an immune complex vasculitis that develops in connection with various underlying diseases or has an allergic cause. This vasculitis thus often follows external stimuli, such as medication. It therefore used to be referred to as "hypersensitivity vasculitis."

10.2 Clinical findings

In cutaneous leukocytoclastic vasculitis, the sole clinical symptom is palpable purpura. Particularly when other symptoms are also present, a primary systemic small-vessel vasculitis (e.g., ANCA-associated vasculitis, cryoglobulinemic vasculitis, Schönlein–Henoch purpura) should be excluded using targeted history and diagnostic testing.

10.3 Diagnosis

In purely cutaneous vasculitis, a detailed patient history (with medications) and laboratory exclusion diagnosis relative to other types of small-vessel vasculitis is required, as the purpura may be the first manifestation of prognostically less favorable diseases in approximately half of the patients. In addition, other diseases possibly contributing to the cutaneous leukocytoclastic angiitis (Table 10-1) also should be excluded, and all medications reviewed and assessed for possible contribution.

A diagnosis of cutaneous leukocytoclastic angiitis can be confirmed histologically via skin biopsy. There are no specific biomarkers for the condition (e.g., autoantibodies). The erythrocyte sedimentation rate (ESR) and C-reactive protein (CRP) level may be elevated. The vasculitis can be classified as cutaneous leukocytoclastic angiitis if three or more criteria are met (sensitivity 71%, specificity 83.9%).

10.4 Treatment

Treatment for cutaneous leukocytoclastic vasculitis is based on the underlying disease or triggering factor and is usually symptomatic (e.g., withdrawal of the causative drug). Glucocorticoids can be administered temporarily. Dapsone is often effective in chronic courses. However, there have been no controlled studies of specific treatments.

10.5 Prognosis and course

In cutaneous leukocytoclastic vasculitis (a purely cutaneous vasculitis), the prognosis is good. The disease has a self-limiting course in most patients following successful treatment of the underlying cause.

Table 10-1 Possible causes of cutaneous leukocytoclastic vasculitis.

4. **Drugs:** allopurinol, aminosalicylate, beta-blockers, insulin, iodine, oral contraceptives, penicillin, phenacetin, propylthiouracil, quinine, streptokinase, streptomycin, sulfonamides, tamoxifen, thiazides, vaccine, vitamins, etc.
5. **Infections:** Candida, cytomegalovirus, Epstein-Barr virus, hepatitis A, B, and C, herpes simplex, histoplasmosis, mycobacteria, streptococci, staphylococci
6. **Malignancies:** T-cell leukemia, chronic lymphocytic leukemia, hairy cell leukemia, lymphoma, plasmacytoma, more rarely solid tumors
7. **Other systemic diseases:** systemic lupus erythematosus, rheumatoid arthritis, Sjögren syndrome, primary biliary cirrhosis, Behçet syndrome, cystic fibrosis, ulcerative colitis

Table 10-2 American College of Rheumatology (ACR) classification criteria for cutaneous leukocytoclastic angiitis.

- Age at first onset > 16 years
- Use of medication at start of disease
- Maculopapular rash
- Biopsy including an arteriole and venule showing perivascular or extravascular leukocytes

11 Schönlein–Henoch purpura

Bernhard Hellmich

11.1 Clinical picture

Schönlein–Henoch purpura (SHP) is characterized by the triad of palpable purpura, abdominal colic, and arthritis. SHP occurs almost exclusively in children. The vasculitis shows IgA-containing immune deposits in situ.

11.2 Clinical findings

Abdominal pain and/or gastrointestinal bleeding are characteristic in Schönlein–Henoch purpura. Half of the patients have glomerulonephritis with microhematuria and mild proteinuria. More rarely, rapidly progressive glomerulonephritis may also occur with Schönlein–Henoch purpura.

11.3 Diagnosis

The diagnosis can be histologically confirmed by evidence of leukocytoclastic vasculitis and/or glomerulonephritis, in each case with immunohistochemical evidence of IgA-containing immune complexes. The focus is on clinical and laboratory monitoring of the visceral manifestations of the condition. In particular, renal function has to be monitored in IgA glomerulonephritis (creatinine, sediment).

11.4 Treatment

There have been no controlled studies on the treatment of Schönlein–Henoch purpura.

In view of the good prognosis and often self-limiting course of the disease, Schönlein–Henoch purpura is initially treated on a purely symptomatic basis, or with glucocorticoids if there is severe renal involvement. If glucocorticoid treatment is necessary—as in cases of rapidly progressive glomerulonephritis, in which cytotoxic agents are used additively—1 mg/kg/d prednisone is administered. The dosage is quickly reduced immediately if there is a response.

11.5 Prognosis

Most patients with Schönlein–Henoch purpura make a complete recovery. Even further treatment is not necessary in some cases. The prognosis is determined by renal involvement, which appears to follow a more aggressive course in adults than in children. Up to 8% of all adults with renal manifestations develop end-stage renal failure.

12 Secondary vasculitides

Bernhard Hellmich

12.1 Clinical picture

Vasculitis for which there is a known triggering factor is called secondary vasculitis. Secondary vasculitides above all occur as side effects of drug treatment and in the context of other autoimmune diseases or tumor diseases (Table 12-1).

Table 12-1 Causes of secondary vasculitides.

Systemic autoimmune diseases
■ Lupus vasculitis, rheumatoid vasculitis, Sjögren syndrome-associated vasculitis, Behçet syndrome
■ Organ-related chronic inflammatory diseases (e.g., ulcerative colitis)
■ Chronic granulomatous diseases (Crohn disease, Boeck disease)
Infections
■ Viruses (HIV, CMV)
■ Bacteria (spirochetes, mycobacteria, streptococci, Tropheryma whippelii)
■ Parasitoses (Ascaris)
■ Fungi (Aspergillus)
Neoplasias
■ Non-Hodgkin lymphoma
■ Myeloproliferative diseases
■ Solid tumors
Intoxication
■ Narcotics (cocaine, morphine)
Drugs
■ Antihypertensive agents (hydralazine)
■ Thyrostatic agents (propylthiouracil)
■ Antibiotics
■ Blood products (antibodies)

CMV, cytomegalovirus; HIV, human immunodeficiency virus.

12.2 Clinical findings

Secondary vasculitides are almost always limited to the skin. Systemic manifestations are rare.

12.3 Diagnosis

Diagnosis of primary vasculitis always involves exclusion of a secondary vasculitis. This mainly involves taking a targeted patient history with attention to potential triggering factors (Table 12-1). Other examinations (e.g., to exclude neoplasia) may then be required.

12.4 Treatment

Basically, the triggering factor should always be eliminated (e.g., withdrawing a drug) or the underlying disease should be treated. Additional immunosuppressive therapy is not then required. Glucocorticoids can be administered temporarily in severe courses.

12.5 Prognosis

The prognosis is determined by the underlying disease, which is often severe. The prognosis in most vasculitides that are limited to the skin is very good.

References for Chapters 1–12

Blockmans D, Stroobants S, Maes A, Mortelmans L. Positron emission tomography in giant cell arteritis and polymyalgia rheumatica: evidence for inflammation of the aortic arch. Am J Med 2000; 108 (3): 246–9.

Both M, Aries PM, Muller-Hulsbeck S, Jahnke T, Schafer PJ, Gross WL, et al. Balloon angioplasty of upper extremity arteries in patients with extracranial giant cell arteritis. Ann Rheum Dis 2006; 7: 7.

Csernok E, Ai M, Gross W, Wicklein D, Petersen A, Lidner B, et al. Wegener's autoantigen induces maturation of dendritic cells and licenses them for Th-1 priming via protease activating receptor-2. Blood 2006; 107: 4440–8.

Csernok E, Holle J, Hellmich B, Cohen Tervaert J, Kallenberg C, Limburg P, et al. Evaluation of capture ELISA for detection of antineutrophil cytoplasmic antibodies against proteinase-3 in Wegener's granulomatosis: first results from a multicenter study. Rheumatology 2004; 43: 174–80.

Csernok E, Luedemann J, Gross W, Bainton D. Ultrastructural localization of proteinase 3, the target of anti-cytoplasmic antibodies circulating in Wegener's granulomatosis. Am J Pathol 1990; 137: 1113–9.

de Groot K, Adu D, Savage C. The value of pulse cyclophosphamide in ANCA-associated vasculitis: meta-analysis and critical review. Nephrol Dial Transplant 2001; 16: 2018–27.

de Groot K, Rasmussen N, Bacon PA, Tervaert JW, Feighery C, Gregorini G, et al. Randomized trial of cyclophosphamide versus methotrexate for induction of remission in early systemic antineutrophil cytoplasmic antibody-associated vasculitis. Arthritis Rheum 2005; 52 (8): 2461–9.

Gross W. Primär systemische Vaskulitiden: Pathogenese und Therapie. Internist 1999; 40: 1194–215.

Guillevin L, Cohen P, Gayraud M, Lhote F, Jarrousse B, Casassus P. Churg-Strauss syndrome. Clinical study and long-term follow-up of 96 patients. Medicine (Baltimore) 1999; 78 (1): 26–37.

Guillevin L, Cohen P, Mahr A, Arene J, Mouthon L, Puechal X, et al. Treatment of polyarteritis nodosa and microscopic polyangiitis with poor prognosis factors: a prospective trial comparing glucocorticoids and six or twelve cyclophosphamide pulses in sixty-five patients. Arthritis Rheum 2003; 49: 93–100.

Guillevin L, Lhote F, Gayraud M, Cohen P, Jarousse B, Lortholary O, et al. Prognostic factors in polyarteritis nodosa and Churg-Strauss syndrome. Medicine 1996; 75: 17–28.

Guillevin L, Mahr A, Cohen P, Larroche C, Queyrel V, Loustaud-Ratti V, et al. Short-term corticosteroids then lamivudine and plasma exchanges to treat hepatitis B virus-related polyarteritis nodosa. Arthritis Rheum 2004; 51 (3): 482–7.

Hellmich B, Ehlers S, Csernok E, Gross WL. Update on the pathogenesis of Churg-Strauss syndrome. Clin Exp Rheumatol 2003; 21 (6 Suppl 32): S69–77.

Hellmich B, Gross WL. Recent progress in the pharmacotherapy of Churg-Strauss syndrome. Expert Opin Pharmacother 2004; 5 (1): 25–35.

Hellmich B, Lamprecht P, Gross WL. Advances in the therapy of Wegener's granulomatosis. Curr Opin Rheumatol 2006; 18 (1): 25–32.

Hellmich B, Merkel F, Weber M, Gross W. Frühdiagnose von chronisch-entzündlichen Systemerkrankungen. Internist 2005; 46: 421–32.

Hellmich B, Metzler C, Gross W. Churg-Strauss Syndrom: Aktueller Stand der Diagnostik und Therapie. Dtsch Med Wochenschr 2006; 131: 2270–4.

Hellmich B, Voswinkel J, Aries P, Gross W. Primäre Systemische Vaskulitiden: Wege zur Diagnose. Dtsch Med Wochenschr 2004; 129: 1322–7.

Hoffman G, Kerr G, Leavitt R, Hallahan C, Lebovics R, Travis W, et al. Wegener's granulomatosis: an analysis of 158 patients. Ann Intern Med 1992; 116: 488–99.

Jayne D, Rasmussen N, Andrassy K, Bacon P, Cohen Tervaert JW, Dadoniene J, et al. A randomized trial of maintenance therapy for vasculitis associated with antineutrophil cytoplasmic autoantibodies. N Engl J Med 2003; 349 (1): 36–44.

Jayne DR, Gaskin G, Rasmussen N, Abramowicz D, Ferrario F, Guillevin L, et al. Randomized trial of plasma exchange or high-dosage methylprednisolone as adjunctive therapy for severe renal vasculitis. J Am Soc Nephrol 2007; 18 (7): 2180–8. Epub 2007 Jun 20.

Jennette J, Andrassy K, Bacon PA, Churg J, Gross WL, Hagen EC, et al. Nomenclature of systemic vasculitides. Proposal of an international consensus conference. Arthritis Rheum 1994; 37: 187–92.

Lamprecht P, Gause A, Gross W. Cryoglobulinemic vasculitis. Arthritis Rheum 1999; 42: 2507–16.

Lamprecht P, Lerin-Lozano C, Merz H, Dennin RH, Gause A, Voswinkel J, et al. Rituximab induces remission in refractory HCV associated cryoglobulinaemic vasculitis. Ann Rheum Dis 2003; 62 (12): 1230–3.

Lamprecht P, Moosig F, Gause A, Herlyn K, Csernok E, Hansen H, et al. Immunological and clinical follow up of hepatitis C virus associated cryoglobulinaemic vasculitis. Ann Rheum Dis 2001; 60: 385–90.

Mahr AD, Jover JA, Spiera RF, Hernandez-Garcia C, Fernandez-Gutierrez B, Lavalley MP, et al. Adjunctive methotrexate for treatment of giant cell arteritis: an individual patient data meta-analysis. Arthritis Rheum 2007; 56 (8): 2789–97.

Metzler C, Hellmich B, Gause A, Gross WL, de Groot K. Churg Strauss syndrome—successful induction of remission with methotrexate and unexpected high cardiac and pulmonary relapse ratio during maintenance treatment. Clin Exp Rheumatol 2004; 22 (6 Suppl 36): S52–61.

Metzler C, Miehle N, Manger K, Iking-Konert C, de Groot K, Hellmich B, et al. Elevated relapse rate under oral methotrexate versus leflunomide for maintenance of remission in Wegener's granulomatosis. Rheumatology (Oxford) 2007; 46 (7): 1087–91. Epub 2007 May 22.

Nesher G, Berkun Y, Mates M, Baras M, Rubinow A, Sonnenblick M. Low-dose aspirin and prevention of cranial ischemic complications in giant cell arteritis. Arthritis Rheum 2004; 50 (4): 1332–7.

Reinhold-Keller E, Beuge N, Latza U, de Groot K, Rudert H, Nolle B, et al. An interdisciplinary approach to the care of patients with Wegener's granulomatosis: long-term outcome in 155 patients. Arthritis Rheum 2000; 43 (5): 1021–32.

Reinhold-Keller E, Herlyn K, Wagner-Bastmeyer R, Gross WL. Stable incidence of primary systemic vasculitides over five years: results from the German vasculitis register. Arthritis Rheum 2005; 53 (1): 93–9.

Savige J, Dimech W, Fritzler M, Goeken J, Hagen EC, Jennette JC, et al. Addendum to the International Consensus Statement on testing and reporting of antineutrophil cytoplasmic antibodies. Quality control guidelines, comments, and recommendations for testing in other autoimmune diseases. Am J Clin Pathol 2003; 120 (3): 312–8.

Schmidt WA, Kraft HE, Vorpahl K, Volker L, Gromnica-Ihle EJ. Color duplex ultrasonography in the diagnosis of temporal arteritis. N Engl J Med 1997; 337 (19): 1336–42.

Schnabel A, Reuter M, Gloeckner K, Muller-Quernheim J, Gross WL. Bronchoalveolar lavage cell profiles in Wegener's granulomatosis. Respir Med 1999; 93 (7): 498–506.

Tatsis E, Schnabel A, Gross W. Interferon-alpha treatment of four patients with the Churg-Strauss syndrome. Ann Intern Med 1998; 129: 370–4.

13 Thromboangiitis obliterans (TAO)
Frans Santosa

13.1 Clinical picture

Thromboangiitis obliterans, also known as Buerger disease, is a rare condition with the clinical symptoms of peripheral arterial and venous occlusions. Although the disease was first reported more than 100 years ago, the pathology underlying TAO is still unclear. Unfortunately, no structured studies have so far been carried out anywhere in the world, and the entire current state of knowledge about the condition is based more or less on descriptive registry data involving highly heterogeneous groups of patients.

The annual incidence rate in North America has been estimated as 8–11.6 per 100,000 population, and similar data have been reported from southwest Poland (8.1 per 100,000 in the year 2000). Asian populations, including Indians, have a much higher tendency to develop TAO than other ethnic groups, and the disease becomes manifest earlier and has a more severe course. In the Tansen Mission Hospital in a mountainous region of Nepal, the 4-year discharge file was investigated for amputations resulting from TAO. An incidence rate of 693 per 100,000 admissions was noted. Consistent risk factors in addition to tobacco consumption were extreme poverty, a diet consisting largely of corn, and living conditions in the foothills of the Himalayas. In Japan, 45 new patients were admitted to Nagoya University Hospital between 1985 and 1989, but only 12 between January 1989 and December 1996. The number of admissions for atherosclerotic peripheral vascular disease did not change substantially during the same period. The prevalence of TAO in Japan thus appears to be generally declining. A similar decline in prevalence has also been observed in Western countries. At the Mayo Clinic in the United States, the prevalence rate of a diagnosis of TAO declined continuously from 104 per 100,000 in 1947 to 13 per 100,000 in 1986.

There are probably various reasons for the declining numbers of patients in individual hospitals. Hygiene standards have improved and diagnostic facilities now often allow more precise classification, so that patients who were formerly assigned to a diagnosis of TAO are now categorized under different clinical pictures.

TAO is a self-limiting disease. The extent to which it reduces patients' life expectancy is not clear. In 2004, Ohta et al. published data on the course of TAO in 106 men and four women (average age 40 years). The cumulative survival rate 25 years after the initial consultation was 84%. Cooper et al. analyzed the survival data for a TAO cohort of 111 patients and compared them with the expected survival rate in the U.S. population, based on age-specific and sex-specific mortality rates. The average age of death in the TAO cohort was 52 ± 9 years, significantly lower than that in the control group. Continuing tobacco consumption had no influence on the figures.

13.2 Diagnosis and differential diagnoses

There are as yet no recognized diagnostic criteria for TAO, although calls for standardized criteria began 30 years ago. In 1960, Papa et al. recommended a scoring system for the diagnosis, taking into account:

- Young age of onset
- Ischemic foot symptoms
- Involvement of the upper extremities
- Superficial venous thrombosis
- Vasospastic phenomena

In 1998, Shionoya listed the following diagnostic criteria for TAO:

- A history of smoking
- Development of the condition under the age of 50 years
- Infrapopliteal arterial occlusions
- Involvement of the upper extremities or migrating phlebitis
- Absence of arteriosclerotic risk factors apart from smoking

A definitive clinical diagnosis of Buerger disease was only possible if all five conditions were met.

In the most recent review, Mills has presented the following criteria:

- History of smoking or tobacco abuse
- Age of onset under 45–50 years
- Infrapopliteal segmental arterial occlusions, not affecting the proximal vascular segments
- Involvement of arteries in the distal upper extremities
- Superficial phlebitis
- Exclusion of arteriosclerosis, diabetes, other types of arteritis, proximal embolic sources, and hypercoagulable conditions

The report that includes the largest number of patients (n = 850) is from Japan. The diagnostic criteria used were established by the Japanese Ministry of Health and Welfare and are presented in Table 13-1.

Exclusion of arteriosclerosis and risk factors for that condition and for other types of vasculitis is a prerequisite for diagnosis required by all authors. However, it has never been specified how, or at what level of intensity, arteriosclerosis and other types of vasculitis should be excluded. The most sensitive method of recognizing early arteriosclerosis is high-resolution ultrasonography. In our experience, most TAO patients diagnosed in the fourth or fifth decades of life have different types of arteriosclerosis. The criterion "exclusion of arteriosclerosis" should therefore only be taken into account if TAO is found in young patients aged 20–30 years.

In contrast to the other criteria mentioned, risk factors for arteriosclerosis do not now automatically exclude TAO. TAO has also been

Table 13-1 Diagnostic criteria for identifying thromboangiitis obliterans published by the Japanese Ministry of Health and Welfare (Sasaki et al. 2000).

Clinical manifestation (at least one or two criteria required)
1. Feeling of cold, paresthesias, Raynaud phenomenon in the hands or feet
2. Intermittent claudication
3. Resting pain in the hands or feet
4. Painful ulcers
5. Migrating phlebitis

Physical tests (at least one or two criteria required)
1. Cold acra in the hands or feet
2. Lack of a distal pulse with preserved proximal pulses
3. Reduced ankle–brachial index (ABI)

Laboratory tests
1. Normal routine laboratory tests

Angiography (at least one or two criteria required)
1. Multiple segmental occlusions of the distal arteries
2. Chronic arterial occlusions
3. No evidence of atherosclerosis with calcification
4. Abrupt occlusions
5. Corkscrew or root-shaped collaterals

No other vascular disease
The following have to be excluded:
1. Arteriosclerosis
2. Traumatic arterial thrombosis
3. Popliteal entrapment syndrome
4. Lupus erythematosus, systemic sclerosis
5. Behçet disease

reported in patients with diabetes and hypercholesterolemia, for example. Lipoprotein Lp(a), a classic risk factor for arteriosclerosis, may also be elevated in patients with TAO. In one study, 40 TAO patients had increased mean lipoprotein Lp(a) values of 21.3 mg/dL, and 316 control individuals had values of 9.4 mg/dL. The authors concluded that lipoprotein Lp(a) may even be an independent risk factor for TAO. Although superficial venous thrombosis is mainly recommended in the literature as a diagnostic criterion, the role of deep venous thrombosis has not been specified. The occurrence of deep venous thrombosis in TAO patients is often due to additional thrombophilia and not due to the specific pathology of TAO.

More than a century after Buerger's original description of TAO, there is still no consensus on the diagnostic criteria for the condition. The lack of a universally accepted method of diagnosis leads to confusion and makes research efforts more difficult. Due to the continuing controversy, it may be better to speak of "Buerger syndrome" rather than "Buerger disease."

13.3 Pathology

TAO can basically affect any of the arteries. Peripheral endothelium-mediated vascular dilation is thus also reduced in unaffected vascular segments. In a study by Makita et al., the increase in blood flow in the lower arm in TAO patients was found to be lower than in healthy controls (22.7 ± 2.9 vs. 14.1 ± 2.8 mL/min per dL tissue volume; $P < 0.01$). By contrast, no significant differences between the groups were seen after sodium nitroprusside infusion or in relation to reactive hyperemia. It can be concluded from this that nonendothelial vascular dilation mechanisms were intact.

Early histological examinations identified a cellular thrombus and cellular infiltration of the vascular wall, with a preserved wall structure. Immunohistochemical examinations in 58 amputated lower extremities and five autopsy controls consistently revealed a primary inflammatory lesion. Lymphocytes, particularly $CD4^+$ T cells, were found more frequently in the affected vessels and their adventitia. The linear arrangement of macrophages and of B and T lymphocytes along the elastic fibers suggests that elastic fibers represent a significant immunogen. Immunohistochemical studies of 33 samples from nine patients showed a generally preserved vascular wall architecture, independent of the stage of the disease, but also cell infiltration in the thrombus and intima. Among the infiltrating cells, $CD3^+$ T cells were numerically superior to $CD20^+$ B cells. $CD68^+$ macrophages and dendritic cells, particularly in the intima, were noted during the acute and subacute phases. All but one case showed infiltration by macrophages carrying the human leukocyte antigen D region (HLA-DR) and dendritic cells in the intima. Immunoglobulins G, A, and M and complement factors 3d and 4c were deposited along the internal elastic lamina. This is a sign that TAO is, strictly speaking, a form of endarteritis in which T cell-mediated cellular immunity and B cell-mediated humoral immunity are triggered in connection with the activation of macrophages or dendritic cells in the intima.

Special HLA genotypes associated with TAO have been reported, but the results are inconsistent due to the heterogeneity of the study populations. Population-specific differences in the HLA system between Asian and Caucasian populations are contributing factors in this problem.

Cardiolipin antibodies have been noted in up to one-third of TAO patients, in comparison with fewer than 10% of patients with arteriosclerosis. Patients with TAO and a high cardiolipin antibody titer were usually younger and had a much higher rate of major amputations than patients without the antibodies (100% vs. 17%; $P = 0.003$). Antineutrophil cytoplasmic antibodies (ANCAs) were identified using indirect immunofluorescence in 15 of 27 TAO patients (56%) and in 16 (59%) using a fixed neutrophil enzyme-linked immunosorbent assay (ELISA). ANCAs were mainly found in patients with severe courses (66.7%; 12 of 18) and less often in those with mild courses (33.3%; three of nine). However, it should be pointed out that no mechanistic role for these antibodies in the pathology of TAO has ever been demonstrated.

A new study has suggested a possible etiological connection between TAO and chronic inflammations such as oral bacterial inflammations. *Treponema denticola* was found in 12 arterial and all oral samples taken in 14 patients. *Campylobacter rectus, Porphyromonas gingivalis, Prevotella intermedia, Tannerella forsythensis,* and *Prevotella nigrescens* were found in 14–43% of arterial samples

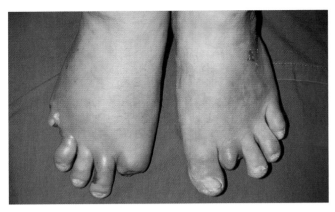

Fig. 13-1 A typical picture in a patient with thromboangiitis obliterans, with multiple lesions in the toes. The extreme painfulness of the wounds, which is disproportionate to their size and appearance, is important and diagnostically suggestive.

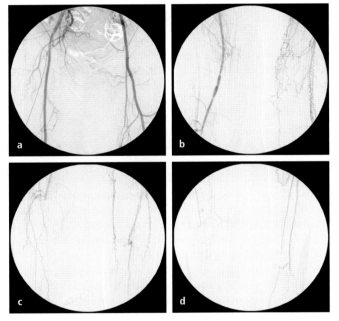

Fig. 13-2a–d Intra-arterial digital subtraction angiography in a patient with thromboangiitis obliterans. There is an occlusion of the distal femoral artery and lower leg arteries on the right. On the left, the occlusion starts in the middle of the thigh, but the fibular artery and posterior tibial arteries are preserved. The striking appearance of bizarre collateral formation is well displayed.

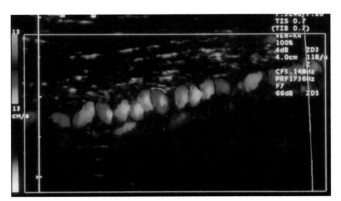

Fig. 13-3 Ultrasound image of tortuous collaterals in a patient with thromboangiitis obliterans.

and 71–100% of oral samples. Histologically, the arterial samples showed the characteristics of a lesion in TAO disease in the chronic intermediate or chronic stage.

Although a few reports have assumed that hypercoagulable states influence the clinical course of TAO, the mechanistic causality underlying this remains unclear. An association with TAO would not be unexpected, as thrombophilic disturbances generally increase the risk of thrombotic occlusion. An elevated hematocrit level and increased blood viscosity in patients with TAO have also only been described in case reports.

The important role played by smoking in the etiology and pathogenesis of TAO should always be emphasized, although no one has succeeded in demonstrating causality. It is still unclear whether smoking itself or specific substances in smoke trigger the development of the disease. Evidence of specific tobacco antigens is anecdotal.

13.4 Clinical manifestation

Few data are available on the very early stages of TAO. Most patients who are referred to vascular specialists already have resting pain (50–89%) or tissue lesions (38–85%). Although involvement of the upper extremity and venous system is important for establishing the diagnosis, the frequency data on this are highly variable (Table 13-2). A systematic analysis reports involvement of the upper extremity in 50% of all patients, with involvement of the venous system in approximately 62% of patients. Overall, the range of patients with TAO appears to be changing, with more women being affected and patients being older at the first onset of the condition.

Table 13-2 Distribution pattern in thromboangiitis obliterans (after Sasaki et al. 2000a)

	Incidence
1. Location	
Only upper extremity	5.1%
Only lower extremity	74.7%
Upper and lower extremities	20.2%
2. Arteries affected	
Ulnar artery	11.5%
Anterior tibial artery	41.4%
Posterior tibial artery	40.4%
3. Initial signs and symptoms	
Paresthesia; cold sensation, cyanosis	37%
Plantar claudication	15%
Sural claudication	16%
Pain at rest	10%
Ulcer/gangrene	19%
4. Signs/symptoms during whole course of disease	
Ulcer/gangrene	72%
Migratory phlebitis	43%
Lesions on upper extremity	90%

Unusual manifestations of TAO may affect the gastrointestinal, cerebrovascular, and coronary arteries. In the gastrointestinal form, there is usually an occlusion of the superior mesenteric artery. The cerebrovascular manifestation is also known as Spatz–Lindenberg disease.

The coronary manifestation has mainly been reported in patients with previous symptoms of peripheral occlusion. Due to the rarity of the cases, there has been critical debate on the etiology of cerebrovascular and coronary manifestations of TAO.

13.5   Treatment

There is no standardized and effective form of treatment that can be offered to patients with TAO to arrest and cure the condition (Table 13-3). The primary and clearly most effective treatment for TAO is discontinuation of all tobacco products and avoidance of all environmental inhalation of tobacco smoke. Independently of the stage of the disease, discontinuation of smoking is absolutely necessary and should be recommended to patients regularly and frequently, with pharmaceutical and psychological support. Despite this, a large proportion of TAO patients do not stop smoking. Unfortunately, the form nicotine ingestion takes in these patients does not appear to materially affect outcomes: switching to chewing tobacco from cigarettes has not averted amputation.

13.5.1   Conservative treatment

The benefit of antiplatelet or lipid-reducing treatment in TAO patients has not been confirmed. Infusions with prostaglandin E_1 or prostacyclin may be successful in a few patients with resting pain and ulcers. In a randomized double-blind study in France, 152 TAO patients with critical leg ischemia were treated either with iloprost or low-dose aspirin for 28 days. After 21–28 days, 43 patients (63%) receiving iloprost treatment were completely free of pain, but only 18 (28%) of those receiving aspirin. The tissue lesions healed completely in 18 of 52 patients (35%) with iloprost, but only in six of 46 (13%) with aspirin. However, these results were not confirmed by the European TAO Study Group in 1998. A total of 319 TAO patients with resting pain and trophic lesions from 23 hospitals in six European countries were included in the study. In a placebo-controlled, double-blind design, 100 or 200 µg iloprost or a placebo were administered twice daily for 8 weeks, with a follow-up examination after 6 months. No differences between the treatment groups were observed relative to the lesion healing rate at any time; however, resting pain improved with iloprost in 63% of the patients.

A series of reports on gene and stem cell therapy have appeared since 1991, particularly from centers in Asia. These techniques appear to provide relief for patients with small-artery disease, but the results are generally still quite preliminary.

Immunosuppressive treatment may be helpful in some TAO patients. A study in Russia including 28 male patients reported that a standardized 3-day regimen with glucocorticoid and cyclophospha-

mide therapy in addition to antiplatelet and vasodilation treatment substantially reduced the amputation rate. In a study in India, 12 TAO patients received 400 mg cyclophosphamide i.v. for 7 days, followed by daily oral administration of cyclophosphamide 100 mg for an additional 7 weeks. The patients' clinical condition started to improve during the third week of treatment, and the maximum benefit was observed at the end of treatment. Histopathological studies of biopsies obtained from the diseased arteries at the end of the treatment showed reduced inflow of lymphocytes and plasma cells into the thrombi and arterial walls in comparison with biopsies taken before the start of treatment.

New insights into the role of lymphocytes and of inflammation caused by tumor necrosis factor-α (TNF-α) in the pathogenesis of TAO suggest new treatment options, such as administration of anti-TNF-α or anti-CD20. Promising results with rituximab have been observed with a number of autoimmune diseases, including rheu-

Table 13-3 Despite the generally unsatisfactory treatment options, therapy in patients with symptomatic thromboangiitis obliterans should include the aspects listed below.

Pain therapy	Pain symptoms are the patient's main concern. Opiates are usually necessary for pain relief, although very few patients become completely free of pain.
Anticoagulation	If it is known that the occlusions have a thrombotic pathogenesis, anticoagulation with low-molecular-weight heparins is useful on an acute basis for several weeks at a therapeutic dosage.
Intravenous prostacyclin administration	The only drug approved for this disease is iloprost. Its effect varies from individual to individual. If no clinical improvement is seen after administration for 3–4 weeks, the drug can be withdrawn again.
Immuno-suppression	When there is no response to prostacyclin, immunosuppression can be tried. Data are available on administration of glucocorticoids and cyclophosphamide.
Individually adjusted wound therapy	Wound therapy should be in accordance with modern methods of wound treatment, mainly moisture.
Intervention	In acute occlusions, intra-arterial fibrinolysis can be attempted—no mechanical recanalization and no stent implantation.
Surgery	In the chronic stage, proximal occlusions of the pelvic and thigh arteries can be surgically recanalized if patent vascular segments are preserved distally.
Sympathectomy	As a last resort for nonhealing wounds that do not respond to iloprost, sympathectomy may be considered. It is not an initial treatment.
Nicotine abstinence	All patients should cease nicotine consumption. This promotes wound healing and prevents long-term deterioration.
Secondary prevention	There is no evidence for the benefit of secondary prevention treatment with antiplatelet medication, lipid reduction, or administration of an angiotensin-converting enzyme inhibitor.

matic arthritis, systemic lupus erythematosus and ANCA-associated vasculitis. No data are currently available with regard to TAO and this type of treatment option.

A pilot study investigated the efficacy of immunoadsorption in 10 patients with advanced thromboangiitis obliterans. The patients received immunoadsorption on each of five consecutive days. The results showed a promising effect; pain intensity on a visual analogue scale fell from 7.7 ± 0.8 (mean $\pm$ SEM) before treatment to 2.0 ± 1.2 on the second day of immunoadsorption. All of the patients were free of pain after 1 month. Their maximum walking distance improved early after immunoadsorption from 301.7 ± 191.4 m to 727.0 ± 192.7 m and increased continuously up to 1811.0 ± 223.7 m within 6 months. The ischemic ulcerations healed in all of the patients.

In stem cell therapy, autologous stem cells are transplanted after being harvested either from bone marrow or from the peripheral blood following administration of granulocyte colony-stimulating factor (G-CSF). This form of treatment may represent a therapeutic option for patients with thromboangiitis obliterans. A recent study investigated the long-term clinical results after transplantation of bone marrow stem cells in 51 patients with chronic critical ischemia, including 25 patients with peripheral arterial occlusive disease (PAOD) and 26 patients with thromboangiitis obliterans. As compared with an untreated control group over 4.8 years, in whom the rates of avoidance of amputation were 0% among the PAOD patients and 6% among those with thromboangiitis obliterans, in the stem cell transplantation group, the rates were 48% and 95%, respectively.

13.5.2   Endovascular therapy

There have only been a few case reports on endovascular treatment for vascular occlusions in TAO patients. Acute ischemia in the lower extremity secondary to Buerger disease in a young patient was successfully treated with thrombolysis and subsequent angioplasty in the popliteal and anterior tibial arteries. An occlusion in the proximal left dorsalis pedis artery was recanalized with a continuous intra-arterial infusion of urokinase using a microcatheter.

13.5.3   Surgical treatment

13.5.3.1   Sympathectomy

Clinical experience suggests that Raynaud phenomenon in the feet can be improved by sympathectomy, although there is only short-term improvement in the hands and no effect on the disease prognosis. Sympathectomy would be indicated in cases of ischemic resting pain if surgical revascularization is not possible. However, there is no reliable evidence that sympathectomy improves the prognosis for the extremity. In 2004, data for 161 patients with a first manifestation of TAO who were treated with sympathectomy in Turkey in 1991–2001 were published. The clinical results after sympathectomy were regarded as improved in 52.3% of the patients, stable in 27.8%, and poorer in 19.8%. Sympathectomy has now largely been abandoned and replaced with pharmacological treatment using prostaglandin.

Electrical spinal cord stimulation was administered to patients with TAO in a larger group of patients with chronic limb ischemia. While only a reduction in pain was achieved in some patients, in others the treatment also led to improved ulcer healing and thus prevented amputation.

13.5.3.2   Revascularization

In Europe and North America, surgical arterial reconstruction is not an accepted strategy, in view of the inflammatory nature of TAO. However, 39 articles on surgical treatment have been published since 1991, particularly from studies in Asia (n = 22), Russia (n = 7), and Turkey (n = 4). Even in these countries, only approximately 10% of patients affected are candidates for reconstructive surgery, due to the distal nature of the disease.

A study in Turkey presented follow-up data for 14 TAO patients who received polytetrafluoroethylene (PTFE) transplants in various anatomic segments over a 10-year period. After a follow-up period of 8 years, the patency rates were: aortofemoral/iliofemoral bypass 80%, femoropopliteal bypass 40%, and femorocrural bypass 50%, with a cumulative patency rate of 57.1% and a limb preservation rate of 88.9%. A report from Japan published in 1993 presented data from 108 patients treated mainly with autologous venous bypasses from 1976 to 1990. The 5-year cumulative patency rates were 88.2% for aortofemoral bypass and 64.8% for infrainguinal bypass. Other authors from these countries have also reported much lower patency rates and large numbers of failures. In 2004, Ohta et al. published follow-up data for 110 TAO patients, 46 of whom underwent bypass surgery. The secondary patency rates were 54% after 1 year, 47% after 5 years, and 39% after 10 years. However, major amputations were only required in 14% of the patients with transplant failure. A follow-up study (mean 141 ± 42 months) in 32 Japanese patients in whom vascular reconstruction had failed also reported a satisfactory rate of limb preservation. It is therefore questionable whether vascular reconstruction was really indicated in each individual patient in the groups described.

Limb preservation depends on bypass patency and on the patient's living conditions. In Russia, TAO patients who lived in the northern Arctic region had poorer results than those in the Moscow area.

Another surgical procedure that has repeatedly been described in the literature is autotransplantation of the greater omentum. The omentum is dissected and anastomosed to the lower extremity either as a pedicled flap or as a free transplant as far distally as possible. Promising results have been reported in small groups of TAO patients. Overall, arterial reconstruction must be considered as a treatment option when there are proximal occlusions and a disease-free target vessel is available.

In distraction osteogenesis, the aim is to achieve secondary bone healing. Surgical transection of the bone creates a fracture cleft that stimulates the formation of callus and bone. In addition, a distractor is used to apply a controlled traction force to the artificially created bone cleft, so that the fracture surfaces are gradually distracted in a controlled fashion (Fig. 13-4). Distraction osteogenesis ultimately also induces desired neoangiogenesis. A research group in Asia has reported on 30 patients with chronic critical ischemia against a background of thromboangiitis obliterans who were treated with this method. However, only 10 of the patients had open wounds. With the treatment, which lasted a mean of 122 ± 23 days, 25 of the patients became free of pain and one had improvement in pain symptoms. In four patients, the treatment led to deterioration that ended with amputation.

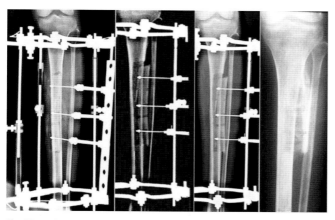

Fig. 13-4 Distraction osteogenesis in the area of the tibia in a patient with thromboangiitis obliterans. The fresh osteotomy can be seen on the left; the middle images show the course of distraction, and the right image shows the final result, with visible osteoneogenesis (from Kulkarni et al. 2008).

References

Baumann G, Stangl V, Klein-Weigel P, Stangl K, Laule M, Enke-Melzer K. Successful treatment of thromboangiitis obliterans (Buerger's disease) with immunoadsorption: results of a pilot study. Clin Res Cardiol. 2011; 100: 683–90.

Bozkurt AK, Besirli K, Koksal C, Sirin G, Yuceyar L, Tuzun H, Sayin AG. Surgical treatment of Buerger's Disease. Vascular 2004; 12: 192–7.

Cooper LT, Tse TS, Mikhail MA, McBane RD, Stanson AW, Ballman KV. Long-term survival and amputation risk in thromboangiitis obliterans. J Am Coll Cardiol 2004; 44: 2410–1.

Idei N, Soga J, Hata T, Fujii Y, Fujimura N, Mikami S, Maruhashi T, Nishioka K, Hidaka T, Kihara Y, Chowdhury M, Noma K, Taguchi A, Chayama K, Sueda T, Higashi Y. Autologous bone-marrow mononuclear cell implantation reduces long-term major amputation risk in patients with critical limb ischemia: a comparison of atherosclerotic peripheral arterial disease and Buerger disease. Circ Cardiovasc Interv 2011; 4: 15–25.

Khazanchi RK, Nanda V, Kumar R, Garg P, Guleria S, Bal S. Omentum autotransplantation in thromboangiitis obliterans: report of three cases. Surg Today 1999; 29: 86–90.

Kobayashi M, Ito M, Nakagawa A, Nishikimi N, Nimura Y. Immunohistochemical analysis of arterial wall cellular infiltration in Buerger's disease. J Vasc Surg 1999; 29: 451–8.

Kulkarni S, Kulkarni G, Shyam AK, Kulkarni M, Kulkarni R, Kulkarni V. Management of thromboangiitis obliterans using distraction osteogenesis: A retrospective study. Indian J Orthop 2011; 45: 459–64.

Lawrence PF, Lund OI, Jimenez JC, Muttalib R. Substitution of smokeless tobacco for cigarettes in Buerger's disease does not prevent limb loss. J Vasc Surg 2008; 48: 210–2.

Matsushita M, Nishikimi N, Sakurai T, Nimura Y. Decrease in prevalence of Buerger's Disease in Japan. Surgery 1998; 124: 498–502.

Mills JL Sr. Buerger's Disease in the 21st century: diagnosis, clinical features, and therapy. Semin Vasc Surg 2003; 16: 179–89.

Naito AT, Minamino T, Tateno K, Nagai T, Komuro I. Steroid-responsive thromboangiitis obliterans. Lancet 2004; 364 (9439): 1098.

Nakajima N. The change in concept and surgical treatment on Buerger's disease—personal experience and review. Int J Cardiol 1998; 66 (Suppl 1): S273–80.

Ohta T, Ishioashi H, Hosaka M, Sugimoto I. Clinical and social consequences of Buerger Disease. J Vasc Surg 2004; 39: 176–80.

Olin JW, Young JR, Graor RA, Ruschhaupt WF, Bartholomew JR. The changing clinical spectrum of thromboangiitis obliterans. Circulation 1990; 82 (5 Suppl): IV3–8.

Sasaki S, Sakuma M, Yasuda K. Current status of thromboangiitis obliterans (Buerger's disease) in Japan. Int J Cardiol 2000a; 75 (Suppl 1): S175–81.

Sasaki S, Sakuma M, Kunihara T, Yasuda K. Distribution of arterial involvement in thromboangiitis obliterans (Buerger's disease): Results of a study conducted by the Intractable Vasculitis Syndromes Research Group in Japan. Surg Today 2000b; 30: 600–5.

Swigris JJ, Olin JW, Mekhail NA. Implantable spinal cord stimulator to treat the ischemic manifestations of thromboangiitis obliterans. J Vasc Surg 1999; 29: 928–35.

Talwar S, Choudhary SK. Omentopexy for limb salvage in Buerger's disease: indications, technique and results. J Postgrad Med 2001; 47: 137–42.

Tanaka K. Pathology and pathogenesis of Buerger's disease. Int J Cardiol 1998; 66 (Suppl 1): S237–42.

Wysokinski WE, Kwiatkowska W, Sapian-Raczkowska B, Czarnacki M, Doskocz R, Kowal-Gierczak B. Sustained classic clinical spectrum of thromboangiitis obliterans. Angiology 2000; 51: 141–50.

D

Congenital vascular diseases

1 Introduction

Siamak Pourhassan

Congenital diseases of the large vessels in children are rare and are usually due to developmental deficiencies, congenital malformations, or disturbances of tissue that later become clinically manifest. Coagulation disturbances that act as promoting factors for the clinical manifestation can also be seen. In the arterial circulation, stenotic processes predominate over aneurysmal changes. Among congenital venous diseases, the major conditions consist of dysgeneses in the iliofemoral segment and in the vena cava.

The treatment of pediatric vascular diseases, particularly congenital ones, has its own unique set of circumstances. The special aspect of reconstruction in infants and children is that there is a lack of adequate material for vascular replacement. In adults, plastic substitutes in all sizes and lengths are available for replacing the aorta and large vessel trunks, and the autologous great saphenous vein provides the ideal vascular replacement for visceral vessels and vessels in the extremities, but in infants very little use of such materials is possible. Plastic does not grow with the child and can therefore only be used in exceptional cases in those under the age of 10 years, to bridge long aortic stenoses (e.g., aortic coarctation, stenosis in the descending thoracic aorta). It also requires a special technique. The great saphenous vein is not mature and is still growing itself, so that it not infrequently undergoes aneurysmal dilation if used as a replacement in the arterial circulation. In brief, a child is not a miniature adult.

2   Arterial malformations
Siamak Pourhassan

2.1   Stenotic arterial malformations

Stenotic processes in the aorta, which may develop juxtarenally or suprarenally, mainly become clinically manifest as a result of epistaxis and headache, due to increased arterial pressure with renovascular hypertension. Symptoms involving intermittent claudication are rare, and abdominal angina is even rarer. In everyday clinical practice, the diagnostic workup is protracted, particularly with abdominal vascular processes, as the disease entity is so rare. When there are repeated nosebleeds, persistent headache, and claudication, blood pressure should be measured in all four extremities to exclude vascular disease and the renal arteries should be evaluated.

2.1.1   Aortic isthmus stenosis

2.1.1.1   Clinical picture

Aortic isthmus stenosis, the typical aortic coarctation, is a congenital stenosis of the proximal descending thoracic aorta. The aortic lumen may be atretic, although continuity between the cranial and caudal aorta is always preserved in aortic coarctation—distinguishing this condition from that of the interrupted aortic arch. Another possibility in the area of the thoracic aorta is coarctation between the left common carotid artery and the left subclavian artery, which is a rare finding.

A topographic distinction is made in aortic isthmus stenosis between preductal (infantile) and postductal (adult) stenosis. The condition is further classified relative to its pathophysiological effects into critical aortic isthmus stenosis, which requires surgery in newborns, and aortic isthmus stenoses that can and should be treated electively either in children or in adults when diagnosed.

Aortic isthmus stenosis causes left ventricular overload due to the increase in arterial pressure in the upper half of the body. In neonates who develop critical aortic isthmus stenosis, an acute deterioration in the clinical condition develops after closure of the ductus arteriosus (Botallo duct).

The situation is different if the ventricle has sufficient time to adapt to the pressure load—e.g., in utero or when there is a slow postnatal increase in the pressure. To compensate for the increased mural stress, the left ventricle becomes hypertrophied, with an increase in coronary resistance and a simultaneous reduction in coronary reserve flow.

2.1.1.2   Diagnosis

The malformation is often noticed prenatally on the color Doppler examination, due to other concomitant cardiac malformations. Postnatally, the clinical examination with auscultation and recording of pulse status is often suggestive, and echocardiography confirms the diagnosis. Magnetic resonance angiography or computed tomographic angiography is used to complete the full diagnosis, particularly when the associated defects are complex.

2.1.1.3   Treatment

Drug treatment

In cases of critical aortic isthmus stenoses in neonates, prostaglandin E is infused to stabilize the child by preventing closure of the ductus arteriosus with the resulting acute pressure load on the heart. Keeping the duct open provides a bridge to early surgical treatment.

Surgical treatment

With critical aortic isthmus stenosis in neonates, corrective surgery must be carried out extremely urgently once the patient has been stabilized. The patients are classified into three groups according to the additional cardiovascular malformations that are present and are treated accordingly: group I, with simple coarctation; group II, with an additional ventricular septal defect; group III, patients with coarctation and associated complex intracardiac malformations.

2.1.2   Coarctation of the abdominal aorta

2.1.2.1   Clinical picture

The synonymous terms abdominal aortic stenosis, abdominal coarctation, atypical coarctation, and mid-aortic syndrome (MAS) refer to a constriction in the distal descending aorta and visceral segment of the aorta. This is rarer than aortic isthmus stenosis (Fig. 2.1-1). Its incidence is 0.5–2.0% of all aortic stenoses. The etiology appears to be varied. It has been suggested that there is abnormal fusion of the paired primordia of the abdominal aorta embryologically. Other hypotheses include possible excess obliterative processes in the area of the ostium of the fourth branchial arch artery, leading to stenosis of the abdominal aorta; or dysmaturity of mesenchymal cells, leading to hypoplasia of the abdominal aorta.

Secondary forms may arise on the basis of inflammatory changes in the vessel walls in the context of Takayasu arteritis (Fig. 2.1-2), giant cell arteritis, or other autoimmune processes. If the condition arises in a setting of neurofibromatosis, Williams–Beuren syndrome, Alagille syndrome, or mucopolysaccharidosis, then a genetic component may be involved in this group of cases. Familial occurrence in father and daughter has also been reported in one case. Fibromuscular changes may also lead to stenosis of the abdominal aorta. Abdominal aortic stenoses have also been reported in individual cases in tuberous sclerosis and after placement of an umbilical ar-

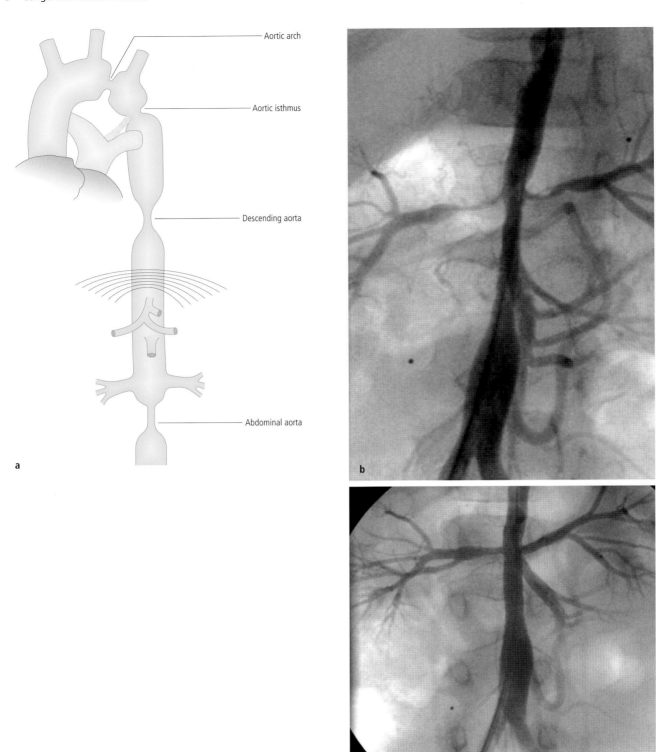

Fig. 2.1-1a–c (a) Atypical locations for aortic coarctation: the aortic arch; arch stenosis; stenosis of the descending aorta; and abdominal coarctation. (b, c) Abdominal coarctation involving both renal arteries in an 8-year-old girl, before and after stent angioplasty in the aorta. (Images courtesy of T. Zeller, Cardiac Center, Bad Krozingen, Germany.)

tery catheter. The first report was by Quain in 1847. Renal artery stenoses are associated with the condition in 80% of the patients. Like aortic isthmus stenosis, the disease leads to increased blood pressure in the upper half of the body and to reduced perfusion distal to the stenosis. Reduced perfusion in the kidneys stimulates renin secretion, which is the main cause of the increased blood pressure.

Different types of abdominal coarctation are distinguished, depending on the location of the stenosis and the extent to which the renal arteries are involved (Fig. 2.1-3). Hallet divides these into the suprarenal, interrenal, and infrarenal types and also describes a group with a mixed distribution of vascular lesions.

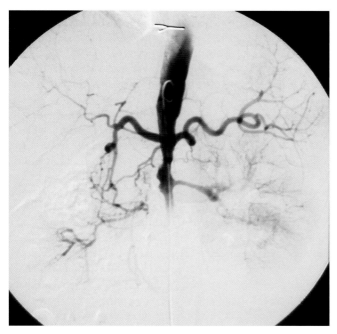

Fig. 2.1-2 A 17-year-old girl with Takayasu arteritis, with involvement of the aortic arch and abdominal aorta. The diagnosis had been established when she was 11 on the basis of vertigo, nausea, severe headache, and renovascular hypertension. She had a single kidney on the left side with a double arterial supply; the right kidney had previously been removed as the alleged cause of the hypertension in her home country (Ukraine), but without effect. The current findings were treated with a 16-mm PTFE stretch prosthesis (using a proximal end-to-side anastomosis between the middle descending aorta and the infrarenal abdominal aorta above the aortoiliac bifurcation, also with an end-to-side technique). The doubled renal artery on the left was debranched, and the distal renal artery was implanted into the aortic prosthesis using a 6-mm PTFE stretch prosthesis. (Image courtesy of W. Sandmann, Department of Vascular Surgery and Kidney Transplantation, University of Düsseldorf, Germany.)

The difficulty, particularly in infants and small children, in assessing blood-pressure measurement often makes early diagnosis difficult, and the mean age at diagnosis is therefore 8–9 years (in our own experience). The characteristic aspect, as in typical aortic isthmus stenosis, is increased blood pressure in the upper half of the body, with a difference in pressure in comparison with the lower extremities. In small children, reluctance to walk and leg pain may also be seen, or classic symptoms of intermittent claudication in older children. Nosebleeds and headache often occur as a result of the increased arterial pressure. Depending on the stenosis type, abdominal angina may also occur. However, these symptoms are usually only seen rarely, due to good collateralization. Renal failure or dilated cardiomyopathy with severe heart failure is observed very rarely.

2.1.2.2   Diagnosis

Up to the end of the 1940s, abdominal coarctation was an autopsy diagnosis. It was only in 1949 that H.T. Bahnson incidentally observed an angiographic image of abdominal coarctation during a cardiac angiogram. As was then the usual practice, the patient underwent a lumbar sympathectomy to allow better peripheral circulation. Further development of radiographic imaging, particularly angiography, made the first correct diagnosis and localization possible.

The major clinical symptom is secondary arterial (renovascular) hypertension, in 80–90% of cases (Fig. 2.1-4).

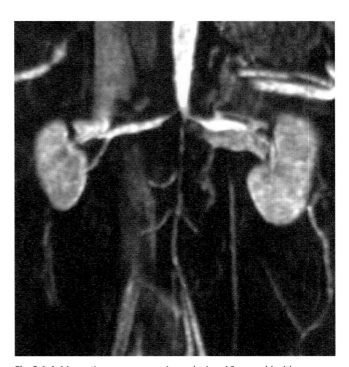

Fig. 2.1-4 Magnetic resonance angiography in a 16-year-old with extended hypoplasia in the infrarenal aorta in abdominal coarctation and bilateral renal artery stenosis. Treatment was carried out with implantation of an aortoiliac bypass (16/8-mm PTFE), and the renal arteries were implanted into the prosthesis limb. (Image courtesy of W. Sandmann, Department of Vascular Surgery and Kidney Transplantation, University of Düsseldorf, Germany.)

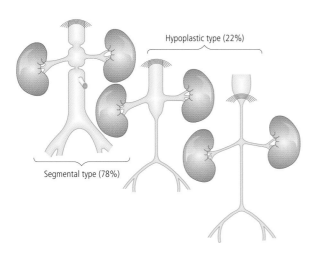

Fig. 2.1-3 The various forms and locations of abdominal coarctation. The aortic constriction is short and segmental in 78% of cases, with the main segment being located suprarenally. In the remaining cases, there is a long hypoplastic stenosis or atresia.

In the *clinical examination,* absent pulses in the lower extremity and possibly enhanced pulses in the arms and carotid arteries may be noted. Depending on the location of the stenosis, it may be possible to auscultate an abdominal, and often paravertebral and thoracolumbar, flow murmur.

The basic diagnostic method is noninvasive *blood-pressure measurement.* To allow better assessment of the severity of the hypertension, 24-h measurement should also be carried out. *Retention parameters* should be assessed to exclude renal function disturbances. Aortic isthmus stenosis, the most important differential diagnosis, should be excluded.

Vascular diseases in childhood can be well assessed using *color duplex ultrasonography.* This reveals stenosis by demonstrating accelerated flow. The threshold values measured in adults appear to be valid in this setting as well. Intrarenal resistance indices (RIs) are markedly reduced after the stenoses and have a typical pulsus tardus and parvus appearance. In abdominal coarctation (with the exception of the infrarenal type), the RIs are reduced in both kidneys, as the pathophysiological model is one of bilateral renal artery stenosis. If it is located cranial to the orifice of the superior mesenteric artery, the stenosis can usually be imaged directly with ultrasound and color Doppler. With stenoses located distally, definite imaging of the aorta is usually difficult due to superimposition of air in the bowel in nonfasting patients. In these cases, the diagnosis may be suspected on Doppler ultrasonography due to the abnormal flow profile in the aorta. Precise morphological imaging should initially be carried out noninvasively using *magnetic resonance angiography* (MRA) (Fig. 2.1-4). In addition to showing the precise extent of the stenotic segment, this also allows clear identification of smaller collateral vessels supplying the organ and the surrounding circulation. Alternatively, direct arteriography can be carried out via femoral artery access. Simultaneous invasive pressure measurement allows precise assessment of the hemodynamics. In infants with hypoplastic vessels, the aorta can be imaged in the levo-phase after venous injection. Magnetic resonance imaging is also suitable for imaging during the postoperative course.

2.1.2.3   Treatment

Drug treatment

Administration of antihypertensive drugs is difficult in affected patients, and rarely leads to lasting success. The aim of invasive treatment is to achieve an effective reduction in arterial pressure.

Endovascular treatment

The topographic classification is very helpful for planning and recommending treatment. Suprarenal or supravisceral stenoses, which are usually circumscribed, can be treated well using endovascular techniques. On the basis of an analysis of the initial and medium-term results, the transluminal endovascular route can be regarded as at least equivalent to surgical procedures. In endovascular procedures in pediatric patients, methodological and technical aspects need to be taken into account when planning the access route, the choice of devices, particularly when adjusting for growth in size. This applies above all to the use of vascular implants, which is why balloon-expandable stents are preferable to self-expanding stents

in principle. Balloon angioplasty is first carried out using balloons with increasing diameters. Stent implantation is indicated in pediatric patients on analogy with the treatment strategy in adults, when there are circumscribed short ostial or truncal stenoses and insufficient primary results after balloon dilation, dissection, or thrombosis.

It is important when choosing the size of balloon-expandable stents to ensure that the stent diameter selected is smaller than the proximal reference vessel diameter, to avoid the risk of perforation. There are few data in the literature on the use of self-expanding nitinol stents. In young patients, implantation of self-expanding stents that are actually slightly larger than the reference vessel diameter has proved to be valuable, as they are able to adapt to the growing size of the aorta. Despite this, repeat procedures may be needed during the course of the disease to dilate the stent further. These implants are not difficult to reexpand to adjust them to age-related increases in the vessel size, and there is little risk of morbidity. In inflammatory vascular pathology, local trauma and the risk of recurrence have been substantially reduced by the use of stents.

Brzezinksa-Rajszys et al. reported a success rate of approximately 70% after stent implantation, although there is a risk of aneurysm formation. Depending on the patient's age, catheter intervention has to be carried out with mask or intubation anesthesia; the standard access route is transfemoral. In any case, the increasing miniaturization of the devices available both makes endovascular management easier and also minimizes the vascular trauma caused by the device.

Surgical reconstruction

In long stenoses and hypoplastic segments, surgical reconstruction of the affected vessels is always indicated, particularly if visceral arteries (renal arteries, celiac trunk, and superior mesenteric artery) are involved in the stenotic process (Fig. 2.1-5a–c).

The first successful vascular reconstructions were carried out by Beatty in 1951 using homologous artery, and by Glenn in 1952 with autologous splenic artery. Until vascular prostheses were introduced in the early 1960s, surgical options in the aorta were limited. It was only the introduction of vascular prostheses that created a breakthrough, as bypass material with adequate lengths and sizes and reliable quality became available for the first time—allowing replacement of long stenotic segments of the aorta, with simultaneous revascularization of the visceral arteries. The reconstruction procedure focuses on correcting the underlying symptoms. In descending order of importance, these consist of renovascular hypertension, abdominal angina, and intermittent claudication. Treatment options thus consist of replacing the affected aortic segment using an interposition graft, or surgery to bypass the stenosis. The decision has to be taken on an individual basis in each case. The choice of the proximal anastomosis in bypass surgery is also not restricted to the ascending or descending aorta, but depends on the individual situation (anatomy and age).

Reconstruction of the renal and other visceral arteries can be done either by direct anastomosis using a bypass or transposition, with an additional bypass or patch angioplasty. In some cases, only a local patch dilation of the aorta is possible. If adequate aortoaortic collateralization is present and there is an absence of clinical symptoms, then only isolated reconstruction of the visceral or renal arteries need to be carried out. To protect the organs and prolong the tol-

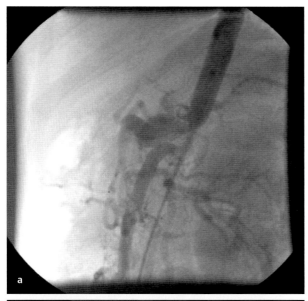

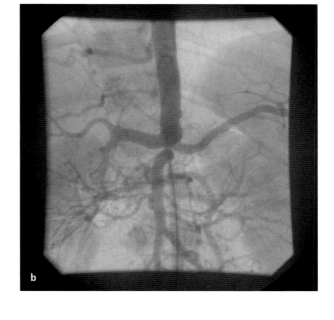

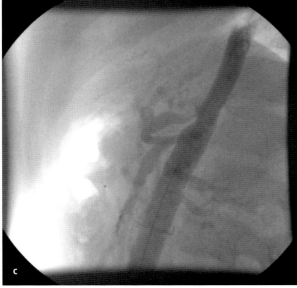

Fig. 2.1-5a–c Lateral (a) and anteroposterior (b) preoperative images and postoperative lateral image (c) in a 12-year-old girl with abdominal coarctation and involvement of the visceral and renal arteries. Treatment was carried out with implantation of a 14-mm PTFE aortoaortic prosthetic bridging graft and reimplantation of the renal arteries into the prosthesis. The stenoses of the visceral arteries were treated at the same time with an enlargement plasty of the proximal anastomosis of the prosthesis graft. (Images courtesy of W. Sandmann, Department of Vascular Surgery and Kidney Transplantation, University of Düsseldorf, Germany.)

erance of ischemia, the visceral and renal arteries can be perfused with 4°C cold Ringer lactate solution with added unfractionated heparin and prostaglandin E$_1$. Homologous reconstruction with a donor vein from the parents has also recently become possible when reconstruction is necessary in children.

2.1.3 Fibromuscular dysplasia

2.1.3.1 Clinical picture

Fibromuscular dysplasia (FMD) is a noninflammatory fibrotic thickening of the arterial wall, which may already occur in children and usually develops in the renal arteries, the extracranial vessels supplying the brain, the mesenteric arteries, and rarely in the arteries of the extremities (Figs. 2.1-6, 2.1-7).

The symptoms are always caused by reduced blood flow due to the stenoses associated with each of the five main types of dysplasia. A histomorphological classification is made, on the basis of the wall layer affected, into intimal, medial, and adventitial fibrosis. Thick-

ening with fibrous tissue rich in collagen and elastin, with proliferated m myocytes, occurs in each layer of the wall, while the elastica always has a fragmented and lamellated appearance. Focal myocyte necrosis is often seen in medial fibroplasia and can lead to aneurysm formation. Stenoses are predominant with the intimal type. Clinically, the children affected have renovascular hypertension. Aneurysms can also follow the vascular dissections that may occur in FMD.

2.1.3.2 Diagnosis

In addition to the physical examination, with inspection (Fig. 2.1-7), palpation, and auscultation, color duplex ultrasonography is available as an initial noninvasive diagnostic method. This method allows examination of all of the important vascular segments, starting with the carotids and continuing to the aortic side branches, although only in the area of the main vessel trunks in FMD. Methods capable of demonstrating the lumen are needed for imaging of the

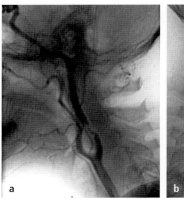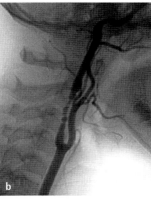

Fig. 2.1-6a, b A 10-year-old girl with fibromuscular dysplasia (FMD) in the internal carotid artery bilaterally (**a, b**), as well as in the celiac trunk, superior mesenteric artery, and renal arteries. Reconstruction of the internal carotid artery, celiac trunk, and renal artery was carried out using autologous venous graft (from the great saphenous vein), and the superior mesenteric artery was transposed infrarenally. (Images courtesy of W. Sandmann, Department of Vascular Surgery and Kidney Transplantation, University of Düsseldorf, Germany.)

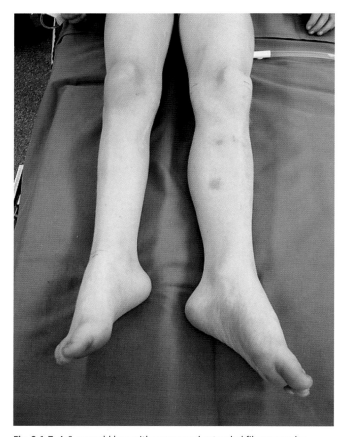

Fig. 2.1-7 A 6-year-old boy with severe and extended fibromuscular dysplasia in the superficial femoral artery and visible differences in the length and circumference of the right leg, with claudication symptoms. Status post failed autologous reconstruction at another institution (with early occlusion). Even with homologous great saphenous vein from the boy's father (femoroperipheral crural reconstruction, with no proximal connecting vessel at the level of the popliteal segment) and subsequent immunosuppression, however, a late re-occlusion still occurred after 1 year. Later revision was planned.

typical stenotic morphology in FMD—ideally MRA, to avoid radiation exposure, or alternatively computed tomographic angiography (CTA) or direct intra-arterial angiography (Fig. 2.1-6). However, radiography should only be used for diagnosis if there are contraindications for MRA.

2.1.3.3   Treatment

Endovascular treatment

Fibromuscular dysplasia in the renal arteries mainly occurs in truncal and intrarenal segmental locations, so that miniaturized low-profile systems and hydrophilic coating on the devices are needed to allow for adequate tracking and dilation. The same applies to stenoses in the course of the celiac trunk and superior mesenteric artery. For planning the access route (femoral or brachial), the patient's age is important, on the one hand (the diameter of the brachial artery in patients under the age of 10 years is usually too small for it to be used as an access artery), and the anatomic course of the vessels on the other. The renal arteries are usually easily treated via a transfemoral access site—e.g., using an IMA-configured 5F sheath (Destination, Terumo)—while a transbrachial route is easier for dilation of the superior mesenteric artery and celiac trunk, due to the steeply caudally directed vessel ostia (see also sections A 3.2.1, A 3.2.2 and Fig. 2.1-8f–h). As balloon dilation without stent implantation is usually sufficient in fibromuscular dysplasia (with clinical success rates of 70–90%), problems with recurrences can be readily managed with repeated percutaneous transluminal angioplasty; only limited experience is available with stent placement. In the pediatric field, vessel growth generally needs to be taken into account, however. The possible need for repeated dilation of the stent to achieve an adequate vascular caliber should be included in treatment planning up to the end of the child's growth period.

Surgical treatment

The choice of procedure needs to be taken into account in general in the treatment strategy for FMD and renal artery stenosis. When the stenosis is located within the truncal artery, the surgical technique consists of an aortorenal autologous venous bypass. When the vascular replacement is carried out with great saphenous vein, patients sometimes require a repeat operation as adults due to aneurysmal degeneration of the transplant, and postoperative outpatient follow-up should therefore be ensured. In addition to anatomic reconstruction, transposition of the splenic artery can also be carried out. The same applies to the visceral arteries, where reconstruction with an internal pelvic artery as a free transplant is possible. In the area of the carotid circulation, autologous great saphenous vein is also the replacement material of choice, and it is also possible to transpose the affected internal carotid artery to the external carotid artery. However, FMD is often associated with excess length, so that resection and end-to-end anastomosis are technically easy to carry out.

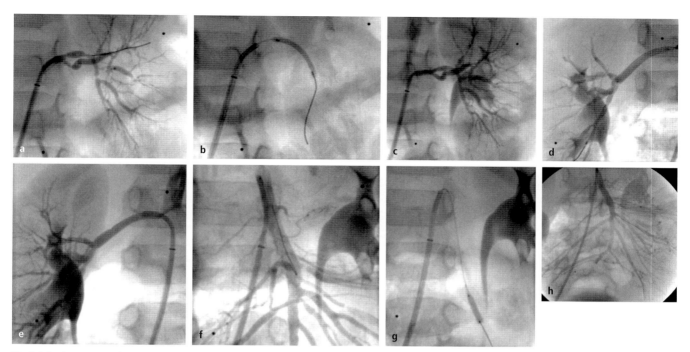

Fig. 2.1-8a–h A 4-year-old boy with secondary hypertension, with typical abdominal angina following normalization of blood pressure with calcium antagonists and angiotensin-converting enzyme inhibitors. Angiography shows multiple segmental artery stenoses in both renal arteries, multiple stenoses in the side branches of the superior mesenteric artery, and stenosis of the gastroduodenal artery and splenic artery. With general anesthesia and transfemoral access using a long 5F sheath, bilateral dilation of multiple intrarenal segmental artery stenoses was carried out in a single session using conventional balloons and an AngioSculpt catheter (each balloon diameter 23 mm; Biotronik), as well as dilation of several side branches of the superior mesenteric artery. After the procedure, blood pressure normalized without medication, and there was no further abdominal angina. (Images courtesy of T. Zeller, Cardiac Center, Bad Krozingen, Germany.)

2.2 Aneurysmal arterial diseases

Aneurysms can occur anywhere in the entire arterial system. They are rare in children, and it is therefore all the more important to consider them as a possibility in order to avoid fatal complications for the child. In contrast to aneurysms in adults, in which the pathogenesis is mainly arteriosclerotic, post-traumatic or postinfectious factors are predominant when aneurysms develop in children—although aneurysms in children can also occur in the context of congenital diseases such as collagenosis, phacomatosis, or vasculitis.

Among the phacomatoses, tuberous sclerosis (Bourneville–Pringle disease), autosomal-dominant neurectodermal dysplasia, and neurofibromatosis (Recklinghausen disease) are particularly liable to cause aneurysm development.

Tuberous sclerosis may have intracranial, thoracic, and abdominal manifestations. Due to the development of vascular hamartomas, obliteration of the vasa vasorum occurs, with subsequent aneurysm development. The early symptoms in the first year of life are cutaneous, lentil-sized, lanceolate hypopigmentations and cerebral convulsions.

Type I *neurofibromatosis*—with the triad of café-au-lait spots, cutaneous neurofibromas, and iris hamartomas—is the type of neurofibromatosis most frequently associated with vascular diseases. Neurofibromatosis has an incidence of one in 3000 births. The vascular changes can lead both to stenoses and to aneurysms. The changes are similar to those seen in FMD, although in contrast to FMD the renal artery ostia and also very peripheral segments may be involved (Fig. 2.2-1). Treatment is mainly surgical, although endovascular procedures may be possible in some cases (see section 2.1.3 on FMD).

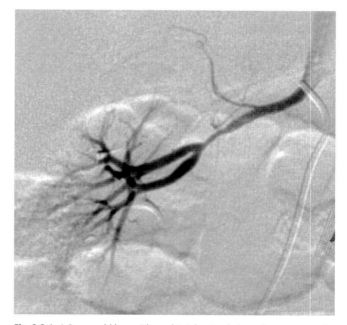

Fig. 2.2-1 A 3-year-old boy with a subtotal extended renal artery stenosis in Recklinghausen disease. Treatment was carried out with a homologous aortorenal venous bypass (with great saphenous vein from the mother as the donor vessel). (Image courtesy of W. Sandmann, Department of Vascular Surgery and Kidney Transplantation, University of Düsseldorf, Germany.

2.2.1   Congenital aneurysms

2.2.1.1   Clinical picture

Aneurysms may become manifest as a result of displacing growth, compression of nerves, pain, peripheral embolization with organ ischemia, and/or rupture. Single arterial aneurysms without a recognizable underlying disease usually develop in children in the area of the extremities, or more rarely in the area of the organ arteries. However, congenital abdominal aortic aneurysms have also been reported; multiple aneurysm formations in pediatric patients are even rarer. The parents usually deny that there is any history of trauma, and histological examination of the resected aneurysm almost always shows a clear tissue disturbance: hypoplasia/aplasia of the muscular layer, poor elastic fiber content, and a narrow collagen layer. This type of aneurysm is not associated with elongation, so that the circulation can only be preserved using a vascular replacement. In addition—in contrast to fibromuscular dysplasia and peripheral Marfan syndrome—thrombi often develop in these aneurysms, which often embolize and lead to the primary symptoms.

2.2.1.2   Diagnosis

Imaging diagnosis supplements the patient history and physical examination. The basic method for all extracranial processes is color duplex ultrasonography. Scout views in addition to color duplex ultrasonography are only rarely necessary, as the aneurysms usually only occur singly. If they are necessary, MRA is preferable as it avoids radiation exposure in these young patients.

2.2.1.3   Treatment

Due to continuing growth in the affected vessels in pediatric patients, endovascular exclusion of the aneurysms can only be considered in exceptional cases. The standard treatment method is open vascular surgery for the condition, although this has some limitations as well. In patients under the age of 10 years, vascular replacement with great saphenous vein is feasible, but usually leads to aneurysmal transformation in the transplant, in most cases followed by embolization and thrombosis. This applies in particular to aneurysms in the area of the large joints (axillary artery, cubital artery, popliteal artery). Plastic replacements are not possible before the age of 14. Technically, transposition can be considered either with an anatomic alteration—for example, transposition of the normal-caliber internal carotid artery to the external carotid artery; or with a free arterial transplant (harvested from an artery that only supplies an organ indirectly, such as the external carotid artery, deep femoral artery, internal iliac artery, or deep brachial artery); or with a free transplant harvested from a straight length of an artery supplying the extremities (e.g., the superficial femoral artery or brachial artery). The defect created can be bridged with narrow-caliber plastic or great saphenous vein. It can be assumed that later correction surgery will be needed, and the patient or relatives should be informed about this.

2.2.2   Aneurysms as a sign of vasculitis

Aneurysms can also occur in association with systemic diseases such as vasculitis. In addition to the coronary artery aneurysms mentioned, iliac aneurysms have also been reported, for example, in children with Kawasaki syndrome. Giant cell arteritis, polyarteritis nodosa, and Takayasu syndrome can also lead to aneurysm formation. Polyarteritis nodosa is quantitatively the most important form of vasculitis in relation to aneurysms. In Takayasu syndrome, the clinical picture may range from dilation to stenosis or occlusion. The aneurysms may be multiple, multifocal, saccular, or fusiform. Disease in the ascending aorta or aortic arch is the most frequent form in Takayasu, but any segment of the aorta or its large orifices may be affected.

In all forms of vasculitis, preventive treatment is required in order to avoid aneurysmal degeneration. Therapy mainly involves anti-inflammatory treatment. If aneurysms do develop, they have to be excluded with reconstruction of vessel continuity.

2.2.3   Pseudoaneurysms and mycotic aneurysms

Although pseudoaneurysms, false aneurysms, and mycotic aneurysms do not in the strict sense belong to the group of congenital aneurysms; due to medical advances they may now occur perinatally or postnatally as a result of procedures required in neonates. They can thus develop iatrogenically due to interventional procedures—e.g., in catheter angiography or large-lumen central access, with resultant damage to the vessel wall and development of a puncture aneurysm or pseudoaneurysm.

The pathogenesis of mycotic aneurysms in children is similar to that in adults. Signs of a vascular lesion develop in the context of systemic bacteremia or septic embolism. This may be caused by bacterial endocarditis. More rarely, aortoiliac (mycotic) aneurysms may develop after a delay following diagnostic catheterization of the umbilical artery. As there is a high risk of rupture, surgery is indicated along with targeted antibiotic therapy, although the most frequent pathogen is *Staphylococcus aureus*. There is controversy regarding the timing of the operation in cases of mycotic aneurysm. The advantage of simultaneous surgical treatment contrasts with potential infection of the reconstruction, and surgery is therefore recommended in such cases after successful antibiotic treatment has been carried out.

References

Adelman RD, Morrell RE. Coarctation of the abdominal aorta and renal artery stenosis related to an umbilical artery catheter placement in a neonate. Pediatrics 2000; 106 (3): E36.

Bahl VK, Chandra S, Taneja K. Self-expanding Wallstent for the management of severe abdominal coarctation due to non-specific aorto-arteritis. Indian Heart J 1997; 49: 189–91.

Bell P, Mantor C, Jacocks MA. Congenital abdominal aortic aneurysm: a case report. J Vasc Surg 2003 Jul; 38 (1): 190–93.

Berger H. Interventionelle Therapie der Nierenarterienstenose und Coarctatio aortae abdominalis. In: Pourhassan S, Sandmann W (eds.). Gefässerkrankungen im Kindes- und Jugendalter. Steinkopff Verlag bei Springer, 2009.

Brzezinska-Rajszys G, Quereshi SA, Ksiazyk J, Zubrzycha M, Kosciesza A, Kubicka K, Tynan M. Middle aortic syndrome treated by stent implantation. Heart 1999; 81 (2): 166–70.

Callicutt CS, Rush B, Eubanks T, Abul-Khoudoud OR. Idiopathic renal artery and infrarenal aortic aneurysms in a 6-year-old child: case report and literature review. J Vasc Surg 2005 May; 41 (5): 893–96.

Connolly JE, Wilson SE, Lawrence PL, Fuhuitani RM. Middle aortic syndrome: distal thoracic and abdominal coarctation, a disorder with multiple etiologies. J Am Coll Surg 2002; 194: 774–81.

Courtel JV, Soto B, Niaudet P, Gagnadoux MF, Carteret M, Quiqnodon JF, Brunelle F. Percutaneous transluminal angioplasty of renal artery stenosis in children. Pediatr Radiol 1998; 28: 59–63.

Criado E et al. Abdominal aortic coarctation, renovascular, hypertension, and neurofibromatosis. Ann Vasc Surg 2002; 16 (3): 363–67.

Dejardin A et al. Severe hypoplasia of the abdominal aorta and its branches in a patient and his daughter. J Intern Med 2004; 255 (1): 130–36.

Delis KT, Gloviczki P. Middle aortic syndrome: from presentation to contemporary open surgical and endovascular treatment. Perspect Vasc Surg Endovasc Ther 2005; 17 (3): 187–203.

Dongen RJAM v. Fibromuskuläre Dysplasie der Nierenarterien – Formen, Varianten und klinische Charakteristika, Bedeutung der angiographischen Morphologie für Behandlung und Prognosestellung. In: Sandmann W, Pfeiffer T. Renovaskuläre Erkrankungen. Aachen: Shaker Verlag, 2003, 133–45.

Flynn PM, et al. Coarctation of the aorta and renal artery stenosis in tuberous sclerosis. Pediatr Radiol 1984; 14 (5): 337–39.

Guzzetta PC. Congenital and acquired aneurysmal disease. Semin Pediatr Surg 1994 May; 3 (2): 97–102.

Hallett JW, Brewster DC, Darling RC. Coarctation of the abdominal aorta: current options in surgical management. Ann Surg 1980; 191: 430–37.

Han M, Criado E. Renal artery stenosis and aneurysms associated with neurofibromatosis. J Vasc Surg 2005; 41: 539–43.

Honjo O et al. Coarctation of the thoraco-abdominal aorta associated with mucopolysaccharidosis VII in a child. Ann Thorac Surg 2005; 80 (2): 729–31.

Jost CJ, Gloviczki P, Edwards WD, Stanson AW, Joyce JW, Pairolero PC. Aortic aneurysms in children and young adults with tuberous sclerosis: report of two cases and review of the literature. J Vasc Surg 2001 Mar; 33 (3): 639–42.

König K, Gellermann J, Querfeld U, Schneider MBE. Treatment of severe renal artery stenosis by percutaneous transluminal renal angioplasty and stent implantation. Pediatr Nephrol 2006; 21: 663–71.

Korbmacher B. Aortenisthmusstenose. In: Pourhassan S, Sandmann W (eds.). Gefässerkrankungen im Kindes- und Jugendalter. Steinkopff Verlag bei Springer, 2009.

Lande A. Takayasu's arteritis and congenital coarctation of the descending thoracic and abdominal aorta: a clinical review. AJR Am J Roentgenol 1976; 127: 227–33.

Lucas A, Kerdiles Y, Guias B, Cardon A, Calon E. Iliac aneurysm in a child complicating umbilical artery catheterization. Ann Vasc Surg 1994 Sep; 8 (5): 500–05.

McLeary, MS, Rouse RA. Tardus-parvus Doppler signals in the renal arteries: a sign of pediatric thoracoabdominal aortic coarctations. AJR Am J Roentgenol 1996; 167 (2): 521–23.

Messina LM, Goldstone J, Ferell LD. Middle aortic syndrome: effectiveness and durability of complex arterial revasculation techniques. Ann Surg 1986; 204: 331–39.

Moresco KP, Shapiro RS. Abdominal aortic coarctation: CT, MRI, and angiographic correlation. Comput Med Imaging Graph 1995; 19 (5): 427–30.

Morrow WR, Palmaz JC, Tio FO, Ehler WJ, VanDellen AF, Mullins CE. Re-expansion of balloon-expandable stents after growth. J Am Coll Cardiol 1993; 22: 2007–13.

Panayiotopoulos YP, et al. Mid-aortic syndrome presenting in childhood. Br J Surg 1996; 83: 235–40.

Pourhassan S, Grotemeyer D, Fokou M, Heinen W, Balzer K, Ramp U, Sandmann W. Extracranial carotid arteries aneurysms in children: single-center experiences in 4 patients and review of the literature. J Pediatr Surg 2007 Nov; 42 (11): 1961–68.

Reiher L, Sandmann W. Coarctation of the thoracoabdominal aorta. Chirurg 1998; 69 (7): 753–58.

Rudolph J, Pourhassan S, Saner F, Zotz RB, Sandmann W. Celiac artery thrombosis in a young patient with multiple platelet receptor polymorphisms and local compression syndrome. J Vasc Surg 2008 Nov; 48 (5): 1335–37.

Shefler AG, Chan MK, Ostman-Smith I. Middle aortic syndrome in a boy with arteriohepatic dysplasia (Alagille syndrome). Pediatr Cardiol 1997; 18 (3): 232–34.

Stadlmaier E, et al. Midaortic syndrome and celiac disease: a case of local vasculitis. Clin Rheumatol 2005; 24 (3): 301–04.

Stanley JC, Zelenock GB, Messina LM, Wakefield TW. Pediatric renovascular hypertension: a thirty year experience of operative treatment. J Vasc Surg 1995; 21: 212–27.

Stiller B, Weng Y, Berger F. Images in cardiology. Mid aortic syndrome: a rare cause of reversible cardiomyopathy. Heart 2006; 92 (5): 640.

Taketani T, et al. Surgical treatment of atypical aortic coarctation complicating Takayasu's arteritis—experience with 33 cases over 44 years. J Vasc Surg 2005; 41 (4): 597–601.

Tyagi S, Kaul UA, Satsanqi DK, Arora R. Percutaneous transluminal angioplasty for reno-vascular hypertension in children: initial and long-term results. J Pediatr 1997; 99: 44–49.

3   Venous malformations
Siamak Pourhassan

3.1   Congenital malformations of the inferior vena cava

Congenital malformations in the inferior vena cava are rare anomalies that are usually discovered during surgery, angiographic and computed tomography (CT) examinations, and at autopsy (Bass et al. 2000). The reported frequency of vascular anomalies in the inferior vena cava varies, relative to the varying extent of the anomaly, between 0.3% and 10% (Bass et al. 2000; Gaynor et al. 2000).

The human inferior vena cava develops in the sixth to eighth gestational week as a result of the genesis and regression of three paired veins—the posterior cardinal vein, the subcardinal vein, and the supracardinal vein. In undisturbed embryonic development, the prerenal part is formed by fusion of the hepatic segment, a derivative of the vitelline vein, and the right subcardinal vein. The pelvic veins arise from the posterior cardinal veins. From this point of view, the inferior vena cava can be divided into a hepatic, renal, and infrarenal segment.

Bass et al. (2000) classified anomalies of the inferior vena cava and renal veins in accordance with morphological and radiographic considerations. The main malformations in the inferior vena cava are:

- Agenesis
- Duplication
- Circumaortic renal veins
- Retrorenal left renal vein
- Left ascending inferior vena cava (Fig. 3.1-1)
- Azygos continuity with the inferior vena cava

Agenesis. The most frequent anomaly of the inferior vena cava is its occlusion, with continuity between the azygos vein and the superior vena cava (Gaber et al. 1998), with the latter and the lumbar veins dilating and thereby ensuring drainage of the lower half of the body (Fig. 3.1-2). The frequency of complete agenesis of the inferior vena cava, with congenital cardiac defects, is reported in the literature as 0.6–2.0% (Gaber et al. 1998). Lin et al. (1998) also described anomalies in the inferior and superior vena cava in connection with Goldenhar syndrome and left-right asymmetry with cardiac defects.

Duplication. Duplicated inferior vena cava—with a prevalence of 0.39–3.0% (Aljabri et al. 2001; Bass et al. 2000)—arises as a result of persistence of the supracardinal veins. The left inferior vena cava typically ends at the left renal vein, which crosses as normal anterior to the aorta and then joins the right inferior vena cava.

Circumaortic renal vein. Circumaortic left renal vein arises as a result of persistence of the posterior branch of the embryonic left renal vein and the posterior arch of the renal pedicle (intersupracardinal anastomosis). Each of the duplicated left renal veins courses ventral and dorsal to the aorta, respectively, and it is therefore

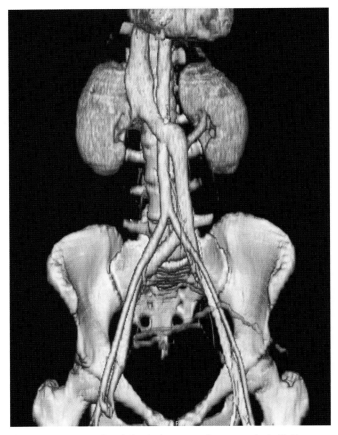

Fig. 3.1-1 Postoperative abdominal computed tomography (with three-dimensional reconstruction) in left ascending inferior vena cava (inferior vena cava transposition). A 24-year-old patient with embolizing thrombosis at several levels, including the left ascending inferior vena cava. The image shows the postoperative status after iliocaval transperitoneal thrombectomy and creation of a right inguinal arteriovenous fistula (resulting in simultaneous imaging of the aorta and inferior vena cava). (Image courtesy of W. Sandmann, Department of Vascular Surgery and Kidney Transplantation, University of Düsseldorf, Germany.)

termed circumaortic. The prevalence of this anomaly is between 0.5% and 8.7% (Aljabri et al. 2001; Bass et al. 2000).

Retrorenal left renal vein. Retrorenal left renal vein is also formally a congenital malformation of the inferior vena cava. It results from persistence of the posterior arch of the renal pedicle. The prevalence is 1.2–3.2% (Aljabri et al. 2001; Bass et al. 2000).

Left ascending inferior vena cava. A persistent left inferior vena cava, ascending on the left, is one of the rarer forms, with a prevalence of 0.2–0.5%, and results from regression of the right supracardinal vein with persistence of the left supracardinal vein.

Azygos continuity with the inferior vena cava. Azygos continuity with the inferior vena cava is also described as an absence of

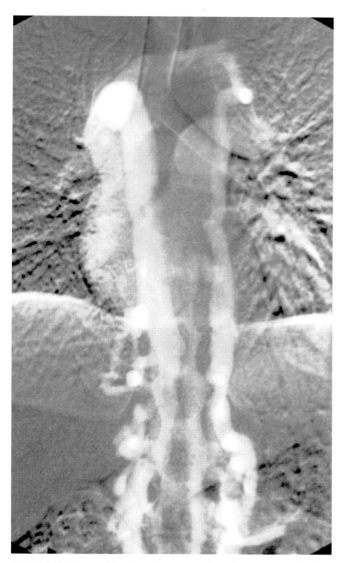

Fig. 3.1-2 A 22-year-old patient with venous thrombosis at several levels and aplasia of the inferior vena cava, with massively dilated paravertebral venous collaterals connected to the azygos system. (Image courtesy of W. Sandmann, Department of Vascular Surgery and Kidney Transplantation, University of Düsseldorf, Germany.)

the hepatic segment of the inferior vena cava with azygos continuity. Embryologically, it is theorized that it may be due to an absent right subcardinal-hepatic anastomosis with resultant atrophy of the right subcardinal vein. The prevalence is 0.6%. The renal segment of the inferior vena cava drains blood from both kidneys and ascends into the thorax behind the crus of the diaphragm as the azygos vein (Ruscazio et al. 1998).

The hepatic segment, often known as the posthepatic segment, is usually not really lacking; instead, it drains directly into the right atrium. As long as the postsupracardinal anastomosis does not contribute to the formation of the inferior vena cava, the gonadal vein drains ipsilaterally into the renal veins. If the infrarenal inferior vena cava is absent and the suprarenal segment is preserved, then complete absence of the hepatic segment indicates that all three of the paired venous systems have not developed.

Persistence of the left lumbar and thoracic supracardinal veins and of the left suprasubcardinal anastomosis, along with agenesis of the

right subcardinal-hepatic anastomosis, is responsible for duplication of the inferior vena cava with a retroaortic right renal vein and hemiazygos continuity with the inferior vena cava. The combination of duplicated inferior vena cava and a retroaortic renal vein and azygos continuity results from persistence of the left supracardinal vein and of the posterior branch of the renal pedicle, with regression of the anterior branch.

Circumcaval ureter is also described as retrocaval ureter. The proximal ureter loops behind the inferior vena cava and then courses on the right of the aorta, before running in front of the right iliac vein. Patients with this anomaly may develop obstructions of the right ureter or recurrent urinary tract infections. Another reason why this anomaly is clinically important is that there is a risk of injury during procedures in the aortoiliac vascular segment.

3.1.1 Clinical findings

If venous backflow from the lower half of the body is adequately ensured via collateral formation, anomalies in the inferior vena cava are of no medical importance. Asymptomatic findings are observed incidentally in 25% of cases (Giordano and Trout 1986). If thrombogenic risk factors are also present, deep venous thrombosis may occur, which often extends bilaterally as far as the pelvis (in 66–75% of cases). The thromboses often occur after extreme physical work or exercise (Dean and Tytle 2006; Obernosterer et al. 2002).

Reduced venous drainage leads to chronic venous obstruction, with a feeling of heaviness, varices, edema, and in some cases very severe skin ulcerations. Other complications include renal vein thromboses and gastrointestinal hemorrhage with ruptured duodenal varices. Systemic symptoms (such as cyanosis, dyspnea, heart failure or cardiac enlargement, and delayed growth in children) may occur if cardiac or visceral malformations, such as tetralogy of Fallot, complicate the case.

3.1.2 Diagnosis

The diagnosis is often based only on incidental findings or is established when the condition becomes symptomatic due to deep vein thrombosis, recurrent thrombophlebitis, or severe cardiovascular insufficiency developing at a young age. The possibility of an inferior vena cava anomaly should be considered particularly in patients with (bilateral) pelvic vein thrombosis, absence of thrombophilia, and/or age under 30 years (Obernosterer et al. 2002) (Fig. 3.1-3). The diagnostic approach is the same as the usual procedure in patients with chronic venous insufficiency or venous thrombosis.

3.1.3 Treatment

3.1.3.1 Conservative treatment

This consists of consistent compression therapy (with compression stockings or preferably tights) and anticoagulation if appropriate.

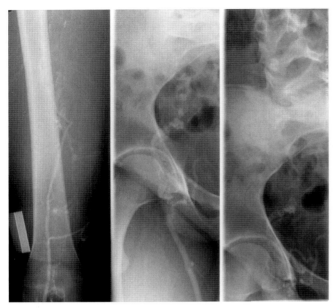

Fig. 3.1-3 A 14-year-old patient with pelvic-leg thrombosis on the right (and left) with aplasia of the inferior vena cava. (Image courtesy of W. Sandmann, Department of Vascular Surgery and Kidney Transplantation, University of Düsseldorf, Germany.)

3.1.3.2   Endovascular treatment

If complications develop during conservative treatment or as an initial manifestation of the disease, catheter-assisted lysis therapy with recombinant tissue plasminogen activator (rTPA), adjusted to the clinical findings, is carried out, combined as needed with stent therapy. Technical details are given in the section on endovascular therapy for deep vein thrombosis. This is indicated when there is raised venous pressure due to outflow obstruction, which can subsequently lead to damage involving post-thrombotic syndrome. Phlegmasia cerulea dolens is an absolute indication. Thrombosis that has already taken place, which often leads to collapse of the collateral system and thus also results in a post-thrombotic syndrome due to increased venous pressure, is also an indication for endovascular treatment, in view of the young age of the patients.

3.1.3.3   Surgical treatment

Surgical treatment depends on the anatomic status. The abdominal transperitoneal access route via a median laparotomy is possible for surgical access—e.g., to expose the inferior vena cava for thrombectomy or replacement. This is carried out with simultaneous inguinal creation of a temporary arteriovenous fistula, usually bilateral, to reduce the recurrent thrombosis rate. If pelvic-leg venous thrombosis is also present, venous thrombectomy using a Fogarty catheter can also be carried out at the same time via the inguinal access site. A bypass can be carried out in addition in cases of agenesis, hypoplasia, or other extended processes (Fig. 3.1-4). Depending on the condition being treated, the bypass can range from placement of a high Palma bypass to replacement of the infrarenal inferior vena cava, to a caval–right atrial bypass. The prosthesis diameter can range from 13–20 mm in such cases. Depending on the findings, a tube or bifurcation prosthesis can be used. In recurrent thrombo-

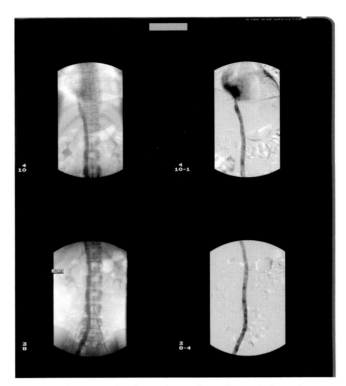

Fig. 3.1-4 Placement of an iliac–right atrial PTFE bypass in the patient shown in Fig. 3.1-2. (Image courtesy of W. Sandmann, Department of Vascular Surgery and Kidney Transplantation, University of Düsseldorf, Germany.)

sis or persistent stricture after catheter-guided lysis treatment with rTPA, consideration should be given to subsequent stent therapy or venous angioplasty (Dean and Tytle 2006).

All patients should receive treatment with oral anticoagulation and compression stockings postoperatively. The duration of anticoagulation therapy should be determined on an individual basis.

The value of surgical, lysis, and anticoagulation treatment options in cases of fresh thrombosis is a matter of controversy. When treatment is being planned, it should be borne in mind that the anomalies become apparent as a result of thrombosis at several levels and that conservative treatment and spontaneous collateralization alone will not be sufficient.

Asymptomatic malformation does not require surgical treatment. Depending on the findings, compression therapy should be carried out.

References

Aljabri B, MacDonald PS, Satin R et al. Incidence of major venous and renal anomalies relevant to aortoiliac surgery as demonstrated by computed tomography. Ann Vasc Surg 2001, 15: 615–8.

Bass JE, Redwine MD, Kramer LA, Huynh PT, Harris JH, Jr. Spectrum of congenital anomalies of the inferior vena cava: cross-sectional imaging findings. Radiographics 2000, 20: 639–52.

Dean SM, Tytle TL. Acute right lower extremity iliofemoral deep venous thrombosis secondary to an anomalous inferior vena cava: a report of two cases. Vascular Medicine 2006; 11: 165–9.

Gaber Y, Schmeller W, Romer C, Heise S, Kummer-Kloess D. Pelvic and leg vein thrombosis in azygous and hemi-azygous vein continuity syndrome and complete agenesis of the inferior vena cava. Vasa 1998 Aug; 27 (3): 187–91.

Gaynor JW, Weinberg PM, Spray TL. Congenital Heart Surgery Nomenclature and Database Project: systemic venous anomalies. Ann Thorac Surg 2000 Apr; 69 (4 Suppl.): 70–6.

Giordano JM, Trout HH. 3rd. Anomalies of the inferior vena cava. J Vasc Surg 1986 Jun; 3 (6): 924–8.

Lin HJ, Owens TR, Sinow RM, Fu PC Jr, DeVito A, Beall MH, Lachman RS. Anomalous inferior and superior venae cavae with oculoauriculovertebral defect: review of Goldenhar complex and malformations of left-right asymmetry. Am J Med Genet 1998 Jan 6; 75 (1): 88–94.

Obernosterer A, Aschauer M, Schnedl W, Lipp RW. Anomalies of the inferior vena cava in patients with iliac venous thrombosis. Annals of Internal Medicine 2002; 136 (1): 37–41.

Ruscazio M, Van Praagh S, Marrass AR, Catani G, Iliceto S, Van Praagh R. Interrupted inferior vena cava in asplenia syndrome and a review of the hereditary patterns of visceral situs abnormalities. Am J Cardiol 1998 Jun 15; 81 (1): 111–6.

E

Diseases of the lymphatic system

1   Diseases of the lymphatic system

Heinrich Hakuba

1.1   Introduction

Edematous swelling—whether unilateral or bilateral, symmetric or asymmetric—occurs very frequently. The many forms of edema, with numerous causes, include lymphedema and lipedema. However, many patients affected by lymphedema or lipedema never receive a correct diagnosis, or only at a very late stage. Lipedema and lymphedema are often still wrongly diagnosed as representing obesity. Many of the patients affected by lymphedema or lipedema thus do not receive adequate treatment, or do not receive it in a timely fashion, and this leads to chronic progression in both conditions. Patients suffer worsening symptoms and their quality of life is increasingly impaired. In addition, patients begin to experience restrictions in relation to clothing and footwear, as well as in mobility, and there is a reduction in self-confidence associated with anxiety and depression.

The purpose of this chapter is to present current findings on the etiology, pathogenesis, and course of these conditions, as well as to suggest recommendations for differential diagnosis and in particular on the treatment of patients with lymphedema and lipedema.

1.2   Etiology and pathogenesis, differential-diagnostic aspects, and course: lymphedema—lipedema

1.2.1   Lymphedema

Without treatment, lymphedema—which can affect both the extremities as well as the face, neck, trunk and genitals—is a progressive, chronic disease resulting from an imbalance between the quantity of substances destined for lymphatic drainage and the transport capacity in the lymphatic system, with primary or secondary causes. It is associated with a subsequent increase and alteration in the interstitial tissue fluid.

Primary lymphedema, which mainly affects females, involves malfunctioning or defective development of the lymphatic vessels and/or lymph nodes, resulting in chronic lymphedema, mainly in the lower extremities. The predominant form (in 97–99% of cases) is sporadic lymphedema (which does not have a clear hereditary cause and is probably due to a developmental disturbance in the lymphatic system during the embryonic period). In the rare cases (1–3% of

patients) of primary lymphedema with a clearly hereditary cause, a distinction is made between two groups: firstly, the more frequently isolated cases of lymphedema such as Nonne–Milroy lymphedema, with autosomal-dominant inheritance, which often appears at birth (type I hereditary lymphedema) and familial Meige lymphedema (type II hereditary lymphedema), which manifests later (usually in puberty); and secondly, lymphedemas that appear in connection with syndromal diseases such as lymphedema distichiasis syndrome (lymphedema in combination with an accessory row of eyelashes), hypotrichosis–lymphedema–telangiectasia syndrome (in which hypotrichosis and telangiectasia develop, mainly on the palms and soles of the feet, in addition to lymphedema), and lymphedema-ptosis syndrome and syndrome-associated lymphedemas such as those occurring in complex Turner syndrome, Klippel–Trenaunay–Weber syndrome, Noonan syndrome, and Down syndrome, etc. The overwhelming majority (roughly more than 80%) of all primary cases of lymphedema, traditionally also called lymphedema praecox, develop between puberty and the age of 35. Women are affected more often than men, with a ratio of approximately 10:1, suggesting that changes in the hormonal metabolism during puberty or pregnancy, particularly in women, have an influence on the pathogenesis of lymphedema. Primary lymphedemas that only manifest after age 35, occurr with a frequency of roughly 10%, are known as lymphedema tarda. The term "congenital lymphedema" is also commonly still used in cases of primary lymphedema (approximately 2% of cases) that have a hereditary cause and manifest in the first two years of life. In these cases, the extremities are also often affected bilaterally. However, primary lymphedema usually starts unilaterally on the toes or feet, with changes also affecting the contralateral leg, developing during the later course in approximately half of the cases (Brunner und Lachat 1989; Ferrell et al. 1998; Finegold et al. 2001; Rockson 2001; Northup et al. 2003; Brice et al. 2005; Bader and Detmar 2006; Herpertz 2004, 2010; Földi et al. 2005a; Carver et al. 2007; Shinawi 2007; Czaika et al. 2008).

Most cases of lymphedema—roughly twice as frequent and usually occurring unilaterally—involve acquired, secondary lymphedema, which in contrast to primary lymphedema often spreads downwards from proximal to distal (e.g., lymphedema related to diagnosis or treatment of malignant tumors. These cases develop relatively often as sequelae of cancer therapy or in the context of diagnosis, particularly after lymphadenectomies such as those carried out in patients with breast cancer or in association with gynecological tumors in the minor pelvis and patients with testicular or prostate cancer, and/or due to radiotherapy at the base of the extremities. The extent to which chemotherapy and hormonal therapy influence the development of lymphedema is as yet unclear. Other frequent causes of secondary lymphedema are associated with parasitic infections including leishmaniasis, schistosomiasis, echinococcosis

Table 1-1 Forms of lymphatic vessels and lymph-node disease and their classification into primary and secondary lymphedema (adapted from AWMF online 2011a).

Primary lymphedema	Secondary lymphedema
Aplasia/atresia	Lymphadenectomy
Hypoplasia	Radiotherapy
Hyperplasia	Malignant processes
Lymph-node fibrosis	Vein harvesting for bypass surgery
Lymph-node agenesis	Post-traumatic
	Post-infectious
	Artificial
	End stage of chronic venous insufficiency (CVI)
	Capillaropathy in internal-medicine diseases

Table 1-2 Stages of lymphedema development (adapted from Földi et al. 2005a; Herpertz 2010; Oberlin 2010; AWMF online 2011a; Deutsche Gesellschaft für Angiologie—Gesellschaft für Gefäßmedizin 2011).

Stage	Characteristics
0 (latency stage)	Transport capacity is reduced on lympho-scintigraphy, but is still sufficient to cope with the quantity of lymph produced, so that no symptoms develop
I (reversible stage)	The protein-rich fluid content of the interstitium is increased. There is slight, soft and painless swelling in which a dent is produced when pressure is applied with the finger or thumb. In addition, raising the legs (e.g., at night) leads to reduced edema
II (non spontaneous irreversible stage)	Pathological cellular changes appear. Due to an increase in connective-tissue fibers, the interstitium also changes. In addition, skin fold dimpling occurs near joints, with subsequent hardening of the tissue consistency. The coarse swelling can no longer be impressed using finger pressure, or only with difficulty, and is no longer influenced by raising the legs
III (final stage, also known as elephantiasis)	Stage II is aggravated, with hard edema up to the level of elephantiasis (i.e., the parts of the body affected are hugely swollen or swollen to the level of shapelessness) and massive changes in the skin, with extensive pachyderma, hyperkeratosis, and papillomatosis. In addition, the skin is often affected by poorly healing ulcers and recurrent infections (particularly erysipelas infections), due to local immunodeficiency in the area of lymphostasis. The infections (such as recurrent erysipelas) can cause extreme proliferation of connective-tissue fibers, leading to an increasingly massive increase in volume. In addition, there is a high risk for malignant degeneration (e.g., lymphangiosarcoma)

and filariasis, the latter of these is considered to be the most frequent cause worldwide. Bacterial and viral infections are also known to disturb lymph transport, namely *streptococcal* and *staphylococcal* infections (the former particularly relating to recurrent erysipelas), borreliosis and tuberculosis, in addition to recurrent herpes simplex infections. However, lymphedema can also be caused by malignancies and metastases, as well as other diseases that lead to chronic recurrent inflammation of lymph vessels and lymph nodes or chronic venous insufficiency, as well as injuries (such as laceration of lymphatic vessels or inflammation caused by mechanical injuries). In addition, factors such as obesity, impared mobility and also physical overexertion and exposure to heat or cold, wearing of tight rings, armbands, or other constrictive clothing, and repeated minor injuries, including injections or acupuncture in the affected parts of the body, can also promote the development of lymphedema (Lee et al. 2001; Rockson 2001; Cornely 2003; Herpertz 2004, 2010; Földi et al. 2005a; Clarc et al. 2005; Tomczak et al. 2005; Pitr et al. 2007; Czaika et al. 2008; AWMF online 2011a; Földi 2011) (Table 1-1).

The plethora of factors that can lead to or contribute to the development of secondary lymphedema may also explain the wide range of data regarding its occurrence reported to date. For example, rates of secondary lymphedema in the arm in patients who have been treated for breast cancer are reported as ranging from 6% to 83% (Lee et al. 2001; Clarc et al. 2005; Földi 2011). However, there is still a lack of epidemiological data regarding both the location and the cause of lymphedema, therefore no further conclusions can be drawn.

Primary lymphedema in particular manifests initially through a positive Stemmer sign (or a severe thickening of the dorsal skin of the toes, which cannot be lifted) (Stemmer 1975) due to early sclerosis of the dorsal skin of the toes. In secondary leg lymphedema, by contrast, the Stemmer sign may be negative initially in the early stage due to the often descending spread of the condition. The subsequent course of the disease in both primary and secondary lymphedema is marked by edema-specific tissue changes, with an increase in connective and adipose tissue and changes in the extracellular matrix (hyaluronic acid, collagen, glycosaminoglycans) (Kasseroller 2001; Cornely 2003; Földi et al. 2005a; Pitr et al. 2007; Schingale 2007; Döller et al. 2008; Kröger 2008; AWMF online 2011a).

As Oberlin (2010) also notes, disease processes either damage the capillary walls and thus increase protein permeability or restrict the transport capacity of the lymphatic vessels which in turn lead to protein-rich fluid collections that alter the interstitium and all its components (such as the ground substance, cell elements, and connective-tissue fibers), so that an "independent clinical picture"—

i.e., lymphedema—arises. Studies by Brenner (2009) are also noteworthy, showing that the increase in subcutaneous tissue in both primary and secondary lymphedema is caused by proteoglycans. According to Brenner's hypothesis, there appears to be a biosignal that initiates increased deposition of hydropexic proteoglycans in the tissue when there is disruption of lymph transport due to damage or disturbance in the lymphatic system. This leads to an increase in the tissue's extent and volume.

However, the current studies on the pathogenesis of lymphedema are still inadequate for clear conclusions to be drawn here. Stages of lymphedema are distinguished depending on its severity (Table 1-2). In the *differential diagnosis*, however, attention should be drawn to the fact that epifascial soft, pitting edema, as in the early stage of lymphedema, can also occur in concomitant forms of edema (e.g., in arthritis, trauma, erysipelas, acrodermatitis chronica atrophicans) and in edema caused by obstructed drainage (as in chronic venous insufficiency and immobilization edema) in forms of edema with systemic causes (as in cardiac decompensation, liver failure, protein deficiency, endocrinological diseases, or associated with drugs). Systemic causes must be considered when bilateral swelling of the legs has already persisted for a considerable time and is symmetrical, while by contrast unilateral swelling that develops acutely with a tender, swollen calf (subfascial edema) is more suggestive of deep venous thrombosis (Forstner et al. 1991; Herpertz 2004, 2010; Czaika et al. 2008; Kröger 2008; Müllegger and Glatz 2008; Partsch 2009; Schindler and Schellong 2009; Taute et al. 2010; Stöberl 2011). Various causes of edema are listed in Table 1-3.

Lymphedema can also be accompanied by numerous other pathological processes that modify the clinical picture (such as those—particularly with inflammation—that alter the permeability of the capillaries or connective tissue). Either substances destined for lymphatic drainage may be pathologically increased when there is limited transport capacity, or lymph formation (i.e., the entrance of tissue fluid into the lymphatic capillaries) or lymph transport may be disturbed as such (Kastenholz 1993; Casley-Smith 1994; Petrek 2000; Herpertz 2004; AWMF online 2011a).

Various forms of edema are often present simultaneously or in combination. One of the examples is combined phlebolymphedema, which develops due to chronic venous insufficiency (CVI). As a result of constant stress, damage to the vascular wall can occur, resulting in a disturbance of lymph transport leading to lymphostasis or

Table 1-3 Various causes of unilateral and bilateral edema (adapted from Stöberl 2011).

Causes of unilateral edema	Causes of bilateral edema
Acute	**Acute**
◾ Deep venous thrombosis, in which subfascial edema is typically found ◾ Ruptured synovial cyst, possibly also with an appearance of subfascial edema—"pseudothrombosis" ◾ Collateral edema after trauma (e.g., after contusion, sprain, muscle laceration), which may be followed by soft epifascial edema, or particularly after severe bleeding into the muscle compartment by collateral edema with a subfascial appearance ◾ Collateral edema in erysipelas ◾ Collateral edema in arthritis/activated arthrosis	◾ Deep venous thrombosis in both legs ◾ Edema with systemic causes, due to acute deterioration in the underlying disease
Chronic	**Chronic**
◾ Chronic venous insufficiency due to post-thrombotic syndrome (PTS) or varicosis ◾ Venous compression syndrome, possibly due to tumor, retroperitoneal fibrosis, synovial cyst, or aneurysm ◾ Primary and secondary lymphedema ◾ Collateral edema in acrodermatitis chronica atrophicans, a progressive skin disease that is a sequela of Borrelia infection that tends to appear on the extensor sides of the distal extremities ◾ Artificial edema—e.g., due to unintentional or intentional ligation of the extremities ◾ Tumors	◾ Bilateral chronic venous insufficiency due to post-thrombotic syndrome (PTS) or varicosis ◾ Bilateral venous compression syndrome—e.g., caused by a tumor or retroperitoneal fibrosis ◾ Lymphedema (more common in primary than in secondary pathogenesis) ◾ Collateral edema in acrodermatitis chronica atrophicans ◾ Lipedema ◾ Immobility edema ◾ Edema with systemic causes: – Cardiac edema, in which the skin is often shiny and there is often symmetrical rubor with blurred borders, sometimes also blistering on the skin on the lower legs as in stasis dermatitis – Hepatogenic edema, the characteristic features of which are often patchy pigmentation extending to the forefoot in the lower leg area, as well as atrichia on the lower legs even in men – Protein deficiency edema (e.g., due to nephrotic syndrome or anorexia, bulimia, cachexia) – Endocrine edema (e.g., due to hypothyroidosis and hyperthyroidosis or hypercorticoidism); pretibial myxedema is typical in hypothyroidosis, with characteristic nodular superficial induration, erythema, coarsening of the skin texture and gaping follicles – Drug-related edema (e.g., due to calcium channel antagonists, methyldopa, minoxidil, dihydralazine, glitazone, nonsteroidal anti-inflammatory drugs, steroids, hormones, saluretic agent abuse, diuretic agent abuse) – Premenstrual edema, mainly occurring in the ankle area and only in the second half of the menstrual cycle, associated with premenstrual weight gain – Idiopathic edema, probably caused by increased capillary permeability, again occurring only in women, mainly perimenopausally. Swelling also occurs in the area of the ankles, as well as the fingers, face, and abdomen. Weight swings are also typical, and a weight increase during the day of at least 1.4 kg may occur

phlebolymphedema. In addition to combined phlebolymphedema, amalgamation such as lipophlebedema, lipophlebolymphedema, and lipolymphedema can also occur. Particularly in its early form, lymphedema is often incorrectly regarded as alimentary obesity, but in contrast to lymphedema and lipedema, the latter can be corrected by dietary measures. Due to obesity, however, lymph drainage may be restricted and venous backflow may occur, leading to what is known as obesity–lymphedema. This develops particularly in the lower half of the body, mainly in both legs, and it is more pronounced in the thighs and calves than in the feet. Abdominal skin lymphedema can also develop when there is a marked fat paunch. In such cases, the Stemmer sign is only slight or not present at all, even in cases of severe obesity lymphedema. Severe skin changes such as those seen in primary or secondary lymphedema are also hardly ever observed (Ludwig and Vetter 1998; Meyer-Dörwald 2003; Herpertz 2004, 2010; Asdonk-Kliniken 2008; Czaika et al. 2008; Döller et al. 2008; Kröger 2008).

1.2.2   Lipedema

Lipedema is a symmetrical disturbance of adipose tissue in the extremities—apparently congenital, not caused by being overweight—that occurs almost exclusively in women (Schingale and Schingale 2002; Cornely 2003, 2004a, 2006a; Schmeller and Meier-Vollrath 2007a, b; Kröger 2008; AWMF online 2011b).

The disease usually starts during a hormonal readjustment phase, in puberty or pregnancy; however, it may also first become manifest in later decades of life (e.g., in menopause) (Marshall and Breu 2002; Herpertz 2004). A peak frequency between the third and fourth decades of life has been reported (Herpertz 2004). There are no confirmed data regarding the epidemiology. Questionnaire surveys in specialist lymphology clinics have shown that 4–20% of in-hospital patients were affected (Herpertz 1997; Meier-Vollrath and Schmeller 2004; Meier-Vollrath et al. 2005).

Typical lipedema changes have been observed in men, only in cases of marked hormonal disturbance such as hypogonadism, alcoholic liver cirrhosis, or after hormonal therapy in connection with cancer (Weissleder and Schuchhardt 1994; Schmeller and Meier-Vollrath 2007b).

In contrast to lymphedema, lipedema is characterized not only by progressive bilateral symmetrical excess of subcutaneous fat deposition, which affects the lower extremities as far as the ankle level more often than the arms, but also by pain developing during the course of the disease (such as tension pain, painful sensation to touch and pressure pain). Additional characteristic features of lipedema are orthostatic edema development, due to increased capillary permeability and an associated increase in fluid collection in the interstitium; a tendency for hematoma to develop due to increased vascular fragility; and resistance to dietary and exercise measures (due to the increase in subcutaneous fat, which basically cannot be altered). A positive finger or thumb test and a positive Stemmer sign are also usually not seen in lipedema. Erysipelas also occurs rarely, in contrast to lymphedema (Wienert and Leeman 1991; Herpertz 1997; Weissleder and Brauer 1997; Cornely 2003, 2004a, 2006a; Schmeller and Meier-Vollrath 2007a, b; Kröger 2008).

The question of why women are almost exclusively affected by lipedema has not yet been explained. Hormonal causes (particularly estrogenic factors) and an underlying genetic predisposition are probable, particularly since several female members of a family are often affected (Wold et al. 1949; Harwood et al. 1996; Meier-Vollrath et al. 2005; Schmeller and Meier-Vollrath 2007b, Kröger 2008). The fat cells in lipedema—the increase in which leads to a noticeable disproportion between the (slim) trunk and (voluminous) lower half of the body, particularly in individuals with normal weight—are formed in a different way from those occurring in increases in fat reserve that occur in obesity for example. As mentioned above, weight reduction is barely possible with lipedema, in contrast to dietary and exercise measures in individuals with obesity. It is also unclear whether lipedema is a sequela of hypertrophy or hyperplasia of the fat cells, or represents a combination of the two (Meier-Vollrath et al. 2005; Schmeller and Meier-Vollrath 2007a, b).

Lipedema is usually classified into the following three stages (Schmeller and Meier-Vollrath 2007b; Herpertz 1997, 2004, 2010):

- Stage I: the surface of the skin is smooth, while the subcutaneous tissue is swollen and the fat structure is finely nodular.
- Stage II: the surface of the skin is uneven, and the subcutaneous tissue is swollen with a coarse nodular structure.
- Stage III: the subcutaneous tissue is swollen with large nodes, and in addition there are large, deforming fat lobes on the inner sides of the thighs and knees, leading to columnar changes in the legs that obstruct walking.

In addition, the lymphatic system is not primarily impaired in lipedema, and initially responds to the increased protein-rich fluid in the interstitium (due to increased capillary permeability) by carrying out increased disposal activity. However, the existing transport capacity in the lymphatic system is not sufficient in the long term to fully remove the increased fluid volume, so that dynamic insufficiency or high-volume insufficiency results in lymphatic congestion and increased pressure in the tissue when the lymphatic vessels are still intact and carry out disproportionately good lymph transport. Due to constant stress on the lymphatic system, inflammation with increasing induration of tissue and changes in the lymphatic vessels, with lymphangiomatic sclerosis and perilymphatic fibrosis, which develop subsequently (particularly in patients with untreated lipedema), leading to reduced transport capacity in the lymphatic vessels (mechanical insufficiency or low-volume insufficiency)—so that lipolymphedema develops in the late stage of lymphedema (Amann-Vesti et al. 2001; Marsch 2001, 2005; Bilancini et al. 2002; Brauer and Weissleder 2002; Brauer and Brauer 2005; Földi et al. 2005b). In addition, lipedema can also occur in combined forms as lipophlebedema or lipophlebolymphedema.

In the differential diagnosis, this condition needs to be distinguished in particular from lipohypertrophy (a variant of body shape, which does not require treatment), in which a disproportionate body shape occurs due to symmetrically accumulated adipose tissue in the hip and/or leg area with a slim trunk. However, women affected by this do not have any orthostatic edema, predisposition to hematoma, tension pain, contact pain, or pressure pain, in contrast to those with lipedema. However, it is suspected that lipohypertrophy may develop into lipedema over several years (Herpertz 1997, 2004, 2010; Marsch 2001). It has not yet been clarified what causes such a transition or whether it exists at all, particularly since a large proportion of cases of lipedema already develop early in puberty without any preliminary stages.

It is also unclear whether adiposis dolorosa (Dercum disease) represents a special form of lipedema occuring late; mainly appearing at the start of the menopause without edema developing, often in connection with alcohol abuse, emotional instability and depression, but as in lipedema it causes painful symmetrical fat deposits mainly on the legs, with the exception of the feet, in the affected women (De Franzo et al. 1990; Steiner et al. 2002). Multiple symmetric lipomatosis (Launois–Bensaude syndrome, Madelung disease) should also be mentioned in this context. In this condition, increased deposition of fat occurs without pain or edema on the neck (type I), in the shoulders (type II), in the pelvic region (type III), or in the abdomen (type IV). Men are affected by this condition more often than women, although increased alcohol consumption with liver damage and/or polyneuropathy, diabetes mellitus, hyperuricemia, hyperlipidemia and other diseases are almost always present (Ruzicka et al. 1987; Sehouli et al. 1997). Similarly to lymphedema, lipedema is still often confused with obesity. However, the characteristic features of obesity are excess of weight with increased adipose tissue over the entire body, which can be reduced using slimming courses or nutritional changes and intensive exercise (Kröger 2008; Herpertz 2010; AWMF online 2011b). Moreover, obesity also develops over the years in approximately half of patients who have lipedema, evidently due to frustration with unsuccessful efforts to diet in order to change the leg shape which may lead to excessive eating (Greer 1974; Meier-Vollrath et al. 2005; Schmeller and Meier-Vollrath 2007b). As mentioned above, concurrent obesity not only makes the diagnosis more difficult, but also promotes the development of secondary lymphatic drainage disturbances.

Additional differential diagnoses that need to be excluded are the forms of leg edema described above and listed in Table 1-3, which may be caused by acute leg vein thrombosis or chronic venous insufficiency (e.g., phlebedema, usually occurring asymmetrically) or with a systemic pathogenesis (e.g., cardiac edema, in which both manual lymph drainage and compression therapy are contraindicated).

1.3 Treatment

1.3.1 Treatment for lymphedema

1.3.1.1 Conservative treatment

If lymphedema is left untreated, its extent can usually be expected to deteriorate. Treatment is more successful the earlier it starts (Földi et al. 1998, 2005a; AWMF online 2011a).

The aim in treatment of lymphedema is ideally to normalize lymph transport. Due to the chronic character of lymphedema, the treatment goal is usually to reverse the disease to its latent stage, meaning limited transport capacity without lymphedema, or at least to lower stages (such as stage I). The long-term treatment often does not lead to cure of lymphedema, but alleviates symptoms and allows to maintain functionality of the lower extremities and prevents progression to elephantiasis. In addition, the treatment can counteract

complications such as deep vein thrombosis, pulmonary embolism, late sequelae of deep vein thrombosis such as post-thrombotic syndrome, chronic venous insufficiency and chronic thromboembolic pulmonary hypertension (Földi et al. 1998, 2005a; Bernas and Witte 2004; Rockson 2008; Fritsch 2009; Seeger et al. 2009; Lüthi et al. 2010).

Depending on the extent of the lymphedema, an individual therapy plan should be drawn up before the start of any treatment (Petrek et al. 2000; Harris et al. 2001; International Society of Lymphology 2003; Hammerl and Döller 2008). In a joint decision-making process including the patient and physician, the patient should receive detailed information about realistic treatment goals, since quality of life and patient satisfaction ultimately depend on setting and achieving realistic treatment goals (AWMF online 2011a).

According to AWMF online (2011a), single or multiple goals that may be considered during treatment planning can be summed up as follows:

- Improving lymphatic drainage
- Softening of fibrosclerotic tissue changes
- Reducing fibrosis
- Improving functional deficits in the extremities to increase the efficacy of muscle pumps and joint pumps
- Providing instruction in methods of self-treatment (skin care, some lymph drainage maneuvers, technique of lymphangiological compression bandaging)
- Returning or reintegrating affected patients into their social environment such as school, college, further studies, or occupation
- Preventing the need for nursing care
- Improving quality of life

Therapeutic measures used include physical edema treatments such as the conventional complex decongestion physiotherapy (CDP) developed by Vodder (1936, 1966) and Asdonk (1979) and device-assisted intermittent compression or intermittent pneumatic compression (IPC), developed more recently as an additional supportive measure. Surgical measures are also used, as well as in some circumstances drug treatment, particularly when complications occur (e.g., use of antibiotics in cases of acute infections such as erysipelas; antihistamines and/or cortisone in cases of allergic skin reaction or congestion dermatosis; and diuretics in cases of extensive drainage obstruction—e.g., by malignant tumors). However, it should be noted that diuretics are usually not appropriate for long-term treatment of lymphedema. Although they remove water from the tissue, they do not remove the proteins that are transported away via the lymphatic vessels. Treatment with diuretics can therefore lead in the longer term to development of fibrosis and thus to thickening of the skin and subcutaneous tissue, which are no longer able to return to normal. Other supportive measures may include diet (fat-reducing and low-salt) and often also psychotherapeutic treatment. Since an active contribution on the part of the lymphedema patient is needed in order to reach the desired treatment goal, it can often be achieved only by taking psychosocial stress factors into account (O'Brien et al. 1977; Franzeck et al. 1997; Sitzia et al. 1997; Földi et al. 1998, 2005a, b; Miller et al. 1998; Gretener et al. 2000; Weissleder and Schuchardt 2001; Brorson 2003; Campisi and Boccardo 2003; Weiss et al. 2002, 2003; Ingianni 2003; Badger et al. 2004; McNeely et al. 2004; Cornely 2006b, 2007; Földi and Strößenreuther 2007; Schingale 2007; Hammerl and Döller 2008; Quendler 2008; Li et

Table 1-4 Stage-appropriate basic therapy for lymphedema using complex decongestive physiotherapy (CDP) with constant skin care (adapted from Földi et al. 1998; Oberlin 2010; AWMF online 2011a; Bringezu and Schreiner 2011; Földi 2011).

Stage	Characteristics	Phase I Decongestion	Phase II (or IIa) Optimization	Phase III (or IIb) Maintenance
0	No swelling, pathological lymphoscintigram	Prevention when risk factors for lymphedema are present		
I	Edema with a soft consistency; elevation reduces the swelling	MLD once daily, compression bandages, exercise, in-patient treatment if needed, duration 14–21 days		MLD in series, compression stockings when needed, or permanently and consistently
II	Edema with secondary tissue changes; elevation has no effect	MLD twice daily, compression bandages, exercise, in-patient treatment, duration 24–28 days	MLD once or twice weekly for 2–5 years, compression stockings and bandages, exercise, repetition of phase I	MLD in series or once weekly, compression stockings permanently and consistently, exercise
III	Elephantiasis-like hard swelling, often with a lobular form with typical skin changes	MLD 2–3 times daily, compression bandages, exercise, in-patient treatment, duration 28–35 days	MLD 2–3 times weekly for 5–10 years, compression stockings and bandages, exercise, repetition of phase I	MLD in series or 1–2 times weekly, compression stockings permanently and consistently, exercise

MLD, manual lymph drainage.

al. 2008; Földi and Földi 2009; Fritsch 2009; Herpertz 2010; AWMF online 2011a; Bringezu and Schreiner 2011).

As mentioned above, complex decongestion physiotherapy (CDP) is the basic treatment for lymphedema, even when surgical procedures are planned. It is also regarded as the most promising physical treatment method and should be integrated into the patient's overall care to ensure lasting treatment success. The coordinated treatment measures used in CDP consist of manual lymph drainage (MLD), compression treatment with compression bandages and stockings, targeted decongestive exercises and physical exercise activities and use of curative and protective skin care with skin-friendly lipids and oils or lotions containing lipids and moisturizing agents. Lotions are particularly important because in lymphedema the skin is often dry, scaly, and fissured—probably due to a disturbance in the balance between moisture and lipid content, often leading to local inflammation and infection (e.g., erysipelas). In addition, the compression materials used may cause further drying or stress in the skin, providing a portal of entry for pathogens. The efficacy of manual lymph drainage, the need for compression therapy and the benefit of decongestive and physical exercise activities have been confirmed (Bertelli et al. 1991; Franzeck et al. 1997; Sitzia et al. 1997; Werner et al. 1997; Földi et al. 1998, 2000, 2005a, b; Gretener et al. 2000; Weissleder and Schuchardt 2001; Badger et al. 2004; McNeely et al. 2004; Gültig 2005; Moffatt et al. 2005; Williams and Keller 2005; Földi and Strößenreuther 2007; Schingale 2007; Hammerl and Döller 2008; Földi and Földi 2009; Herpertz 2010; Földi 2011; AWMF online 2011a; Bringezu and Schreiner 2011).

CDP has two phases (Table 1-4). Phase I (the decongestion phase) involves reducing the extent of the edema as much as possible, mobilizing the congested edematous fluid and reducing fibrosis if present. In phase II, the treatment success achieved in phase I is optimized (phase IIa) and an effort is made to consolidate the results achieved (phase IIb, the maintenance phase). Depending on the severity of the condition, phase I is carried out for 3–5 weeks either on an outpatient or inpatient basis. The procedures should be administered intensively (such as manual lymph drainage at a frequency of one to three times per day, wearing of short-stretch compression

bandages for 12–22 hours per day, as well as decongestive exercises several times per day with the compression bandages on, depending on the severity of the edema and the patient's age). Phase II, usually on an outpatient basis, is started when the best possible decongestion state has been achieved or no further reduction in the extent of the edema can be obtained. Compression therapy (instead of compression bandages) is generally administered on a long-term basis using custom-made flat-knitted compression stockings/clothing, the elasticity and compression pressure of which should be equivalent to those of compression bandages. In addition to careful skin care, decongestive exercises should also be done up to three times per day, and—depending on the severity of the lymphedema—MLD should be either carried out one to three times weekly on a continuous basis or twice weekly in series (Table 1-4).

Manual lymph drainage, which is not comparable with traditional massage, represents a treatment method in which mild mechanical stimuli cause increased pulsation in the lymphatic vessels and thus an improvement in lymph transport. Excessive stimuli (as in classical massage), by contrast, can lead to hyperemia and obstruction of motion in the lymphatics, leading to deterioration in lymphedema. Despite low mechanical stimuli, the skin and subcutaneous tissue are each extensively shifted during MLD, so that the associated lymph vessels are stimulated by transverse and longitudinal stretching stimuli to increase contraction, causing lymph fluid to reach edema-free areas from which it can be transported away. Manual lymph drainage thus represents a circular stretching and shifting technique, based on four basic strokes developed by Vodder (1936, 1966) (stationary circle, pump, scoop, rotary), which are adapted to the various shapes of the body. For example, stationary circles are mainly used for lymph-node collections or when regions of the body need to be treated particularly intensively. Pump strokes are mainly carried out at the extremities from distal to proximal, and scoop strokes in the distal segments of the extremities (lower arm or lower leg). The difference between the pump stroke and the scoop stroke is basically that the pressure movement in the pump stroke leads to deformation of the skin/subcutaneous tissue longitudinal to the axis of the extremity; whereas in the scoop stroke, there is deformation of the skin/subcutaneous tissue diagonal to the axis of the extremity. The rotary technique, consisting of various movement sequences, is a dynamic stroke like the pump and scoop strokes and is mainly carried out on the trunk as well as the extremities, the circumference of which is substantially increased due to the edema formation. Combinations of strokes are often used (such as alternating pump stroke and stationary circle, also known as "combination stroke," "cross-stroke," or "shifting pump stroke") to ensure that treatment is as exhaustive as possible (Vodder 1966; Asdonk 1979; Földi et al. 2005a; Bringezu and Schreiner 2011; Földi and Strößenreuther 2007). Compression treatment should always follow MLD in order to prevent recurrent collections of lymph fluid in the tissue that has been softened by the drainage treatment. A major error leading to treatment failure that is still often made is that even when manual lymph drainage is continuing, compression bandages or stockings are not prescribed (Oberlin 2010).

Depending on the amount of pressure applied, the compression therapy influences the venous, arterial, and lymphatic system and triggers numerous complex physiological and biochemical reactions (Partsch 2003, 2005, 2008; Partsch et al. 2006, 2008a, b; Mosti 2008). However, so far there have been only a few studies on the mechanism of effect of compression therapy (the same applies to other measures such as MLD) and therefore no clear conclusions can be drawn.

At present, possible mechanisms of effect that might explain the success of this compression therapy (with edema reduction, pain relief, and promotion of healing of varicose ulcers due to venous insufficiency) can be summed up as follows (Olszewski 1991; Casley-Smith 2000; Jünger et al. 2000; Levick 2003; Levick and McHale 2003; Partsch 2003, 2005; Földi et al. 2005a, b; Partsch et al. 2006, 2008a, b):

- Displacement of the edematous fluid to uncompressed parts of the body
- Increase in drainage of congested lymph via lymph vessels and improvement in the dynamics of lymph transport, particularly in combination with physical exercise or muscle activity
- Increase in lymph formation due to an increase in inflow of tissue fluid into the lymphatic capillaries
- Reduction of capillary filtration, with an increase in interstitial pressure leading to prevention or reduction of fluid passing from the blood capillary network into the tissue
- Improvement in venous pump activity, with venous reflux being reduced and venous return being promoted, associated with a reduction in venous hypertension. This also reduces pressure in the blood capillaries and consequently the lymph burden
- Regression of tissue with fibrosclerotic changes, due to improved skin perfusion, promoting detachment of leukocytes from the endothelium, and probably also due to positive effects on the release of proinflammatory cytokines

For compression treatment of lymphedema during the intensive phase (decongestion phase), the main recommendation is placement of multilayer bandages, particularly in combination with minimally elastic or nonelastic short-stretch compression bandages. In a multilayer bandage, nonelastic short-stretch compression bandages are usually combined in one or more layers with a cotton tubular bandage as an underlayer to protect the skin and with cushioning materials (Badger et al. 2000; Földi et al. 2005a, b; Gültig

2005; Moffatt et al. 2005; Williams and Keller 2005; Damstra 2008; Damstra et al. 2008; Partsch et al. 2008a, b; AWMF online 2011a).

In comparison with elastic bandages, short-stretch compression bandages have the advantage that the contact pressure during exercise—e.g., during standing up and walking—is much stronger. During walking, short-stretch compression bandages create high intermittent pressure peaks (massage effects), which decline again in the diastolic phase or in resting phases. When the patient is lying down, they therefore exert a comfortable level of resting pressure. Although a similarly high pressure can also be created with elastic bandages as with nonelastic bandages when the patient is standing, if they are placed with sufficient tension, they create an almost constant pressure with only minor deviations during movement and are less comfortable when the patient is supine (Clark 2003; Partsch 2005; Partsch et al. 2006, 2008a, b; Mosti 2008). With elastic bandages, there is also a risk of substantial constriction—which can lead to considerable tissue defects, for example, in patients with (unrecognized) arterial occlusive disease. It has now been confirmed that intermittent compression with high pressure peaks and lower-pressure intervals leads to an increase in arterial inflow. Short-stretch compression bandages have also been found to be better than elastic bandages with regard to improvements in venous pump action (Partsch 2008; Partsch et al. 2008a, b). Mosti (2008) demonstrated that nonelastic compression leads to a significantly greater increase in the venous ejection fraction in both the standing position and in the supine position than elastic compression, with comparable contact pressure. With nonelastic bandages there was also a greater reduction in venous reflux in comparison with elastic bandages, with well tolerable pressure in the supine position and higher pressure in the standing position (Mosti 2008).

Correct placement of a compression bandage is another vital element for successful treatment. The compression bandage has to be firmly placed, with contact pressure declining from distal to proximal, in such a way that it does not slip and applies evenly distributed pressure over the entire cross-section, but without causing pain, restricting natural movement, or damaging the skin and tissue. If the pressure distribution is not adequately graduated, it can lead to renewal of persistent edema due to limited venous and lymphatic flow. The pressure profile may be influenced by the limb shape and circumference, or by the radius of the limb curvature, or by the deformation of the limb shape that is often present in lymphedema patients due to edema distribution, fat deposition, or fibrosclerotic processes. Individually tailored cushioning bandages made of foam plastic or cotton-wool are therefore used in combination to correct the limb shape or achieve an even pressure distribution. Uneven cushioning materials of foam plastic are also used to achieve a micromassage effect during movement (Badger 1997; Badger et al. 2000; Clark 2003; Moffatt et al. 2005; Partsch 2005; Partsch et al. 2006, 2008b; Williams and Keller 2005; AWMF online 2011a).

The Laplace law can be used to calculate a bandage's contact pressure (P [pressure] $\propto$ [proportional to] T [tension in the bandage] / R [radius of the limb curvature]) (Clark 2003; Williams and Keller 2005; Partsch et al. 2006). However, there is still controversy regarding the accuracy of this calculation.

In addition, the level of compression pressure and the profile of a bandage always have to be individually adjusted to the treatment conditions and the patient's needs, taking into account the stage of lymphedema, the underlying pathological processes, concomitant

Table 1-5 General recommendations for compression bandages in phase I (the decongestion phase) of complex decongestion physiotherapy (adapted from AWMF online 2011a).

Patients	Age/stage	Pressure	Cushioning	Wearing period (hours)
Children	6 months–6 years	10–20 mmHg	Smooth: (cushion bandages/foam)	12–16
	2–6 years	20–30 mmHg	Smooth: cushion bandages Uneven: foam	16–20
	6–12 years	20–30 mmHg	Smooth: cushion bandages Uneven: foam	16–20
Adults	Stage I	20–30 mmHg	Smooth: cushion bandages/foam	12–16
	Stage II	30–46 mmHg	Smooth: cushion bandages Uneven: foam	18–22
	Stage III	46 mmHg or more	Smooth: cushion bandages Uneven: foam	18–22
	Lymphedema combination forms	Individual bandages with short-stretch compression	Individual	Individual
Older patients	60–70 years	30–46 mmHg	Smooth: cushion bandages Uneven: foam	18–22
	Over 70 years	20–30 mmHg	Smooth: cushion bandages/foam	12–16

diseases, the condition of the skin and tissue, age, and the patient's degree of mobility and physical activity (Földi et al. 2005b; Moffatt et al. 2005; Williams and Keller 2005; Partsch et al. 2006, 2008b) (Table 1-5).

In general, patients who are not active—such as frail, bedridden, and elderly patients—must receive only low compression pressures. Reduced compression with nonelastic multilayer bandage systems also appears advantageous as a palliative measure in patients with malignancy-associated diseases and patients with concomitant diseases (such as chronic polyarthritis, progressive systemic scleroderma, and those with milder cases of coronary artery stenoses, cardiac arrhythmia and high arterial pressure) whose medical condition does not permit high compression pressures. However, slight compression that does not exceed 25 mmHg also appears to be effective in patients with milder cases of peripheral arterial occlusive disease (PAOD), with a reduced ankle–brachial pressure index (ABPI) of 0.5–0.8 (Marston and Vowden 2003; Moffatt et al. 2005; Partsch et al. 2006, 2008a, b; Partsch 2008).

As mentioned earlier, compression therapy instead of compression bandages should be used on a lifelong basis in phase II in order to prevent relapse. Custom-made flat-knit compression stockings or clothing should be used, with a compression pressure and elasticity corresponding to those of compression bandages. However, the type of compression stocking used and the physical measures for CDP can change over time, depending on the extent to which the lymphedema resolves or swelling reaccumulates and depending on the patient's degree of mobility and occurrence of new diseases (orthopedic, neurological or internal-medical) (Földi et al. 1998, 2005a, b; Partsch 2003; Moffatt et al. 2005; Williams and Keller 2005; Partsch et al. 2006; 2008a, b; Oberlin 2010; AWMF online 2011a; Bringezu and Schreiner 2011). For example, long-term bandaging may be indicated in some patients with lymphedema who are unable to tolerate the pressure of compression stockings/clothing, whose skin is damaged, or who are receiving palliative therapy, or in patients who have only limited dexterity and are unable to put on or take off

compression stockings safely without causing trauma; or in patients in whom compression stockings alone are not sufficient to keep the edema constant (Moffatt et al. 2005). The family physician should always carry out regular examinations in patients with lymphedema during phase II of CDP (or usually permanently?), in order to determine whether changes in the compression treatment are needed with regard to compression stockings or bandaging and to prescribe these changes when needed.

Accompanying decongestive movement exercises during the compression treatment are another important factor for the success of CDP. Targeted movements can activate the muscle pumps and joint pumps, as a result of which contractions of the skeletal musculature lead to an increase in interstitial pressure that is transferred to the lymphatic vessel wall, producing an increase in lymphatic pulsation (Partsch 2003; Partsch et al. 2006, 2008a, b). Other exercise activities are also beneficial, including walking, cross-country skiing, cycling or use of an exercise bike, medical training therapy/strength training (possibly in a fitness studio run by a physiotherapist), or swimming (although in this case appropriate hygiene measures need to be considered). In addition, deep abdominal breathing promotes venous and lymphatic return. On the other hand, overstretching, lacerating, or wrenching movements, as well as overexertion during exercise and other activities (at home or at work) can have unfavorable effects. Exercises which potentially could cause injury should not be advised (such as downhill skiing). Any form of injury in the affected area, with resulting inflammation due to bacterial or fungal infection, should be avoided (e.g., injuries that may occur during various activities such as gardening, blood-pressure measuring, blood sampling, acupuncture, or wearing constrictive clothing, etc.). In addition, prolonged dangling of the affected extremities and exposure to heat or cold are also unfavorable for lymph flow and should be avoided (Rockson 2001; Cornely 2003; Partsch 2003; Partsch et al. 2006, 2008a, b; Herpertz 2010; Földi et al. 2005a; Clarc et al. 2005; Pitr et al. 2007; Asdonk-Kliniken 2008/2011; Czaika et al. 2008; AWMF online 2011a).

1.3.1.2 Surgical treatment

Surgical treatment methods include reconstructive microsurgical procedures (such as microsurgical autologous lymphatic vessel transplantation or flap plasty incorporating lymph vessels, as well as interposition of autologous veins) with which localized lymph vessel interruptions can be restored (Campisi and Boccardo 2003; Weiss et al. 2002, 2003; Li et al. 2008). Diversion procedures to drain lymph extra-anatomically using lymphovenous or lymphonodulovenous anastomoses have also been described (O'Brien et al. 1977; Ingianni 2003). In addition, resection procedures such as various degrees of tissue resection of the skin, subcutaneous tissue, and fascia (Miller et al. 1998), as well as liposuction or liposculpture (a new, refined technique) have been used to remove adipose tissue or subcutaneous tissue (Brorson 2003; Cornely 2006b, 2007). However, surgical treatment is often only carried out when a previous form of conservative therapy (e.g., CDP) has not been successful or when a local interruption of a lymphatic vessel is present. Even when surgical measures of this type are being planned, CDP should be carried out for at least 6 months beforehand so that transient edema can recede (AWMF online 2011a).

1.3.2 Treatment for lipedema

1.3.2.1 Conservative treatment

There is no genuinely curative treatment for lipedema either. The goal of treatment in patients with lipedema thus consists of elimination of the edema process, in order to prevent a transition to combined lipedema/lymphedema or to eliminate or ameliorate symptoms by reducing edema using CDP, as mentioned above or by reducing the adipose tissue using surgical procedures (Herpertz 1997, 2010; Schingale and Schingale 2002; Schmeller and Meier-Vollrath 2007a, b; Fritsch 2009; AWMF online 2011b). As with lymphedema, no diuretic therapy should be advised in patients with lipedema.

Although physical exercise is in principle capable of reducing excess weight, as mentioned above it cannot reduce the disproportional increase in fat in lipedema. The same applies to slimming courses and diet courses. However, weight gains should be avoided and weight reduction should also be aimed for in obese patients, as excess weight generally represents a risk factor for the development of secondary lymph drainage disturbance (Herpertz 1997, 2004; Meyer-Dörwald 2003; Asdonk-Kliniken 2008/2011; Döller et al. 2008; Kröger 2008; Marshall and Schwahn-Schreiber 2008).

CDP has been the established form of conservative treatment since the mid-20th century. In patients with lipedema, particularly if they receive early and consistent long-term compression treatment, CDP leads to a reduction in edema components and thus prevents any progression of edema or transition to lymphedema. It also reduces edema-related pressure, tension and contact pains. Treatment should start with low compression levels, otherwise often lipedema patients would be unable to tolerate the pain caused by the compression (Herpertz 1997, 2010; Meier-Vollrath et al. 2005; Schmeller and Meier-Vollrath 2006, 2007a). Intermittent pneumatic compression can be used as a supportive accompanying measure as well, particularly for pain reduction (Herpertz 1997, 2010).

However, these physical measures alone are not capable of reducing the pathological increase in adipose tissue.

1.3.2.2 Surgical treatment

Surgical procedures that can be used are liposuction or lymphological liposculpture, with tumescent local anesthesia (TLA) using the "wet technique" (Klein 1987; Sattler et al. 1997; Frick et al. 1999; Schingale and Schingale 2002; Cornely 2004b; Schmeller and Meier-Vollrath 2004, 2006, 2007a, 2008; Meier-Vollrath et al. 2005; Rapprich et al. 2011; Stutz 2011). In this method, based on the TLA technique, contour lines are drawn on the patient's skin and a mixture of physiological saline and a local anesthetic is introduced via fine cannulas. During a short application time, the fat cells are softened, so to speak, or swell up and separate from each other (the technique is also known as "water dissection"), so that they can be suctioned away. The blunt vibrating microcannulas that are used (vibration liposuction, power-assisted liposuction, PAL) only remove adipose tissue that lies between the connective-tissue fibers. In contrast to earlier procedures carried out with the patient under general anesthesia with the "dry technique," this avoids injury to the surrounding structures (such as lymph vessels, blood vessels and nerves) (Cornely 2004b, 2006a, b; Hoffmann et al. 2004, 2007; Schmeller and Meier-Vollrath 2006, 2007a, 2008; Rapprich et al. 2011).

Follow-up studies for periods of up to 8 years have shown that liposuction or lymphological liposculpture with the TLA technique not only produces marked improvement in the clinical picture with regard to body shape and symptoms, as well as in the patients' quality of life, but also apparently has a positive effect on high-volume insufficiency. To date the techniques have not been reported to lead to any relevant damage to the nerves, blood vessels, or lymph vessels. The method can therefore be regarded as extremely tissue-conserving and safe, even in lipedema. In particular, these findings contradict the view that the treatment may cause lymphedema due to damage to the lymph vessels (Hanke and Sattler 2003; Hoffmann et al. 2004; Sommer and Sattler 2003; Schmeller et al. 2006; Schmeller and Maier-Vollrath 2006, 2007a, 2008; Bender et al. 2007; Cornely 2007; Stutz and Krahl 2009; Rapprich et al. 2011; Stutz 2011).

As Schmeller and Meier-Vollrath (2007a) already noted, liposuction can sustainably diminish lipedema but is not capable of eliminating it completely. CDP, particularly with compression stockings, is therefore still the main treatment, and should be continued postoperatively, although to a reduced extent. A combination of conservative and surgical measures is therefore able to restore the patients to a quality of life that had previously been unimaginable. However, surgical treatment measures should only be carried out in specialized centers in which there is sufficient experience with the clinical picture of lipedema.

1.3.3 Contraindications to lymph drainage and/or compression bandages

Before the physician takes the decision to treat a patient with lymphedema or lipedema using CDP, it is essential to carry out a precise medical diagnostic work-up to identify any contraindications for compression therapy or lymph drainage (Földi et al. 1998, 2005a, b; Partsch 2003; Moffatt et al. 2005; Oberlin 2010; AWMF online 2011a). Potential contraindications are listed in Tables 1-6 and 1-7. CDP must always be adapted to the patient's individual needs and the individual physical measures should be modified in accordance

Table 1-6 Absolute and relative contraindications for manual lymph drainage (adapted from Oberlin 2010).

	Absolute	Relative
General	■ Acute inflammation with pathogenic bacteria ■ Cardiac edema ■ Acute leg vein disease	■ Malignant lymphedema
Neck	■ Hyperthyroidism ■ Carotid sinus hypersensitivity ■ Cardiac arrhythmia	■ Age
Abdominal/ pelvic region	■ Pregnancy ■ During menstruation ■ Convulsive disorders (epilepsy → beware of tachypnea) ■ Status post intestinal obstruction (ileus) ■ Intestinal diverticulosis ■ Abdominal aortic aneurysm or after surgical aneurysm treatment ■ Extreme arteriosclerotic changes (usually in the context of metabolic disturbances such as diabetes mellitus, hyperlipidemia) ■ Inflammatory bowel disease (ulcerative colitis, Crohn disease) ■ Severe adhesions after surgery ■ Changes after radiotherapy in the abdominal and/or lower abdominal region ■ Radiation cystitis, radiation colitis ■ Status post deep pelvic vein thrombosis	■ Age

Table 1-7 Contraindications for compression treatment (adapted from Oberlin 2010; AWMF online 2011a).

Absolute	Relative*
Cardiac edema	High arterial pressure
Severe arterial occlusive disease	Angina pectoris
Sudeck disease (post-traumatic osteoporosis)	Coronary sclerosis
Scleroderma	Cardiac arrhythmia
	Age > 70 years

* Only under medical supervision.

with the patient's age, degree of mobility, skin and tissue status and relative to any acute inflammations or concomitant diseases (such as chronic venous insufficiency, coronary heart disease, cardiac arrhythmia, high blood pressure, borderline-compensated cardiac, renal, or hepatic failure, peripheral neuropathy or diabetes mellitus, particularly in combination with diabetic neuropathy and microangiopathy or macroangiopathy, malignancy-associated diseases, rheumatic conditions, etc.). To ensure that skin injury is avoided, special considerations in relation to the intensity of CDP administered include existing diabetic polyneuropathy, advanced chronic venous insufficiency with dermatoliposclerosis and possibly fully developed varicose ulcers (Partsch 2003; Földi et al. 2005a, b; Moffatt et al. 2005; Williams and Keller 2005; Partsch et al. 2006, 2008a, b; Oberlin 2010; AWMF online 2011a).

1.4 Conclusions and summary

The various causes of edema may lead to a pathological increase in capillary filtration into the interstitial connective tissue, or may reduce venous resorption and lymph drainage. These can be differentiated with the relevant clinical and technical examinations. If diagnostic problems arise, the "edema consultancy" now established by the German Lymphology Association (*Deutsche Gesellschaft für Lymphologie,* DGL) can be contacted (www.dglymph.de). However, diagnoses of lymphedema or lipedema are still often missed or only made at a late stage.

Without treatment, lymphedema is characterized by a chronic course, with an increase in protein-rich interstitial tissue fluid and changes in all cell elements, connective-tissue fibers, ground substance in the interstitium or a tendency to fibrosclerosis in the tissue. It results in imbalance between substances destined for lymphatic drainage and the lymph transport capacity in the lymphatic system. It may have primary causes (congenital malfunction, defective development of the lymph vessels and/or lymph nodes) or a large number of secondary (acquired) causes. In contrast to secondary forms of lymphedema, the primary forms of lymphedema mainly spread from distal to proximal.

Lipedema is a disturbance of adipose tissue distribution, probably with a hereditary/hormonal etiology, that almost exclusively affects females, with orthostatic edema formation due to increased capillary permeability and the associated protein-rich fluid collection in the interstitium. In contrast to lymphedema, the swelling is painful to touch, with a tendency for hematomas to develop, and it usually arises in a bilateral symmetric form, with contact pressure mainly in the legs, typically with an edema-free forefoot. Lipedema is also a chronic disease, and due to the protein-rich fluid collection in the interstitium, it can lead secondarily to combined lipolymphedema. In addition, combined forms such as lipophlebolymphedema, lipophlebedema, and phlebolymphedema can occur, and this needs to be taken into account in the differential diagnosis. Obesity can also make clear differential-diagnostic classification difficult. In contrast to lymphedema and lipedema, however, obesity is characterized by increased adipose tissue in the entire body and by excess weight that can be reduced using dietary and exercise measures. When obesity is also present, weight loss should be aimed for, as excess weight can promote the development of secondary lymph drainage disturbances.

No curative treatments are available for either lymphedema and lipedema, therefore a complete cure is not currently possible. The longer the edema persists, the less successful the treatment will be.

In both clinical pictures, the most important treatment measure is complex decongestion physiotherapy (CDP)—a combination of compression therapy, manual lymph drainage, decongestive exercises and skin care. The treatment, which is usually lifelong, does not lead to a cure for the disease but can prevent its progression (which in case of lymphedema may advance to the extent of elephantiasis, while in lipedema progressive edema to the extent of combined lipolymphedema may develop) and can improve the symptoms. The most important component of CDP is compression treatment. As it has been shown with lymphedema in particular, this can lead to a reduction in swelling. Prescribing manual lymph drainage as the sole treatment measure should therefore now be obsolete.

In lipedema, however, the excessive fat development, which progresses over the years, is not influenced by compression treatment. The liposuction or lymphological liposculpture methods using tumescent local anesthesia (TLA) that are now available appear very promising in this context. When these are combined with conservative and surgical methods, the affected patients can generally achieve a quality of life not previously imaginable.

In conclusion, it should be emphasized that there is no clear information available regarding the etiology and pathogenesis of lymphedema and lipedema, apart from a few scattered data. Further research is needed.

References

Amann-Vesti BR, Franzeck UK, Bollinger A. Microlymphatic aneurysms in patients with lipedema. Lymphology 2001; 34: 170–5.

Asdonk J. Physikalische Therapie des postmastektomischen Lymphödems. Z Lymphol 1979; 3: 96–8.

Asdonk-Kliniken (Fachkliniken für Lymphologie und Ödemkrankheiten – Feldbergklinik St. Blasien, Seeklinik Zechlin): Informationen über Krankheitsbilder, ambulante und stationäre Behandlung von Ödemkrankheiten, Einweisungsmodalitäten einschl. derer für EU-Bürger sowie Qualitätsmanagement. 2. Aufl. 2008. Online im Internet unter URL: http://www.asdonk-online.de (Stand 02.11.2011).

AWMF online (Arbeitsgemeinschaft der Wissenschaftlichen Medizinischen Fachgesellschaften). Leitlinien der Gesellschaft Deutschsprachiger Lymphologen: Diagnostik und Therapie der Lymphödeme. Online im Internet unter URL: http://www.awmf.org/leitlinien/detail/ll/058-001.html (Stand 05.07.2011a).

AWMF online (Arbeitsgemeinschaft der Wissenschaftlichen Medizinischen Fachgesellschaften). Leitlinien der Deutschen Gesellschaft für Phlebologie (DGP): Lipödem. Online im Internet unter URL: http://www.awmf.org/leitlinien/detail/ll/037-012.html (Stand 08.10.2011b).

Bader C, Detmar M. Hereditäre Lymphödeme. Medgen 2006; 18: 349–54.

Badger CM. A study of the efficacy of multi-layer bandaging and elastic hosiery in the treatment of lymphoedema and their effects on the swollen limb. PhD Thesis. Institute of Cancer Research, London 1997.

Badger CM, Peacock JL, Mortimer PS. A randomized, controlled, parallel group clinical trial comparing multilayer bandaging followed by hosiery versus hosiery alone in the treatment of patients with lymphedema of the limb. Cancer 2000; 88: 2832–7.

Badger C, Preston N, Seers K, Mortimer P. Physical therapies for reducing and controlling lymphoedema of the limbs. Cochrane Database Syst Rev 2004; 4: CD003141.

Bender H, Pleiß C, Cornely ME, Risse JH. Lymphszintigraphie beim Lipödem. Einfluss einer Liposuktion. Vasomed 2007; 19: 60–2.

Bernas M, Witte MH. Consensus and dissent on the ISL consensus document on the diagnosis and treatment of peripheral lymphedema. Lymphology 2004; 37: 165–7.

Bertelli G, Venturini M, Forno G, Macchiavello F, Dini D. Conservative treatment of postmastectomy lymphedema: a controlled, randomized trial. Ann Oncol 1991; 2: 575–8.

Bilancini S, Lucchi M, Tucci S, Eleuteri P. Functional lymphatic alterations in patients suffering from lipedema. Angiology 2002; 46: 333–9.

Brauer WJ, Brauer VS. Altersabhängigkeit des Lymphtransportes bei Lipödem und Lipolymphödem. Lymph Forsch 2005; 9: 6–9.

Brauer WJ, Weissleder H. Methodik und Ergebnisse der Funktionslymphszintigraphie: Erfahrungen bei 924 Patienten. Phlebologie 31: 2002; 118–25.

Brenner E. Plasma – interstitielle Flüssigkeit – Lymphe. Lymph Forsch 2009; 13: 25–7.

Brice G, Child AH, Evans A, Bell R, Mansour S, Burnand K, Sarfarazi M, Jeffery S, Mortimer P. Milroy disease and the VEGFR-3 mutation phenotype. J Med Genet 2005; 42: 98–102.

Bringezu G, Schreiner O. Lehrbuch der Entstauungstherapie, Grundlagen, Beschreibung und Bewertung, Behandlungskonzepte für die Praxis. 3 Aufl., Springer, Berlin, 2011.

Brorson H. Fettabsaugung des Lymphödems am Arm. Handchir Mikrochir Plast Chir 2003; 35: 225–32.

Brunner U, Lachat M. Primary lymphedema and pregnancy. Phlebologie 1989; 42: 481–4.

Campisi C, Boccardo F. Interposition von Venen zur Therapie peripherer Lymphödeme. Handchir Mikrochir Plast Chir 2003; 35: 221–4.

Carver C, Brice G, Mansour S, Ostergaard P, Mortimer P, Jefferey S; Lymphoedema Consortium. Three children with Milroy disease and de novo mutations in VEGFR3. Clin Gen 2007; 71: 187–9.

Casley-Smith JR. Measuring and representing peripheral oedema and its alterations. Lymphology 1994; 27: 56–70.

Casley-Smith JR. Changes in the microcirculation at the superficial and deeper levels in lymphoedema: the effects and results of massage, compression, exercise and benzopyrones on these levels during treatment. Clin Hemorheol Microcirc 2000; 23: 335–43.

Clarc B, Sitia J, Harlow W. Incidence and risk of arm oedema following treatment for breast cancer: a three year follow-up study. Quart J Med 2005; 98: 343–8.

Clark M. Kompressionsverbände: Grundlagen und Definitionen. In: Medical education partnership (ed.). Positionsdokument: Zum Verständnis der Kompressionstherapie. Medical Education Partnership, London UK, 2003.

Cornely ME. Lipödem und Lymphödem. In: Plewig G, Prinz J (Hrsg.). Fortschritte der praktischen Dermatologie und Venerologie. Springer, Berlin, Heidelberg, New York, Tokio, 2003.

Cornely ME. Zur Terminologie bei Lipödem. MÄC 2004a; 4: 4.

Cornely ME. Liposuktion bei Lipödem (Cellulite) – Follow up bei 140 operierten Patienten nach 7 Jahren. Akt Dermatol 2004b; 30 (Abstr).

Cornely ME. Lymphologie. J Dtsch Dermatol Gesellsch 2006a; 6: 564–79.

Cornely ME. Lipedema and lymphatic edema. In: Melvin A, Shiffman MA, Di Guiseppe A (eds.). Liposuction principles and practice. Springer, Berlin, Heidelberg, New York, Tokyo, 2006b.

Cornely ME. Lymphologische Liposculptur. Hautarzt 2007; 58: 653–8.

Czaika VA, Wruck U, Gussmann A. Dicke Beine – und was steckt dahinter? Das primäre Lymphödem frühzeitig erkennen! CME (Springer-Verlag) 2008; 5: 59–67.

Damstra RJ. Volumenreduktion beim Mammakarzinom-bedingten Armlymphödem unter verschieden stark angelegten Kurzzugverbänden. In: Spengler M, Abel M. Medical and Regulatory Affairs, Lohmann & Rauscher GmbH & Co. KG (Hrsg.). Update Kompressionstherapie? Ihr Weg zum Therapie-Erfolg. Zusammenfassung der Präsentationen während der 50. Jahrestagung der Deutschen Gesellschaft für Phlebologie, Bochum, 15.–18.10.2008. Lohmann & Rauscher, Neuwied, 2008.

Damstra RJ, Brouwer ER, Partsch H. Controlled, comparative study of relation between volume changes and interface pressure under short-stretch bandages in leg lymphedema patients. Dermatol Surg 2008; 34: 773–8.

De Franzo AJ, Hall JH, Herring SM. Adipositas dolorosa (Dercum's disease): liposuction is an effective form of treatment. Plast Reconstr Surg 1990; 85: 289–92.

Döller W, Ure C, Lientscher M. Workflow der Lymphödemdiagnostik – Diagnostische Schritte bei Extremitätenschwellung. Eur J Vasc Med (VASA) 2008; 4: 5–10.

Ferrell RE, Levinson KL, Esman JH, Kimak MA, Lawrence EC, Barmada MM, Finegold DN. Hereditary lymphedema: evidence for linkage and genetic heterogeneity. Hum Mol Gen 1998; 7: 2073–8.

Finegold DN, Kimak MA, Lawrence EC, Levinson KL, Cherniske EM, Pober BR, Dunlap JW, Ferrell RE. Truncating mutations in FOXC2 cause multiple lymphedema syndromes. Hum Mol Genet 2001; 10: 1185–9.

Földi E. Das postoperative Lymphödem. Das klinische Problem: Diagnostik und aktuelle Behandlungskonzepte. Phlebologie 2011; 40: 123–6.

Földi E, Baumeister RGH, Bräutigam P, Tiedjen KU. Zur Diagnostik und Therapie des Lymphödems. Dtsch Ärztebl 1998; 95: A-740–7.

Földi E, Sauerwald A, Hennig B. Effect of complex decongestive physiotherapy on gene expression for the inflammatory response in peripheral lymphedema. Lymphology 2000; 33: 19–23.

Földi E, Jünger M, Partsch H. Wissenschaftliche Aspekte zum Lymphödem-Verband. Medical Education Partnership, London UK, 2005b.

Földi M, Földi E. Das Lymphödem und verwandte Krankheiten; Vorbeugung und Behandlung. 9. Aufl., Elsevier, Urban & Fischer, München, 2009.

Földi M, Strößenreuther R. Grundlagen der manuellen Lymphdrainage. 4. Aufl., Elsevier, München, 2007.

Földi M, Földi E, Kubik S (Hrsg.). Lehrbuch der Lymphologie für Mediziner, Masseure und Physiotherapeuten. 6. Aufl., Urban & Fischer, München, Jena, 2005a.

Forstner R, Rendl KH, Dorninger E, Schmoller HJ. Zur Differentialdiagnose des „Dicken Beins" – ein Fallbericht. Eur J Vasc Med (VASA) 1991; 10: 402–5.

Franzeck UK, Spiegel I, Fischer M, Bortzler C, Stahel HU, Bollinger A. Combined physical therapy for lymphedema evaluated by fluorescence microlymphography and lymph capillary pressure measurements. J Vasc Res 1997; 34: 306–11.

Frick A, Hoffmann IN, Baumeister RG, Putz R. Liposuction technique and lymphatic lesions in lower legs: Anatomic study to reduce risks. Plast Reconstruct Surg 1999; 103: 1868–73, 1874–5.

Fritsch P. (Hrsg.). Dermatologie und Venerologie für das Studium. Springer, Berlin, 2009.

Greer KE. Lipedema of the legs. Cutis 1974; 14: 98–100.

Gretener SB, Lauchli S, Leu AJ, Koppensteiner R, Franzeck UK. Effect of venous and lymphatic congestion on lymph capillary pressure of the skin in healthy volunteers and patients with lymph edema. J Vasc Res 2000; 37: 61–7.

Gültig O. Lymphödem-Verbände für Kopf, Brust und Genitalien. Medical Education Partnership, London UK, 2005.

Hammerl B, Döller W. Das sekundäre maligne Lymphödem bei fortgeschrittenen HNO-Tumoren. Wien Med Wochenschr 2008; 158: 695–701.

Hanke CW, Sattler G. Sicherheit der Liposuktionschirurgie. In: Sattler G, Sommer B, Hanke CW (Hrsg.). Lehrbuch der Liposuktion. Thieme, Stuttgart, 2003.

Harris SR, Hugi MR, Olivotto IA, Levine M; for the Steering Committee for Clinical Practice Guidelines for the Care and Treatment of Breast Cancer. Clinical practice guidelines for the care and treatment of breast cancer: 11. Lymphedema. Can Med Assoc J 2001; 164: 191–9.

Harwood CA, Bull RH, Evans J, Mortimer PS. Lymphatic and venous function in lipedema. Br J Dermatol 1996; 134: 1–6.

Herpertz U. Krankheitsspektrum des Lipödems an einer lymphologischen Fachklinik – Erscheinungsformen, Mischbilder und Behandlungsmöglichkeiten. Vasomed 1997; 5: 301–7.

Herpertz U. Entstehungszeitpunkt von Lipödemen. Lymph Forsch 2004; 8: 79–8.

Herpertz U. Ödeme und Lymphdrainage. Diagnose und Therapie von Ödemkrankheiten. 4. überarb. und erw. Aufl., Schattauer, Stuttgart, New York, 2010.

Hoffmann JN, Festmann IT, Baumeister RG, Putz R, Frick A. Tumescent and dry liposuction of lower extremities: differences in lymph vessel injury. Plast Reconstr Surg 2004; 113: 718–26.

Ingianni G. Mikrochirurgische lympho-venöse Anastomose beim sekundären Lymphödem der oberen Extremität. Handchir Mikrochir Plast Chir 2003; 35: 216–20.

International Society of Lymphology. The diagnosis and treatment of peripheral lymphedema. Consensus document of the International Society of Lymphology. Lymphology 2003; 36: 84–91.

Jünger M, Steins A, Hahn M, Häfner HM. Microcirculatory dysfunction in chronic venous insufficiency (CVI). Microcirculation 2000; 7 (6 Pt 2): 3–12.

Kasseroller RG. LVF—Lymphoedema classification of inguinal and axillary lymph flow areas. Lymphol Forsch Prax 2001; 1: 23–6.

Kastenholz A. Representation of flow phenomena in terminal blood vessels and initial lymphatics using fluorescent microbeads. In: Boccalon H (ed.). Vascular medicine. Excerpta Medica, Elsevier Science Publishers BV, Amsterdam, 1993.

Klein JA. The tumescent technique for liposuction surgery. Am J Cosmetic Surg 1987; 4: 248–63.

Kröger K. Lymphoedema and lipoedema of the extremities. Eur J Vasc Med (VASA) 2008; 37: 39–51.

Lee YM, Mak SS, Tse MM, Chan SJ. Lymphoedema care of breast cancer patients in a breast care clinic: a survey of knowledge and health practice. Support Care Cancer 2001; 9: 634–41.

Levick JR. An introduction to cardiovascular physiology. Arnold, London, 2003.

Levick JR, McHale N. The physiology of lymph production and propulsion. In: Browse N, Burnand K, Mortimer P (eds.). Diseases of the lymphatics. Hodder Arnold, London, 2003.

Li S, Cao W, Cheng K, Chang TS. Microvascular transfer of a "lymphatic bearing" flap in the treatment of obstructive lymphedema. Plast Reconstr Surg 2008; 121: 150e–2e.

Ludwig M, Vetter H. Differentialdiagnose des dicken Beins. Schweiz Rundsch Med 1989; 78: 987–92.

Lüthi S, Scholtze D, Husmann M. Das dicke Bein. Praxis 2010; 99: 635–45.

Marsch WCH. Ist das Lipödem ein lymphologisches Krankheitsbild? Z Lymphol 2001; 1: 22–4.

Marsch WCH. Lymphgefäßsystem und Haut. Orthologie, Klinik und Pathologie. Hautarzt 2005; 56: 277–95.

Marshall M, Breu FX. Das Lipödem – ein wenig beachtetes Krankheitsbild. Vasomed 2002; 6: 254–7.

Marshall M, Schwahn-Schreiber Ch. Das Lipödem – ein wenig beachtetes Krankheitsbild. Vasomed 2008; 20: 59–65.

Marston W, Vowden K. Compression therapy: a guide to safe practice. In: EWMA Position Document. Understanding compression therapy. MEP, London, 2003.

McNeely ML, Magee DJ, Lees AW. The addition of manual lymph drainage to compression therapy for breast cancer related lymphoedema: a randomized controlled trial. Breast Cancer Res Treat 2004; 86: 95–106.

Meier-Vollrath I, Schmeller W. Lipödem – aktueller Stand, neue Perspektiven. J Dtsch Dermatol Ges 2004; 2: 181–6.

Meier-Vollrath I, Schneider W, Schmeller W. Lipödem: Verbesserte Lebensqualität durch Therapiekombination. Deutsches Ärzteblatt 2005; 102: A1061–7, B892–7, C840–5.

Meyer-Dörwald I. Wie komplex muss die Physiotherapie bei der Behandlung des phlebolymphostatischen Ödems sein? Lymph Forsch 2003; 7: 94.

Miller TA, Wyatt LE, Rudkin GH. Staged skin and subcutaneous excision for lymphedema: A favourable report of long term results. Plast Reconstr Surg 1998; 102: 1486–98, discussion 1499–501.

Moffatt CJ, Morgan P, Doherty D. Das Lymphödem-Framework: ein Konsens über den Lymphödem-Verband. Medical Education Partnership, London UK, 2005.

Mosti G. Hämodynamische Effekte mit Kurzzug-Kompression. In: Spengler M, Abel M. Medical and Regulatory Affairs, Lohmann & Rauscher GmbH & Co. KG (Hrsg.). Update Kompressionstherapie? Ihr Weg zum Therapie-Erfolg. Zusammenfassung der Präsentationen während der 50. Jahrestagung der Deutschen Gesellschaft für Phlebologie, Bochum, 15.–18.10.2008. Lohmann & Rauscher, Neuwied, 2008.

Müllegger RR, Glatz M. Skin manifestation of Lyme-Borreliosis. Am J Clin Dermatol 2008; 9: 355–68.

Northup KA, Witte MH, Witte CL. Syndromic classification of hereditary lymphedema. Lymphology 2003; 36: 162–89.

Oberlin M. Diagnostik und Therapie des Lymphödems. Tipps und häufige Fallstricke. Ars Medici 2010; 2: 67–70.

O'Brien BM, Sykes P, Threlfall GN, Browning FS. Microlymphaticovenous anastomosis for obstructive lymphedema. Plast Reconstr Surg 1977; 60: 197–211.

Olszewski WG. Lymph pressure and flow in limbs. In: Olszewski WG (ed.). Lymph stasis: pathophysiology, diagnosis and treatment. CRC Press, Boca Raton, Florida, 1991.

Partsch H. Understanding the pathophysiological effects of compression. In: EWMA Position Document. Understanding compression therapy. MEP, London, 2003.

Partsch H. The Static Stiffness Index (SSI). A simple method to assess the elastic property of compression material in vivo. Derm Surg 2005; 31: 625–30.

Partsch H. Experimentelle Nachweise in der Kompressions-Behandlung – ein Überblick. In: Spengler M, Abel M. Medical and Regulatory Affairs, Lohmann & Rauscher GmbH & Co. KG (Hrsg.). Update Kompressionstherapie? Ihr Weg zum Therapie-Erfolg. Zusammenfassung der Präsentationen während der 50. Jahrestagung der Deutschen Gesellschaft für Phlebologie, Bochum, 15.–18.10.2008. Lohmann & Rauscher, Neuwied, 2008.

Partsch H. Varicous veins and chronic venous insufficiency. Eur J Vasc Med (VASA) 2009; 38: 293–301.

Partsch H, Clark M, Bassez S, Becker F, Benigni JP, Blazek V, Caprini J, Cornu-Thénard F, Hafner J, Flour M, Jünger M, Moffatt Ch, Neumann HAM. Measurement of lower leg compression in vivo: Recommendations for the performance of measurements of interface pressure and stiffness: A consensus statement. Dermatol Surg 2006; 32: 229–38.

Partsch H, Clark M, Mosti G, Steinlechner E, Schuren J, Abel M, Benigni JP, Coleridge-Smith P, Cornu-Thénard A, Flour M, Hutchinson J, Gamble J, Issberner K, Juenger M, Moffatt C, Neumann HA, Rabe E, Uhl JF, Zimmet S. Classification of compression bandages: practical aspects. Dermatol Surg 2008a; 34: 600–9.

Partsch H, Flour M, Smith PC, Benigni JP, Cornu-Thénard A, Delis K, Gniadecka M, Mariani F, Mosti G, Neumann HAM, Rabe E, Schuren J, Uhl JF. International Compression Club. Indications for compression therapy in venous and lymphatic disease consensus based on experimental data and scientific evidence. Under the auspices of the IUP. Int Angiol 2008b; 27: 193–219.

Petrek JA, Pressman PI, Smith RA. Lymphedema: Current issues in research and management. CA Cancer J Clin 2000; 50: 292–307.

Pitr K, Treška V, Průcha J, Marková N, Pitrová G. Einfluss der Zeit zwischen Ödemmanifestation und Behandlungsbeginn auf den Therapieerfolg bei Patienten mit sekundärem Lymphödem nach chirurgischer Behandlung von Brustkrebs. Österr Z Phys Med Rehabil 2007; 17: 62–9.

Quendler S. Lebensqualität von Lymphödempatienten und ihre emotionalen und kognitiven Komponenten. Diplomarbeit, Universität Wien, 2008.

Rapprich S, Dingler A, Podda M. Liposuction is an effective treatment for lipedema—results of a study with 25 patients. J Dtsch Dermatol Ges 2011; 9: 33–40.

Rockson SG. Lymphedema. Am J Med 2001; 110: 288–95.

Rockson SG. Diagnosis and management of lymphatic vascular disease. J Am Coll Cardiol 2008; 52: 799–806.

Ruzicka T, Vieluf D, Landthaler M, Braun-Falco O. Benign symmetric lipomatosis Launois-Bensaude. Report of ten cases and review of the literature. J Am Acad Dermatol 1987; 17: 663–74.

Sattler G, Hasche E, Rapprich S, Mössler K, Hagedorn M. Neue operative Behandlungsmöglichkeiten bei benignen Fettgewebserkrankungen. Z Hautkrankh 1997; 72: 579–82.

Schindler C, Schellong M. Drug-induced oedema—pathopysiology, diagnosis and management. Phlebologie 2009; 38: 33–41.

Schingale F-J. Lymphödeme – Lipödeme. Diagnose und Therapie – Ein Ratgeber für Betroffene. 3. überarb. Aufl., Schlütersche Verlagsgesellschaft, Hannover, 2007.

Schingale F-J, Schingale Ph. Das Lipödem – medizinische Grundlagen und Therapie. Orthopädie-Technik 2002; 3: 214–9.

Schmeller W, Meier-Vollrath I. Erfolgreiche operative Therapie des Lipödems mittels Liposuktion. Phlebologie 2004; 33: 23–9.

Schmeller W, Meier-Vollrath I. Anmerkungen zur Therapie des Lipödems. Lymph Forsch 2006; 10: 22–8.

Schmeller W, Meier-Vollrath I. Das Lipödem: neue Möglichkeiten der Therapie. Schweiz Med Forum 2007a; 7: 150–5.

Schmeller W, Meier-Vollrath I. Lipödem – Aktuelles zu einem weitgehend unbekannten Krankheitsbild. Akt Dermatol 2007b; 33: 1–10.

Schmeller W, Meier-Vollrath I. Schmerzen beim Lipödem. Lymph Forsch 2008; 12: 8–12.

Schmeller W, Tronnier M, Kaiserling E. Lymphgefäßschädigung durch Liposuktion? Eine immunhistologische Untersuchung. Lymph Forsch 2006; 9: 81–5.

Seeger H, Asmis L, Husmann M. Management venöser Thromboembolismen. Praxis 2009; 98: 735–46.

Sehouli J, Stengel D, Schauwecker H. Benigne symmetrische Lipomatose. Therapeutisches Dilemma? Langenbecks Arch Chir 1997; 382: 271–3.

Shinawi M. Lymphedema of the lower extremity: Is it genetic or nongenetic? Clin Pediat 2007; 46: 835–41.

Sitzia J, Stanton AWB, Badger C. A review of outcome indicators in the treatment of chronic limb oedema. Clin Rehab 1997; 11: 181–91.

Sommer B, Sattler G. Indikationen und Kontraindikationen der Liposuktion. In: Sattler G, Sommer B, Hanke CW (Hrsg.). Lehrbuch der Liposuktion. Thieme, Stuttgart, 2003.

Steiner J, Schiltz K, Heidenreich F, Weissenborn K. Lipomatosis dolorosa – ein häufig übersehenes Krankheitsbild. Nervenarzt 2002; 73: 183–7.

Stemmer R. Ein klinisches Zeichen zur Früh- und Differentialdiagnose des Lymphödems. Eur J Vasc Med (VASA) 1975; 5: 261–2.

Stöberl C. Klinische Differentialdiagnose der Beinschwellung – Ein Leitfaden für die Praxis. Z Gefäßmedi 2011; 8: 11–8.

Stutz J. Liposuktion beim Lipödem zur Verhinderung von Gelenkspätkomplikationen. Vasomed 2011; 23: 2–6.

Stutz JJ, Krahl D. Water jet-assisted liposuction for patients with lipoedema: histologic and immunohistologic analysis of the aspirates of 30 lipoedema patients. Aesth Plast Surg 2009; 33: 153–62.

Taute B-M, Melnyk H, Podhaisky H. Alternative sonographische Diagnosen bei klinischem Thromboseverdacht. Med Klin 2010; 105: 619–26.

Tomczak H, Nyka W, Lass P. Lymphoedema lymphoscintigraphy versus other diagnostic techniques—a clinical point of view. Nucl Med Rev Cent East Eur 2005; 8: 37–43.

Vodder E. Le drainage lymphatique, une nouvelle méthode thérapeutique. Santé pour tous, 1936.

Vodder E. Die manuelle Lymphdrainage und ihre medizinischen Anwendungsgebiete. Erfahrungsheilkunde 1966; 15: 217–22.

Weissleder H, Brauer WJ. Radiologische Diagnostik beim Lipödem-Syndrom. Lymph Forsch 1997; 1: 26–30.

Weissleder H, Schuchhardt Ch. Erkrankungen des Lymphgefäßsystems. Kagerer Kommunikation, Bonn, 1994.

Weissleder H, Schuchardt C. Diagnose und Therapie des Lymphödems. Viavital, Köln, 2001.

Weiss M, Baumeister RG, Hahn K. Posttherapeutic lymphedema: Scintigraphy before and after autologous lymph vessel transplantation—8 years long-term follow up. Clin Nucl Med 2002; 27: 788–92.

Weiss M, Baumeister RGH, Hahn K. Therapieplanung und Erfolgskontrolle der autologen Lymphgefäß-Transplantation mittels nuklearmedizinischer Lymphabflussszintigraphie. Handchir Mikrochir Plast Chir 2003; 35: 210–5.

Werner GT, Klimczyk K, Rude J. Checkliste Physikalische und Rehabilitative Medizin. Thieme, Stuttgart, 1997.

Wienert V, Leeman S. Das Lipödem. Hautarzt 1991; 42: 484–6.

Williams AF, Keller M. Praktische Anleitung für Lymphödem-Verbände der oberen und unteren Gliedmaßen. Medical Education Partnership, London UK, 2005.

Wold LE, Hines EA, Allen EV. Lipedema of the legs: A syndrome characterized by fat legs and edema. Ann Intern Med 1949; 34: 1243–50.

Index